W9-BZQ-003

HANDBOOK OF
CLINICAL SKILLS

Springhouse Corporation
Springhouse, Pennsylvania

STAFF

Executive Director
Matthew Cahill

Editorial Director
Patricia Dwyer Schull, RN, MSN

Art Director
John Hubbard

Clinical Manager
Judith A. Schilling McCann, RN, MSN

Managing Editor
A.T. McPhee, RN, BSN

Editors
Kathy Goldberg, Peter Johnson,
Michael Lear-Olimpi

Clinical Editors
Clare Brabson, RN, BSN (project manager); Lucille A. Rosso, RN, MSN;
Joanne M. Bartelmo, RN, MSN,
CCRN; Beverly Tscheschlog, RN

Copy Editors
Cynthia C. Breuninger (manager),
Christine Cunniffe, Stacey Ann Follin,
Brenna Mayer, Pamela Wingrod

Designers
Arlene Putterman (associate art director), Donald G. Knauss (book designer), Elaine Ezrow, Susan Hopkins
Rodzewich, Matie Patterson, Mary
Stangl, Lesley Weissman-Cook

Manufacturing
Deborah Meiris (director), Pat
Dorshaw, T.A. Landis, Anna Brindisi

Production Coordinator
Margaret A. Rastiello

Editorial Assistants
Mary Madden, Beverly Lane, Jeanne
Napier

The clinical procedures described and recommended in this publication are based on research and consultation with nursing, medical, and legal authorities. To the best of our knowledge, these procedures reflect currently accepted practice; nevertheless, they can't be considered absolute and universal recommendations. For individual applications, all recommendations must be considered in light of the patient's clinical condition and, before administration of new or infrequently used drugs, in light of the latest package-insert information. The authors and the publisher disclaim any responsibility for any adverse effects resulting from the suggested procedures, from any undetected errors, or from the reader's misunderstanding of the text.

Printed in the United States of America.
HCS-030998

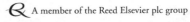 A member of the Reed Elsevier plc group

Library of Congress Cataloging-in-Publication Data

Handbook of clinical skills
   p. cm.
   Includes index.
   1. Nursing — Handbooks, manuals, etc. I. Springhouse Corporation
   [DNLM: 1. Nursing Process — handbooks. 2. Nursing Care — handbooks. WY 49 H234 1997]
RT51.H343 1997
610.73 — dc20
DNLM/DLC   96-28896
ISBN 0-87434-870-6 (alle. paper)   CIP

CONTENTS

Clinical skills (in alphabetical order) 1

Appendices

iii

CONTRIBUTORS

Debra Arnow, RN, BSN, CNA
Nurse Coordinator
Vanderbilt University Medical Center
Nashville, Tenn.

Barbara K. Blue, RN, MSN
Pediatric Pulmonary Nurse Specialist
Phoenix (Ariz.) Children's Hospital

Valeria Brannon, RN, BSN
Health Service Area Manager
Harris County Health Department
Houston

Cynthia Browder, RN,C, BSN
Assistant Director of Nursing
Texas Children's Hospital–Texas Children's
Cancer Center
Houston

Vicki L. Buchda, RN, MS
Nurse Manager, Critical Care and Telemetry Units
Del E. Webb Memorial Hospital
Sun City West, Ariz.

Sherry Buffington, RN, CCRN
Staff Nurse, Critical Care
Doylestown (Pa.) Hospital

Dorothy A. Calabrese, RN, MSN, CURN, OCN
Clinical Nurse Specialist, Urology-Oncology
Cleveland Clinic Foundation

Jeanette K. Chambers, RN, PhD, CS
Renal Clinical Specialist–Education Specialist
Riverside Methodist Hospitals
Adjunct Assistant Professor, College of Nursing
Ohio State University
Columbus

Carla M. Clark, RN, MS
Nurse Research Clinician
Good Samaritan Regional Medical Center
Phoenix

Bonita Gail Largent Cloyd, RN, MSN, CETN
Enterostomal Therapist
Western Baptist Hospital
Paducah, Ky.

Peggy Coleman, RN, MSN, CNA
Senior Occupational Health Consultant
U.S. Public Health Services Corp. HRSA
Bethesda, Md.

Catherine M. Collin, RN, MSN, CANP
Assistant Professor of Clinical Nursing
University of Medicine and Dentistry
of New Jersey, School of Nursing
Newark

Ruth E. Conley, RN, BSN
Nursing Faculty
Indiana Vocational Technical State College
South Bend

Susan Dalton, RN, CCRN
High-Tech Staff Nurse
Home Visiting Nurse
Howell, N.J.

Tina R. Dietrich, RN, BSN, CCRN
Nursing Faculty
Indiana Vocational Technical State College
South Bend

Susan M. DiGiorgio, RN, MSN, ANP
Assistant Clinical Professor
University of Medicine and Dentistry
of New Jersey, School of Nursing
Newark

Jane Dolin, RN, BSN, ET
Patient Education Specialist
Lehigh Valley Hospital Center
Allentown, Pa.

Shirley J. Edwards, RN, MSN, OCN
Clinical Nurse Specialist, Oncology
Saint John's Hospital and Health Center
Santa Monica, Calif.

Marsha L. England, RN, AA, CRNI
Blood and Donor Center
UCLA, Los Angeles

Nancy Evans, RN, BSN, CGRN
Nurse Manager, Gastroenterology Department
Daniel Freeman Memorial Hospital
Inglewood, Calif.

Nina M. Fielden, RN, MSN, CNN
Clinical Instructor, Critical Care Nursing
Department
Cleveland Clinic Foundation

Marina Villano Flecksteiner, RN, BSN, CNN
Clinical Instructor
Lehigh Valley Hospital Center
Allentown, Pa.

Marilyn A. Folcik, RN, MPH, ONC
Nurse Educator, Orthopedics
Hartford (Conn.) Hospital

Ellie Z. Franges, RN, MSN, CCRN, CNRN
Neuroscience Coordinator
Sacred Heart Hospital
Allentown, Pa.

Paul N. Franquist, RN, MSN
Clinical Nurse Specialist
Critical Care Manager, Oncology-HIV
Desert Samaritan Medical Center
Mesa, Ariz.

Jan Fuchs, RN, MS, CNN
Head Nurse
Peritoneal Dialysis Unit
Cleveland Clinic Foundation

Ellen D. Goodner, RN,C, MSN
Education Instructor
Western Baptist Hospital
Paducah, Ky.

JoAnn Gruber, RN, MSN, CCRN
Project Specialist
Lehigh Valley Hospital Center
Allentown, Pa.

Minerva S. Guttman, RN, EdD
Assistant Dean, Central Programs; Associate
Professor
University of Medicine and Dentistry
of New Jersey, School of Nursing
Newark

Connie S. Heflin, RN, MSN
Associate Professor of Nursing
Paducah (Ky.) Community College

Elizabeth A. Henneman, RN, MS, CCRN
Clinical Nurse Specialist
Medical Intensive Care Unit
UCLA Medical Center
Los Angeles

Christy Hoffman, RN
Nurse Manager
Texas Children's Hospital
Houston

Marian J. Hoffman, RN, MSN, CNSN
Clinical-Education Nurse Specialist
Lehigh Valley Hospital Center
Allentown, Pa.

Anna Marie C. Hunsaker, RN, MS, NHA
Associate Director of Training and
Development
Sun Health
Sun City, Ariz.

Flerida A. Imperial, RN, MN
Clinical Nurse Specialist, Cardiothoracic
Intensive Care Unit
UCLA Medical Center
Los Angeles

Marilyn Knoth, RN, MSN
Professor
Paducah (Ky.) Community College

James J. Konzelman, RN, MSN, CCRN
Education and Program Development Specialist
St. Christopher's Hospital for Children
Philadelphia

Laura Kotagal, RN, BSN
Part-time Clinical Nurse Specialist, Pediatric
Neurology
Cleveland Clinic Foundation

Charles F. Krozek, RN, MN
Staff Development Consultant
Santa Monica, Calif.

Jo Ann Maklebust, RN, MSN, CNP, CS
Clinical Nurse Specialist, Wound Care
Case Manager, General and Reconstructive
Surgery
Harper Hospital–Detroit (Mich.) Medical Center

Kathleen M. Malloch, RN, BSN, MBA, PhD-C
Vice President, Patient Care Services
Del E. Webb Memorial Hospital
Sun City West, Ariz.

Clara Martin, RN
Infection Control Assistant
Texas Children's Hospital
Houston

Rebecca M. McCaskey, RN,C, MEd
Nurse Consultant
Athens, Ga.

Karen McCleave, PhD, CIC, FNP-C
Infection Control Practitioner
Riverside Regional Medical Center
Newport News, Va.

Mary Jane McDevitt, RN, BS
Staff Nurse, Oncology Unit
Mercy Catholic Medical Center
Fitzgerald Mercy Division
Darby, Pa.

Kathleen McDonald, RN,C, MSN
Assistant Professor of Clinical Nursing
University of Medicine and Dentistry
of New Jersey, School of Nursing
Stratford

Debra McGeehin, RN, BSN
Clinical Instructor
Lehigh Valley Hospital Center
Allentown, Pa.

M. Kathy McGourty, RN, MA, MS, NP,C
Assistant Clinical Professor
University of Medicine and Dentistry
of New Jersey, School of Nursing
Newark

Kimberly W. McKinney, RN, BSN
Education Instructor
Western Baptist Hospital
Paducah, Ky.

Cheryl Milford, RN, MS, MBA, CCRN
Staff Development Specialist
Ohio State University Medical Center
Columbus

Doris A. Millam, RN, BSN, MS, CRNI
I.V. Therapy Educator–Consultant
I.V. Therapy Resources
Glenview, Ill.

Mary Beth Modic, RN,C, MSN
Clinical Nurse Specialist
Cleveland Clinic Foundation

Deidre P. Mountjoy, RN, BSN, MS, ANPC
Nurse Practitioner
CIGNA
Phoenix

M. Louise Nix, RN,C, MSN, PNP
Staff Development Specialist
Texas Children's Hospital
Houston

Theodora Pappas, RN,C, MS
Assistant Professor
University of Medicine and Dentistry
of New Jersey, School of Nursing
Newark

Tena B. Payne, RN, MSN
Associate Professor
Paducah (Ky.) Community College

Jody Pelusi, RN, MSN, FNP, OCN, RT
Clinical Nurse Specialist, Oncology
Maryvale Samaritan Medical Center
Phoenix

Lois A. Piano, RN,C, MSN
Assistant Professor
Gwynedd Mercy College
Gwynedd Valley, Pa.

Anna M. Pignanelli, RN,C, BSN
Clinical Instructor, Medical-Surgical Nursing
Cleveland Clinic Foundation

Marla J. Prizant-Weston, RN, MS, CCRN
Administrator, Acute Care Services
Paradise Valley Hospital
Phoenix

Frances W. Quinless, RN, PhD
Dean, School of Nursing
University of Medicine and Dentistry
of New Jersey
Newark

vi

Elizabeth M. Rice, RN,C, MSN
Senior Education Specialist
Sun Health
Sun City, Ariz.

Carol F. Robinson, RN, MSN, RRT
Pulmonary Nurse Specialist
Phoenix (Ariz.) Children's Hospital

Teresa Rodriguez-Wargo, RN,C, MSN, PNP
Pediatric Nurse Practitioner
Texas Children's Hospital
Houston

Susan F. Rudy, RN, MSN, CORLN, CRNP
Instructor, Johns Hopkins School of Medicine
Otolaryngology Nurse Practitioner
Johns Hopkins Bayview Medical Center
Baltimore

Sally Russell, RN, MN, CS
Instructor
St. Elizabeth Hospital School of Nursing
Lafayette, Ind.

Pat Sanderson, RN, BSN
Clinical Educator
Saint John's Hospital and Health Center
Santa Monica, Calif.

Rhea C. Sanford, RN, MSN, CS
Clinical Nurse Specialist
John Dempsey Hospital
Farmington, Conn.

Ann Schneidman, RN, MS, NS
Pulmonary Nurse Consultant
Phoenix

Sonya L. Scott, RN, MS, CPN
Nurse Manager
Texas Children's Hospital
Houston

Daniele A. Shollenberger, RN, MSN
Educational Nurse Specialist
Lehigh Valley Hospital Center
Allentown, Pa.

Mary Y. Sieggreen, RN, MSN, CNP, CS
Clinical Nurse Specialist–Case Manager
Harper Hospital–Detroit (Mich.) Medical Center

Susan Simon, RN, MA
Home Care Coordinator
Medical Personnel Pool
Shaker Heights, Ohio

Marian J. Spirk, RN, MSN, CNSN
Clinical Nurse Specialist
Lehigh Valley Hospital Center
Allentown, Pa.

Nancy J. Stefan, RN, BSN
Nurse Consultant–Nursing Systems Specialist
National Institutes of Health
Bethesda, Md.

Jessica Stickley, RN, MSN, CCRN, CNAA
Former Director of Nursing, Critical Care
St. Christopher's Hospital for Children
Philadelphia

Roberta H. Stokes, RN, MSN, CHN, CNN, CS
Clinical Nurse Specialist
Cleveland Clinic Foundation

Susan D. Taylor, RN, MSN
Associate Professor of Nursing
Paducah (Ky.) Community College

Rosemary Theroux, RN,C, MS
Coordinator, Women's Health Network
Leonard Morse Hospital
Natick, Mass.

Freida Thompson, RN, MSN
Education Instructor
Western Baptist Hospital
Paducah, Ky.

Karen J. Vander Laan, RN, MSN, CCRN
Nurse Manager, Burn Center
Detroit (Mich.) Receiving Hospital and
University Health Center

Sarah E. Whitaker, RN,C, MSN
Lecturer
University of Texas
El Paso

Myrtle Taylor Williams, RN, DNS(C)
Director, Center for Nursing Development
Texas Children's Hospital
Houston

FOREWORD

If you're like many nurses, you know there are some procedures you haven't done since nursing school — or maybe haven't done at all. You know you need up-to-date knowledge of complicated procedures and a continuing ability to perform those procedures. And you know you're often too busy to read a bulky procedure manual to find out what you need to do before carrying out a procedure.

Handbook of Clinical Skills offers busy nurses like you — nurses who face increasingly smaller staffs, sicker patients, and shorter length of stays — an easy-to-use, one-stop reference about procedures. Before starting a procedure you haven't done in a while, grab your pocket-sized *Handbook of Clinical Skills* and find the skill you want in a flash.

Each alphabetically arranged skill — whether diagnostic, assessment-related, or another kind — is presented in a consistent, clearly written format that tells you what you need to know. For instance:

Chest physiotherapy opens with an explanation of what the skill is. *Nursing diagnoses and patient outcomes* provide information about specific diagnoses and expected treatment results of the skill.

Equipment tells you what tools you'll need to perform the skill. *Equipment preparation* explains how to get that equipment ready, while *Patient preparation* lets you know how to prepare the patient for the procedure.

Implementation takes you step-by-step through the skill. *Complications* lists problems that may arise and how to prevent or solve them. *Home care* clues you in on how you may need to modify a skill to fit your particular patient's needs at home and assists you with that patient's discharge planning.

Nursing considerations offers tips for caring for the patient before, during, and after the skill is performed. *Documentation* provides guidance on effective, efficient charting.

Handbook of Clinical Skills is the first complete hands-on skills manual available. The book contains more than 250 illustrations, charts, and photographs that clarify the steps to be taken and demonstrate such skills as palpation, auscultation, and the application of medications and dressings. Appendices list common laboratory values, guidelines on minimizing infection, and sources of more information and help.

Three special logos that appear throughout the book present easy-to-read pointers on topics of interest to all nurses. "Problem solver," for instance, identifies specific problems that may occur with equipment or with a patient and offers simple, clear instructions about preventing or solving them.

"Technology update" informs you about the latest equipment, and "Better charting" shows you, with sample progress notes, how to chart better notes.

From basic procedures (such as taking vital signs and administering oxygen) to more advanced skills (such as assisting with the placement of a transcranial Doppler monitor), *Handbook of Clinical Skills* gives you the knowledge and the confidence you'll need to carry out procedures correctly the first time. And you get all that knowledge and confidence in a reference book that fits neatly into your pocket or glove compartment.

Handbook of Clinical Skills is practical, timesaving, and comprehensive. Whether you're being challenged to accept new assignments, perform new procedures, or refine your existing skills, take your trusted *Handbook of Clinical Skills* with you. Feel confident that regardless of the difficulty of the task or the setting, you can meet the challenge.

Linda Honan Pellico, RN, MSN, CCRN, CS
Lecturer and Coordinator, First Year Curriculum
Graduate Entry Program in Nursing
Yale University, School of Nursing
New Haven, Conn.

Abdominal auscultation

When assessing the abdomen, you'll perform the four assessment techniques in this sequence: inspection, auscultation, percussion, palpation. Because percussion and palpation can affect bowel activity — and, as a result, bowel sounds — you'll auscultate *before* percussing and palpating.

When auscultating for bowel sounds, vascular sounds, and friction rubs, establish a regular sequence to use each time you listen for bowel sounds. By using the same sequence every time, you'll ensure a thorough assessment. For instance, start in the right upper quadrant (RUQ) and move clockwise to the right lower quadrant (RLQ), the left lower quadrant (LLQ), and the left upper quadrant (LUQ), listening for at least 2 minutes in each. Note frequency and intensity of sounds. If you don't hear sounds after 5 minutes, record bowel sounds as absent. (See *Assessing for abnormal abdominal and bowel sounds,* page 2.)

≫ Key nursing diagnoses and patient outcomes

Use this nursing diagnosis as a guide when developing your plan of caren.

Knowledge deficit related to lack of exposure to assessment techniques

Based on this nursing diagnosis, you'll establish the following patient outcome. The patient will:
• state understanding of need for assessment.

Equipment
♦ stethoscope.

Patient preparation

• If you can't hear bowel sounds, check that the patient has an empty bladder. A full bladder can obscure bowel sounds.
• If the patient has a nasogastric tube connected to suction, turn it off before auscultating because suctioning noises may obscure or mimic bowel sounds.
• Help the patient into a supine position.
• Explain each procedure before performing it.

Implementation

• Put your stethoscope diaphragm on the RUQ and listen for air and fluid moving through the bowel. Note the character and frequency of sounds. If you don't hear bowel sounds right away, be sure to listen for at least 2 minutes. Keep listening for a total of 5 minutes.
• Normal bowel sounds are soft bubbling or gurgling noises without a pattern. They can last from less than 1 second to several seconds and may occur 5 to 34 times a minute.
• After you hear bowel sounds in the RUQ, move to the other quadrants. The patient may have paralytic ileus or a full bladder may be obscuring the sounds if you don't hear them in a particular quadrant. After 2 minutes without hearing sounds, try gently pressing on the abdomen or flicking a finger against it; then auscultate again. Typically, the light pressure will provoke bowel sounds.
• Next, auscultate for vascular sounds, using the bell of your stethoscope.

Assessing for abnormal abdominal and bowel sounds

ABDOMINAL SOUNDS	WHERE FOUND	POSSIBLE CAUSES
• Friction rub (harsh grating — like two pieces of sandpaper rubbing together)	• Over liver and spleen	• Inflammation of the liver's peritoneal surface, as occurs from a tumor
• Systolic bruits (vascular blowing sounds that resemble cardiac murmurs)	• Over abdominal aorta • Over renal artery • Over iliac artery	• Partial arterial obstruction or turbulent blood flow • Renal artery stenosis • Hepatomegaly
• Venous hum (continuous, medium-pitched tone of blood flowing in a large, engorged vascular organ such as the liver)	• Epigastric and umbilical regions	• Increased collateral circulation between portal and systemic venous systems, as occurs in cirrhosis

BOWEL SOUNDS	WHERE FOUND	POSSIBLE CAUSES
• Hyperactivity (unrelated to hunger)	• Any quadrant	• Diarrhea or early intestinal obstruction
• Hypoactivity to silence	• Any quadrant	• Paralytic ileus or peritonitis
• High-pitched tinkling	• Any quadrant	• Intestinal fluid and air under tension in a dilated bowel
• High-pitched rushing (coinciding with abdominal cramps)	• Any quadrant	• Intestinal obstruction

Auscultate the epigastric and umbilical regions to detect venous hums. Listen in the epigastric region and in each of the quadrants for bruits from the major abdominal arteries. Normally, you won't hear vascular sounds. (See *Auscultating for vascular sounds.*)

• Finally, place the diaphragm of the stethoscope over the liver and spleen and listen for friction rubs.

Nursing considerations
• You can initiate peristalsis and bowel sounds by gently pressing on the surface of the abdomen or by having the patient eat or drink something if eating is allowed.

Documentation
• Document the presence or absence of bowel sounds and vascular sounds in each quadrant.

Auscultating for vascular sounds

After listening to your patient's bowel sounds, use the bell of your stethoscope to auscultate for vascular sounds at the sites shown in this illustration.

Aorta

Right renal artery

Left renal artery

Right iliac artery

Left iliac artery

Right femoral artery

Left femoral artery

• Note whether bowel sounds are *hyperactive* or *hypoactive*. Rapid, high-pitched, loud, and gurgling bowel sounds are hyperactive and may occur normally in a hungry patient. Sounds occurring once a minute or more often are hypoactive and normally occur after bowel surgery or when the colon is filled with feces.

Abdominal inspection

When assessing the abdomen, you'll alter the usual sequence of the four assessment techniques. Perform the examination sequence from inspection and auscultation to percussion and palpation. Because percussion and palpation can affect bowel activity — and, as a re-

sult, bowel sounds — you'll auscultate before percussing and palpating.

The quadrants are the right upper quadrant (RUQ), the right lower quadrant (RLQ), the left upper quadrant (LUQ), and the left lower quadrant (LLQ). (See *Identifying abdominal landmarks*, page 4.)

≫ Key nursing diagnoses and patient outcomes

Use this nursing diagnosis as a guide when developing your plan of care.

Knowledge deficit related to lack of exposure to assessment techniques
Based on this nursing diagnosis, you'll establish the following patient outcome. The patient will:
• state understanding of need for assessment.

Identifying abdominal landmarks

To aid accurate abdominal assessment and documentation of findings, you can mentally divide the patient's abdomen into regions. The quadrant method, the easiest and most commonly used, divides the abdomen into four equal regions by two imaginary lines crossing perpendicularly above the umbilicus.

Right upper quadrant (RUQ)
Liver and gallbladder
Pylorus
Duodenum
Head of pancreas
Hepatic flexure of colon
Portions of ascending and transverse colon

Left upper quadrant (LUQ)
Left liver lobe
Stomach
Body of Pancreas
Splenic flexure of colon
Portions of transverse and descending colon

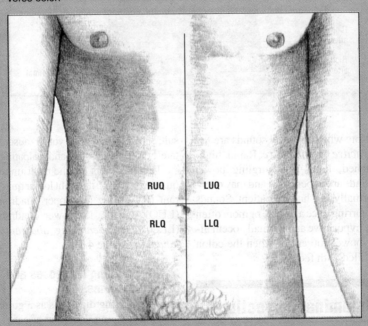

Right lower quadrant (RLQ)
Cecum and appendix
Portion of ascending colon
Lower portion of right kidney
Bladder (if distended)

Left lower quadrant (LLQ)
Sigmoid colon
Portion of descending colon
Lower portion of left kidney
Bladder (if distended)

Equipment
♦ pillows.

Patient preparation
• Make sure the patient has voided before the abdominal examination.
• Prepare him for the examination by placing him in the supine position. A pillow behind his head and another behind his knees will help the patient relax his abdominal muscles.

Implementation
• Begin by inspecting the patient's entire abdomen. A normal abdomen is slightly rounded, or convex, with symmetrical, slightly curved borders, but contours vary with body type. A slender patient, for instance, may have a flat or slightly concave abdomen, and an obese patient may have one that protudes.
• Ask your patient to breathe deeply and inspect his abdomen as he breathes. If the abdomen appears distended, make a mental note to check for ascites when percussing and palpating later in your assessment. Irregular contours or asymmetrical distention will also require further assessment.
• Measure the girth of your patient's abdomen with a tape held at the level of the umbilicus if the abdomen is distended. Mark the abdomen with a felt-tip pen to ensure that subsequent readings accurately reflect changes.
• Observe with your eyes at the level of the patient's abdomen. His skin should be smooth and unbroken, with varying amounts of hair. Note any discoloration, lines, stretch marks, lesions, rashes, dilated veins, or scars.
• Ordinarily, you won't be able to see any abdominal movements except in very thin patients. Some slight, wave-like motion may be visible, but strong contractions crossing the abdomen should be reported because they may signal a bowel obstruction. Note the rate, intensity, and exact location of any aortic pulsations you detect in the epigastric region. Never palpate a visible midline pulsation, which can indicate an abdominal aneurysm.
• Your patient's umbilicus should be concave and midline. Inverted navels are a normal variation. If the umbilicus protrudes when your patient raises his head and shoulders, he may have an umbilical hernia.

Nursing considerations
• To detect abdominal masses or bulges, ask the patient to take a deep breath and hold it. This will lower the diaphragm and compress abdominal organs, causing bulges or masses to appear.
• Then tell him to raise his head to make the rectus abdominis muscles contract and appear more prominent. The increased pressure may force a hernia or other abdominal-wall mass to protrude.

Documentation
• Note any abdominal distention or ascites.
• Note the abdomen's general contour and symmetry as well as any abnormalities of the skin or umbilicus.
• Document any visible pulsations.

Abdominal palpation

You'll use a combination of light and deep palpation and ballottement to assess your patient's abdomen. Start with the right upper quadrant (RUQ) and move clockwise to the right lower

Palpating the spleen

With your patient in the supine position, stand on her right side. Then use your left hand to support her posterior lower rib cage, and ask her to take a deep breath. With your right hand on the abdomen, press up and in toward the spleen, as shown.

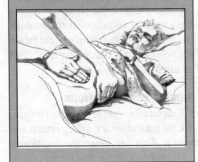

quadrant (RLQ), the left lower quadrant (LLQ), and the left upper quadrant (LUQ). If the patient complains of pain in one quadrant, palpate that one last. As you palpate, check for organ location, masses, muscle resistance, and areas of tenderness.

≫ Key nursing diagnoses and patient outcomes

Use this nursing diagnosis as a guide when developing your plan of care.

Knowledge deficit related to lack of exposure to assessment techniques
Based on this nursing diagnosis, you'll establish the following patient outcome. The patient will:
• state understanding of need for assessment.

Patient preparation
• Ask the patient to keep his abdomen relaxed during the examination.

Implementation
• Begin with light palpation.
• Make sure your hands are warm.
• Palpate one structure at a time.
• Usually, you'll have to use deep palpation to evaluate abdominal masses. Feel for pulsations.

Spleen
• You can't usually palpate the spleen, but unless you think it's ruptured, try to palpate it. Have the patient lie in a supine position. From his right side, support his posterior left lower rib cage with your left hand and tell him to take a deep breath. Use your other hand to press up and in toward the spleen. If you feel the spleen, it's probably enlarged. (See *Palpating the spleen.*)
• When a patient complains of pain or tenderness, try eliciting rebound tenderness, a sign of peritoneal irritation. This maneuver is controversial and considered unnecessary by many practitioners. Wait until the end of the examination if you use it because resulting pain and muscle spasm can interfere with further assessment.
• To try eliciting rebound tenderness, tell the patient to lie in a supine position with his knees flexed. Next, locate McBurney's point (about one-third the distance between the right anterior superior iliac spine and the umbilicus). Press your fingertips slowly and deeply into this area, and then release the pressure in a swift, smooth motion. If the patient complains of pain when the tissue springs back, you've elicited rebound tenderness.
• To lessen the risk of rupturing an inflamed appendix, don't repeat this maneuver. (See *Eliciting rebound tenderness*, and *Causes of acute abdominal pain in children*, page 8.)

Eliciting rebound tenderness

Press your fingertips deeply and gently into the patient's abdomen at McBurney's point, as shown.

Then quickly withdraw your fingertips. If the patient feels pain when the tissue springs back, you've detected rebound tenderness.

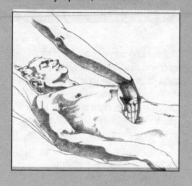
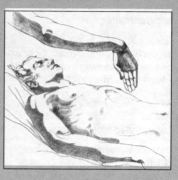

• Use light ballottement to detect areas of muscle resistance or guarding you may have missed on deep palpation. Ballottement can also detect movement or bounce of a freely movable mass.

Liver

• Now try to palpate the liver. You won't be able to feel a normal-sized liver in most patients. You may be able to feel the liver in extremely thin patients or in patients with emphysema. Emphysema patients have a low diaphragm, which may push the liver down, where it may be more easily palpable below the costal margin.

• To palpate the liver, slide your left hand under the patient's back, at the liver's approximate location. Place your right hand below the lower mark you made to indicate the liver's lower border and point your fingers toward the right costal margin. Gently press in and up as the patient inhales. The edge of the liver should feel firm, rounded, and smooth. Note any irregularities or tenderness.

• Try hooking the liver if you can't palpate it. Stand on your patient's right side, near his shoulder. Place your hands side by side below the lower mark you've made. Tell the patient to inhale deeply. Press your fingers in and up to feel the liver with the fingertips of both hands. (See *Palpating and hooking the liver*, page 9.)

Gallbladder

• Employing the same palpation technique you used for the liver, try to palpate the gallbladder, which normally isn't palpable. If the gallbladder is enlarged and distended, however, you'll feel it below the liver margin at the lateral border of the rectus muscle, either medially or laterally. An enlarged, tender gallbladder suggests cholecystitis; an enlarged, nontender gallbladder suggests obstructive disease.

Causes of acute abdominal pain in children

Acute abdominal pain (acute abdomen) occurs frequently in infancy and childhood. This chart details the most common causes of this problem.

DISORDER	ASSESSMENT FINDINGS
Intussusception	
Telescoping of one intestinal segment into another (usually ileum into cecum), leading to acute intestinal obstruction	Colicky abdominal pain, with restlessness and intense crying; passage of bloody, mucoid "currant jelly" stools; palpable, sausage-shaped, tender mass in right upper or lower quadrant
Incarcerated inguinal hernia	
Indirect: weakness in fascial margin of internal inguinal ring *Direct:* weakness in fascial floor of inguinal canal; protrusion of sac (containing intestinal contents) at inguinal opening, with resultant bowel obstruction	Abdominal cramps, vomiting, abdominal distention, lump in inguinal area, palpable, irreducible, tender swelling or lump in inguinal area
Appendicitis	
Obstruction of lumen of appendix, leading to inflammation and possibly perforation with peritonitis	Vomiting common in children under age 8; midabdominal cramps, possibly progressing to right lower quadrant pain; slight fever; request to cough will produce pain over site of peritoneal inflammation; bowel sounds may be depressed; rebound tenderness on palpation (performed by doctor)

Kidneys
• To palpate the right kidney, stand on the patient's right side. Place your left hand under his waist (just below the 12th rib) and place your right hand on his abdomen. Tell him to take a deep breath (so that his kidney will move downward). As he inhales, press up with your left hand and down with your right hand. The kidney should be firm and smooth, not tender.

• To palpate the left kidney, remain at the patient's right side. Reach across him with your left arm, and place your left hand under his back at waist level. Pull up with your left hand to elevate and displace the kidney anteriorly. Ask the patient to take a deep breath. Then try to palpate the lower pole of the left kidney with your right hand. (Note that the left kidney is rarely palpable because it's behind the spleen.)

Palpating and hooking the liver

These illustrations show you the correct hand positions for palpating and hooking the liver.

Liver palpation
Place one hand on the patient's back at the level of the liver and place the other hand below the area of liver dullness, as shown. As the patient inhales deeply, press gently.

Liver hooking
Standing near the patient's right shoulder, place your hands below the area of liver dullness, as shown. As the patient inhales deeply, press your fingers inward and upward.

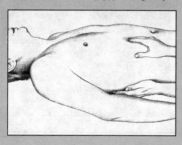
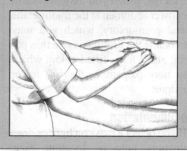

You can palpate the left kidney from the patient's left side: Use the same method described in palpating the right kidney.

Bladder
• Use bimanual technique to palpate the bladder. Begin at midline, 1″ to 2″ (2.5 to 5 cm) above the symphysis pubis, and continue palpating until you feel the bladder's edge. A smooth, rounded, fluctuant suprapubic mass suggests distention; a fluctuant mass extending to the umbilicus indicates extreme distention. A normal bladder may be undetectable.

Abdominal muscles
• To palpate the abdominal muscles, apply light pressure on the umbilical ring and around the umbilicus. The muscle should feel smooth, without bulges, nodules, or soft openings (her-

niations). Use light palpation on all four abdominal quadrants.
• For deep palpation of abdominal muscles, place one hand on top of the other and exert pressure with the top hand. Be alert for tenderness, pulsations, symmetry, mobility, rigidity, guarding, ascites, or pain. Deep palpation may also be used to evaluate abdominal masses.

Nursing considerations
• In a child, the liver is proportionately larger and palpation one to two fingerbreadths below the ribs is considered normal.
• In a normal variation known as Riedel's lobe, the right lobe is elongated down toward the right lower quadrant and is palpable below the right costal margin.
• Don't palpate a pulsating midline mass; it may be a dissecting aneu-

rysm, which can rupture under the pressure of palpation. Report such a mass to the doctor immediately.
• If you can't palpate the spleen, don't press too hard. Manual compression of an enlarged spleen can rupture it.
• Be careful not to mistake a normal finding for a mass during abdominal palpation. It's possible, for instance, to mistake the following for masses: the uterus, which you may palpate in the lower abdomen at the midline; the sacral promontory, which you may feel below the umbilicus in a thin patient; and a feces-filled colon, which you may palpate in the left lower quadrant.

Documentation
• If you detect a mass on light or deep palpation, note its location, size, shape, consistency, type of border, degree of tenderness, presence of pulsations, and degree of mobility (fixed or mobile).

Abdominal percussion

You'll use percussion in your assessment to check size and location of abdominal organs and to detect excessive abdominal fluid and air. Don't percuss (or palpate) a patient who may have an abdominal aortic aneurysm or a patient with an abdominal organ transplant. Percuss cautiously if you suspect appendicitis.

≫ Key nursing diagnoses and patient outcomes
Use this nursing diagnosis as a guide when developing your plan of care.

Abdominal percussion sounds

When you percuss the abdomen, you'll normally hear dull and tympanic percussion sounds over the areas shown here.

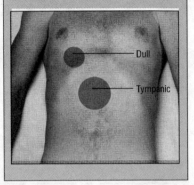

Knowledge deficit related to lack of exposure to assessment techniques
Based on this nursing diagnosis, you'll establish the following patient outcome. The patient will:
• state understanding of need for assessment.

Equipment
♦ felt-tipped pen ♦ tape measure.

Patient preparation
• Have the patient void. Help him into a supine position. Explain each procedure before you perform it.

Implementation
• As with auscultation, start in the right upper quadrant and work clockwise. If your patient has abdominal pain, percuss the painful quadrant last.
• Lightly percuss over the abdomen, identifying tympanic and dull areas. You'll hear tympany when you per-

cuss over a patient's air-filled stomach or intestine. You'll hear dullness over the liver and spleen. As you percuss, note where sounds change from tympanic to dull. Abnormally high-pitched tympanic sounds suggest bowel distention.

• Normally, dull sounds are heard over solid structures, such as the liver, spleen, pancreas, kidneys, and uterus, and over a feces-filled intestine and urine-filled bladder. Be alert for abnormal dullness from solid tumors in the lower abdomen or from ascites. (See *Abdominal percussion sounds.*)

• With the patient in a supine position, note if his flanks bulge, an indication of ascites. Then, percuss for tympany and dullness. You'll detect tympany over the upper abdomen because the bowel rises with the patient in this position. You'll detect dullness in the dependent parts of the abdomen. Check for shifting ascites by having the patient turn to the side and percussing again. If ascites are present, you'll note tympany in the superior portion of the abdomen and dullness in the dependent portion. To detect advanced ascites, place your palm and forearm along the patient's right flank. Next, tap the left flank with your other hand. If a large accumulation of fluid is present, a fluid wave will ripple across the abdomen and cause the patient's right flank to hit against your hand.

• A normal spleen may yield a small area of dullness in the left midaxillary line at about the level of the 10th rib. In most patients, though, you won't hear it because the tympany produced by colonic or gastric air will obscure it. To assess for splenic enlargement, ask the patient to inhale deeply. Then percuss along the 9th and 10th left in-

Differentiating spleen and kidney enlargement

Typically, if you ask the patient to take a deep breath and then you percuss along the 9th and 10th left intercostal spaces, you'll hear tympany produced by colonic or gastric air. If you hear dullness instead, the patient's spleen may be enlarged. If you hear resonance, his left kidney may be enlarged.

tercostal spaces. A change from tympany to dullness as you percuss may indicate splenic enlargement. (See *Differentiating spleen and kidney enlargement.*)

• To estimate the size of the liver, begin percussing the abdomen along the right midclavicular line below the level of the umbilicus. Move upward until the percussion sounds change from tympany to dullness, which typically occurs at or slightly below the costal margin. Mark this point with a felt-tipped pen.

• Next, starting above the nipple, percuss downward along the right midclavicular line until the percussion sounds change from normal lung resonance to dullness. Usually, this occurs between the fifth and seventh intercostal spaces. Again, mark the point where you hear the change. You can estimate the size of your patient's liver by measuring the distance between the two marks. (See *Percussing the liver*, page 12.)

• If you suspect inflammation, hepatitis, or hepatomegaly, use fist percussion, or blunt percussion, to detect tenderness. You should attempt to palpate the liver before using fist percussion.

Percussing the liver

To estimate liver size, percuss along the right midclavicular line, moving upward from below the level of the umbilicus, as shown. Then percuss along the midclavicular line, moving downward from above the level of the nipple.

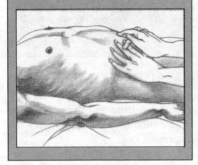

Stop percussing if the patient complains of pain or discomfort. Tenderness on the right side during fist percussion suggests inflammation.

Bladder
• Make sure the patient is properly draped.
• Percuss the area over the bladder, starting about 2″ (5 cm) above the symphysis pubis. Continue percussing downward. A tympanic sound is normal over an empty bladder; a dull sound indicates a distended bladder.

Spleen
• To percuss the spleen, tell the patient to turn onto his right side. Beginning at the sixth rib, percuss posteriorly along the midaxillary line until the sound changes from resonance (from the lungs) to tympany (from colonic or gastric air) over the spleen. Tell the patient to take deep breaths during the

process. Because an enlarged spleen moves forward and downward with inspiration, a descent from tympany to dullness suggests splenic enlargement.

Kidneys
• Use blunt percussion to assess for kidney tenderness. Tell the patient to sit up or lie on his side. Place one hand palm down over the costovertebral angle, between the spine and the 12th rib. Strike this hand lightly with your other fist. A resonant sound indicates your hand is over a kidney. If the patient complains of tenderness during this percussion, suspect kidney, liver, or gallbladder inflammation.

Nursing considerations
• Keep in mind that men normally have a larger liver span than women and tall people a larger liver span than short people.

Airway obstruction management

Sudden airway obstruction may occur when a foreign body lodges in the throat or bronchus; the patient aspirates blood, mucus, or vomitus; the tongue blocks the pharynx; or the patient experiences traumatic injury, bronchoconstriction, or bronchospasm.

An obstructed airway is an emergency; it causes anoxia, which can lead to brain damage and death in 4 to 6 minutes.

Use an upper-abdominal thrust that creates diaphragmatic pressure in the static lung below the foreign body sufficient to expel the obstruction — but use it only on conscious adults.

Use an abdominal thrust on unconscious patients but not on pregnant, markedly obese, and recent abdominal-surgery patients. For these patients use a chest thrust, which forces air out of the lungs to create an artificial cough. The finger-sweep maneuver is then used to manually remove the foreign body from the mouth.

All of these maneuvers are contraindicated in a patient with incomplete or partial airway obstruction or when the patient can maintain adequate ventilation to dislodge the foreign body by effective coughing.

If a person can't speak, cough, or breathe, take immediate action to dislodge the obstruction.

>> Key nursing diagnoses and patient outcomes

Use these nursing diagnoses as a guide when developing your plan of care for someone who has had an obstructed airway.

Inability to sustain spontaneous ventilation related to airway obstruction

Based on this nursing diagnosis, you'll establish the following patient outcomes. The patient will:
• breathe spontaneously after the obstruction is removed or resolved.
• maintain baseline respiratory rate.
• attain baseline arterial blood gas (ABG) levels.
• maintain baseline breathing pattern.
• be free of dyspnea.

Impaired gas exchange related to obstruction

Based on this nursing diagnosis, you'll establish the following patient outcomes. The patient will:
• attain baseline ABG levels.
• maintain baseline breath sounds.
• comfortably maintain air exchange.
• achieve an acceptable baseline respiratory rate.

Anxiety related to acute respiratory distress and fear of impending death

Based on this nursing diagnosis, you'll establish the following patient outcomes. The patient will:
• state that she feels less anxious.
• express knowledge of ways to prevent repeated obstruction.

Equipment

♦ suction equipment ♦ oxygen ♦ hand-held oxygen delivery equipment.

Implementation

• Determine your patient's level of consciousness by tapping her shoulder and asking, "Are you choking?"
• If she has a complete airway obstruction, she won't be able to answer.
• If she makes crowing sounds, her airway is partially obstructed, and you should encourage her to cough, which will clear or completely obstruct the airway.
• For complete obstruction, intervene as follows, depending on whether the patient is conscious or unconscious.

Conscious adult

• Tell her you'll try to dislodge the foreign body.
• Standing behind her, wrap your arms around her waist. Make a fist

with one hand and place the thumb side against her abdomen, slightly above the umbilicus and well below the xiphoid process. Then grasp your fist with the other hand (below).

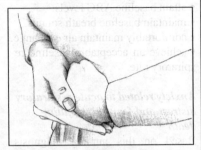

• Squeeze the patient's abdomen 6 to 10 times with quick inward and upward thrusts (as shown below). Each thrust should be a separate movement forceful enough to create an artificial cough that may dislodge an obstruction.

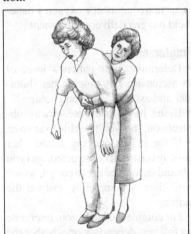

• Make sure you have a firm grasp on the patient because she may lose consciousness and need to be lowered to the floor. Look around the floor for objects that may harm her.
• If she loses consciousness, lower her carefully to the floor. Support her head

and neck to prevent injury, and continue as described below.

Unconscious adult

• If the patient is unconscious, ask any witnesses what happened. Begin cardiopulmonary resuscitation (CPR) if necessary, and try to ventilate the patient. If you're unable to ventilate her, reposition her head and try again.
• If you still can't ventilate the patient or if a conscious patient loses consciousness during abdominal thrusts, kneel astride her thighs. Then place the heel of one of your hands on top of the back of the other oustretched hand, which should be placed palm down. Then rest your hands between the patient's umbilicus and the tip of her xiphoid process at the midline. Push in and up with 6 to 10 quick abdominal thrusts (as shown below).

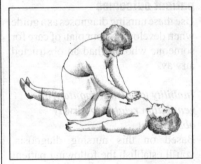

• After the thrusts, open her airway by grasping her tongue and lower jaw between your thumb and fingers. Lift the jaw to draw the tongue away from the back of the throat and away from any foreign body (as shown at the top of the next page).
• If you can see the object, remove it by inserting your index finger deep into the throat at the base of her tongue. Using a hooking motion, remove the obstruction (as shown

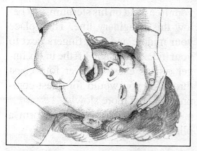

below). *Keep in mind that some clinicians object to a blind finger sweep (using your finger when you can't see the obstruction) because your finger may act as a second obstruction. These clinicians believe that the tongue-jaw lift should dislodge most obstructions.*

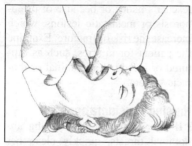

• After removing the object, try to ventilate the patient. Assess for spontaneous respirations and check for a pulse. Proceed with CPR if necessary.
• If the object is not removed, try to ventilate the patient anyway. If you can't, repeat abdominal thrusts until you clear the airway.

Obese or pregnant adult
• If the patient is conscious, stand behind her and place your arms under her armpits and around her chest.
• Place the thumb side of your clenched fist against the middle of the sternum, avoiding the margins of the ribs and the xiphoid process. Grasp your fist with your other hand and

thrust with enough force to expel the foreign body (as shown below). Continue until the patient expels the obstruction or loses consciousness.

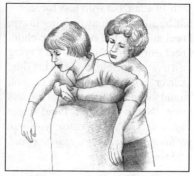

• If the patient loses consciousness, carefully lower her to the floor.
• Kneel near the patient's side and place the heel of one hand just above the bottom of her sternum. The long axis of the heel of your hand should align with the long axis of the patient's sternum. Place the heel of your other hand on top of your hand on the patient's sternum (as shown below), making sure your fingers don't touch the patient's chest. Deliver each thrust forcefully enough to remove the object.

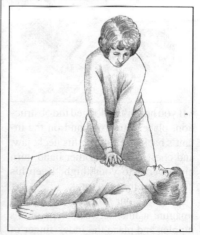

Child

• If the child is conscious and can stand, perform abdominal thrusts using the same technique as you would with an adult, but with less force.

• If he's unconscious or lying down, kneel at his feet; if he's a large child, kneel astride his thighs. If he's lying on a treatment table, stand by his side. Deliver abdominal thrusts as you would for an adult patient, but use less force. (Never perform a blind finger sweep on a child *because you risk pushing the foreign body farther back into the airway.*)

Infant

• Whether the infant is conscious or not, place his face down so he's straddling your arm with his head lower than his trunk. Rest your forearm on your thigh and deliver four back blows with the heel of your hand between his shoulder blades (as shown below).

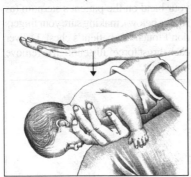

• If you haven't dislodged the obstruction, place your free hand on the infant's back. Supporting his neck, jaw, and chest with your other hand, turn him over onto your thigh. Keep his head lower than his trunk.

• Position your fingers. To do so, imagine a line between the infant's nipples and place the index finger of your free hand on his sternum, just below this imaginary line. Then place your middle and ring fingers next to your index finger and lift the index finger off his chest. Deliver four chest thrusts as you would for chest compression, but more slowly.

• As with a child, never perform a blind finger sweep.

Complications

• Complications may include nausea, regurgitation, and achiness after the patient regains consciousness and can breathe independently.

• The patient may also be injured, possibly from incorrect placement of the rescuer's hands or because of osteoporosis or metastatic lesions, which increase the risk of fracture. Examine the patient for injuries, such as ruptured or lacerated abdominal or thoracic viscera.

Nursing considerations

• If your patient vomits during abdominal thrusts, quickly clean her mouth out with your fingers and resume the maneuver as necessary.

• Even if you can't seem to clear the airway, keep trying. As oxygen deprivation increases, smooth and skeletal muscles relax, making your maneuvers more likely to succeed.

Documentation

• Record the date and time of the procedure, the patient's actions before the obstruction, the approximate length of time it took to clear the airway, and the type and size of the object removed.

• Note her vital signs after the procedure, any complications that occurred and nursing actions taken, and her tolerance of the procedure.

Amniocentesis

This procedure involves transabdominal needle aspiration of amniotic fluid for laboratory analysis and is usually performed between the 16th and 20th weeks of gestation. Amniocentesis can detect neural tube or chromosomal defects and certain metabolic and other disorders. The procedure can also identify the gender of the fetus and aid in the assessment of fetal health. In the final trimester, amniocentesis helps in the evaluation of fetal lung maturity and in the detection of hemolytic disease of the newborn.

Indications for amniocentesis include maternal age over 35 (associated with Down syndrome), a family history of neural tube or chromosomal defects, or inborn errors of metabolism. It's also indicated if miscarriage has occurred in prior pregnancy. Amniocentesis may be performed in a labor and delivery suite, the ultrasonography department, or a doctor's office.

Contraindications for amniocentesis include an anterior uterine wall obscured by the placenta and insufficient amniotic fluid.

Risks must be weighed against expected benefits if the mother tests positive for human immunodeficiency virus, which causes AIDS. (For risks, see "Complications," page 19.)

⟫ Key nursing diagnoses and patient outcomes

Use these nursing diagnoses as a guide when developing your plan of care for a patient having amniocentesis.

Anxiety related to the procedure

Based on this nursing diagnosis, you'll establish the following patient outcomes. The patient will:
• express feelings of anxiety.
• make use of available emotional support.

Knowledge deficit related to amniocentesis

Based on this nursing diagnosis, you'll establish the following patient outcomes. The patient will:
• learn about reasons for amniocentesis.
• recognize that increased knowledge will help her cope better with the procedure.

Equipment

♦ preassembled amniocentesis tray or ♦ hospital gown ♦ two sets of sterile gloves, sterile gowns, and masks ♦ stethoscope ♦ Doppler ultrasound stethoscope and other appropriate ultrasound equipment ♦ fetoscope or electronic fetal monitor ♦ antiseptic solution with sterile container ♦ local anesthetic ♦ alcohol ♦ 10-ml syringe ♦ sterile 20G or 22G 4" spinal needle with stylet ♦ 22G or 25G needle ♦ sterile 20-ml glass syringe ♦ clean amber glass specimen container for Rh sensitization and lecithin-sphingomyelin (L/S) ratio tests ♦ three sterile, glass specimen tubes (for genetic tests) ♦ laboratory request forms ♦ adhesive bandage.

Avoiding bladder puncture

To reduce the risk of bladder puncture, ensure that the patient voids before the procedure if the pregnancy exceeds 20 weeks. (Before 20 weeks, a full bladder may help to hold the uterus steady.)

Equipment preparation
- If you don't have an amber specimen container, cover the outside of a clean test tube or glass container with adhesive tape or aluminum foil. Protecting aspirated amniotic fluid from light prevents the breakdown of such pigments as bilirubin.
- Properly label all specimen containers or tubes.

Patient preparation
- Explain the procedure to the patient. Confirm that she understands the risk of complications. (For risks, see "Complications," page 19.)
- Emphasize that the doctor may need to repeat the procedure and that amniotic fluid analysis can't rule out all birth defects.
- Reaffirm that you have the patient's signed informed consent form.
- Have the patient void before the test to help prevent bladder puncture. (See *Avoiding bladder puncture.*)

Implementation
- Provide privacy and tell the patient to put on a hospital gown.
- Help her to a supine position and obtain baseline maternal vital signs.
- Next, determine baseline fetal heart rate (FHR) with the Doppler ultrasound stethoscope or the fetoscope.

- Tell the patient to fold her hands on her chest or to rest her hands behind her head.
- Remind her to stay still.
- The doctor will use ultrasonography to locate the fetus and the placenta.
- When the doctor identifies an amniotic-fluid pocket, he can determine the appropriate needle-insertion depth.
- Next, the doctor will put on the sterile gown, sterile gloves, and mask and clean the skin at the needle-puncture site with an antiseptic solution.
- If the patient will receive a local anesthetic, clean the diaphragm of the multidose vial of anesthetic solution with alcohol. Provide a 10-ml syringe and 22G or 25G needle. Then invert the bottle *to allow the doctor to withdraw the anesthetic.*
- Scrub your hands, and put on a sterile gown, sterile gloves, and mask to assist the doctor with amniocentesis, an aseptic procedure.
- After the anesthetic takes effect on the patient, the doctor, guided by ultrasound imaging, will advance the 20G spinal needle with a stylet through the abdomen and uterine wall and into the amniotic sac. Then he will remove the stylet. When a drop of amniotic fluid appears, he'll attach the 20-ml glass syringe to the needle and aspirate the fluid.
- When the doctor withdraws the needle, place an adhesive bandage over the insertion site.
- Complete the laboratory request forms, and send the specimens to the laboratory immediately. Speedy transport is important *because if the amniotic fluid contains blood or meconium, immediate centrifuging can preserve the specimen for analysis.*

• If the patient is in the final trimester, tell her to lie on her side *to avoid hypotension from pressure of the gravid uterus on the vena cava.*

• Assess maternal vital signs and FHR at 15 minutes and 30 minutes after the procedure to detect changes from baseline values. FHR changes, such as tachycardia or bradycardia, signal distress. If these signs appear, notify the doctor and continue to monitor FHR.

• Electronically monitor the patient for uterine irritability and the fetus for changes in heart-rate pattern. Monitoring should continue for a few hours after the procedure *to allow early intervention if complications occur.* Normally, maternal vital signs should remain stable.

• Help the patient dress *in preparation for discharge.*

• If the patient is having genetic studies, open the sterile glass specimen tubes. After the doctor transfers amniotic fluid to the tubes, use aseptic technique when closing the tubes *to avoid contamination, which can yield aberrant test results.*

• If the patient is having the Rh sensitization or L/S ratio tests, open the amber or the covered test tube *so the doctor can transfer the amniotic fluid.* Close the container at once *to protect the fluid from light, which may cause pigments in the fluid, such as bilirubin, to break down and skew test results.*

Complications

Although amniocentesis is an invasive procedure, it rarely produces maternal or fetal complications. Maternal complications, which affect fewer than 1% of patients, include:

• amniotic-fluid embolism
• hemorrhage
• infection
• premature labor
• abruptio placentae
• placenta or umbilical-cord trauma
• bladder or intestine puncture
• Rh isoimmunization.

Rare fetal complications include:
• fetal death
• amnionitis
• injury from needle puncture
• amniotic fluid leakage
• bleeding
• spontaneous abortion
• premature birth.

Nursing considerations

• Monitor the patient for signs and symptoms of supine hypotension, such as light-headedness, nausea, and diaphoresis.

• If the patient will receive a dose of Rh₀(D) immunoglobulin (RhoGAM), explain that this passive immunizing agent may help prevent an Rh incompatibility between the patient and the fetus that would cause antibody formation in the mother's blood. This condition is known as erythroblastosis fetalis (hydrops fetalis or hemolytic disease of the newborn).

• Inform the patient, her family, and her support person, as appropriate, that test results should be available in 2 to 4 weeks. Provide emotional support as needed.

Home care

Instruct the patient to report these signs and symptoms of complications.
• vaginal discharge (fluid or blood)
• decreased fetal movement
• contractions
• fever and chills.

Documentation
- Record the name of the doctor and the date and time of the procedure.
- Record baseline maternal vital sign values and the FHR. Note any changes in these baseline data.
- Name the ordered laboratory tests.
- Describe the amount and appearance of the specimen fluid and time of transport to the laboratory.
- Document discharge instructions to the patient.
- Document how the patient tolerated the procedure.

Anaerobic specimen collection

A wound culture is a microscopic analysis of a specimen from a lesion to confirm infection. Normally, there are no pathogens in a clean wound.

An anaerobic culture is for organisms that need little or no oxygen and appear in areas of poor tissue perfusion, such as postoperative wounds, ulcers, or compound fractures. *Clostridium* and *Bacteroides* are among the most common anaerobic pathogens. Indications for wound culture include fever and inflammation, and drainage in damaged tissue.

≫ Key nursing diagnoses and patient outcomes
Use these nursing diagnoses as a guide when developing your plan of care.

Altered (specific) tissue perfusion related to infection
Based on this nursing diagnosis, you'll establish the following patient outcomes. The patient will:
- maintain tissue perfusion and cellular oxygenation.
- express a feeling of comfort or absence of pain at wound site.

Risk for infection related to wound site
Based on this nursing diagnosis, you'll establish the following patient outcomes. The patient will:
- have a temperature that stays in normal limits.
- have all pathogens in anaerobic cultures respond to treatment.

Equipment
♦ sterile cotton-tipped applicators or sterile 10-ml syringe with 21G needle ♦ special culture tube containing carbon dioxide or nitrogen ♦ sterile gloves ♦ alcohol sponges ♦ sterile gauze and povidone-iodine solution ♦ sterile forceps.

Patient preparation
- Explain to the patient that this test is used to identify infectious microbes.
- Describe the procedure, advising him that a drainage specimen from the wound is withdrawn by a syringe or removed on cotton-tipped applicators.
- Tell him who will perform the procedure and when.
- Reassure him that collecting the drainage specimen takes less than 3 minutes.

Implementation
- Wash your hands, prepare a sterile field, and put on sterile gloves.
- With sterile forceps, remove the dressing to expose the wound.
- Dispose of the soiled dressings properly.
- Clean the area around the wound with an alcohol or povidone-iodine sponge to reduce the risk of contaminating the specimen with skin bacteria.
- Allow the area to dry.
- Insert the sterile cotton-tipped applicator deeply into the wound, rotate it gently, remove it, and immediately place it in the anaerobic culture tube. (See *Collecting anaerobic specimens.*)
- You may also insert a sterile 10-ml syringe, without a needle, into the wound and aspirate 1 to 5 ml of exudate into the syringe. Then attach the 21G needle to the syringe and immediately inject the aspirate into the anaerobic-culture tube. If an anaerobic-culture tube isn't available, obtain a rubber stopper, attach the needle to the syringe, and gently push all the air out of the syringe by pressing on the plunger. Stick the needle tip into the rubber stopper, and send the syringe of aspirate to the laboratory immediately with a completed laboratory request form.
- Apply a new dressing to the wound.

Complications
- Rarely, there may be infection from cross-contamination.

Nursing considerations
- Note recent antibiotic therapy on the laboratory request form.

Collecting anaerobic specimens

Because most anaerobes die when exposed to oxygen, they must be transported in tubes filled with carbon dioxide or nitrogen. The anaerobic specimen collector shown here includes a rubber-stoppered tube filled with carbon dioxide, a small inner tube, and a cotton-tipped applicator attached to a plastic plunger.

Before specimen collection, the small inner tube containing the cotton-tipped applicator is held in place with the rubber stopper (as shown on the left). After collecting the specimen, quickly replace the applicator in the inner tube and depress the plunger to separate the inner tube from the stopper (right), forcing it into the larger tube and exposing the specimen to a carbon dioxide–rich environment.

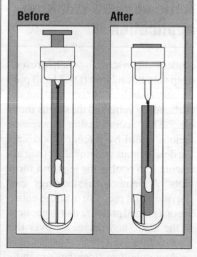

Before   **After**

- Make sure antiseptic doesn't enter the wound because this could cause tissue irritation.

• Obtain exudate from the entire wound, using more than one cotton-tipped applicator if necessary.

• Because some anaerobes die in the presence of even a small amount of oxygen, place the specimen in the culture tube quickly, take care that no air enters into the tube, and check that double stoppers are secure.

• Keep the specimen container upright, and send it to the laboratory within 15 minutes to prevent growth or deterioration of microbes.

Documentation

• Record the time, date, and site of specimen collection and any recent or current antibiotic therapy.

• Make sure that you note whether the specimen has an unusual appearance or odor.

Antiembolism stocking application

Antiembolism stockings help prevent deep vein thrombosis (DVT) and pulmonary embolism by compressing superficial leg veins and the soleus muscle. This compression increases venous return by forcing blood into the deep venous system rather than allowing it to pool in the legs and form clots. Antiembolism stockings can provide equal pressure over the entire leg or a graded pressure that is greatest at the ankle and decreases over the length of the leg.

Antiembolism stockings are indicated for postoperative, bedridden, elderly, or other patients at risk for DVT. They should not, however, be used on patients with dermatoses or open skin lesions, gangrene, severe arteriosclerosis or other ischemic vascular diseases, pulmonary or any massive edema, recent vein ligation, or vascular or skin grafts.

⟫ Key nursing diagnoses and patient outcomes

Use these nursing diagnoses as a guide when developing your plan of care for a patient who is being treated with antiembolism stockings.

Impaired physical mobility related to (specify)
Based on this nursing diagnosis, you'll establish the following patient outcomes. The patient will:

• show no evidence of complications, such as venous stasis or thrombus formation.

• carry out a mobility regimen.

• achieve highest level of mobility quickly to avoid complications.

Risk for peripheral neurovascular dysfunction related to immobility
Based on this nursing diagnosis, you'll establish the following patient outcomes. The patient will:

• maintain circulation in extremities.

• demonstrate correct body-positioning techniques.

• have absence of symptoms of neurovascular compromise.

Equipment

♦ tape measure ♦ antiembolism stockings of correct size and length ♦ talcum powder.

Patient preparation

• Select stocking size according to the manufacturer's specifications. If the patient's measurements are outside

Measuring for antiembolism stockings

Measure the patient carefully to ensure that his antiembolism stockings provide enough compression for adequate venous return.

To choose a *knee-length* stocking of the correct size, measure the circumference of the calf at its widest point (below) and the length of the leg from the bottom of the heel to the back of the knee (bottom left).

To choose a *thigh-length* stocking, measure the calf as for a knee-length stocking and the thigh at its widest point (below). Then measure leg length from the bottom of the heel to the gluteal fold (bottom right).

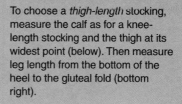

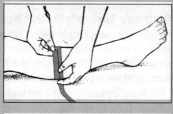

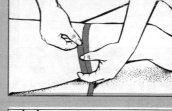

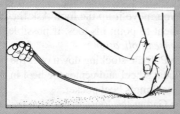

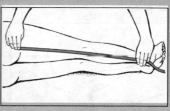

the range indicated by the manufacturer or if the patient's legs are deformed or edematous, ask the doctor if he wants to order custom stockings.

Before applying a knee-length stocking

• Measure the circumference of the calf at its widest point and length of the leg from the bottom of the heel to the back of the knee. (See *Measuring for antiembolism stockings.*)

Before applying a thigh-length stocking

• Measure the circumferences of the calf and thigh at their widest points and the length of the leg from the bottom of the heel to the gluteal fold.

Before applying a waist-length stocking

• Measure the circumference of the calf and thigh at their widest points and the length of the leg from the bottom of the heel to the waist along the side of the body.

Applying antiembolism stockings: Three key steps

Gather the loose part of the stocking at the toes and pull this portion toward the heel.

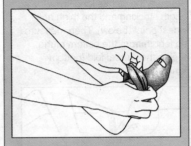

Then gather the loose part of the stocking and bring it over the heel with short, alternating front and back pulls.

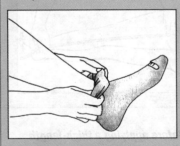

Insert your index and middle fingers into the gathered part of the stocking at the ankle and ease it upward by rocking it slightly up and down.

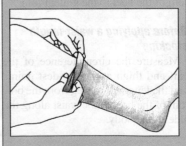

Implementation

• Check the doctor's order and assess the patient's condition. If his legs are cold or cyanotic, notify the doctor before proceeding.

• Explain the procedure to the patient, provide privacy, and wash your hands thoroughly.

• Tell the patient to lie down. Then dust his ankle with talcum powder to ease application.

Applying a knee-length stocking

• With the stocking's heel pocket down, hook the index and middle fingers of both your hands into the foot section, stretching the stocking open.

• Facing the patient, ease the stocking over the toes, stretching it sideways as you move it up the foot. Ask the patient to point his toes, if possible, *to ease application.*

• Pull the stocking down over the patient's heel and center the heel in the stocking's heel pocket.

• Gather the loose material at the ankle and slide the rest of the stocking up over the heel with short pulls, alternating front and back. (See *Applying antiembolism stockings: Three key steps.*)

• Insert your index and middle fingers into the gathered stocking at the ankle and ease the fabric up the leg to the knee.

• Supporting the patient's ankle with one hand, use your other hand to stretch the stocking toward the knee, front and back, *to distribute the material evenly.* The stocking top should be 1″ to 2″ (2.5 to 5 cm) below the bottom of the patella.

• Gently snap the fabric around the ankle *to ensure a tight fit and to eliminate gaps that could reduce pressure.*

• Adjust the foot section of the stocking *for fabric smoothness and toe comfort* by tugging on the toe section. If the stocking has a toe window, make sure it's properly positioned.
• Repeat the procedure for the second stocking if ordered.

Applying a thigh-length stocking
• Follow the procedure for applying a knee-length stocking, taking care to distribute the fabric evenly below the knee before continuing.
• With the patient's leg extended, stretch the rest of the stocking over the knee.
• Flex the patient's knee and pull the stocking over the thigh until the top is 1" to 3" (2.5 to 7.6 cm) below the gluteal fold.
• Stretch the stocking from the top, front and back, *to distribute the fabric evenly over the thigh.*
• Gently snap the fabric behind the knee *to eliminate gaps that could reduce pressure.*

Applying a waist-length stocking
• Follow the procedure for applying knee- and thigh-length stockings, and extend the stocking top to the gluteal fold.
• Fit the patient with the adjustable belt that accompanies the stockings. Make sure that neither the waistband nor the fabric interferes with any incision or with any drainage tube, catheter, or other external device.

Complications
• Some possible complications include obstruction of arterial blood flow, characterized by cold and bluish toes; dusky toenail beds; decreased or absent pedal pulses; leg pain or cramps.
• Less serious complications, such as allergic reaction and skin irritation, can also occur.

Nursing considerations
• Apply the stockings in the morning, if possible, *before edema develops.* If the patient has been walking, ask him to lie down and elevate his legs for 15 to 30 minutes before applying the stockings *to facilitate venous return.*
• Don't allow the stockings to roll or turn down at the top or toe *because the excess pressure could cause venous strangulation.* Have the patient wear the stockings in bed and during ambulation *to provide continuous protection against thrombosis.*
• Check the patient's toes at least once every 4 hours and more often in the patient with a faint pulse or edema. Note skin color and temperature, sensation, swelling, and ability to move. If complications occur, remove the stockings and notify the doctor immediately.
• Be alert for an allergic reaction *because some patients can't tolerate the sizing in new stockings.* Laundering the stockings before applying them reduces this risk. Remove the stockings at least once daily *to bathe the skin and to observe for skin irritation and breakdown.*
• Using warm water and mild soap, wash the stockings when they're soiled. Keep a second pair of stockings handy *for the patient to wear while the other pair is being laundered.*

Home care
- If the patient will require antiembolism stockings after discharge, teach him or a family member how to apply them correctly and explain why it's important that he wear them. Instruct the patient or family member to care for the stockings properly and to replace them when they lose their elasticity.

Documentation
- Record the date and time of stocking application and removal, stocking length and size, condition of the leg before and after treatment, condition of the toes during treatment, any complications, and the patient's tolerance of the treatment.

Apgar scoring

Named for its developer, anesthesiologist Virginia Apgar, the Apgar score quantifies neonatal heart rate, respiratory effort, muscle tone, reflexes, and color. Each category is assessed 1 minute after birth and again 5 minutes later. Scores in each category range from 0 to 2. The highest Apgar score is 10 — the greatest possible sum of the five categories.

The evaluation at 1 minute indicates the neonate's initial adaptation to extrauterine life. The evaluation at 5 minutes gives a clearer picture of overall status. If the neonate doesn't breathe or if his heart beats fewer than 100 times a minute, call for help and begin resuscitation at once. Don't wait for a 1-minute Apgar score.

≫ Key nursing diagnoses and patient outcomes
Use this nursing diagnosis as a guide when developing your plan of care for a neonate who has a low Apgar score.

Altered growth and development related to (specify)
Based on this nursing diagnosis, you'll establish the following patient outcomes. Family members will:
- express realistic expectations for neonate's growth.
- demonstrate understanding of neonate's needs.

After evaluation of neonate's alteration in growth and development, supportive measurements are initiated.

Equipment
♦ Apgar score sheet or neonatal assessment sheet (See *Recording the Apgar score.*) ♦ stethoscope ♦ clock with second hand or two Apgar timers ♦ gloves.

Equipment preparation
- If you use Apgar timers, make sure both timers are on at the instant of birth.

Implementation
- Note the exact time of delivery. Wear gloves *for protection from blood and body fluids.* Dry the neonate *to prevent heat loss.*
- Place the neonate in a 15-degree Trendelenburg's position to promote mucus drainage. Then position his head with the nose slightly tilted upward *to straighten the airway.*
- Assess the neonate's respiratory efforts. If necessary, supply stimulation by rubbing his back or gently flicking his foot.

Recording the Apgar score

Use this chart to record the neonatal Apgar score at 1 minute and at 5 minutes after birth. A score of 7 to 10 indicates good condition; 4 to 6, fair condition — the infant may have moderate central nervous system depression, muscle flaccidity, cyanosis, and poor respirations; 0 to 3, danger — the infant needs immediate resuscitation, as ordered.

APGAR SCORE

SIGN	0	1	2
Heart rate	Absent	Less than 100 beats/minute (slow)	More than 100 beats/minute
Respiratory effort	Absent	Slow, irregular	Good crying
Muscle tone	Flaccid	Some flexion and resistance to extension of extremities	Active motion
Reflex irritability	No response	Grimace or weak cry	Vigorous cry
Color	Pallor, cyanosis	Pink body, blue extremities	Completely pink

• If there are abnormal respiratory responses, begin neonatal resuscitation according to the guidelines of the American Heart Association and the American Academy of Pediatrics. Then, use the Apgar score to judge the progress and success of resuscitation efforts. Should resuscitation efforts prove futile, you'll need to implement measures for dealing with stillbirth. (See *Dealing with a stillbirth*, page 28.)
• If the neonate exhibits normal responses, assign the Apgar score 1 minute after birth.
• Repeat the evaluation and record the score 5 minutes after birth.

To assess neonatal heart rate
• Using a stethoscope, listen to the heartbeat for 30 seconds, and record the rate. To obtain beats/minute, double the rate. You may also palpate the umbilical cord where it joins the abdomen. Monitor pulsations for 6 seconds and multiply by 10 to obtain beats/minute. Assign a 0 for no heart rate, a 1 for a rate under 100 beats/minute, and a 2 for a rate over 100 beats/minute.

To assess respiratory effort
• Count unassisted respirations for 60 seconds, noting quality and regularity (a normal rate is 30 to 50 respirations/minute). Assign a 0 for no respirations; a 1 for slow, irregular, shallow, or gasping respirations; and a 2 for regular respirations and vigorous crying.

Dealing with a stillbirth

A stillbirth occurs when a fetus that's mature enough to survive extrauterine life dies before or during delivery. (Features of maturity include gestational age of 16 weeks or more and length of 6 ¼" [15.8 cm] or more.) Delivery of a less-mature fetus is called a spontaneous abortion.

Nursing interventions

After a stillbirth, your responsibilities include measuring, weighing, identifying, and preparing the stillborn for the morgue. Of course, you must also provide emotional support to the parents. Here are some guidelines to follow.
• If the parents expected the stillbirth, focus on assisting them to continue working through their grief — especially if they delayed grieving while waiting for delivery.
• If the parents didn't expect the stillbirth, help them to express anger and relieve grief in positive ways. Refer them to appropriate support groups.
• Offer bereaved parents the opportunity to hold the stillborn. If possible, provide a photograph, identification bracelet, or other memento. If they refuse these mementos now, file them with the chart so that they may obtain them later if desired.

To assess muscle tone

• Observe the extremities for flexion and resistance to extension by extending the limbs and observing their rapid return to flexion — the neonate's normal state. Assign a 0 for flaccid muscle tone, a 1 for some flexion and resistance to extension, and a 2 for normal flexion of the infant's elbows, knees, and hips, with good resistance to extension.

To assess reflex irritability

• Observe the neonate's response to nasal suctioning or to flicking the sole of his foot. Assign a 0 for no response, a 1 for a grimace or weak cry, and a 2 for a vigorous cry.

To assess color

• Observe skin color, especially at the extremities. Assign a 0 for complete pallor and cyanosis, a 1 for a pink body with blue extremities (acrocyanosis), and a 2 for a completely pink body. To assess color in a dark-skinned neonate, inspect the oral mucous membranes and conjunctiva, the lips, the palms, and the soles.

Nursing considerations

• If the patient and her support person don't know about the Apgar score, discuss it with them during early labor, when they will be more receptive to new knowledge. *To prevent confusion or misunderstanding at delivery*, explain to them what will occur and why. Add that this is a routine procedure.
• If the neonate requires emergency care, make sure that a member of the delivery team offers appropriate support.
• Closely observe the neonate whose mother receives heavy sedation just before delivery. Despite a high Apgar score at birth, he may show secondary effects of sedation in the nursery. Be alert for depression or unresponsiveness.

Documentation

• Record the Apgar score on the Apgar score sheet or the neonatal assessment sheet required by your hospital. Be sure to indicate the total score and the signs for which points were deducted *to guide postnatal care.*

Apnea monitoring

If detected and treated at onset, apneic episodes may be reversed. Using an apnea monitor that signals when breathing rate falls dangerously low may save the life of a neonate who's vulnerable to apnea.

Apnea monitors may be used for vulnerable neonates, such as those who are born prematurely, those who have survived a life-threatening medical emergency, or for those with neurologic disorders, neonatal respiratory distress syndrome, bronchopulmonary dysplasia, congenital heart disease with congestive heart failure, a tracheostomy, a personal history of sleep-induced apnea, a family history of sudden infant death syndrome, or acute drug withdrawal.

≫ Key nursing diagnoses and patient outcomes

Use these nursing diagnoses as a guide when developing a plan of care for a neonate who needs apnea monitoring.

Ineffective family coping related to compromised neonatal health
Based on this nursing diagnosis, you'll establish the following patient outcomes. Family members will:
• communicate feelings regarding neonate's condition.
• become involved in planning and providing neonate's care.
• express feelings of having greater control over their situation.

Knowledge deficit related to apnea monitoring
Based on this nursing diagnosis, you'll establish the following patient outcomes. Family members will:
• set realistic learning goals for developing competence in caring for neonate.
• express understanding of apnea monitoring.
• demonstrate ability to use apnea monitor correctly.
• contact appropriate resource when necessary.

Equipment
♦ monitor unit ♦ electrodes (Prepackaged and pretreated disposable electrodes are available.) ♦ leadwires ♦ electrode belt ♦ electrode gel, if needed ♦ pressure transducer pad, if using apnea mattress ♦ stable surface for monitor placement.

Patient preparation
• Explain the procedure to the parents, as appropriate, and wash your hands.

Implementation
• Plug the monitor's power cord into a grounded wall outlet. Attach the lead wires to the electrodes and attach the electrodes to the belt. If appropriate, apply conduction gel to the electrodes. (Or apply gel to the neonate's chest, place the electrodes on the gel, attach the electrodes to the lead wires, and then secure the belt.)
• To hold the electrodes securely in position, wrap the belt snugly, but not restrictively, around the neonate's chest at the point of greatest movement, optimally at the right and left midaxillary line about $\frac{4}{5}''$ (2 cm) below the axilla. Be sure to position the

TECHNOLOGY UPDATE

Common types of apnea monitors

Two types of apnea monitors are most commonly used. The *thoracic impedance monitor* uses chest electrodes to detect conduction changes caused by respirations. The newest models have alarm systems and memories that record cardiorespiratory patterns.

The *apnea mattress,* or *underpad monitor,* relies on a transducer connected to a pressure-sensitive pad, which detects pressure changes resulting from altered chest movements.

leadwires according to the manufacturer's instructions.

• Follow the color code to connect the lead wires to the patient cable. Then connect the cable to the proper jack at the rear of the monitor.

• Turn the sensitivity controls to maximum to facilitate tuning.

• Set the alarms according to recommendations so that the signal is activated at a set point during an apneic episode.

• Turn the monitor on. If the monitor has two alarms, one to signal apnea and one to signal bradycardia, both will sound until you adjust the monitor and reset the alarms according to the manufacturer's instructions.

• Adjust the sensitivity controls until the indicator lights blink with each breath and heartbeat. (See *Common types of apnea monitors.*)

Complications
Airway obstruction
• An apneic episode resulting from upper airway obstruction may not trigger the alarm if the neonate continues to make respiratory efforts without gas exchange, but the monitor's bradycardia alarm may be triggered by the decreased heart rate resulting from vagal stimulation, which accompanies obstruction.

Bradycardia
• If you're using a thoracic impedance monitor without a bradycardia alarm, you may interpret bradycardia during apnea as shallow breathing. That's because this type of monitor fails to distinguish between respiratory movement and the large cardiac stroke volume associated with bradycardia. In this case, the alarm won't sound until the heart rate drops below the apnea limit.

Nursing considerations
• *To ensure accurate operation,* don't put the monitor on top of any other electrical device. Make sure it is on a level surface and can't be bumped easily.

• Avoid applying lotions, oils, or powders to the neonate's chest, *where they could cause the electrode belt to slip.* Periodically check the alarm by disconnecting the sensor plug. Then listen for the alarm to sound after the preset time delay.

Home care
• To guard against potentially life-threatening apneic episodes in vulnerable neonates, monitoring begins in the hospital and continues at home. Parents need to learn how to operate the monitor, what actions to take when

Using a home apnea monitor

When a neonate in your care will use home apnea monitoring equipment, you'll need to prepare his parents to operate it safely, correctly and confidently.

• First, review the neonate's breathing problem with his parents. Explain that the monitor will warn them of breathing or heart rate changes. Then, offer the following guidelines.

• Advise parents to prepare their home and family for the equipment, for instance by providing a sturdy, flat surface for the monitor and by posting emergency telephone numbers (doctor, nurse, equipment supplier, ambulance) accessibly.

• Teach other responsible family members how to use the monitor safely. Also suggest that older siblings, grandparents, baby-sitters, and other caregivers learn cardiopulmonary resuscitation (CPR).

• Instruct parents to notify local service authorities — police, ambulance, and telephone and electric companies — if their neonate uses an apnea monitor so that alterna-

tive power can be supplied if a failure occurs.

• Explain how a monitor with electrodes works. Teach parents to make sure the respirator indicator goes on each time the neonate breathes. If it doesn't, describe troubleshooting techniques such as moving the electrodes slightly. Tell them to try this technique several times.

• Show parents how to respond to either the apnea or bradycardia alarm. Direct them to check the color of the neonate's oral tissues. If they appear bluish and the neonate isn't breathing, tell them to call loudly and touch him — gently at first, then more urgently as needed. Tell them to stop short of shaking him. If he doesn't respond, urge them to begin CPR.

• Also advise the parents to keep the operator's manual attached to or beside the monitor and to consult it as needed. Explain that an activated loose-lead alarm, for example, may indicate a dirty electrode, a loose electrode patch, a loose belt, or a disconnected or malfunctioning wire or monitor.

---

the alarm sounds, and how to revive a neonate or an infant with cardiopulmonary resuscitation (CPR).

• Crucial steps for using a monitor correctly include: testing the alarm system, positioning the sensor properly, and setting the controls correctly. (See *Using a home apnea monitor*.)

Documentation

• Record all alarm incidents.

• Document the time and duration of apnea. Describe the neonate's color, the stimulation measures implement-

ed, and any other pertinent information.

Arterial pressure monitoring

Direct arterial pressure monitoring permits continuous measurement of systolic, diastolic, and mean pressures. It also allows arterial blood sampling. Because direct measurement reflects systemic vascular resistance and blood flow, it's generally more accurate than indirect methods, such as palpation and auscultation of Korotkoff, or audible pulse, sounds which are based on blood flow.

Direct monitoring is indicated when highly accurate or frequent blood pressure measurements are required, such as in patients with low cardiac output and high systemic vascular resistance. It also may be used for hospitalized patients who are obese or have severe edema, if these conditions make indirect measurement difficult. It may be used, too, for patients who receive titrated vasoactive-drug dosages or who need frequent blood sampling.

Indirect monitoring, which carries few associated risks, is commonly performed by applying pressure to an artery, such as by inflating a blood pressure cuff around the arm, to decrease blood flow. As pressure is released, flow resumes and can be palpated or auscultated. Korotkoff sounds presumably result from a combination of blood flow and arterial wall vibrations; with reduced flow, these vibrations may be less pronounced.

≫ Key nursing diagnoses and patient outcomes

Use these nursing diagnoses as a guide when developing your plan of care.

Decreased cardiac output related to reduced stroke volume as a result of (specify)
Based on this nursing diagnosis, you'll establish the following patient outcomes. The patient will:

• maintain hemodynamic stability: pulse not less than (specify) and not greater than (specify); blood pressure not less than (specify) and not greater than (specify).
• have no complaint of chest pain.
• have adequate cardiac output.

Risk for infection related to arterial line
Based on this nursing diagnosis, you'll establish the following patient outcomes. The patient will:
• have a temperature that stays within normal limits.
• have no evidence of infection at the insertion site; site will be clean and free of purulent drainage.
• have a white blood cell count and differential stay within normal range.

Equipment

For catheter insertion and system setup: ♦ gloves ♦ gown ♦ mask ♦ protective eyewear ♦ sterile gloves ♦ 16G to 20G catheter (type and length depend on the insertion site, patient's size, and other anticipated uses of the line) ♦ preassembled preparation kit if available ♦ sterile drapes ♦ sheet protector ♦ sterile towels ♦ ordered local anesthetic ♦ sutures ♦ pressure bag ♦ preassembled arterial pressure tubing with flush device and disposable pressure transducer (in some units, a reusable transducer may be used; refer to manufacturer's policy for setup) ♦ bedside monitor ♦ cable (to connect the transducer to the bedside monitor) ♦ 500-ml I.V. bag ♦ I.V. flush solution (such as dextrose 5% in water [D_5W] or normal saline solution) ♦ 500 or 1,000 units of heparin (in some hospitals, premixed heparin flush solutions are available)

Performing Allen's test

Rest the patient's arm on the mattress or bedside stand, and support his wrist with a rolled towel. Have him clench his fist. Then, using your index and middle fingers, press on the radial and ulnar arteries. Hold this position for a few seconds.

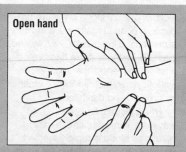

Open hand

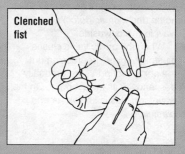

Clenched fist

Release pressure on the patient's ulnar artery. If the hand becomes flushed, which indicates blood filling the vessels, you can safely proceed with the radial artery puncture. If the hand doesn't become flushed, perform the test on the other arm.

Without removing your fingers from the patient's arteries, ask him to unclench his fist and hold his hand in a relaxed position. The palm will be blanched because pressure from your fingers has impaired the normal blood flow.

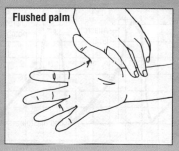

Flushed palm

• syringe and needle (21G to 25G 1″) ◆ I.V. pole ◆ tubing and medication labels ◆ site care kit (containing sterile dressing, antimicrobial ointment, and hypoallergenic tape) ◆ arm board and soft wrist restraint (for a femoral site, an ankle restraint) ◆ optional: shaving kit (for femoral-artery insertion).

Equipment preparation
• Before setting up and priming the monitoring system, wash your hands thoroughly. Maintain asepsis by wear-

ing personal protective equipment throughout preparation.
• When you've completed the equipment preparation, set the alarms on the bedside monitor according to hospital policy.

Implementation
• If the catheter will be inserted into the radial artery, perform Allen's test *to assess collateral circulation in the hand.* (See *Performing Allen's test.*)
• Explain the procedure to the patient and his family, including the purpose

Understanding the arterial waveform

Normal arterial blood pressure produces a characteristic waveform, representing ventricular systole and diastole. The waveform has five distinct components: anacrotic limb, systolic peak, dicrotic limb, dicrotic notch, and end diastole.

The *anacrotic limb* marks the waveform's initial upstroke, which results as blood is rapidly ejected from the ventricle through the open aortic valve into the aorta. The rapid ejection causes a sharp rise in arterial pressure, which appears as the waveform's highest point. This is called the *systolic peak.*

As blood continues into the peripheral vessels, arterial pressure falls, and the waveform begins a downward trend. This part is called the *dicrotic limb.* Arterial pressure usually will continue to fall until pressure in the ventricle is less than pressure in the aortic root. When this occurs, the aortic valve closes. This event appears as a small notch (the *dicrotic notch*) on the waveform's downside.

When the aortic valve closes, diastole begins, progressing until the aortic root pressure gradually descends to its lowest point. On the waveform, this is known as *end diastole.*

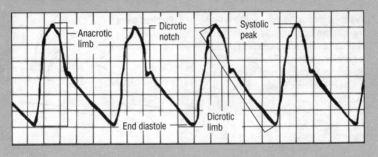

of arterial pressure monitoring and the anticipated duration of catheter placement. Make sure the patient signs a consent form. If he's unable to sign, ask a responsible family member to give written consent.

• Check the patient's history for an allergy or a hypersensitivity to iodine and the ordered local anesthetic.

• Maintain asepsis by wearing personal protection equipment throughout all procedures described below.

• Position the patient for easy access to the catheter insertion site and place a sheet protector under the site.

To insert an arterial catheter

• Using a preassembled preparation kit, the doctor prepares and anesthetizes the insertion site. The doctor then covers the surrounding area with sterile drapes or towels. The catheter is then inserted into the artery and attached to the fluid-filled pressure tubing.

• While the doctor holds the catheter in place, activate the fast-flush release *to flush blood from the catheter.* After each fast-flush operation, observe the drip chamber *to verify that the desired continuous-flush rate has been established.* A waveform should appear on the bedside monitor.

• The doctor may suture the catheter in place or you may secure it with hypoallergenic tape. Apply antimicrobial ointment, and cover the insertion site with a dressing, as specified by hospital policy.

• Immobilize the insertion site. With a radial or brachial site, use an arm board and soft wrist restraint, if the patient's condition requires it. With a femoral site, assess the need for an ankle restraint; maintain the patient on bed rest, with the head of the bed raised no more than 15 to 30 degrees, *to prevent the catheter from kinking.* Level the zeroing stopcock of the transducer with the phlebostatic axis and zero the system to atmospheric pressure.

• Activate monitor alarms, as appropriate.

Complications

Direct arterial-pressure monitoring can cause such complications as:
• arterial bleeding
• infection
• air embolism
• arterial spasm
• thrombosis.

Nursing considerations

• Observing the pressure waveform on the monitor can enhance assessment of arterial pressure. (See *Understanding the arterial waveform.*) An abnormal waveform may reflect an arrhythmia such as atrial fibrillation or other cardiovascular problems,

such as aortic stenosis, aortic insufficiency, pulsus alternans, or pulsus paradoxus. (See *Recognizing abnormal waveforms, pages 36 and 37.*)

• Change the pressure tubing every 2 to 3 days, according to hospital policy. Change the dressing at the catheter site at intervals specified by hospital policy. Regularly assess the site for signs of infection, such as redness and swelling. Notify the doctor immediately if you note any such signs.

• Be aware that erroneous pressure readings may result from a catheter that is clotted, malpositioned, or loose.

• If the catheter lumen clots, the flush system may be improperly pressurized. Regularly assess the amount of flush solution in the I.V. bag, and maintain 300 mm Hg of pressure in the pressure bag.

• False readings may also come from a catheter to which extra stopcocks or extension tubing have been added or a system into which air has leaked.

• Other conditions that may produce erroneous readings are improper calibration, leveling, or zeroing of the monitoring system.

Documentation

• Document the date of system setup *so that all caregivers will know when to change the components.*

• Document systolic, diastolic, and mean pressure readings as well.

• Record circulation in the extremity distal to the site by assessing color, pulses, and sensation.

• Carefully document the amount of flush solution infused *to avoid hypervolemia and volume overload, and to ensure accurate assessment of the patient's fluid status.*

Recognizing abnormal waveforms

Understanding a normal arterial waveform is relatively straightforward, but an abnormal waveform is more difficult to decipher. Abnormal patterns and markings, however, may provide important diagnostic clues to the patient's cardio-

ABNORMALITY	POSSIBLE CAUSES
Alternating high and low waves in a regular pattern 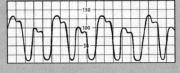	• Ventricular bigeminy
Flattened waveform 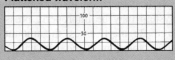	• Overdamped waveform or hypotensive patient
Slightly rounded waveform with consistent variations in systolic height 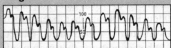	• Patient on ventilator with positive end-expiratory pressure
Slow upstroke 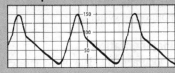	• Aortic stenosis
Diminished amplitude on inspiration 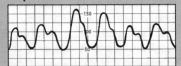	• Pulsus paradoxus, possibly from cardiac tamponade, constrictive pericarditis, or lung disease

vascular status, or they may simply signal trouble in the monitor. Use this chart to help you recognize and resolve waveform abnormalities.

NURSING CONSIDERATIONS

• Check the patient's electrocardiogram (ECG) to confirm ventricular bigeminy. The tracing should reflect premature ventricular contractions every second beat.

• Check the patient's blood pressure with a sphygmomanometer. If you obtain a reading, suspect overdamping. Correct the problem by trying to aspirate the arterial line. If you succeed, flush the line. If the reading is very low or absent, suspect hypotension.

• Check the patient's systolic blood pressure regularly. The difference between the highest and lowest systolic pressure reading should be less than 10 mm Hg. If the difference exceeds that amount, suspect pulsus paradoxus, possibly from cardiac tamponade.

• Check the patient's heart sounds for signs of aortic stenosis. Also notify the doctor, who will document suspected aortic stenosis in his notes.

• Note systolic pressure during inspiration and expiration. If inspiratory pressure is at least 10 mm Hg less than expiratory pressure, call the doctor.
• If you're also monitoring pulmonary artery pressure, observe for a diastolic plateau. This occurs when the mean central venous pressure (right atrial pressure), mean pulmonary artery pressure, and mean pulmonary artery wedge pressure (pulmonary artery obstructive pressure) are within 5 mm Hg of one another.

• Make sure the position of the patient is documented when each blood pressure reading is obtained. *This is important for determining trends.*

Arterial puncture for blood gas analysis

Obtaining an arterial blood sample requires percutaneous puncture of the brachial, radial, or femoral artery or withdrawal of a sample from an arterial line. Once drawn, the sample can be analyzed for arterial blood gases.

Arterial blood gas (ABG) analysis evaluates ventilation by measuring blood pH and the partial pressures of oxygen (PaO_2) and carbon dioxide ($PaCO_2$) in arterial blood. Blood pH measurement reveals the blood's acid-base balance. PaO_2 indicates the amount of oxygen that the lungs deliver to the blood, and $PaCO_2$ indicates the lungs' capacity to eliminate carbon dioxide. ABG samples can also be analyzed for oxygen content and saturation and for bicarbonate values.

ABG analysis is commonly ordered for patients with chronic obstructive pulmonary disease, pulmonary edema, acute respiratory distress syndrome, myocardial infarction, or pneumonia. It's also performed during episodes of shock and after coronary artery bypass surgery, resuscitation from cardiac arrest, changes in respiratory therapy or status, and prolonged anesthesia.

Most ABG samples can be drawn by a respiratory therapist, respiratory technician, or specially trained nurse. Collection from the femoral artery, however, is usually performed by a doctor. Before attempting a radial puncture, Allen's test should be performed to assess the adequacy of the blood supply to the patient's hand. (See *Performing Allen's test*, page 33.)

Normal ABG values fall within these ranges:
• PaO_2, 80 to 100 mm Hg
• $PaCO_2$, 35 to 45 mm Hg
• pH, 7.35 to 7.45
• O_2CT, 15% to 23%
• SaO_2, 94% to 100%
• HCO_3-, 22 to 26 mEq/liter.

Low PaO_2, O_2CT, and SaO_2 levels, in combination with a high $PaCO_2$ value, may stem from conditions that impair respiratory function. Similarly, low readings may result from bronchiole obstruction caused by asthma or emphysema or from an abnormal ventilation-perfusion ratio.

When inspired air contains insufficient oxygen, PaO_2, O_2CT, and SaO_2 also decrease, but $PaCO_2$ may be normal. Such findings are common in pneumothorax, impaired diffusion between alveoli and blood, or in an arteriovenous shunt that permits blood to bypass the lungs. Low O_2CT, with normal PaO_2, SaO_2 and, possibly, $PaCO_2$ values, may result from severe anemia, decreased blood volume, and reduced hemoglobin oxygen-carrying capacity.

≫ Key nursing diagnoses and patient outcomes

Use these nursing diagnoses as a guide when developing your plan of care.

Ineffective breathing pattern related to (specify)
Based on this nursing diagnosis, you'll establish the following patient outcomes. The patient will:
• attain baseline ABG levels.
• maintain baseline breath sounds.

- express a feeling of comfort in maintaining air exchange.
- achieve an acceptable baseline respiratory rate.

Ineffective airway clearance related to (specify)

Based on this nursing diagnosis, you'll establish the following patient outcomes. The patient will:
- breathe spontaneously after the obstruction is removed or resolved.
- maintain baseline respiratory rate.
- attain baseline ABG levels.
- maintain baseline breath sounds.
- be free of dyspnea.

Impaired gas exchange related to (specify)

Based on this nursing diagnosis, you'll establish the following patient outcomes. The patient will:
- attain baseline ABG levels.
- maintain baseline breath sounds.
- express a feeling of comfort in maintaining air exchange.

Equipment

♦ 10-ml glass syringe or plastic luer-lock syringe specially made for drawing blood gases ♦ 1-ml ampule of aqueous heparin (1:1,000) ♦ 20G 1¼″ needle ♦ 22G 1″ needle ♦ alcohol sponge ♦ povidone-iodine sponge ♦ two 2″ × 2″ gauze pads ♦ gloves ♦ rubber cap for syringe hub or rubber stopper for needle ♦ ice-filled plastic bag ♦ label ♦ laboratory request form ♦ adhesive bandage ♦ optional: 1% lidocaine solution.

Equipment preparation

• Many hospitals use commercial ABG kits that contain the equipment listed above (except the adhesive bandage and ice). If your hospital doesn't use such kits, obtain a sterile syringe specially made for drawing blood gases and use a clean emesis basin filled with ice instead of the plastic bag to transport the sample to the laboratory.
• Prepare the collection equipment before entering the patient's room. Wash your hands thoroughly and then open the ABG kit and remove the specimen label and the plastic bag. Record on the label the patient's name and room number, the date and collection time, and the doctor's name. Fill the plastic bag with ice and set it aside.
• You'll need to heparinize the syringe. To do that, first attach the 20G needle to the syringe. Then open the ampule of heparin. Draw all the heparin into the syringe *to prevent the sample from clotting.* Hold the syringe upright and pull the plunger back slowly to about the 7-ml mark. Rotate the barrel while pulling the plunger back *to allow the heparin to coat the inside surface of the syringe.* Then, slowly force the heparin toward the hub of the syringe and expel all but about 0.1 ml of heparin.

To heparinize the needle, first replace the 20G needle with the 22G needle. Then, hold the syringe upright, tilt it slightly, and eject the remaining heparin. *Excess heparin in the syringe alters blood pH and PaO_2 values.*

Implementation

• Tell the patient you need to collect an arterial blood sample and explain the procedure *to help ease anxiety and promote cooperation.* Tell him that the needle stick will cause some discomfort but that he must remain still during the procedure.

Arterial puncture technique

The angle of needle penetration in arterial blood gas sampling depends on the artery to be sampled. For the radial artery, which is most commonly used, the needle should enter bevel up at a 45-degree angle over the artery.

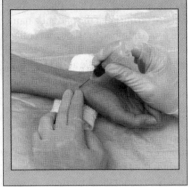

• After washing your hands and donning gloves, place a rolled towel under the patient's wrist for *support*. Locate the artery and palpate it for a strong pulse.

• Clean the puncture site with a povidone-iodine sponge or with an alcohol sponge. Don't wipe off the povidone-iodine with alcohol *because alcohol cancels the effect of povidone-iodine.*

• Using a circular motion, clean the area, starting in the center of the site and spiraling outward *to avoid introducing potentially infectious skin flora into the vessel during the procedure.* If you use alcohol, apply it with friction for 30 seconds or until the final sponge comes away clean. Allow the skin to dry.

• Palpate the artery with the index and middle fingers of one hand while holding the syringe over the puncture site with the other hand.

• Hold the needle bevel up at a 30- to 45-degree angle.

• When puncturing the brachial artery, hold the needle at a 60-degree angle. (See *Arterial puncture technique.*)

• Puncture the skin and the arterial wall in one motion, following the path of the artery.

• Watch for blood backflow in the syringe.

• Don't pull back on the plunger *because arterial blood should enter the syringe automatically.* Fill the syringe to the 5-ml mark.

• After collecting the sample, press a gauze pad firmly over the puncture site until bleeding stops. Keep the pad there for at least 5 minutes. If the patient is receiving anticoagulant therapy or has a blood dyscrasia, apply pressure for 10 to 15 minutes; if necessary, ask a coworker to hold the gauze pad in place while you prepare the sample for transport to the laboratory. Don't ask the patient to hold the pad. *If he fails to apply sufficient pressure, a large, painful hematoma may form, hindering future arterial punctures at that site.*

• Check the syringe for air bubbles *because these can alter PaO₂ values.* If air bubbles appear, remove them by holding the syringe upright and slowly ejecting some of the blood onto a $2'' \times 2''$ gauze pad.

• Insert the needle into a rubber stopper, or remove the needle and place a rubber cap directly on the needle hub. *This prevents the sample from leaking and keeps air out of the syringe.*

• Put the labeled sample in the ice-filled plastic bag or emesis basin. Attach a properly completed laboratory

BETTER CHARTING

Documenting blood withdrawal for ABG analysis

When you must obtain blood for arterial blood gas (ABG) analysis, keep careful records of the following:

- The patient's vital signs and temperature.
- The arterial puncture site.
- The results of Allen's test.
- Any indication of circulatory impairment, such as swelling, discoloration, pain, numbness, or tingling in the bandaged arm or leg, and bleeding at the puncture site.

Also be sure to document the time that the blood sample was drawn, the length of time pressure was applied to the site to control bleeding and, if appropriate, the type and amount of oxygen therapy that the patient received (as shown here).

Filling out a lab request form

When filling out a laboratory request form for ABG analysis, be

1/16/97	1010	Blood drawn from Ⓡ radial artery p̄ + Allen's test c̄ brisk capillary refill. Pressure applied to site for 5 min. and pressure drsg. applied. No bleeding, hematoma, or swelling noted. Hand pink, warm c̄ 2-sec capillary refill. Sample for ABGs placed on ice and taken to lab. Pt. on 40% CAM. T 99.2° F. Hgb 10.2. ———— Pat Mattery RN

sure to include information for laboratory records, including:
- the patient's current temperature and respiratory rate
- his most recent hemoglobin level
- the fraction of inspired oxygen and tidal volume, if he's on mechanical ventilation.

request form, and send the sample to the laboratory immediately.
- When bleeding stops, apply a small adhesive bandage to the site.
- Monitor the patient's vital signs, and observe for signs of circulatory impairment, such as swelling, discoloration, pain, numbness, or tingling in the bandaged arm or leg. Watch for bleeding at the puncture site.

Complications

- If you use too much force when attempting to puncture the artery, the needle may touch the periosteum,

causing the patient considerable pain, or you may advance the needle through the opposite wall of the artery. If this happens, slowly pull the needle back a short distance and check for blood return. If blood still fails to enter the syringe, withdraw the needle completely and start with a fresh heparinized needle. Do not make more than two attempts to withdraw blood from the same site. *Probing the artery may injure it and the radial nerve. Also, hemolysis will alter test results.*
- If arterial spasm occurs, blood will not flow into the syringe and you

won't be able to collect the sample. If this happens, replace the needle with a smaller one and attempt the puncture again. *A smaller-bore needle is less likely to cause arterial spasm.*

Nursing considerations

• If the patient is receiving oxygen, make sure that his therapy has been underway for at least 15 minutes before drawing arterial blood.

• Unless ordered, don't stop oxygen therapy that's underway before drawing arterial blood samples. Be sure, however, to indicate the amount and type of oxygen therapy the patient is receiving on the laboratory request slip.

• If the patient isn't receiving oxygen, indicate that he is breathing room air.

• If the patient has just received a breathing treatment or nebulizer treatment, wait about 20 minutes before drawing the sample.

• If necessary, you may anesthetize the puncture site with 1% lidocaine solution. Consider such use of lidocaine carefully *because it delays the procedure, the patient can be allergic to the drug, and the resulting vasoconstriction can prevent successful puncture.*

• When filling out a laboratory request form for ABG analysis, be sure to include the following information *to help the laboratory staff calibrate the equipment and evaluate the results correctly:* the patient's current temperature, current respiratory rate, most recent hemoglobin level, and fraction of inspired oxygen and tidal volume if the patient is on a ventilator.

Documentation

• Record the results of Allen's test, the time the sample was drawn, the patient's temperature, the site of the ar-

terial puncture, the length of time pressure was applied to the site to control bleeding, and the type and amount of oxygen therapy. (See *Documenting blood withdrawal for ABG analysis,* page 41.)

Arteriovenous hemofiltration, continuous

Continuous arteriovenous hemofiltration (CAVH) is a relatively new procedure used to treat patients who have fluid overload but who don't require dialysis. CAVH filters fluid, solutes, and electrolytes from the patient's blood and infuses a replacement solution.

The hemofilter, composed of about 5,000 hollow-fiber capillaries, filters blood at a rate of about 250 ml/minute and is driven by the patient's arterial blood pressure (a systolic blood pressure of 60 mm Hg is adequate for the procedure). Some of the ultrafiltrate collected during CAVH is replaced with a filter replacement fluid (FRF). This fluid can be lactated Ringer's solution or any solution that resembles plasma. Because the amount of fluid removed is greater than the amount replaced, the patient gradually loses fluid (12 to 15 liters daily).

CAVH carries a much lower risk of hypotension from fluid withdrawal than does conventional hemodialysis because it withdraws the fluid more slowly — at about 200 ml/hour (compared with 1,000 ml/hour for hemodialysis). CAVH can be performed in hypotensive patients who require fluid removal, who can't undergo peritoneal dialysis, or whose requirements for parenteral nutrition would make fluid- volume control problematic. CAVH also reduces the risk of other complications, such as nausea, cramps, vomiting, and headache. And because it withdraws fluid slowly, CAVH allows easier maintenance of stable fluid volume and regulation of fluid and electrolyte balance. The procedure costs less than hemodialysis and the equipment is easier to operate.

A similar procedure, continuous arteriovenous filtration and hemodialysis (CAVH-D), combines hemodialysis with hemofiltration. Like CAVH, it can also be performed in patients with hypotension and fluid overload.

CAVH is often used to treat patients with acute renal failure, fluid overload that doesn't respond to diuretics, and some electrolyte and acid-base disturbances.

>> Key nursing diagnoses and patient outcomes

Use these nursing diagnoses as a guide when developing your plan of care for a patient who is being treated with CAVH.

Altered renal tissue perfusion related to decreased cellular exchange

Based on this nursing diagnosis, you'll establish the following patient outcomes. The patient will:
• maintain fluid balance.
• communicate understanding of medical regimen, medications, diet, and activity restrictions.

Fluid volume excess related to (specify)

Based on this nursing diagnosis, you'll establish the following patient outcomes. The patient will:
• have blood pressure, pulse rate, cardiac rhythm, and breath sounds return to baseline within 24 hours.
• maintain skin integrity.
• not have a weight fluctuation.

Equipment

♦ CAVH equipment. (See *Continuous arteriovenous hemofiltration setup*, page 44.) ♦ heparin flush solution ♦ occlusive dressings for catheter insertion sites ♦ sterile gloves ♦ sterile mask ♦ povidone-iodine solution ♦ sterile 4″ × 4″ gauze pads ♦ tape ♦ FRF as ordered ♦ infusion pump.

Equipment preparation

• Prime the hemofilter and tubing according to the manufacturer's instructions.

Implementation

• Wash your hands.
• Assemble your equipment at the patient's bedside, and explain the procedure.
• If necessary, assist with inserting the catheters into the femoral artery and vein, using strict aseptic technique. (In some cases, an internal arteriovenous fistula or external arteriovenous shunt may be used instead of the femoral route.)
• If ordered, flush both catheters with the heparin flush solution *to prevent clotting.*
• Apply occlusive dressings to the insertion sites, and mark the dressings

Continuous arteriovenous hemofiltration setup

During continuous arteriovenous hemofiltration (CAVH), the patient's arterial blood pressure serves as a natural pump, driving blood through the arterial line. A hemofilter removes water and toxic solutes (ultrafiltrate) from the blood. Filter replacement fluid is infused into a port on the arterial side; this same port can be used to infuse heparin. The venous line carries the replacement fluid, along with purified blood, to the patient. The illustration shows one of several CAVH setups.

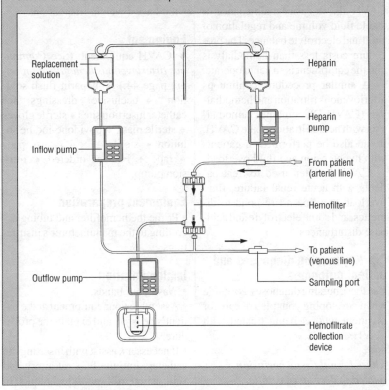

with the date and time. Secure the tubing and connections with tape.
• Assess all pulses in the affected leg every hour for the first 4 hours and then every 2 hours afterward.
• Weigh the patient, take baseline vital signs, and make sure that all necessary laboratory studies have been done (usually, electrolyte levels, coagula-

tion factors, complete blood count, blood urea nitrogen, and creatinine studies). Monitor the patient's weight and vital signs hourly.
• Put on the sterile gloves and mask.
• Prepare the connection sites by cleaning them with povidone-iodine-soaked gauze pads, then connect them to the exit port of each catheter.

- Using aseptic technique, connect the arterial and venous lines to the hemofilter.
- Turn on the hemofilter and monitor the blood-flow rate through the circuit. (See *Correcting flow rate problems.*) The flow rate is usually kept between 500 and 900 ml/hour.
- Inspect the ultrafiltrate during the procedure. It should remain clear yellow, with no gross blood. Pink-tinged or bloody ultrafiltrate may signal a membrane leak in the hemofilter, which would leave the blood compartment open to contamination from bacteria. If a leak occurs, notify the doctor so he can have the hemofilter replaced.
- Assess the affected leg for signs of obstructed blood flow, such as coolness, pallor, and weak pulse. Check the groin area on the affected side for signs of hematoma. Ask the patient if he has pain at the insertion sites.
- Calculate the amount of FRF every hour, or as ordered, according to your hospital's policy. Then infuse the prescribed amount and type of FRF through the infusion pump into the arterial side of the circuit.

Complications
Possible complications include:
- bleeding
- hemorrhage
- hemofilter occlusion
- infection
- thrombosis.

Nursing considerations
- *Because blood flows through an extracorporeal circuit during CAVH,* the blood in the hemofilter may need to be anticoagulated. To do this, infuse heparin in low doses (usually starting at 500 U/hour) into an infusion port

PROBLEM SOLVER

Correcting flow rate problems

If the ultrafiltrate flow rate decreases, raise the patient's bed to increase the distance between the collection device and the hemofilter. Lower the bed to decrease the flow rate. (Clamping the ultrafiltrate line is contraindicated with some types of hemofilters because pressure may build up in the filter, clotting it and collapsing the blood compartment.)

on the arterial side of the setup. Then measure thrombin clotting time or the activated clotting time (ACT). *This ensures that the circuit, not the patient, is anticoagulated.* A normal ACT is 100 seconds; during CAVH, keep ACT between 100 and 300 seconds, depending on the patient's clotting times. If the ACT is too high or too low, the doctor will adjust the heparin dose accordingly.
- Another way to prevent clotting in the hemofilter is not to infuse medications or blood through the venous line. This line may be used in emergencies to infuse I.V. fluids, but it will slow the return of dialyzed blood to the patient, increasing the risk of clotting. Run infusions through another line if possible.
- A third way to help prevent clots in the hemofilter, and to prevent kinks in the catheter, is to make sure the patient doesn't bend the affected leg to more than 30 degrees from the hip.
- *To prevent infection,* perform skin care at the catheter insertion sites every 48 hours, using aseptic technique.

Cover the sites with an occlusive dressing.
• Check the connection sites *to ensure they're taped securely.* Blood loss from a sudden disconnection in the circuit could cause serious complication.

Documentation
• Record the time the treatment began and ended, fluid balance information, times of dressing changes, complications, medications given, and the patient's tolerance of the treatment.

Arteriovenous shunt care

An arteriovenous (AV) shunt consists of two segments of tubing joined (in a U shape) to divert blood from an artery to a vein. Inserted surgically, usually in a forearm or (rarely) an ankle, the AV shunt provides access to the circulatory system for hemodialysis. After insertion, an AV shunt requires regular assessment for patency and examination of the surrounding skin for signs of infection.

AV shunt care also includes aseptically cleaning the arterial and venous exit sites, applying antiseptic ointment, and dressing the sites with sterile bandages. When done just before hemodialysis, this procedure prolongs the life of the shunt, helps prevent infection, and allows early detection of clotting. Shunt-site care is done more often if the dressing becomes wet or nonocclusive.

≫ Key nursing diagnoses and patient outcomes
Use these nursing diagnoses as a guide when developing your plan of care for a patient who has an AV shunt.

Altered renal tissue perfusion related to decreased cellular exchange
Based on this nursing diagnosis, you'll establish the following patient outcomes. The patient will:
• have blood urea nitrogen, creatinine, electrolyte, hemoglobin, and hematocrit levels that remain comparable to baseline levels.
• not have a weight fluctuation.

Risk for infection related to AV shunt
Based on this nursing diagnosis, you'll establish the following patient outcomes.
• Site will remain nonreddened, edematous, or painful, and will be without drainage.
• Vital signs will stay in normal limits.

Equipment
♦ Drape ♦ stethoscope ♦ sterile gloves ♦ sterile 4″ × 4″ gauze pads ♦ sterile cotton-tipped applicators ♦ bulldog clamps ♦ antiseptic (usually povidone-iodine solution) ♦ plasticized or hypoallergenic tape ♦ optional: swab specimen kit, prescribed antimicrobial ointment (usually povidone-iodine), sterile elastic gauze bandage, 2″ × 2″ gauze pads, hydrogen peroxide.

Equipment preparation
• Kits containing all the necessary equipment can be prepackaged and stored for use.

Patient preparation
• Explain the procedure to the patient, provide privacy, and wash your hands.

Implementation
• Place the drape on a stable surface, such as a bedside table, *to reduce the risk of traumatic injury to the shunt site.* Then place the shunted extremity on the draped surface.
• Remove the two bulldog clamps from the elastic gauze bandage and unwrap the bandage from the shunt area.
• Carefully remove the gauze dressing covering the shunt and the $4'' \times 4''$ gauze pad under the shunt.
• Assess the arterial and venous exit sites for signs of infection, such as erythema, swelling, excessive tenderness, or drainage. Obtain a swab specimen of any purulent drainage, and notify the doctor immediately of any signs of infection.
• Check blood flow through the shunt by inspecting the color of the blood and comparing the warmth of the shunt with that of the surrounding skin. The blood should be bright red; the shunt should feel as warm as the skin. (See *Identifying clotting caused by an AV shunt.*)
• Use the stethoscope to auscultate the shunt between the arterial and venous exit sites. A bruit confirms normal blood flow. Palpate the shunt for a thrill, which also indicates normal blood flow. Don't use a Doppler device to auscultate *because it will detect peripheral blood flow as well as shunt-related sounds.*
• Open a few packages of $4'' \times 4''$ gauze pads and cotton-tipped applicators and soak them with the antiseptic.
• Put on the sterile gloves.

Identifying clotting caused by an AV shunt

If the blood is dark purple or black and the temperature of the shunt is lower than the surrounding skin, clotting has occurred. Notify the doctor immediately.

• Using an antiseptic-soaked $4'' \times 4''$ gauze pad, start cleaning the skin at one of the exit sites. Wipe away from the site to remove bacteria and reduce the chance of contaminating the shunt.
• Use the soaked cotton-tipped applicators to remove any crusted material from the exit site *because the encrustations provide a medium for bacterial growth.*
• Clean the other exit site, using fresh, soaked $4'' \times 4''$ gauze pads and cotton-tipped applicators.
• Clean the rest of the skin that was covered by the gauze dressing with fresh, soaked $4'' \times 4''$ gauze pads.
• If ordered, apply antimicrobial ointment to the exit sites *to help prevent infection.*
• Place a dry, sterile $4'' \times 4''$ gauze pad under the shunt. *This prevents the shunt from making contact with the skin, which could cause skin irritation and breakdown.*
• Cover the exit sites with a dry, sterile $4'' \times 4''$ gauze pad, and tape the pad securely *to keep the exit sites clean and protected.*
• For routine daily care, wrap the shunt with an elastic gauze bandage. Leave a small portion of the shunt cannula exposed *so the patient can check*

for patency without removing the dressing.

• Place the bulldog clamps on the edge of the elastic gauze bandage *so the patient can use them quickly to stop hemorrhage in case the shunt separates.*

• For care before hemodialysis, don't re-dress the shunt, but keep the bulldog clamps readily accessible.

Complications

• Hemorrhage and infection are possible complications.

Nursing considerations

• Make sure the AV junction of the shunt is secured with plasticized or hypoallergenic tape. *This prevents separation of the two halves of the shunt, minimizing the risk of hemorrhage.*

• Always handle the shunt and dressings carefully. Don't use scissors or other sharp instruments to remove the dressing *because you may accidentally cut the shunt.* Never remove the tape securing the AV junction during dressing changes.

• When cleaning the shunt exit sites, use each $4'' \times 4''$ gauze pad only once and avoid wiping any area more than once *to minimize the risk of contamination.* When re-dressing the site, make sure the tape doesn't kink or occlude the shunt. If the exit sites are heavily encrusted, place a $2'' \times 2''$ hydrogen peroxide–soaked gauze pad on the area for about 1 hour *to loosen the crust.* Make sure the patient isn't allergic to iodine before using povidone-iodine solution or ointment.

Home care

• Ask the patient how he cares for the shunt at home. Then teach proper home care, if necessary.

Documentation

• Record that shunt care was administered, the condition of the shunt and surrounding skin, any ointment used, and any instructions given to the patient.

Assessment techniques

When performed correctly, the four basic assessment techniques — inspection, palpation, percussion, and auscultation — help elicit valuable information about the patient's condition.

Inspection requires the use of vision, hearing, touch, and smell. Special lighting and various equipment, such as an otoscope, a tongue blade, or an ophthalmoscope, may be used to enhance vision or examine an otherwise hidden area. Inspection begins during the first patient contact and continues throughout the assessment.

Palpation usually follows inspection, except when examining the abdomen or assessing infants and children. Palpation involves touching the body to determine the size, shape, and position of structures; to detect and evaluate temperature, pulsations, and other movement; and to elicit tenderness.

The four palpation techniques include light palpation, deep palpation, light ballottement, and deep ballottement. Ballottement is the palpation technique used to evaluate a floating or movable structure; the nurse gently bounces the structure being assessed by applying pressure against it; she then waits to feel it rebound. This technique may be used, for example, to check the position of an organ or a fetus.

Percussion uses quick, sharp tapping of the fingers or hands against body surfaces to produce sounds, detect tenderness, or assess reflexes. Percussing for sound helps locate organ borders, identify organ shape and position, and determine if an organ is solid or filled with fluid or gas.

Organs and tissues produce sounds of varying loudness, pitch, and duration, depending on their density. For example, air-filled cavities, such as the lungs, produce markedly different sounds from those produced by the liver and other dense tissues. Percussion techniques include indirect percussion, direct percussion, and blunt percussion.

Auscultation involves listening to various body sounds — particularly those produced by the heart, lungs, vessels, stomach, and intestines. Most auscultated sounds result from the movement of air or fluid through these structures.

Usually, the nurse auscultates after performing the other assessment techniques. When examining the abdomen, however, auscultation should occur after inspection but before percussion and palpation, so bowel sounds can be heard before palpation disrupts them. Auscultation is best performed first on infants and young children, who may start to cry when palpated or percussed. Auscultation is most successful when performed in a quiet environment with a properly fitted stethoscope.

≫ Key nursing diagnoses and patient outcomes

Use this nursing diagnosis as a guide when developing your plan of care.

Knowledge deficit related to assessment techniques

Based on this nursing diagnosis, you'll establish the following patient outcomes. The patient will:
• communicate a need to know what to expect.
• cooperate in positioning for assessment.
• remain calm throughout the assessment.

Equipment

♦ flashlight or gooseneck lamp as appropriate ♦ ophthalmoscope ♦ otoscope ♦ stethoscope.

Patient preparation

• Explain the procedure to the patient, have him undress, and drape him appropriately.
• Make sure the room is warm and adequately lit *to make the patient comfortable and aid visual inspection.*
• Warm your hands and the stethoscope.

Implementation

Each of the four basic assessment techniques has its own method of implementation.

Inspection

• Focus on areas related to the patient's chief complaint. Use your eyes, ears, and sense of smell to observe the patient.
• To inspect a specific body area, first make sure the area is sufficiently exposed and adequately lit. Then survey the entire area, noting key landmarks and checking overall condition. Next, focus on specifics — color, shape, texture, size, and movement. Note any unusual findings as well as predictable ones.

Performing palpation

You need to be familiar with four palpation techniques: light palpation, deep palpation, light ballottement, and deep ballottement.

Light palpation
• With the tips of two or three fingers held close together, press gently on the skin to a depth of ½" to ¾" (1 to 2 cm). Use the lightest touch possible; too much pressure blunts your sensitivity.

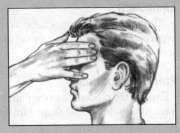

Light ballottement
• Apply light, rapid pressure to the abdomen, moving from one quadrant to another. Keep your hand on the skin surface to detect tissue rebound.

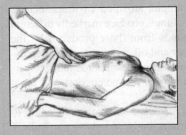

Deep palpation (bimanual palpation)
• Place one hand on top of the other. Then press down about 1 ½" to 2" (4 to 5 cm) with the fingertips of both hands.

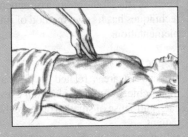

Deep ballottement
• Apply abrupt, deep pressure on the patient's abdomen. Release the pressure completely, but maintain fingertip contact with the skin.

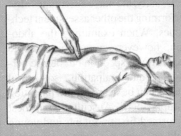

Palpation
• Explain the procedure to the patient, and tell him what to expect, such as occasional discomfort as pressure is applied. Encourage him to relax *because muscle tension or guarding*

can interfere with performance and results of palpation.
• Use the flattened finger pads for palpating tender tissues, feeling for joint crepitus (crackling), and lightly probing the abdomen. Use the thumb and index finger for assessing hair texture,

Identifying percussion sounds

Percussion produces sounds that vary according to the tissue being percussed. This chart lists important percussion sounds along with their characteristics and typical sources.

SOUND	INTENSITY	PITCH	DURATION	QUALITY	SOURCE
Resonance	Moderate to loud	Low	Long	Hollow	Normal lung
Tympany	Loud	High	Moderate	Drumlike	Gastric air bubble, intestinal air
Dullness	Soft to moderate	High	Moderate	Thudlike	Liver, full bladder, pregnant uterus
Hyperresonance	Very loud	Very low	Long	Booming	Hyperinflated lung (as in emphysema)
Flatness	Soft	High	Short	Flat	Muscle

grasping tissues, and feeling for lymph node enlargement. Use the back, or dorsal, surface of the hand when feeling for warmth.

- Provide just enough pressure to assess the tissue beneath one or both hands. Then release pressure and gently move to the next area, systematically covering the entire surface to be assessed. (See *Performing palpation*.)
- To perform light palpation, depress the skin, indenting it ½″ to ¾″ (1 to 2 cm). Use the lightest touch possible *because excessive pressure blunts your sensitivity.*
- If the patient tolerates light palpation and you need to assess deeper structures, palpate deeply by increasing your fingertip pressure, indenting the skin about 1 ½″ (4 cm). Place your

other hand on top of the palpating hand *to control and guide your movements.*

- To perform light ballottement, apply light, rapid pressure from quadrant to quadrant on the patient's abdomen. Keep your hand on the skin to detect tissue rebound.
- To perform deep ballottement, apply abrupt, deep pressure and then release it. Maintain fingertip contact.
- Use bimanual palpation to trap a deep, underlying, hard-to-palpate organ, such as the kidney or the spleen, or to fix or stabilize an organ such as the uterus with one hand while you palpate it with the other.

Percussion

- First, decide which of the percussion techniques best suits your assessment

Performing indirect percussion

To perform indirect percussion, use the middle finger of your nondominant hand as the pleximeter (the mediating device used to receive the taps) and the middle finger of your dominant hand as the plexor (the device used to tap the pleximeter). Place the pleximeter finger firmly against a body surface, such as the upper back. With your wrist flexed loosely, use the tip of your plexor finger to deliver a crisp blow just beneath the distal joint of the pleximeter. Be sure to hold the plexor perpendicular to the pleximeter. Tap lightly and quickly, removing the plexor as soon as you have delivered each blow. Move your nondominant hand to cover the entire area to be percussed.

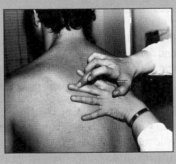

needs. Indirect percussion helps reveal the size and density of underlying thoracic and abdominal organs and tissues. Direct percussion helps assess an adult's sinuses for tenderness and elicits sounds in a child's thorax. Blunt percussion aims to elicit tenderness over organs, such as the kidneys, gallbladder, or liver. When percussing, note the characteristic sounds produced. (See *Identifying percussion sounds*, page 51.)

• To perform indirect percussion, place one hand on the patient and tap the middle finger with the middle finger of the other hand. (See *Performing indirect percussion.*)

• To perform direct percussion, tap your hand or fingertip directly against the body surface.

• To perform blunt percussion, strike the ulnar surface of your fist against the body surface. Or place the palm of one hand against the body, make a fist with the other hand, and strike the back of the first hand.

Auscultation

• First, determine whether to use the bell or diaphragm of your stethoscope. Use the diaphragm to detect high-pitched sounds, such as breath and bowel sounds. Use the bell to detect lower-pitched sounds, such as heart and vascular sounds.

• Place the diaphragm or bell of the stethoscope over the appropriate area of the patient's body. Listen intently to individual sounds and try to identify their characteristics. Determine the intensity, pitch, and duration of each sound, and check the frequency of recurring sounds.

Complications

• Palpation may cause an enlarged spleen or infected appendix to rupture.

Nursing considerations

• Avoid palpating or percussing an area of the body known to be tender at the start of your examination. Instead, work around the area; then gently palpate or percuss it at the end of the examination. *This progression*

TECHNOLOGY UPDATE

At-home patient assessment using Telemedicine

Home care nurses now have another option in assessing their patients. American Telecare of Eden Prairie, Minn., has developed the PTS100 Personal Telemedicine System. The unit, about the size of a microwave oven, stays in the patient's home after he is taught how to use it.

The PTS100 allows the nurse to conduct *video visits*, scheduled like traditional home care visits. The patient must be able to answer the phone and follow instructions. The Telemedicine unit uses an analog phone line (the traditional phone line) and allows for audiovisual interaction between nurse and patient.

Features of the system include:
• video capability, which can be used to examine the patient visually or to see any digital readout, such as blood pressure or pulse oximeter
• freeze-frame to allow fine-tuning of picture resolution to better view a wound

• a telephonic stethoscope for heart, lung, or bowel sounds.

It also features a *close-up* lens attachment with a shelf nearby so small items such as insulin in a syringe can be checked.

Telemedicine has been used with a variety of patients, from those with acquired immunodeficiency syndrome to those on home dialysis. It's a great help when home care visits are precluded such as in distant, rural areas.

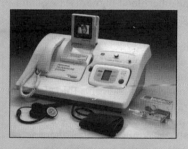

minimizes your patient's discomfort and apprehension.

To pinpoint an inflamed area deep within the patient's body, perform a variation on deep palpation: Press firmly with one hand over the area you suspect is involved and then lift your hand away quickly. If the patient reports that pain increases when you release the pressure, then you have identified rebound tenderness. (Suspect peritonitis if you elicit rebound tenderness when examining the abdomen.)

• If you cannot palpate because the patient fears pain, try distracting him

with conversation. Then perform auscultation and gently press your stethoscope into the affected area *to try to elicit tenderness.*

Home care

• Home care nurses now have another option to help them assess a patient remotely with the aid of a computer. (See *At-home patient assessment using Telemedicine.*)

Documentation

• Document your assessment findings and the technique used to elicit those findings — for example, "right lower quadrant tenderness on deep palpation, no rebound tenderness."

Autologous transfusion

Also called autotransfusion, autologous transfusion is the collection, filtration, and reinfusion of the patient's own blood. Although the technique was developed in the 1920s, it wasn't used widely until the 1960s, when cardiac surgery became common. Today, with concern over acquired immunodeficiency syndrome and other blood-borne diseases, autologous transfusion is on the rise.

Indications for autologous transfusion include:
• elective surgery (blood donated over time)
• nonelective surgery (blood withdrawn immediately before surgery)
• perioperative and emergency blood salvage during and after thoracic or cardiovascular surgery, hip or knee resection, or liver resection, and during surgery for ruptured ectopic pregnancy and hemothorax
• perioperative and emergency blood salvage for traumatic injury of the lungs, liver, chest wall, heart, pulmonary vessels, spleen, kidneys, inferior vena cava, or iliac, portal, or subclavian veins.

Autologous transfusion has several advantages over transfusion of bank blood. Transfusion reactions don't occur, diseases aren't transmitted, anticoagulants aren't added (except in postoperative autotransfusion, when acid citrate dextrose [ACD] or citrate phosphate dextrose [CPD] is added),

and the blood supply isn't depleted. Also, unlike bank blood, autologous blood contains normal levels of 2,3-diphosphoglycerate, which is helpful in tissue oxygenation.

Autologous transfusion is performed before, during, or after surgery and after traumatic injury. The three techniques used are preoperative blood donation, perioperative blood donation, and acute normovolemic hemodilution.

Preoperative blood donation is commonly recommended for patients scheduled for orthopedic surgery, which causes large blood loss. The donation period begins 4 to 6 weeks before surgery.

Perioperative blood donation (sometimes called intraoperative or postoperative) is used in vascular and orthopedic surgery and in treatment of traumatic injury. Blood may be collected during surgery or up to 12 hours afterward. (Considerable bleeding may follow vascular and orthopedic surgery.) The blood is transfused immediately after collection or processed (washed) before infusion. Blood obtained postoperatively may be collected from chest tubes, mediastinal drains, or wound drains (placed in the surgical wound during surgery). Commonly inserted during orthopedic surgery, wound drains can be used when enough uncontaminated blood is recovered from a closed wound to be reinfused.

Acute normovolemic hemodilution is used mainly in open-heart surgery. One or two units of blood are drawn immediately before or after anesthesia induction. The blood is replaced with a crystalloid or colloid solution, such as lactated Ringer's solution or 5% dextran, to produce normovolemic anemia. The blood is reinfused right after surgery. The combination of reduced hemoglobin and the replacement solution causes the patient to lose fewer red blood cells during surgery.

The equipment and procedures presented here are for preoperative and perioperative blood donation only. Acute normovolemic hemodilution is performed the same way as preoperative blood donation, and blood collected this way is reinfused the same way as any other transfusion.

⟫ Key nursing diagnoses and patient outcomes

Use these nursing diagnoses as a guide when developing your plan of care for a patient who is being treated with autologous transfusions.

Fluid volume deficit related to active loss

Based on this nursing diagnosis, you'll establish the following patient outcomes. The patient will:
• have vital signs remain stable.
• have fluid and blood volume return to normal.

Altered tissue perfusion related to decreased cellular exchange

Based on this nursing diagnosis, you'll establish the following patient outcomes. The patient will:
• attain hemodynamic stability.
• pulse (specify) and blood pressure (specify).
• not exhibit arrhythmias.

Equipment

For preoperative blood donation:
◆ ferrous sulfate ◆ povidone-iodine solution ◆ alcohol ◆ tourniquet ◆ rubber ball ◆ large-bore needle for venipuncture ◆ collection bags ◆ I.V. line ◆ in-line filter for reinfusion.

For perioperative blood donation: ◆ autologous transfusion system, such as the Davol or Pleur-evac system ◆ ACD or CPD ◆ collection bottles ◆ vacuum source regulator ◆ suction tubing ◆ 18G needle ◆ blood administration set ◆ 500 ml of normal saline solution ◆ optional: Hemovac and another autologous transfusion system.

Patient preparation

• Explain autologous transfusion to the patient, including what it is, how it's performed, how often he can donate blood (every 7 days), and how much he can donate (one unit every week until 3 to 7 days before surgery).
• At least 1 week before the first donation, give the patient ferrous sulfate or another iron preparation to take three times a day.
• To prevent hypovolemia, tell the patient to drink plenty of fluids before donating blood.
• Warn him that he may feel lightheaded during the donation but that the problem can be treated without further compromise.

Implementation

The steps to take depend on the circumstances of the autologous transfusion.

For preoperative blood donation

• Check the patient's hemoglobin, which must be 11 g/dl or higher to donate blood.
• Check vital signs before blood donation.

• Help the patient into a supine position.
• Clean the needle insertion site (usually the antecubital fossa) with povidone-iodine solution, then with alcohol.
• Apply a tourniquet.
• Insert the large-bore needle into the antecubital vein. Have the patient squeeze a rubber ball while you collect blood.
• Recheck vital signs after the collection.
• If ordered, provide replacement I.V. fluids immediately after the collection.
• Send a blood sample to the hospital laboratory to be tested.
• Before reinfusion, check vital signs again and make sure the I.V. line is patent.
• Administer blood over $1\frac{1}{2}$ to 4 hours, depending on the patient's cardiovascular status and hospital policy.

For perioperative blood donation
• If you know that the patient will leave surgery with a drain to the autologous transfusion device, tell him this beforehand.

For perioperative blood donation using a Davol system
• Open the transfusion unit onto the sterile field. The doctor inserts the drain tube (from the patient) to the connecting tube of the unit.
• He injects 25 to 35 ml of ACD or CPD into the injection port on top of the filter and wets the filter with anticoagulant to keep the blood from clotting.
• Label the collection bag with the patient's name and the time the transfu-

sion was started *so that the reinfusion time is within guidelines.*

After patient arrival in postanesthesia care unit or medical-surgical unit
• Note the amount of blood in the bag and on the postoperative sheet.
• Attach the tube from the suction source to the port on the suction control module.
• Adjust the suction source to between 80 and 100 mm Hg on the wall regulator. Pinch the suction tube. If the regulator exceeds 100 mm Hg, turn the suction down. Suction set at more than 100 mm Hg may cause the collection bag to collapse, resulting in lysis of blood cells. The potential for renal damage renders this blood unsafe. If the collection bag collapses, change the entire collection setup.
• If the doctor orders it, start reinfusing the blood when 500 ml has been collected or 4 hours have passed (whichever comes first). Blood reinfusion must be completed within 6 hours of initiating the collection in the operating room.
• If less than 200 ml is collected in 4 hours, record the amount on the intake and output sheet and the postoperative sheet. Discard the drainage appropriately because the proportion of anticoagulant (inserted in the operating room) to blood is too great to infuse. If this happens, switch from the container to a closed wound suction unit. First remove the suction tube from the suction control unit. Clamp the connecting tubing above the filter. Detach the connecting tubing from the patient's tube and cap the patient's tube. Connect a closed wound suction unit, such as a Hemovac, if you're not going

to collect more blood for reinfusion. If more than 500 ml of blood is collected in the first 4 hours, connect a new autologous transfusion unit to the patient. Then reconnect the unit to suction. Monitor and record the drainage on the intake and output sheet.

To reinfuse the blood
• Prime the blood filter with 500 ml of normal saline solution.
• Twist the suction control module to remove it.
• Remove the hanger assembly from the collection bag.
• Pull the clear cap from the top of the bag, and discard the cap and filter.
• Insert a spike adapter into the large port on top of the bottle.
• Remove the protective seal to expose the filtered vent.
• Attach the blood to the Y-connector of the blood filter.
• Invert the bag and hang it.
• Obtain vital signs and document them.
• Begin the infusion, following hospital policy.
• Be sure to complete the infusion within 2 hours.

For perioperative blood donation using the Pleur-evac system connected to a chest tube
• Establish underwater seal drainage. Following the steps printed on the Pleur-evac unit, connect the patient's chest tube. Inspect the blood collection bag and tubing, making sure that all clamps are open and all connections are airtight.
• Before collection, add an anticoagulant such as heparin or CPD, if prescribed. With CPD, add one part to seven parts blood. Using an 18G (or

smaller) needle, inject the anticoagulant through the red self-sealing port on the autologous transfusion connector. The system is now ready to use. You should see chest cavity blood begin to collect in the bag.
• To collect more than one bag of blood, open a replacement bag when the first one is nearly full. Close the clamps on top of the second bag. Before removing the first collection bag from the drainage unit, reduce excess negativity by using the high-negativity relief valve. Depress the button; then release it when negativity drops to the desired level (watch the water seal manometer).
• Close the white clamp on the patient tubing. Then close the two white clamps on top of the collection bag.
• Disconnect all connectors on the first bag. Attach the red (female) and blue (male) connector sections on top of the autologous transfusion bag.
• Remove the protective cap from the collection tubing on the replacement bag. Connect the collection tubing to the patient's chest drainage tube, using the red connectors.
• Remove the protective cap from the replacement bag's suction tube, and attach the tube to the Pleur-evac unit, using the blue connectors. Make sure all connections are tight. Open all clamps, and inspect the system for airtight connections.
• Spread the metal support arms and disconnect them. Remove the first bag from the drainage unit by disconnecting the foot hook.
• Use the foot hook and support arm to attach the replacement bag.
• To reinfuse blood from the original collection bag, slide the bag off the support frame; then invert it so that the

spike points upward. Reinfuse blood within 6 hours of the start of collection. Never store collected blood.

• Remove the protective cap from the spike port and insert a microaggregate filter into the port, using a twisting motion. Prime the filter by gently squeezing the inverted bag. A new filter should be used with each bag.

• Continue squeezing until the filter is saturated and the drip chamber is half full. Then close the clamp on the reinfusion line and remove residual air from the bag. Invert the bag and suspend it from an I.V. pole. After carefully flushing the I.V. line to remove all air, infuse blood according to hospital policy.

Complications

Autologous transfusion may cause:
• hemolysis
• air and particulate emboli
• coagulation
• thrombocytopenia
• vasovagal reactions (from transient hypotension and bradycardia)
• hypovolemia (especially in elderly patients). (See *Managing problems of autologous transfusion,* pages 59 and 60.)

Nursing considerations

• Autologous transfusion is contraindicated in patients with malignant neoplasms, coagulopathies, excessive hemolysis, and active infections.
• It's also contraindicated in patients taking antibiotics and in those whose blood becomes contaminated by abdominal contents.
• Patients who've recently lost weight because of illness or malnutrition shouldn't donate blood.

For preoperative blood donation

• Monitor the patient closely during and after donation and autologous transfusion. Although vasovagal reactions are usually mild and easy to treat, they can quickly progress to severe reactions, such as loss of consciousness and seizures. Also, make sure the patient isn't bacteremic when he donates blood. Bacteria can proliferate in the collection bag and cause sepsis when reinfused.

• Clearly label the collection bag with: AUTOLOGOUS USE ONLY. This way, the blood won't be subjected to rigorous blood bank testing or be accidentally given to another patient. Before reinfusion, identify the patient and make sure that the collection bag is clearly marked with his name, hospital identification number, and an autologous blood label. If signs of a hemolytic reaction occur, the patient may have received the wrong unit of blood.

• Caution the patient to remain in a supine position for at least 10 minutes after donating blood.

• Encourage him to drink more fluids than usual for a few hours after blood donation and to eat heartily at his next meal.

• Tell him to keep an eye on the needle wound in his arm for a few hours after blood donation. If bleeding occurs, he should apply firm pressure for 5 to 10 minutes. If the bleeding doesn't stop, he should notify the blood bank or his doctor.

• If the patient feels light-headed or dizzy, advise him to sit down immediately and to lower his head between his knees. Or he can lie down with his head lower than the rest of his body until the feeling subsides.

PROBLEM SOLVER

Managing problems of autologous transfusion

PROBLEM	CAUSE	INTERVENTION
Citrate toxicity (rare, unpredictable)	• Chelating effect on calcium of citrate in phosphate dextrose (CPD) • Predisposing factors, including hyperkalemia, hypocalcemia, acidosis, hypothermia, myocardial dysfunction, and liver or kidney problems • Watch for hypotension, arrhythmias, and myocardial contractility.	• Prophylactic calcium chloride may be administered if more than 2,000 ml of CPD-anticoagulated blood is given over 20 minutes. • Stop infusing CPD and correct acidosis. Measure arterial blood gas and serum calcium levels frequently to assess for toxicity.
Coagulation	• Not enough anticoagulant • Blood not defibrinated in mediastinum	• Add CPD or another regional anticoagulant at a ratio of 7 parts blood to 1 part anticoagulant. Keep blood and CPD mixed by shaking collection bottle regularly. • Check for anticoagulant reversal. Strip chest tubes, as needed.
Coagulopathies	• Reduced platelet and fibrinogen levels • Platelets caught in filters • Enhanced levels of fibrin split products	• Patients receiving autologous transfusions of more than 4,000 ml of blood may also need transfusions of fresh frozen plasma or platelet concentrate.
Emboli	• Microaggregate debris • Air	• Don't use equipment with roller pumps or pressure infusion systems. Before reinfusion, remove air from blood bags. • Reinfuse with a 20- to 40-unit microaggregate filter. *(continued)*

Managing problems of autologous transfusion *(continued)*

PROBLEM	CAUSE	INTERVENTION
Hemolysis	• Trauma to blood caused by turbulence or roller pumps	• Don't skim operative field or use equipment with roller pumps. When collecting blood from chest tubes, keep vacuum below 30 mm Hg; when aspirating from a surgical site, keep vacuum below 60 mm Hg.
Sepsis	• Lack of aseptic technique • Contaminated blood	• Give broad-spectrum antibiotics. Use strict aseptic technique. Reinfuse patient within 4 hours. • Don't infuse blood from infected areas or blood with feces, urine, or other contaminants.

• Tell him that he can resume normal activities after resting 15 minutes.

For all donation methods
• Check the patient's laboratory data (coagulation profile and hemoglobin, hematocrit, and calcium levels) after he donates blood and again after reinfusion.
• Be alert for signs and symptoms of a hemolytic reaction: pain at the I.V. site, fever, chills, back pain, hypotension, and anxiety. If these occur, stop the transfusion and call the blood bank and doctor.

Documentation
• Document the amount of blood that the patient donated and had reinfused and how he tolerated each procedure.

Automated external defibrillator operation

Automated external defibrillators (AEDs) are commonly used to provide early defibrillation, which is considered the most effective treatment for ventricular fibrillation. Some hospitals require an AED in every non-critical-care unit. Instruction on using the AED is required as part of basic life support and advanced cardiac life support training.

The AED is equipped with a microcomputer that senses and analyzes a patient's heart rhythm at the push of a button. It then prompts a user audibly or visually to deliver a shock. All AED models have the same basic function but offer different operating options. For example, all AEDs communicate directions via messages on a display screen, give voice commands, or both.

AED training can be enhanced by using a CPR mannequin and AED look-alike devices that can be configured for multiple AED protocols. (See *Using an AED simulator.*)

>> Key nursing diagnoses and patient outcome

Use these nursing diagnoses as a guide when developing your plan of care for a patient being treated for ventricular fibrillation.

Ineffective breathing pattern related to alterations in normal gas exchange

Based on this nursing diagnosis, you'll establish the following patient outcomes. The patient will:
• regain his baseline respiratory rate and maintain stable respiration.
• regain and maintain arterial blood gas values within normal limits.
• demonstrate diaphragmatic pursed-lip breathing.

Decreased cardiac output related to reduced myocardial perfusion

Based on this nursing diagnosis, you'll establish the following patient outcomes. The patient will:
• maintain a normal pulse rate and blood pressure.
• experience no dizziness, syncope, arrhythmias, or chest pain.
• maintain respiratory status within established parameters.

Equipment

♦ automated external defibrillator unit ♦ electrode connector cables
♦ two prepackaged electrode pads.

TECHNOLOGY UPDATE

Using an AED simulator

Training simulators, such as the Lifepak AED trainer, by Physio-Control Corporation, look and feel like an actual AED unit. The trainer provides voice and screen prompts, realistic tones, lighted controls, and reusable electrodes. By varying the amount of hands-on control available to the student, the instructor can tailor the training experience to the student's needs. The unit can also be configured for multiple AED protocols.

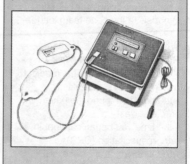

Implementation

• Open the foil packets containing the two electrode pads.
• Attach the white cable connector to one pad and the red cable connector to the other. The pads are not site-specific.

Applying the electrodes

• Expose the patient's chest.
• Remove the plastic backing film from the electrode pads and place the electrode pad attached to the white cable connector on the right upper portion of the patient's chest, just beneath his clavicle.

BETTER CHARTING

Code reporting with the AED

All external defibrillator devices record your interactions with the patient during defibrillation, either on a cassette tape or in a solid-state memory module. Some AEDs have an integral printer for immediate event documentation. Hospital policy defines who is responsible for reviewing all AED interactions; the patient's doctor always has that option. Local and state regulations govern who is responsible for collecting AED data for reporting purposes. After using an AED, give a synopsis to the code team leader.

What to report

Remember to report the following:
- the patient's name, age, medical history and chief complaint
- the time you found the patient in cardiac arrest
- the time you began cardiopulmonary resuscitation (CPR)
- the time you applied the AED
- how many shocks the patient received
- when the patient regained a pulse at any point
- what postarrest care was given, if any
- physical assessment findings.
   Later, be sure to document the code on the appropriate form.

• Place the pad attached to the red cable connector to the left of the heart's apex.
• To help remember where to place the pads, think "white - red, red -ribs." (Placement for both electrode pads is the same as for manual defibrillation or cardioversion.)

Operating the AED

• Firmly press the AED's on button and wait while the machine performs a brief self-test. Most AEDs signal readiness by a computerized voice that says "Stand clear" or by emitting a series of loud beeps. (If the AED were malfunctioning, it would convey the message "Do not use the AED. In that case, remove electrodes and continue CPR.") Remember to report any AED malfunctions in accordance with hospital procedure.
• When the machine is ready to analyze the patient's heart rhythm, ask everyone to stand clear, to avoid the risk of electric shock, and press the ANALYZE button when the machine prompts you to.
• Be careful not to touch or move the patient while the AED is in analysis mode. (If you get the message "Check electrodes," make sure that electrodes are correctly placed and the patient cable is securely attached; then press the analyze button again).

Delivering a shock

• In 15 to 30 seconds, the AED will analyze the patient's rhythm. When the patient needs a shock, the AED will display a "Stand clear" message.
• When an AED is fully charged and ready to deliver a shock, it will prompt you to press the shock button. (Some fully automated AED models automatically deliver a shock within 15 seconds after analyzing the patient's rhythm. If a shock weren't needed, the AED would display the message "No shock indicated" and prompt you to "Check patient.")

• Make sure no one is touching the patient or his bed and call out "Stand clear." Then press the shock button. Most AEDs are ready to deliver a shock within 15 seconds.

• After the first shock, the AED will automatically reanalyze the patient's rhythm. If another shock isn't needed, the machine will prompt you to check the patient.

• If the patient is still in ventricular fibrillation, however, the AED will automatically begin recharging at a higher joule level to prepare for a second shock. Repeat the steps you performed before shocking the patient. The patient can be shocked up to three times at increasing joule levels (200, 200 to 300, and 360 joules).

• If the patient remains in ventricular fibrillation after three shocks, resume CPR for one minute. Then press the ANALYZE button on the AED to identify the heart rhythm. If the patient remains in ventricular fibrillation, continue this sequence until the code-team leader arrives.

Complications

• Defibrillation can cause accidental shock to caregivers.

• Failure to follow the manufacturer's instructions on AED use has rarely (less than one tenth of one percent) resulted in the delivery of inappropriate electrical countershocks.

• There have been occasional failures to deliver shocks to rhythms that may benefit from electrical therapy, such as extremely fine or coarse ventricular fibrillation.

Nursing considerations

• AEDs should be placed in the analysis mode *only* when full cardiac arrest has been confirmed and *only* when all movement, particularly the movement of patient transport, has ceased.

• Agonal respiration poses a problem because some devices may not be able to complete analysis cycles if the patient continues to display gasping respirations.

• Avoid using radio receivers and transmitters during rhythm analysis.

Documentation

• After the code, remove and transcribe the AED's computer memory module or tape, or prompt the AED to print a rhythm strip with the code data.

• Follow hospital policy for analysis and storing of code data. (See *Code reporting with the AED*.)

B

Barium enema

Also called lower-GI examination, barium enema is a diagnostic test that involves the radiographic examination of the large intestine after rectal instillation of barium sulfate (single-contrast technique) or barium sulfate and air (double-contrast technique). It's indicated in patients with histories of altered bowel habits, lower abdominal pain, or passage of blood, mucus, or pus in the stool. It may also be indicated after colostomy or ileostomy; in these patients, barium (or barium and air) is instilled through the stoma.

The single-contrast technique provides a profile view of the large intestine; the double-contrast technique provides profile and frontal views. The latter technique best detects small intraluminal tumors (especially polyps), the early mucosal changes of inflammatory disease, and the subtle intestinal bleeding caused by ulcerated polyps or shallow ulcerations of inflammatory disease.

Barium enema should precede the barium swallow and upper-GI and small-bowel series because barium ingested in the latter procedure may take several days to pass through the GI tract and thus may interfere with subsequent X-ray studies.

Barium enema is contraindicated in patients with tachycardia, fulminant ulcerative colitis associated with systemic toxicity and megacolon, toxic megacolon, or suspected perforation.

This test should be performed cautiously in patients with obstruction; acute inflammatory conditions, such as ulcerative colitis and diverticulitis; acute vascular insufficiency of the bowel; acute fulminant bloody diarrhea; and suspected pneumatosis cystoides intestinalis.

Normally, in the single-contrast enema, the intestine is uniformly filled with barium, and colonic haustral markings are clearly apparent. The intestinal walls collapse as the barium is expelled, and the mucosa has a regular, feathery appearance on the postevacuation film. In the double-contrast enema, the intestine is uniformly distended with air and a thin layer of barium provides excellent detail of the mucosal pattern. As the patient assumes various positions, barium collects on the dependent walls of the intestine by force of gravity.

X-ray films may reveal adenocarcinoma and, rarely, sarcomas occurring higher in the intestine. Carcinoma usually appears as a localized filling defect — an area that isn't fully coated or filled with contrast medium, with a sharp transition between normal and necrotic mucosa.

≫ Key nursing diagnoses and patient outcomes

Use these nursing diagnoses as a guide when developing your plan of care for a patient having a barium enema.

Altered GI tissue perfusion related to (specify)

Based on this nursing diagnosis, you'll establish the following patient outcomes. The patient will have:

- intake equal to output.
- normal bowel function return.
- no nausea, vomiting, or abdominal pain.

Colonic constipation related to (specify)
Based on this nursing diagnosis, you'll establish the following patient outcomes. The patient will:
- have bowel pattern return to normal.
- state understanding of factors causing constipation.

Patient preparation
- Explain to the patient that this test permits examination of the large intestine through X-ray films taken after a barium enema.
- Describe the test, including who will perform it, where it will take place, and how long it will take (30 to 45 minutes).
- Because residual fecal material in the colon obscures normal anatomy on radiographs, carefully follow the prescribed bowel preparation.
- Diet, laxatives, or cleansing enemas may be used. In certain conditions, though, such as ulcerative colitis and active GI bleeding, the use of laxatives or cleansing enemas may be prohibited.
- Stress that accurate test results depend on the patient's cooperation with prescribed dietary restrictions and bowel preparation. A common bowel preparation technique includes restricted intake of dairy products and maintenance of a liquid diet for 24 hours before the test. Encourage the patient to drink five 8-oz glasses of water or clear liquids 12 to 24 hours before the test.

- Administer bowel preparation supplied by the X-ray department. An enema or repeat enemas may be prescribed until return is clear.
- Withhold breakfast before the procedure; if the test is scheduled for late afternoon (or delayed), clear liquids may be allowed.
- Tell the patient that he'll be placed on a tilting X-ray table and adequately draped. During the test, he'll be secured to the table and assisted to various positions.
- Tell the patient that he may experience cramping pains or the urge to defecate as the barium or air is introduced into the intestine. Instruct him to breathe deeply and slowly through his mouth to ease this discomfort.
- Tell him to keep his anal sphincter tightly contracted against the rectal tube; this holds the tube in position and helps prevent leakage of barium. Stress the importance of retaining the barium enema; if the intestinal walls aren't adequately coated with barium, test results may be inaccurate.
- Assure the patient that the barium enema is fairly easy to retain because of its cool temperature.

Implementation
- After the patient is in a supine position on a tilting radiographic table, scout films of the abdomen are taken.
- The patient is assisted to Sims' position and a well-lubricated rectal tube is inserted through the anus. If the patient has anal sphincter atony or severe mental or physical debilitation, a rectal tube with a retaining balloon may be inserted.
- The barium is administered slowly, and the filling process is monitored fluoroscopically. To aid filling, the ta-

ble may be tilted or the patient assisted may be assisted to supine, prone, and lateral decubitus positions.

• As the flow of barium is observed, spot films are taken of significant findings.

• When the intestine is filled with barium, overhead films of the abdomen are taken.

• Withdraw the rectal tube and escort the patient to the toilet or provide a bedpan.

• Instruct the patient to expel as much of the barium as possible.

• After evacuation, an additional overhead film is taken to record the mucosal pattern of the intestine and to evaluate the efficiency of colonic emptying.

• A double-contrast barium enema may directly follow this examination or be performed separately. If it's performed immediately, a thin film of barium remains in the patient's intestine, coating the mucosa, and air is carefully injected to distend the bowel lumen.

• When the double-contrast technique is performed separately, a colloidal barium suspension is instilled, filling the patient's intestine to either the splenic flexure or the middle of the transverse colon. The suspension is then aspirated, and air is forcefully injected into the intestine. The intestine may also be filled to the lower descending colon and then air is forcefully injected, without prior aspiration of the suspension.

• The patient is then assisted to erect, prone, supine, and lateral decubitus positions in sequence.

• Barium filling is monitored fluoroscopically, and spot films are taken of significant findings. After the required films are taken, the patient is escorted to the toilet or provided with a bedpan.

Complications
Complications of barium enema include:

• perforation of the colon
• water intoxication
• barium granulomas
• intraperitoneal and extraperitoneal extravasation of barium and barium embolism (though these are rare).

Nursing considerations
• Make sure further studies haven't been ordered before allowing the patient to eat or drink.

• When studies are completed, encourage extra fluid intake because bowel preparation and the test itself can cause dehydration.

• Encourage rest because this test and the bowel preparation preceding it exhaust most patients.

• Because retention of barium after this test can cause intestinal obstruction or fecal impaction, administer a mild cathartic or a cleansing enema. Tell the patient that stool will be light-colored for 24 to 72 hours.

Documentation
• Document the time and place of the barium enema as well as the patient's tolerance of the procedure.

• Always prepare the patient for the test and document any teaching you've done about the test itself and any follow-up care associated with it.

• Be sure to document the administration or withholding of drugs and preparations, special diets, food or fluid restrictions, enemas, and specimen collection.

• Record and describe any stool passed by the patient in the hospital.

Barium swallow and upper-GI series

The upper-GI and small-bowel series is a diagnostic procedure in which fluoroscopic examination is made of the esophagus, stomach, and small intestine after the patient ingests barium sulfate, a contrast agent. As the barium passes through the digestive tract, fluoroscopy outlines peristalsis and the mucosal contours of the respective organs, and spot films record significant findings. This test is indicated for patients with upper-GI symptoms (difficulty in swallowing, regurgitation, burning or gnawing epigastric pain), signs of small-bowel disease (diarrhea, weight loss), and signs of GI bleeding (hematemesis, melena).

Barium swallow (esophagography) is the cineradiographic, radiographic, or fluoroscopic examination of the pharynx and the fluoroscopic examination of the esophagus after ingestion of thick and thin mixtures of barium sulfate. This test, most commonly performed as part of the upper-GI series, is indicated in patients with histories of dysphagia and regurgitation. More testing is usually required for definitive diagnosis.

The barium swallow, upper-GI and small-bowel series is contraindicated in patients with obstruction or perforation of the digestive tract. Barium may intensify the obstruction or seep into the abdominal cavity. If a perforation is suspected, gastrografin may be used instead of barium.

» Key nursing diagnoses and patient outcomes

Use these nursing diagnoses as a guide when developing a plan of care for a patient having a barium swallow, or upper-GI and small-bowel series.

Altered GI tissue perfusion related to (specify)
Based on this nursing diagnosis, you'll establish the following patient outcomes. The patient will:
• have intake equal to output.
• have normal bowel function return.
• have no nausea, vomiting, or abdominal pain.

Impaired swallowing related to neuromuscular impairment
Based on this nursing diagnosis, you'll establish the following patient outcomes. The patient will:
• show no evidence of aspiration pneumonia.
• maintain weight.
• achieve adequate nutritional intake.

Equipment
♦ Cathartic, if ordered, for after the test.

Patient preparation
• Explain to the patient that this procedure uses ingested barium and X-ray films to examine the esophagus, stomach, and small intestine.
• Tell the patient to maintain a low-residue diet for 2 or 3 days before the test and then to fast and avoid smoking after midnight the night before the test.
• Describe low-residue foods and drinks.
• Describe the test, including who will perform it, where it will take place,

and its expected duration (up to 6 hours).
• Encourage the patient to bring reading material.
• Inform the patient that a rotating X-ray table will be used in vertical, semivertical, and horizontal positions.
• Explain that the patient will be secured to the table and that help will be provided getting into the supine, prone, and side-lying positions required for filming.
• Describe the chalky taste and the milk-shake consistency of the barium mixture. Explain that even though the drink is flavored, it may be unpleasant-tasting, but that 16 to 20 oz (475 to 590 ml) must be consumed to ensure a complete examination.
• Tell the patient that her abdomen may be compressed to ensure proper coating of the stomach or intestinal walls with barium, or to separate overlapping bowel loops.
• As prescribed, withhold most oral medications after midnight and anticholinergics and narcotics for 24 hours because these drugs affect small intestine motility. Antacids are also sometimes withheld for several hours if gastric reflux is suspected.
• Just before the procedure, instruct the patient to put on a hospital gown without snap closures and to remove jewelry, dentures, hair clips, or other objects that might obscure anatomic detail on the X-ray films.

Implementation
The single- or double-contrast technique may be used, depending on the reasons for the test.

Single-contrast technique
• After the patient is secured in a supine position on the table, the table is tilted until the patient is vertical, and the heart, lungs, and abdomen are examined fluoroscopically.
• Tell the patient to take several swallows of the barium suspension, so its route through the esophagus can be observed fluoroscopically.
• When barium enters the stomach, the patient's abdomen is palpated or compressed to ensure adequate coating of the gastric mucosa with barium.

Double-contrast technique
• In a double-contrast examination, tell the patient to sip barium through a perforated straw, which allows some air to enter the stomach. The air permits detailed examination of the gastric rugae.
• After spot films of significant findings are taken, tell the patient to drink the remaining barium suspension, so the filling of the stomach and emptying into the duodenum can be observed fluoroscopically.
• Administer a cathartic, if prescribed.

Complications
• Retention of barium in the intestine may cause obstruction or fecal impaction.

Nursing considerations
• Make sure additional X-rays haven't been ordered before allowing the patient food, fluids, or oral medications.

Documentation
• Document the time and place of the barium swallow or upper-GI and small-bowel series and the patient's tolerance of the procedure.

• Always prepare the patient for the test and document any teaching you've done about the test or follow-up care.
• Be sure to document the administration or withholding of drugs and preparations, special diets, food or fluid restrictions, enemas, and specimen collection.
• Record and describe any stool passed by the patient in the hospital.

Biopsy

Skin biopsy is a diagnostic test in which a small piece of tissue is removed, under local anesthetic, from a lesion suspected of malignant disease or other dermatoses.

One of three techniques may be used: shave biopsy, punch biopsy, or excisional biopsy. Shave biopsy cuts the lesion above the skin line, which allows further biopsy at the site. Punch biopsy removes an oval core from the center of a lesion. Excisional biopsy removes the entire lesion and is indicated for rapidly expanding lesions; for sclerotic, bullous, or atrophic lesions; and for examination of the border of a lesion and surrounding normal skin.

Lesions suspected of being malignant usually have changed color, size, or appearance or have failed to heal properly after injury. Fully developed lesions should be selected for biopsy whenever possible because they provide more diagnostic information than lesions that are resolving or in early stages of development. For example, if the skin shows blisters, bi-

opsy should include the most mature ones.

Normal skin consists of squamous epithelium (epidermis) and fibrous connective tissue (dermis). Histologic examination of the tissue specimen obtained during biopsy may reveal a benign or malignant lesion. Benign growths include cysts, seborrheic keratoses, warts, pigmented nevi (moles), keloids, dermatofibromas, and neurofibromas. Malignant tumors include basal cell carcinoma, squamous cell carcinoma, and malignant melanoma.

⟫ Key nursing diagnoses and patient outcomes

Use these nursing diagnoses as a guide when developing your plan of care.

Impaired skin integrity related to lesion

Based on this nursing diagnosis, you'll establish the following patient outcomes. The patient will:
• exhibit improved or healed lesions.
• have few or no complications.
• explain skin care regimen.

Anxiety related to possible medical diagnoses

Based on this nursing diagnosis, you'll establish the following patient outcomes. The patient will:
• state feeling of anxiety.
• use support systems to assist with coping.
• cope with threat of anxiety by being involved in decisions about care.

Equipment

♦ #15 scalpel for shave or excisional biopsy ♦ local anesthetic ♦ specimen bottle containing 10% formaldehyde solution ♦ 4-O sutures for punch or excisional biopsy ♦ adhesive bandage.

Patient preparation

• Explain to the patient that the biopsy provides a sample of skin for microscopic study.
• Describe the procedure to the patient and answer any questions.
• Inform him that she need not restrict food or fluids.
• Tell him who will perform the procedure.
• Tell him he'll receive a local anesthetic to minimize pain.
• Inform him that the biopsy will take about 15 minutes and that test results are usually available in 1 day.
• Have the patient or an appropriate family member sign a consent form.
• Check patient history for hypersensitivity to the local anesthetic.

Implementation

• Position the patient comfortably, and clean the biopsy site before the local anesthetic is administered.
• *Shave biopsy:* The protruding growth is cut off at the skin line with a #15 scalpel. The tissue is placed immediately in a properly labeled specimen bottle containing 10% formaldehyde solution. Apply pressure to the area to stop the bleeding.
• *Punch biopsy:* The skin surrounding the lesion is pulled taut, and the punch is firmly introduced into the lesion and is rotated to obtain a tissue specimen. The plug is lifted with forceps or a needle and is severed as deeply into

the fat layer as possible. The specimen is placed in a properly labeled specimen bottle containing 10% formaldehyde solution or in a sterile container, if indicated. Closing the wound depends on the size of the punch: A 3-mm punch requires only an adhesive bandage, a 4-mm punch requires one suture, and a 6-mm punch requires two sutures.
• *Excisional biopsy:* A #15 scalpel is used to excise the lesion; the incision is made as wide and as deep as necessary. The tissue specimen is removed and placed immediately in a properly labeled specimen bottle containing 10% formaldehyde solution. Apply pressure to the site to stop the bleeding. The wound is closed using 4-0 suture. If the incision is large, skin graft may be required.
• Check the biopsy site for bleeding.
• If the patient experiences pain, administer medication.

Complications

• Complications may include bleeding and infection of the surrounding tissue.

Nursing considerations

• Send the specimen to the laboratory immediately.

Home care

• Advise the patient with sutures to keep the area clean and as dry as possible.
• Tell the patient that facial sutures will be removed in 3 to 5 days, trunk sutures in 7 to 14 days.
• Instruct the patient with adhesive strips to leave them in place for 14 to 21 days.

Documentation
• Document the time and location where the specimen was obtained, the appearance of the specimen and site, and whether bleeding occurred at the biopsy site.

Bladder irrigation, continuous

Continuous bladder irrigation can help prevent urinary-tract obstruction by flushing out small blood clots that form after prostate or bladder surgery. It may also be used to treat an irritated, inflamed, or infected bladder lining.

This procedure requires placement of a triple-lumen catheter. One lumen controls balloon inflation, one allows irrigant inflow, and one allows irrigant outflow. The continuous flow of irrigating solution through the bladder also creates a mild tamponade that may help prevent venous hemorrhage. (See *Setup for continuous bladder irrigation*, page 72.)

Although the catheter typically is inserted in the operating room after prostate or bladder surgery, it may be inserted at bedside if the patient isn't having surgery.

≫ Key nursing diagnoses and patient outcomes
Use these nursing diagnoses as a guide when developing your plan of care for a patient who requires continuous bladder irrigation.

Altered urinary elimination related to neuromuscular impairment
Based on this nursing diagnosis, you'll establish the following patient outcomes. The patient will:
• maintain fluid balance — intake equal to output.
• voice increased comfort.
• discuss impact of urologic disorder on self and others.

Urinary retention related to neuromuscular impairment
Based on this nursing diagnosis, you'll establish the following patient outcomes. The patient will:
• voice understanding of treatment.
• have few or no complications.

Equipment
♦ One 4,000-ml container or two 2,000-ml containers of irrigating solution (usually normal saline solution) or the prescribed amount of medicated solution ♦ Y-tubing made specifically for bladder irrigation ♦ alcohol or povidone-iodine sponge.

Equipment preparation
• Normal saline solution is usually prescribed for bladder irrigation after prostate or bladder surgery. Large volumes of irrigating solution are usually required during the first 24 to 48 hours after surgery. *This explains the use of Y-tubing, which allows immediate irrigation with reserve solution.*
• Before starting continuous bladder irrigation, double-check the irrigating solution against the doctor's order. If the solution contains an antibiotic, check the patient's chart *to make sure he's not allergic to the drug.*

Setup for continuous bladder irrigation

In continuous bladder irrigation, a triple-lumen catheter allows irrigating solution to flow into the bladder through one lumen and flow out through another, as shown in the inset. The third lumen is used to inflate the balloon that holds the catheter in place.

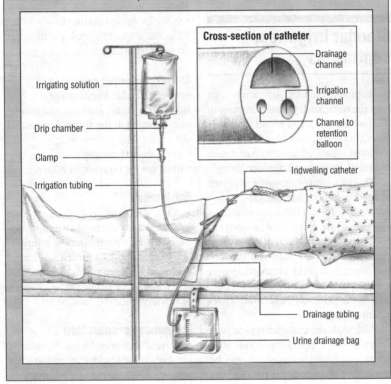

Cross-section of catheter
- Drainage channel
- Irrigation channel
- Channel to retention balloon

Irrigating solution
Drip chamber
Clamp
Irrigation tubing
Indwelling catheter
Drainage tubing
Urine drainage bag

Implementation
- Wash your hands.
- Assemble all equipment at the patient's bedside.
- Explain the procedure and provide privacy.
- Insert the spike of the Y-tubing into the container of irrigating solution. (If you have a two-container system, insert one spike into each container.)
- Squeeze the drip chamber on the spike of the tubing.

- Open the flow clamp and flush the tubing *to remove air, which could cause bladder distention.* Then close the clamp.
- To begin, hang the irrigating solution on the I.V. pole.
- Clean the opening to the inflow lumen of the catheter with the alcohol or povidone-iodine sponge.
- Insert the distal end of the Y-tubing securely into the inflow lumen (third port) of the catheter.

• Make sure the catheter's outflow lumen is securely attached to the drainage bag tubing.

• Open the flow clamp under the container of irrigating solution, and set the drip rate, as ordered.

• *To prevent air from entering the system,* don't allow the primary container to empty completely before replacing it.

• If you have a two-container system, simultaneously close the flow clamp under the nearly empty container and open the flow clamp under the reserve container. *This prevents reflux of irrigating solution from the reserve container into the nearly empty one.* Hang a new reserve container on the I.V. pole, and insert the tubing, maintaining asepsis.

• Empty the drainage bag every 4 hours or as often as needed. Use sterile technique *to avoid the risk of contamination.*

Complications

• Interruptions in a continuous irrigation system can predispose the patient to infection. Obstruction in the catheter's outflow lumen can cause bladder distention.

Nursing considerations

• Check the inflow and outflow lines periodically for kinks *to make sure the solution is running freely.* If the solution flows rapidly, check the lines frequently.

• Measure the outflow volume accurately. It should equal or, allowing for urine production, slightly exceed inflow volume. If inflow volume exceeds outflow volume postoperatively, suspect bladder rupture at the

suture lines or renal damage, and notify the doctor immediately.

• Assess outflow for changes in appearance and for blood clots, especially if irrigation is being performed postoperatively to control bleeding. If drainage is bright red, irrigating solution should usually be infused rapidly *with the clamp wide open* until drainage clears. Notify the doctor immediately if you suspect hemorrhage. If drainage is clear, the solution is usually given at a rate of 40 to 60 drops/minute. The doctor typically specifies the rate for antibiotic solutions.

Documentation

• Each time you finish a container of solution, record the date, time, and amount of fluid given on the intake and output record.

• Record the time and the amount of fluid each time you empty the drainage bag.

• Note drainage appearance and patient complaints.

Blood pressure measurement

Defined as the lateral force exerted by blood on the arterial walls, blood pressure depends on the force of ventricular contractions, arterial wall elasticity, peripheral vascular resistance, and blood volume and viscosity. Systolic, or maximum, pressure occurs during left ventricular contraction and reflects the integrity of the heart, arteries, and arterioles. Diastolic, or minimum, pressure occurs during left ventricular relaxation and directly indicates blood vessel resistance.

Effects of age on blood pressure

AGE	BLOOD PRESSURE (mm Hg)
Neonate	systolic: 50 to 52 diastolic: 25 to 30 mean: 35 to 40
3 years	systolic: 78 to 114 diastolic: 46 to 78
10 years	systolic: 90 to 132 diastolic: 56 to 86
16 years	systolic: 104 to 108 diastolic: 60 to 92
Adult	systolic: 90 to 130 diastolic: 60 to 85
Older adult	systolic: 140 to 160 diastolic: 70 to 90

Pulse pressure, the difference between systolic and diastolic pressures, varies, depending on arterial elasticity. Rigid vessels, incapable of distention and recoil, produce high systolic pressure and low diastolic pressure. Normally, systolic pressure exceeds diastolic pressure by about 40 mm Hg. *Narrowed pulse pressure* — a difference of less than 30 mm Hg — occurs when systolic pressure falls and diastolic pressure remains constant, when diastolic pressure rises and systolic pressure stays constant, or when systolic pressure falls and diastolic pressure rises. These changes reflect reduced stroke volume, increased peripheral resistance, or both. *Widened pulse pressure* — a difference of more than 50 mm Hg between systolic and diastolic blood pressures — occurs when systolic pressure rises and

diastolic pressure remains constant, when diastolic pressure falls and systolic pressure remains constant, or when systolic pressure rises and diastolic pressure falls. These changes reflect increased stroke volume, decreased peripheral resistance, or both.

Blood pressure is measured in millimeters of mercury with a sphygmomanometer and a stethoscope, usually at the brachial artery (less often at the popliteal or radial artery). Lowest in the neonate, blood pressure rises with age, weight gain, prolonged stress, and anxiety.

The sphygmomanometer consists of an inflatable compression cuff linked to a manual air pump and a mercury manometer or an aneroid gauge. The mercury sphygmomanometer is more accurate and requires calibration less frequently than the aneroid model but is larger and heavier. To obtain an accurate reading, you must rest its gauge on a level surface and view the meniscus at eye level; you can rest an aneroid gauge in any position but must view it directly from the front. Some mercury manometers have specially designed cases that open to form a level surface; others must be attached to a wall or to a base unit that stands on the floor.

Hook, bandage, snap, or Velcro cuffs come in six standard sizes ranging from newborn to extra-large adult. Disposable cuffs are available. (See *Effects of age on blood pressure.*)

Frequent blood pressure measurement is critical after serious injury, surgery, or anesthesia and during any illness or condition that threatens cardiovascular stability. (This may be done with an automated vital signs monitor.) Regular measurement is indicated for patients with a history of hypertension or hypotension, and yearly screening is recommended for all adults.

>> Key nursing diagnoses and patient outcomes

Use this nursing diagnosis as a guide when developing your plan of care.

Altered (specify type) tissue perfusion related to decreased cellular exchange

Based on this nursing diagnosis, you'll establish the following patient outcomes. The patient will:
• attain hemodynamic stability: pulse not less than (specify) beats/minute and not greater than (specify) beats/ minute; blood pressure not less than (specify) mm Hg and not greater than (specify) mm Hg.
• maintain adequate cardiac output.

Equipment

♦ mercury or aneroid sphygmomanometer ♦ stethoscope ♦ alcohol sponge ♦ automated vital signs monitor (if available).

Equipment preparation

• Carefully choose a cuff of appropriate size for the patient. *An excessively narrow cuff may cause a false-high pressure reading, an excessively wide one a false-low reading.*
• If you're not using your own stethoscope, disinfect the earpieces with an alcohol sponge before placing them in your ears *to avoid cross-contamination.*
• To use an automated vital signs monitor, collect the monitor, dual air hose, and pressure cuff and then make sure the monitor unit is firmly positioned near the patient's bed. (See *Us-*

ing an electronic vital signs monitor, pages 76 and 77.)

Implementation

• Tell the patient you're going to take his blood pressure.
• The patient can lie in a supine position or sit erect during blood pressure measurement.
• His arm should be extended at heart level and be well supported. *If the artery is below heart level, the blood pressure may read falsely high.*
• Be sure the patient is relaxed and comfortable when you take his blood pressure *so it stays at its normal level.*
• Wrap the deflated cuff snugly around the upper arm.
• If necessary, connect the appropriate tube to the rubber bulb of the air pump and the other tube to the manometer. Then put the stethoscope earpieces into your ears.
• Locate the brachial artery by palpation. Center the bell of the stethoscope over the part of the artery where you detect the strongest beats, and hold it in place with one hand. *The bell of the stethoscope transmits low-pitched arterial-blood sounds more effectively than the diaphragm.*
• Using the thumb and index finger of your other hand, turn the thumbscrew on the rubber bulb of the air pump clockwise to close the valve.
• Then pump air into the cuff while auscultating the sound over the brachial artery *to compress and, eventually, occlude arterial blood flow.* Pump air until the mercury column or aneroid gauge registers 160 mm Hg or at least 10 mm Hg above the level reached at the last audible sound.
• Carefully open the valve of the air pump and slowly deflate the cuff —

TECHNOLOGY UPDATE

 Using an electronic vital signs monitor

An electronic vital signs monitor allows you to track a patient's vital signs continually, without having to reapply a blood pressure cuff each time. What's more, the patient won't need an invasive arterial line to gather similar data. The machine shown here is a Dinamap VS Monitor 8100, but these steps can be followed with most other monitors.

Some automated vital signs monitors, such as the Dinamap, are lightweight and battery-operated, and can be attached to an I.V. pole for continual monitoring, even during patient transfers. Make sure you know the capacity of the monitor's battery, and plug the machine in whenever possible to keep it charged.

Before using any monitor, check its accuracy. Determine the patient's pulse rate and blood pressure manually, using the same arm you'll use for the monitor cuff. Compare your results when you get initial readings from the monitor. If the results differ, call your supply department or the manufacturer's representative.

Preparing the device

• Explain the procedure to the patient. Describe the alarm system *so he won't be frightened if it's triggered.*
• Make sure the power switch is off. Then plug the monitor into a properly grounded wall outlet. Next, secure the dual air hose to the front of the monitor.

• Connect the pressure cuff's tubing into the other ends of the dual air hose, and tighten connections *to prevent air leaks.* Keep the air hose away from the patient *to avoid accidental dislodgment.*
• Squeeze all air from the cuff, and wrap it loosely around the patient's arm or leg, allowing two fingerbreadths between cuff and arm or leg. Never apply the cuff to a limb that has an I.V. line in place. Position the cuff's "artery" arrow over the palpated brachial artery. Then secure the cuff for a snug fit.

Selecting parameters

• When you turn on the monitor, it will default to a manual mode. (In this mode, you can obtain vital signs yourself before switching to the automatic mode.) Press the "auto/manual" button to select the automatic mode. The monitor will give you baseline data for the pulse rate, systolic and diastolic pressures, and mean arterial pressure.
• Compare your previous manual results with these baseline data. If they match, you're ready to set the alarm parameters. Press the "select" button to blank all displays except systolic pressure.
• Use the "high" and "low" limit buttons to set the specific parameters for systolic pressure. (These limits range from a high of 240 to a low of 0.) You'll also do this three more times for mean arterial pressure, pulse rate, and diastolic pressure. After you've set the parameters for diastolic pressure, press the "select"

Using an electronic vital signs monitor *(continued)*

button again to display all current data. Even if you forget to do this last step, the monitor will automatically display current data 10 seconds after you set the last parameters.

Collecting data

• You also need to tell the monitor how often to obtain data. Press the "set" button until you reach the desired time interval in minutes. If you've chosen the automatic mode, the monitor will display a default cycle time of 3 minutes. You can override the default cycle time to set the interval you prefer.

• You can obtain a set of vital signs at any time by pressing the "start" button. Also, pressing the "cancel" button will stop the interval and de-

flate the cuff. You can retrieve stored data by pressing the "prior data" button. The monitor will display the last data obtained along with the time elapsed since then. Scrolling backward, you can retrieve data from the previous 99 minutes.

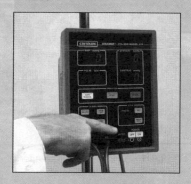

---

no faster than 5 mm Hg/second. While releasing air, watch the mercury column or aneroid gauge and auscultate the sound over the artery.

• When you hear the first beat or clear tapping sound, note the pressure on the column or gauge. This is the systolic pressure. The beat or tapping sound is the first of five Korotkoff sounds. The second sound resembles a murmur or swish; the third sound, crisp tapping; the fourth sound, a soft, muffled tone; and the fifth, the last sound heard.

• Continue to release air gradually while auscultating the sound over the artery.

• Note the diastolic pressure — the fourth Korotkoff sound. If you continue to hear sounds as the column or gauge falls to zero (common in chil-

dren), record the pressure at the beginning of the fourth sound. This is important *because, in some patients, a distinct fifth sound is absent.*

• Rapidly deflate the cuff. Record the pressure, wait 15 to 30 seconds, then repeat the procedure and record the pressures *to confirm your original findings.* After doing so, remove and fold the cuff, and return it to storage.

Complications

You can avoid complications from measuring blood pressure.

• Don't take blood pressure in the arm on the affected side of a mastectomy *because it may decrease already compromised lymphatic circulation, worsen edema, and damage the arm.*

• Don't take blood pressure on the same arm of an arteriovenous fistula

PROBLEM SOLVER

Correcting problems of blood pressure measurement

PROBLEM AND POSSIBLE CAUSE	NURSING ACTION
False-high reading	
Cuff too small	Make sure the cuff bladder is 20% wider than the circumference of the arm or leg being used for measurement.
Cuff wrapped too loosely, reducing its effective width	Tighten the cuff.
Slow cuff deflation, causing venous congestion in the arm or leg	Never deflate the cuff more slowly than 2 mm Hg/heartbeat.
Tilted mercury column	Read pressures with the mercury column vertical.
Poorly timed measurement — after patient has eaten, ambulated, appeared anxious, or flexed arm muscles	Postpone blood pressure measurement, or help the patient relax before taking the reading.
False-low reading	
Incorrect position of arm or leg	Make sure the arm or leg is level with the patient's heart.
Mercury column below eye level	Read the mercury column at eye level.
Failure to notice auscultatory gap (sound fades out for 10 to 15 mm Hg, then returns)	Estimate systolic pressure by palpation before actually measuring it. Then check this pressure against the measured pressure.
Inaudible low-volume sounds	Before reinflating the cuff, instruct the patient to raise the arm or leg to decrease venous pressure and amplify low-volume sounds. After inflating the cuff, tell the patient to lower the arm or leg. Then deflate the cuff and listen. If you still fail to detect low-volume sounds, chart the palpated systolic pressure.

or hemodialysis shunt *because blood flow through the vascular device may be compromised.*

Nursing considerations

• If you can't auscultate blood pressure, you may estimate systolic pressure. To do this, first palpate the brachial or radial pulse. Then inflate the cuff until you no longer detect the pulse. Slowly deflate the cuff and, when you detect the pulse again, record the pressure as the palpated systolic pressure. When measuring blood pressure in the popliteal artery, position the patient on his abdomen; wrap a cuff around the middle of the thigh, and proceed with blood pressure measurement.

• Palpation of systolic blood pressure also may be important *to avoid underestimating blood pressure in patients with an auscultatory gap.* This gap is a loss of sound between the first and second Korotkoff sounds that may be as great as 40 mm Hg. You may find this in patients with venous congestion or hypotension.

• If your patient is crying or anxious, delay blood pressure measurement, if possible, until the patient becomes calm *to avoid false-high readings.*

• If your hospital considers the fourth and fifth Korotkoff sounds as the first and second diastolic pressures, record both pressures.

• Remember that malfunction in an aneroid sphygmomanometer can be identified only by checking it against a mercury manometer of known accuracy. Be sure to check your aneroid manometer this way periodically. Malfunction in a mercury manometer is evident in abnormal behavior of the mercury column. Don't attempt to re-

TECHNOLOGY UPDATE

A new type of telemetry

Multiple parameter telemetry (MPT) from Criticare Systems is a telemetry unit that allows integrated monitoring of ECG, pulse oximetry, and blood pressure, noninvasively. With MPT, patients anywhere in the hospital can be monitored. Antennas for the units can be installed up to 100 feet apart. Information transmitted to a central station can be hardwired or telemetry itself. The system allows trending of data and a clearer signal via a digital pulse oximeter. Blood pressure readings are done on inflation rising to only 10 mm Hg above the systolic reading to increase patient comfort. The ECG is from a 5-lead system. The unit itself includes a readout screen to allow for use as a portable monitor during patient transport if desired.

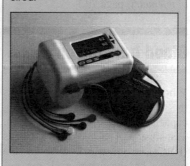

pair either type of sphygmomanometer yourself; instead, send it to the appropriate service department. (See *Correcting problems of blood pressure measurement.*)

• Occasionally, blood pressure must be measured in both arms or with the patient in two different positions (such as lying and standing or sitting and standing). In such cases, observe and record any significant difference between the two readings and record the blood pressure, the extremity, and the position used.

• Measure the blood pressure of patients taking antihypertensive medications while they're in a sitting position *to ensure accurate measurements.*

Documentation

• On the patient's chart, record blood pressure as systolic over diastolic pressures, such as 120/78 mm Hg; if necessary record systolic over the two diastolic pressures such as 120/78/20 mm Hg.

• Chart an auscultatory gap if present.

• If required by your hospital, chart blood pressures on a graph, using dots or check marks

• Document the extremity used and the patient's position. (See *A new type of telemetry,* page 79.)

Blood transfusion

Whole-blood transfusion replenishes the volume and the oxygen-carrying capacity of the circulatory system. Transfusion of packed red blood cells (RBCs), from which 80% of the plasma has been removed, restores only the oxygen-carrying capacity. Both types of transfusion treat decreased hemoglobin and hematocrit levels. Whole blood is usually transfused only when decreased levels result from hemorrhage; packed RBCs are transfused when such depressed levels accompany normal blood vol-ume to avoid possible fluid and circulatory overload. (See *Transfusing blood and selected components,* pages 82 to 85.)

Whole blood and packed RBCs contain cellular debris, necessitating in-line filtration during administration. (Washed packed RBCs — commonly used for patients previously sensitized by transfusions — are rinsed with a special solution that removes white blood cells and platelets, thus decreasing the chance of a transfusion reaction.)

Depending on hospital policy, two nurses may have to identify the patient and blood product before administering a transfusion to prevent errors and a potentially fatal reaction. The procedure also usually requires a signed patient consent form. If the patient is a Jehovah's Witness, a transfusion requires special written permission.

≫ Key nursing diagnoses and patient outcomes

Use these nursing diagnoses as a guide when developing your plan of care for a patient receiving whole-blood transfusions.

Fluid volume deficit related to active loss

Based on this nursing diagnosis, you'll establish the following patient outcomes. The patient will:

• have vital signs remain stable.

• have fluid and blood volume return to normal.

Altered tissue perfusion related to decreased cellular exchange

Based on this nursing diagnosis, you'll establish the following patient outcomes. The patient will:

• attain hemodynamic stability: pulse not < __ and not > __. Blood pressure not < __ and not > __.
• not exhibit arrhythmias.

Equipment

♦ blood recipient set (filter and tubing with drip chamber for blood, or combined set) ♦ I.V. pole ♦ gloves ♦ gown ♦ face shield ♦ multiple-lead tubing ♦ whole-blood or packed RBCs ♦ 250 ml of normal saline solution ♦ venipuncture equipment, if necessary (should include 18G catheter or 19G needle) ♦ optional: ice bag, warm compresses.

Straight-line and Y-type blood administration sets are commonly used. Although filters come in mesh and microaggregate types, the latter type is preferred, especially when transfusing multiple units of blood. New, highly effective leukocyte removal filters are available for use when transfusing blood and packed RBCs. Use of these filters delays a patient from becoming sensitive to transfusion therapy.

Equipment preparation

• Obtain whole-blood or packed RBCs from the blood bank within 30 minutes of the transfusion start time.
• Check the expiration date on the blood bag and observe for abnormal color, RBC clumping, gas bubbles, and extraneous material.
• Return outdated or abnormal blood to the blood bank.
• Prepare to administer packed RBCs with a Y-type set. Using a straight-line set forces you to piggyback the tubing so you can stop the transfusion if necessary but still keep the vein open. Piggybacking increases the chance of

harmful microorganisms entering the tubing as you're connecting the blood line to the established line.
• Multiple-lead tubing minimizes the risk of contamination, especially when transfusing multiple units of blood (a straight-line set would require multiple piggybacking). The Y-type set gives you the option of adding normal saline solution to packed cells — decreasing their viscosity — if the patient can tolerate the added fluid volume.
• Avoid obtaining either whole blood or packed RBCs until you're ready to begin the transfusion *because RBCs deteriorate after 2 hours when stored at room temperature.* Prepare the equipment when you're ready to start the infusion.

Patient preparation

• Explain the procedure.
• Make sure the patient has signed an informed consent form before beginning transfusion therapy.

Implementation

• Record the patient's baseline vital signs.
• Compare the name and number on the patient's wristband with those on the blood bag label.
• Check the blood bag identification number, ABO blood group, and Rh compatibility. Also, compare the patient's blood bank identification number, if present, with the number on the blood bag. Identification of blood and blood products is performed at the patient's bedside by two licensed professionals according to hospital policy.
• Put on gloves, a gown, and a face shield. Using a Y-type set, close all the
(Text continues on page 86.)

Transfusing blood and selected components

BLOOD COMPONENT	INDICATIONS	CROSSMATCHING
Whole blood Complete (pure) blood *Volume:* 500 ml	• To restore blood volume lost from hemorrhaging, trauma, or burns	• ABO identical: Type A receives A; type B receives B; type AB receives AB; type O receives O. • Rh match necessary
Packed red blood cells (RBCs) Same RBC mass as whole blood but with 80% of the plasma removed *Volume:* 250 ml	• To restore or maintain oxygen-carrying capacity • To correct anemia and blood loss that occurs during surgery • To increase RBC mass	• Type A receives A or O. • Type B receives B or O. • Type AB receives AB, A, B, or O. • Type O receives O. • Rh match necessary
Leukocyte-poor RBCs Same as packed RBCs with about 70% of the leukocytes removed *Volume:* 200 ml	• Same as packed RBCs • To prevent febrile reactions from leukocyte antibodies • To treat immunocompromised patients	• Same as packed RBCs • Rh match necessary
White blood cells (WBCs or leukocytes) Whole blood with all the RBCs and about 80% of the supernatant plasma removed *Volume:* usually 150 ml	• To treat sepsis that's unresponsive to antibiotics (especially if patient has positive blood cultures or a persistent fever exceeding 101° F [38.3° C]) and granulocytopenia (granulocyte count usually less than 500/mm^3)	• Same as packed RBCs • Compatibility with human leukocyte antigen (HLA) preferable but not necessary unless patient is sensitized to HLA from previous transfusions • Rh match necessary
Platelets Platelet sediment from RBCs or plasma *Volume:* 35 to 50 ml/ unit; 1 unit of platelets = 7×10^7 platelets	• To treat thrombocytopenia caused by decreased platelet production, increased platelet destruction, or massive transfusion of stored blood • To treat acute leukemia and marrow aplasia • To improve platelet count preoperatively in a patient whose count is 100,000/mm^3 or less	• ABO compatibility unnecessary but preferable with repeated platelet transfusions • Rh match preferred

Transfusing blood and selected components *(continued)*

NURSING CONSIDERATIONS

- Use a straight-line or Y-type I.V. set to infuse blood over 2 to 4 hours.
- Avoid giving whole blood when the patient can't tolerate the circulatory volume.
- Reduce the risk of a transfusion reaction by adding a microfilter to the administration set to remove platelets.
- Warm blood if giving a large quantity.

- Use a straight-line or Y-type I.V. set to infuse blood over 2 to 4 hours.
- Bear in mind that packed RBCs provide the same oxygen-carrying capacity as whole blood without the hazards of volume overload.
- Give packed RBCs, as ordered, to prevent potassium and ammonia buildup, which may occur in stored plasma.
- Avoid administering packed RBCs for anemic conditions correctable by nutritional or drug therapy.

- Use a straight-line or Y-type I.V. set to infuse blood over $1\frac{1}{2}$ to 4 hours.
- Use a 40-micron filter suitable for hard-spun, leukocyte-poor RBCs.
- Other considerations are the same as those for packed RBCs.

- Use a straight line I.V. set with a standard in-line blood filter to provide 1 unit daily for 5 days or until infection resolves.
- As prescribed, premedicate with diphenhydramine.
- Because a WBC infusion induces fever and chills, administer an antipyretic if fever occurs. However, don't discontinue the transfusion; instead, reduce the flow rate, as ordered, for patient comfort.
- Agitate container to prevent WBCs from settling, thus preventing the delivery of a bolus infusion of WBCs.
- Give transfusion with antibiotics (but not amphotericin B) to treat infection.

- Use a component drip administration set to infuse 100 ml over 15 minutes.
- As prescribed, premedicate with antipyretics and antihistamines if the patient's history includes a platelet transfusion reaction.
- Avoid administering platelets when the patient has a fever.
- Prepare to draw blood for a platelet count, as ordered, 1 hour after the platelet transfusion to determine platelet transfusion increments.
- Keep in mind that the doctor seldom orders a platelet transfusion for conditions in which platelet destruction is accelerated, such as idiopathic thrombocytopenic purpura or drug-induced thrombocytopenia.

(continued)

Transfusing blood and selected components *(continued)*

BLOOD COMPONENT	INDICATIONS	CROSSMATCHING
Fresh frozen plasma (FFP) Uncoagulated plasma separated from RBCs and rich in coagulation factors V, VIII, and IX *Volume:* 200 to 250 ml	• To expand plasma volume • To treat postsurgical hemorrhage or shock • To correct an undetermined coagulation factor deficiency • To replace a specific factor when that factor alone isn't available • To correct factor deficiencies resulting from hepatic disease	• ABO compatibility unnecessary but preferable with repeated platelet transfusions • Rh match preferred
Albumin 5% (buffered saline); albumin 25% (salt-poor) A small plasma protein prepared by fractionating pooled plasma *Volume:* 5% = 12.5 g/ 250 ml; 25% = 12.5 g/ 50 ml	• To replace volume lost because of shock from burns, trauma, surgery, or infections • To replace volume and prevent marked hemoconcentration • To treat hypoproteinemia (with or without edema)	• Unnecessary
Factor VIII (cryoprecipitate) Insoluble portion of plasma recovered from FFP *Volume:* About 30 ml (freeze-dried)	• To treat a patient with hemophilia A • To control bleeding associated with factor VIII deficiency • To replace fibrinogen or deficient factor VIII	• ABO compatibility unnecessary but preferable
Factors II, VII, IX, X complex (prothrombin complex) Lyophilized, commercially prepared solution drawn from pooled plasma	• To treat a congenital factor V deficiency and other bleeding disorders resulting from an acquired deficiency of factors II, VII, IX, and X	• ABO and Rh match unnecessary

NURSING CONSIDERATIONS

- Use a straight-line I.V. set and administer the infusion rapidly.
- Keep in mind that large-volume transfusions of FFP may require correction for hypocalcemia because citric acid in FFP binds calcium.

- Use a straight-line I.V. set with rate and volume dictated by the patient's condition and response.
- Remember that reactions to albumin (fever, chills, nausea) are rare.
- Avoid mixing albumin with protein hydrolysates and alcohol solutions.
- Consider delivering albumin as a volume expander until the laboratory completes crossmatching for a whole blood transfusion.
- Keep in mind that albumin is contraindicated in severe anemia and administered cautiously in cardiac and pulmonary disease because congestive heart failure may result from circulatory overload.

- Use the administration set supplied by the manufacturer. Administer factor VIII with a filter. Standard dose recommended for treatment of acute bleeding episodes in hemophilia is 15 to 20 units/kg.
- Half-life of factor VIII (8 to 10 hours) necessitates repeated transfusions at these intervals to maintain normal levels.

- Administer with a straight-line I.V. set, basing dose on desired factor level and patient's body weight.
- Recognize that a high risk of hepatitis accompanies this type of transfusion.
- Arrange to draw blood for a coagulation assay to be performed before administration and at suitable intervals during treatment.
- Keep in mind that this type of transfusion is contraindicated when the patient has hepatic disease resulting in fibrinolysis and when the patient has disseminated intravascular coagulation and isn't undergoing heparin therapy.

clamps on the set. Then insert the spike of the line you're using for the normal saline solution into the bag of saline solution. Next, open the port on the blood bag, and insert the spike of the line you're using to administer the blood or cellular component into the port. Hang the bag of normal saline solution and blood or cellular component on the I.V. pole, open the clamp on the line of saline solution, and squeeze the drip chamber until it's half full. Then remove the adapter cover at the tip of the blood administration set, open the main flow clamp, and prime the tubing with saline solution.

• If you're administering packed RBCs with a Y-type set, you can add saline solution to the bag to dilute the cells by closing the clamp between the patient and the drip chamber and opening the clamp from the blood. Then lower the blood bag below the saline container and let 30 to 50 ml of saline solution flow into the packed cells. Finally, close the clamp to the blood bag, rehang the bag, rotate it gently *to mix the cells and saline solution,* and close the clamp to the saline container.

• If the patient doesn't have an I.V. line in place, perform venipuncture, preferably using an 18G catheter or 19G needle. Avoid using an existing line if the needle or catheter lumen is smaller than 20G. Central venous access devices also may be used for transfusion therapy.

• If you're administering whole blood, gently invert the bag several times *to mix the cells.*

• Attach the prepared blood administration set to the venipuncture device, and flush it with normal saline solution.

• Then close the clamp to the saline solution, and open the clamp between the blood bag and the patient. Adjust the flow clamp closest to the patient to deliver the blood at the calculated drip rate.

• Remain with the patient, and watch for signs of a transfusion reaction. If such signs develop, record vital signs, stop the transfusion, infuse the saline solution at a keep-vein-open rate, and notify the doctor at once. If no signs of a reaction appear within 15 minutes, you'll need to adjust the flow clamp to the ordered infusion rate. *Raising and lowering the blood bag to adjust the rate reduces the risk of hemolysis from pressure on the tubing.* A unit of RBCs may be given over 1 to 4 hours, as ordered.

• After completing the transfusion, you'll need to put on gloves and flush the filter and tubing with normal saline solution, if this is recommended by the manufacturer. Then remember to reconnect the original I.V. fluid or discontinue the I.V. infusion.

• Return the empty blood bag to the blood bank, and discard the tubing and filter.

• Record the patient's vital signs.

Complications

• Despite increasingly accurate cross-matching precautions, transfusion reactions can occur.

• Unlike a transfusion reaction, an infectious disease transmitted during a transfusion may go undetected until days, weeks, or even months later, when it produces signs and symptoms. Measures to prevent disease transmission include laboratory testing of blood products and careful screening of potential donors, neither of which is guaranteed.

• Hepatitis C (non A, non B) accounts for the majority of posttransfusion hepatitis cases. The tests that detect hepatitis B and hepatitis C can produce false-negative results and may allow some hepatitis cases to go undetected.

• When testing for antibodies to human immunodeficiency virus (HIV), keep in mind that antibodies do not appear until about 6 to 12 weeks after exposure. Consequently, blood from a donor exposed to HIV but who has not yet developed antibodies could infect the recipient. The estimated risk of acquiring HIV from blood products varies from 1 in 40,000 to 1 in 153,000, depending on the source.

• Many blood banks screen blood for cytomegalovirus (CMV). Blood with CMV is especially dangerous for an immunosuppressed, seronegative patient. Blood banks also test blood for syphilis, but the routine practice of refrigerating blood kills the syphilis organism and virtually eliminates the risk of transfusion-related syphilis.

• Circulatory overload and hemolytic, allergic, febrile, and pyogenic reactions can result from any transfusion.

• Coagulation disturbances, citrate intoxication, hyperkalemia, acid-base imbalance, loss of 2,3-diphosphoglycerate, ammonia intoxication, and hypothermia can result from massive transfusion.

Nursing considerations

• Although some microaggregate filters can be used for up to 10 units of blood, always replace the filter and tubing if more than 1 hour elapses between transfusions. When administering multiple units of blood under pressure, use a blood warmer *to avoid hypothermia.*

• For rapid blood replacement, you may need to use a pressure bag. Be aware, however, that excessive pressure may develop, leading to broken blood vessels and extravasation, with hematoma and hemolysis of the infusing RBCs.

• If the transfusion stops, take the following steps as needed:

• Check that the I.V. container is at least 3′ (1 m) above the level of the I.V. site.

• Make sure that the flow clamp is open and that the blood completely covers the filter. If it doesn't, squeeze the drip chamber until it does.

• Gently rock the bag back and forth, agitating any blood cells that may have settled on the bottom.

• Untape the dressing over the I.V. site to check needle placement. Reposition the needle if necessary.

• Flush the line with saline solution and restart the transfusion. Using a Y-type set, close the flow clamp to the patient and lower the blood bag. Next, open the saline clamp and allow some saline solution to flow into the blood bag. Rehang the blood bag, open the flow clamp to the patient, and reset the flow rate.

• If a hematoma develops at the I.V. site, immediately stop the infusion. Remove the needle or catheter. Notify the doctor and expect to place ice on the site intermittently for 8 hours; then apply warm compresses. Promote reabsorption of the hematoma by having the patient gently exercise the affected limb. Document your observations and actions.

BETTER CHARTING

Documenting blood transfusions

Whether you administer blood or blood components, you must use proper identification and cross-matching procedures.

After matching the patient's name, medical record number, blood group (or type) and Rh factor (the patient's and the donor's), the cross-match data, and the blood bank identification number with the label on the blood bag, you'll need to clearly document that you did so. The blood or blood component must be identified and documented properly by two health care professionals as well.

On the transfusion record, document:
• date and time the transfusion was started and completed
• name of the health care professional who verified the information
• type and gauge of the catheter
• total amount of the transfusion.

Also record:
• patient's vital signs before and after the transfusion
• any infusion device used
• flow rate
• any blood warming unit used.

If the patient receives his own blood, document in the intake and output records:
• amount of autologous blood retrieved
• reinfused in the intake and output records.

Also monitor and document:
• laboratory data during and after the autotransfusion
• patient's pre- and post-transfusion vital signs.

Pay particular attention to:
• patient's coagulation profile
• hemoglobin and hematocrit values, and arterial blood gas and calcium levels.

• If the blood bag empties before the next one arrives, administer normal saline solution slowly. If you're using a Y-type set, close the blood-line clamp, open the saline-line clamp, and let the saline solution run slowly until the new blood arrives. Decrease the flow rate or clamp the line before attaching the new unit of blood.

Home care
Standards established by the American Association of Blood Banks, in accordance with federal, state, and local regulations, allow a doctor to order

transfusions of blood products (not whole blood) for home care patients. To qualify, a patient must be unable to leave his home without assistance and must have received previous transfusions without difficulties.

Documentation
• Record the date and time of the transfusion, the type and amount of transfusion product, the patient's vital signs, your check of all identification data, and the patient's response.

• Document any transfusion reaction and treatment. (See *Documenting blood transfusions*.)

Bone marrow aspiration and biopsy

You can get a specimen of bone marrow — the major site of blood cell formation — by aspiration or needle biopsy. The procedure allows overall blood-composition evaluation through study of blood elements and precursor cells, and abnormal or malignant cells. An apsiration needle is inserted into the marrow-producing bone cavity; in a biopsy, a small, solid core of marrow tissue is removed through the needle.

Both procedures are usually performed by a doctor, but some hospitals authorize specially trained chemotherapy nurses or nurse clinicians to perform the procedures with the aid of an assistant.

Aspirates are valuable in diagnosing various disorders and cancers, such as oat cell carcinoma and leukemia, and such lymphomas as Hodgkin's disease. This test allows examination of bone marrow to identify the Philadelphia (Ph¹) chromosome, a genetic abnormality present in about 90% of patients with chronic myelogenous leukemia. Biopsies are often performed simultaneously to stage the disease and to monitor response to treatment.

≫ Key nursing diagnoses and patient outcomes
Use these nursing diagnoses as a guide when developing your plan of care for a patient undergoing a bone marrow aspiration and biopsy.

Ineffective individual coping related to personal vulnerability
Based on this nursing diagnosis, you'll establish the following patient outcomes. The patient will:
• communicate feelings.
• become involved in planning care.
• use support systems, such as family and friends, to cope.

Body-image disturbance related to potential medical treatments
Based on this nursing diagnosis, you'll establish the following patient outcomes. The patient will:
• express positive feelings about self.
• acknowledge change in body image.

Equipment
For aspiration: ♦ prepackaged bone marrow set, which includes: povidone-iodine sponges ♦ two sterile drapes (one fenestrated, one plain) ♦ ten 4″ × 4″ gauze pads ♦ ten 2″ × 2″ gauze pads ♦ two 12-ml syringes ♦ 22G 1″ or 2″ needle ♦ a scalpel ♦ sedative ♦ +specimen containers ♦ bone marrow needle ♦ 70% isopropyl alcohol ♦ 1% lidocaine (unopened bottle) ♦ adhesive tape ♦ sterile gloves ♦ glass slides and cover slips ♦ labels.

For biopsy: ♦ all equipment listed above ♦ Vim-Silverman, Jamshidi, Illinois sternal, or Westerman-Jensen needle ♦ Zenker's fixative.

Patient preparation
• Tell the patient the doctor will collect a bone marrow specimen, and explain the procedure *to ease his anxiety and ensure cooperation.*

• Make sure the patient or a responsible family member understands the procedure and implications of this test and signs a consent form.

• Inform the patient that the procedure normally takes 5 to 10 minutes, that test results usually are available in 1 day, and that more than one marrow specimen may be required.

• Check the patient's history for hypersensitivity to the local anesthetic.

• Tell him which bone — sternum or posterior superior or anterior iliac crest — will be sampled.

• Inform him that he'll receive a local anesthetic and will feel heavy pressure from insertion of the biopsy or aspiration needle, plus a brief, pulling sensation on removal of the marrow specimen.

• Tell him the doctor may make a small incision to avoid tearing the skin.

• If the patient has osteoporosis, tell him needle pressure will be minimal; if he has osteopetrosis, inform him a drill may be needed.

Implementation

• Provide a sedative, as ordered, before the test.

• Position the patient according to the selected puncture site. (See *Common sites for bone marrow aspiration and biopsy*.)

• Using sterile technique, clean the puncture site with povidone-iodine solution and allowed to dry; then drape the area.

• To anesthetize the site, the doctor infiltrates it with 1% lidocaine, first injecting a small amount intradermally, and then using a larger 22G 1" or 2" needle to anesthetize the tissue down to the bone.

• When the needle tip reaches the bone, the doctor anesthetizes the periosteum by injecting a small amount of lidocaine in a circular area about $3/4''$ (2 cm) in diameter. The needle should be withdrawn from the periosteum after each injection.

• After allowing about 1 minute for the lidocaine to take effect, a scalpel may be used to make a small stab incision in the patient's skin to accommodate the bone marrow needle. *This technique avoids pushing skin into the bone marrow and also helps avoid unnecessary skin tearing to help reduce the risk of infection.*

Bone marrow aspiration

• The doctor inserts the bone marrow needle at the selected site and lodges it firmly in the bone cortex. If the patient feels sharp pain instead of pressure when the needle first touches bone, the needle was probably inserted outside the anesthetized area. If this happens, the needle should be withdrawn slightly and moved to the anesthetized area.

• The needle is advanced by applying an even, downward force with the heel of the hand or the palm, while twisting it back and forth slightly. A crackling sensation means the needle has entered the marrow cavity.

• Next, the doctor removes the inner cannula, attaches the syringe to the needle, aspirates the required specimen (usually about 1 ml), and withdraws the needle.

• The nurse dons gloves and applies pressure to the aspiration site with a gauze pad for 5 minutes to control bleeding, while an assistant prepares the marrow slides.

Common sites for bone marrow aspiration and biopsy

The posterior superior iliac crest is the preferred site for aspiration because it's free of nearby vital organs or vessels. For aspiration of bone marrow from this site, the patient is placed either in the lateral position with one leg flexed or in the prone position.

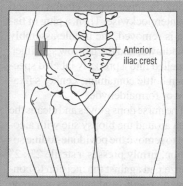

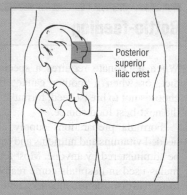

For aspiration or biopsy from the anterior iliac crest, the patient is placed in the supine or side-lying position. This site is used with patient who cannot lie prone because of severe abdominal distention.

Aspiration from the sternum involves the greatest risk but may be used because this site is near the surface, the cortical bone is thin, and the marrow cavity contains numerous cells and relatively little fat or supporting bone. The sternum is rarely used for biopsy, however, because of its small size and proximity to vital organs.

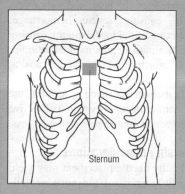

• The area is then cleaned with alcohol to remove the povidone-iodine. The skin is thoroughly dried with a 4″ × 4″ gauze pad, and a sterile pressure dressing applied.

Bone marrow biopsy
• The doctor inserts the biopsy needle into the periosteum and advances it steadily until the outer needle passes through the bone cortex into the marrow cavity.

• The biopsy needle is directed into the marrow cavity by alternately rotating the inner needle clockwise and counterclockwise. Then, a plug of tissue is removed, the needle assembly withdrawn, and the marrow specimen expelled into a properly labeled specimen bottle containing Zenker's fixative or formaldehyde.

• The nurse dons gloves and cleans the area around the biopsy site with alcohol to remove the povidone-iodine solution, firmly presses a sterile $2'' \times 2''$ gauze pad against the incision to control bleeding, and applies a sterile pressure dressing.

Complications
• Potentially life-threatening complications of bone marrow aspiration or biopsy at any site include bleeding and infection.

• Complications of sternal needle puncture are uncommon, but include puncture of the heart and major vessels, causing severe hemorrhage; puncture of the mediastinum, causing mediastinitis or pneumomediastinum; and puncture of the lung, causing pneumothorax.

• If hematoma occurs around the puncture site, apply warm soaks. Give analgesics for site pain or tenderness.

Nursing considerations
• Faulty needle placement may yield too little aspirate. If the procedure fails to produce a specimen, the needle must be withdrawn from the bone (but not from the overlying soft tissue), the stylet replaced, and the needle reinserted in a second site within the anesthetized field.

• Bone marrow specimens should not be collected from irradiated areas *because radiation may have altered or destroyed the marrow.*

Documentation
• Chart the time, date, location, and patient's tolerance of the procedure and the specimen obtained.

• Describe appearance of aspirated specimen and the aspiration site.

Bottle-feeding

When a neonate requires a special diet, or when a mother cannot or chooses not to breast-feed, formula is the next-best food source.

Formula preparations supply all needed vitamins and nutrients and can be administered by anyone. Most formulas used in hospitals come ready-to-feed in disposable containers. Some formulas and equipment, however, may require preparation, such as mixing and sterilization. For the infant's first year, the American Academy of Pediatrics recommends commercially prepared formula over animal milks or homemade preparations.

Because formulas for the neonate must be sterile, they are prepared either by the aseptic method (in which all articles used in formula preparation are sterilized before mixing) or by the terminal-heat method (in which the formula is prepared with clean technique and then sterilized using a home sterilizer). In the United States, some pediatricians recommend clean technique and tap water for formulas because water supplies are clean and safe in most areas.

A normal neonate takes 15 to 20 minutes to consume a 1- to $1\frac{1}{2}$-oz portion of formula. He usually feeds every 3 to 4 hours.

≫ Key nursing diagnoses and patient outcomes

Use these nursing diagnoses as a guide when developing your plan of care for a patient who is bottle-feeding.

Knowledge deficit related to performing bottle feeding

Based on this nursing diagnosis, you'll establish the following patient outcomes. The neonate's parents will:
• express increased confidence to perform appropriate feeding techniques.
• set realistic learning goals for developing bottle-feeding competence.
• report that the neonate gains adequate weight.

Anxiety related to difficulty with bottle-feeding

Based on this nursing diagnosis, you'll establish the following patient outcomes. The neonate's parents will:
• express feelings of anxiety.
• identify cause of anxiety.
• use emotional support.
• show fewer signs of anxiety.

Equipment

♦ commercially prepared formula or ingredients ♦ bottle, nipple, and cap ♦ tissue or cloth ♦ gown.

Hospitals commonly use disposable bottle and nipple units for neonatal feeding.

Equipment preparation

• If you're using commercially prepared formula, uncap the formula bottle and make sure the seal wasn't previously broken *to ensure sterility and freshness.*

• Screw on the nipple and cap.
• Keep the protective sterile cap over the nipple until the neonate is ready to feed.
• If you're preparing formula, follow the manufacturer's instructions or the doctor's prescription.
• Administer the formula at, or slightly below, room temperature.

Implementation

• Wash your hands.
• Invert the bottle and shake some formula on your wrist *to test the patency of the nipple hole and the formula's temperature.* The nipple hole should allow formula to drip freely but not to stream out. *If the hole is too large, the neonate may aspirate formula; if it's too small, the extra sucking effort he expends may tire him before he can empty the bottle.*
• Sit comfortably in a semireclining position, and cradle the neonate in one arm to support his head and back. *This position allows swallowed air to rise to the top of the stomach where it's more easily expelled.* If he can't be held, sit by him and elevate his head and shoulders slightly.
• Place the nipple in the baby's mouth while making sure his tongue is down, but don't insert the nipple so far as to stimulate the gag reflex. He should begin to suck, pulling in as much nipple as is comfortable. If he doesn't start to suck, stroke him under the chin or on his cheek, or touch his lips with the nipple *to stimulate his sucking reflex.*
• As the neonate feeds, tilt the bottle upward *to keep the nipple filled with formula and to prevent him from swallowing air.* Watch for a steady stream of bubbles in the bottle, which indicates proper venting and formula flow.

• If the neonate pushes the nipple out with his tongue, reinsert the nipple. *Expelling the nipple is a normal reflex. It doesn't necessarily mean the neonate is full.*

• Always hold the bottle for a neonate. If left to feed himself, he may aspirate formula or swallow air if the bottle tilts or empties. *Experts link bottle propping with an increased incidence of otitis media and dental caries in older infants.*

• Burp the neonate after each ½ oz of formula because he will typically swallow some air even when fed correctly. Hold the neonate upright in a slightly forward position, supporting his head and chest with one hand. You may also position a clean cloth *to protect your clothing* and hold the neonate upright over your shoulder, or place him face down across your lap. *The change in position helps the gas to rise or "bring up the bubble."* Either way, rub or gently pat his back until he expels the air.

• After you finish feeding and burping the neonate, place him on his back or right side *to prevent aspiration if he regurgitates.* Neonates are prone to regurgitation because of an immature cardiac sphincter.

• Discard any remaining formula, and properly dispose of all equipment.

Complications

Bottle-propping may cause some problems. They include:

• allowing the nipple to block the airway, causing suffocation

• promotion of otitis media or dental caries

• lung infection after aspiration of regurgitated formula

• death after aspiration of regurgitated formula.

Nursing considerations

• Change feeding duration by changing the size of the nipple or nipple hole *because the neonate tires if he feeds too long, and his sucking needs aren't met if he doesn't feed long enough.*

• Note how much formula is in the bottle before and after the feeding. Use calibrations along the side of the container to calculate amount of formula consumed.

• Watch for aspiration in neonates who have a diminished sucking or swallowing reflex and difficulty feeding.

• Take appropriate measures according to hospital policy to feed the neonate with cleft lip and palate.

Home care

• Teach parents to prepare and sterilize (if required) formula, bottles, and nipples properly; feed the neonate; and burp the neonate.

• Although most hospitals have a feeding schedule, advise the parents that they may switch to a more flexible, demand-feeding schedule when at home. Forewarn them that the neonate may not feed well on his first day home because of the new activity and environment. Inform parents about types of formula (ready-to-feed, concentrate, powders), *so they can choose the most convenient kind.*

• Prepare parents to expect the neonate to regurgitate formula. Explain that regurgitation (an overflow that typically follows feeding) shouldn't be confused with vomiting, a more complete emptying of the stomach accompanied by symptoms not associated with feeding.

Documentation
- Record the time of the feeding, the amount of formula consumed, how well the neonate fed, and whether he appeared satisfied.
- Note any regurgitation or vomiting.
- If the mother feeds him, observe and describe their interactions.
- Document any patient teaching.

Breast-feeding assistance

Breast-feeding is the safest, simplest, and least expensive way to provide complete infant nourishment. Components of successful breast-feeding include proper breast care, normal milk flow, and a comfortably positioned mother and infant.

Breast-feeding is contraindicated for a mother with a severe chronic condition, such as active tuberculosis, human immunodeficiency virus (HIV), or hepatitis.

≫ Key nursing diagnoses and patient outcomes
Use these nursing diagnoses as a guide when developing your plan of care for a patient who is breast-feeding.

Effective breast-feeding
Based on this nursing diagnosis, you'll establish the following patient outcomes. The mother will:
- breast-feed infant successfully and experience satisfaction with breast-feeding.
- satisfactorily feed infant on both breasts.
- see the infant grow and develop normally.

- continue breast-feeding after early postpartum period.

Ineffective breast-feeding related to limited maternal experience
Based on this nursing diagnosis, you'll establish the following patient outcomes. The mother will:
- express understanding of breast-feeding techniques and practice.
- display decreased anxiety.
- successfully breast-feed.

Equipment
♦ a chair, bed, or other suitable piece of furniture for the mother ♦ a pillow to support the mother ♦ a blanket or towel for the baby.

Patient preparation
- Explain the procedure to the mother and provide privacy.
- Encourage the mother to drink a beverage before and during or after breast-feeding *to ensure adequate fluid intake, which helps to maintain milk production.*
- Encourage the mother to attend to personal needs and to change the infant's wet or soiled diaper before breast-feeding begins *to avoid interruptions during feeding time.*

Implementation
- Wash your hands.
- Instruct the mother to wash her hands.
- Help the mother find a comfortable position, such as the cradle or side-lying position, *to promote the let-down reflex.* (See *Breast-feeding positions*, pages 96 and 97.)
- Have her expose one breast and rest the nape of the infant's neck at the an-

Breast-feeding positions

Ordinarily, a maternity patient chooses a breast-feeding position that's comfortable and efficient. If the patient experiences discomfort in one position, she can choose another position. In fact, by changing positions periodically, she can alter the infant's grasp on the nipple and thereby avoid constant friction on the same area. As appropriate, suggest these typical breast-feeding positions.

Cradle position

This is the most common position for breast-feeding. The mother sits in a comfortable chair and cradles the infant's head in the crook of her arm. If desired, she can support her elbow with pillows *to minimize tension and fatigue.* She can also tuck the infant's lower arm alongside her body, *so it stays out of the way.* The infant's mouth should remain even with the nipple and his stomach should face and touch the mother's stomach.

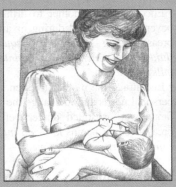

Side-lying position

The mother can choose this position for breast-feeding at night or during recovery from a cesarean section. She lies on her side with her stomach facing the infant and the infant's head near her breast. She then lifts her breast, and as the infant's mouth opens, she pulls him toward her nipple.

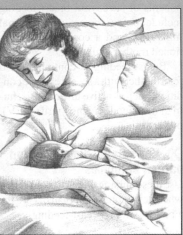

tecubital space of her arm, supporting the back with her forearm.

• Urge the mother to relax during breast-feeding *because relaxation also promotes the let-down reflex,* which causes milk to flow.

• Inform her she may feel a tingling sensation when the let-down reflex occurs and that milk may drip or spray from her breasts.

• Tell her the reflex may also be initiated by hearing the infant's cry.

• Guiding the mother's free hand, have her place her thumb on top of the exposed breast's areola and her first two fingers beneath it, forming a "C" with her hand.

Football position

Often selected by mothers with large breasts or by those who have had a cesarean section, this position is also useful for feeding twins or infants who are small or premature. The mother sits in a comfortable chair with a pillow under her arm on the nursing side. She places her hand under the infant's head and brings it close to the breast, while placing the fingers of her other hand above and below the nipple. As the infant's mouth opens, she pulls his head close to her breast.

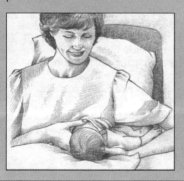

• Turn the infant to face the breast.
• Tell the mother to stroke the infant's cheek nearest her exposed breast or its mouth with the nipple. *This stimulates the rooting instinct*, which will cause the newborn to turn toward the breast and start sucking. Emphasize that she shouldn't touch the infant's other cheek *because he may turn his head toward the touch and away from the breast.*

• When the infant opens his mouth and roots for the nipple, instruct the mother to insert the nipple and as much of the areola as possible into the infant's mouth. *This helps him exert sufficient pressure with his lips, gums, and cheek muscles on the milk sinuses below the areola.*
• Check for occlusion of the infant's nostrils by the mother's breast. If this happens, advise the mother to press her finger on her breast below the infant's nose to give him breathing room.
• Suggest that the mother begin nursing the infant for 15 minutes on each breast.
• To alternate breasts, instruct the mother to slip a finger into the side of the infant's mouth *to break the seal and move him to the other breast.*
• *To burp the infant,* show the mother how to hold him in an upright position tilted forward, with one hand supporting his chest and chin.
• *To expel swallowed air*, tell the mother to gently pat or rub the infant's back. Help her place a protective cover such as a cloth diaper under the infant's chin.
• Tell the mother to feed the infant at the other breast. If she wishes and if the infant remains awake, she may nurse him longer. *A demand-feeding routine, in which the infant feeds according to his hunger and desire, establishes an abundant, steady milk supply appropriate for the infant's requirements (the more the infant feeds, the more milk the mother produces). Frequent nursing also satisfies the infant's need to suck and promotes bonding.*

Breast care for new mothers

If a mother plans to breast-feed her infant, she can prepare her breasts as directed by her doctor. After the infant's birth, she'll need to maintain breast tissue integrity, the keratin layer that builds protectively on the areola, and the natural lubricant that the breast produces as well.

Although postpartum care varies for the breast-feeding and non-breast-feeding mother, both may need a few guidelines.

For the breast-feeding mother
• Instruct the mother to wash the areolae and nipples with water, without soap or a washcloth, to avoid washing away the natural oils and keratin.
• Advise the mother with sore or irritated nipples to apply ice compresses just before breast-feeding. This numbs and firms the nipples, making them less sensitive and easier for the infant to grasp.
• Suggest that lubricating the nipple with a few drops of expressed breast milk before feeding may help prevent tenderness.
• Recommend placing breast pads over the nipples to collect colostrum or milk, which commonly leaks during the first few breast-feeding weeks. Advise replacing pads often to guard against infection.
• Inform the mother that breast milk comes in 2 to 5 days after delivery and is accompanied by a slight temperature elevation and breast

changes — increased size, warmth, and firmness.
• Tell the mother that a well-fitting support bra may help control engorgement.
• Advise the mother with engorged breasts to apply warm compresses, massage the breasts, take a warm shower, or express some milk before feeding. This dilates the milk ducts, promotes the let-down reflex, and makes the nipples more pliable.

For the non-breast-feeding mother
• Instruct the mother to clean her breasts using the same technique as the breast-feeding mother. Add that she may use soap.
• Advise her to wear a support bra to help minimize engorgement and to decrease nipple stimulation.
• Advise her to avoid stimulating the nipples or manually expressing her milk to minimize further milk production. Instead, provide pain medication, as ordered, ice packs, or a breast binder.

• When the mother finishes breast-feeding, tell her to place the infant in a prone position or on his side with a blanket roll at his back *for stability.* Instruct her not to place him in a supine position because he could throw up and aspirate vomitus. If the mother wants to hold the infant longer, encourage her: Touching enhances bonding.

• Instruct the mother to air-dry her nipples for 15 minutes after feeding and teach breast care. (See *Breast care for new mothers.*)
• Check for breast engorgement. If traditional relief measures fail to trigger the let-down reflex, administer an analgesic to relieve discomfort and notify the doctor.

Complications

Possible complications of breast feeding include:
• breast engorgement from venous and lymphatic stasis and alveolar milk accumulation.
• postpartum mastitis (about 1% of mothers), usually from pathogens from the infant's nose or pharynx.

Nursing considerations

• Instruct the mother to use the side-lying position for breast-feeding on the delivery table. *This reduces discomfort from pressure on the episiotomy (if she had one).*
• Furniture can be adjusted to the mother's comfort.
• Stay with the mother during breast-feeding instruction in the hospital because she may be exhausted from delivery or drowsy from medication.
• Inform the mother that infants routinely lose weight (several ounces) during the first days of life.
• Advise her that colostrum, her first milk, is yellow, rich in protein and antibodies, and secreted in small amounts.
• Tell her that her true milk, which is thin and bluish, won't appear until several days after delivery.
• Advise a mother who is breast-feeding twins that using the football position allows her to feed both infants at once. Teach her to alternate breasts and infants at each feeding.
• If the mother prefers to nurse one infant at a time, make sure the nursery and the mother both keep track of which infant came first during each feeding.
• Reassure her that there is no standard schedule for breast-feeding and

that developing a comfortable routine takes time.
• Tell her to expect uterine cramping (contractions) during breast-feeding until her uterus returns to its original size. These contractions result from released oxytocin, a natural hormone that prompts the uterus to return to its prepregnancy state. Oxytocin also initiates the letdown reflex, allowing milk to flow.
• During breast-feeding, milk leakage in the nonnursing breast may be controlled by applying light pressure to the nipple with fingers or the palm.
• If the infant shows little interest in breast-feeding, reassure the mother the infant may need several days to learn and to adjust.
• If the infant is sleepy, encourage the mother to offer the breast frequently but not to force-feed. Instead, advise her to try rubbing the infant's feet, unwrapping his blanket, changing his diaper, changing her position or the infant's, or manually expressing milk and then allowing the infant to suckle. A balky infant may suck eagerly if milk is already flowing.
• If the infant fails to nurse sufficiently and dehydration seems likely, the mother should give him expressed milk with a medicine dropper or small syringe.
• Tell the mother to avoid frequent bottle-feeding *because the infant may become used to the artificial nipple and reject the mother's*. A breast-fed infant rarely needs supplemental glucose and water.
• Advise the mother to start breast-feeding with the breast she used last at the previous feeding *to help avoid engorgement of the breast.* Suggest attaching a safety pin to the bra strap

Comparing breast pumps

Breast pumps are available in battery-operated, electric, and hand-operated models. The pump that's best for your patient depends on such factors as the pump's purpose and the patient's situation. A description of common pumps and their features follows.

Battery-powered pump
Having a battery-powered motor, this pump can be operated with one hand. Easy-to-clean, it's a good choice for mothers who work outside the home or who need a breast pump only for short-term use.

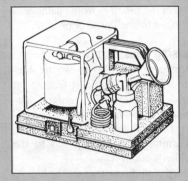

Cylinder pump
This pump operates with two plastic cylinders, one inside the other, that create gentle suction as the outer cylinder is moved back and forth. Because two hands are needed to operate it, it may be tiring to use. Easy-to-clean and portable, however, this pump proves rela-

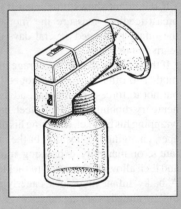

Electric pump
Usually used in hospitals, this efficient, gentle pump plugs into an electrical outlet and can be operated with one hand. It's available as a small, 2-lb model or as a larger model about the size of a small sewing machine. Inform your patient that the larger model can be rented from a pharmacy or medical supply company.

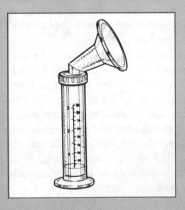

supporting the breast she last used *to serve as a reminder.*

Home care

• Discuss the signs of mastitis — red, tender, or warm breasts and fever, and what to do about them.

• Encourage breast-feeding efforts. *To boost these efforts,* urge her to eat balanced meals, to drink at least eight 8-oz glasses of fluid daily, and to nap daily for at least the first 2 weeks after giving birth.

• Answer questions about breast-feeding and provide instructional materials, if available.

• Before the mother goes home, tell her about local breast-feeding and parenting support groups, such as La Leche League.

• By creating suction, manual and electric breast pumps stimulate lactation. They are indicated for a mother who wants to maintain milk production while she and her infant are separated or while illness temporarily incapacitates one or the other, or both.

• A breast pump also can relieve engorgement or collect milk for a premature infant with a weak sucking reflex (See *Comparing breast pumps.*)

Documentation

• After helping the mother with breast-feeding, note areas in which she needs further instruction and help.

• Document patient teaching.

Breast examination

Whether your patient is male or female, a breast evaluation should be an integral part of your physical assess-ment. To assess the breasts effectively, compile a thorough health history and perform a thorough physical examination. Be sure to explore any breast cancer risk factors such as family history of the disease.

As you proceed, keep basic breast anatomy and function in mind. Recognize that breast size and composition vary among individuals according to age, gender, heredity, and other factors. For example, endocrine changes during pregnancy or throughout the menstrual cycle can affect breast size and composition.

≫ Key nursing diagnoses and patient outcomes

Use these nursing diagnoses as a guide when developing your plan of care.

Knowledge deficit related to self-breast examination
Based on this nursing diagnosis, you'll establish the following patient outcomes. The patient will:

• communicate a need to know about breast examination.

• state or demonstrate understanding of what has been taught.

• state intention to make needed changes in lifestyle, including seeking help from health professionals when needed.

Ineffective individual coping related to personal vulnerability
Based on this nursing diagnosis, you'll establish the following patient outcomes. The patient will:

• express understanding of the relationship between emotional state and behavior.

• become actively involved in care planning.

• identify effective and ineffective coping techniques.

Equipment
♦ a small pillow or a folded towel
♦ glass slide ♦ cytologic fixative spray
♦ optional: nonsterile gloves, a light source, a ruler calibrated in centimeters.

Implementation
• Ask the patient to disrobe to the waist and to sit with her arms resting at each side.
• First, inspect the breasts for size and symmetry.
• Next, examine the breasts for obvious masses, one-sided flattening, or retraction or dimpling (a localized depression). To inspect for hidden dimpling, ask the patient to place her hands on her hips (as shown).

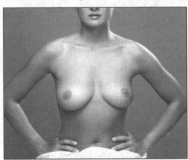

• Evaluate the skin. It should be smooth and soft with a similar venous pattern in both breasts. (Pronounced bilateral venous patterns are normal in obese or fair-skinned people.)
• If you see a skin lesion, ask about its duration and any recent changes.
• Don't be concerned about unchanged, nontender, and long-standing surface lesions such as nevi.
• Ask the patient to raise her hands slowly over her head. Inspect for equal and free breast movement without

dimpling. Repeat this part of the examination if you are unsure of your findings.

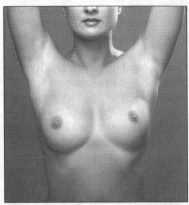

• Ask the patient with large or pendulous breasts to stand and lean forward with her hands or arms outstretched (as shown).

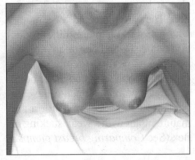

• Support her arms or have her lean on a chair or table. Both breasts should swing forward freely. This position helps reveal breast or nipple asymmetry.
• Inspect the nipples and areolae. Assess their size, shape, and color. (In a lactating patient, assess for signs of mastitis.) Normally, the nipples and areolae are similarly round or oval, of equal size, and free of rashes, fissures, and ulcerations. The nipples usually point in the same direction: outward, slightly upward, or laterally.

• If the patient has had a mastectomy, inspect the scar closely. Malignant changes commonly occur at this site. Look for lumps, color changes, swelling, rash, or irritation. Also assess for muscle loss or lymphedema.

• If the patient has had breast reconstruction, augmentation, or lumpectomy, inspect the breast in the usual manner. Pay close attention to scar tissue or any other new tissue.

Inspecting and palpating the axillae

• While the patient is sitting, inspect the axillae for rashes, signs of infection such as boils, and unusual pigmentation. Both axillae should be free of rashes or lesions and have hair growth if the patient is past puberty.

• For axillae palpation, the patient may lie or sit down, but sitting provides easier access. If the patient has an obvious ulceration or nipple discharge, wear gloves; otherwise, gloves may diminish your sense of feeling. Ask her to relax her arm as you support her elbow or wrist with one hand.

• Keeping the fingers of your other hand together, reach high into the apex of the axilla. Position your fingers so they're directly behind the pectoral muscles, pointing toward the midclavicle. Sweep your fingers downward and against the ribs and the anterior serratus muscle to palpate the midaxillary (central) lymph nodes.

• Assess the anterior pectoral lymph nodes by palpating along the anterior axillary fold (as shown at the top of the next column).

• Use one hand to provide support under the patient's arm. Use the other hand to grasp the axillary fold between your thumb and fingers, palpat-

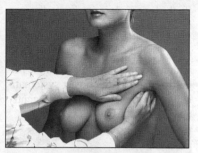

ing inside the borders of the pectoral muscle.

• Palpate the brachial (lateral) lymph nodes by pressing your fingers along the upper inner arm, trying to compress these nodes against the humerus.

• Assess the subscapular (posterior) lymph nodes by palpating along the posterior axillary fold. To do this, stand at the patient's side, and use your fingers to feel inside the muscle of the posterior axillary fold.

• If the axillary lymph node findings appear abnormal, assess the nodes in the clavicular area. Encourage the patient to relax so that her clavicles drop. Direct her to flex her head slightly forward to relax the neck muscles. Then, standing in front of her, hook your fingers over the clavicle beside the sternocleidomastoid muscle. Rotate your fingers deeply into this area to feel the supraclavicular nodes.

Palpating the breasts

• Mentally divide the breasts into four quadrants and a fifth segment, the tail of Spence, so that you can describe your findings according to a quadrant or a segment. It may help to think of the breast as a clock, with the nipple in the center. Specify a lesion's location according to the time (2 o'clock, for example). Whether you use the quadrant or clock method, also specify the lesion's location by its distance in centimeters from the nipple. (See *Supine breast examination.*)

• Using your middle three finger pads, which are more sensitive than the fingertips, palpate the breast systematically, rotating your fingers gently against the chest wall (as shown).

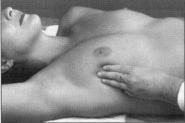

• Palpate each breast circularly from the center out or from the periphery in, making sure to palpate the tail of Spence. Feel for masses or induration (hardness). If you suspect a mass, move or compress the breast gently to look for dimpling. Palpate for consistency and elasticity.

• Alternative methods, especially useful in patients with pendulous breasts, are to palpate across or down the breast. For either procedure, ask the patient to sit up. To palpate across the breast, place a supporting hand under the breast while your other hand sweeps down and across the breast tissue against your supporting hand. Repeat this procedure on the other breast.

• To palpate down the breast, use the finger pads of both hands simultaneously, forming an in-and-out pattern across and down the breast (as shown at the top of the next column).

• Repeat this procedure on the other breast. Also assess for tenderness, which will vary according to the time in the patient's menstrual cycle.

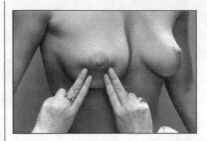

Palpating the areolae

• Palpate the nipple by gently compressing it between your thumb and index finger. The nipple will become erect and the areola will pucker from the tactile stimulation. Gently milk the nipple for discharge by compressing it between the thumb and index finger. Repeat this procedure on the other breast. If a discharge occurs, note the duct or ducts through which it appears.

• Make a cytologic smear of any discharge not explained by pregnancy or lactation. To do this, put on gloves, and then place a glass slide over the nipple and smear the discharge on the slide.

• Immediately spray the slide with fixative, making sure to keep the spray nozzle 6″ (15 cm) from the slide. Label the slide with the patient's name and the date, place it in a slide holder and then in a biohazard bag, and send it to the laboratory for analysis.

Palpating a breast mass

• If you detect a breast mass on palpation, note its size in centimeters, its shape — oval, round, or irregular — and its consistency — firm, cystic, hard, or rubbery.

• Palpate the mass, delineating it from the surrounding tissue by gently pinching the mass between your thumb and index finger to determine its borders.

• Assess the mass for mobility to determine whether it's fixed to the underlying tissue or freely movable. To do so, gently pinch the mass between your thumb and index finger again, attempting to move the mass back and forth (as shown).

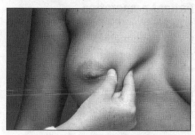

• Ask the patient whether she has any tenderness. Then document the location of the mass by its distance in centimeters from the nipple and its location on the clock (or within the quadrant).

Nursing considerations

• In women, the breasts are normally symmetrical, convex, and similar in appearance. One breast (usually the left) may be slightly larger than the other.
• The male breast may be convex if the patient is overweight or if he's an adolescent with gynecomastia (which typically resolves in about 1 year).
• In pregnant patients, large or pendulous breasts are normal. Other normal inspection findings include enlarged, erectile nipples (flattening or inverting as pregnancy progresses); colostrum secretion; dark, broadened areolae; prominent Montgomery's tubercles; vascular bluish chest veins (from increased estrogen production); and striae from stretching.
• The normal inframammary ridge at the lower edge of the breast is firm and may be mistaken for a tumor.

Supine breast examination

For a supine breast examination, place a small pillow or folded towel under the patient's back on the side being examined. Then place the arm on that same side above her head. This allows the breast tissue to spread more evenly across the chest wall.

• Inspect Montgomery's tubercles for discharge. A manually expressed discharge can occur normally; a spontaneous discharge is an abnormal finding.
• Palpation of one or two small, nontender, freely movable nodes is a normal finding. Hard, large, or tender nodes, however, may be abnormal, as may a suspicious-looking lesion. The breasts are typically tender the week before the menstrual period. Note where the patient is in her menstrual cycle when you document breast assessment data.
• Pregnant or lactating women normally have a discharge during palpation, making milking or squeezing the nipple unnecessary.

Home care

• Be sure to emphasize the patient's own role in breast health, especially in detecting changes that suggest possible disease.
• Show the patient how to perform a breast self-examination.
• If possible, have the patient repeat the demonstration so that you can correct any errors, encourage compliance, and reinforce your teaching.

Documentation
• Document the date and time of the examination.
• Note any abnormal findings, such as the presence of breast cysts or masses, prominent veins, inflammation, nipple retraction, or nipple inversion. Note size, shape, consistency, and location.

Breath sound auscultation

Lung auscultation is an assessment technique to help you detect abnormal fluid or mucus as well as obstructed passages. You can also determine the condition of the alveoli and surrounding pleura. (See *Guide to normal breath sounds* and *Guide to adventitious breath sounds*, page 108.)

❯❯ Key nursing diagnoses and patient outcomes
Use these nursing diagnoses as a guide when developing your plan of care.

Ineffective breathing pattern related to (specify)
Based on this nursing diagnosis, you'll establish the following patient outcomes. The patient will:
• achieve maximum lung expansion with adequate ventilation.
• have arterial blood gas levels within normal limits.
• have respiratory rate stay within plus or minus five of baseline.

Impaired gas exchange related to impaired ventilation due (specify)
Based on this nursing diagnosis, you'll establish the following patient outcomes. The patient will:

• maintain baseline breath sounds.
• express a feeling of comfort in maintaining air exchange.

Equipment
♦ stethoscope.

Patient preparation
• To auscultate the lungs, ask the patient to sit in an upright position. If he can't sit, have him lie on his side. (See *Keeping hair from interfering*, page 109.)

Implementation
• Begin by auscultating the patient's trachea.
• Continue down over the bronchi between the clavicles and midsternum.
• When you reach the mainstem bronchus, the sound will be loud, high-pitched, and longer on expiration than on inspiration.
• Auscultate the anterior thorax in proper sequence (as shown), assessing for changes in normal breath sounds. Listen for a full inspiratory-expiratory phase at each location.

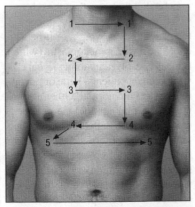

• Auscultate the patient's posterior thorax in a systematic right-to-left pattern.
• Note any abnormal sounds.

Guide to normal breath sounds

The sound of a patient's breathing indicates the condition of his respiratory and other body systems. To help you assess your patient's breathing, you'll need to recognize normal breath sounds.

Air moving through the tracheo-bronchial tree normally produces tracheal, bronchial, bronchovesicular, and vesicular breath sounds.

Tracheal and mainstem bronchial breath sounds are heard over the trachea. Loud, high-pitched, and hollow, they're longer on expiration than inspiration.

Vesicular breath sounds are heard over the anterior thorax and the posterior and lateral thorax. They're longer and louder during inspiration than expiration.

Heard over the mainstem bronchi at the first and second intercostal spaces between the scapulae, bronchovesicular breath sounds have a soft, low-pitched, breezy sound. They're lower pitched than bronchial sounds but higher pitched than vesicular sounds.

Anterior thorax

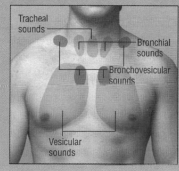

Posterior thorax

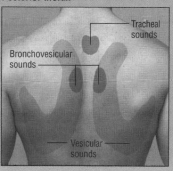

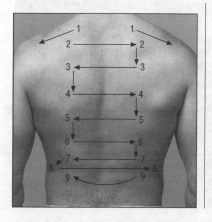

• Have the patient say the phrase "ninety-nine." You should hear a muffled, nondistinct sound through the stethoscope. If you hear "ninety-nine" clearly, the patient has bronchophony. Next, have the patient repeat the sound "ee-ee-ee." You should also perceive a muffled, nondistinct sound. If you hear "ay-ay-ay," the patient has egophony. Next, ask the patient to whisper "ninety-nine" while you auscultate. The sound you hear should be barely audible and nondistinct. If you hear "ninety-nine"

Guide to adventitious breath sounds

Abnormal breath sounds include absent or decreased breath sounds and bronchial breath sounds heard over lung areas other than the mainstem bronchi. Adventitious sounds are also abnormal and may be heard incidental to normal breath sounds. They include crackles, rhonchi, wheezes, and pleural friction rubs. The following information and illustrations will help you recognize the characteristics and location of adventitious sounds.

Crackles

Of the two kinds of crackles, fine crackles can be heard anywhere in the lungs. Typically, you'll first hear them over the lung bases. Their high-pitched, short crackling sounds are heard best on inspiration. Coarse crackles, on the other hand, are loud, low-pitched bubbling and gurgling sounds that start in early inspiration and may last through expiration.

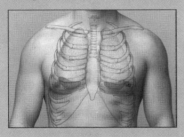

Rhonchi

These abnormal breath sounds are heard over the central airways. They're loud, coarse, low-pitched bubbling sounds heard equally well during inspiration and expiration.

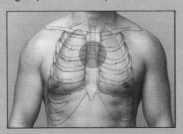

Wheezes

Coming from the large bronchi, wheezes are high-pitched, musical whistling sounds, which may occur during both inspiration and expiration but predominate during expiration.

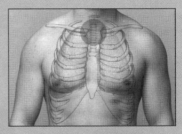

Pleural friction rubs

These coarse, low-pitched abnormal breath sounds are heard at the anterolateral wall during inspiration and expiration.

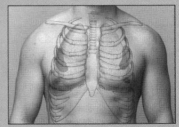

clearly, the patient has whispered pectoriloquy.

Nursing considerations
• Tell the patient to take full, slow breaths through his mouth. (Nose breathing changes the pitch of the breath sounds.) Listen for one full inspiration and expiration before moving the stethoscope. Remember that a patient may try to accommodate you by breathing quickly and deeply with every movement of the stethoscope, which can cause hyperventilation. If your patient becomes light-headed or dizzy, stop auscultation and allow him to breathe normally for a few minutes.

Documentation
• Be alert for crackles, rhonchi, wheezes, and friction rubs, and document their location. Also note any dyspnea, coughing, or chest pain or discomfort that the patient may report.
• As you auscultate, classify normal and abnormal breath sounds according to their location, intensity (amplitude), characteristic sound, pitch (tone), and duration.
• Document whether the abnormal breath sound occurs during inspiration, expiration, or both.

Bronchoscopy

Bronchoscopy is a diagnostic test that allows the doctor to inspect the trachea and bronchi through a flexible fiber-optic or rigid bronchoscope. It enables the doctor to determine the location and extent of pathologic processes, assess resectability of a tumor, diagnose bleeding sites, collect tissue

PROBLEM SOLVER

Keeping hair from interfering

Before you begin auscultation, note whether the patient has excessive chest hair. If so, wet and mat it with a damp washcloth, so the hair won't cause sounds that can be confused with crackles.

or sputum specimens, and remove foreign bodies, mucus plugs, or excessive secretions. Although the rigid bronchoscope allows more room for foreign body removal, it's usually used only in the operating room. On the other hand, the flexible fiber-optic bronchoscope, a slender tube containing fine glass fibers that transmit light, effectively removes mucus plugs and secretions. This device can be used at bedside, in a radiology suite, in a minor-procedures room, or in an operating room.

⟫ Key nursing diagnosis and patient outcomes
Use this nursing diagnosis as a guide when developing your plan of care.

Ineffective airway clearance related to presence of tracheobronchial obstruction or secretions
Based on this nursing diagnosis, you'll establish the following patient outcomes. The patient will:
• maintain a patent airway.
• understand and explain need for bronchoscopy.
• have arterial blood gas levels return to baseline within 24 hours.

Equipment

♦ flexible fiber-optic bronchoscope ♦ lidocaine (2% to 4%) ♦ sterile gloves ♦ an emesis basin ♦ handheld resuscitation bag with face mask ♦ oral and endotracheal airways ♦ laryngoscope ♦ suction equipment ♦ masks ♦ eye protectors ♦ high-flow oxygen source.

If the patient requires controlled mechanical ventilation, obtain a bronchoscopy adapter.

Equipment preparation

• Assemble equipment.

Patient preparation

• Teach your patient about the procedure and answer his questions.

• Reassure the patient that he may experience dyspnea during the test but won't suffocate and that oxygen will be administered through the bronchoscope.

Implementation

• Place the patient in a supine position on a table or bed, though he may need to sit upright in a chair.

• Tell him to remain relaxed, with arms at her sides, and to breathe through his nose during the test.

• As ordered, give medications, such as atropine to decrease secretions and an I.V. barbiturate or narcotic, such as diazepam (Valium), midazolam (Versed), or meperidine (Demerol), to provide sedation or amnesia and allay anxiety.

• The doctor will introduce the bronchoscope tube into the patient's airway through the nose, mouth, or endotracheal or tracheostomy tube. Then, small amounts of anesthetic

will be flushed through the tube to suppress coughing and wheezing.

• Check the patient's vital signs during the procedure and every 15 minutes afterward until they're stable.

• Place him in a semi-Fowler's position.

• Keep resuscitation equipment and a tracheostomy tray available for 24 hours.

• Watch for and immediately report symptoms of respiratory difficulty, such as stridor and dyspnea from laryngeal edema or laryngospasm.

• Watch for bleeding.

• Listen for wheezing, a sign of bronchospasm.

• Monitor for dyspnea and diminished breathing sounds on one side, which may indicate pneumothorax.

• Report any abnormal findings to the doctor and prepare the patient for a chest X-ray, if ordered, to confirm pneumothorax.

• Provide an emesis basin and instruct the patient to spit instead of swallow.

• Expect to find blood-tinged sputum for up to several hours, but report prolonged bleeding or persistent hemoptysis to the doctor.

• Restrict all oral intake until the patient's gag reflex returns.

Complications

Possible complications of bronchoscopy include hypoxemia, hemorrhage (most likely to occur when biopsy is done at the same time), respiratory distress, pneumothorax, bronchospasm, and infection.

Nursing considerations

• If the patient experiences hoarseness or a sore throat, provide medicated lozenges when allowed and encour-

age him not to talk, which will rest his vocal cords. Reassure the patient that hoarseness, sore throat, and a loss of his voice are temporary side effects and will subside with rest and supportive treatment. Emphasize the importance of reporting signs of infection, such as fever or thick, yellow sputum.
• If you assist during the procedure, place specimens in appropriate containers and send them to the laboratory immediately. Failure to treat specimens properly can make accurate diagnosis difficult or impossible.

Documentation
Document the patient's tolerance to the procedure and adverse effects experienced.

Bryant's traction

Also called vertical suspension, Bryant's traction is used mostly to reduce congenital hip dislocations in children. With the patient lying supine in a bed or crib, the traction extends the legs vertically at a 90-degree angle to the body. Even if the disorder affects only one leg, the patient will have traction applied to both legs to prevent hip rotation and to ensure equal stress on the legs and even, bilateral bone growth.

Bryant's traction continues for 2 to 4 weeks. Afterward, the patient may be immobilized in a hip spica cast. Usually chosen for children under age 2 who weigh between 25 and 30 lb (11.3 and 16.3 kg), Bryant's traction is contraindicated for heavier children because the risk of positional hypertension rises with increased weight.

≫ Key nursing diagnoses and patient outcomes
Use these nursing diagnoses as a guide when developing your plan of care for a patient who is being treated with Bryant's traction.

Impaired mobility related to neuromuscular impairment
Based on this nursing diagnosis, you'll establish the following patient outcomes. The patient will:
• maintain muscle strength and joint range of motion.
• show no evidence of complications, such as contractures, venous stasis, thrombus formation, or skin breakdown.

Pain related to physical agents
Based on this nursing diagnosis, you'll establish the following patient outcomes. The patient will:
• express a feeling of comfort and relief from pain.
• state and carry out appropriate interventions for pain relief.

Equipment
♦ traction setup (supplied by the orthopedic department) ♦ moleskin traction straps ♦ elastic bandages ♦ foam rubber padding ♦ cotton balls ♦ compound benzoin tincture ♦ adhesive tape ♦ jacket restraint ♦ optional: safety razor, cotton batting, convoluted foam mattress, sheepskin pad.

Equipment preparation
• Help the doctor and orthopedic technician measure and cut the moleskin straps and assemble the traction equipment.

Patient preparation

• Thoroughly explain the purpose and function of the traction *to enhance learning and alleviate patient and family anxiety.* If possible, use visual aids to illustrate your teaching.

• Keep a diagram handy for parents and a doll in traction for the patient.

• Ask the parents if the patient is sensitive or allergic to rubber or to adhesive tape.

• If the patient has hairy legs, shave or clip the hair with a safety razor *to ensure good contact between the moleskin traction straps and the skin.* Use soap, warm water, and long, downward strokes *to minimize nicking.*

• Apply the compound benzoin tincture, if ordered, to the patient's legs *to protect the skin.*

Implementation

• Assist the doctor or orthopedic technician with placing foam rubber padding and moleskin traction straps against the patient's legs and securing the straps with elastic bandages from foot to thigh. If the patient's allergic to rubber or to adhesive tape, wrap the legs in cotton batting before applying the straps.

• If necessary to keep the patient positioned properly, apply a jacket restraint *to keep the weights from pulling the patient forward and altering the tractional force.*

• Carefully monitor the circulatory status of the patient's legs at 15 minutes and at 30 minutes after applying initial traction. Then check circulatory status every 4 hours *to detect any impairment caused by traction.* Assess capillary refill, skin color, sensation, movement, temperature, peripheral pulses, and bandage tightness. If you detect circulatory compromise, loosen the elastic bandages and notify the patient's doctor.

• Take care to position the elastic bandages precisely. Unless contraindicated, periodically remove the bandages from the unaffected leg to assess circulation and provide skin care. When doing so, have another person hold the traction straps in place *to prevent slipping.* Don't unwrap the affected leg unless ordered to do so by the patient's doctor.

• Check the patient's position regularly *to ensure optimum traction.* Be sure to raise the patient's buttocks high enough off the mattress to allow one hand to slide between the skin and the mattress. Avoid raising the buttocks too high, though, because *this may reduce the effectiveness of traction.*

• Try marking the bed sheet with an "X" at the correct shoulder position as a guide to correct body alignment. Near the patient's bed, post an illustration of the correct alignment to guide other nurses and caregivers. (See *Maintaining body alignment and traction.*)

• Give skin care every 4 hours, focusing especially on the back, buttocks, and elbows. These areas are most prone to breakdown. Place a convoluted foam mattress or a sheepskin pad — or both — beneath the patient *to help prevent or alleviate skin problems.*

• Inspect the traction apparatus at least every 2 hours to ensure the correct weight. Be sure that the weights hang freely, the pulleys glide easily, the ropes aren't frayed, and the knots remain snugly tied and taped.

Maintaining body alignment and traction

Keeping the patient's body in correct position with Bryant's traction requires precision and continual supervision and adjustment.

At the same time that the traction apparatus holds the patient's legs perpendicular to the mattress, you'll need to ensure that the patient's buttocks stay slightly elevated to provide countertraction and that his shoulders stay flat and in the same position on the mattress to maintain body alignment.

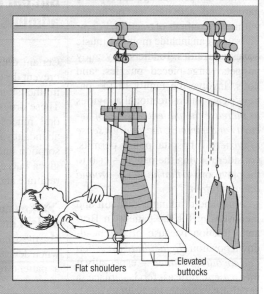

Flat shoulders

Elevated buttocks

• Encourage the patient to take deep breaths at least every 2 hours *to minimize his risk for hypostatic pneumonia.*

• Review the patient's diet to ensure that he consumes enough fiber and fluid *to prevent constipation and urinary stasis.* (Infants should consume about 130 ml of fluid for each kilogram of body weight every 24 hours; toddlers should consume about 115 ml per kilogram.)

• *Promote safety* by keeping the side rails raised on the patient's bed whenever you're not at the bedside.

Complications

• Although generally safe, Bryant's traction may lead to pneumonia from restricted lung expansion resulting from the head-down position.

• Skin necrosis may result from bandages wrapped too tightly.

• Other complications include urinary stasis and constipation.

Nursing considerations

• *To encourage regular deep breathing and guard against pneumonia,* allow the patient to blow a horn, whistle, pinwheel, or bubbles heartily. Or urge him to sing. *This promotes lung expansion and enjoyment at the same time.*

• Because a child can't always tell you that he's in pain, carefully observe his behavior, facial expression, and cry to judge discomfort levels. Besides needing an analgesic or sedative, the patient may need an antispasmodic medication to relieve irritable muscles and muscle spasms.

• *To foster development, diversion, and mobility,* provide age-appropriate games and activities as permitted within the confines of traction. For infants, this can include mobiles, music boxes, and rattles. Toddlers may enjoy puppets, large-pieced puzzles, and dolls. Involve the family in the patient's care and recreational activities *to increase the patient's sense of security and minimize the family's sense of anxiety.* If hospital policy permits, consider moving the patient's crib to the playroom *so that he can be around other children.*

• Eating and drinking is difficult and inconvenient for the patient in Bryant's traction because of the head-down position. *To facilitate digestion and encourage eating* — especially if the patient refuses food — place a small pillow under his head at mealtime. If possible, allow him to choose his own foods, and encourage his family to bring food from home.

• *To minimize patient movement,* change bed linens every other day unless the linens get wet or soiled. Keep sheets taut and wrinkle-free *to help prevent skin breakdown.*

Documentation

• Record the date and time that traction was applied; the amount of weight applied; and the patient's circulatory status, skin condition, and position. Note whether weights hang freely.

• Document changes in the patient's status, and describe the patient's and family's response to the traction.

• Also note the patient's and family's response to any patient teaching.

Buccal drug administration

Certain drugs are given buccally to prevent destruction or transformation in the stomach or small intestine. These drugs act quickly because the oral mucosa's thin epithelium and abundant vasculature allow direct absorption into the bloodstream. Drugs given buccally include erythrityl tetranitrate and methyltestosterone.

≫ Key nursing diagnoses and patient outcomes

Use these nursing diagnoses as a guide when developing your plan of care for a patient receiving buccal medications.

Knowledge deficit related to lack of exposure to procedure

Based on this nursing diagnosis, you'll establish the following patient outcome. The patient will:

• demonstrate proficiency in self-administration of buccal medications.

Risk for injury related to improper technique

Based on this nursing diagnosis, you'll establish the following patient outcomes. The patient will:

• identify factors that increase risk for injury.

• assist in identifying and applying safety measures to prevent injury.

Equipment
♦ patient's medication record and chart ♦ prescribed medication ♦ medication cup.

Patient preparation
• Explain the procedure to the patient if he's never taken a drug buccally.

Implementation
• Verify the order on the patient's medication record by checking it against the doctor's order on his chart.
• Wash your hands with warm water and soap.
• Check the label on the medication before administering it *to make sure you'll be giving the prescribed medication.*
• Confirm the patient's identity by asking his name and checking the name and room and bed number on his wristband.
• Place the tablet in the buccal pouch, between the cheek and gum. (See *Giving drugs buccally.*)
• Instruct the patient to keep the medication in place until it dissolves completely to ensure absorption.
• Caution him against chewing the tablet or touching it with his tongue to prevent accidental swallowing.
• Tell him not to smoke before the drug has dissolved *because nicotine's vasoconstrictive effects slow absorption.*

Complications
• Some buccal medications may irritate the mucosa.
• Alternate sides of the mouth for repeat doses *to prevent continuous irritation of the same site.*

Giving drugs buccally

Buccal administration routes allow some drugs such as methyltestosterone to enter the bloodstream rapidly without being degraded in the GI tract. To give a drug buccally, insert it between the patient's cheek and teeth, as shown here. Ask him to close his mouth and hold the tablet against his cheek until the tablet is absorbed.

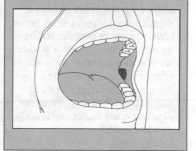

Nursing considerations
• Don't give liquids *because some buccal tablets may take up to 1 hour to be absorbed.* In that case, the patient should rinse his mouth with water *between* doses.

Documentation
• Your employer probably includes a medication administration record (MAR) in your documentation system. Commonly included in a card file (medication Kardex) or on a separate medication administration sheet. The MAR serves as the central record of medication orders and their execution and is part of the patient's permanent record.
• Record the medication administered, the dose, the date and time, and the patient's reaction, if any. (See

BETTER CHARTING

Guidelines for documenting medication administration

When using the medication administration record (MAR), follow these guidelines:

• Know and follow your hospital's policies and procedures for recording drug orders and charting drug administration.

• Make sure that all drug orders include the patient's full name, the date, the drug's name, dose, administration route or method, and frequency. When appropriate include the specific number of doses given or the stop date. When administering a drug dose immediately, or stat, make sure to record the time. Also be certain to include drug allergy information.

• Write legibly.

• Use only standard abbreviations approved by the hospital. When doubtful about an abbreviation, write out the word or phrase.

• After administering the first dose, sign your full name, licensure status, and your initials in the appropriate space on the MAR.

• Record drugs immediately after administration so that another nurse doesn't give the drug again.

• If you document medication administration by computer, chart your information for each drug right after you give it. This is particularly important if you don't use printouts as a backup. By keying in information immediately, you ensure that all health care team members have access to the latest drug administration data for the patient.

• Document the reason the drug was not given (for example, if the patient is having a test, which requires him not to take the drug).

Guidelines for documenting medication administration.)

Burn care

The goals of burn care are to maintain the patient's physiologic stability, repair skin integrity, prevent infection, and promote maximal functioning and psychosocial health. Competent care immediately after a burn occurs can dramatically improve treatment success.

Burn severity is determined by the depth and extent of the burn and other factors, such as age, complications, and coexisting illnesses. (See *Estimating burn surfaces in adults and children*, pages 117 and 118, and *Evaluating burn severity*, page 119.)

To promote stability, carefully monitor your patient's respiratory status, especially if he has inhaled smoke. Remember that patients with burns involving more than 20% of their body area usually need fluid resuscitation, which supports the body's compensatory mechanisms without overwhelming them. Expect to give

Estimating burn surfaces in adults and children

You need to use different formulas to compute burned body surface areas in adults and children because the proportion of body surface areas varies with growth.

Rule of Nines

You can quickly estimate the extent of an adult patient's burn by using the Rule of Nines. This method quantifies body surface area in percentages either in fractions of nine or in multiples of nine. To use this method, mentally assess your patient's burns by the body chart shown below. Add the corresponding percentages for each body section burned. Use the total — a rough estimate of burn extent — to calculate initial fluid replacement needs.

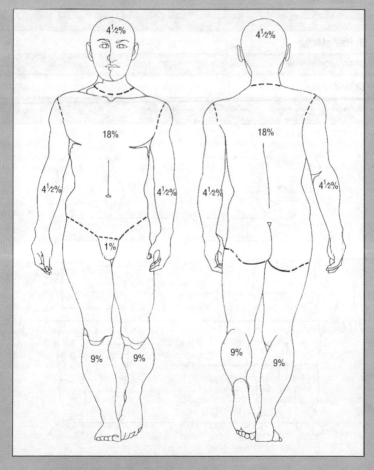

Estimating burn surfaces in adults and children *(continued)*

Lund and Browder
The Rule of Nines isn't accurate for infants and children because their body shapes differ from those of adults. An infant's head, for example, accounts for about 17% of his total body surface area, compared with 7% for an adult. Instead, use the Lund and Browder chart shown here.

Percentage of burned body surface by age

AT BIRTH	0 TO 1 YR	1 TO 4 YR	5 TO 9 YR	10 TO 15 YR	ADULT
A: Half of head					
9½%	8½%	6½%	5½%	4½%	3½%
B: Half of thigh					
2¾%	3¼%	4%	4¼%	4½%	4¾%
C: Half of leg					
2½%	2½%	2¾%–3%	3%	3¼%	3½%

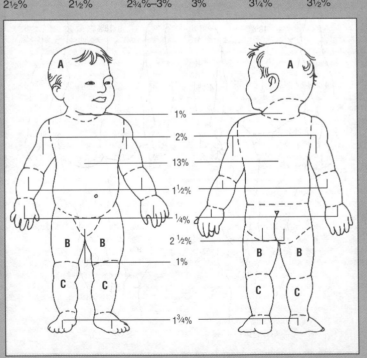

Evaluating burn severity

To judge a burn's severity, assess its depth and extent as well as the presence of other factors.

Superficial partial-thickness (first-degree) burn
Does the burned area appear pink or red with minimal edema? Is the area sensitive to touch and temperature changes? If so, your patient most likely has a superficial partial-thickness, or first-degree, burn affecting only the epidermal skin layer.

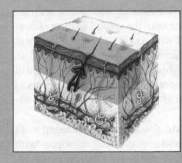

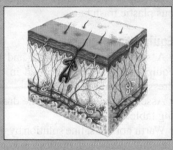

Full-thickness (third-degree) burn
Does the burned area appear red, waxy white, brown, or black? Does red skin remain red with no blanching when you touch it? Is the skin leathery with extensive subcutaneous edema? Is the skin insensitive to touch? Does the hair fall out easily? If so, your patient most likely has a full-thickness, or third-degree, burn that affects all skin layers.

Deep partial-thickness (second-degree) burn
Does the burned area appear pink or red, with a mottled appearance? Do red areas blanch when you touch them? Does the skin have large, thick-walled blisters with subcutaneous edema? Does touching the burn cause severe pain? Is the hair still present? If so, the person most likely has a deep partial-thickness, or second-degree, burn (shown above, at right) affecting the epidermal and dermal layers.

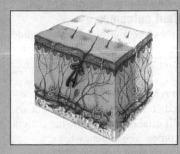

fluids such as lactated Ringer's solution to keep the patient's urine output at 30 to 50 ml/hour, and expect to monitor blood pressure and heart rate. You'll also need to control body temperature because skin loss interferes with temperature regulation. Use warm fluids, heat lamps, and hyperthermia blankets, as appropriate, to keep the patient's temperature above 97° F (36.1° C), if possible. You'll also frequently review laboratory values such as serum electrolyte levels to detect early changes in the patient's condition.

Skin integrity is restored through aggressive wound debridement followed by clean wound-bed maintenance until the wound heals or is covered with a skin graft. Full-thickness burns and some deep partial-thickness burns must be debrided and grafted in the operating room. Surgery occurs as soon after fluid resuscitation as possible.

Most wounds are managed with twice-daily dressing changes with topical antibiotics. Burn dressings encourage healing by barring germ entry and by removing exudate, eschar, and other debris that host infection. After thorough wound cleaning, topical antibacterial agents are applied and the wound is covered with absorptive, coarse mesh gauze. Roller gauze typically tops the dressing and is secured with elastic netting or tape.

≫ Key nursing diagnoses and patient outcomes

Use these nursing diagnoses as a guide when developing your plan of care for a patient who is receiving burn care.

Pain related to burn sites

Based on this nursing diagnosis, you'll establish the following patient outcomes. The patient will:
• identify pain characteristics.
• articulate factors intensifying pain.
• express comfort and pain relief.

Impaired skin integrity related to burns

Based on this nursing diagnosis, you'll establish the following patient outcomes. The patient will:

• demonstrate skin care regimen.
• express feelings about changed body image.

Equipment

♦ normal saline solution ♦ fluffed gauze pads ♦ sterile bowl ♦ scissors ♦ tissue forceps ♦ ordered topical medication ♦ burn gauze ♦ roller gauze ♦ elastic netting or tape ♦ cotton-tipped applicators ♦ ordered pain medication ♦ three pairs of sterile gloves ♦ sterile gown ♦ mask ♦ surgical cap ♦ heat lamps ♦ impervious plastic trash bag.

Equipment preparation

• A sterile field is required, and all equipment and supplies used in the dressing should be sterile.
• Assemble equipment on the dressing table.
• Warm normal saline solution by immersing unopened bottles in warm water.
• Make sure the treatment area has adequate light to allow accurate wound assessment.
• Open equipment packages using aseptic technique.
• Arrange supplies on a sterile field in order of use. To prevent cross-contamination, plan to dress the cleanest areas first and the dirtiest or most contaminated areas last.
• To help prevent excessive pain or cross-contamination, you may need to perform the dressing in stages to avoid exposing all wounds simultaneously.

Implementation

• Administer ordered pain medication about 20 minutes before beginning wound care *to maximize patient comfort and cooperation.*

• Explain the procedure to the patient and provide privacy.
• Turn on overhead heat lamps *to keep the patient warm,* but make sure the lamps don't overheat the patient.
• Pour warmed normal saline solution into the sterile bowl in the sterile field.
• Wash your hands.

To remove a dressing without hydrotherapy

• Put on a gown, mask, and sterile gloves.
• Remove dressing layers down to the innermost by cutting the outer dressings with sterile blunt scissors. Lay open these dressings.
• If the inner layer appears dry, ease removal by soaking the layer with warm normal saline solution.
• Remove the inner dressing with sterile tissue forceps or your sterile gloved hand.
• *Because soiled dressings harbor infectious microorganisms,* dispose of the dressings carefully in an impervious bag according to hospital policy.
• Dispose of your gloves and wash your hands.
• Put on a new pair of sterile gloves.
• Using gauze pads moistened with normal saline solution, gently remove any exudate and old topical medication.
• Carefully remove all loose eschar with sterile forceps and scissors, if ordered.
• Assess wound condition. The wound should appear clean, with no debris, loose tissue, purulence, inflammation, or darkened margins.
• Before applying a new dressing, remove your gown, gloves, and mask. Discard them properly, and put on a

Preventing infection

Infection can increase wound depth, cause rejection of skin grafts, slow healing, worsen pain, prolong hospitalization, and even lead to death. Whenever possible, the health care team should avoid invasive procedures in burn patients because these procedures heighten the risk of infection.

To help prevent infection, use strict aseptic technique during care, dress the burn site as ordered, monitor and rotate I.V. lines regularly, and carefully assess the burn extent, body system function, and the patient's emotional status.

Other interventions, such as careful positioning and regular exercise for burned extremities, help maintain joint function, prevent contractures, and minimize deformity.

clean mask, surgical cap, gown, and sterile gloves.

To apply a wet dressing

• Soak fine-mesh gauze and the elastic gauze dressing in a large sterile basin containing the ordered solution such as silver nitrate.
• Wring out the fine-mesh gauze until it's moist — not dripping — and apply it to the wound. Warn the patient that he may feel transient pain when you apply the dressing. (See *Preventing infection.*)
• Wring out the elastic gauze dressing, and position it to hold the fine-mesh gauze in place.
• Roll an elastic gauze dressing over the dressing *to keep dressings intact.*
• Cover the patient with a cotton bath blanket *to prevent chills.* Change the

blanket if it becomes damp. Use an overhead heat lamp if necessary.

• Change the dressings frequently as ordered, *to keep the wound moist —* especially if you're using silver nitrate. *Silver nitrate becomes ineffective and the silver ions may damage tissue if the dressings become dry.* (To maintain moisture, some protocols call for irrigating the dressing with solution at least every 4 hours through small slits cut into the outer dressing.)

To apply a dry dressing with a topical medication

• Remove old dressings, and clean the wound (as described previously).

• Apply the ordered medication to the wound in a thin layer — about 2 to 4 mm thick — with your sterile gloved hand. Then apply several layers of burn gauze over the wound *to contain the medication but allow exudate to escape.*

• Remember to cut the dressing to fit only the wound areas; do not cover unburned areas.

• Cover the entire dressing with roller gauze, and secure it with elastic netting or tape.

To provide arm and leg care

• Apply the dressings from the distal to the proximal area *to stimulate circulation and prevent constriction.* Wrap the burn gauze once around the arm or leg so the edges slightly overlap. Continue wrapping in this way until the gauze covers the wound.

• Apply a dry roller gauze dressing *to hold the bottom layers in place.* Secure with elastic netting or tape.

To provide hand and foot care

• Wrap each finger separately with a single layer of a $4'' \times 4''$ gauze pad *to allow the patient to use his hands and to prevent webbing contractures.*

• Place the hand in a functional position, and secure this position using a dressing. Apply splints if ordered.

• Put gauze between each toe, as appropriate, *also to prevent webbing contractures.*

To provide chest, abdomen, and back care

• Apply the ordered medication to the wound in a thin layer. Then cover the entire burned area with sheets of burn gauze.

• Wrap with roller gauze or apply a specialty vest dressing *to hold the burn gauze in place.*

• Secure the dressing with elastic netting or tape. Make sure the dressing doesn't restrict respiratory motion, especially in very young or elderly patients or those with circumferential injuries.

To provide facial care

• If the patient has scalp burns, clip or shave the hair around the burn, as ordered. Clip other hair until it's about $2''$ (5 cm) long *to prevent contamination of burned scalp areas.*

• Shave facial hair if it comes in contact with burned areas.

• Typically, facial burns are managed with milder topical agents such as triple antibiotic ointment and are left exposed to air. If dressings are required, make sure they don't cover the eyes, nostrils, or mouth.

To provide ear care
• Clip or shave the hair around the affected ear.
• Remove exudate and crusts with cotton-tipped applicators dipped in saline solution.
• Place a $4'' \times 4''$ layer of gauze behind the auricle *to prevent webbing.*
• Apply ordered topical medication to $4'' \times 4''$ gauze pads, and place the pads over the burned area. Before securing the dressing with a roller bandage, position the patient's ears normally *to avoid damaging the auricular cartilage.*
• Assess the patient's hearing.

To provide eye care
• Clean the area around the eyes and eyelids with a cotton-tipped applicator and normal saline solution every 4 to 6 hours, or as needed, *to remove crusts and drainage.*
• Administer ordered eye ointments or drops.
• If the eyes can't be closed, apply lubricating ointments or drops, as ordered.
• Be sure to close the patient's eyes before applying eye pads *to prevent corneal abrasion.* Don't apply any topical ointments near the eyes without a doctor's order.

To provide nasal care
• Check the nostrils for inhalation injury: inflamed mucosa, singed vibrissae, and soot.
• Clean the nostrils with cotton-tipped applicators dipped in normal saline solution. Remove crusts.
• Apply the ordered ointments.
• If the patient has a nasogastric (NG) tube, use tracheostomy ties to secure the tube. Be sure to check ties frequently for tightness resulting from swelling of facial tissue. Clean the area around the NG tube every 4 to 6 hours.

Complications
• Infection is the most common burn complication.

Nursing considerations
• Thorough assessment and documentation of the wound's appearance is essential to detect infection. A purulent wound or green-grey exudate indicates infection; an overly dry wound suggests dehydration; and a wound with a swollen, red edge suggests cellulitis. Suspect a fungal infection if the wound is white and powdery. Healthy granulation tissue appears clean, pinkish, faintly shiny, and free of exudate.
• *Blisters protect underlying tissue,* so leave them intact unless they impede joint motion, become infected, or cause patient discomfort.
• Keep in mind the patient with healing burns has increased nutritional needs and will require extra protein and carbohydrates *to accommodate an almost doubled basal metabolism.*
• If you must manage a burn with topical medications, exposure to air, and no dressing, watch for such problems as wound adherence to bed linens, poor drainage control, and partial loss of topical medications.

Home care
• Begin discharge planning as soon as the patient enters the hospital *to help him (and his family) make a smooth transition from the hospital to home.*
• *To encourage therapeutic compliance,* prepare him to expect scarring.

Successful burn care after discharge

You can help the patient make a successful transition from hospital to home by encouraging him to follow the wound care and self-care guidelines below.

Wound care

Instruct the patient or a family member to follow this procedure when changing dressings:

• Clean the bathtub, shower, or wash basin thoroughly, and then assemble the required equipment (topical medication, if ordered, and dressing supplies). Open the supplies aseptically on a clean surface.

• Wash your hands. Remove the old dressing and discard it.

• Using a clean washcloth and mild soap and water, wash the wound to remove all the old medication. Try to remove any loose skin, too. Then pat the skin dry with a clean towel.

• Check the burned area for signs of infection — redness, heat, foul odor, increased pain, and difficulty moving the area. If any of these signs is present, notify the doctor after completing the dressing change.

• Wash your hands. If ordered, apply a thin layer of topical medication.

• Cover the area with thin layers of gauze, and wrap it with a roller bandage. Finally, secure it with tape or elastic netting.

Self-care

• To enhance healing, instruct the patient to eat well-balanced meals with adequate carbohydrates and proteins, to eat between-meal snacks, and to include at least one protein source in each meal and snack. Tell him to avoid tobacco, al-

cohol, and caffeine because they constrict peripheral blood flow.

• Advise the patient to wash new skin with mild soap and water. To prevent excessive skin dryness, instruct him to use a lubricating lotion and to avoid lotions containing alcohol or perfume. Caution the patient to avoid bumping or scratching regenerated skin tissue.

• Recommend nonrestrictive, nonabrasive clothing, which should be laundered in a mild detergent. Advise the patient to wear protective clothing during cold weather to prevent frostbite.

• Warn the patient not to expose new skin to strong sunlight and to always use a sunblock with a sun protection factor of 20 or higher. Also tell him not to expose new skin to irritants, such as paint, solvent, strong detergents, or antiperspirants. Recommend cool baths or ice packs to relieve itching.

• To minimize scar formation, the patient may need to wear a pressure garment — usually for 23 hours a day for 6 months to 1 year. Instruct him to remove it only during daily hygiene. Suspect that the garment is too tight if it causes coldness, numbness, or discoloration in the fingers or toes or if its seams and zippers leave deep, red impressions for more than 10 minutes after the garment is removed.

• Teach wound management and pain control.
• Urge following a prescribed exercise regimen.
• Provide encouragement and emotional support.
• Urge the patient to join a burn-survivor support group.
• Teach family or caregivers to encourage, support, and provide care. (See *Successful burn care after discharge.*)

Documentation
• Record the date and time of all care provided.
• Describe wound condition, special dressing-change techniques, topical medications administered, positioning of the burned area, and the patient's tolerance of the procedure.

Burn dressings, biological

Biological burn dressings provide a temporary protective covering for burn wounds and for clean granulation tissue. They also temporarily secure fresh skin grafts and protect graft donor sites. In common use are three organic materials and one synthetic material: pigskin, cadaver skin, amniotic membrane, and Biobrane. (See *Learning about biological dressings,* pages 126 and 127.)

Besides stimulating new skin growth, these dressings act like normal skin: They minimize fluid, electrolyte, and protein losses; reduce heat loss; and block infection.

Amniotic membrane or fresh cadaver skin is usually applied to the pa-

tient in the operating room, although it may be applied in a treatment room. Pigskin or Biobrane may be applied in the operating room or a treatment room. Before applying a biological dressing, the caregiver must clean and debride the wound. The frequency of dressing changes depends on the type of wound and the dressing's specific function.

≫ Key nursing diagnoses and patient outcomes
Use these nursing diagnoses as a guide when developing your plan of care for a patient who is being treated with a biological burn dressing.

Pain related to burn sites
Based on this nursing diagnosis, you'll establish the following patient outcomes. The patient will:
• identify pain characteristics.
• articulate factors that intensify pain.
• express a feeling of comfort and relief from pain.

Impaired skin integrity related to biological burn dressing
Based on this nursing diagnosis, you'll establish the following patient outcomes. The patient will:
• exhibit no signs of rejection.
• demonstrate skin care regimen.
• voice feelings about changed body image.

Equipment
♦ ordered analgesic ♦ cap ♦ mask ♦ two pairs of sterile gloves ♦ sterile or clean gown ♦ shoe covers ♦ biological dressing ♦ normal saline solution ♦ sterile basin ♦ Xeroflo gauze ♦ elastic gauze dressing ♦ stockinette or elastic bandage ♦ sterile for-

Learning about biological dressings

TYPE	DESCRIPTION AND USES	NURSING CONSIDERATIONS
Cadaver (homograft)	• Obtained at autopsy up to 24 hours after death • Applied in the operating room or at the bedside to debrided, untidy wounds • Available as fresh cryopreserved homografts in tissue banks nationwide • Provides protection, especially to granulation tissue after escharotomy • May be used in some patients as a test graft for autografting • Covers excised wounds immediately	• Observe for exudate. • Watch for signs of rejection. • Keep in mind that the gauze dressing may be removed every 8 hours to observe the graft.
Pigskin (heterograft or xenograft)	• Applied in the operating room or at the bedside • Comes fresh or frozen in rolls or sheets • Can cover and protect debrided, untidy wounds, mesh autografts, clean (eschar-free) partial-thickness burns, and exposed tendons	• Reconstitute frozen form with normal saline solution 30 minutes before use. • Watch for signs of rejection. • Cover with gauze dressing or leave exposed to air as ordered. • Note that pigskin dressings are typically changed every 2 to 5 days.
Amniotic membrane (homograft)	• Available from the obstetric department • Must be sterile and come from an uncomplicated birth; serologic tests must be done • Bacteriostatic condition doesn't require antimicrobials • May be used to protect partial-thickness burns or (temporarily) granulation tissue before autografting • Applied by the doctor to clean wounds only	• The membrane will be changed every 48 hours. • Cover the membrane with a gauze dressing or leave exposed as ordered. • If you apply a gauze dressing, change it every 48 hours.

Learning about biological dressings *(continued)*

TYPE	DESCRIPTION AND USES	NURSING CONSIDERATIONS
Biobrane (biosynthetic membrane)	• Comes in sterile, prepackaged sheets in various sizes and in glove form for hand burns • Used to cover donor graft sites, superficial partial-thickness burns, debrided wounds awaiting autograft, or meshed autograft • Provides significant pain relief • Applied by the nurse	• Leave the membrane in place for 3 to 14 days, possibly longer. • Do not use this dressing for preparing a granulation bed for subsequent autografting.

ceps ♦ sterile scissors ♦ sterile hemostats.

Equipment preparation
• Place the biological dressing in the sterile basin containing sterile normal saline solution (or open the Biobrane package).
• Using aseptic technique, open the sterile dressing packages.
• Arrange the equipment on the dressing cart and keep the cart readily accessible.
• Make sure the treatment area has adequate light to allow accurate wound assessment and dressing placement.

Patient preparation
• If this is the patient's first treatment, explain the procedure *to allay fears and promote cooperation.* Provide privacy.
• If ordered, administer an analgesic to the patient 20 minutes before beginning the procedure, or give an I.V. analgesic immediately before the procedure *to increase the patient's comfort and tolerance levels.*

Implementation
• Wash your hands and put on cap, mask, gown, shoe covers, and sterile gloves.
• Clean and debride the wound *to reduce bacteria.*
• Remove and dispose of gloves.
• Wash your hands again and put on a fresh pair of sterile gloves.
• Place the dressing directly on the wound surface. Apply pigskin dermal (shiny) side down; apply Biobrane nylon-backed (dull) side down. Roll the dressing directly onto the skin, if applicable. Place the dressing strips so that the edges touch but don't overlap. Use sterile forceps if necessary. Smooth the dressing. Eliminate folds and wrinkles by rolling out the dressing with the hemostat handle, the forceps handle, or your sterile-gloved hand *to cover the wound completely and ensure adherence.*
• Use the scissors to trim the dressing around the wound, *so the dressing fits the wound without overlapping adjacent areas.*

• Place Xeroflo gauze directly over an allograft, pigskin graft, or amniotic membrane. Place a few layers of gauze on top *to absorb exudate,* and wrap with a roller gauze dressing. Secure the dressing with tape or elastic netting. During daily dressing changes, the dressing will be removed down to the Xeroflo gauze, and the gauze will be replaced after the Xeroflo is inspected for drainage, adherence, and signs of infection.

• Place a nonadhesive dressing such as Exu-dry over the Biobrane *to absorb drainage and provide stability.* Wrap it with a roller gauze dressing, and secure it with tape or elastic netting. During daily dressing changes, the dressing will be removed down to the Biobrane and the site inspected for signs of infection. After the Biobrane adheres (usually 2 to 3 days), it needn't be dressed.

• Position the patient comfortably, elevating the area if possible. *This reduces edema, which may prevent the biological dressing from adhering.*

Complications

• Infection may develop under a biological dressing.

Nursing considerations

• Handle the biological dressing as little as possible.

• Observe the wound carefully during dressing changes for infection signs.

• If wound drainage appears purulent, remove the dressing, clean the area with normal saline solution or another prescribed cleaning solution, as ordered, and apply a fresh biological dressing.

Home care

• Instruct the patient or caregiver to assess the site daily for signs of infection, swelling, blisters, drainage, and separation.

• Make sure the patient knows whom to contact if these complications develop.

Documentation

• Record the time and date of dressing changes.

• Note areas of application, quality of adherence, and purulent drainage or other infection signs.

• Describe the patient's tolerance of the procedure.

C

Cardiac catheterization

This diagnostic test involves passing a catheter into the right or left side of the heart. Catheterization can determine blood pressure and blood flow in the chambers of the heart, permit collection of blood samples, or record films of the heart's ventricles (contrast ventriculography) or arteries (coronary arteriography or angiography). (See *Cardiac catheterization: Two approaches*, page 130.)

Catheterization of the left side of the heart assesses the patency of the coronary arteries, mitral and aortic valve function, and left ventricular function. It aids diagnosis of left ventricular enlargement, aortic stenosis and insufficiency, aortic root enlargement, mitral insufficiency, aneurysm, and intracardiac shunt. (See *Understanding cardiac catheterization findings*, page 131.)

In left-heart catheterization, a catheter is inserted into an artery in the antecubital fossa or into the femoral artery through a puncture or cutdown procedure and, guided by fluoroscopy, the catheter is advanced retrograde through the aorta into the coronary artery orifices and left ventricle. Contrast is then injected into the ventricle, permitting radiographic visualization of the ventricle and coronary arteries and filming (cineangiography) of heart activity.

Catheterization of the right side of the heart assesses tricuspid valve and pulmonic valve functions and pulmonary artery pressures.

In right-heart catheterization, the catheter is inserted into an antecubital vein or into the femoral vein and then advanced through the inferior vena cava or right atrium into the right side of the heart and the pulmonary artery.

Coagulopathy, impaired renal function, or debilitation usually contraindicates catheterization of both heart sides. Unless a temporary pacemaker is inserted to counteract induced ventricular asystole, left bundle-branch block contraindicates catheterization of the right side of the heart.

≫ Key nursing diagnoses and patient outcomes

Use these nursing diagnoses as a guide when developing your plan of care for a patient undergoing a cardiac catheterization.

Activity intolerance related to decreased cardiac output
Based on this nursing diagnosis, you'll establish the following patient outcomes. The patient will:
• maintain blood pressure, pulse, and respiratory rates within prescribed limits during activity.
• demonstrate daily energy-conservation skills at tolerance level.

Knowledge deficit related to heart disease and diagnostic testing
Based on this nursing diagnosis, you'll establish the following patient outcomes. The patient will:
• communicate a need to know.
• state or demonstrate understanding of what has been taught.

Cardiac catheterization: Two approaches

The catheter is inserted through veins to the inferior vena cava and to the right atrium and ventricle for right-side catheterization, and through arteries to the aorta and into the coronary artery orifices or the left ventricle for left-side catheterization. Note that both approaches use the antecubital and femoral vessels.

Right heart

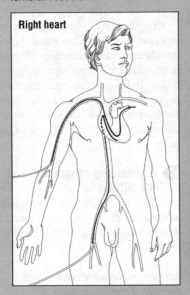

Left heart

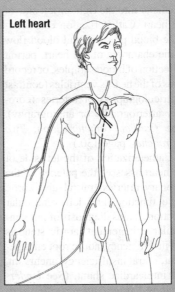

• state intention to make changes in lifestyle, including seeking help from a health professional when needed.

Patient preparation
• Explain that this test evaluates the function of the heart and its vessels.
• Instruct him to restrict food and fluids for at least 6 hours before the test but to continue his prescribed drug regimen unless directed otherwise.
• Describe the test, including who will perform it, where it will take place, and its duration (2 to 3 hours).
• Inform the patient that he may receive a mild sedative but will remain conscious during the procedure. He'll be strapped to a padded table, and the table may be tilted so his heart can be examined from different angles.
• Warn him that the catheterization team will wear gloves, masks, and gowns to protect him from infection and that the changing X-ray plates and advancing film will make clacking noises.
• Inform him he'll have an I.V. needle inserted in his arm to allow administration of medication.
• Assure him that the electrocardiography (ECG) electrodes attached to

Understanding cardiac catheterization findings

Cardiac catheterization provides information on pressures in the heart's chambers and vessels. Higher pressures than normal are clinically significant; lower pressures, except in shock, usually aren't significant.

Cardiac catheterization also provides data used to determine the injection fraction, a comparison of the amount of blood ejected from the left ventricle during systole with the amount of blood remaining in the left ventricle at the end of diastole. A normal ejection fraction (60% to 70%) is a good indicator for successful cardiac surgery.

Normal findings

Cardiac catheterization should reveal no abnormalities of heart chamber size or configuration, wall motion or thickness, direction of blood flow, or valve motion. The coronary arteries should have a smooth and regular outline.

Abnormal findings

• In *coronary artery disease,* catheterization shows constriction of the lumen of the coronary arteries. Constriction greater than 70% is especially significant. Narrowing of the left main coronary artery and occlusion or narrowing high in the left anterior descending artery is often an indication of the need for revascularization surgery.

• Impaired wall motion can indicate *myocardial incompetence* from coronary artery disease, aneurysm, cardiomyopathy, or congenital anomalies. Comparing the size of the left ventricle in systole and diastole helps assess the efficiency of cardiac muscle contraction, segmental wall motion, chamber size, and ejection fraction.

• *Valvular heart disease* is indicated by a gradient, or difference, in pressures above and below a heart valve. The higher the gradient, the greater the stenosis.

• *Septal defects* (atrial and ventricular) can be confirmed by measuring blood oxygen content in both sides of the heart. Elevated blood oxygen on the right side indicates a left-to-right atrial or ventricular shunt; decreased oxygen on the left side indicates a right-to-left shunt.

Measuring cardiac output

Cardiac output can be measured by analyzing blood oxygen levels in the cardiac chambers. This may be accomplished by drawing blood from cardiac chambers or by injecting contrast medium into the venous circulation and measuring its concentration as it moves past a thermodilution catheter.

---

his chest during the procedure will cause no discomfort.

• Tell him the catheter will be inserted into an artery or a vein in his arm or leg; if the skin above the vessel is hairy, it will be shaved and cleaned with antiseptic.

• Explain he'll experience a transient stinging sensation when a local anesthetic is injected to numb the incision site for catheter insertion and that he may feel pressure as the catheter moves along the blood vessel; assure him these sensations are normal.

• Inform him that injection of a contrast medium through the catheter can produce a hot flushing sensation or nausea, but that will quickly pass; instruct him to follow directions to cough or breathe deeply.

• Explain that he'll be given medication if he experiences chest pain during the procedure and that he may also receive nitroglycerin periodically to dilate coronary vessels and aid visualization.

• Assure him that complications, such as myocardial infarction and thromboembolism, are rare.

• Make sure the patient or a responsible family member has signed a consent form.

• Check the patient's history for hypersensitivity to shellfish, iodine, or contrast media used in other diagnostic tests, and notify the doctor of any hypersensitivities.

• If the patient is scheduled for catheterization of the right side of the heart, discontinue any anticoagulant therapy to reduce the risk of complications from venous bleeding.

• If he's scheduled for catheterization of the left side of the heart, begin or continue anticoagulant therapy to reduce the risk of arterial catheter-tip clotting.

• Just before the procedure, tell the patient to void and to put on a hospital gown.

Implementation

• Place the patient in a supine position on a tilt-top table and secure him with restraints.

• Apply ECG leads for continuous monitoring.

• An I.V. line, if not already in place, is started, with dextrose 5% in water or normal saline solution at a keep-vein-open rate.

• After a local anesthetic is injected at the catheterization site, a small incision or percutaneous puncture is made into the artery or vein, and the catheter is passed through the needle into the vessel; the catheter is guided to the cardiac chambers or coronary arteries using fluoroscopy.

• When the catheter is in place, the contrast medium is injected through it.

• The patient may be asked to cough or breathe deeply to help counteract nausea or light-headedness caused by the contrast medium or to correct arrhythmias produced by the medium's depressant effect on the myocardium. Deep breathing can also ease placement of the catheter into the pulmonary artery or the wedge position and moves the diaphragm downward, making the heart easier to see.

• During the procedure, the patient may be given nitroglycerin to eliminate catheter-induced spasm or measure its effect on the coronary arteries. Ergonovine maleate, a vasoconstrictor, may be administered to provoke coronary artery spasm (a risky but valuable test in Prinzmetal's angina).

• Monitor heart rate and rhythm, respiration, pulse rate, and blood pressure frequently during the procedure.

• When the procedure is over, the catheter is removed, and a pressure dressing is applied to the incision site.

• Monitor vital signs every 15 minutes for the first hour after the procedure, then every hour until stable. If unstable, check every 5 minutes and notify the doctor.

• Observe the insertion site for hematoma or blood loss, and reinforce the pressure dressing as needed.
• Check the patient's color, skin temperature, and peripheral pulse below the puncture site every 15 minutes for the first hour. Once the patient is stable, check every hour.
• Enforce bed rest for 8 hours. If the femoral route was used for catheter insertion, keep the patient's leg extended for 6 to 8 hours; if the antecubital fossa was used, keep the patient's arm extended for at least 3 hours.

Complications
• Complications of cardiac catheterization may include endocarditis, arrhythmia, bleeding, and insertion-site hematoma.

Nursing considerations
• If medications were withheld before the test, check with the doctor about resuming administration.
• Administer prescribed analgesics.
• Unless the patient is scheduled for surgery, encourage intake of fluids high in potassium such as orange juice to counteract the diuretic effect of the contrast medium.
• Make sure a posttest ECG is scheduled to check for possible myocardial damage.
• If the patient has valvular heart disease, prophylactic antimicrobial therapy may be indicated to guard against subacute bacterial endocarditis.

Documentation
• Prepare the patient for the test and document any teaching you've done about the test itself and any follow-up care associated with it.

• Be sure to document the administration or withholding of drugs and preparations, special diets, and food or fluid restrictions.

Carbon dioxide monitoring, end-tidal

End-tidal carbon dioxide ($ETCO_2$) monitoring determines the carbon dioxide (CO_2) concentration in exhaled gas. In this technique, a photodetector measures the amount of infrared light absorbed by airway gas during inspiration and expiration. (Light absorption increases along with the CO_2 concentration.) A monitor converts this data to a CO_2 value and a corresponding waveform, or capnogram, if capnography is used. (See *How ETCO_2 monitoring works*, page 134.)

$ETCO_2$ monitoring provides information about the patient's pulmonary, cardiac, and metabolic status, which aids patient management and helps prevent clinical compromise. This technique has become a standard care measure during anesthesia administration and mechanical ventilation.

The sensor, which contains an infrared light source and a photodetector, is positioned at one of two sites in the monitoring setup. With a mainstream monitor, it is positioned directly at the patient's airway with an airway adapter, between the endotracheal (ET) tube and the breathing circuit tubing. With a sidestream monitor, the airway adapter is positioned at the airway (whether or not the patient is intubated) *to allow aspiration of gas from the patient's airway back*

How ETCO$_2$ monitoring works

The optical portion of an end-tidal carbon dioxide (ETCO$_2$) monitor contains an infrared light source, a sample chamber, a special carbon dioxide (CO$_2$) filter, and a photodetector. The infrared light passes through the sample chamber and is absorbed in varying amounts, depending on the amount of CO$_2$ the patient has just exhaled. The photodetector measures CO$_2$ content and relays this information to the microprocessor in the monitor, which displays the CO$_2$ value and waveform.

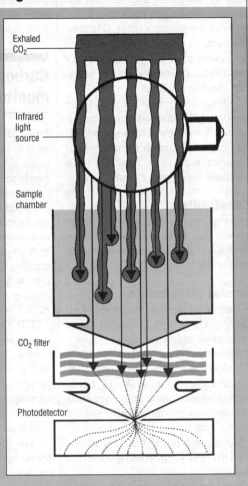

to the sensor, which lies either within or close to the monitor.

Some CO$_2$ detection devices provide semiquantitative indications of CO$_2$ concentrations, supplying an approximate range, rather than a specific value, for ETCO$_2$. Other devices simply indicate whether CO$_2$ is present during exhalation. (See Colorimetric ETCO$_2$ detection.)

For a patient with a stable acid-base balance, ETCO$_2$ monitoring may be used to aid mechanical ventilation weaning. It also reduces the need for frequent arterial blood gas (ABG) measurements, especially when combined with pulse oximetry.

Other uses for $ETCO_2$ monitoring include assessing resuscitation efforts and identifying the return of spontaneous circulation. Because no CO_2 is exhaled when breathing stops, this technique also detects apnea.

When used during ET intubation, $ETCO_2$ monitoring can avert neurologic injury and death by confirming correct ET-tube placement and detecting accidental esophageal intubation, because CO_2 isn't normally produced by the stomach. Ongoing $ETCO_2$ monitoring throughout intubation also can prove valuable because an ET tube may become dislodged during manipulation or patient movement or transport.

≫ Key nursing diagnoses and patient outcomes

Use these nursing diagnoses as a guide when developing your plan of care for a patient who needs end-tidal carbon dioxide monitoring.

Impaired gas exchange related to (specify)

Based on this nursing diagnosis, you'll establish the following patient outcomes. The patient will:
• maintain adequate ventilation.
• have ABG levels within acceptable limits (specify).

Dysfunctional ventilatory weaning response related to (specify)

Based on this nursing diagnosis, you'll establish the following patient outcomes. The patient will:
• maintain respiratory rate within plus or minus 5 breaths/minute of baseline during weaning period.

TECHNOLOGY UPDATE

Colorimetric ETCO₂ detection

A recent innovation in end-tidal carbon dioxide ($ETCO_2$) monitoring, colorimetric $ETCO_2$ detection uses a disposable device that changes color to signal the presence of carbon dioxide in the airway. On exhalation, a color change from purple to yellow or tan reveals the approximate $ETCO_2$ concentration. Color changes may occur for up to 2 hours of monitoring.

Colorimetric $ETCO_2$ detectors are commonly available in code carts, intubation kits, and emergency transport vehicles. They can be used for any intubated patient, especially if electronic $ETCO_2$ monitoring is unavailable.

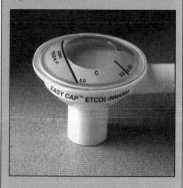

• stabilize mental and emotional states as ventilatory support is gradually withdrawn.

Equipment

♦ mainstream or sidestream CO_2 monitor ♦ CO_2 sensor ♦ airway adapter, as recommended by the manufacturer (a neonatal adapter may have a much smaller dead space, making it appropriate for a smaller patient).

Equipment preparation
• If the monitor you're using isn't self-calibrating, calibrate it as the manufacturer directs.
• If you're using a sidestream CO_2 monitor, be sure to replace the water trap between patients, if directed. *The trap allows humidity from exhaled gases to be condensed into an attached container.* Newer sidestream models don't require water traps.

Implementation
• If the patient requires ET intubation, an $ETCO_2$ detector or monitor is usually applied immediately after the tube is inserted. If he doesn't require intubation or is already intubated and alert, explain the purpose and expected duration of monitoring.
• Tell an intubated patient that the monitor will painlessly measure the amount of carbon dioxide he exhales.
• Inform a nonintubated patient that the monitor will track his carbon dioxide concentration to be sure his breathing is effective.
• Wash your hands.
• After turning on the monitor and calibrating it (if necessary), position the airway adapter and sensor as the manufacturer directs. For an intubated patient, position the adapter directly on the ET tube. For a nonintubated patient, place the adapter at or near the patient's airway. (An oxygen-delivery cannula may have a sample port through which gas can be aspirated for monitoring.)
• Turn on all alarms and adjust alarm settings, as appropriate for your patient.

• Make sure the alarm volume is loud enough to hear.

Complications
• Inaccurate measurements, such as from poor sampling technique, calibration drift, contamination of optics with moisture or secretions, or equipment malfunction, can lead to misdiagnosis and improper treatment.

Nursing considerations
• Be sure to wear gloves when handling the airway adapter to prevent cross-contamination.
• Make sure the adapter is changed with every breathing circuit and ET tube change.
• Place the adapter on the ET tube to avoid contaminating exhaled gases with fresh gas flow from the ventilator.
• If you're using a heat-and-moisture exchanger, you may be able to position the airway adapter between the exchanger and breathing circuit.
• If your patient's $ETCO_2$ values differ from his partial pressure of arterial carbon dioxide values, assess him for factors that can influence $ETCO_2$, especially when the differential between arterial and $ETCO_2$ values (the a-$ADCO_2$ value) is above normal.
• Interpreting the a-$ADCO_2$ value correctly will provide useful information about your patient's state. For example, an increased a-$ADCO_2$ value may mean your patient has worsening dead space, especially if his tidal volume remains constant.
• Remember that $ETCO_2$ monitoring doesn't replace ABG measurements because it doesn't assess oxygenation or blood pH. Supplementing $ETCO_2$ monitoring with pulse oximetry may provide more complete information.

• In a nonintubated patient, use $ETCO_2$ values to establish trends. Be aware that in this patient, exhaled gas is more likely to mix with ambient air, and exhaled CO_2 may be diluted by fresh gas flow from the nasal cannula.

• $ETCO_2$ monitoring is usually discontinued when the patient has been weaned effectively from mechanical ventilation or when he's no longer at risk for respiratory compromise. Carefully assess your patient's tolerance for weaning. After extubation, continuous $ETCO_2$ monitoring may detect the need for reintubation.

Documentation

• Document the initial $ETCO_2$ value and all ventilator settings. Describe the waveform, if one appears on the monitor. If the monitor has a printer, you may want to print out a sample waveform and include it in the patient's medical record.

• Document $ETCO_2$ values at least as often as vital signs, whenever significant changes in waveform or your patient's state occur, and before and after weaning, respiratory, and other interventions.

• Obtain ABG samples for analysis as the patient's condition dictates, and document corresponding $ETCO_2$ values.

Cardiac monitoring

Because it allows continuous observation of the heart's electrical activity, cardiac monitoring is used on patients with conduction disturbances or those at risk for life-threatening arrhythmias.

Like other forms of electrocardiography (ECG), cardiac monitoring uses electrodes placed on the patient's chest to transmit electrical signals that are converted into a tracing of cardiac rhythm on an oscilloscope.

Two types of monitoring may be performed: hardwire or telemetry.

In *hardwire monitoring*, the patient is connected to a monitor at bedside. The rhythm display appears at bedside, but it may also be transmitted to a console at a remote location.

Telemetry uses a small transmitter connected to the ambulatory patient to send electrical signals to a monitor screen for display. Battery-powered and portable, telemetry frees the patient from cumbersome wires and cables and lets him move comfortably and be safely isolated from occasional electrical leakage and accidental hardwire-monitoring electric shock. Telemetry is especially useful for monitoring arrhythmias that occur during sleep, rest, exercise, or stress. Unlike hardwire monitoring, however, telemetry can monitor only cardiac rate and rhythm.

Regardless of the type, cardiac monitors can display the patient's heart rate and rhythm, produce a printed record of cardiac rhythm, and sound an alarm if the patient's heart rate rises above or falls below specified limits. Monitors also recognize and count abnormal heartbeats and changes. For example, a relatively new technique, ST-segment monitoring, helps detect myocardial ischemia, electrolyte imbalance, coronary artery spasm, and hypoxic events. The ST segment represents early ventricular repolarization, and any changes in this waveform component reflect alterations in myocardial oxygenation. Any monitoring lead that views an ischemic heart region will reveal ST-segment changes. The monitor's software establishes a template of the patient's normal QRST pattern from the selected leads; then the monitor displays ST-segment changes. Some monitors display such changes continuously, others only on command.

≫ Key nursing diagnoses and patient outcomes

Use these nursing diagnoses as a guide when developing your plan of care.

Altered cardiopulmonary tissue perfusion related to (specify)

Based on this nursing diagnosis, you'll establish the following patient outcomes. The patient will:
• attain hemodynamic stability: pulse not less than (specify) beats/minute and not more than (specify) beats/minute; blood pressure not less than (specify) mm Hg and not more than (specify) mm Hg.
• not exhibit arrhythmias.
• have his heart rate remain within prescribed limits while he carries out activities of daily living.

Decreased cardiac output related to (specify)

Based on this nursing diagnosis, you'll establish the following patient outcomes. The patient will:
• exhibit no pedal edema.
• experience a diminished heart workload.
• maintain adequate cardiac output.

Equipment

For hardwire monitoring: ♦ cardiac monitor ♦ leadwires ♦ patient cable ♦ disposable pregelled electrodes (number of electrodes varies from three to five, depending on patient's needs) ♦ alcohol sponges ♦ $4'' \times 4''$ gauze pads ♦ optional: shaving supplies, washcloth.

For telemetry: ♦ transmitter ♦ transmitter pouch ♦ telemetry battery pack ♦ leads ♦ electrodes.

Equipment preparation
For hardwire monitoring

• Plug the cardiac monitor into an electrical outlet and turn it on to warm up the unit while you prepare the equipment and the patient.
• Insert the cable into the appropriate socket in the monitor.
• Connect the leadwires to the cable. In some systems, the leadwires are permanently secured to the cable. Each leadwire should indicate the location for attachment to the patient: right arm, left arm, right leg, left leg, chest, and ground. This information should appear on the leadwire, if it's permanently connected — or at the connection of the leadwires and cable to the patient. Then connect an electrode to each of the leadwires, carefully checking that each leadwire is in its correct outlet.

For telemetry

• Insert a new battery into the transmitter. Be sure to match the poles on the battery with the polar markings on the transmitter case. By pressing the button at the top of the unit, test the battery's charge and test the unit to ensure that the battery is operational. If the leadwires aren't permanently affixed to the telemetry unit, attach them securely. If they must be attached individually, be sure to connect each one to the correct outlet.

Implementation

• Explain the procedure to the patient, provide privacy, and ask the patient to expose his chest. Wash your hands.

• Determine electrode positions on the patient's chest, based on the system and lead you're using. (See *Creating monitoring leads*, pages 140 and 141.)

• If the leadwires and patient cable aren't permanently attached, verify that the electrode placement corresponds to the label on the patient cable.

• If necessary for applying monitor leads to a man, shave an area about 4″ (10 cm) in diameter around each electrode site. Clean the area with an alcohol sponge and dry it completely *to remove skin secretions that may interfere with electrode function.* Gently abrade the dried area by rubbing it briskly until it reddens *to remove dead skin cells and to promote better electrical contact with living cells.* (Some electrodes have a small, rough patch for abrading the skin; otherwise, use a dry washcloth or a dry gauze pad.)

• Remove the backing from the electrode, which comes with gel applied. Check the gel for moistness. If it's dry, discard it and replace it with a fresh electrode.

• Apply the electrode to the site and press firmly *to ensure a tight seal.* Repeat with the remaining electrodes.

• When all the electrodes are in place, check for a tracing on the cardiac monitor and assess the quality of the ECG reading. (See *Troubleshooting cardiac monitor problems*, pages 142 and 143.)

• To verify that each beat is being detected by the monitor, compare the digital heart rate display with your count of the patient's heart rate.

• If necessary, use the gain control to adjust the size of the rhythm tracing, and the position control to adjust the waveform position on the recording paper.

• Set the upper and lower limits of the heart rate alarm, based on unit policy. Turn the alarm on.

For telemetry

• Wash your hands.

• Explain the procedure to the patient and provide privacy.

• Expose the patient's chest and select the lead arrangement.

• Remove the backing from one of the gelled electrodes.

• Check the gel for moistness. If it's dry, discard the electrode and obtain a new one.

• Apply the electrode to the appropriate site by pressing one side of the electrode against the patient's skin, pulling gently, and then pressing the other side against the skin. Press your fingers in a circular motion around the electrode *to fix the gel and stabilize the electrode. Repeat for each electrode.*

• Attach an electrode to the end of each leadwire.

• Place the transmitter in the pouch. Tie the pouch strings around the patient's neck and waist, making sure that the pouch fits snugly without causing him discomfort. If no pouch is available, place the transmitter in the patient's bathrobe pocket.

• Check the patient's waveform for clarity, position, and size. Adjust the gain and baseline, as needed. (If necessary, ask the patient to remain rest-

Creating monitoring leads

This chart shows the correct electrode positions for some of the monitoring leads you'll use most often. For each lead, you'll see electrode placement for a five-leadwire system, a three-leadwire system, and a telemetry system.

In the two hardwire systems, the electrode positions for one lead may be identical to the electrode positions for another lead. In this case, you simply change the lead selector switch to the setting that corresponds to the lead you want. In some cases, you'll need to reposition the electrodes.

In the telemetry system, you can create the same lead with two electrodes that you do with three, simply by eliminating the ground electrode.

The chart uses these abbreviations: RA, right arm; LA, left arm; RL, right leg; LL, left leg; C, chest; and G, ground.

FIVE-LEADWIRE SYSTEM	THREE-LEADWIRE SYSTEM	TELEMETRY SYSTEM

Lead I

Lead II

Lead III

Lead MCL$_1$

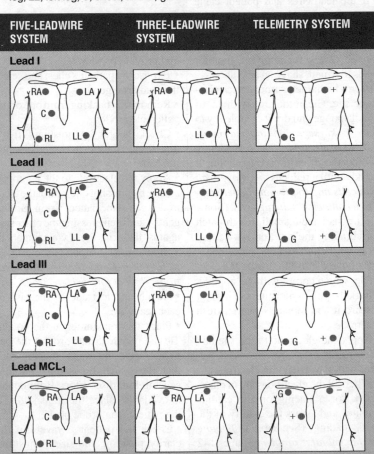

Creating monitoring leads (continued)

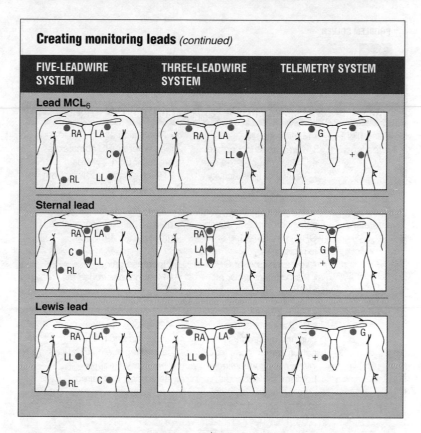

| FIVE-LEADWIRE SYSTEM | THREE-LEADWIRE SYSTEM | TELEMETRY SYSTEM |

ing or sitting in his room while you locate his telemetry monitor at the central station.)
• To obtain a rhythm strip, press the RECORD key at the central station.
• Label the strip with the patient's name, room number, date, and time.
• Identify the rhythm.
• Place the rhythm strip in the appropriate location in the patient's chart.

Nursing considerations
• Make sure all electrical equipment and outlets are grounded *to avoid electric shock and interference (artifacts).*
• Also ensure that the patient is clean and dry *to prevent electric shock.*

• Avoid opening the electrode packages until just before using them *to prevent the gel from drying.*
• Avoid placing the electrodes on bony prominences, hairy areas, areas where defibrillator pads will be placed, or areas for chest compression.
• If the patient's skin is exceptionally oily, scaly, or diaphoretic, rub the electrode site with a dry 4″ × 4″ gauze pad before applying the electrode *to help reduce interference in the tracing.*
• During the procedure, ask the patient to breathe normally. If his respirations distort the recording, ask him

PROBLEM SOLVER

Troubleshooting cardiac monitor problems

PROBLEM	POSSIBLE CAUSES	SOLUTIONS
False high-rate alarm	• Monitor interpreting large T waves as QRS complexes, which doubles the rate • Skeletal muscle activity	• Reposition electrodes to lead where QRS complexes are taller than T waves. • Place electrodes away from major muscle masses.
False low-rate alarm	• Shift in electrical axis from patient movement, making QRS complexes too small to register • Low amplitude of QRS • Poor contact between electrode and skin	• Reapply electrodes. Set gain so height of complex is greater than 1 millivolt. • Increase gain. • Reapply electrodes.
Low amplitude	• Gain dial set too low • Poor contact between skin and electrodes; dried gel; broken or loose leadwires; poor connection between patient and monitor; malfunctioning monitor; physiologic loss of QRS amplitude	• Increase gain. • Check connections on all leadwires and monitoring cable. Replace electrode as necessary. Reapply electrodes, if required.
Wandering baseline	• Poor position or contact between electrodes and skin • Thoracic movement with respirations	• Reposition or replace electrodes. • Reposition electrodes.
Artifact (waveform interference)	• Patient having seizures, chills, or anxiety • Patient movement • Electrodes applied improperly • Static electricity,	• Notify doctor and treat patient as ordered. Keep patient warm and reassure him. • Help patient relax. • Check electrodes and reapply, if necessary. • Make sure cables don't have exposed connectors. Change static-causing bedclothes.

Troubleshooting cardiac monitor problems *(continued)*

PROBLEM	POSSIBLE CAUSES	SOLUTIONS
Artifact *(continued)*	• Electrical short circuit in leadwires or cable	• Replace broken equipment. Use stress loops when applying leadwires.
	• Interference from decreased room humidity	• Regulate humidity to 40%.
Broken leadwires or cable	• Stress loops not used on leadwires	• Replace leadwires and retape them, using stress loops.
	• Cables and leadwires cleaned with alcohol or acetone, causing brittleness	• Clean cable and leadwires with soapy water. *Do not allow cable ends to become wet.* Replace cable as necessary.
60-cycle interference (fuzzy baseline)	• Electrical interference from other equipment in room	• Attach all electrical equipment to common ground. Check plugs to make sure prongs aren't loose.
	• Patient's bed improperly grounded	• Attach bed ground to the room's common ground.
Skin excoriation under electrode	• Patient allergic to electrode adhesive	• Remove electrodes and apply hypoallergenic electrodes and hypoallergenic tape.
	• Electrode on skin too long	• Remove electrode, clean site, and reapply electrode at new site.

to hold his breath briefly *to reduce baseline wander in the tracing.*
• Assess skin integrity and reposition the electrodes every 24 hours, or as necessary.
• If the patient is being monitored by telemetry, show him how the transmitter works.
• If applicable, show him the button that will produce a recording of his ECG at the central station.
• Teach him how to push the button whenever he has symptoms. *This causes the central console to print a rhythm strip.*
• Tell the patient to remove the transmitter if he takes a shower or bath, but stress that he must let you know when he is going to remove the unit.

Home care
• If cardiac monitoring will continue after the patient's discharge, document which caregivers can interpret dangerous rhythms and can perform cardiopulmonary resuscitation.

• Teach troubleshooting techniques to use if the monitor malfunctions.

Documentation
• Record the date and time that monitoring begins and the monitoring lead in your notes.
• Document a rhythm strip at least every 8 hours with any changes in the patient's condition (or as stated by hospital policy).
• Label the rhythm strip with the patient's name and room number and the date and time.
• Document any changes in the patient's condition.
• Document your teaching efforts or referrals, such as to equipment suppliers.

Cardiac output measurement

Measuring a patient's cardiac output — the amount of blood ejected by the heart — helps evaluate cardiac function. The preferred measurement technique is bolus thermodilution. Other means include the Fick method and the dye dilution method.

Thermodilution uses cold as the indicator. Because the thermodilution technique can be performed at the patient's bedside, it's the most practical way to evaluate the cardiac state of critically ill patients or of people believed to have cardiac disease.

To measure cardiac output, a quantity of solution colder than the patient's blood is injected into the right atrium via a port on a pulmonary artery (PA) catheter. This indicator solution mixes with the blood as it trav-

els through the right ventricle into the pulmonary artery, and a thermistor on the catheter registers the change in temperature of the flowing blood. A computer then plots the temperature change over time as a curve and calculates flow based on the area under the curve.

Iced or room-temperature injectate may be used. Choose according to hospital policy and patient status. Accuracy of the bolus thermodilution technique depends on the computer differentiating between the temperature change caused by the injectate in the pulmonary artery and the temperature changes in the pulmonary artery. Because iced injectate is colder than room-temperature injectate, it provides a stronger signal to be detected.

Typically, however, room-temperature injectate is more convenient and provides equally accurate measurements. Iced injectate may be more accurate in patients with high or low cardiac outputs or hypothermia, or when smaller volumes of injectate (3 to 5 ml) must be used, such as in patients with volume restrictions or in children.

≫ Key nursing diagnoses and patient outcomes
Use these nursing diagnoses as a guide when developing a plan of care.

Decreased cardiac output related to reduced stroke volume
Based on this nursing diagnosis, you'll establish the following patient outcomes. The patient will:
• maintain hemodynamic stability: pulse not less than (specify) and not greater than (specify); blood pressure not less than (specify) and not greater than (specify).

• exhibit no signs of arrhythmias.
• not complain of chest pain, dizziness, or syncope.

Altered cardiopulmonary tissue perfusion related to decreased cellular exchange
Based on this nursing diagnosis, you'll establish the following patient outcomes. The patient will:
• maintain adequate cardiac output.
• have clear breath sounds on auscultation.
• have arterial blood gas results within normal limits.

Equipment
For thermodilution: ♦ thermodilution PA catheter in position ♦ output computer and cables (or a module for the bedside cardiac monitor) ♦ closed or open injectate delivery system ♦ 10-ml syringe ♦ 500-ml bag of dextrose 5% in water or normal saline solution ♦ crushed ice and water (if the iced injectate is used). (See *Closed injectate delivery system*, page 146.)

The newer bedside cardiac monitors measure cardiac output continuously, using either an invasive or a noninvasive method. If your bedside monitor doesn't have this capability, you'll need a freestanding cardiac output computer.

Equipment preparation
• Wash your hands thoroughly.
• Assemble the equipment at the patient's bedside.
• Insert the closed injectate system tubing into the 500-ml bag of I.V. solution.
• Connect the 10-ml syringe to the system tubing and prime the tubing with I.V. solution until it's free of air.

Then clamp the tubing. The steps that follow differ, depending on whether you're using a room-temperature or an iced-injectate delivery system.

Room-temperature injectate closed-delivery system
• After clamping the tubing, connect the primed system to the stopcock of the proximal injectate lumen of the PA catheter.
• Connect the temperature probe from the cardiac output computer to the closed injectate system's flow-through housing device.
• Connect the cardiac output computer cable to the thermistor connector on the PA catheter, and verify the blood temperature reading.
• Finally, turn on the cardiac output computer and enter the correct computation constant, as provided by the catheter's manufacturer. The constant is determined by the volume and temperature of the injectate and the size and type of catheter. (With children, you'll need to adjust the computation constant to reflect a smaller volume and a smaller catheter size.)

Iced-injectate closed-delivery system
• After clamping the tubing, place the coiled segment into the plastic foam container and add crushed ice and water to cover the entire coil.
• Let the solution cool for 15 to 20 minutes. The rest of the steps are the same as those for the room-temperature injectate closed-delivery system.

Implementation
• Make sure your patient is in a comfortable position.

Closed injectate delivery system

This illustration shows the equipment needed to measure cardiac output, using a closed injectate delivery system. First, an iced or room-temperature solution is injected into the proximal or right atrial port of the pulmonary artery catheter.

A computer then calculates the cardiac output from temperature changes in the injected material in the proximal lumen and from the temperature at the pulmonary artery, which is measured by the thermistor on the catheter tip. The computer displays the cardiac output as a digital readout.

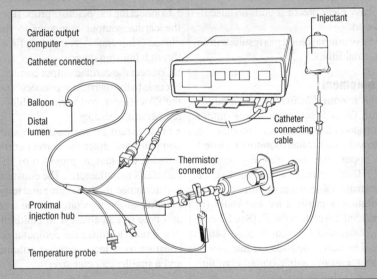

Cardiac output computer

Catheter connector

Balloon

Distal lumen

Thermistor connector

Proximal injection hub

Temperature probe

Injectant

Catheter connecting cable

• Advise him not to move during the procedure *because movement can cause an error in measurement.*
• Explain that the procedure will help determine how well his heart is pumping and that he will feel no discomfort.

To use an iced-injectate closed-delivery system
• Unclamp the I.V. tubing and withdraw 5 ml of solution into the syringe. (With children, use 3 ml or less.)
• Inject the solution to flow past the temperature sensor while observing the injectate temperature that registers on the computer. The injectate temperature is between 43° and 54° F (6° and 12° C).
• Verify presence of a PA waveform on the cardiac monitor.
• Withdraw exactly 10 ml of cooled solution before reclamping the tubing.
• Turn the stopcock at the catheter injectate hub *to open a fluid path between the injectate lumen of the PA catheter and syringe.*

• Press the START button on the cardiac output computer or wait for the INJECT message to flash.
• Inject the solution smoothly within 4 seconds, making sure it doesn't leak at the connectors.
• If available, analyze the contour of the thermodilution washout curve on a strip-chart recorder for a rapid upstroke and a gradual, smooth return to baseline.
• Wait 1 minute between injections and repeat the procedure until three values are within 10% to 15% of the median value. Compute the average, and record the patient's cardiac output.
• Return the stopcock to its original position and make sure the injectate delivery system tubing is clamped.
• Verify the presence of a PA waveform on the cardiac monitor.

To use a room-temperature injectate closed-delivery system

• Verify the presence of a PA waveform on the cardiac monitor.
• Unclamp the I.V. tubing and withdraw exactly 10 ml of solution. Reclamp the tubing.
• Turn the stopcock at the catheter injectate hub *to open a fluid path between the injectate lumen of the PA catheter and the syringe.*
• Press the START button on the cardiac output computer or wait for an INJECT message to flash.
• Inject the solution smoothly within 4 seconds, making sure it doesn't leak at the connectors.
• If available, analyze the contour of the thermodilution washout curve on a strip-chart recorder for a rapid upstroke and a gradual, smooth return to the baseline.

• Repeat these steps until three values are within 10% to 15% of the median value.
• Compute the average, and record the patient's cardiac output.
• Return the stopcock to its original position and make sure the injectate delivery system tubing is clamped.
• Verify the presence of a PA waveform on the cardiac monitor.
• Discontinue cardiac output measurements when the patient is hemodynamically stable and weaned from his vasoactive and inotropic medications. You can leave the PA catheter inserted for pressure measurements.
• Disconnect and discard the injectate delivery system and the I.V. bag. Cover any exposed stopcocks with air-occlusive caps.
• Monitor the patient for signs or symptoms of inadequate perfusion, including restlessness, fatigue, changes in level of consciousness, decreased capillary refill time, diminished peripheral pulses, oliguria, and pale, cool skin.

Complications

Possible complications of cardiac output measurement include:
• pneumothorax (typically on catheter insertion)
• sepsis
• thrombus
• vessel or adjacent organ puncture
• air embolism.

Nursing considerations

• Normal cardiac-output range is 4 to 8 liters/minute. The adequacy of a patient's cardiac output is better assessed by calculating cardiac index (CI), adjusted for body size.

• To calculate the patient's CI, divide his cardiac output by his body surface area (BSA), a function of height and weight. For example, a cardiac output of 4 liters/minute might be adequate for a 65″, 120-lb (165-cm, 48-kg) patient (normally a BSA of 1.59 and a CI of 2.5) but would be inadequate for a 74″, 230-lb (188-cm, 93-kg) patient (normally a BSA of 2.26 and a CI of 1.8). The normal CI for adults ranges from 2.5 to 4.2 liters/minute/m^2. (Normal CI for infants and children is 3.5 to 4 liters/minute/m^2, for pregnant women 3.5 to 6.5 liters/minute/m^2, and for elderly adults 2 to 2.5 liters/minute/m^2.)

• Add the fluid volume injected for cardiac output determinations to the patient's total intake. Injectate delivery of 30 ml/hour will contribute 720 ml to the patient's 24-hour intake.

• After cardiac output measurement, make sure the clamp on the injectate bag is secured. *This will prevent inadvertent delivery of the injectate to the patient.*

Documentation

• Document your patient's cardiac output, CI, and other hemodynamic values and vital signs at the time of measurement.

• Note the patient's position during measurement and any other unusual occurrences, such as bradycardia or neurologic changes.

Cardiopulmonary resuscitation, adult

Cardiopulmonary resuscitation (CPR) is used to restore and maintain a pa-

tient's respiration and circulation after his heartbeat and breathing have stopped. CPR is a basic life-support (BLS) procedure performed on victims of cardiac arrest.

Most adults in sudden cardiac arrest develop ventricular fibrillation and require defibrillation; CPR alone does not improve their chances of survival. Because that's the case, you must assess the victim, and then contact emergency medical services (EMS) or call a code *before* starting CPR. Timing is critical. Early access to EMS, early CPR, and early defibrillation greatly improve chances of survival.

In most instances, you perform CPR to keep the patient alive until advanced cardiac life support (ACLS) can begin. Basic CPR procedure consists of assessing the victim, calling for help, and then following the ABC protocol: opening the airway, restoring breathing, and restoring circulation. After the airway has been opened and breathing and circulation have been restored, drug therapy, diagnosis by electrocardiogram (ECG), or defibrillation may follow. CPR is contraindicated in *no code* patients.

≫ Key nursing diagnoses and patient outcomes

Use these nursing diagnoses as a guide when developing your plan of care for a patient who has received CPR.

Altered cardiopulmonary tissue perfusion related to cardiac arrest
Based on this nursing diagnosis, you'll establish the following patient outcomes. The patient will:

• attain hemodynamic stability: pulse not less than (specify) beats/minute

and not greater than __ beats/minute; blood pressure not less than __ mm Hg and not greater than __ mm Hg.
• maintain cardiac output.
• suffer no CPR complications.

Inability to sustain spontaneous ventilation related to (specify)
Based on this nursing diagnosis, you'll establish the following patient outcomes. The patient will:
• have arterial blood gas levels within normal limits.
• have breathing pattern return to baseline.

Equipment
♦ CPR requires no special equipment except a hard surface on which to place the patient.

Implementation
• The following illustrated instructions provide a step-by-step guide for CPR as currently recommended by the American Heart Association (AHA).

One-person rescue
• If you're the sole rescuer, expect to open the patient's airway, check for breathing, assess for circulation, and call for help before beginning compressions.

Open the airway
• Assess the victim to determine whether he's unconscious. Gently shake his shoulders and shout, "Are you okay?" This helps ensure that you don't start CPR on a person who's conscious.
• Check for injuries, particularly to the head or neck. If you suspect a head or neck injury, move him as little as possible to reduce the risk of paralysis.

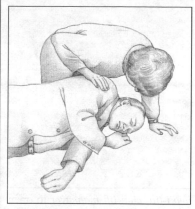

• Call out for help.
• Send someone to contact emergency medical services or call a code, if appropriate.
• Place the victim in a supine position on a hard, flat surface.
• When moving him, roll his head and torso as a unit.
• Avoid twisting or pulling his neck, shoulders, or hips.

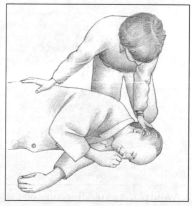

• Kneel near his shoulders to give you easy access to his head and chest.
• In many cases, the muscles controlling the victim's tongue will be relaxed, causing the tongue to obstruct the airway. If the victim doesn't appear to have a neck injury, use the

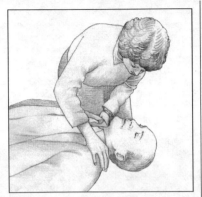

head-tilt, chin-lift maneuver to open his airway. To accomplish this, first place your hand that's closer to the victim's head on his forehead. Then apply firm pressure. The pressure should be firm enough to tilt the victim's head back. Next place the fingertips of your other hand under the bony part of his lower jaw near the chin. Now lift the victim's chin. At the same time, keep his mouth partially open.

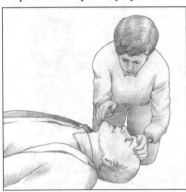

• Avoid placing your fingertips on the soft tissue under the victim's chin *because this maneuver may inadvertently obstruct the airway you're trying to open.*
• If you suspect a neck injury, use the *jaw-thrust maneuver* instead of the *head-tilt, chin-lift maneuver.* Kneel

with your kneecaps pointing toward the top of the victim's head and your elbows on the ground. Rest your thumbs on his lower jaw near the corners of the mouth, pointing your thumbs toward his feet. Then place your fingertips around the lower jaw. To open the airway, lift the lower jaw with your fingertips.

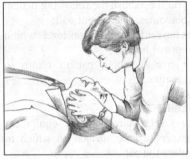

Check for breathing
• While keeping the airway open, place your ear over the victim's mouth and nose and listen for breathing. Note whether his chest rises and falls. You may also feel airflow on your cheek. If he starts to breathe, keep the airway open and continue checking his breathing until help arrives.

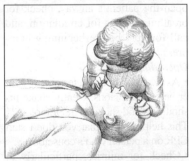

Rescue breathing
• If the victim doesn't start breathing after you open his airway, begin rescue breathing. Pinch his nostrils shut

with the thumb and index finger of the hand you've had on his forehead.

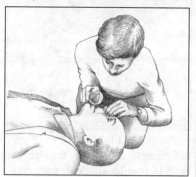

• Take a deep breath and place your mouth over the victim's mouth, creating a tight seal. Give 2 full ventilations, taking a deep breath after each to allow enough time for his chest to expand and relax and to prevent gastric distention. Each ventilation should last $1\frac{1}{2}$ to 2 seconds.

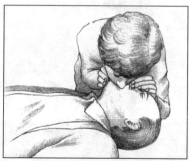

• If the first ventilation isn't successful, reposition the victim's head and try again. If you're still not successful, he may have a foreign-body airway obstruction. Check for loose dentures. If dentures or any other objects are blocking the airway, follow the procedure for clearing an airway obstruction. (See "Airway obstruction management," page 12.)

Assess circulation

• Keep one hand on the victim's forehead so his airway remains open. With your other hand, palpate the carotid artery that's closer to you. To do this, place your index and middle fingers in the groove between the trachea and the sternocleidomastoid muscle. Palpate for 5 to 10 seconds.

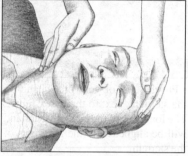

• If you detect a pulse, don't begin chest compressions. Instead, perform rescue breathing by giving the victim 12 ventilations per minute (or one every 5 seconds). After every 12 ventilations, recheck his pulse.
• If there's no pulse, start chest compressions. Make sure your knees are apart for a wide base of support. Using the hand closer to his feet, locate the lower margin of the rib cage and move your fingertips along the margin to the notch where the ribs meet the sternum.

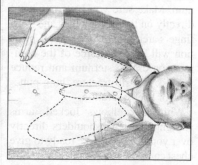

• Place your middle finger on the notch and your index finger next to your middle finger. Your index finger will now be on the bottom of the sternum.

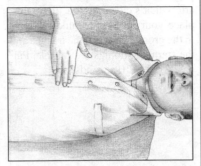

• Put the heel of your other hand on the sternum, next to the index finger. The long axis of the heel of your hand will be aligned with the long axis of the sternum.

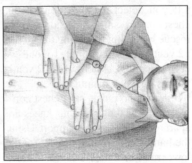

• Take the first hand off the notch and put it on top of the hand on the sternum. Make sure you have one hand directly on top of the other and your fingers aren't on his chest. This position will keep the force of the compression on the sternum and reduce the risk of a rib fracture, lung puncture, or liver laceration.

• With your elbows locked, arms straight, and your shoulders directly over your hands, you're ready to give chest compressions. Using the weight of your upper body, compress the vic-

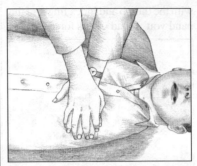

tim's sternum 1 ½" to 2" (3.8 to 5 cm), delivering the pressure through the heels of your hands. After each compression, release the pressure and allow the chest to return to its normal position so that the heart can fill with blood. Don't change your hand position during compressions — you might injure the victim.

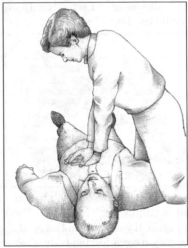

• Give 15 chest compressions at a rate of 80 to 100 per minute. Count, "One and two and three and . . ." up to 15. Open the airway and give 2 ventilations. Then find the proper hand position again and deliver 15 more compressions. Do four complete cycles of 15 compressions and 2 ventilations.

• Palpate the carotid pulse again. If there's still no pulse, continue performing CPR in cycles of 15 compressions and 2 ventilations. Every few minutes, check for breathing and a pulse at the end of a complete cycle of compressions and ventilations. If you detect a pulse but he isn't breathing, give 12 ventilations per minute and monitor his pulse. If he has a pulse and is breathing, monitor his respirations and pulse closely. You should stop performing CPR only when his respirations and pulse return, he's turned over to the EMS, or you're exhausted.

Two-person rescue

If another rescuer arrives while you're giving CPR, follow these steps:

• If the EMS team hasn't arrived, tell the second rescuer to repeat the call for help. If he's not a health care professional, ask him to stand by. Then, if you become fatigued, he can take over one-person CPR.

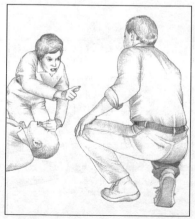

• Have him begin by checking the victim's pulse for 5 seconds after you've given 2 ventilations. If he doesn't feel a pulse, he should give 2 ventilations and begin chest compressions.

• If the rescuer is another health care professional, the two of you can perform two-person CPR. He should start assisting after you've finished a cycle of 15 compressions, 2 ventilations, and a pulse check.

• The second rescuer should get into place opposite you. While you're checking for a pulse, he should be finding the proper hand placement for delivering chest compressions.

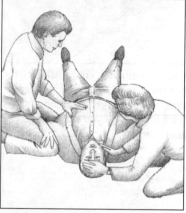

• If you don't detect a pulse, say, "No pulse; continue CPR," and give 1 ventilation. The second rescuer should then begin delivering compressions at a rate of 80 to 100 per minute. Compressions and ventilations should be administered at a ratio of 5 compressions to 1 ventilation. The compressor (at this point, the second rescuer) should count out loud so the ventilator can anticipate when to give ventilations. To ensure that the ventilations are effective, the rescuer performing the chest compressions should stop briefly or at least long enough to observe the victim's chest rise with the air supplied by the rescuer giving ventilations.

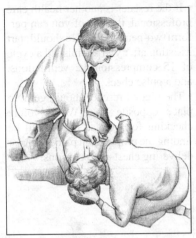

• As the ventilator, you must check for breathing and a pulse. Signal the compressor to stop giving compressions for 5 seconds so you can make these assessments.

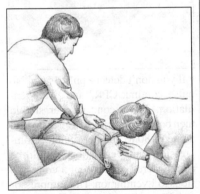

• After a minimum of 10 cycles, the compressor may be tired and call for a switch. When the rescuer is giving a ventilation, the compressor can simply say "change" or "switch." This switch should be done carefully, so that CPR isn't interrupted. You would then give a ventilation and become the compressor by moving down to the victim's chest and placing your hands in the proper position.

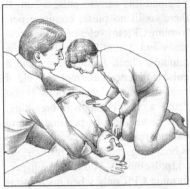

• The second rescuer would become the ventilator and move to the victim's head. He'd check the pulse for 5 seconds. If he found no pulse, he'd say, "No pulse" and give a ventilation. You'd then give compressions at a rate of 80 to 100 per minute, or 5 compressions for each ventilation. Both of you should continue giving CPR until the victim's respirations and pulse return, he's turned over to the EMS, or both of you are exhausted.

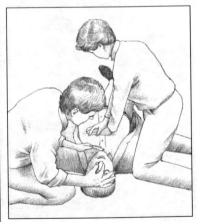

Complications

CPR can cause certain complications, especially if the compressor doesn't

place hands properly on the sternum. Possible complications include:
- gastric distention (a common complication from too much air delivered during ventilation)
- fractured ribs
- lacerated liver
- punctured lungs.

Nursing considerations
- Although acquired human immunodeficiency virus (HIV), which causes AIDS, isn't known to be transmitted in saliva, some health care professionals may hesitate to give rescue breaths, especially if the victim has AIDS or is known to be infected with HIV. For this reason, the AHA recommends that all health care professionals learn how to use disposable airway equipment.
- A second rescuer may instinctively take the victim's pulse without waiting for the end of a cycle. This is *not* part of the AHA's recommendations and may confuse some rescuers. The recommendations are at standardizing rescuers' actions, so time isn't wasted and all efforts help restore respirations and heartbeat.

Documentation
- Whenever you perform CPR, document why you initiated it, whether the victim suffered from cardiac or respiratory arrest, when you found the victim and started CPR, and how long the victim received CPR.
- Note his response and any complications. Also include any interventions taken to correct complications.
- If the victim also received ACLS, document which interventions were performed, who performed them, when they were performed, and what equipment was used.

Cardiopulmonary resuscitation, pediatric

When an adult needs cardiopulmonary resuscitation (CPR), he typically suffers from a primary cardiac disorder or arrhythmia that has stopped his heart. When an infant or child needs CPR, he typically suffers from hypoxia caused by respiratory difficulty or respiratory arrest.

Most pediatric crises requiring CPR are preventable. They include motor vehicle accidents, drowning, burns, smoke inhalation, falls, poisoning, suffocation, and choking (usually from inhaling a plastic bag or small foreign body, such as toys or food). Other causes of cardiopulmonary arrest in children include laryngospasm and edema from upper respiratory infections and sudden infant death syndrome.

In the same way, CPR in adults, children, and infants is aimed at restoring cardiopulmonary function by pumping the victim's heart and ventilating the lungs until natural function resumes. CPR techniques, however, differ depending on whether the patient is an adult, a child, or an infant. (See *Performing infant CPR*, pages 156 and 157.)

For CPR purposes, the American Heart Association defines a patient by age. An infant is under age 1; a child is ages 1 to 8; an adult is over age 8.

Survival chances improve the sooner CPR begins and the faster advanced life support systems are imple-

Performing infant CPR

Although the objective of cardiopulmonary resuscitation (CPR) in an infant is the same as in a child and an adult, the techniques for an infant vary. If bystanders are present, first tell someone to call emergency medical services. If you're alone, perform resuscitation measures for 1 minute; then call for help. You may move an uninjured infant close to a telephone, if necessary.

Clear the airway

• To remove an airway obstruction, place the infant facedown on your forearm, with his head lower than his trunk. Support your forearm on your thigh.

• Use the heel of your free hand to deliver five blows between the infant's shoulder blades. Back blows are safer than abdominal thrusts in infants because of the size of the infant's liver, the close proximity of vital organs, and the poor abdominal muscle tone.

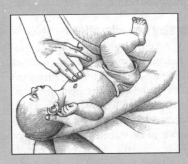

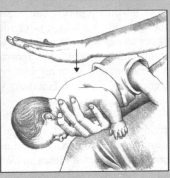

• If the airway remains obstructed, sandwich the infant between your hands and forearms and flip him over onto his back, as shown (top right).

• Keeping the infant's head lower than his trunk, give five midsternal chest thrusts, using your middle and ring fingers only, to raise intrathoracic pressure enough to force a cough that will expel the ob-

struction. Remember to hold the infant's head firmly to avoid injury.

• Repeat this sequence until the obstruction is dislodged or the infant loses consciousness.

Caution: Do not do a blind finger-sweep to discover or remove an obstruction. In an infant, the maneuver may push the object back into the airway and cause further obstruction. Place your fingers in the infant's mouth to remove only an object you can see.

Restore consciousness

• If the infant loses consciousness, position him to open the airway. Deliver two breaths, as described below.

• If he doesn't regain consciousness, reposition his head and try breathing for him again. If this attempt fails, repeat the procedure for removing a foreign object.

• When the foreign object is removed, assess respirations and pulse. Continue revival efforts, if needed.

Performing infant CPR *(continued)*

- Provide ventilation
- Take a breath, and tightly seal your mouth over the infant's nose and mouth.

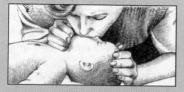

- Deliver a *gentle* puff of air *because an infant's lungs hold less air than an adult's.* If the infant's chest rises and falls, then the amount of air is probably adequate.
- Continue rescue breathing with one breath every 3 seconds (20 breaths/minute) if you can detect a pulse.

Restore heartbeat and circulation

- Assess the infant's pulse by palpating the brachial artery located inside the infant's upper arm between the elbow and the shoulder. If you find a pulse, continue rescue breathing but don't initiate heart compressions.

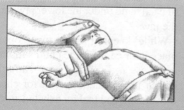

- Begin heart compressions if you find no pulse. To locate the infant's heart, draw an imaginary horizontal line between the infant's nipples. Place three fingers directly below — and perpendicular to — the nipple line. Then lift up your index finger so that the middle and ring fingers lie one finger's width below the nipple line. Use these two fingers to depress the sternum here 1″ to 2″ (1.3 to 2.5 cm) at least 100 compressions/minute.

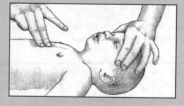

- Supply one breath after every five compressions. Maintain this ratio whether you're the helper or the lone rescuer. This ratio allows for about 100 compressions and 20 breaths/minute for an infant.

mented. But however quickly you begin pediatric CPR, determine whether the patient's respiratory distress results from a mechanical obstruction or an infection, such as epiglottitis or croup, each of which requires imme-

diate medical attention, not CPR. CPR is appropriate only when the child isn't breathing.

≫ Key nursing diagnoses and patient outcomes

Use these nursing diagnoses as a guide when developing your plan of care for a child who has received CPR.

Altered cardiopulmonary tissue perfusion related to (specify)

Based on this nursing diagnosis, you'll establish the following patient outcomes. The patient will:
• maintain hemodynamic stability: pulse not less than (specify) beats/minute and not greater than (specify) beats/minute; blood pressure not less than (specify) mm Hg and not greater than (specify) mm Hg.
• maintain cardiac output.

Ineffective airway clearance related to presence of tracheobronchial obstruction

Based on this nursing diagnosis, you'll establish the following patient outcomes. The patient will:
• cough effectively.
• maintain a patent airway.
• have no adventitious breath sounds.

Equipment

♦ CPR requires no special equipment except a hard surface on which to place the patient.

Implementation

• Gently shake the apparently unconscious child's shoulder and shout at him *to elicit a response.* If the child is conscious but has difficulty breathing, help him into a position that best eases his breathing — if he hasn't naturally assumed this position already.
• Call for help *to alert others and to enlist emergency assistance.* If you're alone and the child isn't breathing,

perform CPR for 1 minute before calling for help.
• Place the child in a supine position on a firm, flat surface (usually the ground). *The surface should provide the resistance needed for adequate heart compression.* If you must turn the child from a prone position, support his head and neck and turn him as a unit *to avoid injuring his spine.*

To establish a patent airway

• Kneel beside the child's shoulder.
• Place one hand on the child's forehead and gently lift his chin with your other hand *to open his airway.* (In infants, this is called the sniffing position.)
• Avoid fingering the soft neck tissue *to avoid obstructing the airway.* Never let the child's mouth close completely.
• If you suspect a neck injury, use the *jaw-thrust maneuver* to open the child's airway *to keep from moving the child's neck.* To do this, kneel at the top of the child's head, with your kneecaps pointing toward it. With your elbows on the ground, rest your thumbs at the corners of the child's mouth, and place two or three fingers of each hand under the lower jaw. Lift the jaw.
• While keeping the airway open, place your ear near the child's mouth and nose *to evaluate his breathing.* Listen for exhalation, look for chest movement, and feel for exhaled air on your cheek.
• If the child is breathing, maintain an open airway and monitor respirations.
• If you suspect that an obstruction is blocking the airway (whether the child's conscious or not), try to clear the airway as you would in an adult with two exceptions: Don't use the

blind finger-sweep maneuver (*which could compound or relodge the obstruction*) and do adjust your technique to the child's size.

To restore ventilation

• If the child isn't breathing, maintain the open airway position and take a breath. Then pinch the child's nostrils shut, and cover the child's mouth with your mouth (top right). Give two slow breaths (1 to 1 ½ seconds/breath), and pause between each.

• If your first attempt at ventilation fails to restore the child's breathing, reposition the child's head to open the airway and try again. If you're still unsuccessful, the airway may be obstructed by a foreign body.

• Repeat the steps for airway clearance.

• Once you free the obstruction, check for breathing and pulse. If absent, proceed with chest compressions.

To restore heartbeat and circulation

• Assess circulation by palpating the carotid artery for a pulse.

• Locate the carotid artery with two or three fingers of one hand. (You'll need the other hand to maintain the head-tilt position that keeps the airway open.) Place your fingers in the center of the child's neck on the side closest to you and slide your fingers into the groove formed by the trachea and the sternocleidomastoid muscles. Palpate the artery for 5 to 10 seconds *to confirm the child's pulse.*

• If you feel the child's pulse, continue rescue breathing, giving one breath every 3 seconds (20 breaths/minute).

• If you can't feel a pulse, begin cardiac compressions.

• Kneel next to the child's chest. Using the hand closest to his feet, locate the lower border of the rib cage on the side nearest you.

• Hold your middle and index fingers together and move them up the rib cage to the notch where the ribs and sternum join. Put your middle finger on the notch and your index finger next to it.

• Lift your hand and place the heel just above the spot where the index finger was. The heel of your hand should be aligned with the long axis of the sternum.

• Using the heel of one hand only, apply enough pressure to compress the child's chest downward 1″ to 1 ½″ (2.5 to 4 cm). Deliver five serial compressions at a rate of 100 compressions/minute.

• After every five compressions, breathe one breath into the child. Deliver one breath for every five compressions whether you're working alone or with a partner.

• After 20 cycles (1 minute) of CPR, feel the pulse for 5 seconds *to detect a heartbeat.* If you can't detect a pulse, continue chest compressions and rescue breathing.

• If you can detect a pulse, check for spontaneous respirations. Without respirations, give one breath every 3 seconds (20 breaths/minute), and continue to monitor the pulse. If the child begins breathing spontaneously, keep the airway open and monitor both the respirations and pulse.

Complications

Possible complications of pediatric CPR include:

• gastric distention (common complication from giving too much air during ventilation)
• fractured ribs
• a lacerated liver
• punctured lungs.

Nursing considerations

• A child's small airway can be easily blocked by his tongue. If this occurs, simply opening the airway may restore breathing.
• Use smooth motions when performing cardiac compressions.
• Keep your fingers off and the heel of your hand on the child's chest at all times.
• Time your motions so the compression and relaxation phases are equal *to promote effective compressions.*
• If the child has difficulty breathing and a parent is present, ask whether the child recently had a fever or an upper respiratory tract infection. If so, suspect epiglottitis. In this instance, do not attempt to manipulate the airway *because laryngospasm may obstruct the airway.* Allow the child to assume a comfortable position and monitor his breathing until help arrives.
• Keep trying to remove an obstruction. As hypoxia develops, the child's muscles will relax, which may allow you to remove the obstruction.
• During resuscitation efforts, make sure someone communicates support and information to the parents.
• If available, a one-way valve mask may be used over the child's nose and mouth when performing CPR.

Documentation

• Document all the events of resuscitation and the names of the individuals present.
• Record whether the child had cardiac or respiratory arrest. Note where the arrest occurred, the time when CPR began, and how long the procedure continued. Note the outcome.
• Note any complications — a fractured rib, bruised mouth, or gastric distention.
• Describe actions taken to correct complications.
• If the child received advanced cardiac life support, document which interventions were performed, who performed them, when they were performed, and what equipment was used.

Cardioversion, synchronized

Used to treat tachyarrhythmias, cardioversion delivers an electric charge to the myocardium at the peak of the R wave. This causes immediate depolarization, interrupting reentry circuits and allowing the sinoatrial node to resume control. Synchronizing the electric charge with the R wave ensures the current won't be delivered on the vulnerable T wave and disrupt repolarization.

Synchronized cardioversion is the treatment of choice for arrhythmias that don't respond to vagal massage or drug therapy, such as atrial tachycardia, atrial flutter, atrial fibrillation, and symptomatic ventricular tachycardia.

Cardioversion may be an elective or urgent procedure, depending on how well the patient tolerates the arrhythmia. For example, if the patient is hemodynamically unstable, he would require urgent cardioversion. Remember, when preparing for cardioversion, the patient's condition can deteriorate quickly, necessitating immediate defibrillation.

Indications for cardioversion include stable paroxysmal atrial tachycardia, unstable paroxysmal supraventricular tachycardia, atrial fibrillation, atrial flutter, and ventricular tachycardia.

≫ Key nursing diagnoses and patient outcomes

Use these nursing diagnoses as a guide when developing your plan of care for a patient who has received synchronized cardioversion.

Altered cardiopulmonary tissue perfusion related to decreased cellular exchange

Based on this nursing diagnosis, you'll establish the following patient outcomes. The patient will:
• attain hemodynamic stability: pulse not less than (specify) beats/minute and not greater than (specify) beats/minute; blood pressure not less than (specify) mm Hg and not greater than (specify) mm Hg.
• not exhibit arrhythmias.
• maintain adequate cardiac output.

Decreased cardiac output related to arrhythmias

Based on this nursing diagnosis, you'll establish the following patient outcomes. The patient will:

• achieve activity within limits of prescribed heart rate.
• have heart's workload diminish.
• exhibit no pedal edema.
• have a balanced intake and output.

Equipment

♦ cardioverter-defibrillator ♦ conductive medium pads ♦ anterior, posterior, or transverse paddles ♦ electrocardiogram (ECG) monitor with recorder ♦ sedative ♦ oxygen therapy equipment ♦ airway ♦ handheld resuscitation bag ♦ emergency pacing equipment ♦ emergency cardiac medications ♦ automatic blood pressure cuff (if available) ♦ pulse oximeter (if available).

Patient preparation

• Explain the procedure to the patient.
• Make sure he's signed a consent form.
• Check the patient's recent serum potassium and magnesium levels and arterial blood gas results.
• Check recent digoxin levels. Although digitalized patients may undergo cardioversion, they tend to require lower energy levels to convert. If the patient takes digoxin, withhold the dose on the day of the procedure.
• Withhold all food and fluids for 6 to 12 hours before the procedure. If the cardioversion is urgent, withhold the meal that would have been eaten before the procedure.
• Obtain a 12-lead ECG for a baseline.
• Check to see if the doctor ordered cardiac drugs before the procedure.
• Verify patency of I.V. site in case drug administration is needed.
• Connect the patient to a pulse oximeter and automatic blood pressure cuff, if available.

• Consider administering oxygen for 5 to 10 minutes before the cardioversion *to promote myocardial oxygenation.* If the patient wears dentures, evaluate whether they support his airway or may cause an airway obstruction. If they may cause an obstruction, remove them.

Implementation
• Place the patient in a supine position and assess vital signs, level of consciousness (LOC), cardiac rhythm, and peripheral pulses.
• Remove any oxygen delivery device just before cardioversion *to avoid possible combustion.*
• Have epinephrine, lidocaine, and atropine at the patient's bedside.
• Administer a sedative, as ordered. The patient should be heavily sedated but still able to breathe adequately.
• Carefully monitor the patient's blood pressure and respiratory rate until he recovers.
• Press the POWER button to turn the defibrillator on.
• Push the SYNC button *to synchronize the machine with the patient's QRS complexes.* Make sure the SYNC button flashes with each of the patient's QRS complexes. You should also see a bright green flag flash on the monitor.
• Turn the energy SELECT dial to the ordered amount of energy. Advanced cardiac life support protocols call for 50 joules for a patient with atrial flutter, 50 to 360 joules for a patient with stable paroxysmal atrial tachycardia, 75 to 360 joules for a patient with unstable paroxysmal supraventricular tachycardia, 100 joules for a patient with atrial fibrillation, 100 to 360 joules for a patient with ventricular

tachycardia with a pulse, and 200 to 360 joules for a patient with pulseless ventricular tachycardia.
• Remove the paddles from the machine, and prepare them as you would if you were defibrillating the patient.
• Place the conductive gel pads or paddles in the same positions as you would to defibrillate.
• Make sure everyone stands away from the bed; then push the discharge buttons.
• Hold the paddles in place and wait for the energy to be discharged — the machine has to synchronize the discharge with the QRS complex.
• Check the waveform on the monitor. If the arrhythmia fails to convert, repeat the procedure two or three more times at 3-minute intervals. Gradually increase the energy level with each additional countershock.
• Record a postcardioversion 12-lead ECG and monitor the patient's ECG rhythm for 2 hours. Check the patient's chest for electric burns.

Complications
Common complications following cardioversion include:
• transient, harmless arrhythmias, such as atrial, ventricular, and junctional premature beats
• serious ventricular arrhythmia such as ventricular fibrillation may also occur, but it's more likely to result from high amounts of electrical energy, digitalis toxicity, severe heart disease, electrolyte imbalance, or improper synchronization with the R wave.

Nursing considerations
• After the cardioversion, frequently assess the patient's LOC and respiratory status, including airway patency,

respiratory rate and depth, and the need for supplemental oxygen. *Because the patient will be heavily sedated, he may require airway support.*
• If the patient is attached to a bedside or telemetry monitor, disconnect the unit before cardioversion. *The electric current it generates could damage the equipment.*
• Be aware that improper synchronization may result if the patient's ECG tracing contains artifact-like spikes, such as peaked T waves or bundle-branch heart blocks when the R wave may be taller than the R wave.
• Although the electric shock of cardioversion won't usually damage an implanted pacemaker, avoid placing the paddles directly over the pacemaker.

Documentation

• Document the procedure, including the voltage delivered with each attempt, rhythm strips before and after the procedure, and how the patient tolerated the procedure.

Casts

A cast is a hard mold that encases a body part, usually an extremity, to immobilize without discomfort. It can be used to treat injuries including fractures, correct orthopedic conditions such as deformities, or promote healing after general or plastic surgery, amputation, or nerve or vascular repair.

Casts can be made of plaster, Fiberglas, or other materials. Plaster, the most commonly used material, is inexpensive, nontoxic, nonflammable, and easy to mold, and it rarely causes allergic reactions or skin irritation. But Fiberglas is lighter, stronger, and more resilient than plaster. Because Fiberglas dries rapidly, it is more difficult to mold, but it can bear body weight immediately if necessary.

Typically, a doctor applies a cast and a nurse prepares the patient and the equipment, and assists with cast application. With special preparation, a nurse may apply or change a standard cast, but an orthopedist must reduce and set the fracture.

Contraindications for casting may include skin diseases, peripheral vascular disease, diabetes mellitus, open or draining wounds, and susceptibility to skin irritations. However, these aren't strict contraindications; the doctor must weigh the potential risks and benefits for each patient.

›› Key nursing diagnoses and patient outcomes

Use these nursing diagnoses as a guide when developing a plan of care for a patient requiring a cast.

Impaired physical mobility related to fracture

Based on this nursing diagnosis, you'll establish the following patient outcomes. The patient will:
• state relief from pain.
• show no evidence of such complications as contractures, venous stasis, thrombus formation, or skin breakdown
• demonstrate mobility regimen.

Altered peripheral tissue perfusion related to fracture

Based on this nursing diagnosis, you'll establish the following patient outcomes. The patient will:
• have strong peripheral pulses.
• have unchanged skin color and temperature.
• have no numbness, tingling, or pain in body parts distal to the cast.

Equipment

♦ tubular stockinette ♦ casting material ♦ plaster rolls ♦ plaster splints if necessary ♦ bucket of water ♦ sink equipped with plaster trap ♦ linensaver pad ♦ sheet wadding ♦ sponge or felt padding if necessary ♦ cast scissors, cast saw, and cast spreader if necessary ♦ pillows or bath blankets ♦ optional: rubber gloves, cast stand, moleskin or adhesive tape.

Gather the tubular stockinette, cast material, and plaster splints in the appropriate sizes. Tubular stockinettes range from 2″ to 12″ (5 to 30.5 cm) wide; plaster rolls, from 2″ to 6″ (5 to 15.2 cm) wide; and plaster splints, from 3″ to 6″ (7.6 to 15.2 cm) wide. Wear rubber gloves, especially if applying a Fiberglas cast.

Equipment preparation

• Gently squeeze the packaged casting material *to make sure the envelopes don't have any air leaks.* Humid air penetrating such leaks can cause plaster to become stale, which could make it set too quickly, form lumps, fail to bond with lower layers, or set as a soft, friable mass. (Baking a stale plaster roll at a medium temperature for 1 hour can make it usable again.)
• Follow the manufacturer's directions for water temperature when preparing plaster. Usually, room temperature or slightly warmer water is best *because it allows the cast to set in about 7 minutes without excessive exothermia.* (Cold water retards the rate of setting and may be used to facilitate difficult molding; warm water speeds the rate of setting and raises skin temperature under the cast.) Place all equipment within the doctor's reach.

Implementation

• *To allay the patient's fears,* explain the procedure. If plaster is being used, make sure she understands that heat will build under the cast because of a chemical reaction between the water and plaster. Also begin explaining some aspects of proper cast care *to prepare for patient teaching and to assess the patient's knowledge level.*
• Cover the appropriate parts of the patient's bedding and gown with a linen-saver pad.
• If the cast is applied to the wrist or arm, remove rings that may interfere with circulation in the fingers.
• Assess the condition of the skin in the affected area, noting any redness, contusions, or open wounds. *This will make it easier to evaluate any complaints the patient may have after the cast is applied.*
• If the patient has severe contusions or open wounds, prepare him for a local anesthetic if the doctor will administer one.
• *To establish baseline measurements,* assess the patient's neurovascular state. Palpate the distal pulses; assess the color, temperature, and capillary refill of the appropriate fingers or toes; and check neurologic function, including sensation and motion in the affected and unaffected extremities.

• Help the doctor position the limb, as ordered. (Commonly, the limb is immobilized in the neutral position.)
• Support the limb in the prescribed position while the doctor applies the tubular stockinette and sheet wadding. The stockinette, if used, should extend beyond the ends of the cast *to pad the edges.* (If the patient has an open wound or a severe contusion, the doctor may not use the stockinette.) He will then wrap the limb in sheet wadding, starting at the distal end, and apply extra wadding to the distal and proximal ends of the cast area, as well as any points of prominence. As he applies the sheet wadding, check for wrinkles.
• If needed, help the doctor place an extra layer of sponge or felt padding over the area where the cast scissors will be used.
• Prepare the various cast materials as ordered.

To prepare plaster casting

• Place a roll of plaster casting on its end in a bucket of water. Make sure to immerse it completely. When air bubbles stop rising from the roll, remove it, gently squeeze out the excess water and hand the casting material to the doctor, who will begin applying it. As the doctor applies the first roll, prepare a second roll the same way. (Stay at least one roll ahead of the doctor during the procedure.)
• After the doctor applies each roll, he'll smooth it to remove wrinkles, spread the plaster into the cloth webbing, and empty air pockets. If he's using plaster splints, he'll apply them in the middle layers of the cast. Before wrapping the last roll, he'll pull the ends of the tubular stockinette over the cast edges *to create padded ends, pre-*

vent cast crumbling, and reduce skin irritation. He will then use the final roll to keep the ends of the stockinette in place.

To prepare cotton and polyester casting

• Open these casting materials one roll at a time *because cotton and polyester casting must be applied within 3 minutes — before humidity in the air hardens the tape.*
• Immerse the roll in cold water and squeeze it four times *to ensure uniform wetness.*
• Remove the dripping wet material from the bucket. Tell the patient that it will be applied immediately. Warn her that the material will feel warm while it sets.

To prepare Fiberglas casting

• If you're using water-activated Fiberglas, immerse the tape rolls in tepid water for 10 to 15 minutes *to initiate the chemical reaction that causes the cast to harden.* Open one roll at a time. Avoid squeezing out excess water before application.
• If you're using light-cured Fiberglas, you can unroll the material more slowly. This casting remains soft and malleable until it's exposed to ultraviolet light, which sets it.

To complete casting

• As necessary, *petal* the cast's edges *to reduce roughness and to cushion pressure points.* (See *How to petal a cast,* page 166.)
• Use a cast stand or the palm of your hand to support the cast in the therapeutic position until it becomes firm to the touch (usually 6 to 8 minutes).

How to petal a cast

Rough cast edges can be cushioned by petaling them with adhesive tape or moleskin. To do this, first cut several $4'' \times 2''$ (10.2 cm x 5 cm) strips. Round off one end of each strip to keep it from curling. Then, making sure the rounded end of the strip is on the outside of the cast, tuck the straight end just inside the cast edge.

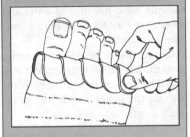

Smooth the moleskin with your finger until you're sure it's secured inside and out. Repeat the procedure, overlapping the moleskin pieces until you've gone all the way around the cast edge.

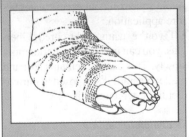

• *To check circulation in the casted limb,* palpate the distal pulse and assess the color, temperature, and capillary refill of the fingers or toes.
• Determine the patient's neurologic state by asking her if she's experiencing paresthesia in the extremity or decreased motion of the extremity's uncovered joints. Assess the unaffected extremity in the same manner and compare findings.
• Elevate the limb above heart with pillows or bath blankets, as ordered, *to facilitate venous return and reduce edema. To prevent molding,* make sure pressure is evenly distributed under the cast.
• The doctor will then send the patient for X-rays *to ensure proper positioning.*
• Instruct the patient to notify the doctor of any pain, foul odor, drainage, or burning sensation under the cast. (After the cast hardens, the doctor may cut a window in it to inspect the painful or burning area.)
• Pour water from the plaster bucket into a sink containing a plaster trap. Don't use a regular sink *because plaster will block the plumbing.*

Complications

Possible complications of improper cast application include:
• compartment syndrome
• palsy
• paresthesia
• ischemia
• myositis
• pressure necrosis.
• misalignment or nonunion of fractured bones (eventually).

Nursing considerations

• A Fiberglas cast dries immediately. A plaster extremity cast dries in approximately 24 to 48 hours; a plaster spica or body cast, in 48 to 72 hours. While it's drying, the cast must be properly positioned to prevent a surface depression that could cause pressure areas or dependent edema. The patient's neurovascular state must be assessed, drainage monitored, and the condition of the cast checked periodically.

After the cast dries completely, it looks white and shiny and no longer feels damp or soft. Care consists of monitoring for changes in the drainage pattern, preventing skin breakdown near the cast, and averting the complications of immobility.

• Patient teaching must begin immediately after the cast is applied and should continue until the patient or a family member can care for the cast.

• Never use the bed or a table to support the cast as it sets *because molding can result, causing pressure necrosis of underlying tissue.* Also, don't use rubber- or plastic-covered pillows before the cast hardens *because they can trap heat under the cast.*

• If a cast is applied after surgery or traumatic injury, remember that the most accurate way to assess for bleeding is to monitor vital signs. A visible blood spot on the cast can be misleading: One drop of blood can produce a circle 3″ (7.6 cm) in diameter.

• The doctor usually removes the cast at the appropriate time, with a nurse assisting. (See *Removing a plaster cast,* page 168.)

• Tell the patient that when the cast is removed, her casted limb will appear thinner and flabbier than the uncasted limb.

• The skin will appear yellowish or gray from the accumulated dead skin and oils from the glands near the skin surface.

• Reassure the patient that with exercise and good skin care, her limb will return to normal.

Home care

• Before the patient goes home, teach her cast care.

• Tell her to keep the casted limb above heart level to minimize swelling.

• Tell the patient to raise casted leg by lying in a supine position and propping the leg on a pillow. Prop a casted arm so the hand and elbow are higher than the shoulder.

• Instruct the patient to call the doctor if she can't move her fingers or toes, if she has numbness or tingling in the affected limb or symptoms of infection, such as a fever, unusual pain, or a foul odor from the cast.

• Instruct the patient to maintain muscle strength by continuing any recommended exercises.

• If the cast needs repair (if it loosens and slips) or if the patient has any questions about cast care, advise her to call her doctor.

• Warn the patient not to get the cast wet because moisture will weaken or destroy it.

• Urge the patient not to insert anything (such as a back scratcher or powder) into the cast to relieve itching. Foreign matter can damage the skin and cause an infection. Tell her she can use alcohol on the skin at the cast edges.

• Warn the patient not to chip, crush, cut, or otherwise break any part of the cast and not to put weight on the cast unless told to by the doctor.

• If the patient must use crutches, instruct him to remove throw rugs from the floor and to rearrange furniture to reduce the risk of tripping and falling.

• If the patient has a cast on her dominant arm, she may need help with bathing, toileting, eating, and dressing.

Removing a plaster cast

Typically a cast is removed when a fracture heals or requires further manipulation. Less common indications include cast damage, a pressure ulcer under the cast, excessive drainage or bleeding, and a constrictive cast.

Explain the procedure to the patient. Tell him he'll feel some heat and vibration as the cast is split with the cast saw. If the patient is a child, tell him the saw is very noisy but will not cut the skin beneath. Warn the patient that when the padding is cut, he'll see discolored skin and signs of poor muscle tone. Reassure him that you'll stay with him. The pictures show how a plaster cast is removed.

First, the doctor cuts one side of the cast, then the other. As he does so, closely monitor the patient's anxiety level.

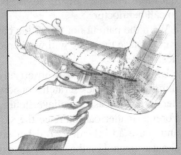

Next, the doctor opens the cast pieces with a spreader.

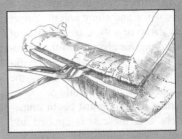

Finally, using the cast scissors, the doctor cuts through the cast padding.

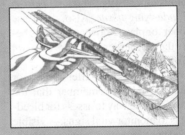

When the cast is removed, give skin care to remove accumulated dead skin and to begin restoring the extremity's normal appearance.

Documentation

• Record the date and time of cast application and skin condition of the extremity before the cast was applied.
• Note any contusions, redness, or open wounds; results of neurovascular checks, before and after application, for the affected and unaffected extremities; location of any special devices, such as felt pads or plaster splints; and any patient teaching.

Central venous line insertion

A central venous (CV) line is a sterile catheter made of polyurethane, polyvinylchloride (PVC), or silicone rubber (Silastic). It's inserted through a major vein, like the subclavian vein or, sometimes, the jugular vein (See *CV catheter pathways*, pages 170 and 171.)

CV therapy offers several benefits. It allows CV pressure monitoring, which indicates blood volume or pump efficiency. It permits aspiration of blood samples for diagnostic tests. It also allows administration of I.V. fluids (in large amounts, if necessary) in emergencies or when decreased peripheral circulation causes peripheral veins to collapse. CV lines help when prolonged I.V. therapy reduces the number of accessible peripheral veins, when solutions must be diluted (for large fluid volumes or for irritating or hypertonic fluids, such as total parenteral nutrition solutions) and when long-term access is needed to patient's venous system. And because repeated blood samples can be drawn through it, the CV line decreases the patient's anxiety and preserves or restores peripheral veins.

A variation of CV therapy, peripheral CV therapy, involves insertion of a catheter into a peripheral vein instead of a central vein, but the catheter tip still lies in the CV circulation. A peripherally inserted central catheter (PICC) usually enters at the basilic vein and terminates in the subclavian vein, the axillary vein, or the superior vena cava. PICCs may be inserted by a specially prepared nurse. New catheters have longer needles and smaller lumens, which makes this procedure easier.

PICCs are commonly used in home I.V. therapy, too, but may also be used with chest injury; chest, neck, or shoulder burns; compromised respiratory function; or a surgery site that's close to a CV insertion site; or

when a doctor's unavailable to insert a CV line.

As with any invasive procedure, however, CV therapy also has its drawbacks. It increases the risk of complications, such as pneumothorax, sepsis, thrombus formation, and vessel and adjacent organ perforation (all life-threatening conditions). Also, the CV line can decrease patient mobility, requires more time and skill to insert than a peripheral I.V. catheter, and costs more than a peripheral I.V. catheter.

⟫ Key nursing diagnoses and patient outcomes

Use these nursing diagnoses as a guide when developing your plan of care for a patient receiving a CV line.

Fluid volume deficit related to (specify)

Based on this nursing diagnosis, you'll establish the following patient outcomes. The patient will:
• have vital signs remain stable.
• have electrolyte levels stay in normal range.
• produce at least 30 ml of urine per hour.

Risk for infection related to presence of CV line

Based on this nursing diagnosis, you'll establish the following patient outcomes. The patient will:
• have no pathogens appear in cultures.
• remain afebrile.
• show no evidence of infection at the insertion site, such as redness, swelling, or drainage.

Equipment

For insertion of a CV line: ♦ shave preparation kit if necessary ♦ sterile

CV catheter pathways

The illustrations below show several common pathways for central venous (CV) catheter insertion. Typically, a CV catheter is inserted into the subclavian vein or the internal jugular vein. The catheter may terminate in the superior vena cava or in the right atrium.

Insertion:
Subclavian vein
Termination:
Superior vena cava

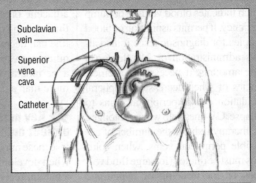

Insertion:
Subclavian vein
Termination:
Right atrium

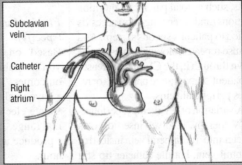

Insertion:
Internal jugular vein
Termination:
Superior vena cava

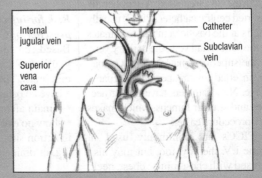

CV catheter pathways *(continued)*

Insertion:
Basilic vein (peripheral)
Termination:
Superior vena cava

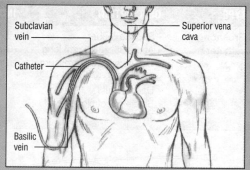

Insertion:
Through a subcutaneous tunnel to the subclavian vein (Dacron cuff helps hold catheter in place)
Termination:
Superior vena cava

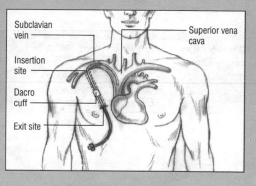

gloves and gowns ◆ blanket ◆ linen-saver pad ◆ sterile towel ◆ sterile drape ◆ masks ◆ povidone-iodine sponges and ointment ◆ alcohol sponges ◆ 70% alcohol solution ◆ hydrogen peroxide ◆ normal saline solution ◆ antibiotic ointment if necessary ◆ 3-ml syringe with 25G 1″ needle ◆ 1% or 2% injectable lidocaine ◆ dextrose 5% in water ◆ syringes for blood samples ◆ suture material ◆ two 14G or 16G CV catheters ◆ I.V. solution with administration set prepared for use ◆ infusion pump or controller as needed ◆ sterile 4″ × 4″ gauze pads ◆ 1″ adhesive tape ◆ sterile scissors ◆ heparin or normal saline flushes as needed ◆ portable X-ray machine ◆ optional: transparent semipermeable dressing.

For flushing a catheter: ◆ normal saline solution or heparin flush solution ◆ alcohol sponge ◆ 70% alcohol solution.

For changing an injection cap: ◆ alcohol sponge or povidone-iodine sponge ◆ injection cap ◆ padded clamp.

The type of catheter selected depends on the type of therapy to be used. (See *Guide to CV catheters*, pages 172 to 175.)

(Text continues on page 176.)

Guide to CV catheters

TYPE	DESCRIPTION	INDICATIONS
Groshong catheter	• Silicone rubber • About 35″ (88.9 cm) long • Closed end with pressure-sensitive two-way valve • Dacron cuff • Single or double lumen • Tunneled	• Long-term central venous (CV) access • Patient with heparin allergy
Short-term, single-lumen catheter	• Polyvinyl chloride (PVC) or polyurethane • About 8″ (20.3 cm) long • Lumen gauge varies • Percutaneously placed	• Short-term CV access • Emergency access • Patient who needs only one lumen
Short-term, multilumen catheter	• PVC or polyurethane • Two, three, or four lumens exiting at ¾″ (2-cm) intervals • Lumen gauges vary • Percutaneously placed	• Short-term CV access • Patient with limited insertion sites who requires multiple infusions

ADVANTAGES AND DISADVANTAGES	NURSING CONSIDERATIONS
Advantages • Less thrombogenic • Pressure-sensitive two-way valve eliminates frequent heparin flushes • Dacron cuff anchors catheter and prevents bacterial migration **Disadvantages** • Requires surgical insertion • Tears and kinks easily • Blunt end makes it difficult to clear substances from its tip	• Two surgical sites require dressing after insertion. • Handle catheter gently. • Check the external portion frequently for kinks or leaks. • Repair kit is available. • Remember to flush with enough saline solution to clear the catheter, especially after drawing or administering blood.
Advantages • Easily inserted at bedside • Easily removed • Stiffness aids central venous pressure (CVP) monitoring **Disadvantages** • Limited functions • PVC is thrombogenic and irritates inner lumen of vessel • Should be changed every 3 to 7 days (Frequency may depend on hospital's CV line infection rate)	• Minimize patient movement. • Assess frequently for signs of infection and clot formation.
Advantages • Same as single-lumen catheter • Allows infusion of multiple (even incompatible) solutions through the same catheter **Disadvantages** • Same as single-lumen catheter	• Know gauge and purpose of each lumen. • Use the same lumen for the same task.

(continued)

Guide to CV catheters *(continued)*

TYPE	DESCRIPTION	INDICATIONS
Hickman catheter	• Silicone rubber • About 35″ (88.9 cm) long • Open end with clamp • Dacron cuff $11\frac{3}{4}$″ (29.8 cm) from hub • Single lumen or multilumen • Tunneled	• Long-term CV access • Home therapy
Broviac catheter	• Identical to Hickman except smaller inner lumen	• Long-term CV access • Patient with small central vessels (pediatric or geriatric)
Hickman/ Broviac catheter	• Hickman and Broviac catheters combined • Tunneled	• Long-term CV access • Patient who needs multiple infusions
Peripherally inserted central catheter (PICC)	• Silicone rubber • 20″ (50.8 cm) long • Available in 16G, 18G, 20G, and 22G • Can be used as midline catheter • Percutaneously placed	• Long-term CV access • Patient with poor CV access • Patient at risk for fatal complications from CV line insertion • Patient who needs CV access but faces or has had head or neck surgery

ADVANTAGES AND DISADVANTAGES	NURSING CONSIDERATIONS
Advantages • Less thrombogenic • Dacron cuff prevents excess motion and migration of bacteria • Clamps eliminate need for Valsalva's maneuver **Disadvantages** • Requires surgical insertion • Open end • Requires doctor for removal • Tears and kinks easily	• Two surgical sites require dressing after insertion. • Handle catheter gently. • Observe frequently for kinks and tears. • Repair kit is available. • Clamp catheter with a nonserrated clamp any time it becomes disconnected or opens.
Advantages • Smaller lumen **Disadvantages** • Small lumen may limit uses • Single lumen	• Check hospital policy before drawing or administering blood or blood products.
Advantages • Double-lumen Hickman catheter allows sampling and administration of blood • Broviac lumen delivers I.V. fluids, including total parenteral nutrition **Disadvantages** • Same as Hickman catheter	• Know the purpose and function of each lumen. • Label lumens to prevent confusion.
Advantages • Peripherally inserted • Easily inserted at bedside with minimal complications • May be inserted by trained registered nurse in some states **Disadvantages** • Catheter may occlude smaller peripheral vessels • May be difficult to keep immobile • Single lumen • Long path to CV circulation	• Check frequently for signs of phlebitis and thrombus formation. • Insert catheter above the antecubital fossa. • Basilic vein is preferable to cephalic vein. • Use arm board if necessary. • Catheter may alter CVP measurements.

Teaching Valsalva's maneuver

Increased intrathoracic pressure reduces the risk of air embolus during insertion and removal of a central venous catheter. A simple way to achieve this is to ask the patient to perform Valsalva's maneuver: forced exhalation against a closed airway. Instruct the patient to take a deep breath and hold it, and then to bear down for 10 seconds. Then tell the patient to exhale and breathe quietly.

Valsalva's maneuver raises intrathoracic pressure from its normal level of 3 to 4 mm Hg to levels of 60 mm Hg or higher. It also slows the pulse rate, decreases the return of blood to the heart, and increases venous pressure.

This maneuver is contraindicated in patients with increased intracranial pressure. It should not be taught to patients who are not alert or cooperative.

Some hospitals have prepared trays containing most of the equipment necessary for catheter insertion.

Equipment preparation

• Before inserting a CV line, confirm catheter type and size with the doctor. Usually, a 14G or 16G catheter is selected.

• Set up the I.V. solution, and prime the administration set, using strict aseptic technique.

• Attach the line to the infusion pump or controller if ordered.

• Recheck all connections to make sure they're tight.

• As ordered, notify the radiology department that a portable X-ray machine will be needed.

Implementation
To insert the catheter

• Wash your hands thoroughly *to prevent the spread of microorganisms.*

• Reinforce the doctor's explanation of the procedure, and answer the patient's questions.

• Ensure that the patient has signed a consent form if necessary, and check his history for hypersensitivity to iodine or the local anesthetic.

• Place the patient in Trendelenburg's position *to dilate the veins and reduce the risk of air embolism.*

• For subclavian insertion, place a rolled blanket lengthwise between the shoulders *to increase venous distention.*

• For jugular insertion, place a rolled blanket under the opposite shoulder *to extend the neck, making anatomic landmarks more visible.*

• Place a linen-saver pad under the appropriate area *to prevent soiling the bed.*

• Turn the patient's head away from the site *to prevent possible contamination from airborne pathogens and to make the site more accessible*, or if dictated by hospital policy place a mask on the patient, unless this increases his anxiety or is contraindicated due to his respiratory state.

• Prepare the insertion site. Make sure the skin is free of hair *because hair can harbor microorganisms.* Infection control practitioners recommend clipping hair close to the skin rather than shaving. *Shaving may cause skin irritation and create multiple small open wounds, increasing the risk of infection.* (If the doctor orders the area to be shaved, try shaving it the evening before catheter insertion; *this allows minor skin irritations to heal partially.*) You may also need to wash the skin with soap and water before the actual skin preparation *to remove surface dirt and body oils.*

• Establish a sterile field on a table, using a sterile towel or the wrapping from the instrument tray.

• Put on a mask and sterile gloves and gown, and clean the area around the insertion site with sponges soaked in povidone-iodine ointment, working in a circular motion outward from the site to avoid reintroducing contaminants. If the patient is sensitive to iodine use a solution of 70% alcohol.

• After the doctor puts on a sterile mask, gown, and gloves and drapes the area to create a sterile field, open the 3-ml syringe and 25G needle packages and present give them to the doctor, using sterile technique.

• Wipe the top of the lidocaine vial with an alcohol sponge and invert it. The doctor then fills the 3-ml syringe and injects the anesthetic into the site.

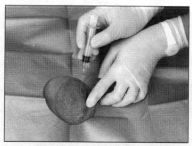

• Open the catheter package and, using sterile technique, give it to the doctor.

• The doctor then inserts the catheter.

• During catheter insertion, prepare the I.V. administration set for imme-

diate attachment to the catheter hub. Ask the patient to perform Valsalva's maneuver while the doctor attaches the I.V. line to the catheter hub. *This increases intrathoracic pressure, reducing the possibility of air embolism.* (See *Teaching Valsalva's maneuver.*)

• After the doctor attaches the I.V. line to the catheter hub, set the flow rate at a keep-vein-open rate to maintain venous access. The doctor then sutures the catheter in place.

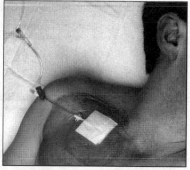

• After an X-ray confirms correct catheter placement, set the flow rate as ordered.

• Use normal saline solution *to remove dried blood that could harbor microorganisms,* and apply povidone-iodine ointment over the site.

• Apply antibiotic ointment to the site, according to hospital policy; secure the catheter with adhesive tape; and apply an occlusive, sterile 4″ × 4″ gauze pad. You may also use a transparent semipermeable dressing (shown above), either alone or placed over the gauze pad. Expect some serosanguineous drainage during the first 24 hours.

• Label the dressing with the time and date of catheter insertion and catheter length (if not imprinted on the catheter).

(Text continues on page 180.)

PROBLEM SOLVER

Risks of CV therapy

PROBLEM	SIGNS AND SYMPTOMS	POSSIBLE CAUSES
Pneumothorax, hemothorax, chylothorax, hydrothorax	• Chest pain • Dyspnea • ICyanosis • Decreased breath sounds on affected side • With hemothorax, decreased hemoglobin because of blood pooling • Abnormal chest X-ray	• Lung puncture by catheter during insertion • Large blood vessel puncture • Lymph node puncture with leakage of lymph fluid • Infusion of solution into chest area through infiltrated catheter
Air embolism	• Respiratory distress • Unequal breath sounds • Weak pulse • Increased central venous pressure • Decreased blood pressure • Churning murmur over precordium • Alteration of consciousness	• Intake of air into central venous (CV) system during catheter insertion or tubing changes, or inadvertent opening, cutting, or breaking of catheter
Thrombosis	• Edema at puncture site • Erythema • Ilpsilateral swelling of arm, neck, and face • Pain along vein • Fever, malaise	• Sluggish flow rate • Catheter composition • Hematopoietic state of patient • Preexisting limb edema • Infusion of irritating solutions • Long-term use of same vein • Cardiovascular disease
Infection	• Redness, warmth, tenderness, swelling • Possible exudate of purulent material • Local rash or pustules • Fever, chills, malaise • Leukocytosis	• Failure to maintain aseptic technique • Failure to comply with dressing change protocol • Wet or soiled dressing site • Immunosuppression • Irritated suture line

NURSING INTERVENTIONS

- Notify doctor, and administer oxygen as ordered.
- Remove catheter or assist with removal.
- Set up and assist with chest tube insertion.
- Document interventions.

Prevention
- Position patient head down with a rolled towel between his scapulae to dilate and expose internal jugular or subclavian vein during catheter insertion.
- Assess for early signs of fluid infiltration (swelling in the shoulder, neck, chest, and arm).
- Ensure that the patient is immobilized and prepared for insertion.
- Minimize patient activity after insertion, especially with a peripheral catheter.

- Clamp catheter immediately.
- Turn patient on left side, head down, so air can enter right atrium and pulmonary artery. Maintain position for 20 to 30 minutes.
- Notify doctor; administer oxygen.

Prevention
- Purge all air from tubing before hookup, and use air-eliminating filter.
- Teach patient to perform Valsalva's maneuver during catheter insertion and tubing changes.
- Use infusion device with air-detection capabilities and luer-lock tubing. Then tape to secure.

- Notify doctor.
- Remove catheter if necessary.
- Apply warm, wet compresses locally.

Prevention
- Maintain steady flow rate with infusion pump, or regularly flush catheter.
- Use catheters made of less thrombogenic materials.
- Use 0.22-micron filter for infusions.

- Monitor vital signs closely.
- Culture the site and the catheter tip if removed.
- Re-dress aseptically.
- Possibly use antibiotic ointment locally.
- Treat systemically with antibiotics or antifungals.
- Catheter may be removed.

(continued)

Risks of CV therapy *(continued)*

PROBLEM	SIGNS AND SYMPTOMS	POSSIBLE CAUSES
Infection *(continued)*	• Nausea and vomiting • Elevated urine glucose level	• Contamination • Frequent opening of catheter or long-term use of single I.V. access site

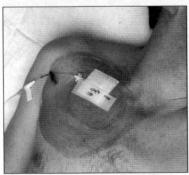

• Put the patient in a comfortable position and reassess his status.

To flush the catheter

• *To maintain patency,* flush the catheter routinely according to your hospital's policy. If the system is being maintained as a heparin lock and the infusions are intermittent, the flushing procedure will vary according to the hospital's policy, medication schedule, and catheter type.

• Typically, a CV catheter with a two-way valve (Groshong catheter) must be flushed weekly with normal saline solution. All lumens of a multilumen catheter (except the Groshong) must be flushed regularly. (No flushing is needed with a continuous infusion through a single-lumen catheter.) Most hospitals use a heparin flush solution available in premixed 10-ml multidose vials. Recommended concentrations vary from 10 units of heparin/ml to 1,000 units of heparin/ml. Some hospitals use normal saline solution instead of heparin flush solution to flush catheters because research suggests that heparin isn't always necessary to keep the line open.

NURSING INTERVENTIONS

- Draw central and peripheral blood cultures; if the same organism appears in both, then catheter is primary source and should be removed.
- If cultures don't match but are positive, the catheter may be removed, or the infection may be treated through the catheter.
- Treat patients with antibiotics as ordered.
- Document interventions.

Prevention
- Maintain sterile technique, and observe dressing-change protocols.
- Teach about restrictions on swimming, bathing, and so on.
- Change dressing more frequently if catheter is located in femoral area or near tracheostomy. Perform tracheostomy care after catheter care.
- Examine solution for cloudiness before infusing; check container for leaks.
- Monitor urine glucose level in patients receiving total parenteral nutrition (TPN) if greater than 2+, suspect early sepsis.
- Use a 0.22-micron filter (or a 1.2-micron filter for 3-In-1 TPN solutions).
- Keep the system closed as much as possible.

- The recommended CV catheter flushing frequency varies from once every 12 hours to once weekly. Most clinicians agree that flushing should be done twice daily for 3 to 4 days after insertion and from once daily to three times a week after that.
- The recommended amount of flushing solution also varies. Most hospitals recommend using 3 to 5 ml of solution to flush the catheter, although some hospital policies call for as much as 10 ml of solution. Different catheters require different amounts of solution, and the volume capacity will be altered if the catheter has been cut to fit the patient.
- To flush, clean the cap with an alcohol sponge (using a 70% alcohol solution).
- Allow it to dry.

- Inject the recommended type and amount of flush solution.
- After flushing the catheter, maintain positive pressure by keeping your thumb on the plunger of the syringe while withdrawing the needle. *This prevents blood backflow and potential clotting in the line.*
- CV catheters used for intermittent infusions have injection caps (short luer-lock devices similar to the heparin lock adapters used for peripheral I.V. infusion therapy). Unlike heparin lock adapters, however, these caps contain a small amount of empty space, so you don't have to preflush the cap before connecting it.

To change the injection cap
- Frequency of cap changes varies according to hospital policy and the number of times the cap is used. Use

strict aseptic technique when changing the cap. Repeated punctures of the injection port increase the risk of infection. Also, pieces of the rubber stopper may break off after repeated punctures, placing the patient at risk for embolism.

• Clean the connection site with an alcohol sponge or a povidone-iodine sponge.

• Instruct the patient to perform Valsalva's maneuver while you quickly disconnect the old cap and connect the new cap, using aseptic technique. If the patient can't perform Valsalva's maneuver, use a padded clamp to prevent air from entering the catheter.

Complications

Complications can occur at any time during the infusion therapy. Possible traumatic complications such as pneumothorax typically occur on catheter insertion but may not be noticed until after the procedure is completed. Systemic complications such as sepsis typically occur later during infusion therapy. Other complications include:

• phlebitis (especially in peripheral CV therapy)

• thrombus formation. (See *Risks of CV therapy*, pages 178 to 181.)

Nursing considerations

• When catheter placement is in doubt, infuse an I.V. solution, such as dextrose 5% in water or normal saline solution, until correct placement is verified. You may also use a heparin lock and flush the line. *Infusing an isotonic solution avoids the risk of vessel wall thrombosis.*

• Watch for such signs of air embolism as sudden onset of pallor, cyano-

sis, dyspnea, coughing, and tachycardia, progressing to syncope and shock. If any of these signs occur, place the patient on his left side in Trendelenburg's position, and notify the doctor.

• After insertion, watch for signs of pneumothorax, such as shortness of breath, uneven chest movement, tachycardia, and chest pain. Notify the doctor immediately if such signs appear.

• Change the dressing at least once a week, according to hospital policy, or whenever it becomes moist, soiled, or nonocclusive.

• Change the tubing and solution every 24 to 48 hours, or according to hospital policy while the CV line is in place.

• Use sterile technique to change dressing, tubing, and solution. (See *Key steps in changing a CV dressing,* page 183.)

• Assess the site for signs of infection, such as discharge, inflammation, and tenderness.

• *To prevent air embolism* have the patient perform Valsalva's maneuver each time the catheter hub is open to air, or close the clamp if the catheter has one. (A Groshong catheter does not require clamping *because it has an internal valve.)*

Home care

• Long-term CV catheters allow patients to receive caustic fluids and blood infusions at home. These catheters have a much longer life because they are less thrombogenic and less prone to infection than short-term devices.

• A candidate for home therapy must have family or friend to safely admin-

Key steps in changing a CV dressing

Expect to change your patient's central venous (CV) dressing at least once a week. Many hospitals specify dressing changes two or three times weekly as well as whenever it becomes soiled, moist, or loose. The following illustrations show the key steps you'll perform.

First, put on clean gloves and remove the old dressing by pulling it toward the exit site of a long-term catheter or toward the insertion site of a short-term catheter. (This technique helps you avoid pulling out the line.) Remove and discard your gloves.

Next, put on sterile gloves and clean the skin around the site three times, using a new alcohol sponge each time. Start at the center and move outward, using a circular motion. Allow the skin to dry and repeat the same cleaning procedure using three swabs soaked in povidone-iodine solution.

After the solution has dried, cover the site with a dressing, such as a gauze dressing or the transparent semipermeable dressing shown here. Write the time and date on the dressing.

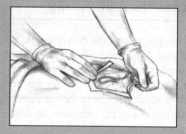

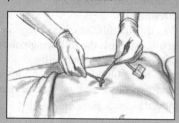

ister I.V. fluids. Also required are a backup helper, a suitable home environment, a telephone, transportation, adequate reading skills, and the ability to prepare, handle, store, and dispose of the equipment. Home care procedures are the same as in the hospital, except that the home therapy patients use clean, instead of sterile, technique.
• The overall goal of home therapy is patient safety, so your patient teaching must begin well before discharge. After discharge, a home therapy coordi-

nator will provide follow-up care until the patient or someone close to him can independently provide catheter care and infusion therapy. Many home-therapy patients learn to care for the catheter themselves and to infuse their own medications and solutions.

Documentation
• Record the time and date of insertion, the length and location of the catheter, the solution infused, the doc-

tor's name, and the patient's response to the procedure.
• Document the time of the X-ray, its results, and your notification of the doctor.
• Other measures to note are time of the X-ray study performed to confirm line placement, X-ray results, and notification of the doctor of the results.

Central venous pressure monitoring

In this procedure, the doctor inserts a catheter through a vein and advances it until the tip is in or near the right atrium. Because there are no major valves at the junction of the vena cava and right atrium, pressure at end diastole reflects back to the catheter. When connected to a manometer, the catheter measures central venous pressure (CVP), an index of right ventricular function.

CVP monitoring helps to assess cardiac function, evaluate venous return to the heart, and gauge indirectly how well the heart is pumping. The central venous (CV) line also provides access to a large vessel for rapid, high-volume fluid administration and allows frequent blood withdrawal for laboratory samples.

CVP monitoring can be done *intermittently* or *continuously*. The catheter is inserted percutaneously or using a cutdown method. Typically, a single CV line is used for intermittent pressure readings. To measure the state of the patient's volume, a disposable plastic water manometer is attached between the I.V. line and the central catheter with a three- or four-way stopcock. CVP is recorded in centimeters of water (cm H_2O) or millimeters of mercury (mm Hg) determined by manometer markings.

Normal CVP ranges from 5 to 10 cm H_2O and any condition that alters venous return, circulating blood volume, or cardiac performance can affect CVP. If circulating volume increases such as with enhanced venous return to the heart CVP rises. If circulating volume decreases such as with reduced venous return CVP drops.

≫ Key nursing diagnoses and patient outcomes

Use these nursing diagnoses as a guide when developing your plan of care for a patient who requires CVP monitoring.

Fluid volume excess related to compromised regulatory mechanisms
Based on this nursing diagnosis, you'll establish the following patient outcomes. The patient will:
• maintain blood pressure: no lower than (specify) and no higher than (specify).
• maintain fluid intake of no more than (specify) and output of no less than (specify).
• maintain CVP reading between 5 and 10 cm H_2O.

Fluid volume deficit related to compromised regulatory mechanisms
Based on this nursing diagnosis, you'll establish the following patient outcomes. The patient will:
• have stable vital signs.
• produce adequate urine volume.
• maintain CVP reading between 5 and 10 cm H_2O.

Equipment

For intermittent CVP monitoring:
♦ disposable CVP manometer set
♦ leveling device, such as a rod from a reusable CVP pole holder or a carpenter's level or rule ♦ additional stopcock (to attach the CVP manometer to the catheter) ♦ extension tubing if needed ♦ I.V. pole ♦ I.V. solution ♦ I.V. drip chamber and tubing ♦ dressing materials ♦ tape.

For continuous CVP monitoring:
♦ pressure monitoring kit with disposable pressure transducer ♦ leveling device ♦ bedside pressure module with oscilloscope ♦ continuous I.V. flush solution ♦ 1 unit-1 to 2 ml of heparin flush solution ♦ pressure bag.

For withdrawing blood samples through the CV line: ♦ appropriate number of syringes for the ordered tests ♦ 5- or 10-ml syringe for the discard sample. (Syringe size depends on the tests ordered.)

If only using the CV line intermittently: ♦ syringe with normal saline solution ♦ syringe with heparin flush solution.

For removing a central venous catheter: ♦ sterile gloves ♦ suture removal set ♦ sterile gauze sponges ♦ iodophor ointment ♦ dressing ♦ tape.

Equipment preparation

• Gather the necessary equipment.
• Familiarize yourself with the equipment before using.
• Obtain separate catheter insertion kits if available and necessary.

Patient preparation

• Explain the procedure to the patient *to reduce her anxiety.*

• Provide emotional support during the procedure *to maintain calm.*

Implementation

• Help the doctor as she inserts the CV catheter. (The procedure is similar to that used for pulmonary artery pressure monitoring, except that the catheter is advanced only as far as the superior vena cava.)

To obtain intermittent CVP readings with a water manometer

• With the CV line in place, position the patient flat. Align the base of the manometer with the previously determined zero reference point by using a leveling device. Because CVP reflects right atrial pressure, you must align the right atrium (the zero reference point) with the zero mark on the manometer. To find the right atrium, locate the fourth intercostal space at the midaxillary line. Mark the appropriate place on the patient's chest, *so all subsequent recordings will be made using the same location.*

• If the patient can't tolerate a flat position, place her in semi-Fowler's position. When the head of the bed is elevated, the phlebostatic axis remains constant but the midaxillary line changes. Use the same degree of head elevation for all subsequent measurements.

• Attach the water manometer to an I.V. pole or place it next to the patient's chest. In either case, make sure the zero reference point is level with the right atrium. (See *Measuring CVP with a water manometer,* page 186.)

• Verify that the water manometer is connected to the I.V. tubing. Typically, markings on the manometer range from 2 to 38 cm H_2O. Markings may

Measuring CVP with a water manometer

To ensure accurate central venous pressure (CVP) readings, make sure the manometer base is aligned with the patient's right atrium (the zero reference point). The manometer set usually contains a leveling rod to allow you to determine this quickly.

After adjusting the manometer's position, examine the typical three-way stopcock, as shown here. By turning it to any position shown, you can control the direction of fluid flow. Four-way stopcocks also are available.

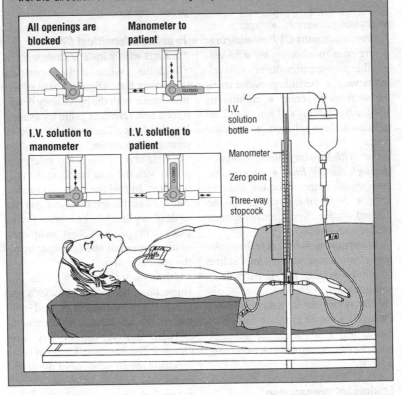

differ from one manufacturer to the next, though, so be sure to read the manufacturer's directions before setting up the manometer and obtaining readings.

• Turn the stopcock off to the patient and slowly fill the manometer with I.V. solution until the fluid level is 10 to 20 cm H_2O higher than the patient's

expected CVP value. Don't overfill the tube *because fluid that spills over the top can become a source of contamination.*

• Turn the stopcock off to the I.V. solution and open to the patient. The fluid level in the manometer will drop. Once the fluid level comes to rest, it will fluctuate slightly with respirations. Expect it to drop during inspiration and to rise during expiration.

• Record CVP at the end of inspiration, when intrathoracic pressure has a negligible effect. Depending on the type of water manometer you're using, note the value either at the bottom of the meniscus or at the midline of the small floating ball.

• After you've obtained the CVP value, turn the stopcock to resume the I.V. infusion. Adjust the I.V. drip rate as required.

• Place the patient in a comfortable position.

To perform continuous CVP monitoring with a water manometer

• Make sure the stopcock is turned so that the I.V. solution port, CVP column port, and patient port are open. Be aware that with the stopcock in this position, infusion of the I.V. solution increases CVP, so expect higher readings than those taken with the stopcock turned off to the I.V. solution. If the I.V. solution infuses at a constant rate, CVP will change as the patient's condition changes, although the initial reading will be higher. Assess the patient closely for changes.

To perform continuous CVP monitoring with a pressure monitoring system

• Make sure the CV line or the proximal lumen of a pulmonary artery catheter is attached to the system. (If the patient has a CV line with multiple lumens, one lumen may be dedicated to continuous CVP monitoring and the other lumens used for fluid administration.)

• Set up the pressure transducer system. Connect noncompliant pressure tubing from the CVP catheter hub to the transducer and then connect the flush solution container to a flush device.

• To obtain values, position the patient flat. If she can't tolerate this position, use semi-Fowler's position. Locate the level of the right atrium by identifying the phlebostatic axis. Zero the transducer, leveling the transducer air-fluid interface stopcock with the right atrium. Read the CVP value from the digital display on the monitor, and note the waveform. Make sure the patient is still when the reading is taken *to prevent artifact.* (See *Correcting common hemodynamic pressure monitoring problems,* pages 188 to 189.)

Use this position for subsequent readings.

To remove a CV line

• You may assist the doctor in removing a CV line. (In some states, a nurse is permitted to remove the catheter with a doctor's order or when acting under advanced collaborative standards of practice.)

• If the head of the bed is elevated, minimize the risk of air embolism during catheter removal by, for instance, placing the patient in Trendelenburg's position if the line was inserted using a superior approach. If she can't tolerate this position, lie her flat.

• Turn the patient's head to the side opposite the catheter insertion site. The doctor removes the dressing and exposes the insertion site. If sutures are in place, she removes them carefully.

• Turn the I.V. solution off.

• The doctor pulls the catheter out in a slow, smooth motion and then applies pressure to the insertion site.

• Clean the insertion site, apply iodophor ointment, and cover it with a dressing, as ordered.

PROBLEM SOLVER

Correcting common hemodynamic pressure monitoring problems

PROBLEM	POSSIBLE CAUSES	INTERVENTIONS
No waveform	• Power supply turned off	• Check power supply.
	• Monitor screen pressure range set too low	• Raise monitor screen pressure range if necessary. • Rebalance and recalibrate equipment.
	• Loose connection in line	• Tighten loose connections.
	• Transducer not connected to amplifier	• Check and tighten connection.
	• Stopcock off to patient	• Position stopcock correctly. • Use fast-flush valve to flush line, or try to aspirate blood from catheter. If the line remains blocked, notify the doctor and prepare to replace the line.
Drifting waveforms	• Improper warm-up	• Allow monitor and transducer to warm up for 10 to 15 minutes.
	• Electrical cable kinked or compressed	• Place monitor's cable where it can't be stepped on or compressed.
	• Temperature change in room air or I.V. flush solution	• Routinely zero and calibrate equipment 30 minutes after setting it up. This allows I.V. fluid to warm to room temperature.
Line fails to flush	• Stopcocks positioned incorrectly	• Make sure stopcocks are positioned correctly.
	• Inadequate pressure from pressure bag	• Make sure pressure bag gauge reads 300 mm Hg.
	• Kink in pressure tubing	• Check pressure tubing for kinks.
	• Blood clot in catheter	• Try to aspirate the clot with a syringe. If the line still won't flush, notify the doctor and prepare to replace the line, if necessary. *Important:* Never use a syringe to flush a hemodynamic line.

Correcting common hemodynamic pressure monitoring problems (continued)

PROBLEM	POSSIBLE CAUSES	INTERVENTIONS
False-high readings	• Transducer balancing port positioned below patient's right atrium	• Position balancing port level with the patient's right atrium.
	• Flush solution flow rate is too fast	• Check flush solution flow rate. Maintain it at 3 to 4 ml/hour.
	• Air in system	• Remove air from the lines and the transducer.
	• Catheter fling (tip of pulmonary artery catheter moving rapidly in large blood vessel or heart chamber)	• Notify the doctor, who may try to reposition the catheter.
False-low readings	• Transducer balancing port positioned above right atrium	• Position balancing port level with the patient's right atrium.
	• Transducer imbalance	• Make sure the transducer's flow system isn't kinked or occluded, and rebalance and recalibrate the equipment.
	• Loose connection	• Tighten loose connections.
Pulmonary artery wedge pressure tracing unobtainable	• Ruptured balloon	• If you feel no resistance when injecting air, or if you see blood leaking from the balloon inflation lumen, stop injecting air and notify the doctor. If the catheter is left in, label the inflation lumen with a warning not to inflate.
	• Incorrect amount of air in balloon	• Deflate the balloon. Check label on catheter for correct volume. Reinflate slowly with correct amount. To avoid rupturing the balloon, never use more than the stated volume.
	• Catheter malpositioned	• Notify the doctor. Obtain chest X-ray.

• Assess the patient for signs of respiratory distress, *which may indicate an air embolism.*

Complications

Possible complications of CVP monitoring include:

• pneumothorax (typically on catheter insertion)

Estimating CVP

To estimate central venous pressure (CVP), place the patient in semi-Fowler's position under a gooseneck lamp, and determine the height from the right atrium to the highest level of visible pulsation in the jugular vein.

To locate the right atrium, first palpate the clavicles where they join the sternum (the suprasternal notch). Place your first two fingers on the suprasternal notch, and slide them down the sternum until you feel a bony protuberance. This is the angle of Louis. The right atrium lies about 2″ (5 cm) below this point.

Then, measure the vertical distance between the highest level of visible pulsation and the angle of Louis. Add 2″ to this figure to estimate the total distance between the highest level of visible pulsation and the right atrium.

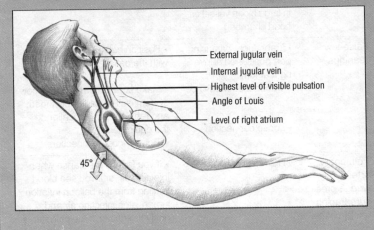

External jugular vein
Internal jugular vein
Highest level of visible pulsation
Angle of Louis
Level of right atrium

45°

- sepsis
- thrombus
- vessel or adjacent organ puncture
- air embolism.

Nursing considerations

- While waiting for the CV catheter to be inserted, you can estimate CVP. (See *Estimating CVP.*)
- Arrange for daily chest X-rays to check catheter placement as ordered.
- Care for the insertion site according to hospital policy. Typically, you'll change the dressing every 24 to 48 hours.
- Be sure to wash your hands before performing dressing changes and to use aseptic technique and sterile gloves when re-dressing the site.
- When removing the old dressing, observe for signs of infection such as redness, and note any patient complaints of tenderness.
- Apply ointment, and then cover the site with a sterile gauze dressing or a clear occlusive dressing.

• After the initial CVP reading, reevaluate readings frequently to establish a baseline for the patient. Authorities recommend obtaining readings at 15-, 30-, and 60-minute intervals *to establish a baseline.* If the patient's CVP fluctuates by more than 2 cm H_2O, suspect a change in his clinical state, and report this finding to the doctor.

• Change the I.V. solution every 24 hours and the I.V. tubing every 48 hours, according to hospital policy.

• Expect the doctor to change the catheter every 72 hours.

Documentation

• Document all dressing, tubing, and solution changes.

• Label the I.V. solution, tubing, and dressing with the date, time, and your initials.

• Document the patient's tolerance of the procedure, the date and time of catheter removal, and the type of dressing applied.

• Note condition of the catheter site and whether a culture specimen was collected.

• Note any complications and actions taken.

Cerebellar function assessment

Signs and symptoms of a neurologic disorder can appear in patients of any age. An elderly patient may show signs of neurologic dysfunction from a cerebrovascular accident (CVA), while a young adult may have neurologic problems from a traumatic brain injury. And patients of all ages can de-velop progressive deterioration of the nervous system.

You can identify such neurologic problems while performing a complete nursing assessment or a neurologic screening while investigating a complaint. With this screening, you can evaluate overall neurologic function and detect abnormalities. One part of this assessment includes testing cerebellar function.

▶ Key nursing diagnoses and patient outcomes

Use these nursing diagnoses as a guide when developing your plan of care.

Impaired physical mobility related to cerebellar dysfunction

Based on this nursing diagnosis, you'll establish the following patient outcomes. The patient will:

• achieve highest level of mobility possible within the confines of the disease.

• make plans to use resources to help maintain level of functioning (physical and occupational therapist, stroke program, National Multiple Sclerosis Society)

Risk for injury related to cerebellar dysfunction

Based on this nursing diagnosis, you'll establish the following patient outcomes. The patient will:

• identify factors that increase potential for injury.

• help identify and observe safety measures to prevent injury.

• identify safety-maintenance strategy.

• optimize activities of daily living within sensorimotor limitations.

Equipment

♦ No special equipment is needed to assess cerebellar function except a place to examine the patient and piece of furniture on which he may sit.

Patient preparation

• Before you test cerebellar function, observe the patient's general balance and coordination. Can he sit upright without support? Can he sit on the edge of the bed? Can he stand at the bedside? Remember that the ability to sit on the edge of the bed and to stand may be diminished by weakness unrelated to cerebellar dysfunction.

Implementation

• Evaluate whole-body coordination and extremity coordination.

Whole-body coordination

• Assessing whole-body coordination includes evaluating the patient as he walks and performs certain other maneuvers.

• Observe the patient as he walks across the room, turns, and walks back.

• Note any imbalance or abnormalities in his gait. He should be able to maintain his posture. His arms should swing in tandem with his leg movements. His movements should be smooth and rhythmic, without hesitation or jerkiness. A patient with cerebellar dysfunction will exhibit a wide-based, unsteady gait. Deviation to one side may indicate a cerebellar lesion on that side.

• Ask the patient to walk heel to toe and observe his balance. He may be slightly unsteady, but should be able to maintain balance while walking forward. (See *Assessing cerebellar function.*)

• Next, perform the Romberg test. Ask the patient to stand with his feet together, his eyes open, and his arms at his side. Hold your outstretched arms on either side of him so you can support him if he sways sideways. Observe his balance, and ask him to close his eyes. Note whether he loses his balance or sways. If he falls to one side, the Romberg test is positive. Patients with cerebellar dysfunction have difficulty maintaining balance with their eyes closed because they cannot use visual cues for upright orientation.

• You can also test whole-body coordination by asking the patient to do deep knee bends or to hop first on one foot and then the other. Keep in mind that patients with arthritis or other musculoskeletal disorders may have difficulty with these tests.

Extremity coordination

• To evaluate the patient's extremity coordination, you'll test point-to-point movements, and rapid skilled and rapid alternating movements.

Point-to-point movements

• Have the patient sit about 2′ (0.6 m) away from you.

• Hold your index finger up, and ask him to touch the tip of his index finger to the tip of yours and then to touch his nose.

• Move your finger and ask him to repeat the maneuver. Gradually, have him increase his speed as you repeat the test.

• Test his other hand. Expect the patient to be more accurate with his dominant hand. A patient with cerebellar dysfunction will overshoot his

Assessing cerebellar function

To evaluate cerebellar function, you'll test the patient's balance and coordination. The illustrations below show you four of the tests you'll use.

Heel-to-toe walking

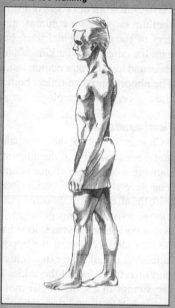

Romberg test

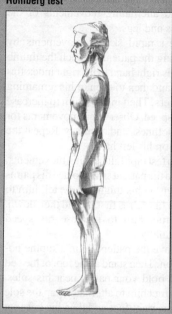

Point-to-point movements

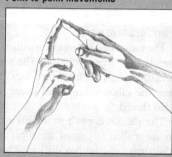

Rapid skilled movements

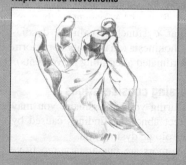

target, and his movements will be jerky.

• Ask the patient to touch the heel of his right foot to his left shin and to run his heel down his shin. Then have him repeat the maneuver with his left foot. If he has cerebellar dysfunction, he'll have difficulty placing his heel on his shin and maintaining the position, and his movements will be jerky.

Rapid skilled and rapid alternating movements
• To further test cerebellar function, observe rapid skilled movements and rapid alternating movements of the arms and legs.
• Test rapid skilled movements by asking the patient to touch the thumb of his right hand to his right index finger and then to each of his remaining fingers. Then instruct him to increase his speed. Observe his movements for smoothness and accuracy. Repeat the test on his left hand.
• To test rapid alternating movements, have the patient sit and place his palms down on his thighs. Now, tell him to turn his palms first up and then down. Instruct him to increase his speed gradually.
• Have the patient lie in a supine position. Then stand at the foot of the bed and hold your palms near his soles. Instruct him to alternately tap the sole of his right foot and then his left foot against your palms. Tell him to increase his speed as you observe his coordination. A patient with cerebellar dysfunction exhibits dysdiadochokinesia (an inability to perform coordinated alternating movements).

Nursing considerations
• During your assessment, you may detect abnormal findings caused by neurologic dysfunction.
• Tremors are involuntary, repetitive movements usually seen in the fingers or wrists and the eyelids, tongue, and legs. They can occur when the affected body part is at rest (resting tremors) or when is voluntarily moved (intention tremors). The patient with cere-

bellar disease has tremors when he voluntarily reaches for an object.
• During your assessment, you may identify one of these four gait abnormalities: hemiparetic, parkinsonian, ataxic, or steppage gait. These gaits may result from disorders of the cerebellum or posterior columns, disorders of the corticospinal tract, basal ganglia defects of Parkinson's disease, and lower motor neuron lesions. The abnormality can reflect both the site and degree of neurologic damage.

Hemiparetic gait
• Characteristics of the hemiparetic gait vary according to the amount of damage to the upper motor neurons. The severely affected patient walks with the affected arm abducted and the elbow, wrist, and fingers flexed. His upper body is somewhat stooped, and he tilts slightly toward the opposite side. As he walks, he extends his leg and inverts his foot at the ankle. The leg swings in a semicircular motion, first away from and then toward the trunk, and the foot drags along the floor.

Parkinsonian gait
• The patient with Parkinson's disease bends over when walking. The neck and thoracic spine are flexed forward, and the elbows, hips, and knees are also flexed.
• The patient doesn't swing his arms as he walks. His steps are short and shuffling, and he has difficulty both initiating and stopping movement.

Ataxic gait
• The patient with cerebellar ataxia has difficulty maintaining balance while standing still and while walk-

ing. Ambulation is characterized by a wide-based, reeling, drunken gait.

• In sensory ataxia, the patient must watch his feet because he can't feel where he is placing them. His legs are partially flexed at the hips, and he lifts his legs up and slaps his feet on the floor with each step.

Steppage gait

• A patient with a steppage gait purposefully lifts his feet up and then slaps them down on the floor. This gait is associated with lower motor neuron disease and is often accompanied by muscle weakness and atrophy, and fasciculations.

Documentation

• Document the time and place of the cerebellar function assessment, noting normal and abnormal findings.

• Charting abnormal findings is essential in ensuring patient safety.

Cerebral blood flow monitoring

Traditionally, caregivers have estimated cerebral blood flow (CBF) in neurologically compromised patients by calculating cerebral perfusion pressure. Modern technology, however, permits continuous regional blood flow monitoring at the bedside.

A sensor placed on the cerebral cortex calculates CBF in the capillary bed by thermal diffusion. Thermistors within the sensor detect the temperature differential between two metallic plates — one heated, one neutral. This differential relates inversely to CBF: As the differential decreases, CBF increases, and vice versa. This monitoring technique yields important information about the effects of different interventions on CBF. It also yields continuous real-time values for CBF, which are essential in conditions that put patients at risk because of compromised blood flow, such as ischemia and infarction.

CBF monitoring is indicated whenever CBF alterations are anticipated. It's used most often in patients with subarachnoid hemorrhage (when a vasospasm may restrict blood flow), trauma associated with high intracranial pressure or vascular tumors. Use of this new technology is likely to grow as practitioners become more familiar with it.

≫ Key nursing diagnoses and patient outcomes

Use these nursing diagnoses as a guide when developing your plan of care for a patient requiring CBF monitoring.

Altered cerebral tissue perfusion related to decreased cellular exchange

Based on this nursing diagnosis, you'll establish the following patient outcomes. The patient will:

• maintain or improve current level of consciousness.

• maintain intracranial pressure between (specify) mm Hg and (specify) mm Hg.

• maintain blood pressure high enough to maintain cerebral perfusion pressure but low enough to prevent increased bleeding or cerebral swelling.

TECHNOLOGY UPDATE

CBF monitoring systems

To monitor cerebral blood flow (CBF) at the patient's bedside, you may use a monitor such as the one shown below. This monitor has a digital display; some also display waveforms. The CBF sensor, placed in the cerebral cortex, continuously measures cortical blood flow.

Bedside CBF monitor

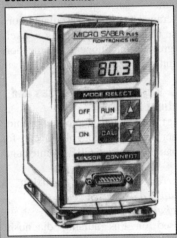

CBF sensor

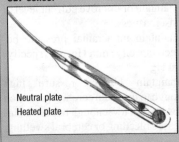

Risk for infection related to CBF sensor

Based on this nursing diagnosis, you'll establish the following patient outcomes. The patient will:
• remain afebrile.
• have white blood cell count and differential stay within normal range.
• present no pathogens in cultures.

Equipment

◆ CBF monitoring requires a special sensor that attaches to a computer data system or to a small battery-powered analog monitor for patient transport. (See *CBF monitoring systems*.)

For care of site: ◆ Linen-saver pad ◆ sterile 4″ × 4″ gauze pads ◆ clean gloves ◆ sterile gloves ◆ povidone-iodine solution or ointment.

For removing sensor: ◆ Sterile suture removal tray ◆ 1″ adhesive tape ◆ sterile 4″ × 4″ gauze pads ◆ clean gloves ◆ sterile gloves ◆ suture material.

Equipment preparation

• Make sure the patient or a family member is understands CBF monitoring procedures.
• Obtain a consent form.
• If the patient will need CBF monitoring after surgery, advise her that a sensor will be in place for about 3 days postoperatively to measure CBF.
• Tell the patient that the insertion site will be covered with a dry, sterile dressing.
• Mention that the sensor may be removed at the bedside.

Setting up the sensor monitor

• Depending on the system you're using, you may need to verify that the monitor has a battery to allow CBF monitoring while the patient is taken to the intensive care unit.

• Assemble the following equipment at the bedside: a monitor and a sensor cable with an attached sensor.

• Attach the distal end of the sensor cable from the patient's head to the SENSOR CONNECT port on the monitor.

• When the sensor cable is securely in place, press the ON key to activate the monitor.

• Calibrate the system by pressing the CAL key. You should see the red light appear on the CAL button. Ideally, you'll begin by calibrating the sensor to 00.0 by pressing the directional arrows. Readouts of plus or minus 0.1 are also acceptable.

Implementation

• The surgeon typically inserts the sensor in the operating room, during or at completion of a craniotomy. (Occasionally, he may place it through a burr hole.) He implants the sensor far from major blood vessels and verifies that the metallic plates have good contact with the brain surface. (See *Placing a CBF sensor*, page 198.)

• Press the RUN key to display the CBF reading. Observe the monitor's digital display, and document the baseline value.

• Record the CBF hourly. Be sure to watch for trends and correlate values with the patient's clinical state.

• Keep in mind that stimulation or activity may cause a 10% increase or decrease in CBF. If you detect a 20% increase or decrease, suspect poor contact between the sensor and the cerebral cortex.

Caring for the insertion site

• Wash your hands.

• Put on clean gloves, and then remove the dressing from the sensor insertion site.

• Observe the site for cerebrospinal fluid (CSF) leakage, a potential complication.

• Remove and discard your gloves.

• Next, put on sterile gloves.

• Using aseptic technique, clean the insertion site with a gauze pad soaked in povidone-iodine solution, starting at the center and working outward in a circular pattern.

• Using a new gauze pad soaked with povidone-iodine, clean the exposed part of the sensor from the insertion site to the end of the sensor.

• Apply povidone-iodine ointment to the insertion site if hospital policy permits.

• Next, place sterile 4″ × 4″ gauze pads over the insertion site to completely cover it.

• Tape all edges securely to create an occlusive dressing.

Removing the sensor

• In most cases, the CBF sensor remains in place for about 3 days when used for postoperative monitoring.

• Explain the procedure to the patient; then wash your hands. Put on clean gloves, remove the dressing, and dispose of the gloves and dressing properly.

• Open the suture removal tray and the package of suture material. The surgeon removes the anchoring sutures and then gently removes the sensor from the insertion site.

• After the surgeon closes the wound with stitches, put on sterile gloves, apply a folded gauze pad to the site, and

Placing a CBF sensor

Typically, the surgeon inserts a cerebral blood flow (CBF) sensor during a craniotomy. He tunnels the sensor toward the craniotomy site and then carefully inserts the metallic plates of the thermistor to make sure that they continuously contact the surface of the cerebral cortex. After closing the dura and replacing the bone flap, he closes the scalp.

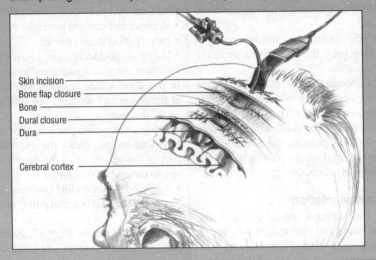

Skin incision
Bone flap closure
Bone
Dural closure
Dura
Cerebral cortex

tape it in place. Observe the condition of the site, including any leakage.

Complications
• Complications include infection and CSF leakage at the insertion site.

Nursing considerations
• CBF fluctuates with the brain's metabolic demands, normally ranging from 60 to 90 ml/100 g/minute, but the patient's neurologic condition dictates the acceptable range. For instance, in a comatose patient, CBF may be half the normal value; in a patient in a barbiturate-induced coma with burst suppression on the electroencephalogram, CBF may be as low as 10 ml/100 g/minute. Vasospasm

secondary to subarachnoid hemorrhage may result in CBF below 40 ml/100 g/minute. In an awake patient, CBF above 90 ml/100 g/minute may indicate hyperemia.
• Document CBF values hourly. Be sure to check for trends, and correlate values with the patient's clinical status.
• Remember that stimulation or activity may cause a 10% increase or decrease in CBF. If you note a 20% increase or decrease, suspect poor contact between the sensor and the cerebral cortex. To correct this, turn the patient toward the side of the sensor or gently wiggle the catheter back and forth (using a sterile-gloved hand). To determine if these maneuvers have

improved contact between the sensor and the cortex, observe the CBF value on the monitor as you perform them.
• If your patient has low CBF but no neurologic symptoms that indicate ischemia, suspect a fluid layer (a small hematoma) between the sensor and the cortex.
• As with ICP monitoring, CBF monitoring may lead to infection. To guard against this complication, administer prophylactic antibiotics as ordered, and maintain a sterile dressing around the insertion site.
• CSF leakage, another potential complication, may occur at the sensor insertion site. To prevent leakage, the surgeon usually places an extra suture at the site.
• To reduce the risk of infection, change the dressing at the insertion site daily.

Documentation
• Document cleaning of the site, appearance of the site, and dressing changes. After sensor removal, document any leakage from the site.

Cerebrospinal fluid drainage

Cerebrospinal fluid (CSF) drainage reduces CSF pressure to desired level and maintains it. Fluid can be withdrawn from the lateral ventricle (ventriculostomy) or lumbar subarachnoid space, depending on the indication and the desired outcome. Ventricular drainage reduces increased intracranial pressure (ICP) lumbar drainage helps healing of the dura mater. External CSF drainage is usually used to manage increased ICP and to facilitate spinal or cerebral dural healing after traumatic injury or surgery. In either case, CSF is drained by a catheter or a ventriculostomy tube in a sterile, closed drainage collection system.

Other therapeutic uses include ICP monitoring via the ventriculostomy; direct instillation of medications, contrast media, or air for diagnostic radiology; and aspiration of CSF for laboratory analysis.

To place the ventricular drain, the doctor inserts a ventricular catheter through a burr hole in the patient's skull. Usually, this is done in the operating room under general anesthesia. To place the lumbar subarachnoid drain, the doctor may administer a local spinal anesthetic at bedside or in the operating room. (See *Methods of CSF drainage*, page 200.)

≫ Key nursing diagnoses and patient outcomes
Use these nursing diagnoses as a guide when developing your plan of care for a patient who requires a CSF drain.

Altered cerebral tissue perfusion related to decreased cellular exchange
Based on this nursing diagnosis, you'll establish the following patient outcomes. The patient will:
• maintain or improve level of consciousness.
• maintain intracranial pressure between (specify) mm Hg and (specify) mm Hg.
• maintain a balanced intake and output.

Methods of CSF drainage

Cerebrospinal fluid (CSF) drainage aims to control intracranial pressure (ICP) during treatment for traumatic injury or other conditions that cause a rise in ICP. Two procedures are commonly used, as detailed below.

For a ventricular drain, the doctor makes a burr hole in the patient's skull and inserts the catheter into the ventricle. The distal end of the catheter is connected to a closed drainage system.

Drainage catheters lead to a sterile, closed collection system affixed securely to the bed or to an I.V. pole. The drip chamber should be set at the level ordered by the doctor.

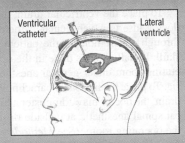

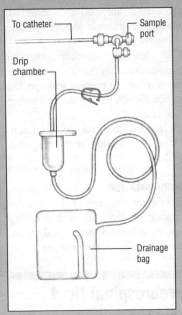

For a lumbar drain, the doctor inserts a catheter beneath the dura into the L3-L4 interspace.

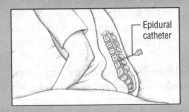

Risk for infection related to presence of CSF drain

Based on this nursing diagnosis, you'll establish the following patient outcomes. The patient will:

• have no pathogens appear in cultures.

• remain afebrile.

• show no evidence of infection at the insertion site, such as redness, swelling, or drainage.

Equipment

♦ overbed table ♦ sterile gloves ♦ sterile cotton-tipped applicators ♦ povidone-iodine solution ♦ alcohol sponges ♦ sterile fenestrated drape ♦ 3-ml syringe for local anesthetic ♦ 25G 4″ needle for injecting anesthetic ♦ local anesthetic (usually 1% lidocaine) ♦ 18G or 20G sterile spinal needle or Tuohy needle ♦ #5 French whistle-tip catheter or ventriculostomy tube ♦ external drainage set (includes drainage tubing and sterile collection bag) ♦ suture material ♦ $4'' \times 4''$ dressings ♦ paper tape ♦ lamp or another light source ♦ I.V. pole ♦ optional: ventriculostomy tray, twist drill, pain medication such as an analgesic, anti-infective agent such as an antibiotic.

Equipment preparation
• Check all packaging for breaks in seals and for expiration dates.
• If equipment packaging is intact and expiration dates have not been met or exceeded, open all equipment using sterile technique.
• After the doctor places the catheter, connect it to the external drainage system tubing. Secure connection points with tape or a connector.
• Place the collection system, including drip chamber and collection bag, on an I.V. pole.

Implementation
• Explain the procedure to the patient and family.
• Document informed consent according to hospital guidelines.
• Wash your hands thoroughly.
• Perform a baseline neurologic assessment, including vital signs, *to help detect alterations or signs of deterioration.*

Inserting a ventricular drain
• Place the patient in a supine position.
• Place the equipment tray on the overbed table, and unwrap the tray.
• Adjust the height of the bed *so that the doctor can perform the procedure comfortably.*

• Illuminate the area of the catheter insertion site.
• The doctor will clean the insertion site and administer a local anesthetic.
• To insert the drain, the doctor will request a ventriculostomy tray with a twist drill. After completing the ventriculostomy, he will connect the drainage system.

Inserting a lumbar subarachnoid drain
• Position the patient in a side-lying position with his chin tucked to his chest and knees drawn up to his abdomen, as for a lumbar puncture.
• Urge the patient to remain as still as possible during the procedure.
• To insert the drain, the doctor attaches a Tuohy needle (or spinal needle) to the whistle-tip catheter. After the doctor removes the needle, he connects the drainage system and sutures or tapes the catheter securely in place.

Monitoring CSF drainage
• Maintain a continuous hourly output of CSF by raising or lowering the drip chamber. To maintain CSF outflow, the drip chamber should be slightly lower than or at the level of the lumbar drain insertion site. Sometimes you may need to carefully raise or lower the drip chamber *to increase or decrease CSF flow.* For ventricular drains, ensure that the flow chamber of the ICP monitoring setup remains positioned as ordered.
• To drain CSF, as ordered, put on gloves; then turn the main stopcock on to drainage. *This allows CSF to collect in the graduated flow chamber.* Document the time and the amount of CSF obtained. Then turn the stopcock off to drainage. To drain the CSF from

this chamber into the drainage bag, release the clamp below the flow chamber. Never empty the drainage bag. Instead, replace it when full, using sterile technique.

• Check the dressing frequently for drainage, which could indicate CSF leakage.

• Check the tubing for patency by watching the CSF drops in the drip chamber.

• Observe CSF for color, clarity, volume, blood, and sediment. CSF specimens for laboratory analysis should be obtained from the collection port attached to the tubing, not from the collection bag.

• Change the collection bag when it's full or every 24 hours, according to your hospital policy.

Complications

Signs of excessive CSF drainage include:

• headache
• tachycardia
• diaphoresis
• nausea.

Acute overdrainage may result in the following:

• collapsed ventricles
• tonsillar herniation
• medullary compression.

Other complications may surface as well:

• If drainage accumulates too rapidly, a neurosurgical emergency may occur. If drainage is too fast, clamp the system and notify the doctor immediately.

• Cessation of drainage may indicate clot formation. If you can't quickly identify the cause of the obstruction, notify the doctor.

• If drainage is blocked, the patient may develop signs of increased ICP. (If the lumbar drain was placed to aid dural wound healing, blockage may cause a CSF leak in the wound area).

• Infection may cause meningitis. Administer antibiotics as ordered to prevent this.

Nursing considerations

• Maintenance of hourly CSF output is essential *to prevent overdrainage or underdrainage.* Underdrainage or lack of CSF may reflect kinked tubing, catheter displacement, or a drip chamber placed higher than the catheter insertion site. Overdrainage can occur if the drip chamber is placed too far below the catheter insertion site.

• Raising or lowering the head of the bed can affect the CSF flow rate. When changing the patient's position, reposition the drip chamber, too.

• Patients often experience chronic headache during continuous CSF drainage. Reassure the patient that this is not unusual; administer analgesics as appropriate.

Documentation

• During drainage, document the time and amount of CSF obtained.

• Record the time and date of the insertion procedure and the patient's response.

• Record routine vital signs and neurologic assessment findings at least every 4 hours.

• Document the color, clarity, and amount of CSF at least every 8 hours.

• Record hourly and 24-hour CSF outputs.

• Describe the condition of the dressing.

Cervical collar

A cervical collar may be used for an acute injury such as strained cervical muscles or for a chronic condition, such as arthritis or cervical metastasis. It may also augment such splinting devices as a spine board to prevent potential cervical spine fracture or spinal cord damage.

Cervical collars are designed to hold the neck straight with the chin slightly elevated and tucked in. Cervical collars immobilize the cervical spine, decrease muscle spasms, and relieve some pain; they also prevent further injury and promote healing. As symptoms of an acute injury subside, the patient may gradually discontinue wearing a cervical collar, alternating periods of wear with more frequent and longer periods without the collar, until it's no longer needed.

>> Key nursing diagnoses and patient outcomes
Use these nursing diagnoses as a guide when developing your plan of care.

Impaired physical mobility related to (specify)
Based on this nursing diagnosis, you'll establish the following patient outcomes. The patient will:
• state relief from pain.
• attain highest degree of mobility possible within the confines of the disease.
• state or demonstrate mobility regimen.

Pain related to cervical injury
Based on this nursing diagnosis, you'll establish the following patient outcomes. The patient will:
• express a relief from pain with proper cervical collar placement and minimal analgesia.
• state satisfaction with pain-management regimen.
• be cooperative with pain-management treatment plan.

Equipment
♦ cervical collar, in the appropriate size. (See *Types of cervical collars,* page 204.)

Patient preparation
• Check the patient's neurovascular status before application.

Implementation
• Instruct the patient to position his head slowly to face directly forward.
• Place the cervical collar in front of the patient's neck *to ensure that the size is correct.*
• Fit the collar snugly around the neck and attach the Velcro fasteners or buckles at the back of the neck.
• Check the patient's airway and his neurovascular status *to ensure that the collar isn't too tight.*

Nursing considerations
• For a sprain or a potential cervical spine fracture, make sure the collar isn't too high in front *because this may hyperextend the neck.* In a neck sprain, such hyperextension may cause ligaments to heal in a shortened position. In a potential cervical spine fracture, hyperextension may cause serious neurologic damage.

Types of cervical collars

Cervical collars are used to support an injured or weakened cervical spine and to maintain alignment during healing.

Made of rigid plastic, the molded cervical collar holds the patient's neck firmly, keeping it straight, with the chin slightly elevated and tucked in.

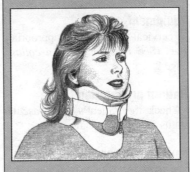

The soft cervical collar, made of spongy foam, provides gentler support and reminds the patient to avoid cervical spine motion.

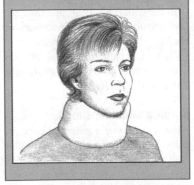

Home care
• Teach the patient how to apply the collar and how to do a neurovascular check.

• Name symptoms to report to the doctor.
• If indicated advise sleeping without a pillow.

Documentation
• Note the type and size of the cervical collar and the time and date of application in your notes.
• Record results of neurovascular checks.
• Document patient comfort, collar snugness, and all patient instruction.

Chemotherapeutic drug administration

Treating cancer with chemotherapy requires skills beyond those involved in giving other kinds of drugs. Some chemotherapeutic drugs, for example, require special equipment or are given by an unusual route. Some quickly become unstable, and others must be protected from light. These drugs are also powerful and require precise dosages to avoid harming patients. For these reasons, only specially trained nurses and doctors should administer drugs for chemotherapy.

I.V. delivery (to a peripheral or central vein) is most common, but chemotherapy may be administered a number of ways, including by mouth, central venous catheter, spinal canal reservoir, or implanted patient-controlled analgesia PCA device.

Chemotherapy also may be administered S.C., I.M., intra-arterially, or into a body cavity. The route depends on the drug's properties and the tumor's characteristics. For a confined tumor, for instance, a drug may be administered through a local or regional method. Regional administration allows high-dose delivery directly into the tumor, which is an advantage in treating solid tumors, many of which don't respond to drug dosages considered safe for systemic administration.

Chemotherapy may be administered when cancer may have been eradicated through surgery or radiation therapy. This treatment, called *adjuvant chemotherapy*, helps ensure that no undetectable metastasis has occurred. A patient may also receive chemotherapy before surgery or radiation therapy, in which case it's called induction chemotherapy (or *neoadjuvant* or *synchronous chemotherapy*). Induction chemotherapy helps improve survival rates by shrinking a tumor before surgical excision or radiation therapy.

In general, higher dosages are more effective than lower ones, but the drugs' adverse effects often limit dosage. One exception is methotrexate. This drug is particularly effective against rapidly growing tumors but toxic to rapidly growing and dividing normal tissues. Fortunately, doctors have discovered they can give a large dose of methotrexate to destroy cancer cells and then, before the drug damages vital organs, give a dose of folinic acid as an antidote.

≫ Key nursing diagnoses and patient outcomes

Use these nursing diagnoses as a guide when developing your plan of care for a patient receiving chemotherapeutic drugs.

Pain related to cancer or chemotherapy

Based on this nursing diagnosis, you'll establish the following patient outcomes. The patient will:
• carry out alternative pain-control measures, such as heat or cold applications.
• express comfort.

Powerlessness related to treatment

Based on this nursing diagnosis, you'll establish the following patient outcomes. The patient will:
• participate in planning care.
• enumerate factors in treatment over which control can be maintained.
• communicate a sense of having gained control.

Equipment

♦ prescribed drug ♦ aluminum foil or a brown paper bag (if the drug is photosensitive) ♦ normal saline solution ♦ syringes and needles ♦ infusion pump or controller ♦ gloves ♦ impervious containers labeled "Caution: Biohazard."

Implementation

• Verify the drug, dosage, and administration route by checking the medication record against the doctor's order. Make sure you know the immediate and delayed adverse effects of the ordered drug.
• Assess the patient's physical condition and review his medical history.
• Make sure you understand the drug to be given and the route.
• Provide instruction and support to the patient and his family.

• Determine the best administration site. When selecting the site, consider the drug's compatibilities, administration frequency, and vesicant potential. For example, if the doctor has ordered intermittent administration of a vesicant drug, you can give it by instilling the drug into the side port of an infusing I.V. line or by direct I.V. push. If, however, the vesicant drug is to be infused continuously, you should administer it only through a central venous line or a vascular-access device. On the other hand, nonvesicant agents (including irritants) may be given by direct I.V. push through the side port of an infusing I.V. line or by continuous infusion.

• Check hospital policy before administering a vesicant. *Because vein integrity decreases with time,* some policies require that vesicants be administered *before* other drugs. Conversely, *because vesicants increase vein fragility,* some policies require that vesicants be given *after* other drugs.

• Evaluate your patient's condition, paying particular attention to results of recent laboratory studies, specifically his complete blood count, blood urea nitrogen level, platelet count, urine creatinine level, and liver function.

• Determine whether the patient has had previous chemotherapy, and note the severity of any adverse effects. Check his drug history for medications that might interact with chemotherapeutic drugs. *As a rule, you shouldn't mix these drugs with other medications.* If you have questions or concerns about giving chemotherapeutic drugs, talk with the doctor first.

• Double-check the patient's chart for the complete chemotherapy protocol order, including the patient's name; the drug's name and dosage; and the route, rate, and frequency of administration. See whether the drug's dosage depends on certain laboratory values. Be aware that some health care facilities require two nurses to read the dosage order and to check the drug and amount to be administered.

• Check whether the doctor ordered an antiemetic, fluids, diuretic, or electrolyte supplement to be given before, during, or after chemotherapy.

• Evaluate the patient's and his family's understanding of chemotherapy, and make sure a consent form has been signed.

• Put on gloves and keep them on through all stages of handling the drug, including preparation, priming the I.V. tubing, and administration.

• Before administering the drug, perform a new venipuncture near the old site (if chemotherapy is ongoing). Avoid administration through an existing I.V. line. To identify an administration site, examine the patient's veins, starting with his hand and proceeding to his forearm.

• Once an appropriate line is in place, infuse 10 to 20 ml of normal saline solution to *test vein patency.* Never use a chemotherapeutic drug to test vein patency.

• Administer the drug — nonvesicants by I.V. push or mixed in a bag of I.V. fluid and vesicants by I.V. push through a piggyback set connected to a rapidly infusing I.V. line.

• During I.V. administration, closely monitor the patient for signs of hypersensitivity or extravasation.

An alternative approach: Intraperitoneal chemotherapy

Administering chemotherapy drugs into the peritoneal cavity has several benefits for patients with malignant ascites or ovarian cancer that has spread to the peritoneum. This technique passes drugs directly to the tumor area in the peritoneal cavity, exposing malignant cells to very high concentrations of chemotherapy — up to 1,000 times what could be safely given systemically. The semipermeable peritoneal membrane also permits prolonged exposure of malignant cells to the drug.

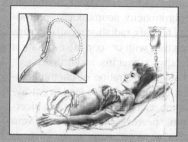

Typically, this therapy is performed using a peritoneal-dialysis kit, but drugs can also be administered to the peritoneal cavity directly, via the Tenckhoff catheter, shown top right.

This method can be performed on an outpatient basis, if necessary, and uses equipment is readily available on most units with oncology patients.

In this technique, the chemotherapy bag is connected directly to the Tenckhoff catheter with a length of I.V. tubing, the solution is infused, and the catheter and I.V. tubing are clamped. Then the patient is asked to change positions every 10 to 15 minutes for 1 hour to move the solution around in the peritoneal cavity. After the prescribed dwell time, the chemotherapy drugs are drained into an I.V. bag. The patient is encouraged to change positions to facilitate drainage. Then the I.V. tubing and catheter are clamped, the I.V. tubing removed, and a new intermittent infusion cap is fitted to the catheter. Finally, the catheter is flushed with a syringe of heparinized saline solution.

• Check for adequate blood return after 5 ml has been infused or according to hospital guidelines.
• After infusion, infuse 20 ml of normal saline solution. Do this between administrations of different chemotherapeutic drugs and before removing the I.V. line.
• Dispose of used needles and syringes carefully. *To prevent aerosol dispersion of chemotherapeutic drugs,* don't clip needles. Place them intact in an impervious container for incineration.

• Dispose of I.V. bags, bottles, gloves, and tubing in a properly labeled and covered trash container.
• Wash your hands thoroughly with soap and warm water after giving any chemotherapeutic drug, even though you have worn gloves.

Complications
• Common adverse effects of chemotherapy include nausea and vomiting, ranging from mild to debilitating; bone marrow suppression, leading to neutropenia and thrombocytopenia.

• Other adverse effects include alopecia, anemia, anorexia, cardiotoxicity, constipation, diarrhea, esophagitis, hearing loss, intestinal irritation, nephrotoxicity, neurotoxicity, pulmonary fibrosis, radiation recall (if drugs are given with or soon after radiation therapy), stomatitis, and urticaria.

• I.V. administration of chemotherapeutic drugs may also lead to extravasation, causing inflammation, ulceration, necrosis, and loss of vein patency.

Nursing considerations

• Observe the I.V. site frequently for signs of extravasation or allergic reaction (swelling, redness, and urticaria). If you suspect extravasation, stop the infusion immediately. Leave the needle in place and notify the doctor. A conservative method for treating extravasation involves aspirating any residual drug from the tubing and needle, instilling an I.V. antidote, and then removing the needle. Afterward, you may apply heat or cold to the site and elevate the affected limb.

• During infusion, some drugs need protection from direct sunlight to avoid breakdown. If this is the case with the drug you're using, cover the vial with a brown paper bag or aluminum foil.

• When giving vesicants, avoid sites where damage to underlying tendons or nerves may occur (veins in the antecubital fossa, near the wrist, or the dorsal surface of the hand).

• If you can't stay with the patient for the entire infusion, use an infusion pump or controller *to ensure drug delivery within the prescribed time and at the prescribed rate.*

• Observe the patient at regular intervals and after treatment for adverse reactions. Monitor his vital signs throughout infusion *to assess any changes during chemotherapy administration.*

• Maintain a list of the types and amounts of drugs the patient has received. This is especially important if he has received drugs that have a cumulative effect and that can be toxic to such organs as the heart or kidneys.

Documentation

• Record the location and description of the I.V. site before treatment or the presence of blood return during bolus administration.

• Record the drugs and dosages administered, sequence of drug administration, needle type and size used, amount and type of flushing solution, and the site's condition after treatment.

• Document any adverse reactions, the patient's tolerance of the treatment, and the topics discussed with the patient and his family.

Chemotherapeutic drug preparation

When preparing chemotherapeutic drugs, take extra care for the patient's safety and your own. The patient and the people preparing and handling these drugs are at risk for teratogenic, mutagenic, or carcinogenic effects. The danger of handling these drugs hasn't been fully determined, but they can increase the handler's risk of reproductive abnormalities. Chemotherapeutic drugs also pose certain environmental threats.

The Occupational Safety and Health Administration (OSHA) has set guideline recommendations for handling chemotherapeutic drugs. Following these recommendations will help ensure your safety.

The OSHA guidelines outline two basic requirements. The first is that all health care workers who handle chemotherapeutic drugs must be educated and trained. A key element of such training involves learning how to reduce exposure when handling the drugs. The second requirement is that the drugs be prepared in a class II biological safety cabinet.

≫ Key nursing diagnoses and patient outcomes

Use these nursing diagnoses as a guide when developing your plan of care for a patient who is receiving chemotherapy.

Pain related to cancer or chemotherapy

Based on this nursing diagnosis, you'll establish the following patient outcomes. The patient will:
• articulate factors that intensify pain and modify behavior accordingly.
• carry out alternative pain-control measures, such as heat or cold applications.
• express comfort.

Powerlessness related to treatment

Based on this nursing diagnosis, you'll establish the following patient outcomes. The patient will:
• participate in planning care.
• enumerate factors in treatment that can be controlled.

• communicate a sense of regained control.

Equipment

♦ prescribed drug or drugs ♦ patient's medication record and chart ♦ long-sleeved gown ♦ latex surgical gloves ♦ face shield or goggles ♦ eyewash ♦ plastic absorbent pad ♦ alcohol sponges ♦ sterile gauze pads ♦ shoe covers ♦ impervious container with the label "Caution: Biohazard" for the disposal of any unused drug or equipment ♦ I.V. solution ♦ diluent (if necessary) ♦ compatibility reference source ♦ medication labels ♦ class II biological safety cabinet ♦ disposable towel ♦ hydrophobic filter or dispensing pin ♦ 18G needle ♦ syringes and needles of various sizes ♦ I.V. tubing with luer-lock fittings ♦ I.V. controller pump (if available).

You should also have available a chemotherapeutic spill kit, which includes: ♦ water-resistant, nonpermeable, long-sleeved gown with cuffs and back closure ♦ shoe covers ♦ two pairs of gloves (for double-gloving) ♦ goggles ♦ mask ♦ disposable dustpan ♦ plastic scraper (for collecting broken glass) ♦ plastic-backed or absorbable towels ♦ container of desiccant powder or granules (to absorb wet contents) ♦ two disposable sponges ♦ puncture-proof, leakproof container labeled "Biohazard waste" ♦ container of 70% isopropyl alcohol for cleaning the spill area.

Implementation

• Wash your hands before and after drug preparation and administration.
• Prepare the drugs in a class II biological safety cabinet.

• Wear protective garments (long-sleeved gown, gloves, and a face shield or goggles), as indicated by hospital policy. Don't wear the garments outside the preparation area.

• Don't eat, drink, smoke, or apply cosmetics in the drug-preparation area.

• Before you prepare the drug (and after you finish), clean the internal surfaces of the cabinet with the alcohol and a disposable towel. Discard the towel in a leakproof chemical-waste container.

• Cover the work surface with a clean plastic absorbent pad *to minimize contamination by droplets or spills.* Change the pad at the end of each shift or whenever a spill occurs.

• You should consider all of the equipment used in drug preparation, and any unused drug, as hazardous waste. Dispose of them according to hospital policy.

• Place all chemotherapy-waste products in leakproof, sealable, plastic bags, or other appropriate container. Make sure the container is appropriately labeled.

Complications

• Some scientific literature suggests that chemotherapeutic drugs are mutagenic. Also, chronic exposure to chemotherapeutic drugs may damage the liver or chromosomes, and direct exposure to the drugs may burn and damage the skin.

Nursing considerations

• Prepare the prescribed drugs according to current product instructions, paying attention to compatibility, stability, and reconstitution technique.

• Take precautions to reduce your exposure to chemotherapeutic drugs. Realize that systemic absorption can occur through ingestion of contaminated materials, contact with the skin, or inhalation. In fact, you can inhale a drug without even realizing it, such as while opening a vial, clipping a needle, expelling air from a syringe, or splashing while discarding leftover drug. You can also absorb a drug from handling contaminated stools or body fluids.

• *For maximum protection,* mix all chemotherapeutic drugs in an approved class II biological safety cabinet. Also, prime all I.V. bags containing chemotherapeutic drugs under the hood. Leave the hood blower on 24 hours a day, 7 days a week.

• If a cabinet isn't available, prepare drugs in a quiet, well-ventilated work space, away from heating or cooling vents and away from other personnel. Vent vials with a hydrophobic filter, or use negative-pressure techniques. Also, use a needle with a hydrophobic filter to remove the solution from vials. To break ampules, wrap a sterile gauze pad or alcohol sponge around the neck of the ampule *to decrease chances of droplet contamination.*

• Make sure the biological safety cabinet is examined every 6 months, or any time the cabinet is moved, by a company specifically prepared for this work. If the cabinet passes certification, the certifying company will affix a sticker to the cabinet attesting to its approval.

• Use only syringes and I.V. sets that have luer-lock fittings.

• Label all chemotherapeutic drugs with a "Chemotherapy hazard" label.

• Don't clip needles, break syringes, or remove the needles from the syringes used in drug preparation. Use a gauze pad when removing chemotherapy syringes and needles from I.V. bags containing chemotherapeutic drugs.

• Place used syringes or needles in a puncture-proof container, along with other sharp or breakable items.

• When mixing chemotherapeutic drugs, wear latex surgical gloves and a gown of low-permeability fabric with a closed front and cuffed long sleeves. When working steadily with chemotherapeutic drugs, change gloves every 30 minutes. If you spill a drug solution, or puncture or tear a glove, remove your gloves immediately. Wash your hands before putting on new gloves and any time you remove your gloves.

• If some of the drug comes in contact with your skin, wash the area thoroughly with soap (not a germicidal agent) and water.

• If eye contact occurs, flood the eye with water or an isotonic eyewash for at least 5 minutes while holding the eyelid open.

• Obtain a medical evaluation as soon as possible after accidental exposure.

• If a major spill occurs, use a chemotherapy-spill kit to clean the area.

• Discard disposable gowns and gloves in an appropriately marked, waterproof receptacle whenever they're contaminated or you leave the work area.

• Don't place food or drinks in the refrigerator that's used for chemotherapeutic drugs.

• Become familiar with drug excretion patterns and take precautions when handling a chemotherapy patient's body fluids.

• Provide male patients with a urinal with a tight-fitting lid.

• Wear disposable latex surgical gloves when handling body fluids.

• Before flushing the toilet, place a waterproof pad over the toilet bowl to avoid splashing.

• Wear gloves and a gown when handling linens soiled with body fluids.

• Place soiled linens in isolation linen bags designated for separate laundering.

• When caring for a patient in her home, empty waste products into the toilet close to the water *to minimize splashing*. Close the lid and flush two or three times. Place soiled linens in a washable pillowcase and launder them twice, separately from other household linens. Wear gloves when handling contaminated linens, bedclothes, or other materials.

• Women who are pregnant, trying to conceive, or breast-feeding should exercise caution when handling chemotherapeutic drugs.

Home care

• When teaching your patient about handling chemotherapeutic drugs, discuss appropriate safety measures.

• If the patient will be receiving chemotherapy at home, teach her how to dispose of contaminated equipment.

• Tell the patient and family to wear gloves when handling chemotherapy equipment or contaminated linens or bedclothes. Instruct them to place soiled linens in a separate washable pillowcase and to launder the pillowcase twice, with the soiled linens inside, separate from other household linens.

• Instruct the patient and family to place all treatment materials in a leakproof container and then take it to a designated disposal area. They should make arrangements with a hospital or waste-disposal company for pickup and disposal of contaminated waste.

Documentation
• Record each incident of exposure according to hospital policy.

Chest drainage

Because negative pressure in the pleural cavity exerts a suction force that keeps the lungs expanded, any chest trauma that upsets this pressure may cause lung collapse. Consequently, one or more chest tubes may be surgically inserted and then connected to a chest drainage system. Chest drainage uses gravity and possibly suction to restore negative pressure and remove any material that collects in the pleural cavity. An underwater seal in the drainage system allows air and fluid to escape from the pleural cavity, but doesn't allow air to reenter. The system may include one, two, or three bottles to collect drainage, create a water seal, and control suction. Or it may be a self-contained, disposable system that combines the features of a multibottle system in a compact, one-piece unit. Because you're less likely to use a bottle system, the procedure here details use of a disposable system. (See *Comparing closed drainage systems*, page 213.)

Chest drainage may be ordered to remove accumulated air, fluids

(blood, pus, chyle, serous fluids, gastric juices), or solids (blood clots) from the pleural cavity; to restore negative pressure in the pleural cavity; or to reexpand a partially or totally collapsed lung.

≫ Key nursing diagnoses and patient outcomes
Use these nursing diagnoses as a guide when developing your plan of care for a patient with chest drainage.

Ineffective breathing pattern related to physical condition
Based on this nursing diagnosis, you'll establish the following patient outcomes. The patient will:
• have a respiratory rate within 5 breaths of baseline.
• have arterial blood gas levels remain normal.

Pain related to physical condition
Based on this nursing diagnosis, you'll establish the following patient outcomes. The patient will:
• express a feeling of comfort and relief from pain.
• state and carry out appropriate interventions for pain relief.

Equipment
♦chest drainage system (Pleur-evac, Argyle, Ohio, or Thora-Klex system, which can function as gravity draining systems or be connected to suction to enhance chest drainage) ♦ sterile distilled water (usually 1 liter) ♦ adhesive tape ♦ sterile clear plastic tubing ♦ bottle or system rack ♦ two rubber-tipped Kelly clamps ♦ sterile 50-ml catheter-tip syringe ♦ suction source, if ordered.

Comparing closed drainage systems

One-bottle system

The one-bottle system is the easiest drainage system to use. It drains by gravity, combining drainage collection and the water-seal chamber. This system is not recommended for excessive drainage.

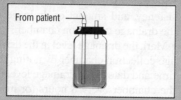

Two-bottle system

The two-bottle system collects drainage in the first bottle and uses the second bottle as the water-seal chamber. This system is not recommended for excessive drainage.

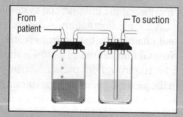

Three-bottle system

In the three-bottle system, the first bottle collects drainage, the second bottle acts as the water-seal chamber, and the third bottle is the suction-control chamber. This system can handle excessive drainage.

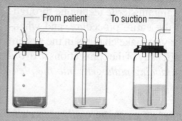

Disposable drainage systems

Commercially prepared disposable systems combine drainage collection, water seal, and suction control in one unit, as shown here. These systems ensure patient safety with positive- and negative-pressure relief valves and have a prominent air-leak indicator. Some systems produce no bubbling sound.

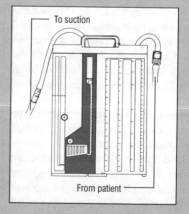

Equipment preparation

• Check the doctor's order to determine the type of drainage system to be used and specific procedural details.

• If appropriate, request the drainage system and suction system from the central supply department.

Collect the appropriate equipment and take it to the patient's bedside.

Patient preparation
• Explain the procedure to the patient.

Implementation
• Wash your hands.
• Maintain sterile technique throughout the entire procedure, and whenever you make changes in the system or alter any of the connections *to avoid introducing pathogens into the pleural space.*

To set up a commercially prepared disposable system
• Open the packaged system and place it on the floor in the rack supplied by the manufacturer *to avoid accidentally knocking it over or dislodging the components.* After the system is prepared, it may be hung from the side of the patient's bed.
• Remove the plastic connector from the short tube that's attached to the water-seal chamber. Using a 50-ml catheter-tip syringe, instill sterile distilled water into the water-seal chamber until it reaches the 2-cm mark, or the mark specified by the manufacturer. The Ohio and Thora-Klex systems are ready to use but, with the Thora-Klex system, 15-ml of sterile water may be added to help detect air leaks. Replace the plastic connector.
• If suction is ordered, remove the cap (also called the muffler or atmosphere vent cover) on the suction-control chamber *to open the vent.* Next, instill sterile distilled water until it reaches the 20-cm mark or the ordered level, and recap the suction-control chamber.
• Using the long tube, connect the patient's chest tube to the closed drainage collection chamber. Secure the connection with tape.

• Connect the short tube on the drainage system to the suction source and turn on the suction. Gentle bubbling should begin in the suction chamber, *indicating that the correct suction level has been reached.*

To manage closed chest underwater seal drainage
• Repeatedly note the character, consistency, and amount of drainage in the drainage collection chamber.
• Mark the drainage level in the drainage collection chamber by noting the time and date at the drainage level on the chamber every 8 hours (or more often) if there is a large amount of drainage.
• Check the water level in the water-seal chamber every 8 hours. If necessary, carefully add sterile distilled water until the level reaches the 2-cm mark indicated on the water-seal chamber of the commercial system.
• Check for fluctuation in the water-seal chamber as the patient breathes. Normal fluctuations of 2″ to 4″ (about 5 to 10 cm) reflect pressure changes in the pleural space during respiration. To check for fluctuation when a suction system is being used, momentarily disconnect the suction system so the air vent is opened, and observe for fluctuation.
• Check for intermittent bubbling in the water-seal chamber. This occurs normally when the system is removing air from the pleural cavity. If bubbling isn't readily apparent during quiet breathing, have the patient take a deep breath or cough. Absence of bubbling indicates that the pleural space has sealed.
• Check the water level in the suction-control chamber. Detach the chamber

or bottle from the suction source; when bubbling ceases, observe the water level. If necessary, add sterile distilled water to bring the level to the -20-cm line, or as ordered.
• Check for gentle bubbling in the suction control chamber *because it indicates that the proper suction level has been reached.* Vigorous bubbling in this chamber increases the rate of water evaporation.
• Periodically check that the air vent in the system is working properly. *Occlusion of the air vent results in a buildup of pressure in the system that could cause the patient to develop a tension pneumothorax.*
• Coil the system's tubing and secure it to the edge of the bed with a rubber band or tape and a safety pin. Avoid creating dependent loops, kinks, or pressure on the tubing *because they may interfere with chest drainage.* Avoid lifting the drainage system above the patient's chest *because fluid may flow back into the pleural space.*
• Be sure to keep two rubber-tipped clamps at the bedside. These are used to clamp the chest tube if a bottle breaks or the commercially prepared system cracks, or to locate an air leak in the system.
• Encourage the patient to cough frequently and breathe deeply *to help drain the pleural space and expand the lungs.*
• Instruct him to sit upright *for optimal lung expansion* and to splint the insertion site while coughing *to minimize pain.*
• Check the rate and quality of the patient's respirations and auscultate his lungs periodically *to assess air exchange in the affected lung.* Diminished or absent breath sounds may in-

dicate that the lung has not reexpanded.
• Tell the patient to report any breathing difficulty immediately. Notify the doctor immediately if the patient develops cyanosis, rapid or shallow breathing, subcutaneous emphysema, chest pain, or excessive bleeding.
• When clots are visible, you may be able to strip (or milk) the tubing, depending on your hospital's policy. This is a controversial procedure because it creates high negative pressure that could suck viable lung tissue into the drainage ports of the tube, with subsequent ruptured alveoli and pleural air leak. Strip the tubing only when clots are visible. Use an alcohol sponge or lotion as a lubricant on the tube and pinch it between your thumb and index finger about 2" (5 cm) from the insertion site. Using the other thumb and index finger, compress the tubing as you slide your fingers down the tube or use a mechanical stripper. After stripping, release the thumb and index finger pinching the tube near the insertion site.
• Check the chest tube dressing at least every 8 hours. Palpate the area surrounding the dressing for crepitus or subcutaneous emphysema, which indicates that air is leaking into the subcutaneous tissue surrounding the insertion site. Change the dressing if necessary or according to hospital policy.
• Encourage active or passive range-of-motion (ROM) exercises for the patient's arm or the affected side if he has been splinting the arm. Usually, the patient splints his arm to decrease his discomfort.
• Give ordered pain medication as needed *for comfort and to help with*

deep breathing, coughing, and ROM exercises.

• Remind the ambulatory patient to keep the drainage system below chest level and to be careful not to disconnect the tubing *to maintain the water seal.* With a suction system, the patient must stay within range of the length of tubing attached to a wall outlet or portable pump.

Complications

• Tension pneumothorax may result from excessive accumulation of air, drainage, or both, and eventually may exert pressure on the heart and aorta, causing a precipitous fall in cardiac output.

Nursing considerations

• Instruct staff and visitors to avoid touching the equipment *to prevent complications from separated connections.*

• If excessive continuous bubbling is present in the water-seal chamber, especially if suction is being used, rule out a leak in the drainage system. Try to locate the leak by clamping the tube momentarily at various points along its length. Begin clamping at the tube's proximal end and work down toward the drainage system, paying special attention to the seal around the connections. If any connection is loose, push it back together and tape it securely. *The bubbling will stop when a clamp is placed between the air leak and the water seal.* If you clamp along the tube's entire length and the bubbling doesn't stop, the drainage unit may be cracked and need replacement.

• If the commercially prepared drainage collection chamber fills, replace it. To do this, double-clamp the tube close to the insertion site (use two clamps facing in opposite directions), exchange the system, remove the clamps, and retape the bottle connection. Never leave the tubes clamped for more than a minute or two *to prevent a tension pneumothorax, which may occur when clamping stops air and fluid from escaping.*

• If the commercially prepared system cracks, clamp the chest tube momentarily with the two rubber-tipped clamps at the bedside (placed there at the time of tube insertion). Place the clamps close to each other near the insertion site; they should face in opposite directions *to provide a more complete seal.*

• Observe the patient for altered respirations while the tube is clamped. Then replace the damaged equipment. (Prepare the new unit before clamping the tube.)

• Instead of clamping the tube, you can submerge the distal end of the tube in a container of normal saline solution *to create a temporary water seal while you replace the bottle.* Check your hospital's policy for the proper procedure.

Documentation

• Record the date and time chest drainage began, type of system used, amount of suction applied to the pleural cavity, presence or absence of bubbling or fluctuation in the water-seal chamber, initial amount and type of drainage, and the patient's respiratory status.

• At the end of each shift, record the frequency of system inspection; how frequently chest tubes were milked or stripped; amount, color, and consistency of drainage; presence or absence of bubbling or fluctuation in the water-seal chamber; the patient's respiratory status; condition of the chest dressings; pain medication, if given; and any complications and the nursing action taken.

Chest physiotherapy

This therapy includes postural drainage, chest percussion and vibration, and coughing and deep-breathing exercises. Together, these techniques move and eliminate secretions, reexpand lung tissue, and promote efficient use of respiratory muscles. Of critical importance to the bedridden patient, chest physiotherapy (PT) helps prevent or treat atelectasis and may help prevent pneumonia.

Postural drainage with percussion and vibration encourages peripheral pulmonary secretions to empty by gravity into the major bronchi or trachea. This is accomplished by sequential repositioning of the patient. Usually, secretions drain best with the patient positioned with bronchi perpendicular to the floor. Lower- and middle-lobe bronchi usually empty best with the patient in the head-down position and upper lobe bronchi in the head-up position.

Percussing the chest with cupped hands dislodges thick, tenacious secretions from the bronchial walls. Vibration can be used with percussion or as an alternative in a patient who is frail, in pain, or recovering from thoracic surgery or trauma.

Candidates for chest PT include patients who expectorate large amounts of sputum, such as those with bronchiectasis and cystic fibrosis. The procedure has not been proven effective in treating patients with status asthmaticus, lobar pneumonia, or acute exacerbations of chronic bronchitis when the patient has scant secretions and is being mechanically ventilated. Chest PT has little value in treating patients with stable, chronic bronchitis.

Contraindications may include active pulmonary bleeding with hemoptysis and immediate posthemorrhage stage, fractured ribs or an unstable chest wall, lung contusions, pulmonary tuberculosis, untreated pneumothorax, acute asthma or bronchospasm, lung abscess or tumor, bony metastasis, head injury, and recent myocardial infarction.

⟫ Key nursing diagnoses and patient outcomes

Use these nursing diagnoses as a guide when developing your plan of care for a patient who is being treated with chest physiotherapy.

Ineffective breathing pattern related to physical condition

Based on this nursing diagnosis, you'll establish the following patient outcomes. The patient will:
• maintain respiratory rate within 5 breaths of baseline.
• report feeling comfortable when breathing.

Impaired gas exchange related to altered oxygen supply

Based upon this nursing diagnosis, you'll establish the following patient outcomes. The patient will:
• cough effectively.

- expectorate sputum.
- have normal breath sounds.

Equipment

♦ stethoscope ♦ pillows ♦ tilt or postural drainage table (if available) or adjustable hospital bed ♦ emesis basin ♦ facial tissues ♦ suction equipment, as needed ♦ equipment for oral care ♦ trash bag ♦ optional: sterile specimen container, mechanical ventilator, supplemental oxygen.

Equipment preparation

- Gather the equipment at the patient's bedside. Set up suction equipment, if needed, and test its function.

Implementation

- Explain the procedure to the patient, provide privacy, and wash your hands.
- Auscultate the patient's lungs *to determine baseline respiratory status.*
- Position the patient as ordered. In generalized disease, drainage usually begins with the lower lobes, continues with the middle lobes, and ends with the upper lobes. In localized disease, drainage begins with the affected lobes and then progresses to the other lobes *to avoid spreading the disease to uninvolved areas.* (See *Positioning patients for postural drainage.*)
- Instruct the patient to remain in each position for 10 to 15 minutes. During this time, perform percussion and vibration, as ordered. (See *Performing percussion and vibration,* page 222.)
- After postural drainage, percussion, or vibration, tell the patient to cough *to remove loosened secretions.* First, tell him to inhale deeply through his nose and exhale in three short puffs. Then have him inhale deeply again and cough through a slightly open

mouth. Three consecutive coughs are highly effective. An effective cough sounds deep, low, and hollow; an ineffective one, high-pitched. Have the patient perform exercises for about 1 minute and then rest for 2 minutes. Gradually progress to a 10-minute exercise period four times daily.

- Provide oral hygiene *because secretions may taste foul or have a stale odor.*
- Auscultate the patient's lungs *to evaluate the effectiveness of therapy.*

Complications

- During postural drainage in the head-down position, pressure on the diaphragm by abdominal contents can impair respiratory excursion and lead to hypoxia or postural hypotension.
- The head-down position also may lead to increased intracranial pressure, which precludes use of chest PT in a patient with acute neurologic impairment.
- Vigorous percussion or vibration can cause rib fracture, especially in the patient with osteoporosis.
- In an emphysematous patient with blebs, coughing could lead to pneumothorax.

Nursing considerations

- For optimal effectiveness and safety, modify chest PT according to the patient's condition. For example, initiate or increase the flow of supplemental oxygen, if indicated.
- Suction the patient who has an ineffective cough reflex.
- If the patient tires quickly during therapy, shorten the sessions *because fatigue leads to shallow respirations and increased hypoxia.*

(Text continues on page 221.)

Positioning patients for postural drainage

The following illustrations show the various postural-drainage positions and the areas of the lungs affected by each.

Lower lobes: Posterior basal segments

Elevate the foot of the bed 30 degrees. Have the patient lie prone with his head lowered. Position pillows under his chest and abdomen. Percuss his lower ribs on both sides of his spine.

Posterior view

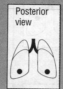

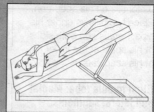

Lower lobes: Lateral basal segments

Elevate the foot of the bed 30 degrees. Tell the patient to lie on his abdomen with his head lowered and his upper leg flexed over a pillow for support. Then have him rotate a quarter turn upward. Percuss his lower ribs on the uppermost portion of his lateral chest wall.

Anterior view

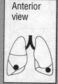

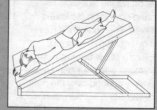

Lower lobes: Anterior basal segments

Elevate the foot of the bed 30 degrees. Instruct the patient to lie on his side with his head lowered. Then place pillows as shown (right). Percuss with a slightly cupped hand over his lower ribs just beneath the axilla. If an acutely ill patient has trouble breathing in this position, adjust the bed to an angle he can tolerate. Then begin percussion.

Anterior view

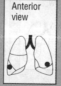

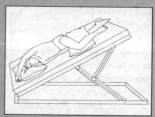

(continued)

Positioning patients for postural drainage *(continued)*

Lower lobes: Superior segments

With the bed flat, have the patient lie on his abdomen. Place two pillows under his hips. Percuss on both sides of his spine at the lower tip of his scapulae.

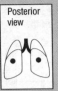

Posterior view

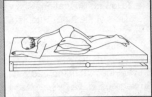

Right middle lobe: Medial and lateral segments

Elevate the foot of the bed 15 degrees. Have the patient lie on his left side with his head down and his knees flexed. Then have him rotate a quarter turn backward. Place a pillow beneath him. Percuss with your hand moderately cupped over the right nipple. For a woman, cup your hand so that its heel is under the armpit and your fingers extend forward beneath the breast.

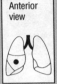

Anterior view

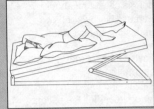

Left upper lobe: Superior and inferior segments, lingular portion

Elevate the foot of the bed 15 degrees. Have the patient lie on his right side with his head down and knees flexed. Then have him rotate a quarter turn backward. Place a pillow behind him, from shoulders to hips. Percuss with your hand moderately cupped over his left nipple. For a woman, cup your hand so that its heel is beneath the armpit and your fingers extend forward beneath the breast.

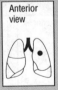

Anterior view

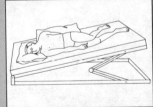

Positioning patients for postural drainage (continued)

Upper lobes: Anterior segments

Make sure the bed is flat. Have the patient lie on his back with a pillow folded under his knees. Then have him rotate slightly away from the side being drained. Percuss between his clavicle and nipple.

Anterior view

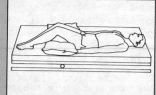

Upper lobes: Apical segments

Keep the bed flat. Have the patient lean back at a 30-degree angle against you and a pillow. Percuss with a cupped hand between his clavicles and the top of each scapula.

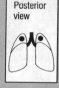

Posterior view

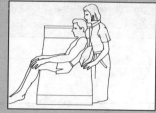

Upper lobes: Posterior segments

Keep the bed flat. Have the patient lean over a pillow at a 30-degree angle. Percuss and clap his upper back on each side.

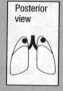

Posterior view

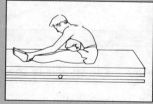

• Maintain adequate hydration in the patient receiving chest PT to prevent mucus dehydration and promote easier mobilization.

• Avoid performing postural drainage immediately before or for up to 1½ hours after meals *to avoid nausea and aspiration of food or vomitus.*

• *Because chest percussion can induce bronchospasm,* any adjunct treatment (intermittent positive-pressure breathing, aerosol, or nebulizer therapy) should precede chest PT.

• Refrain from percussing over the spine, liver, kidneys, or spleen *to avoid injury.*

• Avoid performing percussion on bare skin or a woman's breasts.

• Percuss over soft clothing (but not over buttons, snaps, or zippers) or place a thin towel over the chest wall.

• Remove jewelry that might scratch or bruise the patient.

• Explain coughing and deep-breathing exercises preoperatively, so the patient can practice them when he's

Performing percussion and vibration

To perform percussion, tell the patient to breathe slowly and deeply, using the diaphragm, *to promote relaxation*. Hold your hands in a cupped shape, with fingers flexed and thumbs pressed tightly against your index fingers. Using alternate hands, percuss each segment for 1 to 2 minutes, striking the patient in a rhythmic manner. Listen for a hollow sound on percussion *to verify correct performance of the technique*.

To perform vibration, ask the patient to inhale deeply and then exhale slowly through pursed lips. During exhalation, firmly press your fingers and the palms of your hands against the chest wall. Tense the muscles of your arms and shoulders in an isometric contraction *to send fine vibrations through the chest wall*. Vibrate during five exhalations over each lung segment.

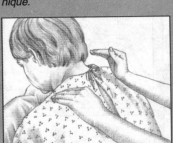
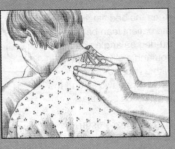

pain-free and better able to concentrate.
• Postoperatively, splint the patient's incision using your hands or, if possible, teach the patient to splint it *to minimize pain during coughing*.

Documentation
• Record the date and time of chest PT; positions for secretion drainage and length of time each is maintained; chest segments percussed or vibrated; color, amount, odor, and viscosity of secretions produced, and presence of any blood; any complications and nursing actions taken; and the patient's tolerance of treatment.

Chest tube insertion

The pleural space normally contains a thin layer of lubricating fluid that allows the lungs to move without friction during respiration. An excess of fluid (hemothorax or pleural effusion), air (pneumothorax), or both, in this space alters intrapleural pressure and causes partial or complete lung collapse.

Insertion of a chest tube permits drainage of air or fluid from the pleural space. Usually performed by a doctor with a nurse assisting, this procedure requires sterile technique. Insertion sites vary, depending on the patient's condition and the doctor's judgment. For pneumothorax, the second intercostal space is the usual site because air rises to the top of the intrapleural space. For hemothorax or pleural effusion, the sixth to the eighth intercostal spaces are common sites because fluid settles to the lower levels of the intrapleural space. For removal of air and fluid, a chest tube is inserted into a high site as well as a low site. Following insertion, one or more chest tubes are connected to a thoracic drainage system that removes air, fluid, or both from the pleural space and prevents backflow into that space, thus promoting lung reexpansion.

≫ Key nursing diagnoses and patient outcomes

Use these nursing diagnoses as a guide when developing your plan of care for a patient who is receiving a chest tube.

Ineffective breathing pattern related to pain

Based on this nursing diagnosis, you'll establish the following patient outcomes. The patient will:
• achieve comfort without experiencing depressed respirations.
• report ability to breathe more comfortably.

Anxiety related to situational crisis

Based on this nursing diagnosis, you'll establish the following patient outcomes. The patient will:
• discuss activities that tend to decrease anxiety.
• cope with current medical situation without demonstrating severe anxiety.

Equipment

♦ two pairs of sterile gloves ♦ sterile drape ♦ povidone-iodine solution ♦ vial of 1% lidocaine ♦ 10-ml syringe ♦ alcohol sponge ♦ 22G 1″ needle ♦ 25G ⅝″ needle ♦ sterile scalpel (usually with #11 blade) ♦ sterile forceps ♦ two rubber-tipped clamps for each chest tube inserted ♦ sterile 4″× 4″ gauze pads ♦ two sterile 4″× 4″ drain dressings (gauze pads with slit) ♦ 3″ or 4″ sturdy, elastic tape ♦ 1″ adhesive tape for connections ♦ chest tube of appropriate size (#16 to 20 French catheter for air or serous fluid; #28 to 40 French catheter for blood, pus, or thick fluid), with or without a trocar ♦ sterile Kelly clamp ♦ suture material (usually 000 silk with cutting needle) ♦ chest drainage system ♦ sterile drainage tubing, 6′ (1.8 m) long, and connector ♦ sterile Y-connector (for two chest tubes on the same side) ♦ optional: antimicrobial ointment, petroleum gauze.

Equipment preparation

• Check the expiration date on the sterile packages and inspect for tears. In a nonemergency situation, make sure the patient has signed the appropriate consent form. Then assemble all equipment in the patient's room, and set up the chest drainage system. Place it next to the patient's bed below the chest level *to facilitate drainage.*

Patient preparation

• Explain the procedure to the patient, provide privacy, and wash your hands.

Implementation

• Record baseline vital signs and respiratory assessment.

TECHNOLOGY UPDATE

Understanding suction regulators

Chest-suction regulators, such as the new Ohmeda Thoracic Suction Regulator (pictured below), are designed specifically for chest drainage. The device shown here is attached to thesuction-control chamber and plugged into the wall suction source. The knob on the device can be used to precisely control the level of negative pressure. The suction is regulated in increments of negative pressure between 5 and 50 cm H_2O, so it may be used for adult and pediatric chest-drainage systems. No water is required in wet suction-control chambers when the thoracic regulator is used with these systems.

As a safety feature, regulators are also able to automatically adjust to changes in the level of negative pressure from the suction source and the patient to maintain original suction settings. They are also equipped with a pressure-relief valve that releases transient positive pressure (which occurs with coughing) and that continues to work when the regulator is turned off.

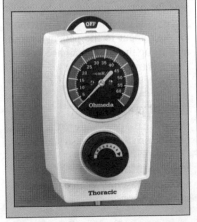

• Position the patient appropriately. If the patient has a *pneumothorax,* place him in the high Fowler's, semi-Fowler's, or the supine position. The doctor will insert the tube in the anterior chest at the midclavicular line in the second or third intercostal space. If the patient has a *hemothorax,* have him lean over the overbed table or straddle a chair with arms dangling over the back. The doctor will insert the tube in the fourth to sixth intercostal space at the mid-axillary line. For either pneumothorax or hemothorax, the patient may lie on his unaffected side with arms extended over his head.

• Once you've positioned the patient properly, place the chest tube tray on the overbed table. Open the tray using sterile technique.

• The doctor puts on sterile gloves and prepares the insertion site by cleaning the area with povidone-iodine solution.

• Wipe the rubber stopper of the lidocaine vial with an alcohol pad, invert the bottle, and hold it for the doctor to withdraw the anesthetic.

• After the doctor anesthetizes the site, he makes a small incision and inserts the chest tube. Then he either immediately connects the chest tube to the chest drainage system or momentarily clamps the tube close to the patient's chest until he can connect it to the drainage system. The doctor orders the appropriate amount of suction to the drainage system. (See *Understanding suction regulators.*) He may then secure the tube to the patient's skin with a suture.

• As the doctor is inserting the chest tube, reassure the patient and assist the doctor as necessary.

• Open the packages containing the $4'' \times 4''$ drain dressings and gauze pads, and put on sterile gloves. If desired, apply antimicrobial ointment to the insertion site. Then place two $4'' \times 4''$ drain dressings around the insertion site, one from the top and the other from the bottom. Place several $4'' \times 4''$ gauze pads on top of the drain dressings. Tape the dressings, covering them completely.

• Tape the chest tube to the patient's chest distal to the insertion site *to help prevent accidental tube dislodgment.*

• Tape the junction of the chest tube and the drainage tube *to prevent separation.*

• Coil the drainage tubing and secure it to the bed linen with a safety pin and tape, providing enough slack for the patient to move and turn. These measures prevent the tubing from getting kinked or dropping to the floor and help prevent accidental dislodgment.

• Immediately after the drainage system is connected, tell the patient to take a deep breath, hold it momentarily, and slowly exhale *to assist drainage of the pleural space and lung reexpansion.*

• A portable chest X-ray is then done *to check tube position.*

• Take the patient's vital signs every 15 minutes for 1 hour and then as his condition indicates. Auscultate his lungs at least every 4 hours following the procedure *to assess air exchange in the affected lung.* Diminished or absent breath sounds indicate that the lung hasn't reexpanded.

Complications

• Tension pneumothorax may result from excessive accumulation of air, drainage, or both, and eventually may exert pressure on the heart and aorta, causing a precipitous fall in cardiac output.

Nursing considerations

• If the patient's chest tube comes out, cover the site with $4'' \times 4''$ gauze pads immediately and tape them in place.

• Stay with the patient and monitor vital signs every 10 minutes.

• Observe the patient for signs of tension pneumothorax (hypotension, distended neck veins, absent breath sounds, tracheal shift, hypoxemia, weak and rapid pulse, dyspnea, tachypnea, diaphoresis, and chest pain).

• Instruct a coworker to notify the doctor and gather equipment needed to reinsert the tube.

• Place the rubber-tipped clamps at the bedside.

• If a drainage bottle breaks, a commercial system cracks, or a tube disconnects, clamp the chest tube momentarily as close to the insertion site as possible.

• *Because no air or liquid can escape from the pleural space while the tube is clamped,* observe the patient closely for signs of tension pneumothorax while the clamp is in place.

• A piece of petroleum gauze may be wrapped around the tube at the insertion site *to make an airtight seal.*

• The tube may be clamped with large, smooth, rubber-tipped clamps for several hours before removal. *This allows time to observe the patient for signs of respiratory distress, an indication that air or fluid remains trapped in the pleural space.*

• A chest tube is usually removed within 7 days of insertion *to prevent infection along the tube tract.* (See *Removing a chest tube,* page 226.)

Removing a chest tube

Once the patient's lung has reexpanded, you may assist the doctor in removing the chest tube. To do so, first obtain the patient's vital signs and perform a respiratory assessment. Then, after explaining the procedure to the patient, you'll administer an analgesic, as ordered, 30 minutes before tube removal. Then follow these steps:
• Place the patient in semi-Fowler's position or on his unaffected side.
• Place a linen-saver pad under the affected side *to protect the linen from drainage and to provide a place to put the chest tube after removal.*
• Put on clean gloves and remove the chest tube dressings, being careful not to dislodge the chest tube.
• Discard soiled dressings.
• The doctor puts on sterile gloves, holds the chest tube in place with sterile forceps, and cuts the suture anchoring the tube.

• Make sure the chest tube is securely clamped, and then instruct the patient to perform Valsalva's maneuver by exhaling fully and bearing down. *Valsalva's maneuver effectively increases intrathoracic pressure.*
• The doctor holds an airtight dressing, usually petroleum gauze over the insertion site *so that he can cover it immediately after removing the tube.*
• After he removes the tube and covers the insertion site, secure the dressing with tape. Be sure to cover the dressing completely with tape *to make it as airtight as possible.*
• Dispose of the chest tube, soiled gloves, and equipment according to hospital policy.
• Take vital signs, as ordered, and assess the depth and quality of the patient's respirations.
• Assess the patient carefully for signs and symptoms of pneumothorax, subcutaneous emphysema, or infection.

Documentation
• Record the date and time of chest tube insertion, the insertion site, drainage system used, presence of drainage and bubbling, vital signs and auscultation findings, any complications, and the nursing action taken.

Clavicle strap

Also called a figure-eight strap, a clavicle strap reduces and immobilizes fractures of the clavicle by elevating, extending, and supporting the shoul-

ders in position for healing, known as the *position of attention.* A commercially available figure-eight strap or a 4″ elastic bandage may serve as a clavicle strap. This strap is contraindicated for an uncooperative patient.

≫ Key nursing diagnoses and patient outcomes
Use these nursing diagnoses as a guide when developing your plan of care for a patient who is being treated with a clavicle strap.

Impaired physical mobility related to pain or discomfort

Based on this nursing diagnosis, you'll establish the following patient outcomes. The patient will:
• attain the highest degree of mobility possible within confines of disease.
• show no evidence of such complications as contractures or skin breakdown.

Pain related to physical condition

Based on this nursing diagnosis, you'll establish the following patient outcomes. The patient will:
• articulate factors that intensify pain and modify behavior accordingly.
• express a feeling of comfort and relief from pain.

Equipment

♦ powder or cornstarch ♦ figure-eight clavicle strap or 4″ elastic bandage ♦ safety pins, if necessary ♦ tape ♦ cotton batting or padding ♦ marking pen ♦ analgesics, as ordered.

Patient preparation

• Explain the procedure to the patient and provide privacy.
• Help the patient take off his shirt.
• Demonstrate the position of attention.

Implementation

• Assess neurovascular integrity by palpating skin temperature; noting the color of the hand and fingers; palpating radial, ulnar, and brachial pulses bilaterally; and then comparing the affected with the unaffected side.
• Ask the patient about any numbness or tingling distal to the injury, and assess his motor function.

• Determine the patient's degree of comfort and administer analgesics, as ordered.
• Tell the patient to sit upright and assume the position of attention gradually *to minimize pain.*
• Gently apply powder or cornstarch, as appropriate, to the axillae and shoulder area *to reduce friction from the clavicle strap.* You can use cornstarch if the patient is allergic to powder.

To apply a figure-eight strap

• Place the apex of the triangle between the scapulae, and drape the straps over the shoulders.
• Bring the strap with the Velcro or buckle end under one axilla and through the loop; then pull the other strap under the other axilla and through the loop. (See *Types of clavicle straps,* page 228.)
• Gently adjust the straps so they support the shoulders in the position of attention.
• Bring the straps back under the axillae toward the anterior chest, making sure the patient maintains the position of attention.

To apply a 4″ elastic bandage

• Roll both ends of the elastic bandage toward the middle, leaving the ends unrolled 12″ to 18″ (30.5 to 45.7 cm).
• Place the unrolled portion diagonally across the patient's back, from right shoulder to left axilla.
• Bring the lower end of the bandage under the left axilla and back over the left shoulder; loop the upper end over the right shoulder and under the axilla.
• Pull the two ends together at the center of the back *so the bandage supports the position of attention.*

Types of clavicle straps

Clavicle straps provide support to the shoulder to help a fractured clavicle heal. They're available ready-made and can be made from a bandage.

Commercially made clavicle straps have a short back panel and long straps that extend around the patient's shoulders and axillae. They have Velcro pads or buckles on the ends for easy fastening.

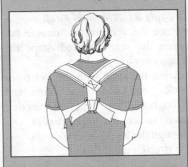

When making a clavicle strap with a wide elastic bandage, start in the middle of the patient's back. After wrapping the bandage around the shoulders, fasten the ends with safety pins.

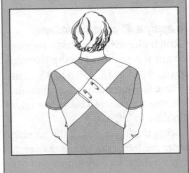

To complete a figure-eight strap or elastic bandage

• Secure the ends using safety pins, Velcro pads, or a buckle, depending on the equipment.
• Make sure a buckle or any sharp edges face away from the skin.
• Tape the secured ends to the underlying strap or bandage.
• Place cotton batting or padding under the straps and under the buckle or pins *to avoid skin irritation.*
• Use a pen to mark the strap at the site of the loop of the figure-eight strap, or the site where the elastic bandage crosses on the patient's back. *If the strap loosens, this mark helps you tighten it to the original position.*
• Assess neurovascular integrity, *which may be impaired by a strap that's too tight.* If neurovascular integrity is compromised when the strap is correctly applied, notify the doctor. *He may want to change the treatment.*

Nursing considerations

• If possible, perform the procedure with the patient standing, although this may not be feasible, *because pain from the fracture can cause syncope.*
• An adult with a clavicle strap made from an elastic bandage may require a triangular sling *to help support the weight of the arm, enhance immobilization, and reduce pain.* (See *Making a sling.*)

For a small child or a confused adult, a well-molded plaster jacket is needed to ensure immobilization. *Inadequate immobilization can cause improper healing.*
• Tell the patient not to remove the clavicle strap.
• Explain that, with assistance, he can maintain proper hygiene by lifting

Making a sling

Place the apex of a triangular bandage behind the patient's elbow on the injured side. Hold one end of the bandage so it extends toward the patient's neck on the uninjured side, and let the other end hang straight down. The bandage's long side should parallel the midline of the patient's body.

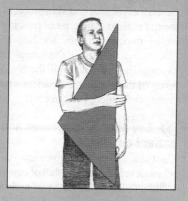

Loop the top corner of the bandage over the shoulder on the uninjured side and around the back of the patient's neck. Then bring the lower end of the bandage over the flexed forearm and up to the shoulder on the injured side.

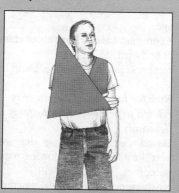

Adjust the bandage so that the forearm and upper arm form an angle of slightly less than 90 degrees *to increase venous return from the hand and forearm* and *to facilitate drainage from swelling.* Then tie the two bandage ends at the side of the patient's neck, rather than at the back, *to prevent neck flexion and to avoid irritation and pressure over a cervical vertebra.*

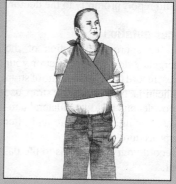

Carefully secure the sling with a safety pin above and behind the elbow. (For a child under age 7, use tape instead of a pin *to avoid the chance of an injury.*)

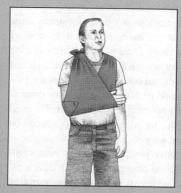

segments of the strap to remove the cotton and by washing and powdering the skin daily. Explain that fresh cotton should be applied after cleaning.
• For a hospitalized patient, monitor the position of the strap by checking the pen markings every 8 hours. Also assess neurovascular integrity.

Home care
• Teach the outpatient how to assess his own neurovascular integrity and to recognize the symptoms that he should report promptly to the doctor.

Documentation
• In the appropriate section of the emergency-department sheet or your notes, record the date and time of strap application, type of clavicle strap, use of powder and padding, bilateral neurovascular integrity before and after the procedure
• Record your instructions to the patient.

Colostomy and ileostomy care

A patient with an ascending or transverse colostomy or an ileostomy must wear an external pouch to collect emerging fecal matter, which will be watery or pasty. The pouch also helps to control odor and to protect the stoma and peristomal skin. Most disposable pouching systems can be used from 2 to 7 days. Some models can be used longer.

Any pouching system needs immediate changing if a leak develops, and every pouch must be emptied when it's one-third to one-half full.

The patient with an ileostomy may need to empty the pouch four or five times daily.
• Naturally, the best time to change the pouching system is when the bowel is least active, usually between 2 and 4 hours after meals. After a few months, most patients can predict the best changing time.
• Pouching-system selection should consider which system provides the best adhesive seal and skin protection for the patient. The type of pouch selected depends on the location and structure of the stoma, the availability of supplies, the wear time, the consistency of the effluent, the patient's personal preference, and the cost.

» Key nursing diagnoses and patient outcomes
Use these nursing diagnoses as a guide when developing your plan of care for a patient with a colostomy or an ileostomy.

Body image disturbance related to presence of colostomy or ileostomy
Based on this nursing diagnosis, you'll establish the following patient outcomes. The patient will:
• acknowledge changes in body image.
• communicate feelings about change in body image.
• express positive feelings about self.

Risk for impaired skin integrity related to presence of colostomy or ileostomy
Based on this nursing diagnosis, you'll establish the following patient outcomes. The patient will:
• experience no skin breakdown.

• communicate understanding of preventive skin care measures.

Equipment

♦ pouching system ♦ stoma measuring guide ♦ stoma paste (if drainage is watery to pasty or stoma secretes excess mucus) ♦ plastic bag ♦ water ♦ washcloth and towel ♦ closure clamp ♦ toilet or bedpan ♦ water or pouch-cleaning solution ♦ gloves ♦ facial tissues ♦ optional: ostomy belt; paper tape; mild, nonmoisturizing soap; skin shaving equipment; liquid skin sealant; pouch deodorant.

Pouching systems may be drainable or closed-bottomed, disposable or reusable, adhesive-backed, and one-piece or two-piece. (See *Comparing ostomy pouching systems,* page 232.)

Patient preparation

• Provide privacy.
• Provide emotional support.

Implementation
To fit the pouch and skin barrier

• *For a pouch with an attached skin barrier,* measure the stoma with the stoma measuring guide. Select the opening size that matches the stoma.
• For an adhesive-backed pouch with a separate skin barrier, measure the stoma with the measuring guide, and select the opening that matches the stoma. Trace the selected size opening onto the paper back of the skin barrier's adhesive side. Cut out the opening. (If the pouch has precut openings, which can be handy for a round stoma, select an opening that's 1/8″ larger than the stoma. If the pouch comes without an opening, cut the hole 1/8″ wider than the measured tracing.) The cut-to-fit

system works best for an irregularly shaped stoma.
• *For guidelines on using a two-piece pouching system,* see *Applying a skin barrier and pouch,* page 233.
• Avoid fitting the pouch too tightly *because the stoma has no pain receptors. A constrictive opening could injure the stoma or skin tissue without the patient becoming aware of any discomfort.* Also avoid cutting the opening too big *because this may expose the skin to fecal matter and moisture.*
• The patient with a descending or sigmoid colostomy who has formed stools and whose ostomy doesn't secrete much mucus may choose to wear only a pouch. In this case, make sure the pouch opening closely matches the stoma size.
• Between 6 weeks and 1 year after surgery, the stoma will shrink to its permanent size. Then, pattern-making preparations will be unnecessary unless the patient gains weight, has additional surgery, or injures the stoma.

To apply or change the pouch

• Collect all equipment.
• Wash your hands, and provide privacy.
• Explain the procedure to the patient. As you perform each step, explain what you are doing and why *because the patient will eventually perform the procedure.*
• Put on gloves.
• Remove and discard the old pouch. Wipe the stoma and peristomal skin gently with a facial tissue.
• Carefully wash and dry the peristomal skin. Inspect the peristomal skin and stoma. If necessary, shave the

(Text continues on page 234.)

Comparing ostomy pouching systems

Manufactured in many shapes and sizes, ostomy pouches are fashioned for comfort, safety, and easy application. For example, a disposable closed-end pouch may meet the needs of a patient who irrigates their colostomy, who wants added security, or who wants to discard the pouch after each bowel movement. Another patient may prefer a reusable, drainable pouch. Some commonly available pouches are described below.

Disposable pouches

The patient who must empty his pouch often (because of diarrhea or a new colostomy or ileostomy) may prefer a one-piece, drainable, disposable pouch with a closure clamp attached to a skin barrier (below, left).

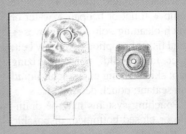

These odorproof, plastic pouches come with attached adhesive or karaya seals. Some have microporous adhesive or belt tabs. The bottom opening allows for easy draining.

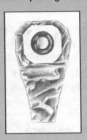 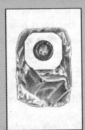

Also disposable and also made of transparent or opaque odorproof plastic, a one-piece disposable closed-end pouch (above, right) may come in a kit with adhesive seal, belt tabs, skin barrier, or carbon filter for gas release. A patient with a regular bowel elimination pattern may choose this style for additional security and confidence.

A two-piece disposable drainable pouch with separate skin barrier, shown at top of next column, permits frequent changes and also minimizes skin breakdown.

Reusable pouches

Typically manufactured from sturdy, opaque, hypoallergenic plastic, the reusable pouch comes with a separate custom-made faceplate and an O-ring, as shown below. Some pouches have a pressure valve for releasing gas. The device has a 1- to 2-month life span, depending on how frequently the patient empties the pouch.

Reusable equipment may benefit a patient who needs a firm faceplate or who wishes to minimize cost. However, many reusable ostomy pouches aren't odorproof.

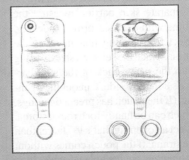

Applying a skin barrier and pouch

Fitting a skin barrier and ostomy pouch properly can be done in a few steps. Shown below is a commonly used two-piece pouching system with flanges.

Measure the stoma using a measuring guide.

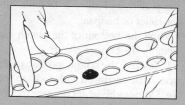

Trace the appropriate circle carefully on the back of the skin barrier.

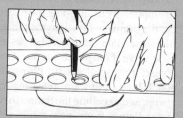

Cut the circular opening in the skin barrier. Bevel the edges to keep them from irritating the patient.

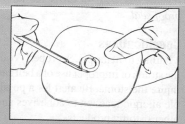

Remove the backing from the skin barrier and moisten it or apply barrier paste, as needed, along the edge of the circular opening.

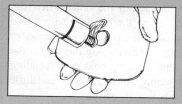

Center the skin barrier over the stoma, adhesive side down, and gently press it to the skin, applying slight pressure for 1 to 2 minutes to help it adhere better.

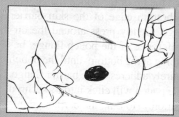

Gently press the pouch opening onto the ring until it snaps into place.

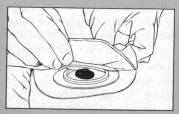

surrounding hair (in a direction away from the stoma) *to promote a better seal and to avoid skin irritation from hair pulling against the adhesive.*
• If applying a separate skin barrier, peel off the paper backing of the prepared skin barrier, center the barrier over the stoma, and press gently to ensure adhesion.
• You may want to outline the stoma on the back of the skin barrier (depending on the product) with a thin ring of stoma paste *to provide extra skin protection.* (Skip this step if the patient has a sigmoid or descending colostomy, formed stools, and little mucus.)
• Remove the paper backing from the adhesive side of the pouching system and center the pouch opening over the stoma. Press gently to secure.
• *For a pouching system with flanges,* align the lip of the pouch flange with the bottom edge of the skin barrier flange. Gently press around the circumference of the pouch flange, beginning at the bottom, until the pouch securely adheres to the barrier flange. (The pouch will click into its secured position.) Holding the barrier against the skin, gently pull on the pouch *to confirm the seal between flanges.*
• Encourage the patient to stay quietly in position for about 5 minutes *to improve adherence. The patient's body warmth also helps to improve adherence and soften a rigid skin barrier.*
• Attach an ostomy belt to secure the pouch, if desired.
• Leave a bit of air in the pouch *to allow drainage to collect at the bottom.*
• Apply the closure clamp, if necessary.

• If desired, apply paper tape in a picture-frame fashion to the pouch edges *for additional security.*

To empty the pouch
• Tilt the bottom of the pouch upward and remove the closure clamp.
• Turn up a cuff on the lower end of the pouch, and allow it to drain into the toilet or bedpan.
• Wipe the bottom of the pouch and reapply the closure clamp.
• If desired, the bottom portion of the pouch can be rinsed with cool tap water. Do not aim water up near the top of the pouch *because this may loosen the seal on the skin.*
• A two-piece flange system can also be emptied by unsnapping the pouch. Let the drainage flow into the toilet.
• Release flatus through the gas-release valve if the pouch has one. Otherwise, release flatus by tilting the pouch bottom upward, releasing the clamp, and expelling the flatus. To release flatus from a system with flanges, loosen the seal between the flanges.
• Never make a pinhole in a pouch to release gas. *This destroys the odor-proof seal.*

Complications
• Failing to fit the pouch properly over the stoma or improper use of a belt can injure the stoma. Be alert for a possible allergic reaction to adhesives and other ostomy products.

Nursing considerations
After performing and explaining the procedure to the patient, encourage the patient's increasing involvement in self-care.

• Use adhesive solvents and removers only after patch-testing the patient's skin because *some products may irritate the skin or produce hypersensitivity reactions.* Consider using a liquid skin sealant, if available, *to give skin tissue additional protection from drainage and adhesive irritants.*

• Remove the pouching system if the patient reports burning or itching beneath it or purulent drainage around the stoma. Notify the doctor of any skin irritation, breakdown, rash, or unusual appearance of the stoma or peristomal area.

• Use commercial pouch deodorants, if desired, but most pouches are odor-free, and odor should be evident only when you empty the pouch or if it leaks. Before discharge, suggest that patient avoid odor-causing foods such as fish, eggs, onions, and garlic.

• If the patient wears a reusable pouching system, suggest that he obtain two or more systems *so he can wear one while the other dries after being cleaned with soap and water or a commercially prepared cleaning solution.*

Documentation

• Record the date and time of the pouching system change; note the character of drainage, including color, amount, type, and consistency.

• Describe the appearance of the stoma and the peristomal skin.

• Document and describe patient teaching.

• Record the patient's response to self-care, and evaluate his learning progress.

Colostomy irrigation

This procedure can serve two purposes: to allow a patient with a descending or sigmoid colostomy to regulate bowel function and to clean the large bowel before and after tests, surgery, or other procedures.

Colostomy irrigation may begin as soon as bowel function resumes after surgery, but most clinicians recommend waiting until bowel movements are more predictable. Initially, the nurse or patient irrigates the colostomy at the same time every day, recording the amount of output and any spillage between irrigations. Between 4 and 6 weeks may pass before colostomy irrigation establishes a predictable elimination pattern.

Depending on the patient's condition, colostomy irrigation may be performed in bed using a bedpan or in the bathroom using the chair and the toilet.

>> Key nursing diagnoses and patient outcomes

Use these nursing diagnoses as a guide when developing your plan of care for a patient who is receiving a colostomy irrigation.

Body image disturbance related to colostomy irrigation

Based on this nursing diagnosis, you'll establish the following patient outcomes. The patient will:

• acknowledge change in body image.

• express positive feelings about self.

Ineffective individual coping related to situational crisis

Based on this nursing diagnosis, you'll establish the following patient outcomes. The patient will:
• communicate feelings about the situation.
• become involved in planning own care.

Equipment

♦ colostomy irrigation set (contains an irrigation drain or sleeve, an ostomy belt [if needed] to secure the drain or sleeve, water-soluble lubricant, drainage pouch clamp, and irrigation bag with clamp, tubing, and cone tip) ♦ 1,000 ml (about 30 oz or 1 quart) of tap water irrigant warmed to about 100° F (37.8° C) ♦ normal saline solution (for cleansing enemas) ♦ I.V. pole or wall hook ♦ wash-cloth and towel ♦ water ♦ ostomy pouching system ♦ linen-saver pad ♦ gloves ♦ optional: bedpan or chair, mild non-moisturizing soap, rubber band or clip, small dressing or bandage, stoma cap.

Equipment preparation

• Set up the irrigation bag with tubing and cone tip. If irrigation will take place with the patient in bed, place the bedpan beside the bed, and elevate the head of the bed between 45 and 90 degrees, if allowed. If irrigation will take place in the bathroom, have the patient sit on the toilet or on a chair facing the toilet, whichever is more comfortable.
• Fill the irrigation bag with warmed tap water (or normal saline solution, if the irrigation is for bowel cleansing). Hang the bag on the I.V. pole or wall hook. The bottom of the bag should be at the patient's shoulder level *to prevent the fluid from entering the bowel too quickly.* Most irrigation sets also have a clamp that regulates the flow rate.
• Prime the tubing with irrigant *to prevent air from entering the colon and possibly causing cramps and gas pains.*

Patient preparation

• Explain every step of the procedure *for teaching purposes because the patient will most likely be irrigating the colostomy himself.*
• Provide privacy.

Implementation

• Wash your hands.
• If the patient's in bed, place a linen-saver pad under him *to protect the sheets from soiling.*
• Put on gloves.
• Remove the ostomy pouch if the patient uses one.
• Place the irrigation sleeve over the stoma. If the sleeve doesn't have an adhesive backing, secure the sleeve with an ostomy belt. If the patient has a two-piece pouching system with flanges, snap off the pouch and save it. Snap on the irrigation sleeve.
• Place the open-ended bottom of the irrigation sleeve in the bedpan or toilet *to promote drainage by gravity.* If necessary, cut the sleeve so it meets the water level inside the bedpan or toilet. *Effluent may splash from a short sleeve and may not drain from a long sleeve.*
• Lubricate your gloved small finger with water-soluble lubricant and insert the finger into the stoma. If you're teaching the patient, have him do this *to determine the bowel angle at which*

to insert the cone safely. Expect the stoma to tighten when the finger enters the bowel and then to relax in a few seconds.

• Lubricate the cone with water-soluble lubricant *to prevent it from irritating the mucosa.*

• Insert the cone into the top opening of the irrigation sleeve and then into the stoma. Angle the cone to match the bowel angle. Insert it gently but snugly.

• Unclamp the irrigation tubing and allow the water to flow slowly. If you don't have a clamp to control the flow rate, pinch the tubing *to control the flow.* The water should enter the colon over 10 to 15 minutes. (If the patient reports cramps, slow or stop the flow, keep the cone in place, and have the patient take a few deep breaths until cramps stop.) Cramping during irrigation may result from a bowel that's ready to empty, water that's too cold, rapid flow rate, or air in the tubing.

• Have the patient remain stationary for 15 or 20 minutes *so the initial effluent can drain.*

• If the patient's ambulatory, he can stay in the bathroom until all effluent empties or he can clamp the bottom of the drainage sleeve with a rubber band or clip and return to bed. Explain that *ambulation and activity stimulate elimination.* Suggest that the non-ambulatory patient lean forward or massage his abdomen *to stimulate elimination.*

• Wait about 45 minutes for the bowel to finish eliminating the irrigant and effluent and then remove the irrigation sleeve.

• If the irrigation was intended to clean the bowel, repeat the procedure

with warm normal saline solution until the return solution appears clear.

• Using a washcloth, mild soap, and water, gently clean the area around the stoma. Rinse and dry the area thoroughly with a clean towel.

• Inspect the skin and stoma for changes in appearance. Usually dark pink to red, stoma color may change with the patient's status. Notify the doctor of marked stoma color changes *because a pale hue may result from anemia, and substantial darkening suggests a change in blood flow to the stoma.*

• Apply a clean pouch or, if the patient has a regular bowel elimination pattern, he may prefer a small dressing, bandage, or commercial stoma cap.

• Discard a disposable irrigation sleeve. Rinse a reusable irrigation sleeve and hang it to dry along with the irrigation bag, tubing, and cone.

Complications

• Bowel perforation may result if a catheter is incorrectly inserted into the stoma.

• Fluid and electrolyte imbalances may result from using too much irrigant.

Nursing considerations

• Irrigating a colostomy to establish a regular bowel elimination pattern doesn't work for all patients.

• If movement in the bowel continues between irrigations, try decreasing the volume of irrigant. *Increasing the irrigant will not help because it serves only to stimulate peristalsis.*

• Keep a record of results.

• Consider irrigating every other day.

• Irrigation may help to regulate bowel function in patients with a descending or sigmoid colostomy *because this is the bowel's stool storage area.* However, a patient with an ascending or transverse colostomy won't benefit from irrigation.

• A patient with a descending or sigmoid colostomy who is missing part of the ascending or transverse colon may not be able to irrigate successfully because his ostomy may function like an ascending or transverse colostomy.

• If diarrhea develops, discontinue irrigations until stools form again. Keep in mind that irrigation alone won't achieve regularity for the patient. He must also observe a complementary diet and exercise regimen.

• If the patient has a strictured stoma that prohibits cone insertion, remove the cone from the irrigation tubing and replace it with a soft silicone catheter. Angle the catheter gently 2″ to 4″ (5 to 10 cm) into the bowel to instill the irrigant. Don't force the catheter into the stoma, and don't insert it farther than the recommended length *because you may perforate the bowel.*

Documentation

• Record the date and time of irrigation and the type and amount of irrigant.

• Note the stoma's color and the character of drainage, including the drainage color, consistency, and amount.

• Record any patient teaching and describe the patient's response to self-care instruction.

• Evaluate the patient's learning progress.

Computed tomography scan

This diagnostic test is an X-ray technique that is far more successful than conventional X-ray films at providing images of internal body structures. As multiple X-ray beams travel through organs on all planes, detectors record body-structure images. A computer reconstructs the information as a three-dimensional image on an oscilloscope screen. Computed tomography (CT) scans may be performed with or without a contrast medium. These scans can examine virtually every part of the body, including the head, orbit of the eye, thorax, biliary tract and liver, pancreas, and kidneys. To study structures, CT scans combine radiologic and computer analysis of tissue density (as determined by the dye absorption). (See *How the CT scanner works.*)

Although the CT scan can't show deep structures clearly, it carries less risk and causes less trauma than studies such as cerebral angiography or brain scanning. Areas of altered density or displaced vasculature and changes in size and shapes of organs may indicate primary tumors or metastases.

A CT scan may help detect contusions; calcifications; atrophy; hydrocephalus; inflammation; space-occupying lesions (such as tumors, hematomas, edema, and abscesses); and vascular changes, such as arteriovenous malformations, infarctions, blood clots, and hemorrhages. A spinal CT scan outlines the vertebral column, allowing the doctor to assess such spinal disorders as herniated disk, spinal cord tumors, and spinal stenosis. Contrast-enhanced CT scans accentuate spinal vasculature and highlight subtle differences in tissue density. Air CT scanning, which involves removing a small amount of cerebrospinal fluid and injecting air via lumbar puncture, intensifies contrast between the subarachnoid space and surrounding tissue.

≫ Key nursing diagnoses and patient outcomes

Use these nursing diagnoses as a guide when developing your plan of care for a patient who is receiving a CT scan.

Anxiety related to situational crisis and physical condition

Based on this nursing diagnosis, you'll establish the following patient outcomes. The patient will:
• identify factors that elicit anxious behaviors.
• cope with current medical situation (specify) without demonstrating signs of severe anxiety (specify for the individual).

Ineffective individual coping related to situational crisis

Based on this nursing diagnosis, you'll establish the following patient outcomes. The patient will:
• communicate feelings about the situation.
• express feeling of having greater control over situation.
• identify at least two coping behaviors.

Equipment

♦ recording equipment ♦ contrast medium (meglumine iothalamate or dia-

How the CT scanner works

The computed tomography (CT) scanner circles the patient's head, taking multiple X-rays that a computer translates into cross-sectional images of the brain. These images clearly define intracranial structures — an improvement on conventional X-rays, which blur the structures into black and white masses.

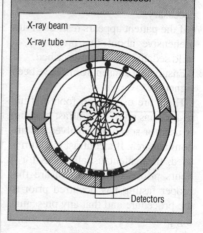

trizoate sodium) ♦ 60-ml syringe ♦ 19G to 21G needle ♦ tourniquet ♦ I.V. equipment ♦ normal saline solution ♦ resuscitation equipment.

Equipment preparation

• Have resuscitation equipment on hand.

Patient preparation

• Explain CT procedure and who will perform the test and where it will take place.
• Describe the CT machine.
• Explain that the patient will be placed on a moving table but will be

secured with seatbelts for safety and to deter patient movement.

• Explain that the patient will be able to breathe and that the machine will move around him to take pictures.

• Inform the patient that he will be asked to remain still during the procedure and will be monitored at all times.

• Ensure that jewelry and other metal devices are removed before the scan.

• Ask the patient to put on a gown, if necessary.

• If the patient appears restless or apprehensive about the procedure, a mild sedative may be prescribed.

• Ensure that consent forms have been signed.

• There are usually no food or fluid restrictions unless a contrast medium is used or scanning involves the abdominal area. If a contrast medium is used, the patient usually fasts for 4 hours prior to the test. Ensure that proper fasting has occurred prior to the procedure and that any prescanning procedures have been performed and required.

• Check for any patient allergies. If the patient is allergic to iodine or shellfish, contrast media may be contraindicated. The doctor may order prophylactic medications or choose not to use contrast enhancement.

• If a contrast medium is used, tell the patient there may be a flushed and warm sensation or transient headache, a salty taste, or nausea and vomiting after the dye is injected.

• If contrast will be used, begin an I.V. of normal saline solution at a keep-vein-open rate.

Intracranial and orbital CT

• Explain that the test will cause minimal discomfort and last 15 to 30 minutes.

• Tell the patient he'll be positioned on a moving CT bed, with his head immobilized and his face uncovered. The head of the table is moved into the scanner, which rotates around his head and makes clacking sounds.

Liver and biliary tract CT

• Instruct the patient to fast after midnight before the test if he is to receive an oral contrast medium.

• Inform him that the test takes approximately 90 minutes.

• Tell him that he'll be asked to hold his breath at certain times.

• If a contrast medium is used, give him the one supplied by the radiology department.

Pancreatic CT

• Tell the patient to fast after midnight before the day of the test.

• Tell the patient the test lasts about 30 minutes.

• Administer the oral contrast medium.

Spinal and skeletal CT

• Tell the patient that the test takes 30 to 60 minutes.

• Reassure him that the procedure is painless, but he may find having to remain still for a prolonged period uncomfortable.

Implementation

• Make sure the patient or a responsible family member has signed an appropriate consent form if needed.

Intracranial and orbital CT scan
• Place the patient in a supine position on a radiographic table, with his head immobilized by straps, and ask him to lie still.
• The head of the table is moved into the scanner, which rotates around the patient's head, taking radiographs at 1-degree intervals in a 180-degree arc.
• Contrast enhancement is performed when the radiographs in the 180-degree arc are completed. Monitor for hypersensitivity reactions, such as urticaria, respiratory difficulty, or rash. Reactions usually develop within 30 minutes.
• After injection of the contrast medium, another series of scans is taken.
• Information from the scans is stored on magnetic tapes, fed into a computer, and converted into images on an oscilloscope screen.
• Photographs of selected views are taken for further study.
• If a contrast medium is used, watch for residual adverse reactions (headache, nausea, and vomiting).
• Inform the patient he may resume his usual diet.

Liver, biliary tract, and renal CT
• Put the patient into a supine position on a radiographic table, and position the table in the opening in the scanning gantry.
• A series of transverse X-ray films is taken and recorded on magnetic tape.
• These images are studied, and selected ones are photographed.
• Contrast enhancement may be performed. After the contrast medium is injected, a second series of films is taken and the patient is carefully observed for allergic reaction.

• After the procedure, tell the patient that he may resume his usual diet.

Pancreatic CT
• Help the patient into the supine position on the radiology table, and position the table within the opening in the scanning gantry.
• A series of transverse X-rays is taken and recorded on magnetic tape. The varying tissue absorption is calculated by computer, and the information is reconstructed through images on a TV screen. These images are studied, and selected ones are photographed.
• After the first series of films is completed, the images are reviewed. Contrast enhancement may then be ordered.
• After the contrast medium is administered, another series of films is taken and the patient is observed for allergic reaction.
• After the procedure, tell the patient he may resume his usual diet.

Spinal, skeletal, and thoracic CT
• Help the patient into a supine position on a table and tell him to lie as still as possible.
• The table slides into the circular opening of the CT scanner, and the scanner revolves around the patient, taking radiographs at preselected intervals.
• After the first set of scans is taken, the patient is removed from the scanner.
• After injection, the patient is moved back into the scanner, and another series of scans is taken. The images obtained from the scan are displayed on a video monitor during the procedure and stored on magnetic tape.

• After testing with contrast enhancement, observe the patient for residual effects, such as headache, nausea, and vomiting, and inform him that he may resume his usual diet.
• Encourage fluids to assist in dye elimination.

Complications

• CT scanning with contrast enhancement is contraindicated in persons who are hypersensitive to iodine or contrast medium.
• Iodine or contrast medium may be harmful or fatal to a fetus, especially during the first trimester.
• CT scanning of the liver, biliary tract, pancreas, and thoracic cavity is usually contraindicated during pregnancy.
• If an I.V. contrast medium is used, the test is contraindicated for patients with hypersensitivity to iodine or with severe renal or hepatic disease.
• Some patients may experience strong feelings of claustrophobia or anxiety when inside the CT body scanner. For such patients, a mild sedative to help reduce anxiety may be ordered.
• For patients with significant back pain, administer prescribed analgesics before the scan.

Nursing considerations

• If the patient is experiencing pain, will be undergoing a prolonged procedure, or is claustrophobic, administer any pain medications or sedatives as prescribed to assist in achieving comfort.
• If contrast medium is administered, observe the patient for signs and symptoms of a hypersensitivity reaction, including pruritus, rash, and re-

spiratory difficulty for 30 minutes after the contrast has been injected.

Documentation

• Record allergies on patient's chart and allergy band clearly, and alert the radiologist and involved doctors of the patient's allergies.
• Record any preparation and instruction given to the patient and his responses.
• Record any premedication given to the patient and its effects.
• Document toleration of procedure and any reactions to the contrast medium or the CT.
• Document type of needle to start I.V., site location, appearance, and the solution used and rate of flow.

Continent ileostomy care

An alternative to conventional ileostomy, a continent, or pouch, ileostomy (also called a Koch ileostomy or an ileal pouch) features an internal reservoir fashioned from the terminal ileum. This procedure may be used for a patient who requires proctocolectomy for chronic ulcerative colitis or multiple polyposis. Other patients may have a traditional ileostomy converted to a pouch ileostomy. This procedure is contraindicated in Crohn's disease or gross obesity. Patients who need emergency surgery and those who cannot care for the pouch also should not have this procedure.

The length of preoperative hospitalization varies with the patient's condition. Nursing responsibilities include providing bowel preparation, antibiotic therapy, and emotional support. After surgery, nursing responsibilities include ensuring patency of the drainage catheter, assessing GI function, caring for the stoma and peristomal skin, managing pain resulting from surgery, and if necessary, perineal skin care.

Usually, daily patient teaching on pouch intubation and drainage begins soon after surgery. Continuous drainage is maintained for about 2 to 6 weeks to allow the suture lines to heal. During this period, a drainage catheter is attached to low intermittent suction. After the suture lines heal, the patient learns how to drain the pouch himself.

≫ Key nursing diagnoses and patient outcomes.

Use these nursing diagnoses as a guide when developing your plan of care for a patient who needs continent ileostomy care.

Knowledge deficit related to lack of exposure to new procedure
Based on this nursing diagnosis, you'll establish the following patient outcomes. The patient will:
• verbalize understanding of procedure for continent ileostomy care.
• show correct procedure for continent ileostomy care.
• verbalize reasons to contact the doctor, nurse, or appropriate caregivers.
• identify appropriate resources for obtaining equipment and local support groups.

Risk for infection related to ileostomy pouch
Based on this nursing diagnosis, you'll establish the following patient outcomes. The patient will:

• maintain normal temperature.
• maintain good personal hygiene at pouch site.
• show no signs of skin breakdown.
• identify signs and symptoms of infection.

Equipment
♦ leg drainage bag ♦ bedside drainage bag ♦ normal saline solution ♦ 50-ml catheter-tip syringe ♦ extra continent ileostomy catheter ♦ 20-ml syringe with adapter ♦ $4'' \times 4'' \times 1''$ foam dressing and Montgomery straps ♦ precut drain dressing ♦ gloves ♦ water-soluble lubricant ♦ graduated container ♦ skin sealant ♦ optional: commercial catheter securing device.

Patient preparation
• Reinforce and, if necessary, supplement the doctor's explanation of a continent ileostomy and its implications for the patient. (See *Understanding pouch construction*.)
• Assess patient and family attitudes related to the operation and to the pending change the patient's body image.
• Provide encouragement and support.

Implementation
Follow the steps below for caring for a patient with a continent, or pouch, ileostomy.

Postoperative care
• When the patient returns to his room, attach the drainage catheter emerging from the ileostomy to continuous gravity drainage.
• A leg drainage bag may be attached to the patient's thigh during ambulation.

Understanding pouch construction

Depending on the patient and related factors during intestinal surgery, the doctor may construct a pouch to collect fecal matter internally. To make such a pouch, the doctor loops about 12″ (30.5 cm) of ileum and sutures the inner sides together.

He opens the loop with a U-shaped cut and seams the inside to create a smooth lining. Then he fashions a nipple or valve between what is becoming the pouch and what will be the stoma.

He folds the open ileum over, sews the pouch closed, and fixes the pouch to the abdominal wall.

Because the pouch holds fecal matter in reserve, the patient benefits from not having to change and empty ostomy equipment. Instead, he empties and irrigates the pouch as needed by inserting a catheter through the stoma and into the pouch.

Initially after surgery, the nurse performs this procedure until the patient can do it himself.

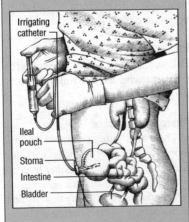

Irrigating catheter

Ileal pouch

Stoma

Intestine

Bladder

• Irrigate the catheter with 30 ml of normal saline solution, as ordered and as necessary, *to prevent catheter obstruction and to allow fluid return by gravity.* During the early postoperative period, keep the pouch empty *to allow the suture lines to heal and to prevent rapid pouch expansion.* At first, drainage will be serosanguineous.

• Monitor fluid intake and output.

• Check the catheter frequently once the patient begins eating solid food *to ensure that mucus or undigested food particles don't block it.*

• If the patient complains of abdominal cramps, distention, and nausea — symptoms of bowel obstruction — the catheter may be clogged. Gently irrigate with 20 to 30 ml of water or normal saline solution until the catheter drains freely. Then move the catheter slightly or rotate it gently *to help clear the obstruction.* Finally, try milking the catheter. If these measures fail, notify the doctor.

• Check the stoma frequently for color, edema, and bleeding. Normally pink to red, a stoma that turns dark red or blue-red may have a compromised blood supply.

• To care for the stoma and peristomal skin, put on gloves. Remove the dressing, gently clean the peristomal area with water, and pat dry. Use a skin sealant around the stoma *to prevent skin irritation.*

• One way to apply a stoma dressing is to slip a precut drain dressing around the catheter to cover the stoma. Cut a hole slightly larger than the lumen of the catheter in the center of a $4″ \times 4″ \times 1″$ piece of foam. Disconnect the catheter from the drainage bag and insert the distal end of the catheter through the hole in the foam. Slide the foam pad onto the dressing. Secure the foam in place with Montgomery straps. Secure the catheter by wrapping the strap ties around it or by using a commercial catheter securing device. Then reconnect the catheter to the drainage bag. (The drainage catheter will be removed by the surgeon when he determines that the suture line has healed.)

• Assess the peristomal skin for irritation from moisture.

• *To reduce discomfort from gas pains,* encourage ambulation. Also recommend that the patient avoid swallowing air (*to minimize gas pains*) by chewing food well, limiting conversation while eating, and not drinking from a straw.

Draining the pouch

• Provide privacy, carefully explain the procedure to the patient, and wash your hands.

• Put on gloves.

• Have the patient with a pouch conversion sit on the toilet *to help him feel more at ease during the procedure.*

• Remove the stoma dressing.

• Encourage the patient to relax his abdominal muscles *to allow the catheter to slide easily into the pouch.*

• Lubricate the tip of the drainage catheter tip with the water-soluble lubricant, and insert it into the stoma.

Gently push the catheter downward. (The direction of insertion may vary depending on the patient.)

• When the catheter reaches the nipple valve of the internal pouch or reservoir (after about 2″ or 2 ½″ [5 or 6.4 cm]), you'll feel resistance. Instruct the patient to take a deep breath as you exert gentle pressure on the catheter to in-

sert it through the valve. If this fails, have the patient lie in a supine position and rest for a few minutes. Then, with the patient still in a supine position, try to insert the catheter again.

• Gently advance the catheter to the suture marking made by the surgeon.

• Let the pouch drain completely. This usually takes 5 to 10 minutes. With thick drainage or a clogged catheter, the process may take 30 minutes.

• If the tube clogs, irrigate using the 50-ml catheter-tip syringe with 30 ml of water or normal saline solution. Also, rotate and milk the tube. If these measures fail, then remove, rinse, and reinsert the catheter.

• Remove the catheter after completing drainage.

• Measure output, subtracting the amount of irrigant used.

• Rinse the catheter thoroughly with warm water.

• Clean the peristomal area and apply a fresh stoma dressing.

Complications

• Common postoperative complications include obstruction, fistula, pouch perforation, nipple valve dysfunction, abscesses, and bacterial overgrowth in the pouch.

Nursing considerations

• Never aspirate fluid from the catheter because the resulting negative pressure may damage inflamed tissue.

• The first few times you intubate the pouch, the patient may be tense, making insertion difficult. Encourage relaxation. To shorten drainage time, have the patient cough, press gently on his abdomen over the pouch, or suddenly tighten his abdominal muscles and then relax them.

• Keep an accurate record of intake and output *to ensure fluid and electrolyte balance.* The average daily output should be 1,000 ml. Report inadequate or excessive output (more than 1,400 ml daily).

Home care
• Be sure the patient can properly intubate and drain the pouch himself.
• Provide the patient with the appropriate equipment. If the postoperative drainage catheter is still in place, teach the patient how to care for it properly.
• Be sure the patient has a pouch-draining schedule, and give him appropriate pamphlets or video instructions on pouch care.
• Make sure he feels comfortable calling the doctor, nurse, or appropriate other caregivers with questions or problems.
• Tell the patient where to obtain supplies.
• Refer the patient to a local ostomy group.
• Provide dietary counseling.

Documentation
• Record the date, time, and all aspects of preoperative and postoperative care, including condition of the stoma and peristomal skin, diet, medications, intubations, patient teaching, and discharge planning.

Cranial nerve assessment

Assessment of the 12 pairs of cranial nerves that transmit motor and sensory messages between the brain and the head and neck is a complicated skill. The cranial nerves are designated by a name and a Roman numeral. The names of the nerves indicate their function. The Roman numerals indicate the order in which the nerves are found in the brain, from anterior to posterior. (See *Reviewing the cranial nerves.*)

Cranial nerve (CN) assessment provides valuable information about the condition of the central nervous system (CNS), particularly the brain stem. Because of their anatomic locations, some cranial nerves are more vulnerable to the effects of increasing intracranial pressure (ICP). Because of that, neurologic screening assessment of the cranial nerves focuses on the optic (II), oculomotor (III), trochlear (IV), and abducens (VI). The cranial nerves are assessed if the patient's history or symptoms indicate a potential cranial nerve disorder or when performing a complete CNS assessment.

≫ Key nursing diagnoses and patient outcomes
Use these nursing diagnoses as a guide when developing your plan of care for a patient receiving a cranial nerve assessment.

Sensory or perceptual alteration (specify) related to physical condition
Based on this nursing diagnosis, you'll establish the following patient outcomes. The patient will:
• discuss impact of loss on lifestyle.
• show interest in external environment.

Reviewing the cranial nerves

The 12 pairs of cranial nerves (CNs) transmit motor or sensory messages, or both, primarily between the brain or brain stem and the head and neck. All cranial nerves, except for the olfactory and optic nerves, exit from the midbrain, pons, or medulla oblongata of the brain stem.

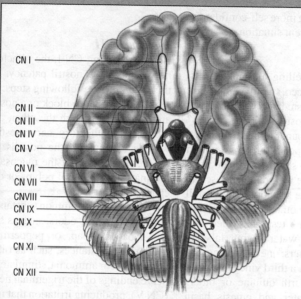

CN I
CN II
CN III
CN IV
CN V
CN VI
CN VII
CN VIII
CN IX
CN X
CN XI
CN XII

Olfactory (CN I) — Sensory: smell

Optic (CN II) — Sensory: vision

Oculomotor (CN III) — Motor: extraocular eye movement (superior, medial, and inferior lateral), pupillary constriction, and upper eyelid elevation

Trochlear (CN IV) — Motor: extraocular eye movement (inferior medial)

Trigeminal (CN V) — Sensory: transmitting stimuli from face and head, corneal reflex
    Motor: chewing, biting, and lateral jaw movements

Abducens (CN VI) — Motor: extraocular eye movement (lateral)

Facial (CN VII) — Sensory: taste receptors (anterior two-thirds of tongue)
    Motor: Facial muscle movement, including muscles of expression (those in the forehead and around the eyes and mouth)

Acoustic (CN VIII) — Sensory: hearing, balance

Glossopharyngeal (CN IX) — Sensory: sensations of throat; taste receptors (posterior one-third of tongue)
    Motor: swallowing movements

Vagus (CN X) — Sensory: sensations of throat, larynx, and thoracic and abdominal viscera (heart, lungs, bronchi, and GI tract)
    Motor: movement of palate, swallowing, gag reflex; activity of the thoracic and abdominal viscera, such as heart rate and peristalsis

Spinal accessory (CN XI) — Motor: shoulder movement, head rotation

Hypoglossal (CN XII) — Motor: tongue movement

Situational low self-esteem
Based on this nursing diagnosis, you'll establish the following patient outcomes. The patient will:
• describe how feelings about self have changed since current health problem began.
• report feeling more self-confident in managing current situation.

Equipment
♦ pungent-smelling substances, such as coffee, tobacco, soap or peppermint ♦ eye chart posted on a wall 20′ away (Snellens is most familiar) ♦ a 3″× 5″ index card or paper folded to that size ♦ penlight ♦ pencil or pen ♦ cotton ball ♦ dull and sharp instrument, such as a disposable ballpoint pen (use cap of a disposable ballpoint pen for dull testing and the other end to test sharp) or a safety pin ♦ test tubes filled with hot and cold water ♦ four labeled, closed containers: one containing salt, another sugar, a third vinegar or lemon, and a fourth quinine or bitters ♦ cup of water and emesis basin ♦ medicine dropper or tongue blade ♦ tuning fork ♦ cotton-tipped applicator ♦ folded gauze pad ♦ ophthalmoscope ♦ large syringe with a small catheter on the tip ♦ 20 to 200 ml of cold or ice water.

Patient preparation
• The patient should refrain from eating, drinking, or smoking during this examination.
• Check the patient's chart for allergies.
• Explain the procedure to patient to enlist cooperation to assist in the assessment.

Implementation
• Ask patient to make himself comfortable; sitting is preferred unless contraindicated by patient's condition.
• Ask patient to respond with open and honest answers for an accurate test.

Assessing CN I
Before assessing CN I, the olfactory nerve, check the nostril patency. Do this by taking the following steps:
• Ask the patient to block one nostril and to inhale through the other, and vice versa. Olfactory nerve testing will be impaired if the nostrils are blocked by edema of the mucosa or turbinates, or by nasal polyps or discharge.
• Use at least two common substances with recognizable odors, such as coffee, tobacco, soap, or peppermint. (Vaporous substances, such as oil of peppermint or ammonia, stimulate the nerve endings of the trigeminal nerve (CN V), producing irritation that may be mistaken for odor perception.)
• Ask the patient to close his eyes.
• Place the container of the first aromatic substance under the patient's nostril and ask her to identify the odor. Repeat this technique with the other nostril. If the patient reports detecting the smell but cannot name it, offer a choice, such as "Do you smell lemon, coffee, or peppermint?" Repeat the procedure with the other substances.

Assessing CN II
You assess CN II, the optic nerve, by assessing visual acuity, visual fields, and retinal structures. Do this in the following way:

• Use the eye chart (Snellen's or similar) and 3″ × 5″ card to cover one eye at a time during testing.

• Using the ophthalmoscope, examine the optic fundi for indications of arteriosclerotic small-vessel disease and diabetic or hypertensive retinopathy.

• Swelling of the optic disk, or papilledema, marked by fuzziness of the disk margins, may indicate an obstruction to venous outflow caused by increased ICP.

• Papilledema also is indicated by the curving of the disk vessels over the edges of the disk and absence of the physiologic cup.

Assessing CN III

To assess CN III, the oculomotor nerve, test pupil size, shape, and response to light following these steps:

• When assessing pupil size, be especially alert for any trends. For example, watch for a gradual increase in the size of one pupil or appearance of unequal pupils in a patient whose pupils were previously equal.

• Next, assess the patient's pupillary reaction to light using the penlight. This reaction depends on the optic nerve's ability to transmit the light stimulus to the visual center and the oculomotor nerve's ability to produce pupillary constriction.

Assessing CN IV and CN VI

Usually, you'll assess CN III (the oculomotor nerve), CN IV (the trochlear nerve), and CN VI (the abducens nerve) together. Begin by evaluating extraocular eye movement. All three nerves control these movements. Here's how to perform the assessment:

• Observe each eye for rapid oscillation (nystagmus), movement not in unison with that of the other eye (strabismus), or inability to move in certain directions (ophthalmoplegia).

• Note any complaint of double vision (diplopia).

Assessing CN V

Here's how to assess CN V, the trigeminal nerve:

• For the sensory portion, gently touch the right and then the left side of the patient's forehead with a cotton ball while his eyes are closed. Instruct him to state the moment the cotton touches the area. Compare his response on both sides.

• Repeat the procedure on the right and left cheek and on the right and the left jaw.

• Next, repeat the entire procedure using a sharp object. The cap of a disposable ballpoint pen can be used to test light touch (dull end) and sharp stimuli (sharp end) or an opened safety pin (sharp) and closed one (dull).

• If an abnormality appears, also test for temperature sensation by touching the patient's skin with test tubes filled with hot and cold water and asking the patient to differentiate between them.

• Ask the patient to clench his jaws. Palpate the temporal and masseter muscles bilaterally, checking for symmetry. Try to open his clenched jaws. Next, watch him opening and closing his mouth for asymmetry.

• Next, test the patient's corneal reflex.

• If he wears contact lenses, have him remove them.

• Tell him to look up and to one side, and lightly touch the cornea with the cotton wisp. Blinking and tearing is the normal corneal reflex response.

Assessing CN VII

To assess CN VII, the facial nerve, proceed in the following manner:
• To test the motor component of the nerve, observe the patient's face for symmetry.
• Compare the lower eyelids and check for drooping.
• Are the nasolabial folds symmetrical? Can the patient shed tears and salivate?
• Ask the patient to wrinkle his forehead, to raise and lower his eyebrows, to smile and show his teeth and puff out his cheeks.
• To test muscle strength, ask the patient to close his eyes tightly and to try to keep them closed while you attempt to force them open.
• Then place your hand against the patient's puffed cheeks and compare the muscle mass and strength of the cheeks.
• To test the sensory portion of the facial nerve, which supplies taste sensation to the anterior two-thirds of the tongue, first prepare four labeled, closed containers, with one containing salt; another sugar; a third, vinegar (or lemon); and a fourth, quinine (or bitters).
• Then, with the patient's eyes closed, place salt on the anterior two-thirds of his tongue using a cotton-tipped applicator or dropper.
• Ask him to identify the taste as sweet, salty, sour, or bitter.
• Rinse his mouth with water.
• Repeat this procedure, alternating flavors and sides tested on both sides.

• Taste sensations to the glossopharyngeal nerve (CN IX) and are usually tested at the same time.

Assessing CN VIII

To assess the acoustic portion of CN VIII, the acoustic nerve, test the patient's hearing acuity. The patient should be able to hear a whispered voice or a watch ticking. If a patient complains of vertigo, dizziness, imbalance, or a gait disturbance, you'll also evaluate the vestibular branch of the acoustic nerve. Follow the procedure below:
• Tell the patient to sit upright on the examination table with his legs and feet resting on the table.
• Ask him to look to the left and hold his head in that position. Observe for nystagmus.
• Then ask him to lie down and turn his head to the left. Have him lower his head to a 45-degree angle below the plane of the table. Keep him in that position for 30 seconds. Again, look for nystagmus, and ask him if he's experiencing vertigo.
• Help him sit up with his head still turned to the left, and assess him again for nystagmus and vertigo.
• Repeat the procedure with the patient's head turned to the right, but only after any sensations from the first test have subsided.
• In an unconscious patient, you can assess brain stem function by testing for the oculocephalic (doll's eyes) reflex and the oculovestibular reflex.

Most likely, you'll assist the doctor in performing these assessment techniques.
• If the patient has a cervical spine injury, expect to use the oculovestibular reflex test as an alternative.

• The oculovestibular reflex test may also be used to determine the status of the vestibular portion of CN VIII.

• The patient should have normal eye movements and balance and no dizziness or vertigo.

Assessing CN IX and CN X

CN IX, the glossopharyngeal nerve, and CN X, the vagus nerve, are usually tested together because their functions overlap. The assessment techniques are outlined in the following steps:

• Begin by listening to the patient's voice for hoarseness or nasal quality. The patient's voice should sound strong and clear.

• Then watch his soft palate while he says "ah." The soft palate and the uvula should rise when he says "ah," and the uvula should remain midline. The palatine arches should remain symmetrical during movement and at rest.

• Next, test the gag reflex after warning him. To evoke this reflex, touch the posterior wall of the pharynx with a cotton-tipped applicator or tongue blade. If the gag reflex diminishes or the pharynx moves asymmetrically, evaluate each side of the posterior pharyngeal wall to confirm integrity of both cranial nerves.

Assessing CN XI

CN XI, the spinal accessory, innervates the sternocleidomastoid and upper portion of the trapezius muscles, which govern shoulder movement and neck rotation. Here's how to assess it:

• Test sternocleidomastoid muscle strength by placing your palm against the patient's cheek and asking him to turn his head against the resistance of your hand.

• Repeat the test on the other side, comparing muscle strength.

• Test the trapezius muscles by placing your hands on the patient's shoulders and asking him to raise or shrug his shoulders against your resistance.

Assessing CN XII

CN XII, the hypoglossal nerve, controls tongue movements involved in swallowing and speech. Assessment steps are listed below:

• To assess this nerve, observe the patient's protruded tongue for any deviation from midline, atrophy, or fasciculations (fine muscle flickering, an indication of lower motor neuron disease).

• Next, instruct the patient to move his tongue rapidly from side to side with the mouth open, to curl his tongue up toward the nose, and to curl his tongue down toward the chin.

• Then, use a tongue blade or folded gauze pad to apply resistance to his protruded tongue.

• Ask him to try to push the tongue blade to one side.

• Repeat this procedure on the other side and note the patient's tongue strength.

• Listen to the patient's speech for the sounds d, l, n, and t, which require use of the tongue to articulate.

• If his general speech suggests a problem, have him repeat a phrase or a series of words containing these sounds, such as "Round the rugged rock the ragged rascal ran."

Complications

• Corneal abrasion may result from too aggressive or frequent testing of CN V with a wisp of cotton.

• Pain may arise when testing temporal and masseter muscles if the patient has trigeminal neuralgia of CN V.

• Nausea, vomiting, or dizziness may occur as a reaction to some of the testing if the patient is very sensitive.

Nursing considerations

• Before assessing the patient, complete history is necessary *to assist in correlation of findings.* If the patient is symptomatic (nauseated, dizzy) prior to testing, don't perform assessments that may prolong those symptoms.

• Keep emesis basin and suction equipment handy.

• In patients with Bell's palsy, CVA, head injury, maxillofacial trauma, or tracheostomy, a complete assessment of the CN may be difficult.

• Never perform taste tests on patients who are unconscious.

• Consult with physician prior to assessing if patient is at any kind of risk.

• Assist physician with evaluating brain stem functioning.

• Correlate findings of assessment with diagnostic testing and history, as applicable.

• Tell the doctor about assessment findings and any changes in subsequent assessments.

• If findings indicate an acute problem that does not correlate with the patients history, such as pupils that are unequal to light reflex or differ in shape, inform the physician immediately upon confirmation as an acute process may be occurring that requires prompt attention.

Documentation

• Chart the time, date, specific testing performed, results obtained, and the patient's tolerance of the procedure.

D

Debridement, mechanical

Debridement involves removing necrotic tissue by mechanical, chemical, or surgical means to allow underlying healthy tissue to regenerate. Mechanical debridement procedures include irrigation, hydrotherapy, and excision of dead tissue with forceps and scissors. The procedure may be done at the bedside or in a specially prepared room.

Burn-wound debridement removes eschar (hardened, dead tissue). This prevents or controls infection, promotes healing, and prepares the wound surface to receive a graft. Ideally, the wound should be debrided daily during the dressing change. Frequent, regular debridement guards against possible hemorrhage resulting from more extensive and forceful debridement. It also reduces the need to conduct extensive debridement under anesthesia.

Depending on the type of burn, a combination of debridement techniques may be used. Besides mechanical methods, treatment may also include chemical debridement (with wound-cleaning beads or topical agents that absorb exudate and debris) or surgical excision and skin grafting (usually reserved for deep burns or ulcers). Typically, the patient receives a local or general anesthetic beforehand.

Closed blisters over partial-thickness burns should not be debrided.

≫ Key nursing diagnoses and patient outcomes

Use these nursing diagnoses as a guide when developing your plan of care for a patient receiving mechanical debridement.

Body image disturbance related to appearance of wounds

Based on this nursing diagnosis, you'll establish the following patient outcomes. The patient will:
• communicate feelings about change in body image.
• express positive feelings about self.
• demonstrate ability to practice two new coping behaviors.

Pain related to physical, biological, or chemical agents

Based on this nursing diagnosis, you'll establish the following patient outcomes. The patient will:
• identify pain characteristics.
• articulate factors that intensify pain and modify behavior accordingly.
• express feelings of comfort and relief from pain.
• state and carry out appropriate interventions for pain relief.

Equipment

♦ ordered pain medication ♦ two pairs of sterile gloves ♦ two gowns or aprons ♦ mask ♦ cap ♦ sterile scissors ♦ sterile forceps ♦ sterile 4″×4″ gauze pads ♦ sterile solutions and medications, as ordered ♦ hemostatic agent, as ordered.

Note: Have the following equipment immediately available to control hemorrhage: ♦ needle holder ♦ gut suture with needle ♦ silver nitrate sticks.

Patient preparation

• Explain the procedure to the patient to allay his fears and promote cooperation.

• Teach distraction and relaxation techniques, if possible, *to minimize his discomfort.*

• Provide privacy.

• Administer an analgesic 20 minutes before debridement begins, or give an I.V. analgesic immediately before the procedure.

• Keep the patient warm.

• Expose only the area to be debrided *to prevent chilling and fluid and electrolyte loss.*

Implementation

• Wash your hands and put on a cap, mask, gown or apron, and sterile gloves.

• Remove the burn dressings and clean the wound. (For detailed directions, see "Burn care," page 116.)

• Remove your gown or apron and dirty gloves, and change to another gown or apron and sterile gloves.

• Lift loosened edges of eschar with forceps.

• Use the blunt edge of scissors or forceps to probe the eschar.

• Cut the dead tissue from the wound with the scissors. Leave a $\frac{1}{4}''$ (0.6-cm) edge on remaining eschar *to avoid cutting into viable tissue.*

• Because debridement removes only dead tissue, bleeding should be minimal.

• If bleeding occurs, apply gentle pressure on the wound with the sterile $4'' \times 4''$ gauze pads. Then apply the hemostatic agent.

• If bleeding persists, notify the doctor, and maintain pressure on the wound until he arrives.

• Excessive bleeding or spurting vessels may require ligation.

• Perform additional procedures, such as application of topical medications and dressing replacements, as ordered.

Complications

• Infection may occur despite aseptic technique and equipment.

• Blood loss is possible if debridement exposes an eroded blood vessel or if you inadvertently cut a vessel.

• Fluid and electrolyte imbalances may result from exudate lost during debridement.

Nursing considerations

• Work quickly with an assistant, if possible, to complete this painful procedure as soon as possible.

• Acknowledge the patient's discomfort and provide emotional support.

• Debride no more than a 4-in^2 (10-cm^2) area at one time.

• Limit procedure time to 20 minutes or less, if possible.

Documentation

• Record date and time of debridement, area debrided, and solutions and medications used.

• Describe wound condition, noting signs of infection or skin breakdown.

• Record the patient's tolerance of and reaction to the procedure.

• Note indications for additional therapy.

Defibrillation

The standard treatment for ventricular fibrillation (VF), defibrillation involves using electrode paddles to direct an electric current through the patient's heart. The current causes the myocardium to depolarize which, in turn, encourages the sinoatrial node to resume control of the heart's electrical activity. The electrode paddles delivering the current may be placed on the patient's chest or, during cardiac surgery, directly on the myocardium.

Because VF leads to death if not corrected, the success of defibrillation depends on early recognition and quick treatment of this arrhythmia. Besides treating VF, defibrillation may also be used to treat ventricular tachycardia (VT) that doesn't produce a pulse.

Patients with a history of VF may be candidates for an implantable cardioverter defibrillator (ICD), a sophisticated device that automatically discharges an electric current when it senses a ventricular tachyarrhythmia. (See *Understanding the ICD*, page 256.)

⟫ Key nursing diagnoses and patient outcomes

Use these nursing diagnoses as a guide when developing your plan of care for a patient who has received defibrillation.

Anxiety related to threat of death

Based on this nursing diagnosis, you'll establish the following patient outcomes. The patient will:
• identify cause of anxiety.
• cope with anxiety by being involved in decision about care.

Decreased cardiac output related to reduced stroke volume as a result of electrophysiologic problems

Based on this nursing diagnosis, you'll establish the following patient outcomes. The patient will:

• have no arrhythmias.
• remain hemodynamically stable as evidenced by: pulse not less than ___ and not greater than ___; blood pressure not less than ___/___ and not greater than ___/___.

Equipment

♦ defibrillator ♦ external paddles ♦ internal paddles (sterilized for cardiac surgery) ♦ conductive medium pads ♦ ECG monitor with recorder ♦ oxygen therapy equipment ♦ handheld resuscitation bag ♦ airway equipment ♦ emergency pacing equipment ♦ emergency cardiac medications.

Implementation

• Assess the patient *to determine the lack of a pulse.*
• Call for help and perform cardiopulmonary resuscitation (CPR) until the defibrillator and emergency equipment arrive.
• If the defibrillator has *quick-look* capability, place the paddles on the patient's chest *to quickly view the cardiac rhythm.* Otherwise, connect the monitoring leads of the defibrillator to the patient, and assess his cardiac rhythm.
• Expose the patient's chest, and apply conductive pads at the paddle placement positions. For anterolateral placement, position one paddle to the right of the upper sternum just below the right clavicle, and the other over the fifth or sixth intercostal space at the left anterior axillary line. For anteroposterior placement, position the anterior paddle directly over the heart at the precordium to the left of the lower sternal border. Place the flat posterior paddle under the patient's body

Understanding the ICD

The implantable cardioverter defibrillator (ICD) is used with patients who have a history of ventricular fibrillation. The device has a pulse generator and lead systems to monitor the heart's activity and deliver shocks as necessary.

The surgeon will position a bipolar lead transvenously in the endocardium of the right ventricle or place two leads $\frac{3}{8}''$ (1 cm) apart on the epicardium of the left ventricle. These leads record the heart rate.

The shocks are delivered by two patch leads sewn onto the heart (as shown) or by one patch lead and a lead (not shown) placed in the right atrium via the superior vena cava. These leads also detect the amount of time the waveform remains at the baseline — called the probability density function.

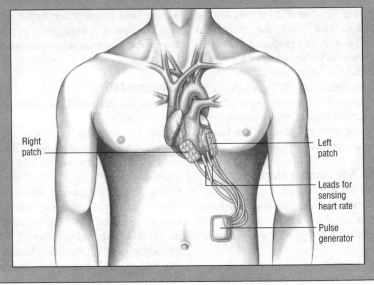

Right patch

Left patch

Leads for sensing heart rate

Pulse generator

beneath the heart and immediately below the scapulae (but not under the vertebral column).
• Turn on the defibrillator and, if performing external defibrillation, set the energy level for 200 joules for an adult patient.
• Charge the paddles by pressing the CHARGE buttons, located either on the machine or on the paddles themselves.

• Place the paddles over the conductive pads and press firmly against the patient's chest, using 25 lb (11 kg) of pressure.
• Reassess the patient's cardiac rhythm.
• If the patient remains in VF or pulseless VT, instruct all personnel to stand clear of the patient and the bed.
• Discharge the current by pressing both paddle CHARGE buttons simultaneously.

• Leaving the paddles in position on the patient's chest, reassess the patient's cardiac rhythm and have someone else assess the pulse.

• If necessary, prepare to defibrillate a second time. Instruct someone to reset the energy level on the defibrillator to 200 to 300 joules.

• Announce that you're preparing to defibrillate, and follow the procedure described above.

• Reassess the patient. If defibrillation is again necessary, instruct someone to reset the energy level to 360 joules. Then follow the same procedure as before.

• Perform the three countershocks in rapid succession, reassessing the patient's rhythm before each defibrillation.

• If the patient still has no pulse after three initial defibrillations, resume CPR, give supplemental oxygen, and begin administering appropriate medications, such as epinephrine. Also consider possible causes for failure of the patient's rhythm to convert, such as acidosis or hypoxia.

• If defibrillation restores a normal rhythm, check the patient's central and peripheral pulses, and obtain a blood-pressure reading and heart and respiratory rate.

• Assess the patient's level of consciousness, cardiac rhythm, breath sounds, skin color, and urine output.

• Obtain baseline arterial blood gas levels and a 12-lead ECG.

• Provide supplemental oxygen, ventilation, and medications, as needed.

• Check the patient's chest for electrical burns and treat them, as ordered, with corticosteroid or lanolin-based creams.

• Prepare the defibrillator for immediate reuse.

Complications
• Those providing care may experience accidental electric shock.

• Insufficient amount of conductive medium may cause skin burns.

Nursing considerations
• *Defibrillators vary from one manufacturer to the next,* so familiarize yourself with your hospital's equipment.

• Defibrillator operation should be checked at least every 8 hours and after each use.

• Defibrillation can be affected by several factors, including paddle size and placement, condition of the patient's myocardium, duration of the arrhythmia, chest resistance, and the number of countershocks.

Documentation
• Document the procedure, including the patient's predefibrillation and postdefibrillation ECG rhythms; the number of times defibrillation was performed; the voltage used with each attempt; whether a pulse returned; the dosage, route, and time of drug administration; whether CPR was used; how the airway was maintained; and the patient's outcome.

Diaphragmatic excursion assessment

Diaphragmatic excursion is a measurement of the distance the diaphragm travels between inhalation and exhalation. Normal diaphragmatic excursion is 1¼″ to 2 ¼″ (3 to 6 cm). Failure of the diaphragm to contract downward may indicate paralysis or muscle flattening, a condition that results from chronic obstructive pulmonary disease.

≫ Key nursing diagnoses and patient outcomes

Use these nursing diagnoses as a guide when developing your plan of care.

Impaired gas exchange related to altered oxygen-carrying capacity of the blood

Based on this nursing diagnosis, you'll establish the following patient outcomes. The patient will:
• carry out activities of daily living without weakness or fatigue.
• maintain adequate ventilation.

Altered cardiopulmonary tissue perfusion related to decreased cellular exchange

Based on this nursing diagnosis, you'll establish the following patient outcomes. The patient will:
• modify lifestyle to minimize risk of decreased tissue perfusion.
• maintain heart rate within prescribed limits while carrying out activities of daily living.

Equipment

♦ felt-tipped marker with water-soluble ink ♦ tape measure or ruler.

Patient preparation

• Explain the procedure.
• Help the patient into sitting position, unless contraindicated by condition.

Implementation

• Instruct the patient to take a deep breath and hold it while you percuss down the right side of the posterior thorax.
• Begin at the lower border of the scapula and continue until the percussion note changes from resonance to dullness, *which locates the diaphragm.*
• Using a felt-tipped pen with water-soluble ink, mark this point with a small line.
• Instruct the patient to take a few normal breaths and then ask him to exhale completely and hold it while you percuss again to locate the point where the resonant sounds become dull. Mark this point with a small line.
• Repeat the procedure on the left side of the posterior thorax.
• Keep in mind that the diaphragm usually sits slightly higher on the right side than on the left because of the position of the liver.
• Next, using a tape measure or ruler, measure the distance between the two marks, as shown here. The distance between these two marks reflects diaphragmatic excursion.

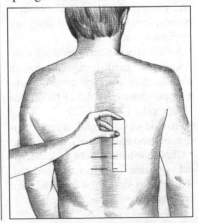

Nursing considerations
• Explain to the patient the importance of the procedure *to assist in attaining information for baseline assessment.*
• Correlate findings with information from the history and physical.

Documentation
• Document patient tolerance of the procedure and the results of nursing assessment.

Drug administration via intermittent infusion device

An intermittent infusion injection device — or heparin lock — eliminates the need for multiple venipunctures or for maintaining venous access with a continuous I.V. infusion. This device allows intermittent administration by infusion or by the I.V. bolus or I.V. push injection methods.

Diluted heparin or normal saline solutions are often injected as the final step in this procedure to prevent clotting in the device. When heparin is used, the device must be flushed with normal saline solution before and after the prescribed medication is administered in case the heparin and the medication are incompatible. The device may then be reflushed with the heparin flush solution.

» Key nursing diagnoses and patient outcomes
Use these nursing diagnoses as a guide when developing your plan of care for a patient receiving medications via an intermittent infusion device.

Knowledge deficit related to lack of exposure
Based on this nursing diagnosis, you'll establish the following patient outcomes. The patient will:
• state or demonstrate understanding of what has been taught.
• demonstrate ability to perform new health related behaviors as they are taught.

Risk for injury related to improper technique
Based on this nursing diagnosis, you'll establish the following patient outcomes. The patient will:
• identify factors that increase risk for injury.
• assist in identifying and applying safety measures to prevent injury.

Equipment
♦ patient's medication record and chart ♦ three 3-ml syringes with 22G or 25G 1″ needles ♦ normal saline solution ♦ alcohol sponges ♦ extra intermittent infusion device ♦ prescribed medication in an I.V. container with administration set and needle (for infusion) or in a syringe with needle (for I.V. bolus or push) ♦ tourniquet ♦ tape ♦ gloves ♦ optional: T-connector, dilute heparin solution, sterile bacteriostatic water.

Equipment preparation
• The concentration of dilute heparin solution ranges from 10 to 100 units/ml. The solution is available in a cartridge-injection system in doses of 10 to 100 units/ml. If this system is used, substitute the supplied syringe

for the 3-ml syringe and the heparin cartridge for the heparin solution. Normal saline solution is available in a similar cartridge system.

• Verify the order on the patient's medication record by checking it against the doctor's order. Wash your hands, put on gloves, and then wipe the tops of the normal saline solution, heparin flush solution, and medication containers with alcohol sponges. Fill two of the 3-ml syringes (with 22G needles) with normal saline solution; if required by hospital policy, draw 1 ml of heparin flush solution into the third syringe. If you'll be infusing medication, insert the administration set spike into the I.V. container, attach the appropriate-sized needle, and prime the line. If you'll be giving an I.V. injection, fill a syringe with the prescribed drug.

Implementation

• Confirm the patient's identity by asking his name and checking the name, room number, and bed number on his wristband. Explain the procedure.

• Wipe the injection port of the intermittent infusion device with an alcohol sponge, and insert the needle of a saline-filled syringe.

• Aspirate the syringe and observe for blood *to verify the patency of the device.* If none appears, apply a tourniquet slightly above the site, keep it in place for about 1 minute, and then aspirate again. If blood still doesn't appear, remove the tourniquet and inject the normal saline solution slowly.

Note: Stop the injection immediately if you feel any resistance *because resistance indicates that the device is occluded.* If this occurs, insert a new intermittent infusion device.

• If you feel no resistance, watch for signs of infiltration (puffiness or pain at the site) as you slowly inject the saline solution. If these signs occur, insert a new intermittent infusion device.

• If blood is aspirated, slowly inject the saline solution and observe for signs of infiltration. *The saline solution flushes out any residual heparin solution that might be incompatible with the medication.*

• Withdraw the syringe of saline solution and needle.

To administer I.V. bolus or I.V. push injections

• Insert the needle and syringe with the medication for the I.V. bolus or I.V. push injection into the injection port of the device.

• Inject the medication at the required rate. Then remove the needle from the injection port.

• Insert the needle of the remaining saline-filled syringe into the injection port and slowly inject the saline solution *to flush all medication through the device.*

• Remove the needle and syringe, and insert and inject the heparin (or saline) flush solution *to prevent clotting in the device.*

To administer an infusion

• Insert and tape the needle attached to the administration set.

• Open the infusion line and adjust the flow rate as necessary.

• Infuse medication for the prescribed time; then flush the device with normal saline solution and heparin flush solution as you would after a bolus or push injection, according to your hospital's policy.

Using a T-connector

A T-connector is a piece of small-bore extension tubing 3″ to 6″ (7.6 to 15.2 cm) long. It's fitted with an injection port near the luer-lock connection. This additional injection site allows simultaneous administration of drugs and fluids or of a primary I.V. solution and a drug that is incompatible with it.

To attach a T-connector, wash your hands and put on gloves to minimize exposure to body fluids. Explain the procedure to the patient.

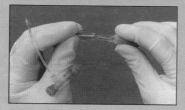

Prime the tubing with I.V. fluid, then attach one end of the T-connector (bottom left). Open the slide clamp, purge the tubing, and close the clamp.

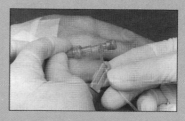

Remove the luer-lock tip-protector cap and insert this tip into the I.V. cannula (above).

Secure this connector in place with tape. Another I.V. needle can be inserted into the latex injection cap of the T connector. Finally, document your actions.

• To administer fluids and drugs simultaneously or to administer a medication incompatible with the primary I.V. solution, you can use a T-connector. (See *Using a T-connector*.)

Complications
• Infiltration and a specific reaction to the infused drug are common.

Nursing considerations
• If you're giving a bolus injection of a drug that's incompatible with normal saline solution, such as diazepam, flush the device with bacteriostatic water.
• Some hospitals use diluted heparin solution (100 units/ml or 10 units/ml) to prevent clotting in the cannula. Other hospitals use 2 to 3 ml of normal saline solution instead. A few hospitals use other solutions or dilutions. Check your hospital's policy.
• Intermittent infusion devices should be changed regularly (usually every 48 to 72 hours), according to universal precautions guidelines and hospital policy.
• If you're unable to rotate injection sites because the patient has fragile veins, document this fact in your notes.

Documentation
• Record the type and amount of drug administered and the times of administration. Include all I.V. solutions used to dilute the medication and flush the line on the intake-and-output record. Also document the use of dilute heparin solution.

Drug administration via a secondary I.V. line

A secondary I.V. line is a complete I.V. set — container, tubing, and microdrip or macrodrip system — connected to the lower Y-port (secondary port) of a primary line instead of to the I.V. catheter or needle. It can be used for continuous or intermittent drug infusion. When used continuously, a secondary I.V. line permits drug infusion and titration while the primary line maintains a constant total infusion rate.

When used intermittently, a secondary I.V. line is commonly called a piggyback set. In this case, the primary line maintains venous access between drug doses. Typically, a piggyback set includes a small I.V. container, short tubing, and a macrodrip system. This set connects to the primary line's upper Y-port, also known as a piggyback port. Antibiotics and histamine-2 receptor antagonists are most commonly administered by intermittent (piggyback) infusion. To make this set work, the primary I.V. container must be positioned below the piggyback container. (The manufacturer provides an extension hook for that purpose.)

Some drugs can be piggybacked with a needle-free system, which consists of a blunt-tipped plastic insertion device and a rubber injection port. The port may be part of a special administration set or an adapter for existing administration sets. This rubber injection port has a preestablished slit that can open and reseal immediately. The needle-free system aims to reduce the risk of accidental needle-stick injuries.

I.V. pumps may be used to maintain constant infusion rates, especially with a drug such as lidocaine. A pump allows more accurate titration of drug dosage and helps maintain venous access because the drug is delivered under sufficient pressure to prevent clot formation in the I.V. cannula.

≫ Key nursing diagnoses and patient outcomes

Use these nursing diagnoses as a guide when developing your plan of care for a patient who is receiving medications via a secondary I.V. line.

Knowledge deficit related to lack of exposure to the procedure
Based on this nursing diagnosis, you'll establish the following patient outcomes. The patient will:
• state or demonstrate understanding of what has been taught.
• demonstrate ability to perform new health-related behaviors as they are taught.

Risk for injury related to improper technique
Based on this nursing diagnosis, you'll establish the following patient outcomes. The patient will:
• identify factors that increase risk for injury.
• assist in identifying and applying safety measures to prevent injury.

Equipment
♦ patient's medication record and chart ♦ prescribed I.V. medication ♦ prescribed I.V. solution ♦ administration set with secondary injection port ♦ 22G 1″ needle ♦ alcohol

sponges ♦ 1" adhesive tape ♦ time tape ♦ labels ♦ infusion pump ♦ extension hook and appropriate solution for intermittent piggyback infusion ♦ optional: normal saline solution for infusion with incompatible solutions.

Equipment preparation

• For intermittent infusion, the primary line typically has a piggyback port with a backcheck valve that stops the flow from the primary line during drug infusion and returns to the primary flow after infusion.

• A volume-control set can also be used with an intermittent infusion line.

• Verify the order on the patient's medication record by checking it against the doctor's order.

• Wash your hands.

• Inspect the I.V. container for cracks, leaks, or contamination, and check drug compatibility with the primary solution.

• Check whether the primary line has a secondary injection port. If it doesn't and the medication will be given regularly, replace the I.V. set with a new one that has a secondary injection port.

• If necessary, add the drug to the secondary I.V. solution. To do so, remove any seals from the secondary container and wipe the main port with an alcohol sponge. Inject the prescribed medication, and gently agitate the solution to mix the medication thoroughly. Properly label the I.V. mixture. Insert the administration set spike and attach the needle. Open the flow clamp and prime the line. Then close the flow clamp.

• Some medications now come in vials suitable for hanging directly on an I.V. pole. Instead of preparing medication and injecting it into a container, you can inject diluent directly into the medication vial. Then you can spike the vial, prime the tubing, and hang the set, as directed.

Implementation

• Confirm the patient's identity by asking his name and checking the name, room number, and bed number on his wristband.

• If the drug is incompatible with the primary I.V. solution, replace the primary solution with a fluid that's compatible with both solutions, such as normal saline, and flush the line before starting the drug infusion. Many hospital protocols require removing the primary I.V. solution and inserting a sterile I.V. plug into the container until you're ready to rehang it. *This will maintain sterility of the solution and prevent someone else from inadvertently restarting the incompatible solution before the line is flushed with normal saline solution.*

• Hang the secondary set's container and wipe the injection port of the primary line with an alcohol sponge.

• Insert the needle from the secondary line into the injection port and tape it securely to the primary line.

• To run the secondary set's container by itself, use an extension hook to lower the primary set's container. To run both containers simultaneously, place them at the same height. (See *Assembling a piggyback set*, page 264.)

• Open the clamp and adjust the drip rate. For continuous infusion, set the secondary solution to the desired drip rate; then adjust the primary solution to achieve the desired total infusion rate.

• For intermittent infusion, adjust the primary drip rate, as required, upon

Assembling a piggyback set

A piggyback set is useful for intermittent drug infusion. To work properly, its drug container must be positioned higher than the primary set's container.

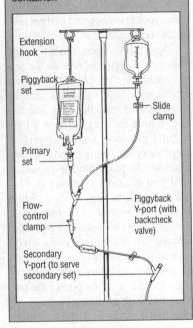

Extension hook

Piggyback set

Slide clamp

Primary set

Flow-control clamp

Piggyback Y-port (with backcheck valve)

Secondary Y-port (to serve secondary set)

completion of the secondary solution. If the secondary solution tubing is being reused, close the clamp on the tubing and follow hospital policy: Either remove the needle and replace it with a new one, or leave it securely taped in the injection port and label it with the time it was first used. In this case, also leave the empty container in place until you replace it with a new dose of medication at the prescribed time. If the tubing won't be reused, discard it appropriately with the I.V. container.

Complications
• Adverse reactions to the infused drug may occur.
• Repeated punctures of the secondary injection port can damage the seal, possibly allowing leakage or contamination.

Nursing considerations
• If hospital policy allows, use a pump for drug infusion. Put a time tape on the secondary container *to help prevent an inaccurate administration rate.*
• When reusing secondary tubing, change it according to hospital policy, usually every 48 to 72 hours. Similarly, inspect the injection port for leakage with each use, and change it more often if needed.
• Unless you're piggybacking lipids, don't piggyback a secondary I.V. line to a total parenteral nutrition line because of the risk of contamination. Check hospital policy for possible exceptions.

Documentation
• Record the amount and type of drug and the amount of I.V. solution on the intake-and-output and medication records.
• Note the date, duration, and rate of infusion, and the patient's response, where applicable.

Drug administration via Z-track injection

This method of I.M. injection prevents leakage, or tracking, into the subcutaneous tissue. Typically, it's used to administer drugs that irritate and discolor subcutaneous tissue, primarily iron preparations, such as iron dextran. It may also be used in elderly patients who have decreased muscle mass. Lateral displacement of the skin during the injection helps to seal the drug in the muscle.

This procedure requires careful attention to technique because leakage into subcutaneous tissue can cause patient discomfort and may permanently stain some tissues.

≫ Key nursing diagnoses and patient outcomes

Use these nursing diagnoses as a guide when developing your plan of care for a patient who is receiving Z-track injection.

Knowledge deficit related to lack of exposure to the procedure

Based on this nursing diagnosis, you'll establish the following patient outcomes. The patient will:
• state or demonstrate understanding of what has been taught.
• demonstrate ability to perform new health related behaviors as they are taught.

Risk for injury related to improper technique

Based on this nursing diagnosis, you'll establish the following patient outcomes. The patient will:
• identify factors that increase risk for injury.
• assist in identifying and applying safety measures to prevent injury.

Equipment

♦ patient's medication record and chart ♦ two 20G 1¼" to 2" needles ♦ prescribed medication ♦ gloves ♦ 3- to 5-ml syringe ♦ two alcohol sponges.

Equipment preparation

• Verify the order on the patient's medication record by checking it against the doctor's order.
• Wash your hands.
• Make sure the needle you're using is long enough to reach the muscle. As a rule of thumb, a 200-pound patient requires a 2" needle; a 100-pound patient, a 1¼" to 1½" needle. Attach one needle to the syringe, and draw up the prescribed medication. Then draw 0.2 to 0.5 cc of air (depending on hospital policy) into the syringe.
• Remove the first needle and attach the second to prevent tracking the medication through the subcutaneous tissue as the needle is inserted.

Implementation

• Confirm the patient's identity, explain the procedure, and provide privacy.
• Place the patient in the lateral position, exposing the gluteal muscle to be used as the injection site. The patient may also be placed in the prone position.
• Clean an area on the upper outer quadrant of the patient's buttock with an alcohol sponge.
• Don gloves. Then displace the skin laterally by pulling it away from the injection site. (See *Displacing the skin for Z-track injection,* page 266.)
• Insert the needle into the muscle at a 90-degree angle.
• Aspirate for blood return; if none appears, inject the drug slowly, followed by the air. *Injecting air after the drug helps clear the needle and prevents tracking the medication through sub-*

Displacing the skin for Z-track injection

By blocking the needle pathway after injection, this technique allows I.M. injection while minimizing the risk of subcutaneous irritation and staining from such drugs as iron dextran. The illustrations below show how to perform a Z-track injection.

Before the procedure begins, the skin, subcutaneous fat, and muscle lie in their normal positions.

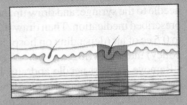

To begin, place your finger on the skin surface, and pull the skin and subcutaneous layers out of alignment with the underlying muscle. You should move the skin about ½″ (1 cm).

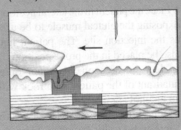

Insert the needle at a 90-degree angle in the site where you initially placed your finger. Inject the drug and withdraw the needle.

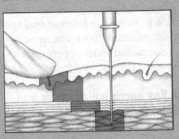

Finally, remove your finger from the skin surface, allowing the layers to return to their normal positions. The needle track (shown by the dotted line) is now broken at the junction of each tissue layer, trapping the drug in the muscle.

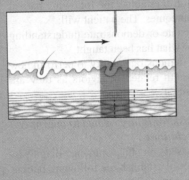

---

cutaneous tissues as the needle is withdrawn.
• Wait 10 seconds before withdrawing the needle *to ensure dispersion of the medication.*
• Withdraw the needle slowly. Then release the displaced skin and subcutaneous tissue *to seal the needle track.* Don't massage the injection site or al-

low the patient to wear a tight-fitting garment over the site *because it could force the medication into subcutaneous tissue.*
• Encourage the patient to walk or to move about in bed *to facilitate absorption of the drug from the injection site.*

• Discard the needles and syringe in an appropriate sharps container. Do not recap needles *to avoid needle-stick injuries.*
• Remove and discard your gloves.

Complications
• Discomfort and tissue irritation may result from drug leakage into subcutaneous tissue.

Nursing considerations
• Never inject more than 5 ml of solution into a single site using the Z-track method.
• Alternate gluteal sites for repeat injections.
• If the patient is on bed rest, encourage active range-of-motion (ROM) exercises or perform passive ROM exercises *to facilitate absorption from the injection site.*

Documentation
• Record the medication, dosage, date, time, and site of injection on the patient's medication record.
• Also record the patient's response to the injected drug.

Drug implants

A newer method of advanced drug delivery involves implanting drugs beneath the skin, subdermally or subcutaneously, and by targeting specific tissues with radiation implants.

With subcutaneous implants, drug pellets are injected into the skin's subcutaneous layer. The drug is then stored in one area of the body, called a *depot.* A newer treatment for prostate cancer is implanted goserelin ac-

etate, a synthetic form of luteinizing hormone. By inhibiting pituitary gland secretion, goserelin implants reduce serum testosterone to levels previously achieved only through castration. This reduction causes tumor regression and suppression of symptoms.

With subdermal implants, flexible capsules are placed under the skin. The drug most commonly administered by this method is levonorgestrel, a synthetic hormone used for long-term contraception. Small Silastic capsules filled with the hormone are placed under the skin of the patient's upper arm. The drug then continuously diffuses through the walls of the capsule.

Implanted radioactive drugs with short half-lives may be placed inside a body cavity, in a tumor or on its surface, or in the area from which a tumor has been removed. These drugs include: iodine 125 for lung and prostate tumors; gold 198 for oral and ocular tumors, with radium 226 and cesium 137 for tongue and lip therapy; and radium 226 and cesium 137 for skin therapy. These implants are usually inserted by a doctor, with a nurse assisting. Some specially-trained nurses may insert or inject intradermal implants. Radiation implants are usually put in place in an operating room or a radiation oncology suite.

≫ Key nursing diagnoses and patient outcomes
Use these nursing diagnoses as a guide when developing your plan of care for a patient receiving drug implants.

Knowledge deficit related to lack of exposure to the procedure
Based on this nursing diagnosis, you'll establish the following patient outcomes. The patient will:
• state or demonstrate understanding of what has been taught.
• demonstrate ability to perform new health related behaviors as they are taught.

Risk for injury related to improper technique
Based on this nursing diagnosis, you'll establish the following patient outcomes. The patient will:
• identify factors that increase risk for injury.
• assist in identifying and applying safety measures to prevent injury.

Equipment
For subdermal implants: ◆ sterile surgical drapes ◆ sterile gloves ◆ antiseptic solution ◆ local anesthetic ◆ set of implants ◆ needles ◆ syringe ◆ scalpel (#11) ◆ trocar (#10) ◆ forceps ◆ sutures ◆ sterile gauze ◆ tape.

For subcutaneous implants: ◆ alcohol sponge ◆ drug implant in a preloaded syringe ◆ local anesthetic (for some patients).

For radiation implants: ◆ RADIATION PRECAUTION sign for the patient's door ◆ warning labels for his wristband and personal belongings ◆ film badge or pocket dosimeter ◆ lead-lined container ◆ long-handled forceps ◆ masking tape ◆ portable lead shield.

Implementation
Subdermal implants
• Before the procedure, tell the patient what will happen, and let her see a set of implants. Also explain to her the benefits and risks of the procedure. Then assist her into a supine position on the examination table. Stay with her during the procedure and provide support, as necessary.
• After anesthetizing the upper portion of the nondominant arm, the doctor will use a trocar to insert each capsule through a 2-mm incision. After positioning the capsules correctly, he'll remove the trocar and palpate the area. He'll then close the incision and cover it with a dry compress and sterile gauze.

The steps below describe how levonorgestrel subdermal contraceptive implants are inserted:
• Have the patient lie supine on the examination table and flex the elbow of her nondominant arm so that her hand is opposite her head.
• Swab the insertion site with antiseptic solution. (The ideal insertion site is inside the upper arm about 3″ to 4″ [7.5 to 10 cm] above the elbow.)
• Cover the arm above and below the insertion site with sterile surgical drapes.
• The doctor fills a 5-ml syringe with a local anesthetic, inserts the needle under the skin, and injects a small amount of anesthetic into several areas, each about 1½″ to 2″ (4 to 5 cm) long, in a fanlike pattern.
• The doctor makes a small, shallow incision (about 2 mm) through the skin using the scalpel.
• Next, he inserts the tip of the trocar through the incision at a shallow angle beneath the skin. He makes sure the trocar bevel is up so he can place the capsules in a superficial plane. To avoid placing the capsules too deep, he tents the skin with the trocar. He

advances the trocar slowly to the first mark near the hub of the trocar. The tip of the trocar should now be about $1\frac{1}{2}''$ to $2''$ from the incision site. The doctor then removes the obturator and loads the first capsule into the trocar.
• He gently advances the capsule with the obturator toward the tip of the trocar until he feels resistance. Next, he inserts each succeeding capsule beside the last one in a fanlike pattern. With the forefinger and middle finger of his free hand, he fixes the position of the previous capsule, advancing the trocar along the tips of his fingers. *This ensures a suitable distance of about 15 degrees between capsules and keeps the trocar from puncturing any of the previously inserted capsules.*

Subcutaneous implants
• Help the patient into the supine position, and drape him so that his abdomen is accessible. Remove the syringe from the package, and make sure you can see the drug in the chamber. Clean a small area on the patient's upper abdominal wall with the alcohol sponge.
• As you stretch the skin at the injection site with one hand, grip the needle with the fingers of your other hand around the barrel of the syringe. Insert the needle into subcutaneous fat. Don't attempt to aspirate. If blood appears in the syringe, withdraw the needle and inject a new, preloaded syringe and new needle at another site.
• Next, change the direction of the needle so it's parallel to the abdominal wall. With the barrel hub touching the patient's skin, push the needle in. Then withdraw it about $\frac{1}{2}''$ (1 cm), creating a space in which to discharge the drug. Depress the plunger. Withdraw the needle and bandage the site.

• Inspect the tip of the needle. If you can see the metal tip of the plunger, the drug has been discharged.

Radiation implants
• To prepare for radiation-implant insertion, first place the lead-lined container and long-handled forceps in a corner of the patient's room. With masking tape, mark a safe line on the floor 6' (2 m) from the patient's bed to warn visitors of the danger of radiation exposure. Also place the portable lead shield in the back of the room to wear when providing care.
• Place an emergency tracheotomy tray in the room if an implant will be inserted in the patient's mouth or neck.
• To insert the implant, the doctor makes a small incision in the skin and creates a pocket in the tissue. He puts the implant in position and closes the incision. If the patient is being treated for tonsillar cancer, he'll undergo a bronchoscopy, during which radioactive pellets will be implanted in tonsillar tissue.
• Your role in the implant procedure is to explain the treatment and its goals to the patient. Review radiation-safety procedures and visitation policies. Talk with the patient about long-term physical and emotional aspects of the therapy, and discuss home care.

Complications
Subdermal implants
• Possible complications of levonorgestrel include hyperpigmentation at the insertion site, menstrual irregularities, headache, nervousness, nausea, dizziness, adnexal enlargement, dermatitis, acne, appetite changes, weight

changes, mastalgia, hirsutism, and alopecia.
• Some women suffer more serious reactions, including breast abnormalities and mammographic changes, diabetes, elevated cholesterol or triglyceride levels, hypertension, seizures, depression, or gallbladder, heart, or kidney disease.

Subcutaneous implants
• Goserelin implants may cause anemia, lethargy, pain, dizziness, insomnia, anxiety, depression, headache, chills, fever, edema, congestive heart failure, arrhythmias, cerebrovascular accident, hypertension, peripheral vascular disease, nausea, vomiting, diarrhea, decreased number of erections, renal insufficiency, urinary obstruction, rash, sweating, hot flashes, gout, hyperglycemia, weight increase, and breast swelling and tenderness.

Radiation implants
• Depending on the implant site and radiation dosage, complications may include dislodgment of the implant, tissue fibrosis, xerostomia, radiation pneumonitis, muscle atrophy, sterility, vaginal dryness or stenosis, fistulas, altered bowel habits, hypothyroidism, infection, airway obstruction, diarrhea, cystitis, myelosuppression, neurotoxicity, and secondary cancers.
• If an implant becomes dislodged, collect it with long-handled forceps and place it in a lead-lined container.

Nursing considerations
Subdermal implants
• Tell the patient that she can resume her normal activities after the implantation, although she should use extra caution during the first few days.

• Advise her not to bump the insertion site and to keep the area dry and covered with a gauze bandage for 3 days.
• Tell the patient to report signs of bleeding or infection at the insertion site.

Subcutaneous implants
• Be aware that if an implant must be removed, a doctor will order an X-ray to locate it.
• Tell your patient to check the administration site between injections for signs of infection or bleeding.

Radiation implants
• Know that if laboratory work is required during treatment, a technician wearing a film badge will obtain the specimen, affix a RADIATION PRECAUTION label to the specimen container, and alert laboratory personnel.
• If urine tests are needed, ask the radiation oncology department or laboratory technician how to transport the specimens safely.
• Minimize your own exposure to radiation. Wear a personal, nontransferable film badge or dosimeter at waist level during your entire shift. Turn in the film badge regularly. (Pocket dosimeters measure immediate exposures.)
• Use the three principles of time, distance, and shielding as follows. *Time:* Plan to give care in the shortest time possible. Less time equals less exposure. *Distance:* Work as far away from the radiation source as possible. Give care from the side opposite the implant or from a position allowing the greatest working distance possible. Prepare the patient's meal trays outside his room. *Shielding:* Wear a portable shield, if necessary.

• Ensure that the patient's room is monitored daily by the radiation oncology department and that disposable items are monitored and removed according to hospital policy.

• Keep staff members and visitors who are pregnant or trying to conceive or father a child away from the patient. *The gonads and a developing embryo or fetus are highly susceptible to the damaging effects of ionizing radiation.*

• If you must take the patient out of his room, notify the appropriate department of the patient's status *to allow time for the necessary preparations.*

• Be aware that a patient with a permanent implant may not be released until his radioactivity level is less than 5 millirem/hour at a distance of about 3′ (1 m).

Documentation
Subdermal implants
• Document the name of the drug, the insertion site, the date and time of insertion, and the patient's response to the procedure.

• Note the date the implants should be removed and a new set inserted.

Subcutaneous implants
• Document the name of the drug, the dose, the date, the administration site, and the date of the next administration.

Radiation implants
• Document radiation precautions taken during treatment, adverse reactions to therapy, instructions given to the patient and family and their responses, the patient's tolerance of isolation procedures and the family's compliance with procedures, and referrals to local cancer services.

E

Ear irrigation

Irrigating the ear involves washing the external auditory canal with a stream of solution to clean the canal of discharges, to soften and remove impacted cerumen, or to dislodge a foreign body. Sometimes, irrigation aims to relieve localized inflammation and discomfort. The procedure must be performed carefully to avoid causing patient discomfort or vertigo and to avoid increasing the risk of otitis externa. Because irrigation may contaminate the middle ear if the tympanic membrane is ruptured, an otoscopic examination always precedes ear irrigation.

This procedure is contraindicated when a vegetable foreign body (such as a pea) obstructs the auditory canal. These foreign bodies attract and absorb moisture. In contact with an irrigant or other solution, they swell, causing intense pain and complicating removal of the object by irrigation. The procedure also is contraindicated if the patient has a cold, a fever, an ear infection, or an injured or ruptured tympanic membrane. Obstruction by small foreign bodies from batteries also contraindicates irrigation because battery acid could leak and irrigation would spread caustic material throughout the canal.

» Key nursing diagnoses and patient outcomes

Use these nursing diagnoses as a guide when developing your plan of care for a patient who is receiving ear irrigations.

Knowledge deficit related to lack of exposure to the procedure

Based on this nursing diagnosis, you'll establish the following patient outcomes. The patient will:
• state or demonstrate understanding of what has been taught.
• demonstrate ability to perform new health related behaviors as they are taught.

Risk for injury related to improper technique

Based on this nursing diagnosis, you'll establish the following patient outcomes. The patient will:
• identify factors that increase risk for injury.
• assist in identifying and applying safety measures to prevent injury.

Equipment

♦ ear irrigation syringe (rubber bulb)
♦ otoscope with aural speculum
♦ prescribed irrigant ♦ large basin
♦ linen-saver pad and bath towel
♦ emesis basin ♦ cotton balls or cotton-tipped applicators ♦ $4'' \times 4''$ gauze pad ♦ optional: adjustable light (such as a gooseneck lamp), container for irrigant, tubing, clamp, or syringe with ear tip.

Equipment preparation

• Select the appropriate syringe, and obtain the prescribed irrigant.
• Put the container of irrigant into the large basin filled with hot water *to warm the solution to body temperature:* 98.6° F (37° C).
• Avoid extreme temperature changes *because they can affect inner ear fluids, causing nausea and dizziness.*

• Test the temperature of the solution by sprinkling a few drops on your inner wrist.
• Inspect equipment (syringe or catheter tips) for breaks or cracks; inspect all metal tips for roughness.

Patient preparation
• Explain the procedure to the patient, and provide privacy.
• Wear gloves if you expect contact with infected matter.

Implementation
• Wash your hands, and put on gloves (if necessary).
• If you haven't already done so, use the otoscope to inspect the auditory canal to be irrigated.
• Help the patient to a sitting position. *To prevent the solution from running down his neck,* tilt his head slightly forward and toward the affected side. If he can't sit, have him lie on his back and tilt his head slightly forward and toward the affected ear.
• Make sure that you have adequate lighting.
• If the patient is sitting, place the linen-saver pad (covered with the bath towel) on his shoulder and upper arm, under the affected ear. If he's lying down, cover his pillow and the area under the affected ear.
• Have the patient hold the emesis basin close to his head under the affected ear.
• *To avoid getting foreign matter into the ear canal,* clean the auricle and the meatus of the auditory canal with a cotton ball or cotton-tipped applicator moistened with normal saline or the prescribed irrigating solution.
• Draw the irrigant into the syringe and expel any air.

• Straighten the auditory canal; then insert the syringe tip and start the flow. (See *How to irrigate the ear canal,* page 274.)
• During irrigation, observe the patient for signs of pain or dizziness. If he reports either, stop the procedure, recheck the temperature of the irrigant, inspect the patient's ear with the otoscope, and resume irrigation, as indicated.
• Keep in mind that forceful irrigation can rupture the tympanic membrane.
• When the syringe is empty, remove it and inspect the return flow. Then, refill the syringe, and continue the irrigation until the return flow is clear. Never use more than 500 ml of irrigant during this procedure.
• Remove the syringe, and inspect the ear canal for cleanliness with the otoscope.
• Dry the patient's auricle and neck.
• Remove the bath towel and linen-saver pad. Help the seated patient lie on his affected side with the 4″× 4″ gauze pad under his ear *to promote drainage of residual debris and solution.*

Complications
• Possible complications include vertigo, nausea, otitis externa, and otitis media (if the patient has a perforated or ruptured tympanic membrane).

Nursing considerations
• Avoid dropping or squirting irrigant on the tympanic membrane. *This may startle the patient and cause discomfort.*
• If you're using an irrigating catheter instead of a syringe, adjust the flow of solution to a steady, comfortable rate with a flow clamp. Don't raise the container more than 6″ (15.2 cm) above

How to irrigate the ear canal

Follow these guidelines for irrigating the ear canal:

• Gently pull the auricle up and back to straighten the ear canal. (For a child, pull the ear down and back.)

• Have the patient hold an emesis basin beneath the ear to catch returning irrigant. Position the tip of the irrigating syringe at the meatus of the auditory canal. Don't block the meatus *because you'll impede backflow and raise pressure in the canal.*

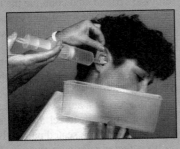

• Tilt the patient's head toward you, and point the syringe tip upward and toward the posterior ear canal. This angle prevents damage to the tympanic membrane and guards against pushing debris farther into the canal.

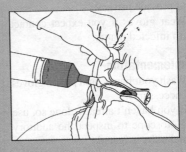

• Direct a steady stream of irrigant against the upper wall of the ear canal, and inspect return fluid for cloudiness, cerumen, blood, or foreign matter.

the ear. *If the container is higher, the resulting pressure may damage the tympanic membrane.*

• If the doctor directs you to place a cotton pledget in the ear canal to retain some of the solution, pack the cotton loosely. Instruct the patient not to remove it.

• If irrigation doesn't dislodge impacted cerumen, the doctor may order you to instill several drops of glycerin, carbamide peroxide, or a similar preparation two to three times daily for 2 to 3 days, and then to irrigate the ear again.

Documentation

• Record the date and time of irrigation.

• Note which ear you irrigated.

• Note the volume and the solution used, the appearance of the canal before and after irrigation, the appearance of the return flow, the patient's tolerance of the procedure, and any comments he made about his condition, especially related to his hearing acuity.

Eardrop instillation

Eardrops may be instilled to treat infection and inflammation, to soften cerumen for later removal, to produce local anesthesia, or to facilitate removal of an insect trapped in the ear by immobilizing and smothering it. Instillation of ear drops is usually contraindicated if the patient has a perforated eardrum; however, it may be permitted with certain medications and adherence to sterile technique. Other conditions may also prohibit instillation of certain medications into the ear. For instance, instillation of drops containing hydrocortisone is contraindicated if the patient has herpes, another viral infection, or a fungal infection.

>> Key nursing diagnoses and patient outcomes

Use these nursing diagnoses as a guide when developing your plan of care for a patient who is receiving eardrops.

Knowledge deficit related to lack of exposure to the procedure

Based on this nursing diagnosis, you'll establish the following patient outcomes. The patient will:
• state or demonstrate understanding of what has been taught.
• demonstrate ability to perform new health related behaviors as they are taught

Risk for injury related to improper technique

Based on this nursing diagnosis, you'll establish the following patient outcomes. The patient will:
• identify factors that increase risk for injury.
• assist in identifying and applying safety measures to prevent injury.

Equipment

♦ prescribed eardrops ♦ patient's medication record and chart ♦ light source ♦ facial tissue or cotton-

tipped applicator ♦ optional: cotton ball, bowl of warm water.

Equipment preparation

• *To avoid adverse effects (such as vertigo, nausea, and pain) resulting from instillation of eardrops that are too cold,* warm the medication to body temperature in the bowl of warm water or carry it in your pocket for 30 minutes before administration.
• If necessary, test the temperature of the medication by placing a drop on your wrist. *If the medication is too hot, it may burn the patient's eardrum.*
• Before using a glass dropper, make sure it's not chipped *to avoid injuring the ear canal.*

Patient preparation

• Provide privacy, if possible.
• Explain the procedure to the patient.

Implementation

• Verify the order on the patient's medication record by checking it against the doctor's order.
• Wash your hands.
• Confirm the patient's identity by asking his name and checking the name, room number, and bed number on his wristband.
• Have the patient lie on the side opposite the affected ear.
• Straighten the patient's ear canal. For an adult, pull the auricle of the ear up and back. For an infant or child under age 3, gently pull the auricle down and back because the ear canal is straighter at this age. (See *Positioning the patient for eardrop instillation,* page 276.)
• Using a light source, examine the ear canal for drainage. If you find any, clean the canal with the cotton-tipped

Positioning the patient for eardrop instillation

Before instilling eardrops, have the patient lie on his side. Then straighten the patient's ear canal to help the medication reach the eardrum. In an adult, gently pull the auricle *up and back;* in an infant or young child, gently pull *down and back,* as shown.

Adult

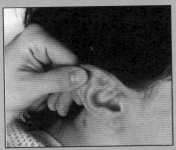

Child

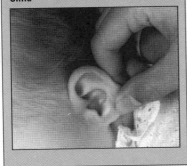

applicator or tissue *because drainage can reduce the medication's effectiveness.*

• Compare the label on the eardrops with the order on the patient's medication record. Check the label again while drawing the medication into the dropper. Check the label for the final time before returning the eardrops to the shelf or drawer.

• *To avoid damaging the ear canal with the dropper,* gently support the hand holding the dropper against the patient's head. Straighten the patient's ear canal once again and instill the ordered number of drops. *To avoid patient discomfort,* aim the dropper so that the drops fall against the sides of the ear canal, not on the eardrum. Hold the ear canal in position until you see the medication disappear down the canal. Then release the ear.

• Instruct the patient to remain on his side for 5 to 10 minutes *to allow the medication to run down into the ear canal.*

• If ordered, loosely tuck the cotton ball into the opening of the ear canal to prevent the medication from leaking out. Be careful not to insert it too deeply into the canal *because this would prevent drainage of secretions and increase pressure on the eardrum.*

• Clean and dry the outer ear.

• If ordered, repeat the procedure in the other ear after 5 to 10 minutes.

• Assist the patient into a comfortable position.

• Wash your hands.

Nursing considerations

• Remember that some conditions make the normally tender ear canal even more sensitive, so be especially gentle when performing this procedure.

• Wash your hands before and after caring for the patient's ear and between caring for each ear.

• *To prevent injury to the eardrum,* never insert a cotton-tipped applicator into the ear canal past the point where you can see the tip. After applying ear-

drops to soften cerumen, irrigate the ear as ordered *to facilitate its removal.*
• If the patient has vertigo, keep the side rails of his bed up and assist him during the procedure, as necessary. Also, move slowly and unhurriedly *to avoid exacerbating his vertigo.*
• Teach the patient to instill the eardrops correctly so that he can continue treatment at home, if necessary. Review the procedure and let the patient try it himself while you observe.

Documentation
• Record the medication, the ear treated, and the date, time, and number of eardrops instilled.
• Note any signs or symptoms that arise during the procedure, such as drainage, redness, vertigo, nausea, or pain.

Echocardiography

This noninvasive diagnostic imaging technique records the reflection of ultra-high frequency sound waves directed at the patient's heart. It enables the doctor to visualize heart size and shape, myocardial wall thickness and motion, and cardiac valve structure and function. It also helps evaluate overall left ventricular function and detect some MI complications; mitral valve prolapse; mitral, tricuspid, or pulmonary valve insufficiency; cardiac tamponade; pericardial diseases; cardiac tumors; prosthetic valve function; subvalvular stenosis; ventricular aneurysms; cardiomyopathies; and congenital abnormalities.

To create an "acoustic window," you may apply conductive jelly to the patient's chest in the third or fourth intercostal space just left of the sternum. A transducer placed on the patient's chest sends ultrasound waves to the heart; the waves reflect back to the transducer, which reabsorbs them. These ultrasonic echoes, translated into electrical signals, appear on an oscilloscope for viewing and recording. Echocardiography is useful for evaluating patients with chest pain, enlarged cardiac silhouettes on X-ray films, electrocardiographic changes unrelated to coronary artery disease, and abnormal heart sounds on auscultation. Results are correlated with clinical history, physical examination, and findings from additional tests.

The techniques most commonly used in echocardiography are M-mode (motion-mode), for recording the motion and dimensions of intracardiac structures, and two-dimensional (cross-sectional), for recording lateral motion and providing the correct spatial relationship between cardiac structures.

≫ Key nursing diagnoses and patient outcomes
Use these nursing diagnoses as a guide when developing your plan of care.

Decreased cardiac output related to reduced stroke volume as a result of mechanical or structural problems
Based on this nursing diagnosis, you'll establish the following patient outcomes. The patient will:
• exhibit no arrhythmias.
• maintain hemodynamic stability; pulse not under __ or over __ beats/minute; blood pressure not below __/__ or above __/__.

Altered cardiopulmonary tissue perfusion related to decreased cellular exchange

Based on this nursing diagnosis, you'll establish the following patient outcomes. The patient will:
• not exhibit arrhythmias.
• maintain adequate cardiac output.

Equipment

♦ echocardiograph machine ♦ conductive gel.

Patient preparation

• Explain that this test is used to evaluate the size, shape, and motion of various cardiac structures.
• Inform him that he need not restrict food or fluids before the test.
• Tell him who will perform the test and where, that it usually takes 15 to 30 minutes, and that it is safe and painless.
• Explain that the room may be darkened slightly to aid visualization on the oscilloscope screen and that other procedures (ECG and phonocardiography) may be performed simultaneously to time events in the cardiac cycle.
• Describe the procedure and instruct the patient to remain still during the test *because movement may distort results.*
• Inform the patient that he may be asked to inhale a gas with a sweet odor (amyl nitrite), while changes in heart function are recorded; describe the possible adverse effects of amyl nitrite (dizziness, flushing, and tachycardia), but assure the patient that such symptoms quickly subside.

Implementation

• The patient is placed in supine position.
• Conductive jelly is applied to the third or fourth intercostal space to the left of the sternum, and the transducer is placed directly over it.
• The transducer is systematically angled to direct ultrasonic waves at specific parts of the patient's heart.
• Significant oscilloscopic findings are recorded on a strip chart recorder (M-mode echocardiography) or on a videotape recorder (two-dimensional echocardiography).
• For a different view of the heart, the transducer is placed beneath the xiphoid process or directly above the sternum.
• For a left lateral view, the patient may be positioned on his left side.
• To record heart function under various conditions, the patient is asked to inhale and exhale slowly, to hold his breath, or to inhale amyl nitrite.
• Remove conductive jelly from the skin.

Nursing considerations

• Reassure the patient that this 15- to 30-minute test doesn't cause pain or pose any risks. Mention that he may undergo other tests, such as ECG and phonocardiography simultaneously.
• Explain to the patient that he may have to breathe in and out slowly, to hold his breath, or to breathe in a gas with a slightly sweet odor (amyl nitrate) during the procedure. Amyl nitrate may cause dizziness, flushing, and tachycardia, but these effects quickly subside. The patient must sit still during the test *because movement may distort results.*

• Assist the patient into a position most favorable for the echocardiograph.
• Provide privacy and a darkened environment for the test to be completed.

Documentation
• Document patient tolerance to procedure, date and time of the test.

Electrocardiography

One of the most valuable and frequently used diagnostic tools, electrocardiography (ECG) measures the heart's electrical activity as waveforms. Impulses moving through the heart's conduction system create electric currents that can be monitored on the body's surface. Electrodes attached to the skin can detect these electric currents and transmit them to an instrument that produces a record (an ECG) of cardiac activity.

ECG can be used to identify myocardial ischemia and infarction, rhythm and conduction disturbances, chamber enlargement, electrolyte imbalances, and drug toxicity.

The standard 12-lead ECG uses a series of electrodes placed on the extremities and the chest wall to assess the heart from 12 different views (leads). The 12 leads consist of 3 standard bipolar limb leads (designated I, II, III), 3 unipolar augmented leads (aV_R, aV_L, aV_F), and 6 unipolar precordial leads (V_1 to V_6). The limb leads and augmented leads show the heart from the frontal plane. The precordial leads show the heart from the horizontal plane.

The ECG device measures and averages the differences between the electrical potential of the electrode sites for each lead and graphs them over time. This creates the standard ECG complex, called P-QRS-T. The P wave represents atrial depolarization; the QRS complex, ventricular depolarization; and the T wave, ventricular repolarization. (See *Reviewing ECG waveform components,* page 280.)

Variations of the standard ECG include exercise ECG (stress ECG) and ambulatory ECG (Holter monitoring). Exercise ECG monitors heart rate, blood pressure, and ECG waveforms as the patient walks on a treadmill or pedals a stationary bicycle. For ambulatory ECG, the patient wears a portable Holter monitor to record heart activity continuously over 24 hours.

Today, ECG is typically accomplished using a multichannel method. All electrodes are attached to the patient at once and the machine prints a simultaneous view of all leads.

≫ Key nursing diagnoses and patient outcomes
Use these nursing diagnoses as a guide when developing your plan of care.

Knowledge deficit related to lack of exposure to the procedure
Based on this nursing diagnosis, you'll establish the following patient outcomes. The patient will:
• communicates a need to know reasons for the procedure.
• state understanding of the procedure and the reasons for it.

Equipment
♦ ECG machine ♦ recording paper
♦ pre-gelled disposable electrodes

Reviewing ECG waveform components

An electrocardiogram (ECG) waveform has three basic components:
P wave, QRS complex, and T wave. These elements can be further divided
into a PR interval, J point, ST segment, U wave, and QT interval.

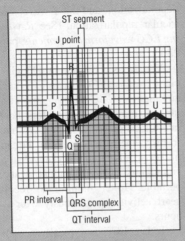

takes for the impulse to travel
through the bundle branches to the
Purkinje fibers).

The Q wave appears as the first
negative deflection in the QRS complex; the R wave, as the first positive deflection. The S wave appears
as the second negative deflection
or the first negative deflection after
the R wave.

J point and ST segment
Marking the end of the QRS complex, the J point also indicates the
beginning of the ST segment. The
ST segment represents part of ventricular repolarization.

P wave and PR interval
The P wave represents atrial depolarization. The PR interval represents the time it takes an impulse
to travel from the atria through the
atrioventricular node and bundle of
His. The PR interval measures from
the beginning of the P wave to the
beginning of the QRS complex.

QRS complex
The QRS complex represents ventricular depolarization (the time it

T wave and U wave
Usually following the same deflection pattern as the P wave, the
T wave represents ventricular
repolarization. The U wave follows
the T wave but is not always evident.

QT interval
The QT interval represents ventricular depolarization and repolarization. It extends from the beginning
of the QRS complex to the end of
the T wave.

◆ 4″ × 4″ gauze pads ◆ optional:
shaving supplies, marking pen.

Equipment preparation
• Place the ECG machine close to the
patient's bed, and plug the cord into
the wall outlet.

• If the patient is already connected to
a cardiac monitor, remove the electrodes to accommodate the precordial
leads and minimize electrical interference on the ECG tracing.
• Keep the patient away from electrical fixtures and power cords.

Patient preparation

• Explain the procedure, telling the patient that the test records the heart's electrical activity and that it may be repeated at certain intervals.

• Emphasize that no electrical current will enter his body.

• Tell him that the test typically takes about 5 minutes.

Implementation

• Have the patient lie in a supine position in the center of the bed with his arms at his sides. You may raise the head of the bed *to promote his comfort.* Expose his arms and legs, and drape him appropriately. His arms and legs should be relaxed *to minimize muscle trembling, which can cause electrical interference.*

• If the bed is too narrow, place the patient's hands under his buttocks *to prevent muscle tension.* Also use this technique if the patient is shivering or trembling. Make sure his feet aren't touching the bed board.

• Select flat, fleshy areas to place the electrodes. Avoid muscular and bony areas. If the patient has an amputated limb, choose a site on the stump.

• If an area is excessively hairy, shave it. Clean excess oil or other substances from the skin *to enhance electrode contact.*

• Apply the electrode paste or gel or the disposable electrodes to the patient's wrists and to the medial aspects of his ankles. If you're using paste or gel, rub it into the skin. If you're using disposable electrodes, peel off the contact paper and apply them directly to the prepared site, as recommended by the manufacturer's instructions. *To guarantee the best connection to the leadwire,* position disposable elec-

trodes on the legs with the lead connection pointing superiorly.

• If you're using paste or gel, secure electrodes promptly after you apply the conductive medium. *This prevents drying of the medium, which could impair ECG quality.* Never use alcohol or acetone pads in place of the electrode paste or gel *because they impair electrode contact with the skin and diminish the transmission quality of electrical impulses.*

• Connect the limb leadwires to the electrodes. Make sure the metal parts of the electrodes are clean and bright. *Dirty or corroded electrodes prevent a good electrical connection.*

• You'll see that the tip of each leadwire is lettered and color coded for easy identification. The white or RA leadwire goes to the right arm; the green or RL leadwire, to the right leg; the red or LL leadwire, to the left leg; the black or LA leadwire, to the left arm; and the brown or V_1 to V_6 leadwire, to the chest.

• Now, expose the patient's chest. Put a small amount of electrode gel or paste or a disposable electrode at each electrode position. (See *Positioning chest electrodes,* page 282.)

If your patient is a woman, be sure to place the chest electrodes below the breast tissue. In a large-breasted woman, you may need to displace the breast tissue laterally.

• Check to see that the paper speed selector is set to the standard 25 mm/second and that the machine is set to full voltage. The machine will record a normal standardization mark — a square that's the height of two large squares or 10 small squares on the recording paper. Then, if necessary, enter the appropriate patient identification data.

Positioning chest electrodes

To ensure accurate test results, position chest electrodes as shown:

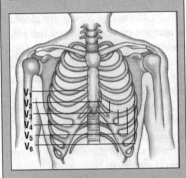

V_1: Fourth intercostal space at right border of sternum

V_2: Fourth intercostal space at left border of sternum

V_3: Halfway between V_2 and V_4

V_4: Fifth intercostal space at midclavicular line

V_5: Fifth intercostal space at anterior axillary line (halfway between V_4 and V_6)

V_6: Fifth intercostal space at midaxillary line, level with V_4

• If any part of the waveform extends beyond the paper when you record the ECG, adjust the normal standardization to half-standardization. Note this adjustment on the ECG strip *because this will need to be considered in interpreting the results.*

• Now you're ready to begin the recording. Ask the patient to relax and breathe normally. Tell him to lie still and not to talk when you record his ECG. Then press the AUTO button. Observe the quality of the tracing. The machine will record all 12 leads automatically, recording three consecutive leads simultaneously. Some machines have a display screen so you can preview waveforms before the machine records them on paper.

• When the machine finishes recording the 12-lead ECG, remove the electrodes and clean the patient's skin. After disconnecting the leadwires from the electrodes, dispose of or clean the electrodes, as indicated.

Nursing considerations

• Small areas of hair on the patient's chest or extremities may be shaved, but this usually isn't necessary.

• If the patient's skin is exceptionally oily, scaly, or diaphoretic, rub the electrode site with a dry $4'' \times 4''$ gauze pad or alcohol before applying the electrode to help reduce interference in the tracing. During the procedure, ask the patient to breathe normally.

• If his respirations distort the recording, ask him to hold his breath briefly *to reduce baseline wander in the tracing.*

• If the patient has a pacemaker, you can perform an ECG with or without a magnet. Be sure to note the presence of a pacemaker and the use of the magnet (to turn off the pacemaker) on the strip.

Documentation

• Label the ECG recording with the patient's name, room number, and hospital identification number. This can be done by hand or electronically by entering patient information in the machine.

• Document in your notes the test's date and time and significant responses by the patient as well.

• Record the date, time, patient's name, and room number on the ECG itself.

• Note any appropriate clinical information on the ECG.

Electrocardiography, signal-averaged

Signal-averaged electrocardiography (ECG) helps to identify patients at risk for sustained ventricular tachycardia (VT). Because this cardiac arrhythmia can be a precursor of sudden death after a myocardial infarction (MI), the results of signal-averaged ECG can allow appropriate preventive measures.

Signal averaging detects low-amplitude signals or late electrical potentials, which reflect slow conduction or disorganized ventricular activity through abnormal or infarcted regions of the ventricles that's detected by a computer-based ECG. The signal-averaged ECG is developed by recording the noise-free surface ECG in three specialized leads for several hundred beats. Signal averaging enhances signals that would otherwise be missed because of increased amplitude and sensitivity to ventricular activity. For instance, on the standard 12-lead ECG, "noise" created by muscle tissue, electronic artifacts, and electrodes masks late potentials, which have a low amplitude. This procedure identifies the risk for sustained VT in patients with malignant VT, a history of MI, unexplained syncope, nonischemic congestive cardiomyopathy, or nonsustained VT.

» Key nursing diagnoses and patient outcomes

Use these nursing diagnoses as a guide when developing your plan of care.

Knowledge deficit related to lack of exposure to the procedure
Based on this nursing diagnosis, you'll establish the following patient outcomes. The patient will:
• communicates a need to know reasons for the procedure.
• state understanding of the procedure and the reasons for it.

Equipment
♦ signal-averaged ECG machine ♦ signal-averaged computer ♦ record of patient's surface ECG for 200 to 300 QRS complexes ♦ three bipolar electrodes or leads ♦ alcohol sponges ♦ shaving supplies.

Patient preparation
• Inform the patient that this procedure will take 10 to 30 minutes and will help the doctor determine his risk for a certain type of arrhythmia.
• If appropriate, mention that it may be done along with other tests, such as echocardiography, Holter monitoring, and a stress test.
• Place the patient in a supine position.
• Tell him to lie as still as possible.
• Tell him he shouldn't speak.
• Tell him he should breathe normally during the procedure.
• If the patient has hair on his chest, shave the area, rub it with alcohol, and dry it before placing the electrodes.

Implementation
• Place the leads in the X, Y, and Z orthogonal positions. (See *Placing electrodes for signal-averaged ECG*, page 284.)
• The ECG machine gathers information from these leads and amplifies, filters, and samples the signals. The

Placing electrodes for signal-averaged ECG

To prepare your patient for signal-averaged electrocardiography (ECG), place the electrodes in the X, Y, and Z orthogonal positions, as shown here. These positions bisect one another to provide a three-dimensional, composite view of ventricular activation.

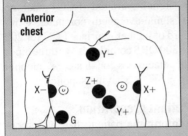

Anterior chest

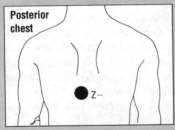

Posterior chest

X+ Fourth intercostal space, mid-axillary line, left side
X– Fourth intercostal space, mid-axillary line, right side
Y+ Standard V_3 position (or proximal left leg)
Y– Superior aspect of manubrium
Z+ Standard V_2 position
Z– V_2 position, posterior
G Ground; eighth rib on right side

computer collects and stores data for analysis. The crucial values are those showing QRS complex duration, duration of the portion of the QRS complex with an amplitude under 40 microvolts, and the root mean square voltage of the last 40 msec.

Nursing considerations
• Proper electrode placement and skin preparation are essential to this procedure.
• Because muscle movements may cause a false-positive result, patients who are restless or in respiratory distress are poor candidates for signal-averaged ECG.
• Results indicating low-amplitude signals include a QRS complex duration greater than 110 milliseconds (msec); a duration of more than 40 msec for the amplitude portion under 40 microvolts; and a root mean square voltage of less than 25 microvolts during the last 40 msec of the QRS complex. However, all three factors needn't be present to consider the result positive or negative. The final interpretation hinges on individualized patient factors.
• Results of signal-averaged ECG help the doctor determine whether the patient is a candidate for invasive procedures, such as electrophysiologic testing or angiography.
• Keep in mind that the significance of signal-averaged ECG findings in patients with bundle-branch heart block is unknown because myocardial activation doesn't follow the usual sequence in these patients.

Documentation
• Document the time of the procedure, why the procedure was done, and how the patient tolerated it.

Electroencephalography

In this diagnostic test, electrodes attached to areas of the patient's scalp record a portion of the brain's electrical activity and transmit this information to an electroencephalography (EEG) machine, which records the resulting brain waves on recording paper. (See *Understanding basic waveforms of the EEG*, page 286.)

The procedure may be performed in a special laboratory or by a portable unit at the bedside.

By recording the brain's continuous electrical activity, EEG can help identify seizure disorders, head injury, intracranial lesions (such as abscesses and tumors), transient ischemic attacks, and cerebrovascular accidents, to evaluate the brain's electrical activity in metabolic disease, head injury, meningitis, encephalitis, mental retardation, and psychological disorders, or to confirm brain death.

≫ Key nursing diagnoses and patient outcomes

Use these nursing diagnoses as a guide when developing your plan of care.

Knowledge deficit related to lack of exposure to the procedure

Based on this nursing diagnosis, you'll establish the following patient outcomes. The patient will:
• communicates a need to know reasons for the procedure.
• state understanding of the procedure and the reasons for it.

Equipment

♦ EEG machine ♦ electrodes ♦ EEG electrode paste ♦ chloral hydrate or other sedative for sleep EEG ♦ diazepam or other anticonvulsant ♦ suction equipment ♦ acetone.

Patient preparation

• Explain to the patient that this test records the brain's electrical activity.
• Describe the procedure to the patient and family members, and answer all questions
• Tell him that he must forgo caffeine prior to the test; other than this, there are no food or fluid restrictions.
• Thoroughly wash and dry his hair to remove hair sprays, creams, or oils.
• Explain that during the test, he'll relax in a reclining chair or lie on a bed, and that electrodes will be attached to his scalp with a special paste. Assure him that the electrodes won't shock him.
• If needle electrodes are used, explain that he'll feel a pricking sensation as they're inserted; however, flat electrodes are usually used.
• Tell the patient it's important for him to remain still during the test.
• Do your best to allay the patient's fears *because nervousness can affect brain-wave patterns.*
• Check his medication history for drugs that may interfere with test results — for example, anticonvulsants, sedative-hypnotics, antianxiety agents, and antidepressants — and withhold these medications for 24 to 48 hours before the test.
• A patient with a seizure disorder may require a "sleep EEG." In this case, keep the patient awake the night before the test, and administer a sedative (such as chloral hydrate) *to help him sleep during the test.*

Understanding basic waveforms of the EEG

Electroencephalography (EEG) record a portion of the brain's electrical activity as waves; some are irregular, whereas others demonstrate frequent patterns. Among the basic waveforms are the alpha, beta, theta, and delta rhythms.

Alpha waves occur at a frequency of 8 to 12 cycles/second in a regular rhythm. They're present only in the waking state when the patient's eyes are closed but he's mentally alert; usually, they disappear with visual activity or mental concentration.

Beta waves (13 to 30 cycles/second) — generally associated with anxiety, depression, or use of sedatives — are seen most readily in the frontal and central regions of the brain.

Theta waves (4 to 7 cycles/second) are most common in children and young adults and appear in the frontal and temporal regions.

Delta waves (0.5 to 3.5 cycles/second) normally occur only in young children and during sleep.

Implementation

• Position the patient on the bed or in a reclining chair.

• Reassure the patient as electrodes are attached to his scalp.

• Before the recording procedure begins, instruct the patient to close his eyes, relax, and remain still.

• During the recording, observe the patient carefully; note blinking, swallowing, talking, or other movements that may cause artifacts on the tracing.

• The recording may be stopped at intervals to let the patient rest or reposition himself. *This is important because restlessness and fatigue can alter brain-wave patterns.*

• After an initial baseline recording, the patient may be tested under various stress-producing conditions to elicit patterns not observable while he is at rest. For example, he may be asked to breathe deeply and rapidly for 3 minutes (hyperventilation), which may elicit brain wave patterns typical of seizure disorders or other abnormalities. This technique is commonly used to detect absence seizures. Also, photic stimulation tests central cerebral activity in response to bright light, accentuating abnormal activity in absence or myoclonic seizures.

• Review carefully the reinstatement of anticonvulsant medication or other drugs withheld before the test.

• Carefully observe the patient for seizure activity and provide a safe environment.

• Help the patient remove electrode paste from his hair.

Nursing considerations

• Observe the patient carefully for seizure activity. If seizure activity occurs, record seizure patterns and be prepared to provide assistance.

• Have suction equipment and diazepam for I.V. injection available.

• If the patient received a sedative before the test, take safety precautions, such as raising the bed's side rails.

• Tell the patient to wash his hair and to resume his usual activities afterward.

• If the test is performed to confirm brain death, provide family members with emotional support.

Documentation
• Record date, time, and tolerance to procedure and the safety precautions used.

Electrolyte testing via vascular intermittent access device

The vascular intermittent access system measures electrolyte levels automatically in patients who have an indwelling arterial or venous line. In just 1 minute, it obtains such critical indices as potassium, calcium, sodium, glucose, hematocrit, and arterial blood gas levels. Then it reinfuses the blood sample into the patient.

By detecting changes in electrolyte levels almost as they occur, this system allows you to respond quickly to any abnormalities. The arterial or venous line can be accessed as often as every 3 minutes. This avoids the need to draw blood manually for laboratory samples and eliminates problems that an indwelling sensor sometimes causes. Easily transported with the patient from one area to another, the device can be used in the operating room, intensive care unit, emergency department, and other special care units.

Abnormal electrolyte values measured by this system indicate electrolyte imbalances, which can disrupt various body systems and cause serious health problems.

≫ Key nursing diagnoses and patient outcomes
Use these nursing diagnoses as a guide when developing your plan of care for a patient who is receiving electrolyte testing via a vascular intermittent access device.

Risk for fluid volume deficit related to excessive loss
Based on this nursing diagnosis, you'll establish the following patient outcomes. The patient will:
• have vital signs remain stable.
• have electrolyte values within the normal range.

Altered cardiopulmonary tissue perfusion related to decreased cellular exchange
Based on this nursing diagnosis, you'll establish the following patient outcomes. The patient will:
• attain hemodynamic stability with pulse not under ___ or over ___ beats/minute; blood pressure not below __/__ and not above __/__.
• exhibit no arrhythmias.

Equipment
♦ vascular intermittent access system with monitor and sensor array ♦ isotonic I.V. solution (lactated Ringer's solution) ♦ tubing and calibration additives ♦ printer ♦ automatic timer to automatically initiate the process at predetermined intervals. (See *Vascular intermittent access system,* page 288.)

Implementation
• Set up the vascular intermittent access system, following the manufacturer's directions. Place the sensor array at the distal end of the I.V. administration set by twisting the luer-lock connection.
• Turn on the monitor by pressing the ON/OFF key. Choose the appropriate

Vascular intermittent access system

Used to measure electrolyte levels automatically, the vascular intermittent access system includes a sensor array, an I.V. administration set, I.V. solution with additives for sensor calibration, and a monitor that processes signals from the sensors. A pumping mechanism infuses the solution and withdraws blood samples.

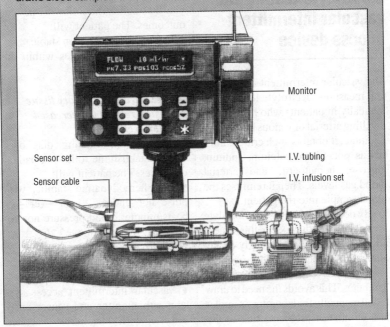

mode by pressing the up or down arrow.
• Press the star (*) key to advance the instructions. The monitor screen will display cues (or prompts) for continuing.
• Open the door on the monitor. Then pull the anti-free-flow lever down to open the pump mechanism.

Setting up the pump
• Holding the silicone portion of the tubing, place the tubing adapter into the top of the tubing retainer in the pump compartment.

• Hold the sensor disk so that the flat side faces the monitor. Pull down slightly and hook the disk under its retainer in the monitor.
• Holding the sensor disk in place, push the anti-free-flow lever up to close the pump. Now shut the monitor door.

Programming the sensor system
• Open the regulating clamp on the I.V. tubing all the way. Check the drip chamber to make sure the solution isn't flowing.

• Continue to advance the programming instructions by pressing the star key. When the previously infused volume appears on the screen, you may clear it by pressing the CLEAR VOL INFUSED key for 1 second.

• Select the intended infusion volume (in 50-ml increments from 50 to 1,000) by pressing the up and down arrows until the desired total appears. Simultaneously press the SET VOL TO BE INFUSED key. *To prevent the system from running dry and to give yourself adequate time to prepare a new I.V. solution,* enter a volume that's 50 ml less than the volume in the I.V. bag. This accounts for fluid in the tubing and fluid lost in priming. Once the selected volume infuses, an alarm will sound. The solution will continue to infuse at a rate of 10 ml/hour — the keep-vein-open rate.

Connecting the system to the patient

• Before connecting the system to the patient, perform an initial two-point calibration check of the sensor. Remember to perform this check each time you use a new sensor. (See the operator's manual for complete instructions.) Use a four-way stopcock to connect the end of the tubing from the sensor set to the patient's arterial line. Secure all luer-lock connections, and be careful not to introduce air into the line.

• Press the star key. This starts the infusion and maintains the flow rate at 10 ml/hour. The display screen will alternately present two messages — one identifying the flow rate and the other, the measurable values. The actual values will follow the equal signs when the blood is tested.

• Connect the monitor's sensor cable to the sensor set of the infusion tubing by lining up the cable with the sensor set and sliding it in place.

• Position the sensor upright and horizontal on the patient's arm, as indicated by the label on the sensor cable, and secure it with surgical tape.

• Secure all of the tubing and the cable lines to the patient's wrist *so that they won't accidentally dislodge or fall out.* As needed, use an armboard to stabilize the patient's wrist. Also, remind the patient to keep his wrist on top of his bed linens at all times.

Testing blood

• To start a sampling cycle and measure an electrolyte level, press the SAMPLE key. During the sampling cycle, the following steps occur automatically: The system calibrates its sensors, and the word *Calibrating* and a countdown time appear on the screen (until the system segregates and analyzes a blood sample). After 8 seconds, the pumping system reverses its action and withdraws about 1.2 ml of blood, and the word *Sampling* appears. As the patient's blood comes in contact with the sensors, the word *Analyzing* appears on the screen. The word *Purging* will appear on the screen when the system returns the blood and I.V. solution to the patient.

• Finally, blood chemistry values appear on the alternating screens. To hold the display for 30 seconds, press the DISPLAY FREEZE key. To resume the alternating display, press the same key again. Promptly record the results because they appear for only 5 minutes, after which they automatically clear from the system. If your monitor has an attached printer, however, you can print the results along with the date and time.

Nursing considerations

• Be aware that the vascular intermittent access system doesn't require long-term compatibility between the sensors and the patient's blood. Except for the few seconds during which the measurement is being made, the sensors are exposed only to the I.V. solution, not the blood.

• Because the system is closed, blood handling by caregivers is avoided and blood loss in the patient is prevented.

Documentation

• Document the entire procedure and the patient's tolerance of it.

Endotracheal drug administration

When an I.V. line isn't readily available, drugs can be administered into the respiratory system through an endotracheal (ET) tube. This route allows uninterrupted resuscitation efforts and avoids such complications as coronary artery laceration, cardiac tamponade, and pneumothorax, which can occur when emergency drugs are administered intracardially.

When given endotracheally, drugs usually have a longer duration of action than when given I.V. because of absorption in the alveoli. For this reason, repeat doses and continuous infusions must be adjusted to prevent adverse effects. Drugs commonly given by this route include naloxone, atropine, diazepam, epinephrine, and lidocaine.

Endotracheal drugs are usually administered in an emergency situation by a doctor, an emergency medical technician, or a critical care nurse. Although guidelines may vary depending on state, county, or city regulations, the basic administration method is the same. (See *Administering endotracheal drugs.*)

Endotracheal drugs may be given by the syringe or adapter method. Usually used for bronchoscopy suctioning, the swivel adapter can be placed on the end of the tube and, while ventilation continues through a bag-valve device, the drug can be delivered with a needle through the closed stopcock.

≫ Key nursing diagnoses and patient outcomes

Use these nursing diagnoses as a guide when developing your plan of care for a patient who is receiving drugs endotracheally.

Knowledge deficit related to lack of exposure

Based on this nursing diagnosis, you'll establish the following patient outcomes. The patient will:

• state or demonstrate understanding of what has been taught.

• demonstrate ability to perform new health related behaviors as they are taught.

Risk for injury related to improper technique

Based on this nursing diagnosis, you'll establish the following patient outcomes. The patient will:

• identify factors that increase injury risk.

Administering endotracheal drugs

In an emergency, some drugs may be given through an endotracheal (ET) tube if I.V. access isn't available. They may be given using the syringe method or the adapter method.

Before injecting any drug, however, check for proper placement of the ET tube, using your stethoscope. Make sure that the patient is supine and his head is level with, or slightly higher than, his trunk.

Using the syringe method
Remove the needle before injecting medication into the ET tube. Insert the tip of the syringe into the ET tube, and inject the drug deep into the tube, as shown below.

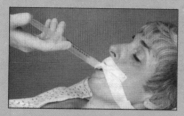

Adapter method
A recently developed device for endotracheal drug administration, shown below, provides a more closed system of drug delivery than the syringe method. A special adapter placed on the end of the ET tube allows needle insertion and drug delivery through the closed stopcock.

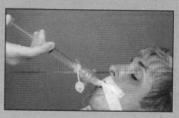

• help identify and apply safety measures to prevent injury.

Equipment
♦ ET tube ♦ gloves ♦ stethoscope ♦ handheld resuscitation bag ♦ ordered drug ♦ syringe or adapter ♦ sterile water or normal saline solution.

Equipment preparation
• Calculate the drug dose. Adult Advanced Cardiac Life Support guidelines recommend that drugs be administered at twice to two-and-one-half times the recommended I.V. dose. Next, draw the drug up into a syringe. Dilute it in 10 ml of sterile water or normal saline solution. Dilution increases drug volume and contact with lung tissue.

Implementation
• Verify the order on the patient's medication record by checking it against the doctor's order.
• Wash your hands.
• Check ET tube placement by using a handheld resuscitation bag and stethoscope.
• Put on gloves.
• The patient should be lying in a supine position with his head level with, or slightly higher than, his trunk.

BETTER CHARTING

Reporting adverse events and product problems to the FDA

As a health care professional, you play a key role in reporting adverse events and product problems. Reporting such problems helps ensure the safety of products that the Food and Drug Administration (FDA) regulates.

What to report

Complete a *MedWatch* form when you suspect that a drug, a medical device, a special nutritional prod-uct, or other product regulated by the FDA is responsible for:

- a death

(continued)

Reporting adverse events and product problems to the FDA (continued)

- a life-threatening illness
- initial or prolonged hospitalization
- a disability
- congenital anomaly
- the need for any medical or surgical intervention to prevent permanent impairment or an injury.

Also inform the FDA promptly of product quality problems, such as:
- defective devices
- inaccurate or unreadable labels
- packaging or product mix-ups
- contamination or stability problems
- particulates in injectable drugs.

Your responsibility in reporting
When filing a form, keep the following points in mind:

- You're not expected to establish a connection between the product and the problem, so don't include many details: Report only the adverse event or problem with the drug or product.
- Send completed forms to the FDA by using the fax number or mailing address on the form.
- File a separate form for each patient and attach additional pages, if needed.
- If appropriate, report product problems to the manufacturer.
- Comply with your health care facility's protocols for reporting adverse events associated with drugs and medical devices.

- Ventilate the patient three to five times with the resuscitation bag. Then remove the bag.
- Remove the needle from the syringe, and insert the tip of the syringe into the ET tube.
- Inject the drug deep into the tube.
- After injecting the drug, reattach the resuscitation bag and ventilate the patient briskly five or six times. *This propels the drug into the lungs, oxygenates the patient, and clears the tube.* Briefly place your thumb over the tube opening *to prevent drug reflux.*
- Discard the syringe in an appropriate sharps container.
- Remove and discard your gloves.

Complications
Potential complications of endotracheal drug administration result from the prescribed drug, not the administration route.

Nursing considerations
Be aware that the drug's onset of action may be quicker than it would be by I.V. administration. If the patient doesn't respond quickly, the doctor may order a repeat dose.

Documentation
- Record the date and time of drug administration, the drug administered, and the patient's response.
- Occasionally, you may suspect a connection between a patient's medication and an adverse event, such as illness, injury or death. In such a case, report this information to the Food and Drug Administration (FDA) on a *MedWatch* form issued by the FDA. (See *Reporting adverse events and product problems to the FDA,* pages 292 and 293.)

Endotracheal tube care

The intubated patient requires meticulous care to ensure airway patency and prevent complications until he can maintain independent ventilation. This care includes frequent assessment of airway status, maintenance of proper cuff pressure to prevent tissue ischemia and necrosis, careful repositioning of the endotracheal (ET) tube to avoid traumatic manipulation, and constant monitoring for complications. ET tube repositioning is done for patient comfort or when a chest X-ray shows improper placement. Move the tube from one side of the mouth to the other to prevent pressure ulcers.

≫ Key nursing diagnoses and patient outcomes

Use these nursing diagnoses as a guide when developing your plan of care for a patient who has an ET tube.

Risk for aspiration related to absence of protective mechanisms
Based on this nursing diagnosis, you'll establish the following patient outcomes. The patient will:
• show no signs of aspiration.
• reveal no adventitious breath sounds on auscultation.

Ineffective airway clearance related to presence of secretions
Based on this nursing diagnosis, you'll establish the following patient outcomes. The patient will:
• cough effectively.
• expectorate sputum.
• keep airway patent.

Equipment

For maintaining the airway: ♦ stethoscope ♦ suction equipment ♦ gloves.

For repositioning the ET tube: ♦ 10-cc syringe ♦ compound benzoin tincture ♦ stethoscope ♦ adhesive or hypoallergenic tape or Velcro tube holder ♦ suction equipment ♦ sedative or 2% lidocaine ♦ gloves ♦ handheld resuscitation bag with mask in case of accidental extubation ♦ equipment for measuring cuff pressure (listed below).

For measuring cuff pressure: ♦ 10-cc syringe ♦ three-way stopcock ♦ cuff pressure manometer ♦ stethoscope ♦ suction equipment ♦ gloves.

For removing the ET tube: ♦ 10-cc syringe ♦ suction equipment ♦ supplemental oxygen source with mask ♦ cool-mist large-volume nebulizer ♦ handheld resuscitation bag with mask ♦ gloves ♦ equipment for reintubation.

Equipment preparation
For repositioning the ET tube
• Assemble all equipment at the patient's bedside.
• Using sterile technique, set up the suction equipment.

For measuring cuff pressure
• Assemble all equipment at the patient's bedside.
• If measuring with a blood pressure manometer, attach the syringe to one stopcock port; then attach the tubing from the manometer to another port of the stopcock.
• Turn off the stopcock port where you'll be connecting the pilot balloon cuff so that air can't escape from the cuff.

• Use the syringe to instill air into the manometer tubing until the pressure reading reaches 10 mm Hg. This will prevent sudden cuff deflation when you open the stopcock to the cuff and the manometer.

For removing the ET tube

• Assemble all equipment at the patient's bedside.

Set up the suction and supplemental oxygen equipment. Have ready all equipment for emergency reintubation.

Patient preparation

• Explain the procedure to the patient even if he doesn't appear to be alert.
• Provide privacy, wash your hands thoroughly, and put on gloves.

Implementation
To maintain airway patency

• Auscultate the patient's lungs at any sign of respiratory distress. If you detect an obstructed airway, determine the cause and treat accordingly. If secretions are obstructing the lumen of the tube, suction the secretions from the tube. (See "Tracheal Suction," page 866.)
• If the tube has slipped from the trachea into the right or left main stem bronchus, breath sounds will be absent over one lung. As ordered, obtain a chest X-ray to verify tube placement and, if necessary, reposition the tube.

To reposition the ET tube

• Get help from a respiratory therapist or another nurse *to prevent accidental extubation during the procedure if the patient coughs.*
• Suction the patient's trachea through the ET tube to remove any se-

cretions, *which can irritate the bronchi and cause the patient to cough during the procedure. Coughing increases the risk of traumatic injury to the vocal cords and the likelihood of dislodging the tube.* Then suction the patient's pharynx *to remove any secretions that may have accumulated above the tube cuff. This helps to prevent aspiration of secretions during cuff deflation.*
• *To prevent traumatic manipulation of the tube,* instruct the assisting nurse to hold it as you carefully untape the ET tube or unfasten the Velcro tube holder. When freeing the tube, be sure to locate any identifying landmark, such as a number on the tube, or measure the distance from the patient's mouth to the top of the tube *so you have a reference point when moving the tube.*
• Next, deflate the cuff by attaching a 10-cc syringe to the pilot balloon port and aspirating air until you meet resistance and the pilot balloon deflates. Deflate the cuff before moving the tube *because the cuff forms a seal within the trachea and movement of an inflated cuff can damage the tracheal wall and vocal cords.*
• Reposition the tube as necessary, noting new landmarks or measuring the length. Then immediately reinflate the cuff. To do this, instruct the patient to inhale, and slowly inflate the cuff using a 10-cc syringe attached to the pilot balloon port. As you do this, use your stethoscope to listen to the patient's neck *to determine the presence of an air leak.* Once air leakage ceases, stop cuff inflation and, while still listening to the patient's neck with your stethoscope, aspirate a small amount of air until you detect a slight

leak. *This creates a minimal air leak, which indicates that the cuff is inflated at the lowest pressure possible to create an adequate seal.* If the patient is being mechanically ventilated, aspirate to create a minimal air leak during the inspiratory phase of respiration *because the positive pressure of the ventilator during inspiration will create a larger leak around the cuff.* Note the number of cubic centimeters of air required to inflate the cuff to achieve a minimal air leak.

• Measure cuff pressure and compare the reading with previous pressure readings *to prevent overinflation.* (See *How to measure tracheal cuff pressure.*) Then use benzoin and tape to secure the tube in place, or refasten the Velcro tube holder.

• Make sure the patient is comfortable and the airway patent. Properly clean or dispose of equipment.

To measure cuff pressure

• Once the cuff is inflated, measure its pressure at least every 8 hours *to avoid overinflation.*

To remove the ET tube

• When you're authorized to remove the tube, obtain another nurse's assistance *to prevent traumatic manipulation of the tube when it's untaped or unfastened.*

• Elevate the head of the patient's bed to approximately 90 degrees.

• Suction the patient's oropharynx and nasopharynx *to remove any secretions that may have accumulated above the cuff and to help prevent aspiration of secretions when the cuff is deflated.*

• Using a handheld resuscitation bag or the mechanical ventilator, give the patient several deep breaths through the ET tube *to hyperinflate his lungs and increase his oxygen reserve.*

• Attach a 10-cc syringe to the pilot balloon port and aspirate air until you meet resistance and the pilot balloon deflates. If you fail to detect an air leak around the deflated cuff, notify the doctor immediately, and *do not* proceed with extubation. *Absence of an air leak may indicate marked tracheal edema and can result in total airway obstruction if the ET tube is removed.*

• If you detect the proper air leak, untape or unfasten the ET tube while the assisting nurse stabilizes the tube.

• Insert a sterile suction catheter through the ET tube. Then apply suction and ask the patient to take a deep breath and to open his mouth fully and pretend to cry out. *This causes abduction of the vocal cords and reduces the risk of laryngeal trauma during withdrawal of the tube.*

• Simultaneously remove the ET tube and the suction catheter in one smooth, outward and downward motion, following the natural curve of the patient's mouth. *Suctioning during extubation removes secretions retained at the end of the tube and prevents aspiration.*

• Give the patient supplemental oxygen. For highest humidity, use a cool-mist, large-volume nebulizer *to help decrease airway irritation, patient discomfort, and laryngeal edema.*

• Encourage the patient to cough and deep breathe. Remind him that a sore throat and hoarseness are to be expected and will gradually subside.

• Make sure the patient is comfortable and the airway is patent. Clean or dispose of equipment properly.

How to measure tracheal cuff pressure

An endotracheal (ET) or tracheostomy cuff provides a closed system for mechanical ventilation, allowing a desired tidal volume to be delivered to the patient's lungs. To function properly, the cuff must exert enough pressure on the tracheal wall to seal the airway without compromising the blood supply to the tracheal mucosa. The ideal pressure — known as minimal occlusive volume — is the lowest amount needed to seal the airway. Many authorities recommend maintaining a cuff pressure lower than venous perfusion pressure — usually about 16 to 24 cm H_2O. (More than 24 cm H_2O may exceed venous perfusion pressure.) Actual cuff pressure will vary with each patient, however. To keep pressure within safe limits, measure minimal occlusive volume at least once each shift or as directed by hospital policy. Cuff pressure can be measured by a respiratory therapist or by the nurse.

Taking the measurement

To measure cuff pressure, gather a cuff-pressure manometer, gloves, and a stethoscope. You'll also need suctioning equipment.

Explain the procedure to the patient. Put on gloves and suction the ET or tracheostomy tube and the patient's oropharynx to remove accumulated secretions above the cuff. Then attach the cuff-pressure manometer to the pilot balloon port, as shown below.

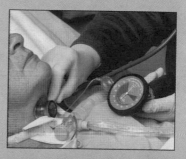

If you don't hear an air leak, press the red button under the dial of the cuff-pressure manometer to slowly release air from the balloon on the tracheal tube. Auscultate for an air leak.

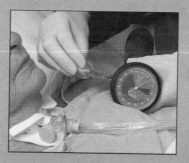

Place the diaphragm of the stethoscope over the trachea and listen for an air leak (as shown at top right). Keep in mind that a smooth, hollow sound indicates a sealed airway; a loud, gurgling sound indicates an air leak.

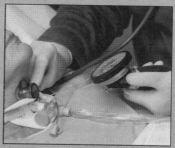

(continued)

How to measure tracheal cuff pressure *(continued)*

As soon as you hear an air leak, release the red button and gently squeeze the handle of the cuff-pressure manometer to inflate the cuff. Continue to add air to the cuff until you no longer hear an air leak.

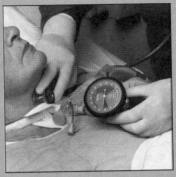

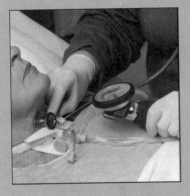

When the air leak ceases, read the dial on the cuff-pressure manometer. This is the minimal pressure required to effectively occlude the trachea around the tracheal tube. In many cases, this pressure will fall within the green area (16 to 24 cm H_2O) on the manometer dial.

Disconnect the cuff-pressure manometer from the pilot balloon port. Document the pressure value.

Special consideration
Keep in mind that some patients require less pressure in the cuff, whereas others (for example, those with tracheal malacia [abnormal softening of the tracheal tissue]) — require more pressure. Maintaining cuff pressure at the lowest possible level will minimize cuff-related problems.

• After extubation, auscultate the patient's lungs frequently and watch for signs of respiratory distress. Be especially alert for stridor or other evidence of upper airway obstruction. If ordered, draw an arterial sample for blood gas analysis.

Complications
• Traumatic injury to the larynx or trachea may result from manipulation of the tube, accidental extubation, or slippage of the tube into the right bronchus.

• Aspiration of upper airway secretions, underventilation, or coughing spasms may occur if a leak is created during cuff pressure measurement. Ventilatory failure and airway obstruction, caused by laryngospasm or marked tracheal edema, are the gravest complications of extubation.

Nursing considerations
• When repositioning a tube, be especially careful in patients with highly sensitive airways. Sedation or direct instillation of 2% lidocaine to numb

the airway may be indicated in such patients. *Because the lidocaine is absorbed systemically,* you must have a doctor's order to use it.

• After extubation of a patient who's been intubated for an extended time, keep reintubation supplies available for at least 12 hours, or until you're sure the patient can tolerate extubation.

• Never extubate a patient unless someone skilled at intubation is available.

• When measuring cuff pressure, keep the connection between the measuring device and the pilot balloon port tight *to avoid an air leak that could compromise cuff pressure.* If you're using a stopcock, do not leave the manometer in the off position *because air will leak from the cuff if the syringe accidentally comes off.* Also note the volume of air needed to inflate the cuff. A gradual increase in this volume indicates tracheal dilatation or erosion. A sudden increase in volume indicates rupture of the cuff and requires immediate reintubation if the patient is being ventilated, or if he requires continuous cuff inflation to maintain a high concentration of delivered oxygen.

• If you inadvertently cut the pilot balloon on the cuff, immediately call the person responsible for intubation in your hospital, who will remove the damaged ET tube and replace it with one that's intact. Don't remove the tube yourself before assistance arrives *because a tube with an air leak is better than no airway.*

Documentation

• After tube repositioning, record the date and time of the procedure, reason for repositioning (such as malposition shown by chest X-ray or prevention of pressure ulcers around the mouth), new tube position, total amount of air in the cuff after the procedure, any complications and the nursing action taken, and the patient's tolerance of the procedure.

• After cuff-pressure measurement, record the date and time of the procedure, cuff pressure, total amount of air in the cuff after the procedure, any complications and the nursing action taken, and the patient's tolerance of the procedure.

• After extubation, record the date and time of extubation, presence or absence of stridor or other signs of upper airway edema, type of supplemental oxygen administered, any complications and required subsequent therapy, and the patient's tolerance of the procedure.

Endotracheal tube insertion

This procedure involves the oral or nasal insertion of a flexible tube through the larynx into the trachea for the purposes of controlling the airway and mechanically ventilating the patient. Performed by a doctor, anesthetist, respiratory therapist, or nurse educated in the procedure, endotracheal (ET) tube insertion usually occurs during emergency situations, such as cardiopulmonary arrest, or in diseases, such as epiglottitis. However, intubation may also occur under more controlled circumstances, such as just before surgery. In these instances, ET intubation requires patient teaching and preparation.

Advantages of the procedure are that it establishes and maintains a patent airway, protects against aspiration by sealing off the trachea from the digestive tract, permits removal of tracheobronchial secretions in patients who can't cough effectively, and provides a route for mechanical ventilation. Disadvantages are that it bypasses normal respiratory tract defenses against infection, reduces cough effectiveness, and prevents verbal communication.

Oral ET intubation is contraindicated in patients with acute cervical spinal injury and degenerative spinal disorders, while nasal intubation is contraindicated in patients with apnea, bleeding disorders, chronic sinusitis, or nasal obstructions.

≫ Key nursing diagnoses and patient outcomes

Use these nursing diagnoses as a guide when developing your plan of care for a patient who is being treated with an ET tube.

Risk for aspiration related to absence of protective mechanisms

Based on this nursing diagnosis, you'll establish the following patient outcomes. The patient will:
• show no signs of aspiration.
• reveal no adventitious breath sounds on auscultation.

Ineffective airway clearance related to presence of secretions

Based on this nursing diagnosis, you'll establish the following patient outcomes. The patient will:
• cough effectively.

• expectorate sputum.
• keep airway patent.

Equipment

♦ two ET tubes (one spare) in the appropriate size ♦ 10-cc syringe ♦ stethoscope ♦ gloves ♦ lighted laryngoscope with a handle and blades of various sizes, curved and straight ♦ sedative ♦ local anesthetic spray, such as xylocaine (for conscious patients) ♦ mucosal vasoconstricting agent (for nasal intubation) ♦ overbed or other table ♦ water-soluble lubricant ♦ adhesive or other strong tape or Velcro tube holder ♦ compound benzoin tincture ♦ transparent adhesive dressing, if necessary ♦ gloves ♦ oral airway or bite block (for oral intubation) ♦ suction equipment ♦ handheld resuscitation bag with sterile swivel adapter ♦ humidified oxygen source ♦ optional: prepackaged intubation tray, sterile gauze pad, stylet, Magill forceps, sterile water, and sterile basin.

Equipment preparation

• Quickly gather the individual supplies or use a prepackaged intubation tray, which will contain most of the necessary supplies.
• Select an ET tube of the appropriate size. Typically, this will be size 2.5 to 5.5 mm, uncuffed, for children. Adult sizes range from 6 to 10 mm and are cuffed. The typical size for oral intubation in women is 7.5 mm and in men, 9 mm. Select a sightly smaller tube for nasal intubation.
• Check the light in the laryngoscope by snapping the appropriate size blade into place; if the bulb doesn't light, replace the batteries or the laryngoscope (whichever will be quicker).

• Using sterile technique, open the package containing the ET tube and, if desired, the other supplies as well, on an overbed table. Pour the sterile water into the basin. *To ease insertion,* lubricate the first inch (2.5 cm) of the distal end of ET tube with the water-soluble lubricant, using aseptic technique. Do this by either placing some of the lubricant on the gauze pad and wiping it on the tube or by squeezing the lubricant directly onto the tube. Use only water-soluble lubricant *because it can be absorbed by mucous membranes.*

• Attach the syringe to the port on the tube's exterior pilot cuff. Slowly inflate the cuff, observing for uniform inflation. If desired, submerge the tube in the sterile water and watch for air bubbles, *which would indicate a leak.* Then use the syringe to deflate the cuff.

• A stylet may be used on oral intubations *to stiffen the tube.* Lubricate the entire stylet *so that it can be easily removed after intubation.* Insert the stylet into the tube so that its distal tip lies about ½" (1.3 cm) inside the distal end of the tube. Make sure that the stylet does not protrude from the tube *to avoid vocal cord trauma.* Prepare the humidified oxygen source and the suction equipment for immediate use. If the patient is in bed, remove the headboard *to provide easier access.*

Patient preparation

• Administer medication, as ordered, *to decrease respiratory secretions, induce amnesia or analgesia, and help calm and relax the conscious patient.*

• Remove dentures and bridgework, if present.

Implementation

• Administer oxygen until the tube is inserted *to prevent hypoxia.*

• Place the patient supine in the sniffing position so that his mouth, pharynx, and trachea are extended. For a blind intubation, place the patient's head and neck in a neutral position.

• Put on gloves.

• For oral intubation, spray local anesthetic (such as xylocaine) deep into the patient's posterior pharynx *to diminish the gag reflex and reduce patient discomfort.* For nasal intubation, spray a local anesthetic and a mucosal vasoconstricting agent into the patient's nasal passages *to anesthetize and shrink the nasal turbinates and reduce the chance of bleeding.*

• If necessary, suction the patient's pharynx just before tube insertion *to improve visualization of the patient's pharynx and vocal cords.*

• Time each intubation attempt, limiting attempts to less than 30 seconds *to prevent hypoxia.*

Intubation with direct visualization

• Stand at the head of the patient's bed. Using your right hand, hold the patient's mouth open by crossing your index finger over your thumb, placing your thumb on the patient's upper teeth and your index finger on his lower teeth. This technique *provides greater leverage.*

• Grasp the laryngoscope handle in your left hand and gently slide the blade into the right side of the patient's mouth. Center the blade and push the patient's tongue to the left. Hold the patient's lower lip away from his teeth *to prevent the lip from being traumatized.*

• Advance the blade *to expose the epiglottis.* When using a straight blade, insert the tip under the epiglottis; when using a curved blade, insert the tip between the base of the tongue and the epiglottis.

• Lift the laryngoscope handle upward and away from your body at a 45-degree angle *to reveal the vocal cords.* Avoid pivoting the laryngoscope against the patient's teeth to prevent damaging them.

• If desired, have an assistant apply pressure to the cricoid ring *to occlude the esophagus and minimize gastric regurgitation.*

• When performing an oral intubation, insert the ET tube into the right side of the patient's mouth. When performing a nasotracheal intubation, insert the ET tube through the nostril and into the pharynx. Then use Magill forceps *to guide the tube through the vocal cords.*

• Guide the tube into the vertical openings of the larynx between the vocal cords, being careful not to mistake the horizontal opening of the esophagus for the larynx. If the vocal cords are closed because of a spasm, wait a few seconds for them to relax, and then gently guide the tube past them *to avoid traumatic injury.*

• Advance the tube until the cuff disappears beyond the vocal cords. Avoid advancing the tube farther *to avoid occluding a major bronchus and precipitating lung collapse.*

• Holding the ET tube in place, quickly remove the stylet, if present.

Blind nasotracheal intubation

• Pass the ET tube along the floor of the nasal cavity. If necessary, use gentle force to pass the tube through the nasopharynx and into the pharynx.

• Listen and feel for air movement through the tube as it's advanced *to ensure that the tube is properly placed in the airway.*

• Slip the tube between the vocal cords when the patient inhales *because the vocal cords separate on inhalation.*

• Once the tube is past the vocal cords, the breath sounds should become louder. If, at any time during tube advancement, breath sounds disappear, withdraw the tube until they reappear.

After intubation

• Inflate the tube's cuff with 5 to 10 cc of air until you feel resistance. Once the patient is mechanically ventilated, you'll use the minimal-leak technique or the minimal occlusive volume technique to establish correct inflation of the cuff.

• Remove the laryngoscope. If the patient was intubated orally, insert an oral airway or bite block *to prevent the patient from obstructing airflow or puncturing the tube with his teeth.*

• *To ensure correct tube placement,* observe for chest expansion and auscultate for bilateral breath sounds. If the patient is unconscious or uncooperative, use a handheld resuscitation bag while observing for upper chest movement and auscultating for breath sounds. Feel the tube's tip for warm exhalations and listen for air movement. Observe for condensation forming inside the tube.

• If you don't hear any breath sounds, auscultate over the stomach while ventilating with the resuscitation bag. Stomach distention, belching, or a gurgling sound indicates esophageal intubation. Immediately deflate the cuff and remove the tube. After reoxygenating the patient *to prevent hypoxia,* repeat insertion using a sterile tube *to prevent contamination of the trachea.*

• Auscultate bilaterally *to exclude the possibility of endobronchial intubation.* If you fail to hear breath sounds on both sides of the chest, you may have inserted the tube into one of the main stem bronchi (usually the right one because of its wider angle at the bifurcation); such insertion occludes the other bronchus and lung and results in atelectasis on the obstructed side. Or the tube may be resting on the carina, resulting in dry secretions that obstruct both bronchi. (The patient's coughing and fighting the ventilator will alert you to the problem.) *To correct these situations,* deflate the cuff, withdraw the tube 1 to 2 mm, auscultate for bilateral breath sounds, and reinflate the cuff.

• Once you've confirmed correct tube placement, administer oxygen or initiate mechanical ventilation, and suction if indicated.

• *To secure tube position,* apply compound benzoin tincture to each cheek and let it dry *for enhanced tape adhesion.* Tape the tube firmly with adhesive or other strong tape, or use a Velcro tube holder. (See *Three methods to secure an ET tube,* pages 304 and 305.)

• Inflate the cuff with the minimal-leak technique or the minimal occlusive volume technique. For the *minimal-leak technique,* attach a 10-cc syringe to the port on the tube's exterior pilot cuff, and place a stethoscope on the side of the patient's neck. Inject small amounts of air with each breath until leaking can no longer be heard. Then aspirate 0.1 cc of air from the cuff *to create a minimal air leak.* Record the amount of air needed to inflate the cuff *for subsequent monitoring of tracheal dilatation or erosion.* For the *minimal occlusive volume technique,* follow the first two steps of the minimal-leak technique, placing your stethoscope over the trachea instead of the side of the neck. Then aspirate until you hear a small leak on inspiration, and add just enough air to stop the leak. Record the amount of air needed to inflate the cuff for subsequent monitoring of tracheal dilatation or erosion.

• Clearly note the centimeter marking on the tube at the point where the tube exits the patient's mouth or nose. *By periodically monitoring this mark, you can detect tube displacement.*

• Make sure that a chest X-ray is taken *to verify tube position.*

• Place a swivel adapter between the tube and the humidified oxygen source *to allow for intermittent suctioning and to reduce tube tension.*

• Place the patient on his side with his head in a comfortable position *to avoid tube kinking and airway obstruction.*

• Auscultate both sides of the chest and watch chest movement as indicated by the patient's condition *to ensure correct tube placement and full lung ventilation.* Give frequent oral care to the orally intubated patient and position the ET tube *to prevent formation of pressure ulcers and to avoid excessive pressure on the sides of the mouth.* Give frequent nasal and oral care to the nasally intubated patient *to prevent formation of pressure ulcer*

(Text continues on page 306.)

Three methods to secure an endotracheal tube

Before taping an endotracheal (ET) tube in place, make sure the patient's face is clean, dry, and free of beard stubble. If possible, suction his mouth and dry the tube just before taping. Also check the reference mark on the tube to ensure correct placement. After taping, always check for bilateral breath sounds to ensure that the tube hasn't been displaced by manipulation.

To tape the tube securely, use one of the following three methods.

Method 1

Cut two 2″ (5-cm) strips and two 15″ (38-cm) strips of 1″ (2.5-cm) cloth adhesive tape. Then cut a 13″ (33-cm) slit in one end of each 15″ strip, as shown.

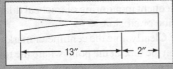

Apply compound benzoin tincture to the patient's cheeks. Place the 2″ strips on his cheeks, creating a new surface on which to anchor the tape securing the tube. *When frequent retaping is necessary, this helps preserve skin integrity.* If the patient's skin is excoriated or at risk, you can use a transparent semipermeable dressing to protect the skin.

Apply the benzoin tincture to the tape on the patient's face and to the part of the tube where you will be applying the tape.

On the side of the mouth where the tube will be anchored, affix the unslit end of the long tape to the top of the tape on the patient's cheek.

Wrap the top half of the tape around the tube twice, pulling the tape as tight as possible around the tube. Then, directing the tape over the patient's upper lip, place the end of the tape on the patient's other cheek. Cut off any excess tape. Use the lower half of the tape to secure an oral airway, if necessary, as shown.

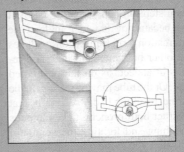

Or twist the lower half of the tape around the tube twice, and attach it to the original cheek. *Taping in opposite directions places equal traction on the tube.*

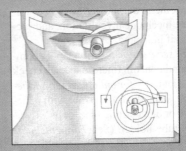

If you've taped an oral airway on or are concerned about the tube's stability, apply the other 15″ strip of tape in the same manner as the first, starting on the other side of the patient's face. If the tape around the tube is too bulky, use only the upper part of the tape and cut off the lower

Three methods to secure an endotracheal tube *(continued)*

part. If the patient has copious oral secretions, seal the tape by cutting a 1″ piece of paper tape, coating it with benzoin tincture, and placing the paper tape over the adhesive tape.

Method 2

Cut one piece of 1″ cloth adhesive tape long enough to wrap around the patient's head and overlap in front. Then cut an 8″ (20-cm) piece of tape and center it on the longer piece, sticky sides together. Next, cut a 5″ (12-cm) slit in each end of the longer tape, as shown.

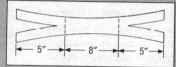

Apply benzoin tincture to the patient's cheeks, under his nose, and lower lip. (Don't spray benzoin directly on the patient's face because the vapors can be irritating if inhaled and can also harm the eyes.)

Place the top half of one end of the tape under the patient's nose and wrap the lower half around the ET tube. Place the lower half of the other end of the tape across the upper lip and wrap the top half around the tube.

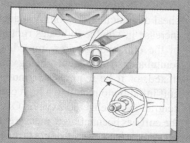

Method 3

Cut a tracheostomy tie in two pieces, one a few inches longer than the other, and cut two 6″ (15.2-cm) pieces of 1″ cloth adhesive tape. Then cut a 2″ slit in one end of both pieces of tape. Fold back the other end of the tape ½″ so the sticky sides are together and cut a small hole in it, as shown.

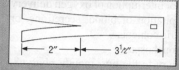

Apply benzoin tincture to the part of the ET tube that will be taped. Wrap the split ends of each piece of tape around the tube, one piece on each side. Overlap the tape to secure it.

Apply the free ends of the tape to both sides of the patient's face. Then insert tracheostomy ties through the holes in the tape and knot the ties.

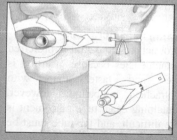

Bring the longer tie behind the patient's neck. *Knotting the ties on the side prevents the patient from lying on the knot and developing a pressure ulcer.*

and drying of oral mucous membranes.
• Suction secretions through the ET tube as the patient's condition indicates *to clear secretions and prevent mucus plugs from obstructing the tube.*

Complications

Possible complications of ET intubation include:
• apnea caused by reflex breath holding or interruption of oxygen delivery
• aspiration of blood, secretions, or gastric contents
• bronchospasm
• injury to the lips, mouth, pharynx, or vocal cords
• laryngeal edema and erosion
• tooth damage or loss
• tracheal stenosis, erosion, and necrosis.

Nasotracheal intubation can result in:
• nasal bleeding
• laceration
• sinusitis
• otitis media.

Nursing considerations

• Orotracheal intubation is preferred in emergencies because insertion is easier and faster than with nasotracheal intubation. However, maintaining exact tube placement is more difficult, and the tube must be well secured *to avoid kinking and prevent bronchial obstruction or accidental extubation.* Orotracheal intubation is also poorly tolerated by the conscious patient because it stimulates salivation, coughing, and retching.
• Nasotracheal intubation is preferred for elective insertion when the patient is capable of spontaneous ventilation for a short period. Blind intubation is typically used in conscious patients who risk imminent respiratory arrest or who have cervical spinal injury.
• Although nasotracheal intubation is more comfortable than oral intubation, it's also more difficult to perform. Because the tube passes blindly through the nasal cavity, the procedure causes greater tissue trauma, increases the risk of infection by nasal bacteria introduced into the trachea, and risks pressure necrosis of the nasal mucosa. However, exact tube placement is easier and the risk of dislodgment is lower. The cuff on the ET tube maintains a closed system that permits positive-pressure ventilation and protects the airway from aspiration of secretions and gastric contents.
• Although low-pressure cuffs have significantly reduced the incidence of tracheal erosion and necrosis caused by cuff pressure on the tracheal wall, overinflation of a low-pressure cuff can negate this benefit. Use the minimal-leak technique to avoid these complications. Inflating the cuff a bit more to make a complete seal with the least amount of air is the next most desirable method.
• Always record the volume of air needed to inflate the cuff. A gradual increase in this volume indicates tracheal dilatation or erosion. A sudden increase in volume indicates rupture of the cuff and requires immediate reintubation if the patient is being ventilated, or if he requires continuous cuff inflation to maintain a high concentration of delivered oxygen. Once the cuff has been inflated, measure its pressure at least every 8 hours *to avoid*

overinflation. Normal cuff pressure is about 18 mm Hg.

Documentation

• Record the date and time of the procedure; its indication and success or failure; tube type and size; cuff size, amount of inflation and inflation technique; administration of medication; initiation of supplemental oxygen or ventilation therapy; and results of chest auscultation and of the chest X-ray.

• Record any complications and the nursing action taken.

• Note the patient's reaction to the procedure.

Epidural analgesic administration

In this procedure, the doctor injects or infuses medication into the epidural space, which lies just outside the subarachnoid space where cerebrospinal fluid (CSF) flows. The drug diffuses slowly into the subarachnoid space of the spinal canal and then into the CSF, which carries it directly into the spinal area—bypassing the blood-brain barrier. In some cases, the doctor injects drugs directly into the subarachnoid space. (See *Understanding intrathecal injections.*)

Epidural analgesia helps manage acute or chronic pain, including moderate to severe postoperative pain. It's especially useful in patients with cancer or degenerative joint disease. This procedure works well because opiate receptors are located along the spinal cord. Narcotic drugs act directly on the receptors of the dorsal horn to pro-

Understanding intrathecal injections

An intrathecal injection allows the doctor to inject medication into the subarachnoid space of the spinal canal. Certain drugs — such as anti-infectives or antineoplastics used to treat meningeal leukemia— are administered by this route because they do not travel through the bloodstream and thus don't penetrate the blood-brain barrier. Intrathecal injection may also be used to deliver anesthetics, such as lidocaine hydrochloride, to achieve regional anesthesia (as in spinal anesthesia or epidural block).

An invasive procedure performed by a doctor under sterile conditions with the nurse assisting, intrathecal injection requires informed patient consent. The injection site is usually between L3 and L4, well below the spinal cord, to avoid the risk of paralysis. This procedure may be preceded by aspiration of spinal fluid for laboratory analysis.

Contraindications to intrathecal injection include inflammation or infection at the puncture site, septicemia, and spinal deformities (especially when considered as an anesthesia route).

duce localized analgesia without motor blockade. Narcotics, such as morphine, fentanyl, and hydromorphone are administered as either an I.V. bolus dose or by continuous infusion, either alone or in combination with bupivacaine (a local anesthetic). The infusion, given via an epidural catheter, is preferable because it allows a smaller drug dosage to be given continuously. The epidural catheter, inserted near

Placement of a permanent epidural catheter

An epidural catheter is implanted under the patient's skin and inserted near the spinal cord at the L1 interspace.

For temporary analgesic therapy (less than 1 week), the catheter may exit directly over the spine and be taped along the patient's back up to the shoulder. For prolonged therapy, however, the catheter may be tunneled subcutaneously to an exit site on the patient's side or abdomen or over his shoulder.

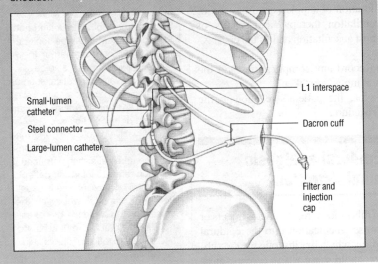

the spinal cord, eliminates the risks of multiple I.M. injections, minimizes adverse cerebral and systemic effects, and eliminates the analgesic peaks and valleys that usually occur with intermittent I.M. injections. (See *Placement of a permanent epidural catheter.*)

Typically, epidural-catheter insertion is performed by an anesthesiologist using aseptic technique. Once the catheter has been inserted, the nurse is responsible for monitoring the infusion and assessing the patient.

Epidural analgesia is contraindicated in patients who have local or systemic infection, neurologic disease, anticoag-

ulant therapy, coagulation disorders, spinal arthritis or deformity, hypotension, marked hypertension, or allergy to the prescribed drug.

≫ Key nursing diagnoses and patient outcomes

Use these nursing diagnoses as a guide when developing your plan of care for a patient who is being treated with epidural medications.

Knowledge deficit related to lack of exposure to the procedure
Based on this nursing diagnosis, you'll establish the following patient outcomes. The patient will:

• state or demonstrate understanding of what has been taught.
• demonstrate ability to perform new health related behaviors as they are taught.

Risk for injury related to improper technique

Based on this nursing diagnosis, you'll establish the following patient outcomes. The patient will:
• identify factors that increase risk of injury.
• assist in identifying and applying safety measures to prevent injury.

Equipment

♦ volume infusion device and epidural infusion tubing (depending on hospital policy) ♦ patient's medication record and chart ♦ prescribed epidural solutions ♦ transparent dressing or sterile gauze pads ♦ epidural tray ♦ labels for epidural infusion line ♦ silk tape ♦ optional: monitoring equipment for blood pressure and pulse, apnea monitor.

Have the following drugs and equipment on hand for emergency use: naloxone 0.4 mg I.V., ephedrine 50 mg I.V., oxygen, intubation set, handheld resuscitation bag.

Equipment preparation

• Prepare the infusion device according to the manufacturer's instructions and hospital policy.
• Obtain an epidural tray.
• Be sure the pharmacy has been notified ahead of time regarding the medication order *because epidural solutions require special preparation.*
• Check the medication concentration and infusion rate against the doctor's order.

Implementation

• Explain the procedure and its possible complications to the patient.
• Tell the patient she'll feel some pain as the catheter is inserted.
• Answer any questions.
• Make sure that a consent form has been properly signed and witnessed.
• Position the patient on her side in the knee-chest position, or have her sit on the edge of the bed and lean over a bedside table.
• After the catheter is in place, prime the infusion device, confirm the appropriate medication and infusion rate, and adjust the device for the correct rate.
• Help the anesthesiologist connect the infusion tubing to the epidural catheter and then connect the tubing to the infusion pump.
• Bridge-tape all connection sites and label the catheter, infusion tubing, and infusion pump with EPIDURAL INFUSION *to prevent accidental infusion of other drugs into the epidural lines.*
• Start the infusion.
• Tell the patient to immediately report any feeling of pain, using a pain scale from 0 to 10, with 0 denoting no pain and 10 denoting the worst pain imaginable. A response of 3 or less typically indicates tolerable pain. If the patient reports a higher pain score, the infusion rate may need to be increased. Call the doctor or change the rate within prescribed limits.
• If ordered, place the patient on an apnea monitor for the first 24 hours after beginning the infusion.
• Change the dressing over the catheter's exit site every 24 to 48 hours, or as needed. The dressing is usually transparent to allow inspection of

drainage and commonly appears moist or slightly blood-tinged.
• Change the infusion tubing every 48 hours, or as specified by hospital policy.

To remove an epidural catheter
• Typically, the anesthesiologist orders analgesics and removes the catheter, but hospital policy may allow a specially trained nurse to remove the catheter.
• If you feel resistance when removing the catheter, stop and call the doctor for further orders.
• The doctor will want to examine the catheter tip to rule out any damage during removal, so be sure to save the catheter.

Complications
• The most common complication of epidural infusion is numbness and leg weakness, which may occur after the first 24 hours and is drug- and concentration-dependent. Identifying the dosage level that provides adequate pain control without causing excessive numbness and weakness requires that the doctor titrate the dosage.
• Respiratory depression, which usually occurs during the first 24 hours, may be treated with naloxone, 0.2 to 0.4 mg I.V.
• Pruritus, which may also occur, may be treated with nalbuphine, 5 mg I.V., or diphenhydramine, 25 mg I.V.
• Nausea and vomiting, other adverse effects, are treated with prochlorperazine, 5 to 10 mg I.V., or metoclopramide, 10 mg I.V.

Nursing considerations
• Assess the patient's respiratory rate and blood pressure every 2 hours for 8 hours, then every 4 hours for 8 hours, during the first 24 hours after starting the infusion. Then, assess the patient once per shift, depending on her condition or unless ordered otherwise.
• Notify the doctor if the patient's respiratory rate is less than 10 breaths/minute or if her systolic blood pressure is less than 90 mm Hg.
• Assess the patient's sedation level, mental status, and pain relief status every hour initially, then every 2 to 4 hours, until adequate pain control is achieved.
• Notify the doctor if the patient appears drowsy or experiences nausea and vomiting, refractory itching, or inability to void, which are adverse effects of certain narcotic analgesics, or if he complains of unrelieved pain.
• Assess lower-extremity motor strength every 2 to 4 hours. If sensory and motor loss occurs, large motor nerve fibers have been affected and dosage may need to be decreased.
• Keep in mind that drugs given epidurally diffuse slowly and may cause adverse effects, including excessive sedation, up to 12 hours after epidural infusion has been discontinued.
• The patient should always have a peripheral I.V. line (either continuous infusion or intermittent infusion device) open *to allow immediate administration of emergency drugs.*
• If CSF leaks into the dura mater during removal of an epidural catheter, the patient usually experiences headache. This postanalgesia headache worsens with postural changes, such as standing or sitting. The headache can be treated with a " blood patch," in which the patient's own blood (about 10 ml) is withdrawn from a pe-

ripheral vein and then injected into the epidural space. When the epidural needle is withdrawn, the patient is instructed to sit up. Because the blood clots seal off the leaking area, the blood patch should relieve the patient's headache immediately.
• The patient need not restrict his activity after this procedure.

Home care
• Home use of epidural analgesia is possible only if the patient or her family is willing and able to learn the care needed. The patient also must be willing and able to abstain from alcohol and "street drugs" *because these substances potentiate opiate action.*

Documentation
• Record the patient's response to treatment, catheter patency, condition of the dressing and insertion site, vital signs, and assessment results.
• Document the labeling of the epidural catheter, changing of the infusion bags, ordered analgesics, if any, and the patient's response.

Esophageal airway insertion and removal

Esophageal airways, such as the esophageal gastric tube airway (EGTA) and the esophageal obturator airway (EOA), are used temporarily (for up to 2 hours) to maintain ventilation in the comatose patient during cardiac or respiratory arrest. These devices avoid tongue obstruction, prevent air from entering the stomach, and keep stomach contents from entering the tra-

chea. They can be inserted only after a patent airway is established.

Although health care providers must have special training to insert an EGTA or EOA, insertion of these airways is much simpler than endotracheal intubation. One reason is that these devices do not require visualization of the trachea or hyperextension of the neck. This makes them useful for treating patients with suspected spinal cord injuries.

Because conscious and semiconscious patients will reject an esophageal airway, one should not be used unless the patient is unconscious and not breathing. These airways are also contraindicated if facial trauma prevents a snug mask fit or if the patient has an absent or weak gag reflex, has recently ingested toxic chemicals, has esophageal disease, or has taken an overdose of narcotics that can be reversed by naloxone. In addition, because pediatric sizes aren't currently available, these airways should not be used in patients under age 16.

≫ Key nursing diagnoses and patient outcomes
Use these nursing diagnoses as a guide when developing your plan of care for a patient who is being treated with an esophageal airway.

Risk for aspiration related to absence of protective mechanisms
Based on this nursing diagnosis, you'll establish the following patient outcomes. The patient will:
• show no signs of aspiration.
• reveal no adventitious breath sounds on auscultation.

Ineffective airway clearance related to presence of secretions
Based on this nursing diagnosis, you'll establish the following patient outcomes. The patient will:
• cough effectively.
• expectorate sputum.
• keep airway patent.

Equipment

♦ esophageal tube ♦ face mask ♦ #16 or 18 French nasogastric (NG) tube (for EGTA) ♦ 35-cc syringe ♦ intermittent gastric suction equipment ♦ oral suction equipment ♦ optional: handheld resuscitation bag, water-soluble lubricant.

Equipment preparation

• Gather the equipment. (See *Types of esophageal airways.*)
• Fill the face mask with air *to check for leaks.*
• Inflate the esophageal tube's cuff with 35 cc of air *to check for leaks*; then, deflate the cuff.
• Connect the esophageal tube to the face mask (the lower opening on an EGTA) and listen for the tube to click *to determine proper placement.*

Implementation

• Lubricate the first inch (2.5 cm) of the tube's distal tip with a water-soluble lubricant, I.V. fluid, the patient's saliva, or tap water. With an EGTA, also lubricate the first inch of the NG tube's distal tip.

To insert an esophageal airway

• Assess the patient's condition *to determine if he's a safe candidate for an esophageal airway.*
• If the patient's condition permits, place him in the supine position with

his neck in a neutral or semiflexed position. *Hyperextension of the neck may cause the tube to enter the trachea instead of the esophagus.* Remove his dentures, if applicable.
• Insert your thumb deeply into the patient's mouth behind the base of his tongue. Place your index and middle fingers of the same hand under the patient's chin, and lift his jaw straight up.
• With your other hand, grasp the esophageal tube just below the mask in the same way you'd grasp a pencil. *This promotes gentle maneuvering of the tube and reduces the risk of pharyngeal trauma.*
• Still elevating the patient's jaw with one hand, insert the tip of the esophageal tube into the patient's mouth. Gently guide the airway over the tongue into the pharynx and then into the esophagus, following the natural pharyngeal curve. No force is required for proper insertion; the tube should easily seat itself. If you encounter resistance, withdraw the tube slightly and readvance it. When the tube is fully advanced, the mask should fit snugly over the patient's mouth and nose. When this is accomplished, the cuff will lie below the level of the carina. If the cuff is above the carina, it may, when inflated, compress the posterior membranous portion of the trachea and cause tracheal obstruction.
• *Because the tube may enter the trachea,* deliver positive-pressure ventilation before inflating the cuff. Watch for chest rise *to confirm that the tube is in the esophagus.*
• Once the tube is properly in place in the esophagus, draw 35 cc of air into the syringe, connect the syringe to the tube's cuff-inflation valve, and inflate

Types of esophageal airways

Gastric tube airway

This airway consists of an inflatable mask and an esophageal tube, as shown below. The transparent face mask has two ports: a lower one for insertion of an esophageal tube and an upper one for ventilation, which can be maintained with a handheld resuscitation bag. The inside of the mask is soft and pliable; it molds to the patient's face and makes a tight seal, preventing air loss.

The proximal end of the esophageal tube has a one-way, nonrefluxing valve that blocks the esophagus. This valve prevents air from entering the stomach, thus reducing the risk of abdominal distention and aspiration. The distal end of the tube has an inflatable cuff that rests in the esophagus just below the tracheal bifurcation, preventing pressure on the noncartilaginous tracheal wall.

During ventilation, air is directed into the upper port in the mask and, with the esophagus blocked, it enters the trachea and lungs.

Obturator airway

This airway consists of an adjustable, inflatable, transparent face mask with a single port, attached by a snap lock to a blind esophageal tube.

When properly inflated, the transparent mask prevents air from escaping through the nose and mouth, as shown below.

The esophageal tube has 16 holes at its proximal end through which air or oxygen introduced into the port of the mask is transferred to the trachea. The tube's distal end is closed and circled by an inflatable cuff. When the cuff is inflated, it occludes the esophagus, preventing air from entering the stomach and acting as a barrier against vomitus and involuntary aspiration.

Esophageal gastric tube airway

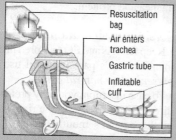

Resuscitation bag
Air enters trachea
Gastric tube
Inflatable cuff

Esophageal obturator airway

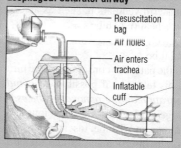

Resuscitation bag
Air holes
Air enters trachea
Inflatable cuff

the cuff. Avoid overinflation *because this can cause esophageal trauma.*
• If you've inserted an EGTA, insert the NG tube through the lower port on the face mask and into the esophageal tube, and advance it to the second

marking so it reaches 6″ (15.2 cm) beyond the distal end of the esophageal tube. Suction stomach contents using intermittent gastric suction *to decompress the stomach.* This is particularly necessary after mouth-to-mouth resuscitation, which introduces air to the stomach. Leave the tube in place during resuscitation.

• For both airways, attach a handheld resuscitation bag or a mechanical ventilator to the face-mask port (upper port) on the EGTA. Up to 100% of the fraction of inspired oxygen can be delivered this way.

• Monitor the patient *to ensure adequate ventilation.* Watch for chest movement, and suction the patient if mucus blocks the EOA tube perforations or in any way interrupts respiration.

To remove an esophageal airway

• Assess the patient's condition *to determine if it's appropriate to remove the airway.* The airway may be removed if respirations are spontaneous and number 16 to 20 breaths/minute. If 2 hours have elapsed since airway insertion and respirations are not spontaneous and at the normal rate, the patient must be switched to an artificial airway that can be used for long-term ventilation, such as an endotracheal (ET) tube.

• Detach the mask from the esophageal tube.

• If the patient is conscious, place him on his left side, if possible, *to avoid aspiration during removal of the esophageal tube.* If he's unconscious and requires an ET tube, insert it or assist with its insertion and inflate the cuff of the ET tube before removing the esophageal tube. *With the esophageal tube in place, the ET tube can be easily guided into the trachea, and stomach contents are less likely to be aspirated when the esophageal tube is removed.*

• Deflate the cuff on the esophageal tube by removing air from the infla-

tion valve with a syringe. Don't try to remove the tube with the cuff inflated *because it may perforate the esophagus.*

• Turn the patient's head to the side, if possible, *to avoid aspiration.*

• Remove the EGTA or EOA in one swift, smooth motion, following the natural pharyngeal curve *to avoid esophageal trauma.*

• Perform oropharyngeal suctioning *to remove any residual secretions.*

• Assist the doctor as required in monitoring and maintaining adequate ventilation for the patient.

Complications

• EOAs may be inferior to ET intubation in providing adequate oxygenation and ventilation.

• Esophageal airways may cause esophageal injuries, including rupture and, in semiconscious patients, may cause laryngospasm, vomiting, and aspiration. *Note:* The EOA does not prevent aspiration of foreign material from the mouth and pharynx into the trachea and bronchi.

Nursing considerations

• Keep EGTAs and EOAs stored in the manufacturer's package until use *to preserve their natural curve.*

• To ease insertion, you may prefer to direct the airway along the right side of the patient's mouth *because the esophagus is located to the right of and behind the trachea.* Or you may advance the tube tip upward toward the hard palate; then invert the tip and glide it along the tongue surface and into the pharynx. *This keeps the tube centered, avoids snagging it on the sides of the throat, and eases insertion in the patient with clenched jaws.*

• Watch the unconscious patient as he regains consciousness. Restrain his hands *if he tries to remove the airway.* Explain the procedure to him, if possible, *to reduce his apprehension.* Observe also for retching and, if it occurs, remove the airway immediately because the accumulation of vomitus blocked by the airway cuff may perforate the esophagus. *To help prevent complications,* do not leave the EOA in place for more than 2 hours.

• A mechanical ventilator attached to an ET or tracheostomy tube maintains a more precise tidal volume than a mechanical ventilator attached to an esophageal airway.

Documentation

• Record the date and time of the procedure, type of airway inserted, patient's vital signs and level of consciousness, removal of the airway, and any alternative airway inserted after extubation.

• Record any complications and the nursing action taken.

Esophageal tube care

Although the doctor inserts an esophageal tube, the nurse cares for the patient during and after intubation. Typically, the patient is in the intensive care unit for close observation and constant care. The environment may help to increase the patient's tolerance for the procedure and may help to control bleeding. Sedatives may be contraindicated, especially for a patient with portal systemic encephalopathy.

Most important, the patient who has an esophageal tube in place to control variceal bleeding (typically from portal hypertension) must be observed closely for possible esophageal rupture because varices weaken the esophagus. Additionally, possible traumatic injury from intubation or esophageal balloon inflation increases the chance of rupture. Usually, emergency surgery is performed if a rupture occurs. The operation has a low success rate.

≫ Key nursing diagnoses and patient outcomes

Use these nursing diagnoses as a guide when developing your plan of care for a patient who has an esophageal tube.

Risk for aspiration related to absence of protective mechanisms

Based on this nursing diagnosis, you'll establish the following patient outcomes. The patient will:

• show no signs of aspiration.

• reveal no adventitious breath sounds on auscultation.

Ineffective airway clearance related to presence of secretions

Based on this nursing diagnosis, you'll establish the following patient outcomes. The patient will:

• cough effectively.

• expectorate sputum.

• keep airway patent.

Equipment

♦ manometer ♦ two 2-liter bottles of normal saline solution ♦ irrigation set ♦ water-soluble lubricant ♦ several cotton-tipped applicators ♦ mouthcare equipment ♦ nasopharyngeal suction apparatus ♦ several #12

French suction catheters ◆ intake-and-output record sheets ◆ gloves ◆ goggles ◆ sedatives ◆ traction weights or football helmet ◆ foam noseguard.

Patient preparation

• *To ease the patient's anxiety,* explain the care you'll give.
• Provide privacy.

Implementation

• Wash your hands and put on gloves and goggles.
• Monitor the patient's vital signs every 5 minutes to 1 hour, as ordered. *A change in vital signs may signal complications or recurrent bleeding.*
• If the patient has a Sengstaken-Blakemore or a Minnesota tube, check the pressure gauge on the manometer every 30 to 60 minutes *to detect any leaks in the esophageal balloon and to verify the set pressure.*
• Maintain drainage and suction on gastric and esophageal aspiration ports, as ordered. This is important because *fluid accumulating in the stomach may cause the patient to regurgitate the tube, and fluid accumulating in the esophagus may lead to vomiting and aspiration.*
• Irrigate the gastric aspiration port, as ordered, using the irrigation set and normal saline solution. *Frequent irrigation keeps the tube from clogging. Obstruction in the tube can lead to regurgitation of the tube and vomiting.*
• *To prevent pressure ulcers,* clean the patient's nostrils, and apply water-soluble lubricant frequently. Use warm water to loosen crusted nasal secretions before applying the lubricant with cotton-tipped applicators.

• Give mouth care often *to rid the patient's mouth of foul-tasting matter and to relieve dryness from mouth breathing.*
• Use #12 French catheters to provide gentle oral suctioning, if necessary, *to help remove secretions.*
• Offer emotional support. Keep the patient as quiet as possible, and administer sedatives, if ordered.
• Be sure that the traction weights hang from the foot of the bed at all times. Never rest them on the bed. Instruct housekeepers and other co-workers not to move the weights *because reduced traction may change the position of the tube.*
• Elevate the head of the bed about 25 degrees *to ensure countertraction for the weights.*
• Keep the patient on complete bed rest because exertion, such as coughing or straining, increases intra-abdominal pressure, which may trigger further bleeding.
• Keep the patient in semi-Fowler's position *to reduce blood flow into the portal system and to prevent reflux into the esophagus.*
• Monitor intake and output, as ordered.

Complications

• Esophageal rupture, the most life-threatening complication associated with esophageal balloon tamponade, can occur at any time but is most likely to occur during intubation or inflation of the esophageal balloon.
• Asphyxia may result if the balloon moves up the esophagus and blocks the airway. Aspiration of pooled esophageal secretions may also complicate this procedure.

Nursing considerations

• Observe the patient carefully for esophageal rupture indicated by signs and symptoms of shock, increased respiratory difficulties, and increased bleeding. Tape scissors to the head of the bed *so you can cut the tube quickly to deflate the balloons if asphyxia develops.* When performing this emergency intervention, hold the tube firmly close to the nostril before cutting.

• If using traction, be sure to release the tension before deflating any balloons. If weights and pulleys supply traction, remove the weights. If a football helmet supplies traction, untape the esophageal tube from the face guard before deflating the balloons. *Deflating the balloon under tension triggers a rapid release of the entire tube from the nose, which may injure mucous membranes, initiate recurrent bleeding, and obstruct the airway.*

• If the doctor orders an X-ray study to check the tube's position or to view the chest, lift the patient in the direction of the pulley, and then place the X-ray film behind his back. Never roll him from side to side *because pressure exerted on the tube in this way may shift the tube's position.* Similarly lift the patient to make the bed or to assist him with the bedpan.

Documentation

• Read the manometer hourly, and record the esophageal pressures.

• Note when the balloons are deflated and by whom.

• Document vital signs, the condition of the patient's nostrils, routine care, and any drugs administered.

• Note the color, consistency, and amount of gastric returns.

• Record any signs and symptoms of complications and the nursing actions taken.

• Document gastric port and nasogastric tube irrigations. Maintain accurate intake and output records.

Esophageal tube insertion and removal

Used to control hemorrhage from esophageal or gastric varices, an esophageal tube is inserted nasally or orally and advanced into the esophagus or stomach. Ordinarily, a doctor inserts and removes the tube. In an emergency, a nurse may remove it.

Once the tube is in place, a gastric balloon secured at the end of the tube can be inflated and drawn tightly against the cardia of the stomach. The inflated balloon secures the tube and exerts pressure on the cardia. The pressure against the varices in turn controls the bleeding.

Most tubes also contain an esophageal balloon to control esophageal bleeding. (See *Types of esophageal tubes*, pages 318 and 319.)

Usually, gastric or esophageal balloons are deflated after 24 hours. If the balloon remains inflated longer than 24 hours, pressure necrosis may develop and cause further hemorrhage or perforation.

• Other procedures to control bleeding include irrigation with tepid or iced saline solution and drug therapy with a vasopressor. Used with the esophageal tube, these procedures

(Text continues on page 319.)

Types of esophageal tubes

When working with patients who have an esophageal tube, keep in mind the advantages of the most common types, described below.

Sengstaken-Blakemore tube

This triple-lumen, double-balloon tube has a gastric aspiration port, which allows you to obtain drainage from below the gastric balloon and also to instill medication.

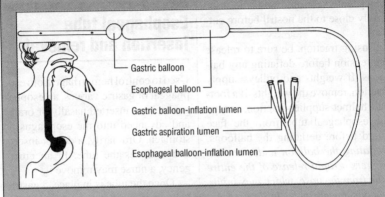

Gastric balloon
Esophageal balloon
Gastric balloon-inflation lumen
Gastric aspiration lumen
Esophageal balloon-inflation lumen

Linton tube

This triple-lumen, single-balloon tube has a port for gastric aspiration and one for esophageal aspiration, too. Additionally, the Linton tube reduces the risk of esophageal necrosis because it doesn't have an esophageal balloon.

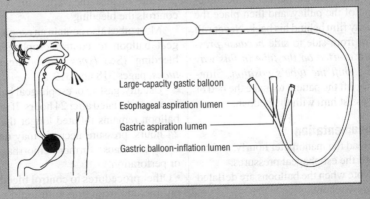

Large-capacity gastic balloon
Esophageal aspiration lumen
Gastric aspiration lumen
Gastric balloon-inflation lumen

Types of esophageal tubes *(continued)*

Minnesota esophagogastric tamponade tube

This esophageal tube has four lumens and two balloons. The device provides pressure-monitoring ports for both balloons without the need for Y-connectors. One port is used for gastric suction, the other for esophageal suction.

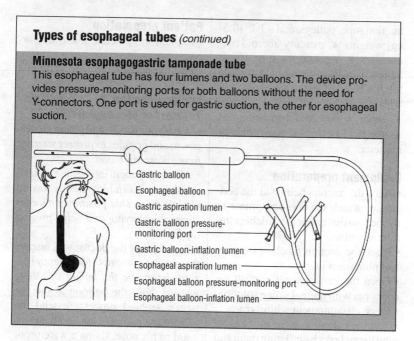

Gastric balloon
Esophageal balloon
Gastric aspiration lumen
Gastric balloon pressure-monitoring port
Gastric balloon-inflation lumen
Esophageal aspiration lumen
Esophageal balloon pressure-monitoring port
Esophageal balloon-inflation lumen

provide effective, temporary control of acute variceal hemorrhage.

▶▶ Key nursing diagnoses and patient outcomes

Use these nursing diagnoses as a guide when developing your plan of care for a patient who is being treated with an esophageal tube.

Risk for aspiration related to absence of protective mechanisms

Based on this nursing diagnosis, you'll establish the following patient outcomes. The patient will:
• show no signs of aspiration.
• reveal no adventitious breath sounds on auscultation.

Ineffective airway clearance related to presence of secretions

Based on this nursing diagnosis, you'll establish the following patient outcomes. The patient will:
• cough effectively.
• expectorate sputum.
• keep airway patent.

Equipment

♦ esophageal tube ♦ nasogastric (NG) tube (if using a Sengstaken-Blakemore tube) ♦ two suction sources ♦ basin of ice ♦ irrigation set ♦ 2 liters (or quarts) of normal saline solution ♦ two 60-ml syringes ♦ water-soluble lubricant ♦ ½" or 1" adhesive tape ♦ stethoscope ♦ foam noseguard ♦ four rubber-shod clamps (two clamps and two plastic plugs for a Minnesota tube) ♦ anesthetic spray (as ordered) ♦ traction equipment (football helmet or a basic frame with traction rope, pulleys, and a 1-lb [0.5-kg] weight) ♦ mercury aneroid manometer ♦ Y-connector tube (for a Sengstaken-Blakemore or a Linton tube) ♦ basin of water ♦ cup of water with straw ♦ scissors ♦ gloves ♦ gown ♦ waterproof marking pen ♦ goggles ♦ tape ♦ sphygmomanometer.

Equipment preparation

• Keep the traction helmet at the bedside or attach traction equipment to the bed, so that either is available after tube insertion.

• Place the suction machines nearby and plug them in.

• Open the irrigation set and fill the container with normal saline solution.

• Place all equipment within reach.

• Test the balloons on the esophageal tube for air leaks by inflating them and submerging them in the basin of water. If no bubbles appear in the water, the balloons are intact. Remove them from the water and deflate them. Clamp the tube lumens, so that the balloons stay deflated during insertion.

• To prepare the Minnesota tube, connect the mercury manometer to the gastric-pressure monitoring port. Note the pressure when the balloon fills with 100, 200, 300, 400, and 500 cc of air.

• Check the aspiration lumens for patency, and make sure that they are labeled according to their purpose. If they aren't identified, label them carefully with the marking pen.

• Chill the tube in a basin of ice. *This will stiffen it and facilitate insertion,* as ordered.

Patient preparation

• Explain the procedure and its purpose to the patient.

• Provide privacy.

Implementation
To insert an esophageal tube

• Wash your hands, and put on gloves, gown, and goggles *to protect yourself from splashing blood.*

• Assist the patient into semi-Fowler's position and turn him slightly toward his left side. *This position promotes stomach emptying and helps prevent aspiration.*

• Explain that the doctor will inspect the patient's nostrils (for patency).

• *To determine the length of tubing needed,* hold the balloon at the patient's xiphoid process; extend the tube to the patient's ear and then forward to his nose. Using a waterproof pen, mark this point on the tubing.

• Inform the patient that the doctor will spray the patient's posterior pharynx (throat) and nostril with an anesthetic *to minimize discomfort and gagging during intubation.*

• After lubricating the tip of the tube with water-soluble lubricant *to reduce friction and to facilitate insertion,* the doctor will pass the tube through the more patent nostril. As he does, he will direct the patient to tilt his chin toward his chest and to swallow when he senses the tip of the tube in the back of his throat. *Swallowing helps to advance the tube into the esophagus and prevents intubation of the trachea.* (If the doctor introduces the tube orally, he will direct the patient to swallow immediately.) As the patient swallows, the doctor quickly advances the tube at least 1½″ (1.3 cm) beyond the previously marked point on the tube.

- *To confirm tube placement,* the doctor will aspirate stomach contents through the gastric port. He will also auscultate the stomach with a stethoscope as he injects air. After partially inflating the gastric balloon with 50 to 100 cc of air, he will order an X-ray of the abdomen *to confirm correct placement of the balloon.* Before fully inflating the balloon, he will use the 60-ml syringe to irrigate the stomach with normal saline solution and empty the stomach as completely as possible. *This helps the patient avoid regurgitating gastric contents when the balloon inflates.*
- After confirming tube placement, the doctor fully inflates the gastric balloon (250 to 500 cc of air for the Sengstaken-Blakemore tube; 700 to 800 cc of air for the Linton tube) and clamps the tube. If he's using the Minnesota tube, he connects the pressure-monitoring port for the gastric balloon lumen to the mercury manometer and then inflates the balloon in 100-cc increments until it holds 500 cc of air. As he introduces the air, he monitors the intragastric balloon pressure *to make sure the balloon stays inflated.* Then, he clamps the ports. For the Sengstaken-Blakemore or Minnesota tube, the doctor gently pulls on the tube until he feels resistance, *which indicates that the gastric balloon is inflated and exerting pressure on the cardia of the stomach.* When he senses that the balloon is engaged, the doctor places the foam noseguard around the area where the tube emerges from the nostril.
- Be ready to tape the noseguard in place around the tube. *This helps to minimize pressure on the nostril from*

Securing an esophageal tube

To reduce the risk of the gastric balloon's slipping down or away from the cardia of the stomach, secure an esophageal tube to a football helmet. Tape the tube, as shown, to the face guard, and fasten the chin strap.

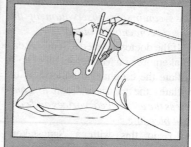

To remove the tube quickly, unfasten the chin strap and pull the helmet slightly forward. Cut the tape and the gastric balloon and esophageal balloon lumens. Be sure to hold onto the tube near the patient's nostril.

the traction and decreases the risk of necrosis.
- With the noseguard secured, traction can be applied to the tube with a traction rope and a 1-lb weight, or the tube can be pulled gently and taped securely to the face guard of a football helmet. (See *Securing an esophageal tube.*)
- With pulley-and-weight traction, lower the head of the bed to about 25 degrees *to produce countertraction.*
- Lavage the stomach through the gastric aspiration lumen with normal sa-

line solution (iced or tepid) until the return fluid is clear. *The vasoconstriction thus achieved stops the hemorrhage; the lavage empties the stomach. Any blood detected later in the gastric aspirate indicates that bleeding remains uncontrolled.*

• Attach one of the suction sources to the gastric aspiration lumen. *This empties the stomach, helps prevent nausea and possible vomiting, and allows continuous observation of the gastric contents for blood.*

• If the doctor inserted a Sengstaken-Blakemore or a Minnesota tube, he'll inflate the esophageal balloon as he inflates the gastric balloon *to compress the esophageal varices and control bleeding.*

• To do this with a Sengstaken-Blakemore tube, attach the Y-connector tube to the esophageal lumen. Then, attach a sphygmomanometer inflation bulb to one end of the Y-connector and the manometer to the other end. Inflate the esophageal balloon until the gauge shows a pressure between 30 and 40 mm Hg. Then clamp the tube.

• To do this with a Minnesota tube, attach the mercury manometer to the esophageal pressure-monitoring outlet. Then, using the 60-ml syringe and pushing the air slowly into the esophageal balloon port, inflate the balloon until the gauge indicates a pressure between 35 and 45 mm Hg.

• Set up esophageal suction *to prevent accumulation of secretions that may cause vomiting and pulmonary aspiration.* This is important *because swallowed secretions can't pass into the stomach if the patient has an inflated esophageal balloon in place.* If the patient has a Linton or a Minnesota tube, attach the suction source to the

esophageal aspiration port. If the patient has a Sengstaken-Blakemore tube, advance an NG tube through the other nostril into the esophagus to the point where the esophageal balloon begins, and attach the suction source as ordered.

To remove an esophageal tube

• The doctor deflates the esophageal balloon by aspirating the air with a syringe. (He may order the esophageal balloon to be deflated at 5 mm Hg increments every 30 minutes for several hours.) Then if bleeding does not recur, he will remove the traction from the gastric tube and deflate the gastric balloon (also by aspiration). The gastric balloon is always deflated just before removing the tube *because the balloon may ride up into the esophagus or pharynx and obstruct the airway or, possibly, cause asphyxia or rupture.*

• After disconnecting all suction tubes, the doctor gently removes the esophageal tube. If he feels resistance, he aspirates the balloons again. (To remove a Minnesota tube, he grasps it near the patient's nostril and cuts across all four lumens approximately 3″ [7.6 cm] below that point. This ensures deflation of all balloons.)

• After the tube is removed, assist the patient with mouth care.

Complications

• Erosion and perforation of the esophagus and gastric mucosa may result from the tension placed on these areas by the balloons during traction.

• Esophageal rupture may result if the gastric balloon accidentally inflates in the esophagus.

• Acute airway occlusion may result if the balloon dislodges and moves upward into the trachea.

• Other erosions, nasal tissue necrosis, and aspiration of oral secretions may also complicate the patient's condition.

Nursing considerations

• If the patient appears cyanotic or if other signs of airway obstruction develop during tube placement, remove the tube immediately *because it may have entered the trachea instead of the esophagus.*

• After intubation, keep scissors taped to the head of the bed. If respiratory distress occurs, cut across all lumens while holding the tube at the nares, and remove the tube quickly.

• Unless contraindicated, the patient can sip water through a straw during intubation *to facilitate tube advancement.*

• Remember: Intraesophageal-balloon pressure varies with respirations and esophageal contractions. Baseline pressure is the important pressure.

• The balloon on the Linton tube should stay inflated no longer than 24 hours *because necrosis of the cardia may result.* To check for rebleeding, the doctor usually removes the tube only after a trial period (at least 12 hours) with the esophageal balloon deflated or with the gastric-balloon tension released from the cardia. In some centers, the doctor may deflate the esophageal balloon for 5 to 10 minutes every hour to temporarily relieve pressure on the esophageal mucosa.

Documentation

• Record the date and time of insertion and removal, the type of tube used, and the name of the doctor who performed the procedure.

• Document the intraesophageal balloon pressure (for the Sengstaken-Blakemore or Minnesota tubes), the intragastric balloon pressure (for the Minnesota tube), or the amount of air injected (for the Linton and the Sengstaken-Blakemore tubes).

• Record the amount of fluid used for gastric irrigation and the color, consistency, and amount of gastric returns, both before and after lavage.

Eye care, neonatal (Credé's treatment)

Named for its developer, Credé's treatment prevents damage and blindness from conjunctivitis caused by Neisseria gonorrhoeae and transmitted during birth by a mother who has gonorrhea. It's also used to treat chlamydial conjunctivitis transmitted during birth.

Required by law in all states in the United States, the treatment consists of instilling 1% silver nitrate solution into the neonate's eyes. Most states permit alternative treatment with 1% tetracycline ointment or 0.5% erythromycin ophthalmic ointment. By this method, the neonate may avoid chemical irritation from silver nitrate, yet benefit from the antimicrobial effects of broad-spectrum antibiotics.

The nurse instills the solution or ointment in the conjunctival sac (from the eye's inner canthus to its outer canthus). The treatment, which may cause conjunctival swelling, may also disturb the typically quiet but alert neonate at birth. So, although silver ni-

How to instill medication for Credé's treatment

Using your nondominant hand, gently raise the neonate's upper eyelid with your index finger, and pull down the lower eyelid with your thumb.

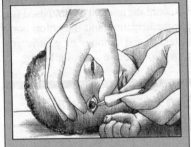

Using your dominant hand, instill two drops of silver nitrate solution into the lower conjunctival sac, or apply the ordered ophthalmic antibiotic ointment in a line along the lower conjunctival sac.

Repeat the procedure for the other eye.

trate treatment is usually given at delivery, it can be delayed for up to 1 hour to allow initial parent-child bonding.

Silver nitrate prophylaxis may be ineffective if the neonate acquires the infection *in utero* after premature rupture of the membranes.

≫ Key nursing diagnoses and patient outcomes

Use this nursing diagnosis as a guide when developing your plan of care for a patient who is receiving Credé's treatment.

Risk for injury related to improper technique

Based on this nursing diagnosis, you'll establish the following patient outcomes. The patient will:
• identify factors that increase risk for injury.
• assist in identifying and applying safety measures to prevent injury.

Equipment

♦ silver nitrate ampule or ophthalmic antibiotic ointment, as ordered ♦ sterile needle or pin supplied by silver nitrate manufacturer ♦ gloves ♦ gauze pads.

Equipment preparation

• Puncture one end of the wax silver nitrate ampule with the needle or pin.
• If you're administering ophthalmic antibiotic ointment, remove the cap from the ointment container.
• A single-dose ointment tube should be used *to prevent contamination and spread of infection.*

Implementation

• If the parents are present for the procedure, explain that state law mandates Credé's treatment. Forewarn them that the neonate may cry and that the treatment may irritate his eyes. Reassure them that these are temporary effects.
• Put on gloves. *For comfort and effectiveness,* shield the neonate's eyes from direct light, tilt his head slightly to the side of the intended treatment, and instill the medication. (See *How to instill medication for Credé's treatment.*)
• Close the eyelids and gently massage them *to spread the medication over the eye.*

• Wait 15 seconds after instilling the medication. Then, *to prevent staining the skin,* remove excess silver nitrate with a gauze pad.

Complications
Especially after silver nitrate instillation, chemical conjunctivitis may cause redness, swelling, and drainage.

Nursing considerations
• Instill another drop if the silver nitrate solution touches only the eyelid or eyelid margins *to ensure complete prophylaxis.*
• If chemical conjunctivitis occurs or if the skin around the neonate's eyes discolors, reassure the parents that these temporary effects will subside within a few days.

Documentation
• If you perform Credé's treatment in the delivery room, record the treatment on the delivery room form.
• If you perform Credé's treatment in the nursery, document it in your notes.

Eye care, routine

When paralysis or coma impairs or eliminates the corneal reflex, frequent eye care aims to keep the exposed cornea moist, preventing ulceration and inflammation. Application of saline-saturated gauze pads over the eyelids moistens the eyes. Commercially available eye ointments and artificial tears also lubricate the corneas, but a doctor's order is required for their use.

Although eye care isn't a sterile procedure, asepsis should be maintained as much as possible.

⟫ Key nursing diagnoses and patient outcomes
Use these nursing diagnoses as a guide when developing your plan of care for a patient who is receiving routine.

Knowledge deficit related to lack of exposure to the procedure
Based on this nursing diagnosis, you'll establish the following patient outcomes. The patient will:
• state or demonstrate understanding of what has been taught.
• demonstrate ability to perform new health-related behaviors as they are taught.

Risk for injury related to improper technique
Based on this nursing diagnosis, you'll establish the following patient outcomes. The patient will:
• identify factors that increase risk for injury.
• assist in identifying and applying safety measures to prevent injury.

Equipment
♦ sterile basin ♦ gloves ♦ sterile towel ♦ sterile normal saline solution ♦ sterile cotton balls ♦ mineral oil ♦ artificial tears or eye ointment (if ordered) ♦ gauze or eye pads ♦ hypoallergenic tape.

Equipment preparation
• Assemble the equipment at the patient's bedside.
• Pour a small amount of saline solution into the basin.

Implementation
• Wash your hands thoroughly, put on gloves, and tell the patient what you're

about to do, even if he is comatose or appears unresponsive.

• *To remove secretions or crusts adhering to the eyelids and eyelashes,* first soak a cotton ball in sterile normal saline solution. Then gently wipe the patient's eye with the moistened cotton ball, working from the inner canthus to the outer canthus *to prevent debris and fluid from entering the nasolacrimal duct.*

• *To prevent cross-contamination,* use a fresh cotton ball for each wipe until the eye is clean. To prevent irritation, avoid using soap for cleaning the eyes. Repeat the procedure for the other eye.

• After cleaning the eyes, instill artificial tears or apply eye ointment, as ordered, *to keep them moist.*

• Close the patient's eyelids. Dab a small amount of mineral oil on each lid *to lubricate and protect fragile skin.*

• Soak gauze or eye pads in sterile normal saline solution, place them over the eyelids, and secure with hypoallergenic tape. Change gauze pads, as necessary, *to keep them well saturated.*

• After giving eye care, cover the basin with a sterile towel and dispose of gloves. Change the setup (basin, towel, and normal saline solution) at least daily.

Nursing considerations

• *For comfort and to avoid startling the patient,* place the closed bottle of normal saline solution under a stream of warm (not hot) water.

Documentation

• Record the time and type of eye care in your notes.

• If applicable, chart administration of eyedrops or ointment in the patient's medication record.

• Document unusual crusting or excessive or colored drainage.

Eye medication application

Eye medications — drops, ointments, and disks — serve diagnostic and therapeutic purposes. During an eye examination, eyedrops can be used to anesthetize the eye, dilate the pupil to facilitate examination, and to stain the cornea to identify corneal abrasions, scars, or other anomalies. Eye medications can also be used to lubricate the eye, treat certain eye conditions (such as glaucoma and infections), protect the vision of neonates, and lubricate the eye socket for insertion of a prosthetic eye.

Understanding the ocular effects of medications is important because certain drugs may cause eye disorders or have serious ocular effects. For example, anticholinergics, which are often used during eye examinations, can precipitate acute glaucoma in patients with a predisposition to the disorder.

›› Key nursing diagnoses and patient outcomes

Use these nursing diagnoses as a guide when developing your plan of care for a patient who is receiving eye medications.

Knowledge deficit related to lack of exposure to the procedure

Based on this nursing diagnosis, you'll establish the following patient outcomes. The patient will:

• state or demonstrate understanding of what has been taught.

• demonstrate ability to perform new health related behaviors as they are taught.

Risk for injury related to improper technique

Based on this nursing diagnosis, you'll establish the following patient outcomes. The patient will:

• identify factors that increase the risk for injury.

• assist in identifying and applying safety measures to prevent injury.

Equipment

♦ prescribed eye medication ♦ patient's medication record and chart ♦ gloves ♦ warm water or normal saline solution ♦ sterile gauze pads ♦ facial tissues ♦ optional: ocular dressing.

Equipment preparation

• Make sure the medication is labeled for ophthalmic use. Then check the expiration date.

• Date the container the first time you use the medication.

• After it's opened, an eye medication may be used for a maximum of 2 weeks *to avoid contamination.*

• Inspect ocular solutions for cloudiness, discoloration, and precipitation, but remember that some eye medications are suspensions and normally appear cloudy.

• Don't use any solution that appears abnormal.

• If the tip of an eye ointment tube has crusted, turn the tip on a sterile gauze pad *to remove the crust.*

Implementation

• Verify the order on the patient's medication record by checking it against the doctor's order.

• Wash your hands.

• Check the medication label against the medication record.

• Make sure you know which eye to treat *because different medications or doses may be ordered for each eye.*

• Confirm the patient's identity by asking him his name and then checking the name, room number, and bed number on his wristband.

• Explain the procedure to the patient and provide privacy. Put on gloves.

• If the patient is wearing an eye dressing, remove it by gently pulling it down and away from his forehead. Be careful not to contaminate your hands.

• Remove any discharge by cleaning around the eye with sterile gauze pads moistened with warm water or normal saline solution. With the patient's eye closed, clean from the inner to the outer canthus, using a fresh sterile gauze pad for each stroke.

• *To remove crusted secretions around the eye,* moisten a gauze pad with warm water or normal saline solution. Ask the patient to close the eye, and then place the gauze pad over it for a minute or two. Remove the pad, and then reapply moist sterile gauze pads, as necessary, until the secretions are soft enough to be removed without traumatizing the mucosa.

• Have the patient sit or lie in the supine position. Instruct him to tilt his head back and toward the side of the affected eye *so excess medication can*

Instilling eye medications

To instill eyedrops, pull the lower lid down to expose the conjunctival sac. Have the patient look up and away, and squeeze the prescribed number of drops into the sac. Release the patient's eyelid and have him blink to distribute the medication.

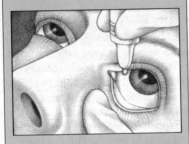

If using an ointment, gently apply a thin strip of the medication along the conjunctival sac from the inner canthus to the outer canthus. Avoid touching the tip of the tube to the patient's eye. Then, release the eyelid and have the patient roll his eye behind closed lids to distribute the medication.

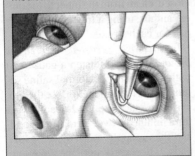

flow away from the tear duct, minimizing systemic absorption through the nasal mucosa.
• Remove the dropper cap from the medication container, if necessary,

and draw the medication into it. Be careful to avoid contaminating the dropper tip or bottle top.
• Before instilling the eyedrops, instruct the patient to look up and away. *This moves the cornea away from the lower lid and minimizes the risk of touching the cornea with the dropper if the patient blinks.*

Instilling eyedrops
• You may steady the hand in which you're holding the dropper by resting it against the patient's forehead. Then, with your other hand, gently pull down the lower lid of the affected eye and instill the drops in the conjunctival sac. Try to avoid placing the drops directly on the eyeball. (See *Instilling eye medications.*)

Applying eye ointment
• Squeeze a small ribbon of medication on the edge of the conjunctival sac from the inner to the outer canthus.
• Cut off the ribbon by turning the tube. If you want, steady the hand holding the medication tube against the patient's forehead or cheek.

Using a medication disk
• A medication disk can release medication in the eye for up to 1 week. Pilocarpine, for example, can be administered this way to treat glaucoma. (For specific instructions, see *How to insert and remove an eye medication disk.*)

After instilling eyedrops or eye ointment
• Instruct the patient to close his eyes gently, without squeezing the lids shut.

How to insert and remove an eye medication disk

Small and flexible, an oval eye medication disk consists of three layers: two soft outer layers and a middle layer containing the medication. Floating between the eyelids and the sclera, the disk stays in the eye while the patient sleeps and even during swimming and athletic activities. The disk frees the patient from having to remember to instill his eyedrops. Once the disk is in place, ocular fluid moistens it, releasing the medication. Eye moisture or contact lenses don't adversely affect the disk. The disk can release medication for up to 1 week before replacement is needed. Pilocarpine, for example, can be administered this way to treat glaucoma.

Contraindications include conjunctivitis, keratitis, retinal detachment, and any condition where constriction of the pupil should be avoided.

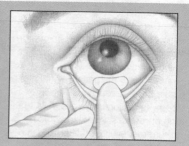

To insert an eye medication disk

Arrange to insert the disk before the patient goes to bed. *This minimizes the blurring that usually occurs immediately after disk insertion.*

• Wash your hands and don gloves.

• Press your fingertip against the oval disk so it lies lengthwise across your fingertip. It should stick to your finger. Lift the disk out of its packet.

• Gently pull the patient's lower eyelid away from the eye and place the disk in the conjunctival sac (as shown above right). It should lie horizontally, not vertically. The disk will adhere to the eye naturally.

• Pull the lower eyelid out, up, and over the disk. Tell the patient to blink several times. If the disk is still visible, pull the lower lid out and over the disk again. Tell the patient that once the disk is in place, he can adjust its position by *gently* pressing his finger against his closed lid. Caution him against rubbing his eye or moving the disk across the cornea.

• If the disk falls out, wash your hands, rinse the disk in cool water, and reinsert it. If the disk appears bent, replace it.

• If both of the patient's eyes are being treated with medication disks, replace both disks at the same time *so that both eyes receive medication at the same rate.*

• If the disk repeatedly slips out of position, reinsert it under the upper eyelid. To do this, gently lift and evert the upper eyelid and insert the disk in the conjunctival sac. Then, gently pull the lid back into position and tell the patient to blink several times. Again, the patient may press gently on the closed eyelid to reposition the disk. The more the patient uses the disk, the easier it should be for him to retain it. If he can't, notify the doctor.

• If the patient will continue therapy with an eye medication disk after

(continued)

How to insert and remove an eye medication disk *(continued)*

discharge, teach him to insert and remove it himself. To check his mastery of these skills, have him demonstrate insertion and removal techniques for you.

• Also, teach the patient about possible adverse reactions. Foreign-body sensation in the eye, mild tearing or redness, increased mucous discharge, eyelid redness, and itching can occur with the use of disks. Blurred vision, stinging, swelling, and headaches can occur with pilocarpine, specifically. Mild symptoms are common but should subside within the first 6 weeks. Tell the patient to report persistent or severe symptoms to his doctor.

To remove an eye medication disk

You can remove an eye medication disk with one or two fingers. To use one finger, put on gloves and evert the lower eyelid to expose the disk. Then use the forefinger of your other hand to slide the disk onto the lid and out of the patient's eye. To use two fingers, evert the lower lid with one hand to expose the disk. Then pinch the disk with the thumb and forefinger of your other hand and remove it from the eye.

• If the disk is located in the upper eyelid, apply long circular strokes to the patient's closed eyelid with your finger until you can see the disk in the corner of the patient's eye. Once the disk is visible, you can place your finger directly on the disk and move it to the lower sclera. Then remove it as you would a disk located in the lower lid.

• If you instilled drops, tell the patient to blink.

• If you applied ointment, tell him to roll his eyes behind closed lids *to help distribute the medication over the surface of the eyeball.*

• Use a clean tissue to remove any excess solution or ointment leaking from the eye. Use a fresh tissue for each eye *to prevent cross-contamination.*

• Apply a new eye dressing if necessary.

• Return the medication to the storage area. Make sure you store it according to the label's instructions.

• Wash your hands.

Complications

• Instillation of some eye medications may cause transient burning, itching, and redness.

• Systemic effects rarely occur.

Nursing considerations

• When administering an eye medication that may be absorbed systemically (such as atropine), gently press your thumb on the inner canthus for 1 to 2 minutes after instilling drops while the patient closes his eyes. *This helps prevent medication from flowing into the tear duct.*

• *To maintain the drug container's sterility,* never touch the tip of the bottle or dropper to the patient's eyeball, lids, or lashes.

• Discard any solution remaining in the dropper before returning the dropper to the bottle. If the dropper or bottle tip has become contaminated, discard it and obtain another sterile dropper.

• *To avoid cross-contamination,* never use a container of eye medication for more than one patient.

• Teach the patient to instill eye medications *so that he can continue treatment at home, if necessary.* Review the procedure and ask for a return demonstration.

Documentation

• Record the medication instilled or applied, the eye or eyes treated, and the date, time, and dose.

• Note any adverse effects and the patient's response.

Eye compress application

Whether applied hot or cold, eye compresses are soothing and therapeutic. Hot compresses may be used to relieve discomfort. Because heat increases circulation, which enhances absorption and decreases inflammation, hot compresses promote drainage of superficial infections. On the other hand, cold compresses reduce swelling or bleeding and relieve itching. Because cold numbs sensory fibers, cold compresses may be ordered to ease periorbital discomfort between prescribed doses of pain medication. Typically, a hot or cold compress should be applied for 20-minute periods, four to six times a day. Ocular

infection calls for the use of aseptic technique.

≫ Key nursing diagnoses and patient outcomes

Use these nursing diagnoses as a guide when developing your plan of care for a patient who is receiving eye compresses.

Sensory or perceptual alterations (specify) related to visual changes
Based on this nursing diagnosis, you'll establish the following patient outcomes. The patient will:

• maintain orientation to person, place, and time.

• remain free from injury.

Body image disturbance related to visual impairment
Based on this nursing diagnosis, you'll establish the following patient outcomes. The patient will:

• communicate feelings about change in body image.

• participate in self-care procedures.

Equipment

For hot compresses: ◆ gloves ◆ prescribed solution, usually sterile water or normal saline solution ◆ sterile bowl ◆ sterile $4'' \times 4''$ gauze pads ◆ towel.

For cold compresses: ◆ small plastic bag (such as a sandwich bag) or glove ◆ ice chips ◆ $\frac{1}{2}''$ (1.3 cm) hypoallergenic tape ◆ towel ◆ sterile $4'' \times 4''$ gauze pads ◆ sterile water, normal saline solution, or prescribed ophthalmic irrigant ◆ gloves.

Equipment preparation

For hot compresses: Place a capped bottle of sterile water or normal saline solution in a bowl of hot water or under a stream of hot, tap water. Allow the solution to become warm, not hot (no higher than 120° F [49° C]). Pour the warm water or saline solution into a sterile bowl, filling the bowl about halfway. Place some sterile gauze pads in the bowl.

For cold compresses: Place ice chips in a plastic bag (or a glove if necessary) to make an ice pack. Keep the ice pack small to avoid excessive pressure on the eye. Remove excess air from the bag or glove and knot the open end. Cut a piece of hypoallergenic tape to secure the ice pack. Place all equipment on the bedside stand near the patient.

Patient preparation

• Explain the procedure to the patient, make him comfortable, and provide privacy.

• When applying hot compresses, have the patient sit, if possible. When applying cold compresses, have the patient lie in a supine position. Support his head with a pillow, and turn his head slightly to the unaffected side. This position will help to hold the compress in place.

• If the patient has an eye patch, remove it.

• Drape a towel around the patient's shoulders *to catch any spills.* Wash your hands, and put on gloves.

Implementation

Follow the steps below to apply hot or cold compresses.

To apply hot compresses

• Take two 4″ × 4″ gauze pads from the basin. Squeeze out the excess solution.

• Instruct the patient to close his eyes. Gently apply the pads — one on top of the other — to the affected eye. (If the patient complains that the compress feels too hot, remove it immediately.)

• Change the compress every few minutes, as necessary, for the prescribed length of time. After removing each compress, check the skin for signs that the compress solution is too hot.

To apply cold compresses

• Moisten the middle of one of the sterile 4″ × 4″ gauze pads with the sterile water, normal saline solution, or ophthalmic irrigating solution. *This helps to conduct the cold from the ice pack.* Keep the edges dry *so that they can absorb excess moisture.*

• Tell the patient to close his eyes; then place the moist gauze pad over the affected eye.

• Place the ice pack on top of the gauze pad and tape it in place. If he complains of pain, remove the ice pack. Some patients may have an adverse reaction to cold.

• After 15 to 20 minutes, remove the tape, ice pack, and gauze pad and discard them.

To conclude the procedure

• Use the remaining sterile 4″ × 4″ gauze pads to clean and dry the patient's face.

• If ordered, apply ophthalmic ointment or an eye patch. (See *Applying an eye patch.*)

Nursing considerations

• When applying hot compresses, change the prescribed solution as fre-

Applying an eye patch

With a doctor's order, you may apply an eye patch for various reasons: to protect the eye after injury or surgery, to prevent accidental damage to an anesthetized eye, to promote healing, to absorb secretions, or to prevent the patient from touching or rubbing his eye.

A thicker patch, called a pressure patch, may be used to help corneal abrasions heal, compress postoperative edema, or control hemorrhage from traumatic injury. Application requires an ophthalmologist's prescription and supervision.

To apply a patch, choose a gauze pad of appropriate size for the patient's face, place it gently over the closed eye.

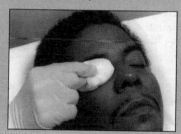

Secure the patch with two or three strips of tape. Extend the tape from midforehead across the eye to below the earlobe. A pressure patch, which is markedly thicker than a single-thickness gauze patch, exerts extra tension against the closed eye. After placing the initial gauze

pad, you'll need to build it up with additional gauze pieces (as shown below). Tape it firmly so that the patch exerts even pressure against the closed eye.

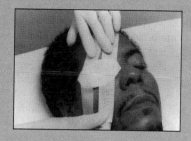

For increased protection of an injured eye, you should place a plastic or metal shield (as shown below) on top of the gauze pads and apply tape over the shield.

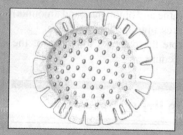

Occasionally, you may use a head dressing to secure a pressure patch. The dressing applies additional pressure or, in burn patients, holds the patch in place without tape.

quently as necessary to maintain a constant temperature.
• If ordered to apply moist, cold compresses directly to the patient's eyelid, fill a bowl with ice and water and soak $4'' \times 4''$ gauze pads in it. Place a compress directly on the lid; change compresses every 2 to 3 minutes.
• Cold compresses are contraindicated in treating eye inflammation, such as keratitis or iritis, *because the cap-*

illary constriction inhibits delivery of nutrients to the cornea.

Home care
• When teaching a patient to apply warm compresses at home, explain that he can substitute a clean bowl and washcloth for the sterile equipment.
• If both eyes are infected, emphasize the importance of using separate equipment for each eye.
• Inform the patient that this will keep him from passing infection back and forth between eyes.
• Direct the patient to wash his hands thoroughly after treating each eye.

Documentation
• Record the time and duration of the procedure.
• Describe the eye's appearance before and after treatment.
• Name any ointments (and amounts) or dressings applied to the eye.
• Note the patient's tolerance of the procedure.

Eye irrigation

Used mainly to flush secretions, chemicals, and foreign bodies from the eye, eye irrigation also provides a way to administer medications for corneal and conjunctival disorders. In an emergency, tap water may serve as an irrigant.

The amount of solution needed to irrigate an eye depends on the contaminant. Secretions require a moderate volume; major chemical burns require a copious amount. Usually, an I.V. bottle or bag of normal saline solution (with I.V. tubing attached) supplies enough solution for continuous irrigation of a chemical burn. (See *Three devices for eye irrigation.*)

≫ Key nursing diagnoses and patient outcomes
Use these nursing diagnoses as a guide when developing your plan of care for a patient who's undergoing eye irrigation.

Risk for infection related to (specify)
Based on this nursing diagnosis, you'll establish the following patient outcomes. The patient will:
• be free from temperature elevation.
• identify signs and symptoms of infection.

Risk for injury related to (specify)
Based on this nursing diagnosis, you'll establish the following patient outcomes. The patient will:
• be free from injury.
• practice safety and take safety precautions.

Equipment
♦ gloves ♦ goggles ♦ towels ♦ eyelid retractor ♦ cotton balls or facial tissues ♦ optional: litmus paper, proparacaine hydrochloride topical anesthetic.

For moderate-volume irrigation: ♦ prescribed sterile ophthalmic irrigant ♦ cotton-tipped applicators.

For copious irrigation: ♦ one or more 1,000-ml bottles or bags of normal saline solution ♦ standard I.V. infusion set without needle.

Commercially prepared bottles of sterile ophthalmic irrigant are available. All solutions should be at body temperature: 98.6° F (37° C).

Three devices for eye irrigation

Depending on the type and extent of injury, the patient's eye may need to be irrigated using different devices.

Squeeze bottle

For moderate-volume irrigation — to remove eye secretions, for example — apply sterile ophthalmic irrigant to the eye directly from the squeeze bottle container. Direct the stream at the inner canthus and position the patient so the stream washes across the cornea and exits at the outer canthus.

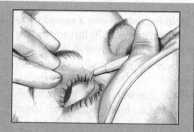

Morgan lens

Connected to irrigation tubing, a Morgan lens permits continuous lavage and also delivers medication to the eye. Use an adapter to connect the lens to the I.V. tubing and the solution container. Begin the irrigation at the prescribed flow rate. To insert the device, ask the patient to look down as you insert the lens under the upper eyelid. Then have her look up as you retract and release the lower eyelid over the lens.

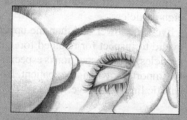

I.V. tube

For copious irrigation — to treat chemical burns, for example — set up an I.V. bag and tubing without a needle. Use the procedure described for moderate irrigation to flush the eye for at least 15 minutes.

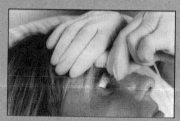

Equipment preparation

• Read the label on the sterile ophthalmic irrigant. Double-check its sterility, strength, and expiration date.

• *For moderate-volume irrigation:* Remove the cap from the irrigant container, and place the container within easy reach. (Be sure to keep the tip of the container sterile.)

• *For copious irrigation:* Use sterile technique to set up the I.V. tubing and the bag or bottle of normal saline solution. Hang the container on an I.V. pole, fill the I.V. tubing with the solution, and adjust the drip regulator valve *to ensure an adequate but not forceful flow.* Place all other equipment within easy reach.

Patient preparation

• Explain the procedure to the patient.

• If the patient has a chemical burn, ease his anxiety by explaining that irrigation prevents further damage.
• Help the patient into a supine position. Turn his head slightly toward the affected side *to prevent solution flowing over his nose and into the other eye.*
• Place a towel under the patient's head, and let him hold another towel against his affected side *to catch excess solution.*

Implementation

• Wash your hands, and put on gloves and goggles.
• Using the thumb and index finger of your nondominant hand, separate the patient's eyelids.
• If ordered, instill proparacaine hydrochloride eyedrops *as a comfort measure.* Use them only once *because repeated use retards healing.*
• *To irrigate the conjunctival cul-de-sac,* continue holding the eyelids apart with your thumb and index finger.
• *To irrigate the upper eyelid (the superior fornix)* use an eyelid retractor. Steady the hand holding the retractor by resting it on the patient's forehead. *The retractor prevents the eyelid from closing involuntarily when solution touches the cornea and conjunctiva.*

Moderate irrigation

• Holding the bottle of sterile ophthalmic irrigant about 1″ from the eye, direct a constant, gentle stream at the inner canthus *so that the solution flows across the cornea to the outer canthus.*
• Evert the lower eyelid and then the upper eyelid to inspect for retained foreign particles.

• Remove any foreign particles by gently touching the conjunctiva with sterile, wet, cotton-tipped applicators. Do not touch the cornea.
• Resume irrigating the eye until it's clean of all visible foreign particles.

Copious irrigation

• Hold the control valve on the I.V. tubing about 1″ above the eye, and direct a constant, gentle stream of normal saline solution at the inner canthus so that the solution flows across the cornea to the outer canthus.
• Ask the patient to rotate his eye periodically while you continue the irrigation. This action may dislodge foreign particles.
• Evert the lower and then the upper eyelid to inspect for retained foreign particles. (This inspection is especially important when the patient has caustic lime in his eye.)

Aftercare

• After eye irrigation, gently dry the eyelids with cotton balls or facial tissues, wiping from the inner to the outer canthus. Use a new cotton ball or tissue for each wipe. *This reduces the patient's need to rub his eye.*
• Remove and discard your gloves and goggles.
• When indicated, arrange for follow-up care.
• Wash your hands *to avoid burning from residual chemical contaminants.*

Nursing considerations

• When irrigating both eyes, have the patient tilt his head toward the side being irrigated to avoid cross-contamination.
• For chemical burns, irrigate each eye for at least 15 minutes with normal

saline solution *to dilute and wash out the harsh chemical.* If the patient can't identify the specific chemical, use litmus paper *to determine if the chemical is acidic or alkaline, or to be sure that the eye has been irrigated adequately.* (After irrigating any chemical, note the time, date, and chemical for your own reference *in case you develop contact dermatitis.*)

Documentation

• Note the duration of irrigation, the type and amount of solution, and characteristics of the drainage.
• Record your assessment of the patient's eye before and after irrigation.
• Note the patient's response to the procedure.

F

Fecal impaction removal

Fecal impaction—large, hard, dry mass of stool in the folds of the rectum and, at times, in the sigmoid colon—results from prolonged retention and accumulation of stool. Common causes include poor bowel habits, inactivity, dehydration, improper diet (especially inadequate fluid intake), constipation-inducing drugs, and incomplete bowel cleaning after a barium enema or barium swallow. Digital removal of fecal impaction, which is used when oil retention and cleansing enemas, suppositories, and laxatives fail to clear the impaction, may require a doctor's order.

This procedure is contraindicated during pregnancy; after rectal, genitourinary, abdominal, perineal, or gynecologic reconstructive surgery; in patients with myocardial infarction, coronary insufficiency, pulmonary embolus, congestive heart failure, heart block, or Stokes-Adams syndrome (without pacemaker treatment); and in patients with GI or vaginal bleeding, hemorrhoids, rectal polyps, or blood dyscrasia.

>> Key nursing diagnoses and patient outcomes

Use these nursing diagnoses as a guide when developing your plan of care for a patient needing digital removal of fecal impaction.

Constipation related to (specify)
Based on this nursing diagnosis, you'll establish the following patient outcomes. The patient will:
• experience return of normal elimination.
• experience bowel movements every (specify) days without laxatives, enemas, or suppositories.
• state understanding of causative factors of constipation.
• describe changes in personal habits to maintain normal elimination patterns.

Knowledge deficit related to lack of exposure to digital removal of fecal impaction
Based on this nursing diagnosis, you'll establish the following patient outcome. The patient will:
• state understanding of procedure.

Equipment

♦ gloves (2 pairs) ♦ linen-saver pad ♦ bedpan ♦ plastic disposal bag ♦ soap ♦ water-filled basin ♦ towel ♦ water-soluble lubricant ♦ washcloth.

Patient preparation

• Explain the procedure to the patient and provide privacy.
• Position the patient on his left side and flex his knees *to allow easier access to the sigmoid colon and rectum.*
• Drape the patient, and place a linen-saver pad beneath the buttocks *to prevent soiling the bed linens.*

Implementation

• Put on gloves, and moisten an index finger with water-soluble lubricant *to reduce friction during insertion, thereby avoiding injury to sensitive tissue.*

• Instruct the patient to breathe deeply *to promote relaxation.* Then gently insert the lubricated index finger beyond the anal sphincter until you touch the impaction. Rotate the finger gently around the stool *to dislodge and break it into small fragments.* Then work the fragments downward to the end of the rectum, and remove each one separately.

• Before removing the finger, gently stimulate the anal sphincter with a circular motion two or three times *to increase peristalsis and encourage evacuation.*

• Remove the finger and change your gloves. Then clean the anal area with soap, rinse with water, and lightly pat dry with a towel.

• Offer the patient the bedpan or commode *because digital manipulation stimulates the urge to defecate.*

• Place disposable items in the plastic bag, and discard properly. If necessary clean the bedpan, and return it to the bedside stand.

• Wash your hands.

Complications

Digital removal of fecal impaction can stimulate the vagus nerve and may decrease heart rate and cause syncope.

Nursing considerations

• If the patient experiences pain, nausea, rectal bleeding, changes in pulse rate or skin color, diaphoresis, or syncope, stop immediately and notify the doctor.

Documentation

• Record the time and date of the procedure, the patient's response, and stool color, consistency, and odor.

Fecal occult blood tests

Fecal occult blood tests are valuable for determining the presence of occult blood (hidden GI bleeding) and for distinguishing between true melena and melena-like stools. Certain medications, such as iron supplements and bismuth compounds, can darken stools so that they resemble melena.

Two common occult blood screening tests are the Hemoccult slide (filter paper impregnated with guaiac) and the Hematest (an orthotolidin reagent tablet). Both tests produce a blue reaction in a fecal smear if occult blood loss exceeds 5 ml in 24 hours. A newer test, Colocare, requires no fecal smear.

Occult blood tests are particularly important for early detection of colorectal cancer because 80% of patients with this disorder test positive. A single positive test result, however, does not necessarily confirm GI bleeding or indicate colorectal cancer. For a confirmed positive result, the test must be repeated at least three times while the patient follows a meatless, high-residue diet. Still, a confirmed positive test doesn't necessarily indicate colorectal cancer. It does indicate the need for further diagnostic studies; GI bleeding can result from many causes other than cancer, such as ulcers and diverticula. These tests are easily performed on collected specimens or smears from digital rectal examination.

≫ Key nursing diagnoses and patient outcomes

Use these nursing diagnoses as a guide when developing your plan of care for a patient needing fecal occult blood tests.

Knowledge deficit related to lack of exposure to fecal occult blood tests
Based on this nursing diagnosis, you'll establish the following patient outcome. The patient will:
• state the need for performing fecal occult blood tests.

Anxiety related to results of fecal occult blood tests
Based on this nursing diagnosis, you'll establish the following patient outcomes. The patient will:
• verbalize feelings about potential outcome of procedure.
• use available support systems, such as family and significant others.

Equipment
♦ test kit ♦ glass or porcelain plate ♦ tongue blade or other wooden applicator ♦ gloves.

Implementation
• Put on gloves and collect a stool specimen.

Hemoccult slide test
• Open the flap on the slide packet, and use a wooden applicator to apply a thin smear of the stool specimen to the guaiac-impregnated filter paper exposed in box A. Or, after performing a digital rectal examination, wipe the finger you used for examination on a square of the filter paper.
• Apply a second smear from another part of the specimen to the filter paper exposed in box B *because some parts of the specimen may not contain blood.*
• Allow the specimen to dry for 3 to 5 minutes.
• Open the flap at the rear of the slide package, and place two drops of Hemoccult developing solution on the paper over each smear. A blue reaction will appear in 30 to 60 seconds if the test is positive.
• Record the results, and discard the slide package.
• Remove and discard your gloves, and wash your hands thoroughly.

Hematest reagent tablet test
• Use a wooden applicator to smear a bit of the stool specimen on the filter paper supplied with the kit. Or, after performing a digital rectal examination, wipe the finger you used for examination on a square of the filter paper.
• Place the filter paper with the stool smear on a glass plate.
• Remove a reagent tablet from the bottle, and immediately replace the cap tightly. Then, place the tablet in the center of the stool smear on the filter paper.
• Add one drop of water to the tablet, and allow it to soak in for 5 to 10 seconds. Add a second drop, letting it run from the tablet onto the specimen and filter paper. If necessary, tap the plate gently to dislodge any water from the top of the tablet.
• After 2 minutes, the filter paper will turn blue if the test is positive. Do not read the color that appears on the tab-

let itself or develops on the filter paper after the 2-minute period.
• Note the results, and discard the filter paper.
• Remove and discard your gloves, and wash your hands thoroughly.

Nursing considerations
• Make sure stool specimens aren't contaminated with urine, soap solution, or toilet tissue, and test them as soon as possible after collection.
• Test samples from several different portions of the same specimen *because occult blood from the upper GI tract isn't always evenly dispersed throughout the formed stool; likewise, blood from colorectal bleeding may occur mostly on the outer stool surface.*
• Check the condition of the reagent tablets, and note their expiration date. Use only fresh tablets and discard outdated ones. Protect Hematest tablets from moisture, heat, and light.
• If repeated testing is necessary after a positive screening test, explain the test to the patient. Instruct him to maintain a high-fiber diet and to refrain from eating red meat, poultry, fish, turnips, and horseradish for 48 to 72 hours before the test as well as throughout the collection period *because these substances may alter test results.*
• As ordered, have the patient discontinue use of iron preparations, bromides, iodides, rauwolfia derivatives, indomethacin, colchicine, salicylates, potassium, phenylbutazone, oxyphenbutazone, bismuth compounds, steroids, and ascorbic acid for 48 to 72 hours before the test and during it *to ensure accurate test results and to*

Home tests for fecal occult blood

Most fecal occult blood tests require the patient to collect a sample of his stool and smear some of it on a slide. In contrast, some new tests don't require the patient to handle stool, making the procedure safer and simpler. One example is a test called Colocare.

Tell the patient to avoid red meat and vitamin C supplements for 2 days before performing the Colocare test at home. He should check with his doctor about discontinuing any medications before the test. Drugs that may interfere with test results include aspirin, indomethacin, corticosteroids, phenylbutazone, reserpine, dietary supplements, anticancer drugs, and anticoagulants.

Tell the patient to flush the toilet twice just before performing the test to remove any toilet-cleaning chemicals from the tank. Tell him to defecate into the toilet but to throw no toilet paper into the bowl. Within 5 minutes, he should remove the test pad from its pouch and float it printed side up on the surface of the water. Tell him to watch the pad for 15 to 30 seconds for any evidence of blue or green color changes, and have him record the result on the reply card.

Emphasize that he should perform this test with three consecutive bowel movements and then send the completed card to his doctor. However, he should call his doctor immediately if he notes a positive color change in the first test.

avoid possible bleeding that some of these compounds may cause.

Home care
• If the patient will be using the Hemoccult slide packet at home, advise him to complete the label on the slide packet before specimen collection.
• If he'll be using a Colocare test packet, advise him that this test is a preliminary screen for occult blood in his stool. Tell him he won't have to obtain a stool specimen to perform the test, but that he should follow your instructions carefully. (See *Home tests for fecal occult blood*, page 341.)

Documentation
• Record the time and date of the test, the result, and any unusual characteristics of the stool tested.
• Report positive results to the doctor.

Feeding button care

The gastrostomy feeding button serves as an alternative feeding device for an ambulatory patient receiving long-term enteral feedings. Approved by the Food and Drug Administration for 6-month implantation, the feeding button can be used to replace the gastrostomy tube if necessary.

The button has a mushroom dome at one end and two wing tabs and a flexible safety plug at the other. When inserted into an established stoma, the button lies almost flush with the skin, with only the top of the safety plug visible.

The button can usually be inserted into a stoma in less than 15 minutes.

Besides its cosmetic appeal, the device is easily maintained, reduces skin irritation and breakdown, and has a smaller risk of dislodgment and migration than an ordinary feeding tube. A one-way, antireflux valve mounted just inside the mushroom dome prevents accidental leakage of gastric contents. The device usually requires replacement after 3 to 4 months, most often because the antireflux valve wears out.

≫ Key nursing diagnoses and patient outcomes
Use these nursing diagnoses as a guide when developing your plan of care for a patient who needs feeding button care.

Altered nutrition: less than body requirements related to (specify)
Based on this nursing diagnosis, you'll establish the following patient outcomes. The patient will:
• consume at least (specify) calories daily.
• gain (specify) lb weekly or maintain normal body weight.

Impaired skin integrity related to the feeding button
Based on this nursing diagnosis, you'll establish the following patient outcomes. The patient will:
• experience no evidence of skin breakdown at feeding button site.
• communicate understanding of skin care at feeding button site.

Knowledge deficit related to lack of exposure to feeding button care
Based on this nursing diagnosis, you'll establish the following patient outcomes. The patient will:

• verbalize understanding of care of feeding button.

• demonstrate correct procedure for insertion of feeding button.

• verbalize care of skin around feeding button.

• identify available resources that can provide assistance.

Equipment

♦ gastrostomy feeding button of the correct size (all three sizes, if the correct one isn't known) ♦ obturator ♦ water-soluble lubricant ♦ gloves ♦ feeding accessories, including adapter, feeding catheter, food syringe or bag, and formula ♦ catheter clamp ♦ cleaning equipment, including water, a syringe, cotton-tipped applicator, pipe cleaner, and mild soap or povidone-iodine solution ♦ optional: pump to provide continuous infusion over several hours.

Patient preparation

• Explain the insertion, reinsertion, and feeding procedure to the patient.

• Tell him the doctor will perform the initial insertion.

Implementation

• Wash your hands and put on gloves. (See *How to reinsert a gastrostomy feeding button*, page 344.)

• Attach the adapter and feeding catheter to the syringe or feeding bag. Clamp the catheter and fill the syringe or bag and catheter with formula. Refill the syringe before it's empty. *These steps prevent air from entering the stomach and distending the abdomen.*

• Open the safety plug and attach the adapter and feeding catheter to the button. Elevate the syringe or feeding bag above stomach level, and gravity-feed the formula for 15 to 30 minutes, varying the height as needed *to alter the flow rate.* Use a pump for continuous infusion or for feedings lasting several hours.

• After feeding, flush the button with 10 ml of water and clean the inside of the feeding catheter with a cotton-tipped applicator and water *to preserve patency and to dislodge formula or food particles.* Then lower the syringe or bag below stomach level *to allow burping.* Remove the adapter and feeding catheter. The antireflux valve should prevent gastric reflux. Then snap the safety plug in place *to keep the lumen clean and prevent leakage if the antireflux valve fails.* If the patient feels nauseated or vomits after feeding, vent the button with the adapter and feeding catheter *to control emesis.*

• Wash the catheter and syringe or feeding bag in warm soapy water and rinse thoroughly. Clean the catheter and adapter with a pipe cleaner. Rinse well before using for the next feeding. Soak the equipment once a week according to manufacturer's recommendations.

Nursing considerations

• If the button pops out while feeding, reinsert it, estimate the formula already delivered, and resume feeding.

• Once daily, clean the peristomal skin with mild soap and water or povidone-iodine, and let the skin air-dry for 20 minutes, *to avoid skin irritation.* Also clean the site whenever spillage from the feeding bag occurs.

How to reinsert a gastrostomy feeding button

If your patient's gastrostomy feeding button pops out (with coughing for instance), either you or he will need to reinsert the device. Here are some steps to follow.

Prepare the equipment

Collect the feeding button, an obturator, and water-soluble lubricant. Wash the button with soap and water, and rinse it thoroughly if it will be reinserted.

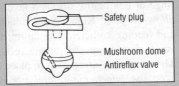

Safety plug
Mushroom dome
Antireflux valve

Insert the button

• Check the depth of the patient's stoma *to make sure you have a feeding button of the correct size*. Then, clean around the stoma.
• Lubricate the obturator with a water-soluble lubricant, and distend the button several times *to ensure patency of the antireflux valve within the button*.
• Lubricate the mushroom dome and the stoma. Gently push the button through the stoma into the stomach.

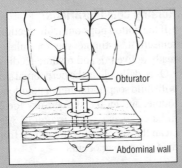

Obturator
Abdominal wall

• Remove the obturator by gently rotating it as you withdraw it, *to keep the antireflux valve from adhering to it*. Gently push the obturator back into the button until the valve closes if the valve sticks.
• After removing the obturator, check the valve to make sure it's closed. Then close the flexible safety plug, which should be relatively flush with the skin surface.

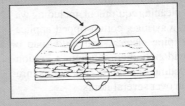

• Open the safety plug and attach the feeding adapter and feeding tube if you need to administer a feeding right away. Deliver the feeding as ordered.

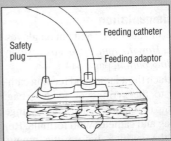

Feeding catheter
Safety plug
Feeding adaptor

Home care
• Before discharge, be sure the patient can insert and care for the gastrostomy feeding button.
• Teach him or a family member how to reinsert the button by first practicing on a model, if necessary.
• Offer written instructions, and answer his questions on obtaining replacement supplies.

Documentation
• Record feeding time and duration, amount and type of feeding formula used, and patient tolerance.
• Maintain intake and output records, as necessary.
• Note the appearance of the stoma and surrounding skin.

Feeding tube insertion and removal

Inserting a feeding tube nasally or (sometimes) orally into the stomach or duodenum allows a patient who can't or won't eat to receive nourishment. The feeding tube also permits supplemental feedings in a patient who has exceptionally high nutritional requirements — an unconscious patient or one with extensive burns, for example. Typically, the procedure is done by a nurse as ordered. The preferred feeding tube route is nasal, but the oral route may be used for patients with such conditions as a deviated septum or a head or nose injury.

The doctor may order duodenal feeding when the patient can't tolerate gastric feeding or when he expects gastric feeding to produce aspiration. Absence of bowel sounds or possible intestinal obstruction contraindicates using a feeding tube.

Feeding tubes differ somewhat from standard nasogastric tubes. Made of silicone, rubber, or polyurethane, feeding tubes have small diameters and great flexibility. This reduces oropharyngeal irritation, necrosis from pressure on the tracheoesophageal wall, distal esophageal irritation, and discomfort from swallowing. To facilitate passage, some feeding tubes are weighted with tungsten, and some need a guide wire to keep them from curling in the back of the throat.

These small-bore tubes usually have radiopaque markings and a water-activated coating, which provides a lubricated surface.

≫ Key nursing diagnoses and patient outcomes
Use these nursing diagnoses as a guide when developing your plan of care for a patient who requires feeding tube insertion and removal.

Altered nutrition: less than body requirements related to (specify)
Based on this nursing diagnosis, you'll establish the following patient outcomes. The patient will:
• tolerate (specify) milliliters of tube feeding.
• avoid aspiration.
• avoid episodes of diarrhea.
• gain (specify) lb weekly.
• communicate understanding of special dietary needs.

Knowledge deficit related to lack of exposure to procedure
Based on this nursing diagnosis, you'll establish the following patient outcomes. The patient will:

- communicate a need to know.
- state understanding of procedure.

Anxiety related to lack of exposure to procedure
Based on this nursing diagnosis, you'll establish the following patient outcomes. The patient will:
- communicate feelings of anxiety about procedure.
- use available support systems, such as family and significant others.

Equipment
For insertion: ♦ feeding tube (#6 to #18 French, with or without guide) ♦ linen-saver pad ♦ gloves ♦ hypoallergenic tape ♦ water-soluble lubricant ♦ cotton-tipped applicators ♦ skin preparation (such as tincture of benzoin) ♦ facial tissues ♦ penlight ♦ small cup of water with straw, or ice chips ♦ emesis basin ♦ 60-ml syringe ♦ stethoscope.
  During use: ♦ mouthwash or saltwater solution ♦ toothbrush.
  For removal: ♦ linen-saver pad ♦ tube clamp ♦ bulb syringe.

Equipment preparation
- Have the proper size tube available. Usually, the doctor orders the smallest-bore tube that will allow free passage of the liquid feeding formula.
- Read the instructions on the tubing package carefully *because tube characteristics vary according to the manufacturer.* (For example, some tubes have marks at the appropriate lengths for gastric, duodenal, and jejunal insertion.)
- Examine the tube *to make sure it's free of defects, such as cracks or rough or sharp edges.* Next, run water through the tube. *This checks for pa-tency, activates the coating, and allows for easier removal of the guide.*

Patient preparation
- Explain the procedure to the patient and show him the tube, *so he knows what to expect and can cooperate more fully.*
- Provide privacy and wash your hands. Put on gloves.
- Assist the patient into semi-Fowler's (or high Fowler's) position.
- Place a linen-saver pad across the patient's chest *to protect him from spills.*
- *To determine the tube length needed to reach the stomach,* first extend the distal end of the tube from the tip of the patient's nose to his earlobe. Coil this portion of the tube around your fingers *so the end will remain curved until you insert it.* Then extend the uncoiled portion from the earlobe to the xiphoid process. Use a small piece of hypoallergenic tape to mark the total length of these two portions.

Implementation
Follow the steps below for inserting or removing a feeding tube.

To insert the tube nasally
- Using the penlight, assess nasal patency.
- Inspect nasal passages for a deviated septum, polyps, or other obstructions. As the patient breathes through his nose, occlude one nostril, then the other, *to determine which has the better airflow.*
- Assess the patient's history of nasal injury or surgery.
- Lubricate the curved tip of the tube (and the feeding tube guide, if appropriate) with a small amount of water-

soluble lubricant *to ease insertion and prevent tissue injury.*

• Ask the patient to hold the emesis basin and facial tissues in case he needs them.

• *To advance the tube,* insert the curved, lubricated tip into the more patent nostril and direct it along the nasal passage toward the ear on the same side. When it passes the nasopharyngeal junction, turn the tube 180 degrees *to aim it downward into the esophagus.* Instruct the patient to lower his chin to his chest *to close the trachea.* Then, give him a small cup of water with a straw or ice chips. Direct him to sip the water or suck on the ice and swallow frequently. *This will ease the tube's passage.* Advance the tube as he swallows.

To insert the tube orally

• Have the patient lower his chin *to close his trachea,* and ask him to open his mouth.

• Place the tip of the tube at the back of the patient's tongue, give water, and instruct the patient to swallow, as above. Remind him to avoid clamping his teeth down on the tube. Advance the tube as he swallows.

To position the tube

• Keep passing the tube until the tape marking the appropriate length reaches the patient's nostril or lips.

• *To check tube placement,* attach the syringe filled with 10 cc of air to the end of the tube. Gently inject the air into the tube as you auscultate the patient's abdomen with the stethoscope about 3″ (7.6 cm) below the sternum. Listen for a whooshing sound, *which signals that the tube has reached its target in the stomach.* If the tube re-

mains coiled in the esophagus, you'll feel resistance when you inject the air, or the patient may belch.

• If you hear the whooshing sound, gently try to aspirate gastric secretions. Successful aspiration confirms correct tube placement. (In some cases, X-rays may be ordered to verify tube placement.) If no gastric secretions return, the tube may be in the esophagus. You'll need to advance the tube or reinsert it before proceeding.

• After confirming proper tube placement, remove the tape marking the tube length.

• Tape the tube to the patient's nose and remove the guide wire.

• *To advance the tube to the duodenum,* especially a tungsten-weighted tube, position the patient on his right side. *This lets gravity assist tube passage through the pylorus.* Move the tube forward 2″ to 3″ (5 to 7.6 cm) hourly until X-ray studies confirm duodenal placement. (An X-ray film must confirm placement before feeding begins *because duodenal feeding can cause nausea and vomiting if accidentally delivered to the stomach.*)

• Apply a skin preparation to the patient's cheek before securing the tube with tape. *This helps the tube adhere to the skin and also prevents irritation.*

• Tape the tube securely to the patient's cheek *to avoid excessive pressure on his nostrils.*

To remove the tube

• Protect the patient's chest with a linen-saver pad.

• Flush the tube with air, clamp or pinch it *to prevent fluid aspiration during withdrawal,* and withdraw it gently but quickly.

• Promptly cover and discard the used tube.

Complications

Prolonged intubation may lead to:
• skin erosion at the nostril.
• sinusitis.
• esophagitis.
• esophagotracheal fistula.
• gastric ulceration.
• pulmonary infection.
• oral infection.

Nursing considerations

• Flush the feeding tube every 8 hours with up to 60 ml of normal saline solution or water *to maintain patency.* Retape the tube at least daily and as needed. Alternate taping the tube toward the inner and outer side of the nose *to avoid constant pressure on the same nasal area.* Inspect the skin for redness and breakdown.

• Provide nasal hygiene daily using the cotton-tipped applicators and water-soluble lubricant *to remove crusted secretions.* Assist the patient with oral hygiene at least twice daily. Help him brush his teeth, gums, and tongue with mouthwash or a mild saltwater solution.

• If the patient can't swallow the feeding tube, use a guide *to aid insertion.*

• Precise feeding tube placement is especially important *because small-bore feeding tubes may slide into the trachea without causing immediate signs or symptoms of respiratory distress, such as coughing, choking, gasping, or cyanosis.* However, the patient will usually cough if the tube enters the larynx. To be sure that the tube clears the larynx, ask the patient to speak. If he can't, the tube is in the larynx. Withdraw the tube at once and reinsert.

• When aspirating gastric contents to check tube placement, pull gently on the syringe plunger *because negative pressure may traumatize the stomach lining or bowel.* If you meet resistance during aspiration, stop the procedure *because resistance may result simply from the tube lying against the stomach wall.* If the tube coils above the stomach, you'll be unable to aspirate stomach contents. To rectify this, change the patient's position or withdraw the tube a few inches, readvance it, and try to aspirate again. If the tube was inserted with a guide wire, do not use the guide wire to reposition the tube. The doctor may do so, using fluoroscopic guidance.

Home care

• If your patient will use a feeding tube at home, make appropriate home care nursing referrals, and teach the patient and caregivers how to use and care for a feeding tube. Help them understand how to obtain equipment, insert and remove the tube, prepare and store feeding formula, and troubleshoot tube position and patency.

Documentation

• For tube insertion, record the date, time, tube type and size, site of insertion, area of placement, and confirmation of proper placement.

• Record the name of the person performing the procedure. For tube removal, record the date and time and describe the patient's tolerance of the procedure.

Fetal monitoring, external

An indirect, noninvasive procedure, external fetal monitoring uses two devices strapped to the mother's abdomen to evaluate fetal well-being during labor.

One device, an ultrasound transducer, transmits high-frequency sound waves through soft body tissues to the fetal heart. The waves rebound from the heart through the abdominal wall, where the transducer relays them to a monitor. The other, a pressure-sensitive tocotransducer, responds to the pressure exerted by uterine contractions and simultaneously records their duration and frequency. (See *Applying external fetal monitoring devices*, page 350.)

The monitoring apparatus traces fetal heart rate (FHR) and uterine contraction data onto the same printout paper.

Indications for external fetal monitoring include high-risk pregnancy, oxytocin-induced labor, and antepartal nonstress and contraction stress tests. Many labor and delivery units use external fetal monitoring for all patients. The procedure has no contraindications, but may be difficult to perform on patients with hydramnios, on obese patients, or on hyperactive or premature fetuses.

≫ Key nursing diagnoses and patient outcomes

Use these nursing diagnoses as a guide when developing your plan of care for a patient who needs external fetal monitoring.

Anxiety related to procedure
Based on this nursing diagnosis, you'll establish the following patient outcomes. The patient will:
• communicate feelings of anxiety.
• utilize available emotional support.
• show decreased signs of anxiety.

Knowledge deficit related to lack of exposure to procedure
Based on this nursing diagnosis, you'll establish the following patient outcomes. The patient will:
• verbalize understanding of procedure.
• recognize that increased knowledge will help her cope better with the procedure.

Equipment
♦ electronic fetal monitor ♦ ultrasound transducer ♦ tocotransducer ♦ conduction gel ♦ transducer straps ♦ damp cloth ♦ printout paper.

Monitoring devices, such as phonotransducers and abdominal electrocardiogram transducers, are commercially available. However, hospitals use these devices less frequently than the ultrasound transducer.

Equipment preparation
• Because fetal monitor features vary, review the operator's manual before proceeding. If the monitor has two paper speeds, select the slower speed (typically 1.2 inches/minute [3 cm/minute]) *to ensure an easy-to-read tracing.* At higher speeds (for example, ¼ inch/minute [1 cm/minute]), the printed tracings are condensed, making results difficult *to decipher and interpret accurately.*
• Next, plug the tocotransducer cable into the uterine activity jack and the

Applying external fetal monitoring devices

To ensure clear tracings that define fetal status and labor progress, be sure to precisely position external monitoring devices, such as an ultrasound transducer and a tocotransducer.

Fetal heart monitor
Palpate the uterus to locate the fetus's back. Place the ultrasound transducer over this site where the fetal heartbeat sounds the loudest, if possible. Then tighten the belt. Use the fetal heart tracing on the monitor strip to validate the transducer's position.

Labor monitor
A tocotransducer records uterine motion during contractions. Place the tocotransducer over the uterine fundus where it contracts, either midline or slightly to one side. Place your hand on the fundus and palpate a contraction to verify proper placement. Secure the tocotransducer's belt; then adjust the pen set so that the baseline values read between 5 and 15 mm Hg on the monitor strip.

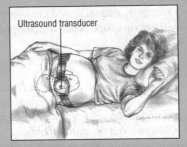

Ultrasound transducer

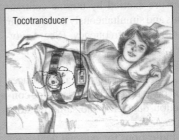

Tocotransducer

ultrasound transducer cable into the phono-ultrasound jack. Attach the straps to the tocotransducer and the ultrasound transducer.

• Label the printout paper with the patient's hospital number or birth date and name, the date, maternal vital signs and position, the paper speed, and the number of the strip paper *to maintain accurate, consecutive monitoring records.*

Patient preparation
• Explain the procedure to the patient, and provide emotional support.

• Inform her that the monitor may make noise if the pen set tracer moves above or below the grids on the printout paper.

• Reassure her that this doesn't indicate fetal distress. As appropriate, explain other aspects of the monitor *to help reduce maternal anxiety about fetal well-being.*

• Make sure the patient has signed a consent form if required.

• Wash your hands, and provide privacy.

Implementation

• Assist the patient to a semi-Fowler's or a left-lateral position with her abdomen exposed. Don't let her lie in a supine position *because pressure from the gravid uterus on the maternal inferior vena cava may cause maternal hypotension, decrease uterine perfusion, and induce fetal hypoxia.*

• Palpate the patient's abdomen to locate the fundus — the area of greatest muscle density in the uterus. Then, using transducer straps, secure the tocotransducer over the fundus.

• Adjust the pen set tracer controls so that the baseline values read between 5 and 15 mm Hg on the monitor strip. *This prevents triggering the alarm that indicates the tracer has dropped below the paper's margins.* The proper setting varies among tocotransducers.

• Apply conduction gel to the ultrasound transducer crystals *to promote an airtight seal and optimal soundwave transmission.*

• Use Leopold's maneuvers to palpate the fetal back, through which fetal heart tones resound most audibly.

• Start the monitor. Then apply the ultrasound transducer directly over the site having the strongest heart tones.

• Activate the control that begins the printout. On the printout paper, note any coughing, position changes, drug administration, vaginal examinations, and blood pressure readings, which can affect interpretation of the tracings.

• Explain to the patient and her support person how to time and control contractions with the monitor. To time contractions, inform them that the distance from one dark vertical line to the next on the printout grid represents 1 minute. The support person can use this information to prepare the patient for the onset of a contraction and to guide and slow her breathing as the contraction subsides.

To monitor the patient

• Observe the tracings *to identify frequency and duration of uterine contractions,* but palpate the uterus *to determine intensity of contractions.*

• Mentally note the baseline FHR — the rate between contractions — *to compare with suspicious-looking deviations.* FHR normally ranges from 120 to 160 beats/minute.

• Assess periodic accelerations or decelerations from the baseline FHR. Compare the FHR patterns with those of the uterine contractions. Note the time relationship between the onset of an FHR deceleration and the onset of a uterine contraction, the time relationship of the lowest level of an FHR deceleration to the peak of a uterine contraction, and the range of FHR deceleration. *These data help distinguish fetal distress from benign head compression.*

• Move the tocotransducer and the ultrasound transducer *to accommodate changes in maternal or fetal position.* Readjust both transducers every hour and assess the patient's skin for reddened areas caused by the strap pressure. Document skin condition.

• Clean the ultrasound transducer periodically with a damp cloth *to remove dried conduction gel that can interfere with ultrasound transmission.* Apply fresh gel, as necessary. After use, place the cover over the ultrasound transducer.

TECHNOLOGY UPDATE

Portable Doppler stethoscope monitors fetal heart sounds

Monitoring fetal heart sounds is easier with this Doppler ultrasound unit, the Sonicaid 121 from Oxford Instruments. Self-contained, the palm-sized unit requires no attachments such as cables. Two standard AA penlight batteries give the unit enough power for 1,500 two-minute tests.

The device provides a digital display of fetal heart rate, a "freeze" button to hold the reading until it's recorded, and an automatic shutoff to save power. A 10-second manual count mode can also be used. The Sonicaid 121 filters out background noise to provide a clear sound that both the mother and examiner can hear. A waterproof model is also available.

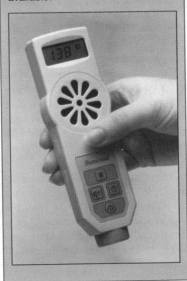

Nursing considerations

• If the monitor fails to record uterine activity, palpate for contractions.

• Check for equipment problems as the manufacturer directs and readjust the tocotransducer.

• If the patient reports discomfort in the position that provides the clearest signal, try to obtain a satisfactory 5- or 10-minute tracing with the patient in this position before assisting her to a more comfortable position.

• As the patient progresses through labor and abdominal pressure increases, the pen set tracer may exceed the alarm boundaries.

• Be aware that a new device, the portable ultrasound stethoscope, allows easier monitoring of fetal heart sounds. (See *Portable Doppler stethoscope monitors fetal heart sounds.*)

Documentation

• Check to be sure you numbered each monitor strip in sequence and labeled each printout sheet with the patient's hospital number or birth date and name, the date, the time, and the paper speed.

• Record the time of any vaginal examinations, membrane rupture, drug administration, and maternal or fetal movements.

• Record maternal vital signs and the intensity of uterine contractions.

• Document each time that you moved or readjusted the tocotransducer and ultrasound transducer, and summarize this information in your notes.

Fetal monitoring, internal electronic

Also called direct fetal monitoring, this sterile, invasive procedure uses a spiral electrode and an intrauterine catheter to evaluate fetal status during labor. By providing an electrocardiogram (ECG) of the fetal heart rate (FHR), internal electronic fetal monitoring (EFM) assesses fetal response to uterine contractions more accurately than does external EFM. It precisely measures intrauterine pressure, tracks labor progress, and allows evaluation of short- and long-term FHR variability.

Internal EFM is indicated whenever direct, beat-to-beat FHR monitoring is required. Specific indications include maternal diabetes or hypertension, fetal postmaturity, suspected intrauterine growth retardation, and meconium-stained fluid. However, internal EFM is performed only if the amniotic sac has ruptured, the cervix is dilated at least 2 cm, and the presenting part of the fetus is at least at the −1 station.

Contraindications of internal EFM include maternal blood dyscrasia, suspected fetal immune deficiency, placenta previa, face presentation or uncertainty about the presenting part, and cervical or vaginal herpetic lesions.

A spiral electrode is the most commonly used device for internal EFM. Shaped like a corkscrew, the electrode is attached to the presenting fetal part (usually the scalp). It detects the fetal heartbeat and then transmits it to the monitor, which converts the signals to a fetal ECG waveform.

A pressure-sensitive catheter, called an Intran catheter, though not as widely used as the tocotransducer, is the most accurate method of determining the true intensity of contractions. It's especially helpful in dysfunctional labor and in preventing or rapidly determining the need for a cesarean section, but the risk of infection or uterine perforation associated with this device is high.

⟫ Key nursing diagnoses and patient outcomes

Use these nursing diagnoses as a guide when developing your plan of care for a patient who needs internal electronic fetal monitoring.

Anxiety related to invasive procedure and potential outcomes
Based on this nursing diagnosis, you'll establish the following patient outcomes. The patient will:
• verbalize feelings of anxiety.
• use available emotional support.
• show fewer signs of anxiety.
• identify positive aspects of her efforts to cope during childbirth.

Knowledge deficit related to lack of exposure to invasive procedure
Based on this nursing diagnosis, you'll establish the following patient outcomes. The patient will:
• verbalize understanding of invasive procedure.
• demonstrate ability to perform skills needed for coping with labor.

Equipment
♦ electronic fetal monitor and operator's manual   ♦ spiral electrode and

a drive tube ♦ disposable leg plate pad or reusable leg plate with Velcro belt ♦ conduction gel ♦ antiseptic solution ♦ hypoallergenic tape ♦ two pairs of sterile gloves ♦ Intran catheter connection cable and pressure-sensitive catheter ♦ graph paper.

Equipment preparation

• Be sure to review the operator's manual before using the equipment.
• If the monitor has two paper speeds, set it at 3 cm/minute *to ensure a readable tracing.* A tracing at 1 cm/minute is more condensed and harder to interpret accurately.
• Connect the Intran cable to the uterine activity outlet on the monitor.
• Wash your hands and open the sterile equipment, maintaining aseptic technique.

Patient preparation

• Describe the procedure to the patient and her partner, if present, and explain how the equipment works. Tell the patient that a doctor or specially trained nurse will perform a vaginal examination to identify the position of the fetus.
• Before internal EFM, make sure that the patient is fully informed about the procedure, and obtain a signed consent form.

Implementation

• Label the printout paper with the patient's hospital number or name and birth date, the date, the paper speed, and the number on the monitor strip.

To monitor contractions

• Assist the patient into the lithotomy position for a vaginal examination. The doctor puts on sterile gloves.

• Attach the connection cable to the outlet on the monitor marked UA (uterine activity). Connect the cable to the Intran catheter. Next, zero the catheter with a gauge provided on the distal end of the catheter. *This will help determine the resting tone of the uterus, usually 5 to 15 mm Hg.*
• Cover the patient's perineum with a sterile drape, if hospital policy so dictates. Then clean the perineum with antiseptic solution, according to hospital policy. Using aseptic technique, the doctor inserts the catheter into the uterine cavity while performing a vaginal examination. The catheter is advanced to the black line on the catheter and secured with hypoallergenic tape along the inner thigh.
• Observe the monitoring strip *to verify proper placement of the catheter guide and to ensure a clear tracing.* Periodically evaluate the monitoring strip to determine the exact amount of pressure exerted with each contraction. Note all such data on the monitoring strip and on the patient's medical record.
• The Intran catheter is usually removed during the second stage of labor or at the doctor's discretion. Dispose of the catheter, and clean and store the cable according to hospital policy. (See *Applying an internal electronic fetal monitor.*)

To monitor FHR

• Apply conduction gel to the leg plate. Then secure the leg plate to the patient's inner thigh with Velcro straps or 2″ tape. Connect the leg plate cable to the ECG outlet on the monitor.
• Inform the patient that she'll undergo a vaginal examination to identify the fetal presenting part (which is usu-

Applying an internal electronic fetal monitor

During internal electronic fetal monitoring, a spiral electrode monitors the fetal heart rate (FHR), and an internal catheter monitors uterine contractions.

Monitoring FHR

The spiral electrode is inserted after a vaginal examination determines the position of the fetus. As shown below, the electrode is attached to the presenting fetal part, usually the scalp or buttocks.

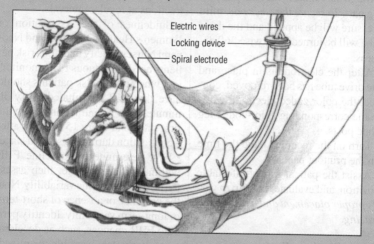

Electric wires
Locking device
Spiral electrode

Monitoring uterine contractions

The intrauterine catheter is inserted up to a premarked level on the tubing and then connected to a monitor that interprets uterine contraction pressures.

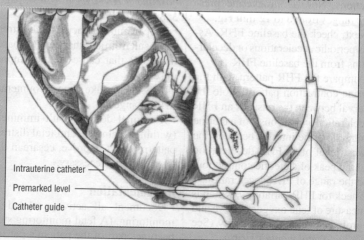

Intrauterine catheter
Premarked level
Catheter guide

ally the scalp or buttocks), to determine the level of fetal descent, and to apply the electrode. Explain that this examination is done to ensure that the electrode is not attached to the suture lines, fontanels, face, or genitalia of the fetus. The spiral electrode will be placed in a drive tube and advanced through the vagina to the fetal presenting part. *To secure the electrode,* mild pressure will be applied and the drive tube will be turned clockwise 360 degrees.

• After the electrode is in place and the drive tube has been removed, connect the color-coded electrode wires to the corresponding color-coded leg plate posts.

• Turn on the recorder. Note the time on the printout paper.

• Assist the patient to a comfortable position, and evaluate the strip *to verify proper placement and a clear FHR tracing.*

To monitor the patient

• Begin by noting the frequency, duration, and intensity of uterine contractions. Normal intrauterine pressure ranges from 8 to 12 mm Hg.

• Next, check the baseline FHR. Assess periodic accelerations or decelerations from the baseline FHR.

• Compare the FHR pattern with the uterine contraction pattern. Note the interval between the onset of an FHR deceleration and the onset of a uterine contraction; the interval between the lowest level of an FHR deceleration and the peak of a uterine contraction; and the range of FHR deceleration.

• Check for FHR variability, which is a measure of fetal oxygen reserve and neurologic integrity and stability. (See *Reading a fetal monitor strip.*)

Complications

• Maternal complications of internal EFM may include uterine perforation and intrauterine infection.

• Fetal complications may include abscess, hematoma, and infection

Nursing considerations

• Interpret the FHR and uterine contractions at regular intervals.

• Guidelines of the Association of Women's Health, Obstetric, and Neonatal Nurses specify that high-risk patients need continuous FHR monitoring, whereas low-risk patients should have the FHR auscultated every 30 minutes after a contraction during the first stage and every 15 minutes after a contraction during the second stage.

• First determine the baseline FHR within 10 beats/minute; then assess the degree of baseline variability. Note the presence or absence of short-term or long-term variability. Identify periodic FHR changes, such as decelerations (early, late, variable, or mixed) or nonperiodic changes such as a sinusoidal pattern. (See *Identifying baseline FHR irregularities,* pages 358 to 361.)

• Keep in mind that acute fetal distress can result from any change in the baseline FHR that causes fetal compromise.

• If necessary, take steps to counteract FHR changes.

• If vaginal delivery isn't imminent (within 30 minutes) and fetal distress patterns don't improve, cesarean delivery will be necessary.

Documentation

• Document all activity related to monitoring. (A fetal monitoring strip becomes part of the patient's perma-

Reading a fetal monitor strip

Presented in two parallel recordings, the fetal monitor strip records the fetal heart rate (FHR) in beats/minute in the top recording and uterine activity (UA) in mm Hg in the bottom recording. You can obtain information on fetal status and labor progress by reading the strips horizontally and vertically.

Reading horizontally on the FHR or the UA strip, each small block represents 10 seconds. Six consecutive small blocks, separated by a dark vertical line, represent 1 min-

ute. Reading vertically on the FHR strip, each block represents an amplitude of 10 beats/minute. Reading vertically on the UA strip, each block represents 5 mm Hg of pressure.

Assess the baseline FHR — the "resting" heart rate — between uterine contractions when fetal movement diminishes. This baseline FHR (normal range: 120 to 160 beats/minute) pattern serves as a reference for subsequent FHR tracings produced during contractions.

Baseline fetal heart rate

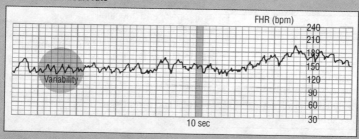

Uterine activity

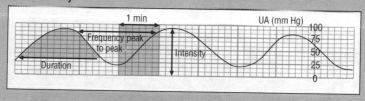

nent record, so it's considered a legal document.)
• Be sure to document the type of monitoring your patient receives and all interventions.
• Identify the monitoring strip with the patient's name, her doctor's name, your name, and the date and time.
• Note the paper speed.

• Record the patient's vital signs at regular intervals.
• Note her pushing efforts and record any change in her position.
• Document any I.V. line insertion and any changes in the I.V. solution or infusion rate.
• Note the use of oxytocin, regional anesthetics, or other medications.

Identifying baseline FHR irregularities

IRREGULARITY	POSSIBLE CAUSES
Baseline tachycardia beats/minute 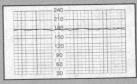	• Early fetal hypoxia • Maternal fever • Parasympathetic agents, such as atropine and scopolamine • Beta-adrenergics, such as ritodrine and terbutaline • Amnionitis (inflammation of inner layer of fetal membrane, or amnion) • Maternal hyperthyroidism • Fetal anemia • Fetal heart failure • Fetal arrhythmias
Baseline bradycardia beats/minute 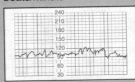	• Late fetal hypoxia • Beta-adrenergic blocking agents such as propranolol and anesthetics • Maternal hypotension • Prolonged umbilical cord compression • Fetal congenital heart block
Early decelerations beats/minute 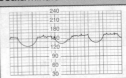 mm Hg 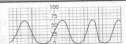	• Fetal head compression
Late decelerations beats/minute 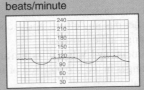	• Uteroplacental circulatory insufficiency (placental hypoperfusion) caused by decreased intervillous blood flow during contractions or a structural placental defect, such as abruptio placentae • Uterine hyperactivity caused by excessive oxytocin infusion • Maternal hypotension • Maternal supine hypotension

Identifying baseline FHR irregularities *(continued)*

CLINICAL SIGNIFICANCE	NURSING INTERVENTIONS
Persistent tachycardia without periodic changes usually doesn't adversely affect fetal well-being — especially when associated with maternal fever. However, tachycardia is an ominous sign when associated with late decelerations, severe variable decelerations, or lack of variability.	Intervene to alleviate the cause of fetal distress and provide supplemental oxygen, as ordered. Also administer I.V. fluids as prescribed. Discontinue oxytocin infusion to reduce uterine activity. Turn the patient onto her left side and elevate her legs. Continue to observe the fetal heart rate (FHR). Document your interventions and their outcomes. Notify the doctor; further medical intervention may be necessary.
Bradycardia with good variability and no periodic changes doesn't signal fetal distress if FHR remains above 80 beats/minute. But bradycardia caused by hypoxia and acidosis is an ominous sign when associated with loss of variability and late decelerations.	Intervene to correct the cause of fetal distress. Administer supplemental oxygen as ordered. Start an I.V. line and administer fluids as prescribed. Discontinue oxytocin infusion to reduce uterine activity. Turn the patient onto her left side and elevate her legs. Continue observing the FHR. Document interventions and outcomes. Notify the doctor.
Early decelerations are benign, indicating fetal head compression at dilation of 4 to 7 cm.	Reassure the patient that the fetus isn't at risk. Observe the FHR. Document the frequency of decelerations.
Late decelerations indicate uteroplacental circulatory insufficiency and may lead to fetal hypoxia and acidosis if the underlying cause isn't corrected.	Turn the patient onto her left side to increase placental perfusion and decrease contraction frequency. Increase the I.V. fluid rate to boost intravascular volume and placental perfusion as prescribed. Administer oxygen by mask to increase fetal oxygenation as ordered. Assess for signs of the underlying cause, such as hypotension or *(continued)*

Identifying baseline FHR irregularities *(continued)*

IRREGULARITY	POSSIBLE CAUSES
Late decelerations *(continued)* mm Hg 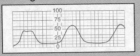	
Variable decelerations beats/minute 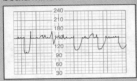 mm Hg 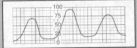	• Umbilical cord compression causing decreased fetal oxygen perfusion

• After a vaginal examination, document cervical dilation and effacement as well as fetal station, presentation, and position.

• Document membrane rupture, including the time it occurred and whether it was spontaneous or artificial. Note the amount, color, and odor of the fluid.

• If internal EFM was used, document electrode placement.

Foot care

Daily bathing of feet and regular trimming of toenails promotes cleanliness, prevents infection, stimulates peripheral circulation, and controls odor by removing debris from between toes and under toenails. It's particularly important for bedridden patients and those especially susceptible to foot infection. Increased susceptibility may be caused by peripheral vascular disease, diabetes mellitus,

CLINICAL SIGNIFICANCE	NURSING INTERVENTIONS
	uterine tachysystole. Take other appropriate measures such as discontinuing oxytocin as prescribed. Document interventions and outcomes. Notify the doctor; further medical intervention may be necessary.
Variable decelerations are the most common deceleration pattern in labor because of contractions and fetal movement.	Help the patient change position. No other intervention is necessary unless you detect fetal distress. Assure the patient that the fetus tolerates cord compression well. Explain that cord compression affects the fetus the same way that breath-holding affects her. Assess the deceleration pattern for reassuring signs: a baseline FHR that's not increasing, short-term variability that's not decreasing, abruptly beginning and ending decelerations, and decelerations lasting less than 50 seconds. If assessment doesn't reveal reassuring signs, notify the doctor. Start I.V. fluids and administer oxygen by mask at 7 liters/minute, as prescribed. Document interventions and outcomes. Discontinue oxytocin infusion to decrease uterine activity.

poor nutritional status, arthritis, or any condition that impairs peripheral circulation. In such patients, proper foot care should include meticulous cleanliness and regular observation for signs of skin breakdown. (See *Foot care for diabetic patients*, page 362.)

Toenail trimming is contraindicated in patients with toe infections, diabetes mellitus, neurologic disorders, renal failure, or peripheral vascular disease, unless performed by a doctor or podiatrist.

≫ Key nursing diagnoses and patient outcomes

Use these nursing diagnoses as a guide when developing your plan of care for a patient who needs foot care.

Impaired skin integrity related to (specify)

Based on this nursing diagnosis, you'll establish the following patient outcomes. The patient will:
• experience no skin breakdown.
• maintain muscle strength.

Foot care for diabetic patients

Because diabetes mellitus can reduce blood supply to the feet, minor foot injuries can lead to dangerous infection. When caring for a diabetic patient, keep these foot care guidelines in mind.

Promote exercise
• Exercising the feet daily can improve circulation. While the patient is sitting on the edge of the bed, ask him to point his toes upward, then downward, 10 times. Then have him make a circle with each foot 10 times.

Teach about foot and skin care
• A diabetic's shoes must fit properly. Instruct the patient to break in new shoes gradually by increasing wearing time by 30 minutes each day. Also tell him to check his old shoes frequently in case they develop rough spots in the lining.
• Tell the patient to wear clean socks daily and to avoid socks with holes, darned spots, or rough, irritating seams.
• Advise the patient to see a doctor if he has corns or calluses.

• Tell the patient to wear warm socks or slippers and use extra blankets to avoid cold feet. He should not use heating pads or hot water bottles on his feet.
• Teach the patient to regularly inspect the skin on his feet for cuts, cracks, blisters, or red, swollen areas. Tell him to wash cuts thoroughly, apply a mild antiseptic, then call the doctor. Urge him to avoid harsh antiseptics such as iodine because they can damage tissue.

Other instructions
• Advise the patient to avoid tight-fitting garments or activities that impede circulation. He should especially avoid wearing elastic garters, sitting with knees crossed, picking at sores or rough spots on the feet, walking barefoot, or applying adhesive tape to his feet.

Risk for infection related to (specify)
Based on this nursing diagnosis, you'll establish the following patient outcomes. The patient will:
• have a normal body temperature.
• have normal white blood cell and differential counts.
• show no evidence of skin breakdown.
• remain free of all signs and symptoms of infection.
• state infection risk factors.
• communicate understanding of signs and symptoms of infection.

• be able to identify early signs and symptoms of infection.

Knowledge deficit related to lack of exposure to procedure for foot care.
Based on this nursing diagnosis, you'll establish the following patient outcomes. The patient will:
• verbalize understanding of procedure for foot care.
• return demonstrate correct procedure for foot care.
• identify risk factors and health seeking behaviors.

Equipment

- bath blanket ◆ large basin ◆ soap
- towel ◆ linen-saver pad ◆ pillow
- washcloth ◆ toenail clippers ◆ orangewood stick ◆ emery board ◆ cotton-tipped applicator ◆ cotton ◆ lotion ◆ water-absorbent powder ◆ bath thermometer ◆ gloves, if the patient has open lesions.

Equipment preparation

• Assemble equipment at the patient's bedside.

• Fill the basin halfway with warm water.

• Test water temperature with a bath thermometer *because patients with diminished peripheral sensation could burn their feet in excessively hot water (over 105° F [40.6° C]) without feeling any warning pain.* If a bath thermometer is unavailable, test the water by inserting your elbow.

• The water should feel comfortably warm.

Patient preparation

• Wash your hands, and put on gloves, if necessary.

• Tell the patient that you'll wash his feet and provide foot and toenail care.

• Cover the patient with a bath blanket. Fanfold the top linen to the foot of the bed.

• Place a linen-saver pad and a towel under the patient's feet *to keep the bottom linen dry.* Then position the basin on the pad.

• Insert a pillow beneath the patient's knee *to provide support,* and cushion the rim of the basin with the edge of the towel *to prevent pressure.*

Implementation

• Immerse one foot in the basin. Wash it with soap, then allow it to soak for about 10 minutes. *Soaking softens the skin and toenails, loosens debris under toenails, and comforts and refreshes the patient.*

• After soaking the foot, rinse it with a washcloth, remove it from the basin, and place it on the towel.

• Dry the foot thoroughly, especially between the toes, *to avoid skin breakdown.* Blot gently to dry *because harsh rubbing may damage the skin.*

• Empty the basin, refill it with warm water, and clean and soak the other foot.

• While the second foot is soaking, give the first one a pedicure. Using the cotton-tipped applicator, carefully clean the toenails. Using an orangewood stick, gently remove any dirt beneath the toenails; avoid injuring subungual skin.

• Trim nails with toenail clippers, if needed, by cutting straight across *to prevent ingrown toenails.* Clip small sections of the nail at a time, starting at one edge and working across. File trimmed toenails with an emery board to smooth rough edges. *Keeping toenails trimmed and filed prevents scratching and injury to the skin on the opposite leg.*

• Rinse the foot that has been soaking, dry it thoroughly, and give it a pedicure.

• Apply lotion *to moisten dry skin,* or lightly dust water-absorbent powder between the toes *to absorb moisture.*

• Remove and clean all equipment and dispose of gloves.

Nursing considerations

• While providing foot care, observe the color, shape, and texture of the toenails. If you see redness, drying, cracking, blisters, discoloration, or other signs of traumatic injury, especially in patients with impaired peripheral circulation, notify the doctor. *Because such patients are vulnerable to infection and gangrene,* they need prompt treatment.

• If a patient's toenail grows inward at the corners, tuck a wisp of cotton under it *to relieve pressure on the toe.*

• When giving the bedridden patient foot care, unless contraindicated, perform range-of-motion exercises *to stimulate circulation and prevent foot contractures or muscle atrophy.* Tuck folded 2″ × 2″ gauze pads between overlapping toes *to protect the skin from the toenails.* Apply heel protectors *to prevent skin breakdown.*

Home care

• Instruct the patient in the correct procedure for foot care.

• Instruct him to call the doctor with any signs and symptoms of infection.

• Provide written guidelines.

Documentation

• Record the date and time of bathing and toenail trimming in your notes.

• Record and report any abnormal findings and any nursing actions you take.

G

Gastric lavage

After poisoning or a drug overdose, especially in patients who have central nervous system depression or an inadequate gag reflex, gastric lavage flushes the stomach and removes ingested substances through a gastric lavage tube. For patients with gastric or esophageal bleeding, lavage with tepid or iced water or normal saline solution may be used to stop bleeding. However, some controversy exists over the effectiveness of iced lavage for this purpose. (See *Is iced lavage effective?*, page 366)

Gastric lavage can be continuous or intermittent. Typically, this procedure is done in the emergency department or intensive care unit by a doctor, gastroenterologist, or nurse, although the wide-bore lavage tube is almost always inserted by a gastroenterologist.

Gastric lavage is contraindicated after ingestion of a corrosive substance (such as lye, ammonia, or mineral acids) because the lavage tube may perforate the already compromised esophagus.

Correct lavage tube placement is essential for patient safety because accidental misplacement (in the lungs, for example) followed by lavage can be fatal. Other complications of gastric lavage include bradyarrhythmias and aspiration of gastric fluids.

≫ Key nursing diagnoses and patient outcomes

Use these nursing diagnoses as a guide when developing your plan of care for a patient who needs gastric lavage.

Risk for poisoning related to (specify)

Based on this nursing diagnosis, you'll establish the following patient outcomes. The patient will:
• be free from effects of poisoning.
• communicate an understanding of self-protection.
• state method for safekeeping of dangerous or potentially dangerous products.

Anxiety related to lack of exposure to gastric lavage

Based on this nursing diagnosis, you'll establish the following patient outcomes. The patient will:
• verbalize understanding of need for procedure.
• use available support systems.
• exhibit decreased or no signs of anxiety.

Equipment

♦ lavage setup (two graduated containers for drainage, three pieces of large-lumen rubber tubing, Y-connector, and a clamp or hemostat) ♦ 2 to 3 L of normal saline solution or tap water as ordered ♦ I.V. pole ♦ basin of ice if ordered ♦ Ewald tube or any large-lumen gastric tube, typically #36 to #40 French (see *Using wide-bore gastric tubes*, page 367) ♦ water-soluble lubricant or anesthetic ointment ♦ stethoscope ♦ ½″ hypoallergenic tape ♦ 50-ml bulb or cath-

Is iced lavage effective?

Some experts question the effectiveness of using an iced irrigant for gastric lavage to treat GI bleeding. Here's why.

Iced irrigating solutions stimulate the vagus nerve, which triggers increased hydrochloric acid secretion. In turn, this stimulates gastric motility, which can irritate the bleeding site.

Some clinicians prefer using unchilled normal saline solution (which may prevent rapid electrolyte loss) or even water if the patient must avoid sodium. These clinicians point out that no research exists to support the use of iced irrigant to stop acute GI bleeding.

eter-tip syringe ♦ gloves ♦ face shield ♦ linen-saver pad or towel ♦ tonsillar suction device ♦ suction apparatus ♦ labeled specimen container ♦ laboratory request form ♦ norepinephrine ♦ optional: patient restraints, charcoal tablets.

A prepackaged, syringe-type irrigation kit may be used for intermittent lavage. For poisoning or a drug overdose, however, the continuous lavage setup may be more appropriate to use because it's a faster and more effective means of diluting and removing the harmful substance.

Equipment preparation

• Set up the lavage equipment. (See *Preparing for continuous gastric lavage,* page 368.)
• If iced lavage is ordered, chill the desired irrigant (water or normal saline solution) in a basin of ice.

• Lubricate the end of the lavage tube with the water-soluble lubricant or anesthetic ointment.

Patient preparation

• Explain the procedure to the patient, provide privacy, and wash your hands.
• Put on gloves and a face shield.
• Drape the towel or linen-saver pad over the patient's chest *to protect him from spills.*

Implementation

• The doctor inserts the lavage tube nasally and advances it slowly and gently *because forceful insertion may injure tissues and cause epistaxis.* He then checks the tube's placement by injecting about 30 cc of air into the tube with the bulb syringe and then auscultating the patient's abdomen with a stethoscope. If the tube is in place, he'll hear the sound of air entering the stomach.
• *Because the patient may vomit when the lavage tube reaches the posterior pharynx during insertion,* be prepared to suction the airway immediately with a tonsillar suction device.
• Once the lavage tube passes the posterior pharynx, assist the patient into Trendelenburg's position, and turn him toward his left side in a three-quarter prone posture. *This position minimizes passage of gastric contents into the duodenum and helps prevent the patient from aspirating vomitus.*
• After securing the lavage tube nasally or orally and making sure the irrigant inflow tube on the lavage setup is clamped, connect the unattached end of this tube to the lavage tube. Allow the stomach contents to empty into the drainage container before instilling any irrigant. *This confirms proper*

Using wide-bore gastric tubes

If you need to deliver a large volume of fluid rapidly through a gastric tube (when irrigating the stomach of a patient with profuse gastric bleeding or poisoning, for example), a wide-bore gastric tube usually serves best. Typically inserted orally, these tubes remain in place only long enough to complete the lavage and evacuate stomach contents.

Ewald tube
In an emergency, using this single-lumen tube with several openings at the distal end allows you to aspirate large amounts of gastric contents quickly.

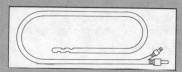

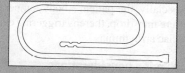

Edlich tube
This single-lumen tube has four openings near the closed distal tip. A funnel or syringe may be connected at the proximal end. Like the Ewald tube, the Edlich tube lets you withdraw large quantities of gastric contents quickly.

Levacuator tube
This tube (above right) has two lumens. Use the larger lumen for evacuating gastric contents, the smaller for instilling an irrigant.

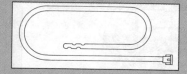

tube placement and decreases the risk of overfilling the stomach with irrigant and inducing vomiting. If you're using a syringe irrigation set, aspirate stomach contents with a 50-ml bulb or catheter-tip syringe before instilling the irrigant.

• Once you confirm proper tube placement, begin gastric lavage by instilling about 250 ml of irrigant *to assess the patient's tolerance and prevent vomiting.* If you're using a syringe, instill about 50 ml of solution at a time until you've instilled between 250 and 500 ml.

• Clamp the inflow tube and unclamp the outflow tube *to allow the irrigant to flow out.* If you're using the syringe irrigation kit, aspirate the irrigant with the syringe and empty it into a calibrated container. Measure the outflow amount to make sure that it equals at least the amount of irrigant you instilled. *This prevents accidental stomach distention and vomiting.* If the drainage amount falls significantly short of the instilled amount, reposition the tube until sufficient solution flows out. Gently massage the abdomen over the stomach to promote outflow.

• Repeat the inflow-outflow cycle until returned fluids appear clear. *This signals that the stomach no longer*

Preparing for continuous gastric lavage

Prepare the lavage setup as follows:
• Connect one of the three pieces of large-lumen tubing to the irrigant container.
• Insert the Y-connector stem in the other end of the tubing.
• Connect the remaining two pieces of tubing to the free ends of the Y-connector.
• Place the unattached end of one of the tubes into one of the drainage containers. (Later, you'll connect the other piece of tubing to the patient's gastric tube.)
• Clamp the tube leading to the irrigant.
• Suspend the entire setup from the I.V. pole, hanging the irrigant container at the highest level.

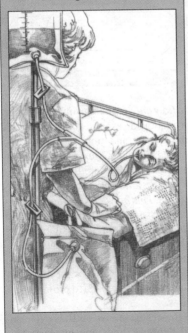

holds harmful substances or that bleeding has stopped.
• Assess the patient's vital signs, urine output, and level of consciousness (LOC) every 15 minutes. Notify the doctor of any changes.
• If ordered, remove the lavage tube.

Complications

• Vomiting and subsequent aspiration, the most common complication of gastric lavage, occurs more often in a groggy patient. Bradyarrhythmias also may occur. After iced lavage especially, the patient's body temperature may drop, thereby triggering cardiac arrhythmias.

Nursing considerations

• *To control GI bleeding,* the doctor may order continuous irrigation of the stomach with an irrigant and a vasoconstrictor such as norepinephrine. After the stomach absorbs norepinephrine, the portal system delivers the drug directly to the liver, where it's metabolized. *This prevents the drug from circulating systemically and initiating a hypertensive response.* Or the doctor may use an alternate drug-delivery method, directing you to clamp the outflow tube for a prescribed period after instilling the irrigant and the vasoconstrictive medication and before withdrawing it. This allows the mucosa time to absorb the drug.
• Never leave a patient alone during gastric lavage. Observe continuously for any changes in his LOC, and monitor vital signs frequently *because the natural vagal response to intubation can depress the patient's heart rate.*
• If you need to restrain the patient, secure restraints on the same side of the bed or stretcher *so that you can*

free them quickly without moving to the other side of the bed. Avoid restraining the patient in a "spread eagle" position, *which would prevent him from turning and leave him at risk for aspirating vomitus.*

• Remember also to keep tracheal suctioning equipment nearby and watch closely for airway obstruction caused by vomiting or excess oral secretions. Throughout gastric lavage, you may need to suction the oral cavity frequently *to ensure an open airway and prevent aspiration.* For the same reasons, and if he doesn't exhibit an adequate gag reflex, the patient may require an endotracheal tube before the procedure.

• When aspirating the stomach for ingested poisons or drugs, be sure to save the contents in a labeled container to send to the laboratory for analysis. If ordered, after lavage to remove poisons or drugs, mix charcoal tablets with the irrigant (whether it's water or normal saline solution) and administer the mixture through the nasogastric tube. The charcoal will absorb remaining toxic substances. The tube may be clamped temporarily, allowed to drain via gravity, attached to intermittent suction, or removed.

• When performing gastric lavage to stop bleeding, keep precise intake and output records *to determine the amount of bleeding.* When the patient has large volumes of fluid instilled and withdrawn, serum electrolyte or arterial blood gas levels (or both) may be measured during or at the end of lavage.

Documentation

• Record the date and time of lavage, the size and type of NG tube used, the volume and type of irrigant, and the amount of drained gastric contents. Record this information on the intake and output record sheet, and include your observations, noting, for example, color and consistency of drainage.

• Keep precise records of the patient's vital signs and LOC, any drugs instilled through the tube, the time the tube was removed, and how well the patient tolerated the procedure.

Gavage feeding of the neonate

Gavage feeding involves passing nutrients directly to the neonate's stomach by a tube advanced nasally or orally. If a neonate can't suck (because of prematurity, illness, or congenital deformity) or if a neonate risks aspiration (because of gastroesophageal reflux, ineffective gag reflex, or easy tiring), gavage feeding may supply nutrients until he can take food by mouth.

Unless the neonate has problems with the feeding tube, the nurse usually inserts it orally before each feeding and withdraws it after the feeding. This intermittent method stimulates the sucking reflex. If the neonate can't tolerate this, the nurse advances the tube nasally and leaves it in place for 24 to 72 hours.

Tube feeding is contraindicated for neonates without bowel sounds or with suspected intestinal obstruction, severe respiratory distress, or massive gastroesophageal reflux.

>> Key nursing diagnoses and patient outcomes

Use these nursing diagnoses as a guide when developing your plan of care for a neonate who's receiving gavage feedings.

Ineffective infant feeding pattern related to (specify)

Based on this nursing diagnosis, you'll establish the following patient outcomes. The patient will:
• not lose more than 10% of birth weight within first week of life.
• gain 4 to 7 oz (113 to 198 g)/week after the first week of life.
• not experience dehydration.
• receive adequate nutrition until able to suckle sufficiently.

Ineffective family coping: compromised, related to compromised neonatal health

Based on this nursing diagnosis, you'll establish these family outcomes. The family will:
• communicate feelings regarding neonate's condition.
• become involved in planning and providing neonate's care.
• express feeling of having greater control over the situation.

Equipment

♦ feeding tube (#3 ½ up to #6 French for nasogastric feeding of premature neonate; #8 French for others) ♦ feeding reservoir or large (20- to 50-ml) syringe ♦ prescribed formula or breast milk ♦ sterile water ♦ tape measure ♦ tape ♦ stethoscope ♦ gloves ♦ optional: bowl and pacifier. A commercial feeding reservoir is available.

Equipment preparation

• Allow the formula or breast milk to warm to room temperature, if necessary.
• Wash your hands and open the sterile water, if it comes in a small-sized disposable container.
• Remove the syringe or reservoir and the feeding tube from the packaging

Patient preparation

• Identify the neonate, and verify the doctor's orders.
• Using a tape measure, determine the length of tubing needed to ensure placement in the stomach. You'll usually measure from the tip of the nose to the tip of the earlobe to the xiphoid process. Mark the tube at the appropriate distance with a piece of tape. Measure from the bottom.
• Position the neonate in a supine position. Elevate the head of his mattress one notch. Otherwise, place him in a supine position or tilted slightly to his right with head and chest slightly elevated.

Implementation

• Put on gloves.
• Stabilize the neonate's head with one hand, and lubricate the feeding tube with sterile water with the other hand.
• Insert the tube smoothly and quickly up to the premeasured tape mark. For oral insertion, pass the tube toward the back of the throat. For nasal insertion, pass the tube toward the occiput in a horizontal plane.
• Synchronize tube insertion with throat movement if the neonate swallows *to facilitate tube passage into the stomach*. During insertion, watch for choking and cyanosis, signs that a

tube has entered the trachea. If these occur, remove the tube and reinsert it. Also watch for bradycardia and apnea resulting from vagal stimulation.

• If the tube will remain in place, tape it flat to the neonate's cheek. *To prevent possible nasal skin breakdown,* don't tape the tube to the bridge of his nose.

• Make sure the tube is in the stomach (and not the lungs) by aspirating residual stomach contents with the syringe. Check the content's pH because gastric contents are highly acidic. This helps confirm tube placement. Note the volume obtained, and then reinject it *to avoid altering the neonate's buffer system and electrolyte balance.* Or, as ordered, reduce the feeding volume by the residual amount, or prolong the interval between feedings.

• Alternatively, or additionally, check placement of the feeding tube in the stomach by injecting 0.5 to 1 cc of air into the tube while listening with the stethoscope for air sounds in the stomach and on each side of the anterior chest.

• If you suspect that the tube is displaced, advance it several centimeters farther and test again. *Don't* begin feeding until you're certain the tube is in the stomach.

• When the tube is in place, fill the feeding reservoir or syringe with formula or breast milk. Connect the feeding reservoir or syringe to the top of the tube, and start the feeding.

• If the neonate is on your lap, hold the container about 4″ (10 cm) above his abdomen. If he's lying down, hold it between 6″ and 8″ (15 to 20 cm) above his head. When using a commercial feeding reservoir, look for air bubbles in the container, an indicator of formula passage.

• Regulate flow by raising and lowering the container, so that the feeding takes 15 to 20 minutes, the average time for a bottle-feeding. *To prevent stomach distention, reflux, and vomiting,* don't let the feeding proceed too rapidly.

• When the feeding is finished, pinch off the tubing before air enters the neonate's stomach. *This helps prevent distention, fluid leakage into the pharynx during tube removal, and consequent aspiration.*

• Withdraw the tube smoothly and quickly. If the tube will remain in place, flush it with several milliliters of sterile water if ordered.

• Burp the neonate *to decrease abdominal distention.* Hold him upright or in a sitting position. Let your one hand support his head and chest and your other hand gently rub or pat his back until he expels the air.

• Place him on his stomach or right side for 1 hour after feeding *to facilitate gastric emptying and to prevent aspiration if he regurgitates.*

• Don't perform postural drainage and percussion until 1 hour or more after feeding.

Complications

• Gagging with regurgitation causes loss of nutrients. An indwelling nasogastric tube can irritate mucous membranes and cause nasal airway obstruction, epistaxis, and stomach perforation.

• A feeding tube may kink, coil, or knot and become obstructed, preventing feeding.

Nursing considerations

• Use the nasogastric approach for the neonate who must keep the feeding tube in place *because this approach holds the tube more securely than the orogastric approach.*

• Alternate the nostril used at each insertion *to prevent skin and mucosal irritation.*

• Observe the premature neonate for indications that he's ready to begin bottle- or breast-feeding: strong sucking reflex, coordinated sucking and swallowing, alertness before feeding, and sleep after it.

• Provide the neonate with a pacifier during feeding *to soothe him, to help prevent gagging, and to promote an association between sucking and the full feeling that follows feeding.*

Documentation

• Record the amount of residual fluid and the amount currently taken.

• Note the type and amount of any vomitus, and any adverse reactions to tube insertion or feeding.

Glucose and hemoglobin testing at bedside

Increasingly, nurses are monitoring blood glucose and hemoglobin levels at the patient's bedside. The fast, accurate results obtained this way allow immediate intervention, if necessary. It allows faster determination of results than traditional monitoring methods, in which blood samples must be sent to the laboratory for interpretation. A blood sample that sits at room temperature for an hour may undergo glycolysis, which reduces glucose concentration by 3% to 30%, leading to inaccurate test results.

Numerous testing systems are available for bedside monitoring. Bedside systems are also convenient for patient home use.

HemoCue, a widely used system, gives accurate results without having to dispense, pipette, or mix blood and reagents for readings, which eliminates risk of leakage, broken tubes, and splattered blood. A plastic, disposable microcuvette functions as a combination pipette, test tube, and measuring vessel. It contains a reagent that produces a precise chemical reaction as soon as it makes contact with blood. The photometer is powered by a battery or an AC adapter. One model is calibrated at the factory and rarely needs to be recalibrated, returning to 0 between tests. Use the control cuvette included with each system to test photometer function.

Normal glucose values range from 70 to 100 mg/dl; normal hemoglobin values range from 12.5 to 15 g/dl.

An above-normal glucose level (hyperglycemia) may indicate diabetes mellitus or the use of steroid drugs. A below-normal glucose level may indicate overly rapid glucose use, which may occur with strenuous exercise or infection, resulting in tissues receiving insufficient glucose.

A below-normal hemoglobin value may indicate anemia, recent hemorrhage, or fluid retention, causing hemodilution. An elevated hemoglobin value suggests hemoconcentration from polycythemia or dehydration.

≫ Key nursing diagnoses and patient outcomes

Use these nursing diagnoses as a guide when developing your plan of care for a patient who needs bedside blood glucose and hemoglobin testing.

Knowledge deficit related to lack of exposure to procedure

Based on this nursing diagnosis, you'll establish the following patient outcome. The patient will:
• verbalize understanding of need for procedure.

Anxiety related to lack of exposure to procedure

Based on this nursing diagnosis, you'll establish the following patient outcome. The patient will:
• communicate to the nurse any feelings of anxiety related to procedure.

Equipment

For the HemoCue system: ♦ microcuvette ♦ photometer ♦ sterile gloves ♦ alcohol sponges ♦ gauze pads.

Equipment preparation

• Take the equipment to the patient's bedside.
• Plug the AC adapter into the photometer power inlet and then plug the other end of the adapter into the wall outlet.
• Turn the photometer on. If it hasn't been used recently, insert the control cuvette to make sure that it's working properly.

Patient preparation

• Explain the test purpose to the patient.
• Tell him that he'll feel a pinprick in his finger during blood sampling.

Implementation

• Wash your hands and put on sterile gloves.
• Select an appropriate puncture site. You'll usually use the fingertip or earlobe for an adult, or the heel or great toe for an infant. For an adult, the middle and fourth fingers are the best choices. The second finger is usually the most sensitive, and the thumb may have thickened skin or calluses. Blood should circulate freely in the finger from which you're drawing blood, so avoid using a ring-bearing finger.
• Keep the patient's finger straight and ask him to relax it. Holding his finger between the thumb and index finger of your nondominant hand, gently rock the patient's finger as you move your fingers from his top knuckle to his fingertip. This causes blood to flow to the sampling point.
• Use an alcohol wipe to clean the puncture site, wiping in a circular motion from the center of the site outward. Dry the site thoroughly with a gauze pad.
• Pierce the skin quickly and sharply with the microcuvette, which automatically draws a precise amount of blood.
• Place the microcuvette into the photometer. Results appear on the photometer screen within 40 seconds to 4 minutes. (See *How to use a bedside blood glucose and hemoglobin monitor,* page 374.)
• Place a gauze pad over the puncture site until the bleeding stops.
• Dispose of the microcuvette according to your hospital's policy. Take off your gloves and wash your hands. Notify the doctor if the patient's result is outside the expected parameters.

How to use a bedside blood glucose and hemoglobin monitor

Monitoring blood glucose and hemoglobin levels at the patient's bedside is a straightforward procedure. A photometer, such as the HemoCue analyzer featured below, relies on capillary action to draw blood into a disposable microcuvette. This method of obtaining blood minimizes a health care worker's exposure to the patient's blood and decreases the risk of cross-contamination. Follow the three steps shown here when using the HemoCue system.

After you pierce the skin, the microcuvette draws blood automatically.

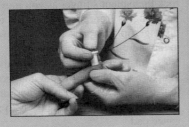

Next, place the microcuvette into the photometer.

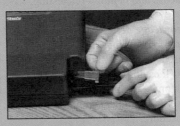

The photometer screen displays the blood glucose and hemoglobin levels.

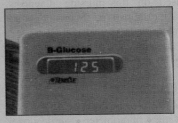

Nursing considerations
• Before using a microcuvette, note its expiration date. Microcuvettes can be stored for up to 2 years. However, after the microcuvette vial is opened, the shelf life is 90 days.
• Before taking a blood sample, operate the photometer with the control cuvette to check for proper function. To ensure an adequate blood sample, don't use a cold, cyanotic, or swollen area as the puncture site. The middle and fourth fingers are the best choice for puncture site. The second finger is usually the most sensitive, and the thumb may have thickened skin or cal-

luses. Blood should circulate freely in the finger from which you're drawing blood, so avoid using a ring-bearing finger.

Documentation
• Document the values obtained from the photometer.
• Document any interventions.

Glucose testing

Rapid, easy-to-perform reagent strip tests (such as Glucostix, Chemstrip bG, or Multistix) use a drop of capillary blood obtained by fingerstick, heelstick, or earlobe puncture as a sample. These tests can detect or monitor elevated blood glucose levels in patients with diabetes, screen for diabetes mellitus and neonatal hypoglycemia, and help distinguish diabetic coma from nondiabetic coma.

In these tests, a reagent patch on the tip of a hand-held plastic strip changes color in response to the amount of glucose in the blood sample. Comparing the color change with a standardized color chart provides a semiquantitative measurement of blood glucose levels; inserting the strip in a portable blood glucose meter (such as a Glucometer II, Accu-Chek II, or One Touch) provides quantitative measurements that compare in accuracy with other laboratory tests. Some meters store successive test results electronically to help determine glucose patterns.

These tests can be performed in the hospital, the doctor's office, or the patient's home.

⟫ Key nursing diagnoses and patient outcomes

Use these nursing diagnoses as a guide when developing your plan of care.

Knowledge deficit related to lack of exposure to blood glucose testing

Based on this nursing diagnosis, you'll establish the following patient outcomes. The patient will:
• verbalize understanding of procedure.
• return demonstrate correct procedure for blood glucose testing.
• identify parameters for reporting results to doctor or health care professional.

Health seeking behaviors related to elevated blood glucose levels

Based on this nursing diagnosis, you'll establish the following patient outcomes. The patient will:
• identify risk factors for elevated blood glucose levels.
• verbalize effects of elevated blood glucose levels.
• verbalize measures to increase control over blood glucose levels.

Equipment

♦ reagent strips ♦ gloves ♦ portable blood glucose meter, if available ♦ gauze pads ♦ alcohol sponges ♦ disposable lancets ♦ small adhesive bandage ♦ watch or clock with a second hand.

Patient preparation

• Explain the procedure to the patient or to the infant's parents.

Implementation

• Next, select the puncture site — usually the fingertip or earlobe for an adult or the heel or great toe for an infant.
• Wash your hands and don gloves.
• If necessary, dilate the capillaries by applying warm, moist compresses to the area for about 10 minutes.
• Wipe the puncture site with an alcohol sponge, and dry it thoroughly with a gauze pad.
• To draw a sample from the patient's fingertip with a disposable lancet (smaller than 2 mm), make the puncture on the side of the fingertip and position the lancet perpendicular to the lines of the patient's fingerprints. Pierce the skin sharply and quickly *to minimize the patient's anxiety and pain, and to increase blood flow.*

Glucose tolerance tests

For monitoring trends in glucose metabolism, two tests may offer benefits over testing blood with reagent strips.

Oral glucose tolerance test

The most sensitive test for detecting borderline diabetes mellitus, the oral glucose tolerance test (OGTT) measures carbohydrate metabolism after ingestion of a challenge dose of glucose. The body absorbs this dose rapidly, causing plasma glucose levels to rise and peak within 30 minutes to 1 hour. The pancreas responds by secreting insulin, causing glucose levels to return to normal within 2 to 3 hours. During this period, plasma and urine glucose levels are monitored to assess insulin secretion and the body's ability to metabolize glucose.

Although you may not collect the blood and urine specimens (usually five of each) required for this test, you will be responsible for preparing the patient for the test and monitoring his physical condition during the test.

Begin by explaining the OGTT to the patient. Then, tell him to maintain a high-carbohydrate diet for 3 days and to fast for 10 to 16 hours before the test, as ordered. The patient must not smoke, drink coffee or alcohol, or exercise strenuously for 8 hours before or during the test. Inform him that he will then receive a challenge dose of 100 g of carbohydrate (usually a sweetened carbonated beverage or gelatin).

Tell the patient who will perform the venipunctures and when, and that he may feel slight discomfort from the needle punctures and the pressure of the tourniquet. Reassure him that collecting each blood sample usually takes less than 3 minutes. As ordered, withhold drugs that may affect test results. Remind him not to discard the first voided urine specimen on waking.

During the test period, watch for signs and symptoms of hypoglycemia — weakness, restlessness, nervousness, hunger, and sweating — and report these to the doctor immediately. Encourage the patient to drink plenty of water to promote adequate urine excretion. Provide a bedpan, urinal, or specimen container when necessary.

I.V. glucose tolerance test

This test may be chosen for patients unable to absorb an oral dose of glucose — for example, those with malabsorption disorders, short-bowel syndrome, or those who have had a gastrectomy. The I.V. glucose tolerance test measures blood glucose after an I.V. infusion of 50% glucose over 3 or 4 minutes. Blood samples are then drawn after 30 minutes, 1 hour, 2 hours, and 3 hours. After an immediate glucose peak of 300 to 400 mg/dl (accompanied by glycosuria), the normal glucose curve falls steadily, reaching fasting levels within 1 to 1¼ hours. Failure to achieve fasting glucose levels within 2 to 3 hours typically confirms diabetes.

Alternatively, you may want to use a mechanical bloodletting device, such as an Autolet, which uses a spring-loaded lancet.

• After puncturing the finger, make sure you don't squeeze the puncture site *to avoid diluting the sample with tissue fluid.*

• Touch a drop of blood to the reagent patch on the strip; make sure you cover the entire patch.

• After collecting the blood sample, briefly apply pressure to the puncture site *to prevent painful extravasation of blood into subcutaneous tissues.* Ask the adult patient to hold a gauze pad firmly over the puncture site until bleeding stops.

• Make sure you leave the blood on the strip for exactly 60 seconds.

• Compare the color change on the strip with the standardized color chart on the product container. If you're using a blood glucose meter, follow the manufacturer's instructions. Meter designs vary, but they all analyze a drop of blood placed on a reagent strip that comes with the unit, and they provide a digital display of the resulting glucose level.

• After bleeding has stopped, you may apply a small adhesive bandage to the puncture site.

Nursing considerations

• Before using reagent strips, check the expiration date on the package and replace outdated strips.

• Check for special instructions related to the specific reagent.

• The reagent area of a fresh strip should match the color on the "0" block on the color chart.

• Protect the strips from light, heat, and moisture.

• Before using a blood glucose meter, calibrate it and run it with a control sample *to ensure accurate test results.*

• Make sure you follow the manufacturer's instructions for calibration.

• Avoid selecting cold, cyanotic, or swollen puncture sites *to ensure an adequate blood sample.*

• If you can't obtain a capillary sample, perform venipuncture and place a large drop of venous blood on the reagent strip.

If you want to test blood from a refrigerated sample, remember to allow the blood to return to room temperature before testing it.

• To help detect abnormal glucose metabolism and diagnose diabetes mellitus, the doctor may order other blood glucose tests. (See *Glucose tolerance tests.*)

Home care

• If the patient will be using the reagent strip system at home, teach him the proper use of the lancet or Autolet, the reagent strips and color chart, and the portable blood glucose meter, as necessary.

• Provide written guidelines.

Documentation

Record the reading from the reagent strip (using a portable blood glucose meter or a color chart) in your notes or on a special flowchart, if available.

• Record the time and date of the test.

H

Halo-vest traction

Halo-vest traction immobilizes the head and neck after traumatic injury to the cervical vertebrae, the most common of all spinal injuries. This procedure, which can prevent further injury to the spinal cord, is performed by an orthopedic surgeon, with nursing assistance, in the emergency department, a specially-equipped room, or in the operating room after surgical reduction of vertebral injuries. The halo-vest traction device consists of a metal ring that fits over the patient's head and metal bars that connect the ring to a plastic vest that distributes the weight of the entire apparatus around the chest. (See *Comparing halo-vest traction devices*.)

Once in place, halo-vest traction allows the patient greater mobility than does traction with skull tongs. It also carries less risk of infection, because it doesn't require skin incisions and drill holes to position skull pins.

≫ Key nursing diagnoses and patient outcomes

Use these nursing diagnoses as a guide when developing your plan of care for a patient who is receiving halo vest traction.

Ineffective coping related to personal vulnerability
Based on this nursing diagnosis, you'll establish the following patient outcomes. The patient will:
• become actively involved in planning own care.

• identify effective and ineffective coping techniques.

Knowledge deficit related to lack of exposure
Based on this nursing diagnosis, you'll establish the following patient outcomes. The patient will:
• communicate a need to know.
• state or demonstrate understanding of what has been taught.

Equipment
♦ halo-vest traction unit ♦ halo ring ♦ cervical collar or sandbags (if needed) ♦ plastic vest ♦ board or padded headrest ♦ tape measure ♦ halo ring conversion chart ♦ scissors and razor ♦ 4″ × 4″ gauze pads ♦ povidone-iodine solution ♦ sterile gloves ♦ Allen wrench ♦ four positioning pins ♦ multiple-dose vial of 1% lidocaine (with or without epinephrine) ♦ alcohol sponges ♦ 3-ml syringe ♦ 25G needles ♦ five sterile skull pins (one more than needed) ♦ torque screwdriver ♦ sheepskin liners ♦ cotton-tipped applicators ♦ ordered cleaning solution ♦ medicated powder or cornstarch ♦ sterile water or normal saline solution. Optional: hair dryer, pain medication (such as an analgesic).

Most hospitals supply packaged halo-vest traction units that include software (jacket and sheepskin liners), hardware (halo, head pins, upright bars, and screws), and tools (torque screwdriver, two conventional wrenches, Allen wrench, and screws and bolts). These units don't include sterile gloves, povidone-iodine solution, sterile drapes, cervical collars, or

Comparing halo-vest traction devices

TYPE	DESCRIPTION	ADVANTAGES
Low profile (standard) 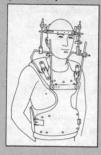	• Traction and compression are produced by threaded support rods on either side of the halo ring. • Flexion and extension are obtained by moving the swivel arm to an anterior or posterior position, depending on the location of the skull pins.	• Immobilizes cervical spine fractures while allowing patient mobility • Facilitates surgery of the cervical spine and permits flexion and extension • Allows airway intubation without losing skeletal traction • Facilitates necessary alignment by an adjustment at the junction of the threaded support rods and horizontal frame
Mark II (type of low profile) 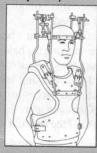	• Traction and compression are produced by threaded support rods on either side of the halo ring. • Flexion and extension are obtained by swivel clamps, which allow the bars to intersect and hold at any angle.	• Enables doctors to assemble the metal framework more quickly • Allows unobstructed access for anteroposterior and lateral X-rays of the cervical spine • Allows patient to wear his usual clothing because uprights are shaped closer to the body
Mark III (update of Mark II) 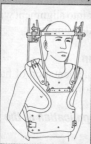	• Traction and compression are produced by threaded support rods on either side of the halo ring. • Flexion and extension are accommodated by a serrated split articulation coupling attached to the halo ring, which can be adjusted in 4-degree increments.	• Simplifies application while promoting patient comfort • Eliminates shoulder pressure and discomfort by using a flexible padded strap instead of the vest's solid plastic shoulder • Accommodates the tall patient with modified hardware and shorter uprights and allows unobstructed access for medial and lateral X-rays *(continued)*

Comparing halo-vest traction devices *(continued)*

TYPE	DESCRIPTION	ADVANTAGES
Trippi-Wells tongs 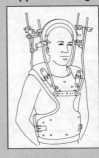	• Traction is produced by four pins that compress the skull. • Flexion and extension are obtained by adjusting the midline vertical plate.	• Applies tensile force to the neck or spine while allowing patient mobility • Makes it possible to change from mobile to stationary traction without interrupting traction • Adjusts to three planes for mobile and stationary traction • Allows unobstructed access for medial and lateral X-rays

equipment for injection of local anesthetic.

Obtain a halo-vest traction unit with halo rings and plastic vests in several sizes. Check the expiration date of the prepackaged tray, and check the outside covering for damage *to ensure the sterility of the contents.* Then assemble the equipment at the patient's bedside.

Patient preparation
• Explain the procedure.
• Check the support that was applied to the patient's neck on the way to the hospital. If necessary, apply the cervical collar immediately or immobilize the head and neck with sandbags. Keep the cervical collar or sandbags in place until the halo is applied. This support will then be carefully removed *to facilitate application of the vest. Because the patient is likely to be frightened,* try to reassure him.
• Remove the headboard and any furniture at the head of the bed *to provide ample working space.* Then carefully

place the patient's head on a board or on a padded headrest that extends beyond the edge of the bed.

Note. Never put the patient's head on a pillow before applying the halo *to avoid further injury to the spinal cord.*
• Elevate the bed to a working level that gives the doctor easy access to the front and back of the halo unit.
• Stand at the head of the bed and see whether the patient's chin lines up with his midsternum, *indicating proper alignment.* If ordered, support the patient's head in your hands and gently rotate the neck into alignment without flexing or extending it.

Implementation
Steps in the implementation of halo-vest traction follow.

To assist with application of the halo
• Ask another nurse to help you with the procedure.
• Explain the procedure to the patient, wash your hands, and provide privacy.

• Have the assisting nurse hold the patient's head and neck stable while the doctor removes the cervical collar or sandbags. Maintain this support until the halo is secure, while you assist with pin insertion.

• The doctor first measures the patient's head with a tape measure and refers to the halo ring conversion chart to determine the correct ring size. (The ring should clear the head by 1.5 cm and fit 1 cm above the bridge of the nose.)

• The doctor selects four pin sites: 1 cm above the lateral one-third of each eyebrow and 1 cm above the top of each ear in the occipital area. He also takes into account the degree and type of correction needed to provide proper cervical alignment.

• Trim and shave the hair at the pin sites with scissors or a razor *to facilitate subsequent care and help prevent infection.* Then, use 4″ × 4″ gauze pads soaked in povidone-iodine solution to clean the sites.

• Open the halo-vest unit using sterile technique *to avoid contamination.* The doctor puts on the sterile gloves and removes the halo and the Allen wrench. He then places the halo over the patient's head and inserts the four positioning pins *to hold the halo in place temporarily.*

• Help the doctor prepare the anesthetic. First, clean the injection port of the multiple-dose vial of lidocaine with the alcohol sponge. Then, invert the vial so the doctor can insert a 25G needle attached to the 3-ml syringe and withdraw the anesthetic.

• The doctor injects the anesthetic at the four pin sites. He may change needles on the syringe after each injection.

• The doctor removes four of the five skull pins from the sterile setup and

firmly screws in each pin at a 90-degree angle to the skull. When the pins are in place, he removes the positioning pins. He then tightens the skull pins with the torque screwdriver.

To apply the vest
• After the doctor measures the patient's chest and abdomen, he selects a vest of appropriate size.

• Place the sheepskin liners inside the front and back of the vest *to make it more comfortable to wear and to help prevent pressure ulcers.*

• Help the doctor carefully raise the patient while the other nurse supports the head and neck. Slide the back of the vest under the patient and gently lay him down. The doctor then fastens the front of the vest on the patient's chest using Velcro straps.

• The doctor attaches the metal bars to the halo and vest and tightens each bolt in turn, *to avoid tightening any single bolt completely, causing maladjusted tension.* Once halo-vest traction is in place, X-rays should be taken immediately *to check the depth of the skull pins and verify proper alignment.*

To care for the patient
• Take routine and neurologic vital signs at least every 2 hours for 24 hours (preferably every hour for 48 hours) and then every 4 hours until stable.

• Notify the doctor immediately if you observe any loss of motor function or any decreased sensation, *which could indicate spinal cord trauma.*

• Put on gloves. Gently clean the pin sites every 4 hours with cotton-tipped applicators dipped in cleaning solution. Rinse the sites with sterile water or normal saline solution *to remove any excess cleaning solution.* Then clean the pin sites with povidone-iodine solution or other ordered solution. *Meticulous pin site care prevents infection and removes debris that might block drainage and lead to abscess formation.* Watch for signs of infection — a loose pin, swelling or redness, purulent drainage, pain at the site — and notify the doctor if these signs develop.

• The doctor retightens the skull pins with the torque screwdriver 24 and 48 hours after the halo is applied. If the patient complains of a headache after the pins are tightened, obtain an order for an analgesic. If pain occurs with jaw movement, notify the doctor because this may indicate that pins have slipped onto the thin temporal plate.

• Examine the halo-vest unit every shift to make sure that everything is secure and that the patient's head is centered within the halo. If the vest fits correctly, you should be able to insert one or two fingers under the jacket at the shoulder and chest when the patient is lying supine.

• Wash the patient's chest and back daily. First, place the patient on his back. Loosen the bottom Velcro straps so you can get to the chest and back. Then, reaching under the vest, wash and dry the skin. Check for tender, reddened areas or pressure spots that may develop into ulcers. If necessary, use a hair dryer to dry damp sheepskin because moisture predisposes the skin to pressure ulcer formation. Lightly dust the skin with medicated powder or cornstarch to prevent itching. If itching persists, check to see if the patient is allergic to sheepskin and if any drug he's taking might cause a skin rash. If the hospital's policy allows, change the vest lining, as necessary.

• Turn the patient on his side (less than 45 degrees) to wash his back. Then close the vest.

• Be careful not to put any stress on the apparatus, *which could knock it out of alignment and lead to subluxation of the cervical spine.*

Complications

• Manipulating the patient's neck during application of halo-vest traction may cause subluxation of the spine, or could push a bone fragment into the spinal cord, possibly compressing the cord and causing paralysis below the break.

• Inaccurate positioning of the skull pins can lead to a puncture of the dura mater, causing a loss of cerebrospinal fluid and a serious central nervous system infection. Nonsterile technique during application of the halo or inadequate pin site care can also lead to infection at the pin sites. Pressure ulcers can develop if the vest fits poorly or chafes the skin.

Nursing considerations

• Keep two conventional wrenches available at all times. In the event of cardiac arrest, use the wrenches to remove the distal anterior bolts. Pull the two upright bars outward. Unfasten the Velcro straps and remove the front of the vest. Use the sturdy back of the vest as a board for cardiopulmonary resuscitation (CPR). *To prevent subluxating the cervical injury,* start CPR with the jaw thrust, which avoids hyperextension of the neck. Pull the patient's mandible forward, while maintaining proper head and neck alignment. *This pulls the tongue forward to open the airway.*

• Never lift the patient up by the vertical bars. *This could strain or tear the skin at the pin sites, or misalign the traction.*

• To prevent falls, walk with the ambulatory patient. Remember, he'll have trouble seeing objects at or near his feet, and the weight of the halovest unit (about 10 lb [4.5 kg]) may throw him off balance. If the patient is in a wheelchair, lower the leg rests *to prevent the chair from tipping backward.*

• *Because the vest limits chest expansion,* routinely assess pulmonary function, especially in a patient with pulmonary disease.

Home care

• Teach the patient to turn slowly — in small increments — to avoid losing his balance.

• Remind him to avoid bending forward *because the extra weight of the halo apparatus may cause him to fall.*

• Teach him to bend at the knees, rather than the waist.

• Have a physical therapist teach him how to use assistive devices to extend his reach and to help him put on socks and shoes.

• Suggest wearing shirts or blouses that button in front and that are larger than usual to accommodate the halovest.

• Most importantly, teach the patient about pin site care and about shampooing and hair care.

Documentation

• Record the date and time that the halo-vest traction was applied.

• Note the length of the procedure and the patient's response.

• After application, record routine and neurologic vital signs.

• Document pin site care and note any signs of infection.

Head and neck inspection

Typically, you'll assess the head and neck to uncover clues to physical problems in the integumentary, musculoskeletal, cardiovascular, respiratory, and neurologic systems. You'll also learn about the patient's nutritional status and sensory problems.

You'll need a clear understanding of head and neck structures to help you detect abnormalities. (See *Anatomy of the head and neck,* page 384.)

You'll also need to take a health history that focuses on the patient's specific head or neck problem. (See *Asking the right questions,* page 385.)

≫ Key nursing diagnoses and patient outcomes

Use these nursing diagnoses as a guide when developing your plan of care.

Knowledge deficit related to lack of exposure to assessment techniques
Based on this nursing diagnosis, you'll establish the following patient outcomes. The patient will:

• verbalize reason for assessment of head and neck.

• verbalize understanding of procedures to be performed during assessment of head and neck.

Anatomy of the head and neck

A clear understanding of head and neck structures will help you detect abnormalities when assessing this area. Use the illustration below to review normal anatomy of the head and neck.

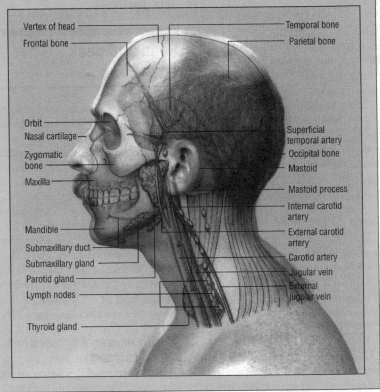

Anxiety related to assessment techniques

Based on this nursing diagnosis, you'll establish the following patient outcomes. The patient will:
• communicate feelings of anxiety.
• remain calm and relaxed during assessment procedure.

Equipment

♦ stethoscope ♦ flashlight or gooseneck lamp if needed.

Patient preparation

• Ensure patient privacy.
• Explain the procedure to the patient.
• Make sure the head and neck area is sufficiently exposed and the room temperature is comfortable and lighting is adequate.
• Warm your hands and the stethoscope.

Asking the right questions

When obtaining the health history of a patient with a head or neck problem, you may need to elicit information on diverse topics. Here are some questions to use as a guide.

Medical-surgical history
☐ Have you noticed any lump or growth on your head or neck? If so, when did you first notice it? Has it changed recently? Is it painful?
☐ Have you ever had an operation on your head or neck? If so, when and for what condition?
☐ Have you ever had a problem with your thyroid gland? If so, how was it treated?

Headaches
☐ Do you have headaches? If so, what do you think causes them? How do you relieve the pain?
☐ Do the headaches affect your vision?
☐ Do you ever feel dizzy or faint?

Mobility
☐ Do you have any problems moving your head or neck?
☐ Does moving your head or neck cause you pain? If so, what relieves the pain?

Hair and scalp
☐ Do you have any problems with your scalp, such as itching, dandruff, or sores? If so, has any treatment helped?
☐ Have you changed your shampoo recently?
☐ Have you experienced hair loss? If so, for how long? Is it generalized or localized? Does your family have a history of baldness?

Implementation
Follow these steps when inspecting the head and neck.

Examining the head
• Inspect your patient's head, noting its general size and shape and the skull's contour. Normally, the skull is symmetrical and round. Although skull size varies from one patient to another, a disproportionately large or small skull is abnormal.
• Next, palpate the skull. It should feel hard and smooth. Note any deformities, lumps, or areas of tenderness.
• Gently palpate the temporal artery area with your fingertips. Note the character of the pulse, which should be steady.

• Inspect the patient's hair. Assess thickness, distribution, and texture. Separate the hair into sections with a comb to inspect the scalp. Look for lesions, cuts, scales, and nits.
• Inspect the patient's face, noting the symmetry of his facial structures. Look for abnormalities, such as drooping eyelids or mouth. Note any involuntary movements, such as facial tics. Inspect the skin for lesions or altered integrity.
• With your fingertips, palpate the facial bones lightly for lumps, tenderness, and edema.
• Palpate over the frontal sinuses for tenderness. Press upward from under the bony brow on each side of the face. Avoid pressing on the eyeball.

• Now, using your thumbs, press upward on each maxillary sinus. Note any tenderness.

• Lightly percuss over the frontal and maxillary sinus areas. Note any tenderness.

Examining the neck

Working downward, inspect the patient's neck for symmetry and tracheal deviation, jugular vein distention, and carotid artery prominence. Have the patient demonstrate his neck's range of motion by asking him to flex, extend, and rotate his head and touch his ear to his shoulder. Movement should be unrestricted and painless.

• Gently locate and palpate the carotid artery to check the patient's pulse rate and blood flow. Repeat this procedure on the carotid artery on the opposite side. Never palpate both carotid arteries at the same time; this could impede blood flow.

• Direct the patient to take a deep breath and hold it. Auscultate over the carotid artery with the bell of the stethoscope, listening for abnormal sounds, such as a bruit. Repeat this procedure on the carotid artery on the other side.

• Using the finger pads of both hands, palpate bilaterally under the patient's chin and under and behind the ears. Be alert for lymph node abnormalities. Assess the nodes for size, shape, mobility, hardness, and tenderness.

• Palpate the trachea, which is normally positioned midline in the neck. Place your thumbs along each side of the trachea near the lower portion of the neck. Determine whether the distance between the trachea's outer edge and the sternocleidomastoid muscle is equal on both sides.

• Now feel the thyroid, also to detect deviation or displacement from the midline. Inspect the trachea while the patient swallows. It should move symmetrically during swallowing. Then position yourself behind the patient. Place two fingers from each hand on the sides of the trachea, and ask the patient to swallow. Expect to feel the thyroid move freely.

• Displace the thyroid to the right and ask the patient to swallow again. Palpate the right lobe, noting enlargement, nodules, tenderness, or a gritty sensation. Displace the thyroid to the left and palpate the left lobe as the patient swallows.

• If you detect an enlarged thyroid, auscultate the area with the bell of your stethoscope. Listen for a bruit or a soft, rushing sound indicating a hypermetabolic state.

Nursing considerations

• Wear gloves for palpation if the patient has scalp lesions.

• Avoid palpating an area of the head or neck known to be tender at the start of your examination. Instead, work around the area; then gently palpate it at the end of the examination. This progression minimizes your patient's discomfort and apprehension.

Documentation

• Document any significant normal and abnormal findings from inspection of head, skull, hair, face, facial bones, sinuses, and neck.

• Document patient response during the inspection as well as any complaints specific to the head and neck.

Heart sound auscultation

No body system wears out, breaks down, or otherwise malfunctions so often, in so many people, as the cardiovascular system. Cardiovascular disease, after all, affects people of all ages and can take many forms. It can be congenital or acquired, and it can develop suddenly or insidiously. (Atherosclerosis, for example, can be far advanced or even life-threatening before signs and symptoms appear.) Among hospitalized patients, cardiovascular disease causes the majority of serious complications, including pulmonary embolism, thrombophlebitis, congestive heart failure, shock, and cardiac arrhythmias.

The cardiovascular system requires more auscultation than any other body system. Performed correctly, auscultation for heart sounds helps identify and evaluate changes in the patient's cardiac function—changes that may disrupt or threaten his life. Baseline information obtained during auscultation will help guide your intervention and follow-up care.

≫ Key nursing diagnoses and patient outcomes

Use these nursing diagnoses as a guide when developing your plan of care.

Anxiety related to lack of knowledge about purpose and procedure of heart auscultation
Based on this nursing diagnosis, you'll establish the following patient outcomes. The patient will:
• state feelings of anxiety.

• identify heart sound auscultation as cause of his anxiety.
• learn more about heart sound auscultation.

Knowledge deficit related to purpose and procedure of heart sound auscultation
Based on this nursing diagnosis, you'll establish the following patient outcomes. The patient will:
• state purpose of heart sound auscultation.
• explain procedure for heart sound auscultation.
• demonstrate skill in conserving energy while carrying out daily activities to tolerance level.

Decreased cardiac output related to (specify)
Based on this nursing diagnosis, you'll establish the following patient outcomes. The patient will:
• achieve activity within limits of prescribed heart rate.
• experience a decrease in heart workload.
• state understanding of signs and symptoms, prescribed activity level, diet, and medications.

Equipment
♦ stethoscope.

Equipment preparation
• Select a stethoscope with a chestpiece size appropriate for the patient's chest.

Patient preparation
• Explain the procedure to the patient. Maintain patient privacy. If the patient has special equipment, such as oxygen nebulizer or suction device, per-

form auscultation with equipment off if possible.

• Clothing and surgical dressings will muffle heart sounds or render them inaudible — open the front of the patient's gown, and drape the patient appropriately.

• Help the patient into a supine position, either flat or at a comfortable elevation.

Implementation

• Make sure that the room remains as quiet as possible.

• If you're right-handed, stand at the patient's right side — this will allow you to manipulate the stethoscope with your dominant hand.

• Use alternate positions as needed to improve heart sound auscultation (See *Alternate auscultation positions.*)

Auscultating the heart

• Keep the patient covered and in a supine position, with his head level or slightly elevated. Expose the area to be auscultated. Then warm your stethoscope between your hands. Have the patient inhale normally through his nose and exhale by mouth.

• To measure the apical pulse rate, place the diaphragm of the stethoscope over the point of maximal impulse (this normally appears in the fifth intercostal space at, or just medial to, the left midclavicular line).

• Count the heartbeats for 1 minute. Note the heart rhythm during this time. Is it regular or irregular? If it is irregular, does the rhythm have a pattern? If so, note the pattern.

• Mentally identify the four cardiac auscultation sites (See *Auscultation sites,* page 390.)

• Listen at each site in this sequence: Aortic area, pulmonic area, tricuspid area, and mitral area. Because the opening and closing of the hear valves create most normal heart sounds, auscultation sites lie close together in the chest, behind or to the left of the sternum. Auscultation sites are not located directly over the valves; they lie over the pathways the blood takes as it flows through them.

• Listen to several cardiac cycles at each site to become familiar with the rate and rhythm of S_1 and S_2. (See *Understanding normal heart sounds in the cardiac cycle,* page 391.)

• Once you're familiar with the rate and rhythm of normal heart sounds, listen for the heart sounds in each of the four areas following the sequence described previously. First, pressing firmly, use the diaphragm of the stethoscope. Then, pressing lightly, use the bell.

Note. In the aortic and pulmonic areas, S_1 is normally quieter than S_2. A split S_2 may be heard during inspiration in the pulmonic area. In the tricuspid and mitral areas, S_1 is normally louder than S_2. A split S_2 may be heard in the tricuspid area.

Auscultating additional heart sounds

When auscultating for S_1 and S_2, you may hear additional heart sounds: S_3, S_4, or both. (See *Where extra heart sounds occur in the cardiac cycle.*) Listen for S_3 (also called a ventricular gallop) when the patient is in the left lateral recumbent position. Place the bell of the stethoscope at the tricuspid and mitral areas. Expect to hear S_3 during early to mid-diastole, just after S_2, at the end of ventricular filling. The rhythm of S_3 resembles a horse gal-

Alternate auscultation positions

If heart sounds seem faint or undetectable, you may have to reposition the patient. Alternate positioning may enhance the sounds or make them seem louder by bringing the heart closer to the chest's surface. Common positions include a seated, forward-leaning position and the left-lateral decubitus position.

Forward-leaning position

Use this position when listening for high-pitched sounds related to semilunar valve problems, such as aortic and pulmonary valve murmurs. After helping the patient to the forward-leaning position, place the stethoscope's diaphragm over the aortic and pulmonary areas at the right and left second intercostal spaces.

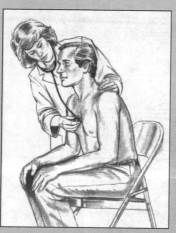

Left-lateral decubitus position

This position proves especially helpful when listening for low-pitched sounds related to atrioventricular valve problems, such as mitral valve murmurs and extra heart sounds. After helping the patient to the left-lateral decubitus position, place the stethoscope's bell over the apical area.

If these positions don't amplify heart sounds, try auscultating with the patient standing or squatting.

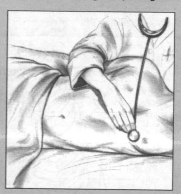

loping; its cadence resembles the word *ken-tuc-ky* or *lub-dub-by*. If the right ventricle is noncompliant, you'll hear the sound in the tricuspid area; if the left ventricle is noncompliant, you'll hear the sound in the mitral area.

• Listen for S_4 (also called atrial or presystolic gallop) with the patient in the supine position. Place the bell of the stethoscope on the patient's chest over the tricuspid and mitral areas. Expect to hear this heart sound late in diastole, immediately before the S_1 of the next cycle. S_4 has the same cadence as the word *ten-nes-see* or *le-lub-dub*. S_4 is associated with the acceleration and deceleration of blood entering a chamber that resists additional filling. In right ventricular dys-

Auscultation sites

When auscultating for heart sounds, place the stethoscope over four different sites. Follow the same auscultation sequence during every cardiovascular assessment.

• Place the stethoscope in the second intercostal space along the right sternal border, as shown. In the aortic area, blood moves from the left ventricle during systole, crossing the aortic valve and flowing through the aortic arch.
• Move to the pulmonary area, located in the second intercostal space at the left sternal border. In the pulmonary area, blood ejected from the right ventricle during systole crosses the pulmonary valve and flows through the main pulmonary artery.
• Assess in the third auscultation site, the tricuspid area, which lies in the fifth intercostal space along the left sternal border. In the tricuspid area, sounds reflect blood movement from the right atrium across the tricuspid valve, filling the right ventricle during diastole.
• Finally, listen in the mitral area, located in the fifth intercostal space near the midclavicular line. The mitral area may be closer to the anterior axillary line if the patient's heart is enlarged. In the mitral, or apical, area, sounds represent blood flow across the mitral valve and left ventricular filling during diastole.

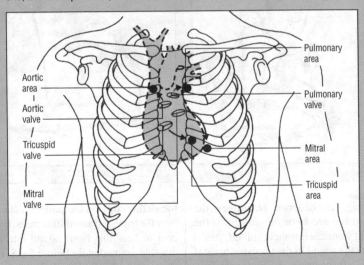

function, you'll hear S_4 in the tricuspid area; in left ventricular dysfunction, you'll hear it in the mitral area.

• To detect a pericardial friction rub, have the patient sit upright and lean forward or exhale. This enhances the sound of the friction rub. Then use the

Understanding normal heart sounds in the cardiac cycle

The cardiac cycle has two phases: systole, when the ventricles contract, increasing blood pressure and ejecting blood into the aorta and the pulmonary artery, and diastole, when the ventricles relax and blood pressure decreases, thereby contracting the atria. Using your stethoscope, you can hear each phase reverberate distinctively as the heart's valves open and close.

Sounds of systole

At the beginning of systole, increasing ventricular pressure forces the mitral and tricuspid valves to shut. The closing of these atrioventricular (AV) valves produces the first heart sound (S_1), or the *lub* of the *lub-dub.* The ventricular pressure builds until it exceeds that in the pulmonary artery and the aorta. Then the aortic and pulmonic (semilunar) valves open and the ventricles eject blood into the arteries (see arrows below).

Sounds of diastole

As the ventricles empty and relax, ventricular pressure falls below that in the pulmonary artery and the aorta. The semilunar valves close, producing the second heart sound (S_2), or the *dub* of *lub-dub* and marking the end of systole. As the ventricles relax during diastole, the pressure in the ventricles is less than that in the atria. The AV valves open, and blood begins to flow into the ventricles from the atria (see arrows below). When the ventricles become full near the end of diastole, the atria contract to send the rest of the blood to the ventricles. Ventricular pressure is now greater than atrial pressure. The AV valves close, marking the beginning of systole and repetition of the cardiac cycle.

Note: Events on the right side of the heart occur a fraction of a second after events on the left side because the pressure is lower on the right side of the heart.

Systole

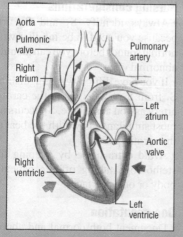

Aorta
Pulmonic valve
Right atrium
Pulmonary artery
Left atrium
Aortic valve
Right ventricle
Left ventricle

Diastole

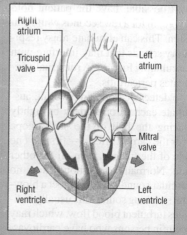

Right atrium
Tricuspid valve
Left atrium
Mitral valve
Right ventricle
Left ventricle

Where extra heart sounds occur in the cardiac cycle

To understand where the extra heart sounds fall in relation to systole, diastole, and the normal heart sounds, compare these illustrations representing normal and extra heart sounds.

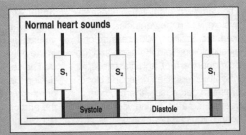

Normal heart sounds

S_1 S_2 S_1

Systole   Diastole

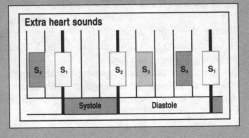

Extra heart sounds

S_4 S_1 S_2 S_3 S_4 S_1

Systole   Diastole

diaphragm of the stethoscope to auscultate at the third left intercostal space along the lower left sternal border. Listen for a harsh, scratchy, scraping, or squeaking sound.

If possible, have the patient hold his breath for a few seconds while you listen. This can eliminate noisy respiratory sounds that may interfere with auscultating for rubs. A rub usually indicates pericarditis.

• To detect a carotid artery bruit, auscultate each carotid artery by lightly placing the bell of the stethoscope over the carotid artery — first on one side of the trachea, then on the other side. Normally, you should hear no vascular sounds. If you detect a blowing, swishing sound, this usually indicates turbulent blood flow, which may occur in persons who have cardiovascular disease.

Ask the patient to hold his breath, if he can. This will eliminate respiratory sounds that may interfere with your findings.

Nursing considerations
• Always identify S_1 and S_2 first because you need to be familiar with normal sounds before you can identify abnormal ones.
• If you have difficulty distinguishing S_1 from S_2, try palpating the carotid artery as you auscultate. S_1 occurs almost simultaneously with the beat of the carotid pulse.
• Avoid extra noise by keeping the stethoscope tubing off the patient's body or other surfaces.

Documentation
• Document both normal and abnormal heart sounds.

Heat application

Heat applied directly to the patient's body raises tissue temperature and enhances the inflammatory process by causing vasodilation and increasing local circulation. This promotes leukocytosis, suppuration, drainage, and healing. Heat also increases tissue metabolism, reduces pain caused by muscular spasm, and decreases congestion in deep visceral organs.

Direct heat may be dry or moist. Dry heat can be delivered at a higher temperature and for a longer time. Devices for applying dry heat include the hot water bottle, electric heating pad, K pad, and chemical hot pack.

Moist heat softens crusts and exudates, penetrates deeper than dry heat, doesn't dry the skin, produces less perspiration, and usually is more comfortable for the patient. Devices for applying moist heat include warm compresses for small body areas and warm packs for large areas.

Direct heat treatment can't be used on a patient at risk for hemorrhage. It's also contraindicated if the patient has a sprained limb in the acute stage (because vasodilation would increase pain and swelling) or if he has a condition associated with acute inflammation such as appendicitis. Direct heat should be applied cautiously to pediatric and elderly patients and to patients with impaired renal, cardiac, or respiratory function; arteriosclerosis or atherosclerosis; and impaired sensation. It should be applied with extreme caution to heat-sensitive areas, such as scar tissue or stomas.

≫ Key nursing diagnoses and patient outcomes

Use these nursing diagnoses as a guide when developing your plan of care for a patient needing direct heat application.

Risk for injury related to heat application

Based on this nursing diagnosis, you'll establish the following patient outcomes. The patient will:
• experience no injury from application of heat.
• identify factors that increase potential for injury.
• verbalize understanding of safety measures to prevent injury from application of heat.

Pain related to (specify)

Based on this nursing diagnosis, you'll establish the following patient outcomes. The patient will:
• identify specific characteristics of pain.
• express relief from pain after application of heat.
• use available resources to understand pain phenomenon.

Risk for impaired skin integrity related to direct heat application

Based on this nursing diagnosis, you'll establish the following patient outcomes. The patient will:
• experience no skin breakdown.
• communicate understanding of preventive skin care measures.

Equipment

♦ patient thermometer ♦ towel ♦ adhesive tape or roller gauze ♦ gloves if the patient has an open lesion.

For a hot water bottle: ♦ hot tap water ♦ pitcher ♦ bath (utility) thermometer ♦ absorbent, protective cloth covering.

For an electric heating pad: ♦ absorbent, protective cloth covering.

For a K pad: ♦ distilled water ♦ temperature-adjustment key ♦ absorbent, protective cloth covering.

For a chemical hot pack (disposable): ♦ absorbent, protective cloth covering.

For a warm compress or pack: ♦ basin of hot tap water or container of sterile water, normal saline solution, or other solution as ordered ♦ hot-water bottle, K pad, or chemical hot pack ♦ linen-saver pad.

The following items may be sterile or nonsterile, depending on the type of procedure required: ♦ compress material (flannel, $4'' \times 4''$ gauze pads) or pack material (absorbent towels, ABD pads) ♦ petroleum jelly ♦ cotton-tipped applicators ♦ forceps ♦ bowl or basin ♦ bath (utility) thermometer ♦ waterproof covering ♦ towel ♦ dressing.

Equipment preparation

• *Hot-water bottle:* Fill the bottle with hot tap water to detect leaks and warm the bottle, and then empty it. Run hot tap water into a pitcher, and measure the water temperature with the bath thermometer. Adjust the temperature as ordered, usually to 115° to 125° F (46.1° to 51.7° C) for adults and 105° to 115° F (40.6° to 46.1° C) for children under age 2 and elderly patients. Next, pour hot water into the bottle, filling it one-half to two-thirds full. *Partially filling the bottle keeps it lightweight and flexible to mold to the*

treatment area. Squeeze the bottle until the water reaches the neck *to expel any air that would make the bottle inflexible and reduce heat conduction.* Fasten the top, and cover the bag with an absorbent, protective cloth *to provide insulation and absorb perspiration.* Secure the cover with tape or roller gauze.

• *Electric heating pad:* Check the cord for frayed or damaged insulation. Then plug in the pad and adjust the control switch to the desired setting. Wrap the pad in a protective cloth covering, and secure the cover with tape or roller gauze.

• *K pad:* Check the cord for safety, as above, and fill the control unit two-thirds full with distilled water. Do not use tap water *because it leaves mineral deposits in the unit.* Check for leaks, and then tilt the unit in several directions *to clear the pad's tubing of air, which could interfere with even heat conduction.* Tighten the cap, and then loosen it a quarter turn *to allow heat expansion within the unit.* After making sure the hoses between the control unit and the pad are free of tangles, place the unit on the bedside table, slightly above the patient *so gravity can assist water flow.* If the central supply department has not preset the temperature on the control unit, use the key provided to make this adjustment. The usual temperature is 105° F. Then, place the pad in a protective cloth covering and secure the cover with tape or roller gauze. Plug in the unit, turn it on, and allow the pad to warm for 2 minutes.

• *Chemical hot pack:* Select a pack of the correct size. Then, follow the manufacturer's directions (strike, squeeze, or knead) *to activate the heat-produc-*

ing chemicals. Place the pack in a protective cloth covering and secure the cover with tape or roller gauze.

• *Sterile warm compress or pack:* Warm the container of sterile water or solution by setting it in a sink or basin of hot water. Measure the solution's temperature with a sterile bath thermometer. If a sterile thermometer is unavailable, pour some heated sterile solution into a clean container, check the temperature with a regular bath thermometer, and then discard the tested solution. Adjust the temperature of the sterile solution by adding hot or cold water to the sink or basin until the solution reaches 131° F (55° C) for adults or 105° F for children and elderly patients and for an eye compress. Pour the heated solution into a sterile bowl or basin. Then, using sterile technique, soak the compress or pack in the heated solution. If necessary, prepare a hot water bottle, K pad, or chemical hot pack *to keep the compress or pack warm.*

• *Nonsterile warm compress or pack:* Fill a bowl or basin with hot tap water or other solution, and measure the temperature of the fluid with a bath thermometer. Adjust the temperature as ordered, usually to 131° F (55° C) for adults or 105° F (40.6° C) for children and elderly patients and for an eye compress. Then soak the compress or pack in the hot liquid. If necessary, prepare a hot water bottle, K pad, or chemical hot pack *to keep the compress or pack warm.*

Patient preparation
• Check the doctor's order, and assess the patient's condition.
• Explain the procedure to the patient, and tell him not to lean or lie directly

on the heating device *because this reduces air space and increases the risk of burns.* Warn the patient against adjusting the temperature of the heating device or adding hot water to a hotwater bottle. Advise him to report pain or discomfort immediately and to remove the device himself if necessary.
• Provide privacy and make sure the room is warm and free of drafts. Wash your hands thoroughly.
• Take the patient's temperature, pulse, and respirations *to serve as a baseline.* If heat treatment is being applied to raise the patient's body temperature, monitor temperature, pulse, and respirations throughout the application.
• Expose only the treatment area *because vasodilation will make the patient feel chilly.*

Implementation
To apply a hot-water bottle, an electric heating pad, a K pad, or a chemical hot pack:
• Before applying the heating device, press it against the inner aspect of your forearm *to test its temperature and heat distribution.* If it heats unevenly, obtain a new device.
• Apply the device to the treatment area, and if necessary, secure it with tape or roller gauze. Begin timing the application.
• Assess the patient's skin condition frequently, and remove the device if you observe increased swelling or excessive redness, blistering, maceration, or pronounced pallor, or if the patient reports pain or discomfort. Refill the hot-water bottle as necessary *to maintain the correct temperature.*
• Remove the device after 20 to 30 minutes, or as ordered.

• Dry the patient's skin with a towel and re-dress the site, if necessary. Take the patient's temperature, pulse, and respirations *for comparison with the baseline*. Position him comfortably in bed.

• If the treatment is to be repeated, store the equipment in the patient's room, out of his reach; otherwise, return the equipment to its proper place.

To apply a warm compress or pack

• Place a linen-saver pad under the treatment area. Spread petroleum jelly (sterile, if necessary) over the affected area. Avoid applying it directly to any areas of skin breakdown or to eye tissues. (You may use sterile cotton-tipped applicators for a sterile procedure.) *The petroleum jelly reduces maceration and the risk of burns by decreasing the rate of heat penetration.*

• Remove the warm compress or pack from the bowl or basin. (Use sterile forceps for a sterile procedure.)

• Wring excess solution from the compress or pack, using sterile forceps for a sterile procedure. *Excess moisture increases the risk of burns.*

• Apply the compress gently to the affected site, using forceps if warranted. After a few seconds, lift the compress with forceps if needed, and check the skin for excessive redness, maceration, or blistering. When you're sure the compress isn't causing a burn, mold it firmly to the skin *to keep out air, which reduces the temperature and effectiveness of the compress*. Work quickly, *so the compress retains its heat.*

• Apply a waterproof covering (sterile, if warranted) to the compress. Secure the covering with tape or roller gauze *to prevent it from slipping.*

• Place a hot-water bottle, K pad, or chemical hot pack over the compress and waterproof covering *to maintain the correct temperature*. Begin timing the application.

• Check the patient's skin every 5 minutes for signs of tissue intolerance. Remove the device if the skin shows excessive redness, maceration, or blistering or if the patient feels pain or discomfort. Change the compress as necessary to maintain the correct temperature.

• After 15 or 20 minutes or as ordered, remove the compress. (Use forceps, if warranted.) Discard the compress into a waterproof trash bag.

• Dry the patient's skin with a towel (sterile, if necessary). Note the condition of the skin and re-dress the area, if necessary. Take the patient's temperature, pulse, and respiration *for comparison with the baseline*. Then make sure the patient is comfortable.

Complications

• Because tissue damage may result from direct heat application, monitor the temperature of the compress carefully.

• Assess frequently the condition of the patient's skin under the heat application device

Nursing considerations

• If the patient is unconscious, anesthetized, irrational, neurologically impaired, or insensitive to heat for any reason, stay with him throughout the treatment.

• When direct heat is ordered to decrease congestion within internal organs, the application must cover a large enough area *to increase blood volume at the skin's surface*. For relief of pelvic organ congestion, for example, apply heat over the patient's lower abdomen, hips, and thighs. To achieve local relief, you may concentrate heat only over the specified area. (See *Using moist heat to relieve muscle spasm.*)

• As an alternative method of applying sterile moist compresses, use a bedside sterilizer to sterilize the compresses. Saturate the compress with tap water or another solution and wring it dry. Then place it in the bedside sterilizer at 275° F (135° C) for 15 minutes. Remove the compress with sterile forceps or sterile gloves, and wring out the excess solution. Then place the compress in a sterile bowl and measure its temperature with a sterile thermometer.

Home care

• Tell patients to choose moist heat rather than dry heat when attempting to ease muscle tension or spasm. Moist heat is less drying to the skin, less apt to cause burns, less likely to cause excessive fluid and salt loss through sweating, and more likely to penetrate deeper tissues.

Instruct the patient to apply heat for 20 to 30 minutes, as follows:
• Place a moist towel over the painful area.
• Cover the towel with a hot-water bottle properly filled and at the correct temperature.
• Remove the hot-water bottle and wet pack after 20 to 30 minutes. Don't continue application for longer than 30 minutes because therapeutic value decreases after that time.

Using moist heat to relieve muscle spasm

Tell patients to use moist heat rather than dry heat when attempting to ease muscle tension or spasm. Moist heat is less drying to the skin, less apt to cause burns, less likely to cause excessive fluid and salt loss through sweating, and more likely to penetrate deeper tissues. Instruct the patient to apply heat for 20 to 30 minutes, as follows:
• Place a moist towel over the painful area.
• Cover the towel with a hot water bottle properly filled and at the correct temperature.
• Remove the hot water bottle and wet pack after 20 to 30 minutes. Don't continue application for longer than 30 minutes because therapeutic value decreases after that time.

Documentation

• Record the time and date of heat application; the type, temperature or heat setting, duration, and site of application; the patient's temperature, pulse, respirations, and skin condition before, during, and after treatment; signs of complications; and the patient's tolerance of and reaction to treatment.

Height and weight measurement, adult

Height and weight are routinely measured for most patients during admission to the hospital. An accurate record of the patient's height and weight is essential for calculating dosages of drugs, anesthetics, and contrast agents; assessing the patient's nutritional status; and determining the height-weight ratio. And because body weight provides the best overall picture of fluid status, monitoring it daily proves important for patients receiving sodium-retaining or diuretic medications. Rapid weight gain may signal fluid retention; rapid weight loss may indicate diuresis.

Weight can be measured with a standing scale, chair scale, or bed scale; height can be measured with the measuring bar on a standing scale or with a tape measure for a patient in a supine position.

≫ Key nursing diagnoses and patient outcomes

Use these nursing diagnoses as a guide when developing your plan of care.

Knowledge deficit related to lack of exposure to assessment techniques

Based on this nursing diagnosis, you'll establish the following patient outcome. The patient will:
• verbalize understanding of procedure for height or weight measurement, or both.

Altered nutrition: more than body requirements related to (specify)

Based on this nursing diagnosis, you'll establish the following patient outcomes. The patient will:
• identify internal and external cues that increase food consumption.
• lose at least (specify) lb weekly.
• plan menus appropriate to prescribed diet.

Altered nutrition: less than body requirements related to (specify)

Based on this nursing diagnosis, you'll establish the following patient outcomes. The patient will:
identify emotional and psychological factors that interfere with eating.
• gain (specify) lb weekly.
• consume at least (specify) calories daily.

Equipment

♦ standing (with measuring bar), chair, or bed scale ♦ wheelchair (if needed to transport patient) ♦ tape measure if needed.

Equipment preparation

• Select the appropriate scale — usually, a standing scale for an ambulatory patient or a chair or bed scale for an acutely ill or debilitated patient. (See *Types of scales.*)
• Then check scale balance. Standing scales and, to a lesser extent, bed scales may become unbalanced when transported.

Patient preparation

• Explain the procedure to the patient. Refer to a chart of suggested healthy weight ranges *to determine norms for your patient's height and weight.* (See *Suggested weights for adults,* page 400.)

Implementation

Follow the steps below for using different methods of weight measurement.

Using a standing scale

• Place a paper towel on the scale's platform.
• Tell the patient to remove his robe and slippers or shoes to ensure accu-

Types of scales

For ambulatory patients

Standing scale

For acutely ill or debilitated patients

Chair scale

Bed scale

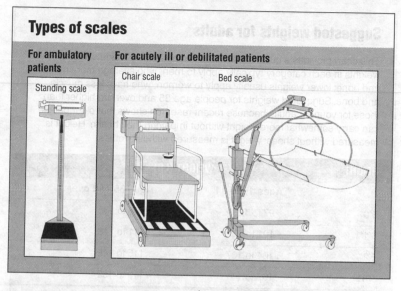

rate measurement of height and weight. If the scale has wheels, lock them before the patient steps on. Assist the patient onto the scale *to prevent falls.* Remain close to the patient *so you can steady him if necessary.*
• If you're using an upright balance (gravity) scale, slide the lower rider to the groove representing the largest increment below the patient's estimated weight. Grooves represent 50, 100, 150, and 200 lb (23, 45, 68, and 91 kg). Then slide the small upper rider until the beam balances. Add the upper and lower rider figures to determine the weight. (The upper rider is calibrated to eighths of a pound.)
• If you're using a multiple-weight scale, move the appropriate ratio weights onto the weight holder to balance the scale; ratio weights are labeled 50, 100, and 200 lb. Add ratio weights until the next weight causes the main beam to fall. Then adjust the main beam poise until the scale bal-

ances. Next, add the sum of the ratio weights to the figure on the main beam to obtain the patient's weight.
• Return ratio weights to their rack and the weight holder to its proper place.
• If you're using a scale with a digital display, make sure the display reads 0 before use. Read the display with the patient on the scale and standing as still as possible.
• If you're measuring height, tell the patient to stand erect on the platform of the scale. Raise the measuring bar beyond the top of the patient's head, extend the horizontal arm, and lower the bar until it touches the top of the patient's head. Then read the patient's height.
• Help the patient off the scale, and give him his robe and slippers or shoes. Then return the measuring bar to its initial position.

Suggested weights for adults

This chart provides a guideline for determining healthy weights. Higher weights in each category typically apply to men, who average more muscle and bone; lower weights usually apply to women, who have less muscle and bone. Suggested weights for people age 35 and over are higher than those for younger adults because recent research shows that older people can carry somewhat more weight without impairing their health. Height is measured without shoes; weight is measured without clothes.

HEIGHT	WEIGHT (LB)	
	Ages 19 to 34	Ages 35 and over
5'0"	97 to 128	108 to 138
5'1"	101 to 132	111 to 143
5'2"	104 to 137	115 to 148
5'3"	107 to 141	119 to 152
5'4"	111 to 146	122 to 157
5'5"	114 to 150	126 to 162
5'6"	118 to 155	130 to 167
5'7"	121 to 160	134 to 172
5'8"	125 to 164	138 to 178
5'9"	129 to 169	142 to 183
5'10"	132 to 174	146 to 188
5'11"	136 to 179	151 to 194
6'0"	140 to 184	155 to 199
6'1"	144 to 189	159 to 205
6'2"	148 to 195	164 to 210
6'3"	152 to 200	168 to 216
6'4"	156 to 205	173 to 222
6'5"	160 to 211	177 to 228
6'6"	164 to 216	182 to 234

Source: U.S. Department of Agriculture, U.S. Department of Health and Human Services. *Nutrition and Your Health: Dietary Guidelines for Americans,* 3rd ed. Washington, D.C., 1990.

Using a chair scale

• Transport the patient to the weighing area or the scale to the patient's bedside.

• Lock the scale in place *to prevent it from moving accidentally.*

• If you're using a scale with a swing-away chair arm, unlock the arm. When unlocked, the arm swings back 180 degrees to permit easy patient access.

• Position the scale beside the patient's bed or wheelchair with the chair arm open. Transfer the patient onto the scale, swing the chair arm to the front of the scale, and lock it in place.

• Weigh the patient by adding ratio weights and adjusting the main beam poise. Then unlock the swing-away chair arm as before, and transfer the patient back to his bed or wheelchair.

• Lock the main beam *to avoid damaging the scale during transport.* Unlock the wheels and remove the scale from the patient's room.

Using a multiple-weight bed scale

• Provide privacy, and tell the patient that you're going to weigh him on a special bed scale.

• Position the scale next to the patient's bed and lock the scale's wheels. Then turn the patient on his side, facing away from the scale.

• Release the stretcher frame to the horizontal position, and pump the hand lever until the stretcher is positioned over the mattress. Lower the stretcher onto the mattress, and roll the patient onto the stretcher.

• Raise the stretcher 2″ (5 cm) above the mattress. Then add ratio weights, and adjust the main beam poise as for the standing and chair scales.

• After weighing the patient, lower the stretcher onto the mattress, turn the patient on his side, and remove the stretcher. Be sure to leave the patient in a comfortable position.

Using a digital bed scale

• Provide privacy, and tell the patient that you're going to weigh him on a special bed scale. Demonstrate the scale's operation if the patient is being weighed for the first time.

• Release the stretcher to the horizontal position, then lock it in place. Turn the patient on his side, facing away from the scale.

• Roll the base of the scale under the patient's bed. Adjust the lever *to widen the base of the scale, providing stability.* After doing so, lock the scale's wheels.

• Center the stretcher above the bed, lower it onto the mattress, and roll the patient onto the stretcher. Then position the circular weighing arms of the scale over the patient, and attach them securely to the stretcher bars.

• Pump the handle with long, slow strokes *to raise the patient a few inches off the bed.* Ensure that the patient doesn't lean on or touch the headboard, side rails, or other bed equipment *because this will affect weight measurement.*

• Depress the operate button, and read the patient's weight on the digital display panel. Then press in the scale's handle *to lower the patient onto the bed.*

• Detach the circular weighing arms from the stretcher bars, roll the patient off the stretcher and remove it, and position him comfortably in bed.

• Release the wheel lock and withdraw the scale. Return the stretcher to its vertical position for storage.

Nursing considerations

• Reassure and steady patients who are at risk for losing their balance on a scale.

• Weigh the patient at the same time each day (usually before breakfast), in similar clothing, and with the same scale. If the patient uses crutches, weigh him with the crutches; then weigh the crutches and any heavy clothing and subtract their weight from the total to determine the patient's weight. If the patient is markedly obese, check scale capacity. (Although some newer scales can measure up to 600 lb [272 kg], most scales can measure a maximum of 250 lb [113 kg].) You may have to weigh the patient on a large commercial scale (usually located on the loading dock or in the dietary department).

• Before using a bed scale, cover its stretcher with a drawsheet *to avoid stains from perspiration, drainage, or excretions.* Balance the scale with the drawsheet in place *to ensure accurate weighing.*

• When rolling the patient onto the stretcher, be careful not to dislodge I.V. lines, indwelling catheters, and other supportive equipment.

Documentation

• Record the patient's height and weight on the nursing assessment form and other medical records, as required by your hospital.

Height and weight measurement, neonatal

A beginning point for many neonatal assessments, measuring anthropometric dimensions and weight establishes the baseline for accurately monitoring normal growth. Size and weight measurements help detect such disorders as failure to thrive, small for gestational age, hydrocephalus, and intracranial bleeding. The nurse takes the measurements in the nursery during routine checkups and sometimes at the neonate's home. She then compares the results with previous measurements and with normal values.

Normally the neonate's head circumference measures the same as or more than his chest circumference. The exception is the first 24 hours after birth when head molding leaves the head circumference slightly smaller than chest circumference. The head's contour usually returns to normal in 2 to 3 days.

The neonate's weight varies with sex, gestational age, heredity, and other factors. A firstborn usually weighs less at birth than his siblings. The neonate with a diabetic mother tends to be large. Because of an erratic feeding pattern and passage of urine and meconium, the normal neonate loses between 5% and 10% of his birth weight during the first few days. However, he usually regains this weight in 10 days. Normal weight gain for the neonate is 5 to 7 oz (142 to 198 g) weekly. (See *Baby scale monitors breast milk intake, too.*)

›› Key nursing diagnoses and patient outcomes

Use these nursing diagnoses as a guide when developing your plan of care.

Altered growth and development related to (specify)

Based on this nursing diagnosis, you'll establish the following patient outcomes. The patient and family will:

• exhibit normal growth and development for age.

• express realistic expectations for neonate's growth.

• demonstrate understanding of neonate's special needs.

• accept referrals to available community resources.

Ineffective infant feeding pattern related to (specify)

Based on this nursing diagnosis, you'll establish the following patient outcomes. The patient or family will:

• not lose more than 10% of birth weight within first week of life.

• gain 4 to 7 oz (113 to 198 g)/week after the first week of life.

• identify factors that interfere with the neonate establishing an effective feeding pattern.

• express increased confidence in their ability to perform appropriate feeding techniques.

Equipment

♦ crib or examination table with a firm surface ♦ scale with tray ♦ scale paper if necessary ♦ tape measure ♦ length board ♦ gloves if the neonate hasn't been bathed yet.

Disposable paper tape measures are available. Cloth tapes aren't rec-

TECHNOLOGY UPDATE

Baby scale monitors breast milk intake, too

A new mother often worries if her baby is receiving sufficient nutrients during breast-feeding. One way of assessing nutritional status is to monitor weight gain and loss. A new baby scale (Medela, Inc.) calculates breast milk intake based on the baby's weight gain during feedings.

To determine breast milk intake, the baby is weighed before and after feeding. A microprocessor in the scale calculates milk intake with an accuracy of plus or minus 0.07 oz (2 g). The scale can be rented for home use.

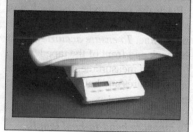

ommended because they can stretch, leading to inaccurate measurements.

Equipment preparation

• Put clean paper on the scale to promote warmth and prevent cold stress.

• Balance the scale at zero as directed by the manufacturer.

Patient preparation

• Explain the procedure to the parents, if present.

• Wash your hands, and put on gloves if you haven't bathed the neonate yet.

• To begin, position the neonate in a supine position in the crib or on the examination table.

• Remove all clothing but his diaper (if he has one). Be sure to record all measurements. (See *Average neonatal size and weight.*)

Implementation

Here's how to measure a neonate's dimensions and weight.

To measure head circumference

• Slide the tape measure under the neonate's head at the occiput. *To arrive at the greatest circumference,* draw the tape snugly around, just above the eyebrows.

To measure chest circumference

• Place the tape under the back and wrap it snugly around the chest at the nipple line. *To ensure accuracy,* keep the back and front of the tape level.

• Take the measurement after the neonate inspires and before he begins to exhale.

To measure head-to-heel length

• Fully extend the neonate's legs with the toes pointing up. Measure the distance from the heel to the top of the head. If possible, have someone extend the legs by pressing down gently on the knees. Or use a length board, if available.

To measure crown-to-rump length

• Place the neonate on his side and measure from the crown of his head to his buttocks. This measurement should approximate the head circumference.

To weigh the neonate

• Take this measurement before, not after, a feeding. Remove the neonate's diaper before placing him in the middle of the scale tray.

• Note the neonate's weight. Keep one hand poised over him at all times to prevent accidents. Work quickly to avoid having the scale become soiled or wet and to prevent neonatal heat loss.

• Return the neonate to the crib or examination table.

• Be sure to record if the neonate has clothing or equipment (such as an I.V. armband) on him.

• Clean the scale tray *to prevent cross-contamination between neonates.*

To measure abdominal girth

• Place the neonate in a supine position, and measure his girth just above the umbilicus. Though not an anthropometric measurement, *the size of this expanse may suggest abnormalities such as an obstruction.*

• When you finish, dress and diaper the neonate. Return him to his crib, if necessary, or give him to a parent who can hold and comfort him.

Nursing considerations

• Keep in mind that head swelling or molding after delivery may skew initial head circumference measurements.

• Length can also be measured by placing the neonate on paper such as that used on examination tables. Mark the paper at the heel, with the toes pointing straight up, and at the head. Then measure the distance between the marks.

• Various scale models are available. Be sure to learn how to read and operate the one available to you. If you use a model that measures metrically,

Average neonatal size and weight

Besides weight, anthropometric measurements include head and chest circumferences, crown-to-rump length, and head-to-heel length (as shown below). These measurements serve as a baseline and show whether neonatal size is within normal ranges or whether there may be a significant problem or anomaly — especially if values stray far from the mean. Initial average anthropometric ranges for a neonate follow:

• Head circumference: 13″ to 14″ (33 to 35.6 cm)
• Chest circumference: 12″ to 13″ (30.5 to 33 cm)
• Crown to rump: about the same as head circumference
• Head to heel: 18″ to 21″ (45.7 to 53.3 cm)
• Weight: 5 lb 8 oz to 8 lb 13 oz (2,500 to 4,000 g)

Head circumference

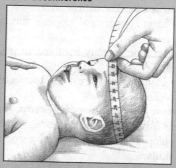

Chest circumference

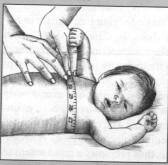

Crown to rump

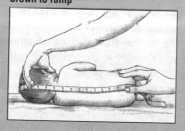

Head to heel

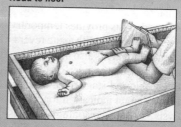

supply the parents with a table of metric equivalents for use at home.

Documentation

• Record each weight and dimension measurement in your notes or neonatal assessment sheet.

• During routine checkups, remember to share information with the parents, who may carry a booklet in which they also document weight and dimensions.

Hemodialysis

Hemodialysis is performed to remove toxic wastes from the blood of patients in renal failure. This potentially life-saving procedure removes blood from the body, circulates it through a purifying dialyzer, and then returns the blood to the body. Various access sites can be used for this procedure. (See *Hemodialysis access sites*.)

The most common access device for long-term treatment is an arteriovenous (AV) fistula.

The underlying mechanism in hemodialysis is differential diffusion across a semipermeable membrane, which extracts by-products of protein metabolism, such as urea and uric acid as well as creatinine and excess body water. This process restores or maintains the balance of the body's buffer system and electrolyte level. Hemodialysis thus promotes a rapid return to normal serum values and helps prevent complications associated with uremia.

Hemodialysis provides temporary support for patients with acute reversible renal failure. It's also used for regular long-term treatment of patients with chronic end-stage renal disease. A less common indication for hemodialysis is acute poisoning, such as barbiturate or analgesic overdose. The patient's condition (rate of urea generation, weight gain) determines the number and duration of hemodialysis treatments.

Specially prepared personnel usually perform this procedure in a hemodialysis unit. However, if the patient is acutely ill and unstable, hemodialysis can be done at bedside in the intensive care unit.

Special hemodialysis units are also available for home use.

≫ Key nursing diagnoses and patient outcomes

Use these nursing diagnoses as a guide when developing your plan of care for a patient needing hemodialysis.

Ineffective individual coping related to hemodialysis

Based on this nursing diagnosis, you'll establish the following patient outcomes. The patient will:
• identify personal coping mechanisms.
• become actively involved in planning own care.
• identify effective and ineffective coping techniques.
• use available support systems, such as family and significant others, to develop and maintain effective coping skills.

Ineffective management of therapeutic regimen: individual related to (specify)

Based on this nursing diagnosis, you'll establish the following patient outcomes. The patient will:
• express personal beliefs about illness and its management.
• identify dietary modifications.
• develop plan for integrating components of therapeutic regimen into pattern of daily living.

Risk for infection related to hemodialysis

Based on this nursing diagnosis, you'll establish the following patient outcomes. The patient will:

Hemodialysis access sites

Hemodialysis requires vascular access. The site and type of access may vary, depending on the expected duration of dialysis, the surgeon's preference, and the patient's condition.

Subclavian vein catheterization
Using the Seldinger technique, the doctor or surgeon inserts an introducer needle into the subclavian vein. He then inserts a guide wire through the introducer needle and removes the needle. Using the guide wire, he then threads a 5″ to 12″ (12.7- to 30.5-cm) plastic or Teflon catheter (with a Y-hub) into the patient's vein.

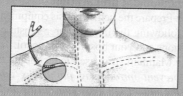

Femoral vein catheterization
Using the Seldinger technique, the doctor or surgeon inserts an introducer needle into the left or right femoral vein. He then inserts a guide wire through the introducer needle and removes the needle. Using the guide wire, he then threads a 5″ to 12″ plastic or Teflon catheter with a Y-hub or two catheters, one for inflow and another placed about ½″ (1.3 cm) distal to the first for outflow.

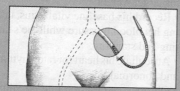

Arteriovenous fistula
To create a fistula, the surgeon makes an incision into the patient's wrist or lower forearm, then a small incision in the side of an artery and another in the side of a vein. He sutures the edges of these incisions together to make a common opening 3 to 7 mm long.

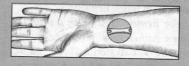

Arteriovenous shunt
To create a shunt, the surgeon makes an incision in the patient's wrist, lower forearm, or (rarely) an ankle. He then inserts a 6″ to 10″ (15.2- to 25.4-cm) transparent Silastic cannula into an artery and another into a vein. Finally, he tunnels the cannulas out through stab wounds and joins them with a piece of Teflon tubing.

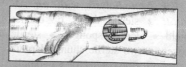

Arteriovenous graft
To create a graft, the surgeon makes an incision in the patient's forearm, upper arm, or thigh. He then tunnels a natural or synthetic graft under the skin and sutures the distal end to an artery and the proximal end to a vein.

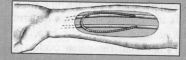

• remain free from elevated temperature.
• remain free of all signs and symptoms of infection.

Equipment

For preparing the hemodialysis machine: ◆ hemodialysis machine with appropriate dialyzer ◆ I.V. solution, administration sets, lines, and related equipment ◆ dialysate ◆ optional: heparin, 3-ml syringe with needle, medication label, hemostats.

For hemodialysis with a double-lumen catheter: ◆ povidone-iodine sponges ◆ two sterile $4'' \times 4''$ gauze pads ◆ two 3-ml and two 5-ml syringes ◆ tape ◆ heparin bolus syringe ◆ clean gloves.

For hemodialysis with an AV fistula: ◆ two winged fistula needles (each attached to a 10-ml syringe filled with heparinized normal saline solution) ◆ linen-saver pad ◆ povidone-iodine sponges ◆ sterile $4'' \times 4''$ gauze pads ◆ tourniquet ◆ clean gloves ◆ adhesive tape.

For hemodialysis with an AV shunt: ◆ sterile drape or barrier shield ◆ alcohol sponges ◆ sterile gloves ◆ two sterile shunt adapters ◆ sterile Teflon connector ◆ two bulldog clamps ◆ two 10-ml syringes ◆ normal saline solution ◆ four short strips of adhesive tape ◆ optional: sterile shunt spreader.

For discontinuing hemodialysis with a double-lumen catheter: ◆ two sterile $4'' \times 4''$ gauze pads ◆ povidone-iodine sponge ◆ precut gauze dressing ◆ clean gloves ◆ normal saline solution ◆ sterile gauze sponges ◆ heparin flush solution ◆ luer-lock injection caps ◆ optional: transparent occlusive

dressing, skin barrier preparation, tape, materials for culturing drainage.

For discontinuing hemodialysis with an AV fistula: ◆ clean gloves ◆ sterile $4'' \times 4''$ gauze pads ◆ two adhesive bandages ◆ povidone-iodine ointment ◆ hemostats ◆ optional: sterile absorbable gelatin sponges (Gelfoam).

For discontinuing hemodialysis with an AV shunt: ◆ sterile gloves ◆ two bulldog clamps ◆ two hemostats ◆ povidone-iodine solution ◆ sterile $4'' \times 4''$ gauze pads ◆ alcohol sponges ◆ elastic gauze bandages.

Equipment preparation

• Prepare the hemodialysis equipment following the manufacturer's instructions and your hospital's protocol.
• Maintain strict aseptic technique *to prevent introducing pathogens into the patient's bloodstream during dialysis.*
• Be sure to test the dialyzer and dialysis machine for residual disinfectant after rinsing.
• Test all the alarms.

Patient preparation

• Weigh the patient.
• To determine ultrafiltration requirements, compare his present weight to his weight after the last dialysis and his target weight.
• Record his baseline vital signs, taking his blood pressure while he's sitting and standing.
• Auscultate his heart for rate, rhythm, and abnormalities.
• Observe respiratory rate, rhythm, and quality.
• Assess for edema.
• Check his mental status and the condition and patency of the access site.

• Check for problems since the last dialysis, and evaluate previous laboratory data.

• Help the patient into a comfortable position (supine or sitting in recliner chair with feet elevated). Be sure the access site is well supported and resting on a clean drape.

• If the patient is undergoing hemodialysis for the first time, explain the procedure in detail.

• Use standard precautions in all cases *to prevent transmission of infection.*

Implementation

• Wash your hands before beginning.

To begin hemodialysis with a double-lumen catheter

• Prepare venous access. If extension tubing isn't already clamped, clamp it *to prevent air from entering the catheter.* Then clean each catheter extension tube, clamp, and luer-lock injection cap with povidone-iodine sponges *to remove contaminants.* Next, place a sterile $4'' \times 4''$ gauze pad under the extension tubing, and place two 5-ml syringes and two sterile gauze pads on the drape.

• Prepare anticoagulant regimen as ordered.

• Identify arterial and venous blood lines, and place them near the drape.

• *To remove clots and ensure catheter patency,* remove catheter caps, attach syringes to each catheter port, open one clamp, and aspirate 1.5 to 3 ml of blood. Close the clamp and repeat the procedure with the other port. Flush each port with 5 ml of heparinized saline.

• Attach blood lines to patient access. First, remove the syringe from the arterial port, and attach the line to the arterial port. Then administer the heparin according to protocol. *This prevents clotting in the extracorporeal circuit.*

• Grasp the venous blood line and attach it to the venous port. Open the clamps on the extension tubing, and secure the tubing to the patient's extremity with tape *to reduce tension on the tube and minimize trauma to the insertion site.*

• Begin hemodialysis according to your unit's protocol.

To begin hemodialysis with an AV fistula

• Flush the fistula needles, using attached syringes containing heparinized saline solution, and set them aside.

• Place a linen-saver pad under the patient's arm.

• Using aseptic technique, clean a $3'' \times 10''$ (7.5×25.1 cm) area of skin over the fistula with povidone-iodine sponges. Discard each pad after one wipe. (If the patient is sensitive to iodine, use chlorhexidine gluconate [Hibiclens] or alcohol instead.)

• Apply a tourniquet above the fistula *to distend the veins and facilitate venipuncture.* Make sure you avoid occluding the fistula.

• Put on clean gloves. Perform the venipuncture with a fistula needle. Remove the needle guard and squeeze the wing tips firmly together. Insert the arterial needle at least $1''$ (2.5 cm) above the anastomosis, being careful not to puncture the fistula.

• Release the tourniquet and flush the needle with heparinized normal saline solution *to prevent clotting.* Clamp the arterial needle tubing with a hemostat, and secure the wing tips of the needle

to the skin with adhesive tape *to prevent it from dislodging within the vein.*
• Perform another venipuncture with the venous needle a few inches above the arterial needle. Flush the needle with heparinized saline solution. Clamp the venous needle tubing, apply ointment, and secure the wing tips of the arterial needle as you did the arterial needle.
• Remove the syringe from the end of the arterial tubing, uncap the arterial line from the hemodialysis machine, and connect the two lines. Tape the connection securely *to prevent it from separating during the procedure.* Repeat these two steps for the venous line.
• Release the hemostats and start hemodialysis.

To begin hemodialysis with an AV shunt
• Remove the bulldog clamps and place them within easy reach of the sterile field. Remove the shunt dressing, and clean the shunt, using aseptic technique, as you would for daily care. Clean the bulldog clamps with an alcohol sponge.
• Assemble the shunt adapters according to the manufacturer's directions.
• Clean the arterial and venous shunt connection with povidone-iodine sponges *to remove contaminants.* Use a separate sponge for each tube, and wipe in one direction only, from the insertion site to the connection sites. Allow the tubing to air-dry.
• Put on sterile gloves.
• Clamp the arterial side of the shunt with a bulldog clamp *to prevent blood from flowing through it.* Clamp the venous side *to prevent leakage when the shunt is opened.*

• Open the shunt by separating its sides with your fingers or with a sterile shunt spreader, if available. Both sides of the shunt should be exposed. Always inspect the Teflon connector on one side of the shunt *to see if it's damaged or bent.* If necessary, replace it before proceeding. Note which side contains the connector *so you can use the new one to close the shunt after treatment.*
• *To adapt the shunt to the lines of the machine,* attach a shunt adapter and 10-ml syringe filled with about 8 ml of normal saline solution to the side of the shunt containing the Teflon connector. Attach the new Teflon connector to the other side of the shunt with the second adapter. Attach the second 10-ml syringe filled with about 8 ml of normal saline solution to the same side.
• Flush the shunt's arterial tubing by releasing its clamp and gently aspirating it with the normal saline solution–filled syringe. Then flush the tubing slowly, observing it for signs of fibrin buildup. Repeat the procedure on the venous side of the shunt.
• Secure the shunt to the adapter connection with adhesive tape *to prevent separation during treatment.*
• Connect the arterial and venous lines to the adapters and secure the connections with tape. Tape each line to the patient's arm *to prevent unnecessary strain on the shunt during treatment.*
• Begin hemodialysis according to your unit's protocol.

To discontinue hemodialysis with a double-lumen catheter
• Wash your hands.
• Clamp the extension tubing *to prevent air from entering the catheter.*

Clean all connection points on the catheter and blood lines as well as the clamps *to reduce the risk of systemic or local infections.*

• Place a clean drape under the catheter, and place two sterile 4″ × 4″ gauze pads on the drape beneath the catheter lines. Soak the pads with povidone-iodine solution. Then prepare the catheter flush solution with normal saline or heparin-saline solution, as ordered.

• Put on clean gloves. Then grasp each blood line with a gauze pad and disconnect each line from the catheter.

• Flush each port with saline solution *to clean the extension tubing and catheter of blood.* Administer additional heparin flush solution as ordered *to ensure catheter patency.* Then attach luer-lock injection caps *to prevent entry of air or loss of blood.*

• Clamp the extension tubing.

• When hemodialysis is complete, re-dress the catheter insertion site; also re-dress it if it's occluded, soiled, or wet. Place the patient in a supine position with his face turned away from the insertion site *so he doesn't contaminate the site by breathing on it.*

• Wash your hands, and remove the outer occlusive dressing. Then put on sterile gloves, remove the old inner dressing, and discard the gloves and the inner dressing.

• Set up a sterile field, and observe the site for drainage. Obtain a drainage sample for culture if necessary. Notify the doctor if the suture appears to be missing.

• Put on sterile gloves and clean the insertion site with an alcohol sponge *to remove skin oils.* Then clean the site with a povidone-iodine sponge and allow it to air-dry. Then apply povidone-iodine ointment to the insertion site and the suture site.

• Put a precut gauze dressing over the ointment and under the catheter, and place another gauze dressing over the catheter.

• Apply a skin barrier preparation to the skin surrounding the gauze dressing. Then cover the gauze and catheter with a transparent occlusive dressing.

• Apply a 4- to 5-inch piece of 2-inch tape over the cut edge of the dressing *to reinforce the lower edge.*

To discontinue hemodialysis with an AV fistula

• Wash your hands. Turn the blood pump on the hemodialysis machine to 50 to 100 ml/minute.

• Put on clean gloves and remove the tape or disc luer-lock from the connection site of the arterial lines. Clamp the needle tubing with the hemostat and disconnect the lines. The blood in the machine's arterial line will continue to flow toward the dialyzer, followed by a column of air. Just before the blood reaches the point where the saline solution enters the line, clamp the blood line with another hemostat.

• Unclamp the saline solution *to allow a small amount to flow through the line.* Unclamp the hemostat on the machine line. *This allows all blood to flow into the dialyzer where it passes through the filter and back to the patient through the venous line.*

• After blood is retransfused, clamp the venous needle tubing and the machine's venous line with hemostats. Turn off the blood pump.

• Remove the tape or disc luer-lock from the connection site of the venous lines and disconnect the lines.

• Remove the venipuncture needle and apply pressure to the site with a folded 4″ × 4″ gauze pad until all bleeding stops, usually within 10 minutes. Apply an adhesive bandage. Repeat the procedure on the arterial line.

• When hemodialysis is complete, assess the patient's weight, vital signs (including standing blood pressure) and mental status. Then compare your findings with your predialysis assessment data. Document your findings.

• Disinfect and rinse the delivery system according to the manufacturer's instructions.

To discontinue hemodialysis with an AV shunt

• Wash your hands. Turn the blood pump on the hemodialysis machine to 50 to 100 ml/minute.

• Put on the sterile gloves and remove the tape from the connection site of the arterial lines. Clamp the arterial cannula with a bulldog clamp, and then disconnect the lines. The blood in the machine's arterial line will continue to flow toward the dialyzer, followed by a column of air. Just before the blood reaches the point where the normal saline solution enters the line, clamp the blood line with a hemostat.

• Unclamp the saline solution *to allow a small amount to flow through the line.* Reclamp the saline solution line and unclamp the hemostat on the machine line. *This allows all blood to flow into the dialyzer where it's circulated through the filter and back to the patient through the venous line.*

• Just before the last volume of blood enters the patient, clamp the venous cannula with a bulldog clamp and the machine's venous line with a hemostat.

• Remove the tape from the connection site of the venous lines. Turn off the blood pump and disconnect the lines.

• Reconnect the shunt cannula. Remove the older of the two Teflon connectors and discard it. Connect the shunt, taking care to position the Teflon connector equally between the two cannulas. Remove the bulldog clamps.

• Secure the shunt connection with plasticized or hypoallergenic tape *to prevent accidental disconnection.*

• Clean the shunt and its site with the gauze pads soaked with povidone-iodine solution. When the cleaning procedure is finished, remove the povidone-iodine with alcohol sponges.

• Make sure blood flows through the shunt adequately.

• Apply a dressing to the shunt site and wrap it securely, but not too tightly, with elastic gauze bandages. Attach the bulldog clamps to the outside dressing.

• When hemodialysis is complete, assess the patient's weight, vital signs, and mental status. Then compare your findings with your predialysis assessment data. Document your findings.

• Disinfect and rinse the delivery system according to the manufacturer's instructions.

Complications

• Bacterial endotoxins in the dialysate may cause fever.

• Rapid fluid removal and electrolyte changes during hemodialysis can cause early dialysis dysequilibrium syndrome.

• Signs and symptoms include headache, nausea, vomiting, restlessness, hypertension, muscle cramps, backache, and seizures.

• Excessive removal of fluid during ultrafiltration can cause hypovolemia and hypotension.

• Diffusion of the sugar and sodium content of the dialysate solution into the blood can cause hyperglycemia and hypernatremia. These conditions, in turn, can cause hyperosmolarity.

• Cardiac arrhythmias can occur during hemodialysis as a result of electrolyte and pH changes in the blood. They can also develop in patients taking antiarrhythmic drugs because the dialysate removes these drugs during treatment. Angina may develop in patients with anemia or preexisting arteriosclerotic cardiovascular disease because of the physiologic stress on the blood during purification and ultrafiltration.

• Reduced oxygen levels resulting from extracorporeal blood flow or membrane sensitivity may require increasing oxygen administration during hemodialysis.

• Some complications of hemodialysis can be fatal. For example, an air embolism can result if the dialyzer retains air, if tubing connections become loose, or if the saline solution container empties. Symptoms include chest pain, dyspnea, coughing, and cyanosis.

• Hemolysis can result from obstructed flow of the dialysate concentrate or from incorrect setting of the conductivity alarm limits. Symptoms include chest pain, dyspnea, cherry red blood, arrhythmias, acute decrease in hematocrit, and hyperkalemia.

• Hyperthermia, another potentially fatal complication, can result if the dialysate becomes overheated. Exsanguination can result from separations of the blood lines or from rupture of the blood lines or dialyzer membrane.

Nursing considerations

• Obtain blood samples from the patient, as ordered. Samples are usually drawn before beginning hemodialysis.

Nursing alert. To avoid pyrogenic reactions and bacteremia with septicemia resulting from contamination, use strict aseptic technique during preparation of the machine. Discard equipment that has fallen on the floor or that has been disconnected and exposed to the air.

• Immediately report any machine malfunction or equipment defect.

• Avoid unnecessary handling of shunt tubing. However, be sure to inspect the shunt carefully for patency by observing its color. Also look for clots and serum and cell separation, and check the temperature of the Silastic tubing. Assess the shunt insertion site for signs of infection, such as purulent drainage, inflammation, and tenderness, which may indicate the body's rejection of the shunt. Also check to see if the shunt insertion tips are exposed.

• Make sure you complete each step in this procedure correctly. *Overlooking a single step or performing it incorrectly can cause unnecessary blood loss or inefficient treatment from poor clearances or inadequate fluid removal.* For example, never allow a saline solution bag to run dry while priming and soaking the dialyzer. *This can cause air to enter the patient portion of the dialysate system.* Ultimately, failure to perform accu-

rate hemodialysis therapy can lead to patient injury and even death.
• If bleeding continues after you remove an AV fistula needle, apply pressure with a sterile, absorbable gelatin sponge. If bleeding persists, apply a similar sponge soaked in topical thrombin solution.
• Throughout hemodialysis, carefully monitor the patient's vital signs. Read blood pressure at least hourly or as often as every 15 minutes, if necessary. Monitor the patient's weight before and after the procedure *to ensure adequate ultrafiltration during treatment.* (Many dialysis units are equipped with bed scales.)
• Perform periodic tests for clotting time on the patient's blood samples and samples from the dialyzer. If the patient receives meals during treatment, make sure they're light.
• Continue necessary drug administration during dialysis, unless the drug would be removed in the dialysate; if so, administer the drug after dialysis.

Home care
• Before the patient leaves the hospital, teach him how to care for his vascular access site. Instruct him to keep the incision clean and dry *to prevent infection* and to clean it daily until it heals completely and the sutures are removed (usually 10 to 14 days after surgery). He should notify the doctor of pain, swelling, redness, or drainage in the accessed arm. Teach him how to use a stethoscope to auscultate for bruits and how to palpate a thrill.
• Explain that once the access site heals, he may use the arm freely. In

fact, exercise is beneficial because it helps stimulate vein enlargement. Remind him not to allow any treatments or procedures on the accessed arm, including blood pressure monitoring or needle punctures. Also tell him to avoid putting excessive pressure on the arm. He shouldn't sleep on it, wear constricting clothing on it, or lift heavy objects or strain with it. He also should avoid getting wet for several hours after dialysis.
• Teach the patient exercises for the affected arm *to promote vascular dilation and enhance blood flow.* He may start by squeezing a small rubber ball or other soft object for 15 minutes, when advised by the doctor.
• If the patient will be performing hemodialysis at home, thoroughly review all aspects of the procedure with the patient and his family. Give them the phone number of the dialysis center. Emphasize that training for home hemodialysis is a complex process requiring 2 to 3 months *to ensure that the patient or family member performs it safely and competently.* Keep in mind that this procedure is stressful.

Documentation
• Record the time treatment began and any problems with it.
• Note the patient's vital signs and weight before and during treatment.
• Note the time blood specimens were taken for testing, the test results, and treatment for complications.
• Record the time the treatment was completed and the patient's response to it.

Home parenteral nutrition

Home parenteral nutrition (HPN) makes possible prolonged or indefinite I.V. total parenteral nutrition (TPN). This technique has dramatically improved the health of patients with such chronic conditions as Crohn's disease and malabsorption syndrome, those with such acute conditions as incomplete bowel obstruction, and those receiving chemotherapy. It has also shortened hospital stays. Although peripheral parenteral nutrition may be administered at home, long-term TPN is the primary home care therapy. Preparation for HPN usually necessitates extensive patient teaching and, when possible, instructions for the patient's family.

Typically, patients receiving HPN can ingest part of their caloric requirements during the day and receive 10 to 14 hours of infusion nightly to supply the remaining nutrients. If all the patient's nutrition must be received I.V., a continuous infusion may be necessary. For intermittent and continuous infusion, patient teaching must include techniques for proper care.

≫ Key nursing diagnoses and patient outcomes

Use these nursing diagnoses as a guide when developing your plan of care for a patient who needs home parenteral nutrition.

Knowledge deficit related to lack of exposure to new procedure

Based on this nursing diagnosis, you'll establish the following patient outcomes. The patient will:

• express interest in learning new procedure.
• return demonstrate correct procedure for home parenteral nutrition.
• develop realistic plan for maintaining new skills at home.
• identify appropriate available resources for after discharge.

Altered nutrition: less than body requirements related to (specify)

Based on this nursing diagnosis, you'll establish the following patient outcomes. The patient will:

• show no evidence of weight loss.
• tolerate parenteral feedings without adverse effects.
• gain (specify) lb weekly.
• communicate understanding of special dietary needs.

Risk for infection related to I.V. line

Based on this nursing diagnosis, you'll establish the following patient outcomes. The patient will:

• maintain normal temperature.
• show no signs or symptoms of infection.
• verbalize understanding of signs and symptoms of infection and notify doctor if they occur.
• change I.V. dressing every (specify).

Equipment

◆ teaching aids (including audiovisual teaching aids and mannequins), as available ◆ I.V. infusion apparatus ◆ dressings ◆ TPN solution ◆ volumetric infusion pump ◆ portable I.V. pole or ambulatory TPN vest ◆ HPN supplies (including tubing, dressings, TPN solution).

Patient preparation

• Assess the patient's ability to perform the care routines necessary for HPN, and determine if family members or friends can assist with or perform them. Consider the patient's motivation, mental aptitude, job or other daily activities, and home environment as well as the accessibility of hospitals, home nursing services, and other health care support systems.

• Formulate a patient-teaching plan based on your assessment and on the patient's expectations. Make sure the plan incorporates goals, specifies criteria for meeting them, and proceeds from simple to complex tasks *to allow the patient to develop confidence.* Avoid placing time limits on goals *because learning ability and mastery of tasks requiring manual dexterity vary from patient to patient.*

• If desired, develop a written contract between you and the patient that specifies the goals of HPN and the means to achieve them. Revise the contract, as necessary, to reflect changes in the patient's needs and performance. *A contractual relationship enhances the patient's independence, minimizes conflict and frustration between patient and nurse, encourages open communication, and promotes a cooperative patient-nurse relationship.*

• Conduct patient-teaching sessions in a quiet area and, if possible, arrange to have a family member present. *When the family member understands the patient's pathophysiology, medical management, and progress, he tends to be less anxious, more satisfied with the quality of health care, and more able to acknowledge the limitations and constraints of HPN.*

Implementation

• Use a variety of teaching aids *to accommodate differences in the patient's ability.* When teaching the mature patient, use an extensively illustrated manual (if available) that includes goals, equipment, procedures with rationales, suggested learning activities, and evaluations of HPN equipment. Give demonstrations with mannequins (if available) and real equipment *to involve the patient actively and reduce anxiety about performing the HPN tasks.* Stimulate his interest with audiovisual teaching aids.

• Offer positive feedback during all teaching phases.

• Before discharge, critically evaluate the patient's ability to perform HPN tasks and ensure that all essential learning goals have been met.

• Remind the patient to change the catheter site dressing, as ordered (usually every 2 to 3 days) or whenever it becomes soiled or nonocclusive, and to change administration tubing as scheduled. Tell the patient to wash gently around the site and to take only sponge baths. Tell him he may be allowed to remove his dressing and bathe or shower after the implanted catheter has been in place for 1 month or longer.

• Also remind the patient to prevent contact between the catheter and granular or lint-producing surfaces *to avoid local tissue reaction from airborne particles and surface contaminants.*

• Discuss a suitable TPN schedule with the patient, considering his nutritional needs as well as his lifestyle. Emphasize his adherence to the prescribed schedule and volume *to prevent glucose imbalance.*

• Arrange for a home care agency to help the patient adjust to HPN and resolve any difficulties (including how to obtain supplies), or notify the hospital's discharge planner *so the appropriate referrals can be made.*

Nursing considerations

• Suggest that the patient wear a medical identification bracelet or subscribe to a medical alert service.

• Tell the patient that a nurse from the home health care team will always be available in case of emergency.

• To preserve as much patient mobility as possible, equipment such as the ambulatory TPN vest is available. This vest is made from lightweight materials and is adjustable to individual specifications. Breast pockets accommodate bags of nutrient solution, which are attached to the front of each shoulder. The pockets vary with the size of the nutrient bags. Y-tubing connects these bags to a portable volumetric pump, located in a zippered pocket. To provide balance and enhance patient comfort, the pump empties both bags at the same rate. When the patient is wearing the vest, the administration tubing is coiled in one of the pockets. When the patient isn't wearing the vest, the nutrient bags can hang from a clothes hanger.

Because the financial burden of long-term or permanent HPN can be devastating — even for the patient with health insurance — make a social service referral. Inform the elderly patient that Medicare may assume the cost of supplies and pharmaceuticals if he meets eligibility requirements.

Documentation

• Record your patient-teaching measures and the patient's learning progress in your notes.

Humidifiers

Humidifiers, which deliver a maximum amount of water vapor without producing particulate water, are used to prevent drying and irritation of the upper airway in conditions where the upper airway is inflamed such as in croup. They're also used when secretions are particularly thick and tenacious.

Some humidifiers heat the water vapor, which raises the moisture-carrying capacity of gas and thus increases the amount of humidity delivered to the patient. Room humidifiers add humidity to an entire room, while humidifiers added to gas lines humidify only the air being delivered to the patient. (See *Comparing humidifiers,* page 418.)

≫ Key nursing diagnoses and patient outcomes

Use these nursing diagnoses as a guide when developing your plan of care for a patient needing humidification.

Risk for infection related to humidification equipment

Based on this nursing diagnosis, you'll establish the following patient outcomes. The patient will:

• be free from signs and symptoms of infection.

• verbalize understanding of potential risk for infection with home use.

Comparing humidifiers

TYPE	DESCRIPTION AND USES	ADVANTAGES AND DISADVANTAGES
Bedside	• Spinning disc splashes water against baffle, creating small drops and increasing evaporation; motor disperses mist to humidify room air directly	*Advantages* • May be used with all oxygen masks and nasal cannulas • Easy to operate • Inexpensive *Disadvantages* • Produces humidity inefficiently • Can't be used for patient with bypassed upper airway • May harbor bacteria and molds
Heated vaporizer	• Directly humidifies room air by heating the water in the reservoir	*Advantages* • May be used with all oxygen masks and nasal cannulas • Easy to operate • Inexpensive *Disadvantages* • Can't guarantee the amount of humidity delivered • Poses a risk of burn injury if the machine is knocked over
Diffusion head	• In-line humidifier most commonly used with low-flow oxygen delivery systems; gas flows through porous diffuser in reservoir to increase gas-liquid interface; provides humidification to patients using a nasal cannula or oxygen mask (except the Venturi mask)	*Advantages* • Easy to operate • Inexpensive *Disadvantages* • Provides only 20% to 30% humidity at body temperature • Can't be used for a patient with bypassed upper airway
Cascade bubble diffusion	• Gas is forced through plastic grid in reservoir of warmed water to create fine bubbles; commonly used in patients receiving mechanical ventilation or continuous positive airway pressure therapy	*Advantages* • Delivers 100% humidity at body temperature • The most effective of all evaporative humidifiers *Disadvantages* • Mucosa can become irritated if correct water level isn't maintained

• return demonstrate correct procedure for preventing bacterial buildup with home use.

Ineffective airway clearance related to (specify)

Based on this nursing diagnosis, you'll establish the following patient outcomes. The patient will:
• maintain a patent airway.
• drink 3 to 4 qt (3 to 4 L) of fluid daily (if not contraindicated).
• cough effectively to expectorate sputum.
• demonstrate correct procedure for breathing exercises.
• perform activities of daily living to level of tolerance.

Equipment

♦ humidifier ♦ bottled distilled water, or tap water if the unit has a demineralizing capability ♦ container for waste water ♦ bleach ♦ white vinegar.

Equipment preparation

• *For a bedside humidifier:* Open the reservoir and add sterile distilled water to the fill line; then close the reservoir. Keep all room windows and doors closed tightly to maintain adequate humidification. Then plug the unit into the electrical outlet.

• *For a heated vaporizer:* Remove the top and fill the reservoir to the fill line with tap water. Replace the top securely. Then place the vaporizer about 4 feet from the patient, directing the steam toward but not directly onto the patient. Place the unit in a spot where it can't be overturned *to avoid hot water burns.* This is especially important if children will be in the room.

Plug the unit into an electrical outlet. Steam should soon rise from the unit into the air. Close all windows and doors to maintain adequate humidification.

• *For a diffusion head humidifier:* Unscrew the humidifier reservoir and add sterile distilled water to the appropriate level. (If using a disposable unit, screw the cap with the extension onto the top of the unit.) Then screw the reservoir back onto the humidifier and attach the flowmeter to the oxygen source.

Screw the humidifier onto the flowmeter until the seal is tight. Then set the flowmeter at a rate of 2 L/minute, and check for gentle bubbling. Next, check the positive-pressure release valve by occluding the end valve on the humidifier. The pressure should back up into the humidifier, signaled by a high-pitched whistle. If this doesn't occur, tighten all connections and try again.

• *For a cascade bubble diffusion humidifier:* Unscrew the cascade reservoir, and add sterile distilled water to the fill line. Screw the top back onto the reservoir. Then plug in the heater unit, and set the temperature between 95° F (35° C) and 100.4° F (38° C).

Patient preparation

• Explain the procedure to the patient and wash your hands.

Implementation

• Check to make sure that the humidifier or vaporizer has been prepared properly.

For a bedside humidifier

• Direct the humidifier unit's nozzle away from the patient's face (but toward the patient) for effective treatment. Check for a fine mist emission from the nozzle, which indicates proper operation.

• Check the unit every 4 hours for proper operation, the water level every 8 hours. When refilling, unplug the unit, discard any old water, wipe with a disinfectant, rinse the reservoir container, and refill with sterile distilled water as necessary.

• Keep the unit cleaned and refilled with sterile water *to reduce the risk of bacterial growth.* Replace the unit every 7 days and send used units for proper decontamination.

For a heated vaporizer

• Check the unit every 4 hours for proper functioning.

• If steam production seems insufficient, unplug the unit, discard the water, and refill with half distilled water and half tap water, or clean the unit well.

• Check the water level in the unit every 8 hours. To refill, unplug the unit, discard any old water, wipe with a disinfectant, rinse the reservoir container, and refill with tap water as necessary.

For a diffusion head humidifier

• Attach the oxygen delivery device to the humidifier and then to the patient. Then adjust the flowmeter to the appropriate oxygen flow rate.

• Check the reservoir every 4 hours. If the water level drops too low, empty the remaining water, rinse the jar, and refill it with sterile water. (As the reservoir water level decreases, the evaporation of water in the gas decreases, reducing humidification of the delivered gas.)

• Change the humidification system regularly *to prevent bacterial growth and invasion.*

• Periodically assess the patient's sputum; *if too thick, it can hinder mobilization and expectoration.* If this occurs, the patient requires a device that can provide higher humidity.

For a cascade bubble diffusion humidifier

• Assess the temperature of the inspired gas near the patient's airway every 2 hours when used in critical care and every 4 hours when used in general patient care. If the cascade becomes too hot, drain the water and replace it. *Overheated water vapor can cause respiratory tract burns.*

• Check the reservoir's water level every 2 to 4 hours, and fill as necessary. *If the water level falls below the minimum water level mark, humidification will decrease to that of room air.*

• Be alert for condensation buildup in the tubing, which can result from the very high humidification produced by the cascade.

• Check the tubing frequently, and empty the condensate as necessary *so it can't drain into the patient's respiratory tract, encourage growth of microorganisms, or obstruct dependent sections of tubing.* To do so, disconnect the tubing, drain the condensate into a container, and dispose of it properly. Never drain the condensate into the humidification system.

• Change the cascade regularly according to your hospital's policy.

Complications

• Cascade humidifiers can cause aspiration of tubal condensation and, if the air is heated, can cause pulmonary burns. Humidifiers, if contaminated, can cause infection.

Nursing considerations

• Because it creates a humidity level comparable to that of ambient air, the diffusion head humidifier is only used for oxygen flow rates that are greater than 4 L/minute.

• Because the bedside humidifier doesn't deliver a precise amount of humidification, assess the patient regularly *to determine the effectiveness of therapy.* Ask him if he's noticed any improvement and evaluate his sputum.

• Like the bedside humidifier, the heated vaporizer doesn't deliver a precise amount of humidification, so assess the patient regularly by asking if he's feeling better and by examining his sputum.

• Keep in mind that a humidifier, if not kept clean, can cause or aggravate respiratory problems, especially for people allergic to molds. Refer to your hospital's policy for changing and disposing of humidification equipment.

Home care

• Make sure that the patient and his family understand the reason for using a humidifier and that they know how to use the equipment. Give the patient specific, written guidelines concerning all aspects of home care.

• Instruct a patient using a bedside humidifier at home to fill it with plain tap water and to use sterile distilled water periodically *to prevent mineral buildup.* Also advise him to run white vinegar through the unit *to help clean it, prevent bacterial buildup, and dissolve deposits.*

• Tell the patient to rinse a heated vaporizer unit with bleach and water every 5 days. Also run white vinegar through it *to help clean it, prevent bacterial buildup, and dissolve any deposits.*

Documentation

• Record the date and time when humidification began and was discontinued; the type of humidifier; the flow rate (of a gas system); thermometer readings (if heated); any complications and the nursing action taken; and the patient's reaction to humidification.

Hyperthermia-hypothermia blanket

A blanket-sized aquamatic K pad, the hyperthermia-hypothermia blanket raises, lowers, or maintains body temperature through conductive heat or cold transfer between the blanket and the patient. It can be operated manually or automatically.

In manual operation, the nurse or doctor sets the temperature on the unit. The blanket reaches and maintains this temperature, regardless of the patient's temperature. The temperature setting must be manually adjusted to reach a different temperature setting. The nurse monitors the patient's body temperature using a conventional thermometer.

In automatic operation, the unit directly and continually monitors the patient's temperature by means of a thermistor probe (rectal, skin, or esophageal) and alternates heating and cooling cycles as necessary to achieve and maintain the desired body temperature. The thermistor probe may also be used in conjunction with manual operation but is not essential. The unit is equipped with an alarm to warn of abnormal temperature fluctuations, and a circuit breaker that protects against current overload.

The blanket is most commonly used to reduce high fever when more conservative measures — such as baths, ice packs, and antipyretics — are unsuccessful. Its other uses include maintaining normal temperature during surgery or shock; inducing hypothermia during surgery to decrease metabolic activity and thereby reduce oxygen requirements; reducing intracranial pressure; controlling bleeding and intractable pain in patients with amputations, burns, or cancer; and providing warmth in cases of severe hypothermia.

≫ Key nursing diagnoses and patient outcomes

Use these nursing diagnoses as a guide when developing your plan of care for a patient who needs hyperthermia-hypothermia blanket.

Hypothermia related to (specify)

Based on this nursing diagnosis, you'll establish the following patient outcomes. The patient will:
- maintain a normal body temperature.
- not shiver.
- express feelings of comfort.
- maintain a heart rate and blood pressure within normal limits.
- exhibit warm and dry skin.
- show no complications associated with hypothemia, such as soft-tissue

injury, fracture, dehydration, hypovolemic shock if warmed too quickly.

Hyperthermia related to (specify)

Based on this nursing diagnosis, you'll establish the following patient outcomes. The patient will:
- maintain a normal body temperature.
- experience no seizure activity.
- state increased comfort.

Knowledge deficit related to lack of exposure to hyperthermia-hypothermia blanket

Based on this nursing diagnosis, you'll establish the following patient outcomes. The patient will:
- verbalize understanding of use for blanket.
- communicate feelings of anxiety and verbalize questions during treatment.

Equipment

♦ hyperthermia-hypothermia control unit ♦ operation manual ♦ fluid for the control unit (distilled water or distilled water and 20% ethyl alcohol) ♦ thermistor probe (rectal, skin, or esophageal) ♦ one or two hyperthermia-hypothermia blankets ♦ one or two disposable blanket covers (or one or two sheets or bath blankets) ♦ lanolin or a mixture of lanolin and cold cream ♦ patient thermometer (for manual mode) ♦ adhesive tape ♦ towel ♦ sphygmomanometer ♦ gloves if necessary ♦ optional: protective wraps for the patient's hands and feet.

Disposable hyperthermia-hypothermia blankets are available for single-patient use.

Equipment preparation

• Read the operation manual.
• Inspect the unit and each blanket for leaks and the plugs and the connecting wires for broken prongs, kinks, and fraying.
• If you detect or suspect malfunction, don't use the equipment.
• Review the doctor's order, and prepare one or two blankets by covering them with disposable covers (or use a sheet or a bath blanket when positioning the blanket on the patient). *The cover absorbs perspiration and condensation, which could cause tissue breakdown if left on the skin.*
• Connect the blanket to the control unit, and set the controls for manual or automatic operation and for the desired blanket or body temperature.
• Make sure the machine is properly grounded before plugging it in.
• Turn on the machine, and add liquid to the unit reservoir, if necessary, as fluid fills the blanket. Allow the blanket to preheat or precool *so the patient receives immediate thermal benefit.* Place the control unit at the foot of the bed.

Patient preparation

• Assess the patient's condition and explain the procedure to him.
• Provide privacy, and make sure the room is warm and free of drafts.
• Check hospital policy and, if necessary, make sure the patient or a responsible family member has signed a consent form.
• Wash your hands thoroughly. If the patient is not already wearing a hospital gown, ask him to put one on. Use a gown with cloth ties, not metal snaps or pins *because these could cause heat or cold injury.*

• Take the patient's temperature, pulse, respirations, and blood pressure *to serve as a baseline,* and assess level of consciousness, pupil reaction, limb strength, and skin condition.
• Keeping the bottom sheet in place and the patient recumbent, roll him to one side and slide the blanket halfway under him, so its top edge aligns with his neck. Then roll the patient back, and pull and flatten the blanket across the bed. Place a pillow under the patient's head. Make sure the patient's head doesn't lie directly on the blanket *because the blanket's rigid surface may be uncomfortable and the heat or cold may lead to tissue breakdown.* Use a sheet or bath blanket as insulation between the patient and the blanket, if necessary.

Implementation

• Apply lanolin or a mixture of lanolin and cold cream to the patient's skin where it touches the blanket *to help protect the skin from heat or cold sensation.*
• In automatic operation, insert the thermistor probe in the patient's rectum and tape it in place *to prevent accidental dislodgment.* If rectal insertion is contraindicated, tuck a skin probe deep into the axilla, and secure it with tape. If the patient is comatose or anesthetized, insert an esophageal probe. Plug the other end of the probe into the correct jack on the unit's control panel.
• Place a sheet or, if ordered, the second hyperthermia-hypothermia blanket over the patient. *This increases thermal benefit by trapping cooled or heated air.*
• Wrap the patient's hands and feet, if he wishes, *to minimize chilling and*

promote comfort. Monitor vital signs, and perform a neurologic assessment every 5 minutes until the desired body temperature is reached; then every 15 minutes until temperature is stable or as ordered.

• Check fluid intake and output hourly or as ordered. Observe the patient regularly for color changes in skin, lips, and nail beds, and for edema, induration, inflammation, pain, or sensory impairment. If these occur, discontinue the procedure and notify the doctor.

• Reposition the patient every 30 minutes to 1 hour, unless contraindicated, *to prevent skin breakdown.* Keep the patient's skin, bedclothes, and blanket cover free of perspiration and condensation, and reapply cream to exposed body parts as needed.

• After turning off the machine, follow the manufacturer's directions. *Some units must remain plugged in for at least 30 minutes to allow the condenser fan to remove water vapor from the mechanism.* Continue to monitor the patient's temperature until it stabilizes *because body temperature can fall as much as 5° F (2.8° C) after this procedure.*

• Remove all equipment from the bed. Dry the patient and make him comfortable. Supply a fresh hospital gown, if necessary. Cover the patient lightly.

• Continue to perform neurologic checks and monitor vital signs, fluid intake and output, and general condition every 30 minutes for 2 hours and then hourly or as ordered.

• Return the equipment to the central supply department for cleaning, servicing, and storage.

Complications

• Use of a hyperthermia-hypothermia blanket can cause shivering, marked changes in vital signs, increased intracranial pressure, respiratory distress or arrest, cardiac arrest, oliguria, and anuria.

Nursing considerations

• If the patient shivers excessively during hypothermia treatment, discontinue the procedure and notify the doctor immediately. *By increasing metabolism, shivering elevates body temperature.*

• Avoid lowering the temperature more than 1° every 15 minutes *to prevent premature ventricular contractions.*

• Don't use pins to secure catheters, tubes, or blanket covers *because an accidental puncture can result in fluid leakage and burns.*

• With hyperthermia or hypothermia therapy, the patient may experience a secondary defense reaction (vasoconstriction or vasodilation, respectively), which causes body temperature to rebound and thus defeat the treatment's purpose.

• If the patient requires isolation, place the blanket, blanket cover, and probe in a plastic bag clearly marked with the type of isolation *so the central supply department can give it special handling.* If the blanket is disposable, discard it using appropriate precautions.

• To avoid bacterial growth in the reservoir or blankets, always use sterile distilled water and change it monthly. Check to see if hospital policy calls for adding a bacteriostatic agent to the water. Avoid using deionized water *because it may corrode the system.*

Documentation

• Record the patient's pulse, respirations, blood pressure, neurologic signs, fluid intake and output, skin condition, and position change.

• Record the patient's temperature and that of the thermal pad every 30 minutes while the pad is in use.

• Note the type of hyperthermia-hypothermia unit used; control settings (manual or automatic, and temperature settings); date, time, duration, and patient's tolerance of treatment; and any signs of complications.

I

Incontinence management

In elderly patients, incontinence commonly follows any loss or impairment of urinary or anal sphincter control. The incontinence may be transient or permanent. In all, about 10 million adults experience some form of urinary incontinence; this includes about 50% of the 1.5 million people in extended care facilities. And fecal incontinence affects up to 10% of the patients in such facilities.

Contrary to popular opinion, urinary incontinence is not a disease and not part of normal aging. It may be caused by confusion, dehydration, fecal impaction, or restricted mobility. It's also a sign of various disorders, such as prostatic hyperplasia, bladder calculus, bladder cancer, urinary tract infection (UTI), cerebrovascular accident, diabetic neuropathy, Guillain-Barré syndrome, multiple sclerosis, prostatic cancer, prostatitis, spinal cord injury, and urethral stricture. It may also result from urethral sphincter damage after prostatectomy. What's more, certain drugs, including diuretics, hypnotics, sedatives, anticholinergics, antihypertensives, and alpha antagonists, may trigger urinary incontinence.

Urinary incontinence is classified as acute or chronic. Acute urinary incontinence results from disorders that are potentially reversible, such as delirium, dehydration, urine retention, restricted mobility, fecal impaction, infection or inflammation, drug reactions, and polyuria. Chronic urinary incontinence occurs as four distinct types: stress, overflow, urge, or functional incontinence. With *stress incontinence,* leakage results from a sudden physical strain, such as a sneeze, cough, or quick movement. In *overflow incontinence,* urine retention causes dribbling because the distended bladder cannot contract strongly enough to force a urine stream. In *urge incontinence,* the patient cannot control the impulse to urinate. Finally, *functional (total) incontinence* results when urine leakage occurs even though the bladder and urethra function normally. This condition is usually related to cognitive or environmental factors, such as mental impairment or lack of appropriate or timely care.

Fecal incontinence, the involuntary passage of feces, may occur gradually (as it does in dementia) or suddenly (as it does in spinal cord injury). It most commonly results from fecal stasis and impaction secondary to reduced activity, inappropriate diet, or untreated painful anal conditions. It can also result from chronic laxative use, reduced fluid intake, and neurologic deficit. Pelvic, prostatic, or rectal surgery can also cause fecal incontinence as can medications, including antihistamines, psychotropics, and iron preparations. Not usually a sign of serious illness, fecal incontinence can seriously impair an elderly patient's physical and psychological well-being.

Patients with urinary or fecal incontinence should be carefully assessed for underlying disorders. Most can be treated — some can be cured. Treatment aims to control the condition through bladder or bowel retraining or other behavior management techniques, diet modification, drug therapy, and possibly surgery. Corrective surgery for urinary incontinence includes transurethral resection of the prostate in men, repair of the anterior vaginal wall or retropelvic suspension of the bladder in women, urethral sling, and bladder augmentation.

≫ Key nursing diagnoses and patient outcomes

Use these nursing diagnoses as a guide when developing your plan of care for a patient who is being treated for incontinence.

Functional incontinence related to (specify)

Based on this nursing diagnosis, you'll establish the following patient outcomes. The patient will:
• void in appropriate situation using suitable receptacle.
• void at specific times.
• have no wet episodes.
• demonstrate skill in managing incontinence.
• discuss impact of incontinence on self and significant other.
• identify resources to assist with care following discharge.

Bowel incontinence related to (specify)

Based on this nursing diagnosis, you'll establish the following patient outcomes. The patient will:
• establish and maintain a regular pattern of bowel care.
• state understanding of bowel care routine.

• demonstrate skill in carrying out bowel care routine.
• participate in social activities.

Social isolation related to incontinence

Based on this nursing diagnosis, you'll establish the following patient outcomes. The patient will:
• express feelings associated with social isolation.
• participate in developing a plan for increasing social activity.
• indicate social relationships have improved and negative feelings have diminished.
• achieve expected state of wellness.

Equipment

♦ bladder retraining record sheet ♦ gloves ♦ stethoscope (to assess bowel sounds) ♦ lubricant ♦ moisture barrier cream ♦ antidiarrheal or laxative suppository ♦ incontinence pads ♦ bedpan ♦ specimen container ♦ label ♦ laboratory request form ♦ optional: stool collection kit, urinary catheter.

Patient preparation

• Whether the patient reports urinary or fecal incontinence or both, you'll need to perform initial and continuing assessments to plan effective interventions. (See *Correcting urinary incontinence with bladder retraining,* page 428.)

Implementation

Deal with incontinence by following the steps listed below.

For urinary incontinence

• Ask the patient when he first noticed urine leakage and whether it began

Correcting urinary incontinence with bladder retraining

The incontinent patient typically feels frustrated, embarrassed, and sometimes hopeless. Fortunately, his problem can usually be corrected by bladder retraining — a program that aims to establish a regular voiding pattern. To implement such a program, follow these guidelines.

Assess elimination patterns
First assess the patient's intake pattern, voiding pattern, and reason for each accidental voiding (for example, a coughing spell).

Establish a voiding schedule
Encourage the patient to void regularly — every 2 hours, for example. Once he can stay dry for 2 hours, increase the time between voidings by 30 minutes each day until he achieves a 3- to 4-hour voiding schedule.

Teach the patient to practice relaxation techniques such as deep breathing, *which helps decrease the sense of urgency.*

Record results and remain positive
Keep a record of continence and incontinence for about 5 days — *this may reinforce your patient's efforts to remain continent.*

Remember, both your positive attitude and your patient's are crucial to his successful bladder retraining.

Take steps for success
Here are some additional tips to help boost the patient's success:
• Be sure to locate the patient's bed near a bathroom or portable toilet. Leave a light on at night. Promptly answer the call for help if the patient needs assistance getting out of a bed or a chair.
• Encourage the patient to wear his usual clothing. *This confirms your confidence in his ability to stay dry.* Use high quality incontinence products *to decrease the risk of skin breakdown if necessary.*
• Encourage the patient to drink 1,500 to 2,000 ml of fluid each day. Lowering fluid intake will not reduce or prevent incontinence; it will promote infection. Limiting fluid intake after 6 p.m., however, will help the patient remain continent during the night.
• Reassure your patient that periodic incontinent episodes don't signal failure of the program. Encourage persistence, tolerance, and a positive attitude.

suddenly or gradually. Have him describe his typical urinary pattern: Does incontinence usually occur during the day or at night? Ask him to rate his urinary control: Does he have moderate control, or is he completely incontinent? If he sometimes urinates with control, ask him to identify when and how much he usually urinates.

• Evaluate related problems, such as urinary hesitancy, frequency, urgency, nocturia, and decreased force or interrupted urine stream. Ask the patient to describe any previous treatment he had for incontinence or measures he performed by himself. Also ask about medications, including nonprescription drugs.

• Assess the patient's environment. Is a toilet or commode readily available, and how long does the patient take to reach it? Once the patient is in the bathroom, assess manual dexterity — for example, how easily does he manipulate his clothes?

• Evaluate the patient's mental status and cognitive function.

• Quantify the patient's normal daily fluid intake.

• Review the patient's medication and diet history for drugs and foods that affect digestion and elimination.

• Review or obtain the patient's medical history, noting especially number and route of births and any incidence of UTI, prostate disorders, spinal injury or tumor, cerebrovascular accident, or bladder, prostate, or pelvic surgery. Also assess for disorders, such as delirium, dehydration, urine retention, restricted mobility, fecal impaction, infection, inflammation, or polyuria.

• Inspect the urethral meatus for obvious inflammation or anatomic defects. Have the female patient bear down while you note any urine leakage. Gently palpate the abdomen for bladder distention, signaling urine retention. Have the patient examined by a urologist, if possible.

• Obtain specimens for appropriate laboratory tests as ordered. Label each specimen container, and send it to the laboratory with a request form.

• Begin incontinence management by implementing an appropriate bladder retraining program.

• *To manage stress incontinence,* implement an exercise program to help strengthen the pelvic floor muscles. (See *Strengthening pelvic floor muscles,* page 430.)

• *To manage functional incontinence,* frequently assess the patient's mental and functional status. Regularly remind the patient to void. Respond to his calls promptly, and help him get to the bathroom as quickly as possible. Provide positive reinforcements.

• *To ensure healthful hydration and to prevent UTI,* be sure the patient maintains adequate daily fluid intake (six to eight 8-oz glasses of fluid). Restrict fluid intake after 6 p.m.

For fecal incontinence

• Ask the patient with fecal incontinence to identify its onset, duration, and severity. Also have him identify discernible incontinence patterns — for instance, determine whether it occurs at night or with diarrhea. Focus the history on GI, neurologic, and psychological disorders.

• Note the frequency, consistency, and volume of stool passed within the last 24 hours and obtain a stool specimen, if ordered. Protect the patient's bed with an incontinence pad.

• Assess the patient for chronic constipation, GI and neurologic disorders, and laxative abuse. Also inspect the abdomen for distention, and auscultate for bowel sounds. If not contraindicated, check for fecal impaction (which may be a factor in overflow incontinence).

• Assess the patient's medication regimen. Check for medications that affect bowel activity, such as aspirin, some anticholinergic antiparkinson agents, aluminum hydroxide, calcium carbonate antacids, diuretics, iron preparations, opiates, tranquilizers, tricyclic antidepressants, and phenothiazines.

Strengthening pelvic floor muscles

Stress incontinence is the most common kind of urinary incontinence in women and usually results from weakening of the urethral sphincter. In men, it may sometimes occur after a radical prostatectomy.

You can help a patient prevent or minimize stress incontinence by teaching about pelvic floor (Kegel) exercises to strengthen the pubococcygeal muscles. Here's how.

Learning the exercises

First, teach the patient how to locate the muscles of the pelvic floor. Instruct the patient to tense the muscles around the anus, as if to retain stool or intestinal gas.

Next, teach the patient to tighten the muscles of the pelvic floor to stop the flow of urine while urinating and then to release the muscles to restart the flow.

Once learned, these exercises can be done anywhere at any time.

Establishing a regimen

Suggest starting out by contracting the muscles and holding the contraction for 10 seconds. Then direct the patient to relax for 10 seconds before slowly tightening the muscles and then releasing them. Stress that contraction and relaxation exercises are essential to muscle retraining.

Typically, the patient starts with 15 contractions in the morning and afternoon and 20 at night. Or the patient may exercise for 10 minutes, three times a day, working up to 25 contractions at a time as strength improves.

Advise the patient not to use stomach, leg, or buttock muscles. Also discourage leg crossing or breath holding during these exercises.

• For the neurologically capable patient with chronic incontinence, provide bowel retraining.

• Advise the patient to consume a fiber-rich diet, with raw, leafy vegetables (such as carrots and lettuce), unpeeled fruits (such as apples), and whole grains (such as wheat or rye breads and cereals). If the patient has a lactase deficiency, suggest calcium supplements to replace calcium lost by eliminating dairy products from the diet.

• Encourage adequate fluid intake.

• Teach the elderly patient to gradually stop using laxatives, if necessary. Point out, as needed, that using laxatives to promote regular bowel movement may have the opposite effect — producing either constipation or incontinence over time. Suggest using natural laxatives, such as prunes or prune juice, instead.

• Promote regular exercise by explaining how it helps to regulate bowel motility. Even a nonambulatory patient can perform some exercises while sitting or lying in bed.

Complications

• Skin breakdown and infection may result from incontinence. Psychological problems resulting from incontinence include social isolation, loss of independence, lowered self-esteem, and depression.

Nursing considerations

• To rid the bladder of residual urine, teach the patient to perform Valsalva's or Credé's maneuver. Or institute clean intermittent catheterization. Use an indwelling urinary catheter only as a last resort *because of the risk of UTI.*

• For fecal incontinence, maintain effective hygienic care *to increase the patient's comfort and prevent skin breakdown and infection.* Clean the perineal area frequently, and apply a moisture barrier cream. Control foul odors as well.

• Schedule extra time to provide encouragement and support for the patient. After all, he may feel shame, embarrassment, and powerlessness from loss of control.

Documentation

• Record all bladder and bowel retraining efforts, noting scheduled bathroom times, food and fluid intake, and elimination amounts, as appropriate.

• Record duration of continent periods. Note any complications, including emotional problems, and signs of skin breakdown and infection. Document treatment given for complications.

Intermittent infusion device insertion

Also called a heparin lock, an intermittent infusion device consists of either a steel, winged-tip needle with tubing that ends in a resealable rubber injection port or a catheter with an injection cap attached. Filled with dilute heparin flush solution or normal saline solution to prevent blood clot formation, the device maintains venous access in patients who are receiving I.V. medication regularly or intermittently but who don't require a continuous fluid infusion. It's superior to a keep-vein-open line because it minimizes the risk of fluid overload and electrolyte imbalance. It also cuts costs, reduces the risk of contamination by eliminating I.V. solution containers and administration sets, increases patient comfort and mobility, reduces patient anxiety and, if inserted in a large vein, allows collection of multiple blood samples without repeated venipuncture.

>> Key nursing diagnoses and patient outcomes

Use these nursing diagnoses as a guide when developing your plan of care for a patient who needs insertion of an intermittent infusion device.

Risk for infection related to intermittent infusion device

Based on this nursing diagnosis, you'll establish the following patient outcomes. The patient will:

• maintain a normal body temperature.

• show no signs of infection at the I.V. puncture site.

• remain free of all signs and symptoms of infection.

Knowledge deficit related to lack of exposure to intermittent infusion device

Based on this nursing diagnosis, you'll establish the following patient outcomes. The patient will:

• communicate a need to know.

• state understanding of what has been taught.
• verbalize questions related to therapy with an intermittent infusion device.

Equipment

♦ intermittent infusion device ♦ 25G needle ♦ heparin flush solution in a 1-ml syringe ♦ normal saline solution ♦ povidone-iodine sponges ♦ tourniquet ♦ alcohol sponges ♦ venipuncture equipment, sterile dressing, and tape ♦ optional: transparent semipermeable dressing, stretch net protective sleeve.

Some hospitals use a 100 U/ml or 10 U/ml heparin flush solution, and others use normal saline solution instead of heparin. Prefilled heparin or saline cartridges are available in both dosages for use in a syringe cartridge holder.

Patient preparation

• Wash your hands thoroughly *to prevent contamination of the venipuncture site.*
• Explain the procedure to the patient, and describe the purpose of the intermittent infusion device.

Implementation

• Remove the set from its packaging, wipe the port with an alcohol sponge, and inject a heparin flush solution or normal saline solution to fill the tubing and 25G needle. *This removes air from the system, preventing formation of an air embolus.*
• Select a venipuncture site, and clean it first with povidone-iodine sponges, wiping outward from the site in a circular motion. Do not wipe off the povidone-iodine with alcohol *because doing so negates its effect.*
• Perform the venipuncture and ensure correct needle placement in the vein. Then release the tourniquet. (See "Venipuncture," page 982.)
• Tape the set in place, using the chevron method or an accepted alternative. Loop the tubing, if applicable, so the injection port is free and easily accessible.
• Apply a sterile dressing. On the last piece of tape used to secure the dressing, write the time, date, and your initials.
• Inject heparin flush solution or normal saline solution every 8 to 24 hours or according to hospital policy *to maintain the patency of the intermittent infusion device.* Inject the heparin slowly *to prevent stinging.*
• If the doctor orders an I.V. infusion discontinued and an intermittent infusion device inserted it its place, convert the existing line by disconnecting the I.V. tubing and inserting a male adapter plug into the device. (See *Converting an I.V. line to an intermittent infusion device.*)

Complications

• Intermittent infusion device complications that can result from the needle or catheter are infection, phlebitis, and embolism.

Nursing considerations

• Whenever inserting or removing a needle from a heparin lock, be sure to stabilize the device to prevent dislodging it from the vein. (See *Stabilizing an intermittent infusion device,* page 434.)
• If ordered, obtain a blood sample for activated partial thromboplastin time

before inserting the intermittent infusion set *because small amounts of heparin can alter the results of this test.*

• If the patient has a clotting disorder, use 1 to 2 ml of normal saline solution, according to hospital policy, instead of a heparin flush.

• If the patient feels a burning sensation during injection of heparin, stop the injection and check needle placement. If the needle is in the vein, inject the heparin at a slower rate *to minimize irritation.* If the needle isn't in the vein, remove and discard it. Then select a new venipuncture site and, using fresh equipment, restart the procedure.

• Change the sterile dressing every 24 to 48 hours and the intermittent infusion device every 72 hours, according to hospital policy, using a new venipuncture site. Some hospitals use a transparent semipermeable dressing or a stretch net protective sleeve to cover the entire device. *This allows more patient freedom and better observation of the injection site.*

Home care

• Most patients receiving I.V. therapy at home will have a central venous line. But if you care for a patient who will be going home with a peripheral line, you should teach the patient how to care for the I.V. site and how to identify complications.

• If the patient must observe movement restrictions, make sure he understands which movements to avoid.

• Because the patient may have special drug delivery equipment that differs from the hospital's, be sure to demonstrate the equipment and have

Converting an I.V. line to an intermittent infusion device

Two types of adapter plugs (shown below) allow you to convert an existing I.V. line into an intermittent infusion device. To make the conversion, follow these steps:

• Prime the adapter plug with heparin flush solution or normal saline solution, as appropriate.

• Clamp the I.V. tubing and remove the administration set from the catheter or needle hub.

• Insert the male adapter plug.

Inject the remaining heparin flush solution or normal saline solution to fill the line and to prevent clot formation.

Long male adapter
This long adapter plug slides into place.

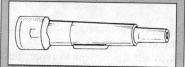

Short male adapter
This short luer-lock adapter plug twists into place.

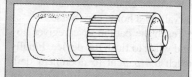

the patient give a return demonstration.

• Teach the patient to examine the site and to notify the doctor if the dressing becomes moist, if blood appears in the

Stabilizing an intermittent infusion device

Before inserting or removing a needle from an intermittent infusion device, you must stabilize the device. To do this, grasp it just below the injection cap with the thumb and index finger of your nondominant hand, as shown, and hold the device steady during needle insertion and withdrawal.

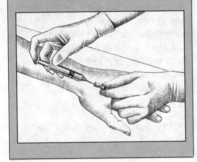

tubing, or if redness, swelling, or discomfort develops.

• Also tell the patient to report any problems with the I.V. line — for instance, if the solution stops infusing or if an alarm goes off on the infusion pump controller. Explain that the I.V. site will be changed at established intervals by a home care nurse.

• Teach the patient or caregiver how and when to flush the device. Finally, teach the patient to document daily whether the I.V. site is free from pain, swelling, and redness.

Documentation

• Record the date and time of insertion, the type and gauge of needle, and the date and time of each saline or heparin flush.

Intermittent positive-pressure breathing

Intermittent positive-pressure breathing (IPPB) delivers room air or oxygen into the lungs at a pressure higher than atmospheric pressure. This delivery ceases when pressure in the mouth or in the breathing circuit tube increases to a predetermined airway pressure.

IPPB was once the mainstay of pulmonary therapy, with its proponents claiming that the device delivered aerosolized medications deeper into the lungs, decreased the work of breathing, and assisted in the mobilization of secretions. Studies now show that IPPB has no clinical benefit over handheld nebulizers. However, IPPB may be useful in helping asthmatics with hypercapnia and impending respiratory failure avoid intubation and mechanical ventilation. Although IPPB easily inflates healthy alveoli, it may have little effect on alveoli with thickened or obstructed wall — the walls most difficult to inflate.

Typically, personnel from the respiratory therapy department deliver these treatments.

⟫ Key nursing diagnoses and patient outcomes

Use these nursing diagnoses as a guide when developing your plan of care for a patient who needs intermittent positive-pressure breathing.

Impaired gas exchange related to (specify)

Based on this nursing diagnosis, you'll establish the following patient outcomes. The patient will:
• maintain adequate ventilation.
• cough effectively.
• expectorate sputum.
• maintain respiratory rate within +/- 5 of baseline.
• perform activities of daily living (ADLs) to level of tolerance.
• have normal breath sounds.
• express feeling of comfort in maintaining air exchange.

Ineffective breathing pattern related to (specify)

Based on this nursing diagnosis, you'll establish the following patient outcomes. The patient will:
• demonstrate diaphragmatic pursed-lip breathing.
• achieve maximum lung expansion with adequate ventilation.
• demonstrate skill in conserving energy while carrying out ADLs.

Anxiety related to difficulty breathing

Based on this nursing diagnosis, you'll establish the following patient outcomes. The patient will:
• verbalize feelings of anxiety.
• use support systems to assist with coping.
• perform relaxation techniques every 4 hours.

Equipment

♦ IPPB machine ♦ breathing circuit tubing ♦ other necessary tubing (usually one or two sections) ♦ mouthpiece or mask ♦ noseclips if necessary ♦ source of pressurized gas at 50 psi if necessary ♦ oxygen if desired ♦ prescribed medication, such as isoetharine hydrochloride (Bronkosol) and normal saline solution ♦ 3-ml syringe with needle ♦ sphygmomanometer ♦ stethoscope ♦ facial tissues and waste bag, or specimen cup ♦ optional: suction equipment.

Equipment preparation

• Follow the manufacturer's instructions to set up the equipment properly.

Patient preparation

• Explain the procedure to the patient *to ensure his cooperation.*
• Tell him to sit erect in a chair, if possible, *to allow for optimal lung expansion.* Otherwise, place him in semi-Fowler's position. Wash your hands.
• Take baseline blood pressure and heart rate, especially if a bronchodilator will be administered, and listen to breath sounds for posttreatment comparisons.
• Instruct the patient to breathe deeply and slowly through his mouth as if sucking on a straw. Encourage the patient to let the machine do the work.
• During treatment, instruct the patient to hold his breath for a few seconds after full inspiration *to allow for greater distribution of gas and medication.* Then instruct him to exhale normally.

Implementation

• During treatment, take the patient's blood pressure and heart rate. *IPPB treatment increases intrathoracic pressure and may temporarily decrease cardiac output and venous return, resulting in tachycardia, hypotension, or headache. Monitoring also detects reactions to the broncho-*

dilator. If you find a sudden change in blood pressure or increase in heart rate by 20 or more beats, stop the treatment and notify the doctor.

• If the patient is tolerating the treatment, continue until the medication in the nebulizer is exhausted, usually about 10 minutes.

• After treatment, or as needed, have the patient expectorate into tissues or a specimen cup, or suction him as necessary. Listen to his breath sounds and compare them to the pretreatment assessment.

• Shake excess moisture from the nebulizer and the mouthpiece or mask. After 24 hours of use, either discard the equipment or clean it with warm, soapy water. After washing, rinse with warm water and immerse in gluteraldehyde solution (Control III) for 10 minutes. Then remove the equipment, rinse in warm water, and air dry. Once it's dry, store in a clean plastic bag.

Complications

• Gastric insufflation may result from swallowed air and occurs more commonly with a mask than with a mouthpiece.

• Dizziness can result from hyperventilation.

• The work of breathing can be increased, especially if the patient is uncomfortable with or frightened by the machine.

• Decreased blood pressure can result from decreased venous return, especially in the patient with hypovolemia or cardiovascular disease.

• Increased intracranial pressure can result from impeded venous return from the brain.

• Spontaneous pneumothorax may result from increased intrathoracic pressure; this complication is rare but is most likely to occur in patients with emphysematous blebs.

Nursing considerations

• If possible, avoid administering IPPB treatment immediately before or after a meal *because the treatment may induce nausea and because a full stomach reduces lung expansion.*

• Never give IPPB treatment without medication in the nebulizer *because this could dry the patient's airways and make secretions more difficult to mobilize.* If the purpose of treatment is to mobilize secretions, use a specimen cup to measure the secretions obtained.

• If the patient wears dentures, leave them in place *to ensure a proper seal,* but remove them if they slide out of position. If the patient has an artificial airway, use a special adapter, such as mechanical ventilation tubing, to give IPPB treatments. When using a mask to administer treatments, allow the patient frequent rest periods, and observe for gastric distention *because this is more likely to occur with a mask.*

• If the patient's blood pressure is stable during the initial treatment, you may not need to check it during subsequent treatments unless he has a history of cardiovascular disease, hypotension, or sensitivity to any drug delivered in the treatment.

Documentation

• Record the date, time, and duration of treatment; medication administered; pressure used; vital signs; breath sounds before and after treatment; amount of sputum produced; any complications and nursing actions taken; and the patient's tolerance of the procedure.

Intra-aortic balloon counterpulsation care

Providing temporary support for the heart's left ventricle, intra-aortic balloon counterpulsation (IABC) mechanically displaces blood within the aorta by means of an intra-aortic balloon attached to an external pump console. It monitors myocardial perfusion and the effects of drugs on myocardial function and perfusion. When used correctly, IABC improves two key aspects of myocardial physiology: It increases the supply of oxygen-rich blood to the myocardium, and it decreases myocardial oxygen demand. (See *How the intra-aortic balloon pump works,* page 438, and *Interpreting intra-aortic balloon waveforms,* pages 439 and 440.)

The balloon is usually inserted through the common femoral artery and positioned with its tip just distal to the left subclavian artery.

IABC is recommended for patients with a wide range of low-cardiac-output disorders or cardiac instability, including refractory anginas, ventricular arrhythmias associated with ischemia, and pump failure caused by cardiogenic shock, intraoperative myocardial infarction (MI), or low cardiac output after bypass surgery. IABC is also indicated for patients with low cardiac output secondary to acute mechanical defects after MI (such as ventricular septal defect, pap-

illary muscle rupture, or left ventricular aneurysm).

Perioperatively, the technique is used to support and stabilize patients with a suspected high-grade lesion who are undergoing such procedures as angioplasty, thrombolytic therapy, cardiac surgery, and cardiac catheterization.

IABC is contraindicated in patients with severe aortic regurgitation, aortic aneurysm, or severe peripheral vascular disease.

≫ Key nursing diagnoses and patient outcomes

Use these nursing diagnoses as a guide when developing your plan of care for a patient who needs intra-aortic balloon counterpulsation.

Decreased cardiac output related to (specify)

Based on this nursing diagnosis, you'll establish the following patient outcomes. The patient will:
• maintain hemodynamic stability as evidenced by a normal pulse rate and blood pressure.
• experience no dizziness, syncope, or arrhythmias.
• experience a decrease in heart's workload.
• maintain respiratory status within established parameters.

Anxiety related to invasive monitoring and treatment

Based on this nursing diagnosis, you'll establish the following patient outcomes. The patient will:
• verbalize feelings of anxiety.
• use support systems to assist with coping.

How the intra-aortic balloon pump works

Made of polyurethane, the intra-aortic balloon is attached to an external pump console by means of a large-lumen catheter. These illustrations show the direction of blood flow when the pump inflates and deflates the balloon.

Balloon inflation
The balloon inflates as the aortic valve closes and diastole begins. Diastole increases perfusion to the coronary arteries.

Balloon deflation
The balloon deflates before ventricular ejection, when the aortic valve opens. This permits ejection of blood from the left ventricle against a lowered resistance. As a result, aortic end-diastolic pressure and afterload decrease and cardiac output rises.

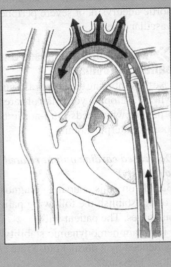

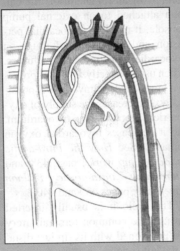

• cope with threat of anxiety by being involved in decisions about care.
• demonstrate abated physical symptoms of anxiety.

Equipment
♦ IABC console and balloon catheters ♦ Dacron graft (for surgically inserted balloon) ♦ electrocardiogram (ECG) monitor and electrodes ♦ I.V. solution and infusion set ♦ sedative ♦ pain medication ♦ arterial line catheter ♦ heparin flush solution, transducer, and flush setup ♦ pulmonary artery (PA) catheter setup ♦ temporary pacemaker setup ♦ 18G angiography needle ♦ sterile drape ♦ sterile gloves ♦ gown ♦ mask ♦ sutures ♦ povidone-iodine and saline solution or sterile water for irrigation and suction setup ♦ oxygen setup and respirator if necessary ♦ defibrillator and emergency medications ♦ fluoroscope ♦ indwelling catheter ♦ uri-

Interpreting intra-aortic balloon waveforms

During intra-aortic balloon counterpulsation, you can use electrocardiogram and arterial pressure waveforms to determine whether the balloon pump is functioning properly.

Normal timing

Balloon inflation occurs after aortic valve closure, deflation during isovolumetric contraction, just before the aortic valve opens. In a properly timed waveform, like the one shown at right, the inflation point lies at or slightly above the dicrotic notch. Both inflation and deflation cause a sharp V. Peak diastolic pressure exceeds peak systolic pressure; peak systolic pressure exceeds assisted peak systolic pressure.

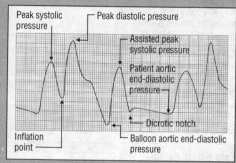

Early inflation

With *early inflation*, the inflation point lies before the dicrotic notch. Early inflation dangerously increases myocardial stress and decreases cardiac output.

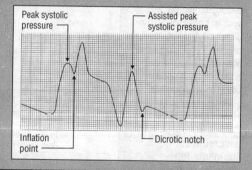

Early deflation

With *early deflation*, a U shape appears, and peak systolic pressure is less than or equal to assisted peak systolic pressure. This will not decrease afterload or myocardial oxygen consumption.

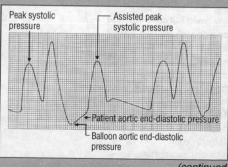

(continued)

Interpreting intra-aortic balloon waveforms (continued)

Late inflation

With *late inflation,* the dicrotic notch precedes the inflation point, and the notch and the inflation point create a W shape. This can lead to a reduction in peak diastolic pressure, coronary and systemic perfusion augmentation time, and augmented coronary perfusion pressure.

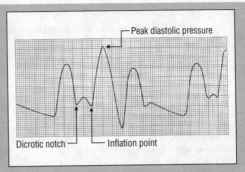

Late deflation

With *late deflation,* balloon aortic end-diastolic pressure increases and peak systolic pressure exceeds assisted peak systolic pressure. This increases afterload, myocardial oxygen consumption, cardiac workload, and preload. It occurs when the balloon has been inflated for too long.

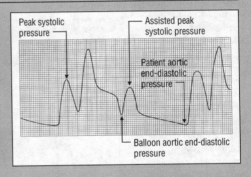

Proper timing with reduced augmentation

Sometimes, inflation and deflation are properly timed but the balloon doesn't inflate enough. When this happens, peak diastolic pressure equals or drops below peak systolic pressure. You'll need to evaluate the patient's condition to determine the cause of reduced augmentation.

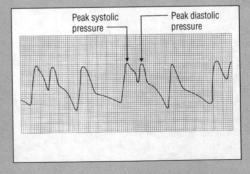

meter ♦ arterial blood gas (ABG) kits and tubes for laboratory studies ♦ povidone-iodine swabs and ointment ♦ dressing materials ♦ 4″ × 4″ gauze pads ♦ shaving supplies ♦ optional: defibrillator, atropine, I.V. heparin, low-molecular-weight dextran.

Equipment preparation

• Depending on hospital policy, you or a perfusionist must balance the pressure transducer in the external pump console and calibrate the oscilloscope monitor to ensure accuracy.

Patient preparation

• Explain to the patient that the doctor will place a special balloon catheter in the aorta *to help his heart pump more easily.*
• Briefly explain the insertion procedure, and mention that the catheter will be connected to a large console next to his bed.
• Tell the patient that the balloon will temporarily reduce the heart's workload *to promote rapid healing of the ventricular muscle.*
• Let him know that it will be removed after his heart can resume an adequate workload.
• Make sure the patient or a family member understands and signs a consent form. Verify that the form is attached to his chart.

Implementation

To prepare for intra-aortic balloon insertion
• Obtain the patient's baseline vital signs, including pulmonary artery pressure (PAP). (A PA line should already be in place.) Attach the patient to an ECG machine for continuous monitoring. Be sure to apply chest electrodes in a standard lead II position — or in whatever position produces the largest R wave — *because the R wave triggers balloon inflation and deflation.* Obtain a baseline ECG.
• Attach another set of ECG electrodes to the patient unless the ECG pattern is being transmitted from the patient's bedside monitor to the balloon pump monitor through a phone cable. Administer oxygen as ordered and as necessary.
• Make sure the patient has an arterial line, a PA line, and a peripheral I.V. line in place. *The arterial line is used for withdrawing blood samples, monitoring blood pressure, and assessing the timing and effectiveness of therapy. The PA line allows measurement of PAP, aspiration of blood samples, and cardiac output studies.* Increased PAP indicates increased myocardial workload and ineffective balloon pumping. Cardiac output studies are usually performed with and without the balloon *to check the patient's progress.* The central lumen of the intra-aortic balloon, used to monitor central aortic pressure, produces an augmented pressure waveform that allows you to check for proper timing of the inflation-deflation cycle and demonstrates the effects of counterpulsation, elevated diastolic pressure, and reduced end-diastolic and systolic pressures.
• Insert an indwelling catheter *so you can measure the patient's urine output and assess his fluid balance and renal function. To reduce the risk of infection,* shave or clip hair bilaterally from the lower abdomen to the lower thigh, including the pubic area.
• Observe and record the patient's peripheral leg pulse and document sen-

sation, movement, color, and temperature of the legs.
• Administer a sedative as ordered.

To insert the intra-aortic balloon percutaneously

• The doctor may insert the balloon percutaneously through the femoral artery into the descending thoracic aorta, using a modified Seldinger technique. First, he accesses the vessel with an 18G angiography needle and removes the inner stylet.
• Then he passes the guide wire through the needle and removes the needle.
• After passing a #8 French vessel dilator over the guide wire into the vessel, he removes the vessel dilator, leaving the guide wire in place.
• Next, the doctor passes an introducer (dilator and sheath assembly) over the guide wire into the vessel until 1″ (2.5 cm) remains above the insertion site. He then removes the inner dilator, leaving the introducer sheath and guide wire in place.
• After passing the balloon over the guide wire into the introducer sheath, the doctor advances the catheter into position, 3/8″ to 3/4″ (1 to 2 cm) distal to the left subclavian artery.
• The doctor attaches the balloon to the control system to initiate counterpulsation. The balloon catheter then unfurls.

To insert the intra-aortic balloon surgically

• If the doctor chooses not to insert the catheter percutaneously, he usually inserts it through a femoral arteriotomy.
• After making an incision and isolating the femoral artery, the doctor at-

taches a Dacron graft to a small opening in the arterial wall.
• He then passes the catheter through this graft. With fluoroscopic guidance, as needed, he advances the catheter up the descending thoracic aorta and positions the catheter tip between the left subclavian artery and the renal arteries.
• The doctor sews the Dacron graft around the catheter at the insertion point and connects the other end of the catheter to the pump console. (See *Surgical insertion sites for the intra-aortic balloon.*)
• If the balloon can't be inserted through the femoral artery, the doctor inserts it in an antegrade direction through the anterior wall of the ascending aorta. He positions it 3/8″ to 3/4″ (1 to 2 cm) beyond the left subclavian artery and brings the catheter out through the chest wall.

To monitor the patient after balloon insertion

• If the control system malfunctions or becomes inoperable, don't let the balloon catheter remain dormant for more than 30 minutes. Get another control system and attach it to the balloon; then resume pumping. In the meantime, inflate the balloon manually, using a 60-cc syringe and room air a minimum of once every 5 minutes, *to prevent thrombus formation in the catheter.*
• Obtain a chest X-ray *to determine correct balloon placement.*
• Assess and record pedal and posterior tibial pulses as well as color, sensation, and temperature in the affected limb every 15 minutes for 1 hour, then hourly. Notify the doctor immediately

Surgical insertion sites for the intra-aortic balloon

The doctor will insert the intra-aortic balloon surgically, using a femoral or transthoracic approach, if it can't be inserted percutaneously.

Femoral approach
Insertion through the femoral artery requires a cutdown and an arteriotomy. The doctor passes the balloon through a Dacron graft that has been sewn to the artery.

successful. He inserts the balloon in an antegrade direction through the subclavian artery and then positions it in the descending thoracic aorta.

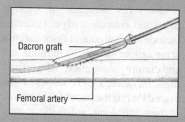

Dacron graft

Femoral artery

Transthoracic approach
The doctor may use a transthoracic approach if femoral insertion is un-

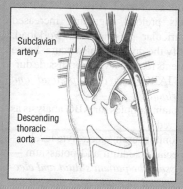

Subclavian artery

Descending thoracic aorta

if you detect circulatory changes; *the balloon may need to be removed.*
• Observe and record the patient's baseline arm pulses, arm sensation and movement, and arm color and temperature every 15 minutes for 1 hour after balloon insertion, then every 2 hours while the balloon is in place. Loss of left arm pulses may indicate upward balloon displacement. Notify the doctor of any changes.
• Monitor the patient's urine output every hour. Note baseline blood urea nitrogen (BUN) and serum creatinine levels, and monitor these levels daily. Changes in urine output, BUN, and serum creatinine levels may signal reduced renal perfusion from downward balloon displacement.

• Auscultate for and record bowel sounds every 4 hours. Check for abdominal distention and tenderness as well as changes in the patient's elimination patterns.
• Measure the patient's temperature every 1 to 4 hours. If it's elevated, obtain blood samples for a culture, send them to the laboratory immediately, and notify the doctor. Culture any drainage at the insertion site.
• Monitor the patient's hematologic status. Observe for bleeding gums, blood in the urine or stools, petechiae, and bleeding at the insertion site. Monitor his platelet count, hemoglobin levels, and hematocrit daily. Expect to administer blood products *to maintain hematocrit at 30%.* If the

platelet count drops, expect to administer platelets.

• Monitor partial thromboplastin time (PTT) every 6 hours while the heparin dose is adjusted *to maintain PTT at 1.5 to 2 times the normal value,* then every 12 to 24 hours while the balloon remains in place.

• Measure PAP and pulmonary artery wedge pressure (PAWP) every 1 to 2 hours as ordered. A rising PAWP reflects preload, signaling increased ventricular pressure and workload; notify the doctor if this occurs. Some patients require I.V. nitroprusside during IABC *to reduce preload and afterload.*

• Obtain samples for ABG analysis as ordered.

• Monitor serum electrolyte levels — especially sodium and potassium — *to assess the patient's fluid and electrolyte balance and help prevent arrhythmias.*

• Watch for signs and symptoms of a dissecting aortic aneurysm: a blood pressure differential between the left and right arms, elevated blood pressure, syncope, pallor, diaphoresis, dyspnea, a throbbing abdominal mass, a reduced red blood cell count with an elevated white blood cell count, and pain in the chest, abdomen, or back. Notify the doctor immediately if you note any of these findings.

To wean the patient from the intra-aortic balloon

• Assess the cardiac index, systemic blood pressure, and PAWP *to help the doctor evaluate the patient's readiness for weaning* — usually about 24 hours after balloon insertion.

• To begin weaning, gradually decrease the frequency of balloon aug-

mentation to 1:2, 1:4, and 1:8, as ordered. Although your hospital has its own weaning protocol, be aware that assist frequency is usually maintained for an hour or longer. If the patient's hemodynamic indices remain stable during this time, weaning may continue.

• Avoid leaving the patient on a low augmentation setting for more than 2 hours to prevent embolus formation.

• Assess his tolerance of weaning. Signs and symptoms of poor tolerance include confusion and disorientation, urine output below 30 ml/hour, cold and clammy skin, chest pain, arrhythmias, ischemic ECG changes, and elevated PAP. If the patient develops any of these problems, notify the doctor at once.

To remove the intra-aortic balloon

• The balloon is removed when the patient can tolerate counterpulsation in 1:4 or 1:8 and no longer needs augmentation. The control system is turned off and the connective tubing is disconnected from the catheter *to ensure balloon deflation.*

• The doctor withdraws the balloon until the proximal end of the catheter contacts the distal end of the introducer sheath.

• The doctor then applies pressure below the puncture site and removes the balloon and introducer sheath as a unit, allowing a few seconds of free bleeding *to prevent thrombus formation.*

• *To promote distal bleedback,* the doctor applies pressure above the puncture site.

• Apply direct pressure to the site for 30 minutes or until bleeding stops. (In

some hospitals, this is the doctor's responsibility.)
• If the balloon was inserted surgically, the doctor will close the Dacron graft and suture the insertion site. The cardiologist usually removes a percutaneous catheter.
• After balloon removal, provide wound care according to hospital policy. Record the patient's pedal and posterior tibial pulses, and the color, temperature, and sensation of the affected limb. Enforce bed rest as appropriate (usually for 24 hours).

Complications

IABC may cause numerous complications.
• The most common, arterial embolism, stems from clot formation on the balloon surface.
  Other potential complications include:
• extension or rupture of an aortic aneurysm
• femoral or iliac artery perforation
• femoral artery occlusion
• sepsis.
  Bleeding at the insertion site may be aggravated by pump-induced thrombocytopenia caused by platelet aggregation around the balloon.

Nursing considerations

• Before using the IABC control system, make sure you know what the alarms and messages mean and how to respond to them.
  Note: You must respond immediately to alarms and messages.
• Change the dressing at the balloon insertion site every 24 hours or as needed, using strict sterile technique. Don't let povidone-iodine solution come in contact with the catheter.

• Make sure the head of the bed is elevated no more than 30 degrees.
• Watch for pump interruptions, which may result from loose ECG electrodes or leadwires, static or 60-cycle interference, catheter kinking, or improper body alignment.

Documentation

• Document all aspects of patient assessment and management, including the patient's response to therapy.
• If you're responsible for the IABC device, document all routine checks, problems, and troubleshooting measures.
• If a technician is responsible for the IABC device, record only when and why the technician was notified as well as the result of his actions on the patient, if any.
• Document any teaching of the patient, family, or close friends as well as their responses.

Intracranial pressure monitoring

This procedure measures pressure exerted by the brain, blood, and cerebrospinal fluid (CSF) against the inside of the skull. Indications for monitoring intracranial pressure (ICP) include head trauma with bleeding or edema, overproduction or insufficient absorption of CSF, cerebral hemorrhage, and space-occupying brain lesions. ICP monitoring can detect elevated ICP early, before clinical danger signs develop. Prompt intervention can then help avert or diminish neurologic damage caused by cerebral hypoxia and shifts of brain mass.

The four basic ICP monitoring systems feature ventricular catheter, subarachnoid bolt, epidural sensor, and intraparenchymal pressure monitoring. (See *Understanding ICP monitoring*.)

Regardless of the system used, the procedure is always performed by a neurosurgeon in the operating room, emergency department (ED), or critical care unit. Insertion of an ICP monitoring device requires sterile technique to reduce the risk of central nervous system (CNS) infection. Setting up equipment for the monitoring systems also requires strict asepsis.

≫ Key nursing diagnoses and patient outcomes

Use these nursing diagnoses as a guide when developing your plan of care for a patient who needs intracranial pressure monitoring.

Decreased adaptive capacity: intracranial related to (specify)

Based on this nursing diagnosis, you'll establish the following patient outcomes. The patient will:
• experience a decrease in intracranial pressure.
• show signs of improving level of consciousness.

Risk for infection related to invasive monitoring procedure

Based on this nursing diagnosis, you'll establish the following patient outcomes. The patient will:
• maintain a normal body temperature.
• show no signs or symptoms of infection from invasive procedure.

Equipment

♦ monitoring unit and transducers, as ordered ♦ 16 to 20 sterile 4″ × 4″ gauze pads ♦ linen-saver pads ♦ shave preparation tray or hair scissors ♦ sterile drapes ♦ povidone-iodine solution ♦ sterile gown ♦ surgical mask ♦ two pairs of sterile gloves ♦ povidone-iodine ointment ♦ head dressing supplies (two rolls of 4″ elastic gauze dressing, one roll of 4″ roller gauze, adhesive tape) ♦ optional: suction apparatus, a yardstick.

Equipment preparation

• Monitoring units and setup protocols are varied and complex and differ among hospitals. Check your hospital's guidelines for your particular unit and its preparation.
• Various models of preassembled ICP monitoring units are available, each with its own setup protocols. These units are designed to reduce the risk of infection by eliminating the need for multiple stopcocks, manometers, and transducer dome assemblies. Some hospitals use units that have miniature transducers rather than transducer domes.

Patient preparation

• Explain the procedure to the patient or his family.
• Make sure the patient or a responsible family member has signed a consent form.
• Determine whether the patient is allergic to iodine preparations.
• Provide privacy if the procedure is being done in an open ED or intensive care unit.
• Obtain baseline routine and neurologic vital signs to aid in prompt de-

Understanding ICP monitoring

Intracranial pressure (ICP) can be monitored using one of four systems.

Intraventricular catheter monitoring

In this procedure, which monitors ICP directly, the doctor inserts a small polyethylene or silicone rubber catheter into the lateral ventricle through a burr hole.

Although this method measures ICP most accurately, it carries the greatest risk of infection. This is the only type of ICP monitoring that allows evaluation of brain compliance and drainage of significant amounts of cerebrospinal fluid (CSF).

Contraindications usually include stenotic cerebral ventricles, cerebral aneurysms in the path of catheter placement, and suspected vascular lesions.

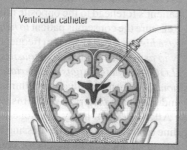

Ventricular catheter

Subarachnoid bolt monitoring

This procedure involves insertion of a special bolt into the subarachnoid space through a twist-drill burr hole that's positioned in the front of the skull behind the hairline.

Placing the bolt is easier than placing an intraventricular catheter, especially if a computed tomography scan reveals that the cerebrum has shifted or the ventricles have collapsed. This type of monitoring carries less risk of infection and pa-

renchymal damage because the bolt doesn't penetrate the cerebrum.

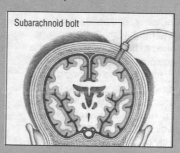

Subarachnoid bolt

Epidural or subdural sensor monitoring

ICP can be monitored from the epidural or the subdural space. For epidural monitoring, a fiber-optic sensor is inserted into the epidural space through a burr hole, as shown. This system's main drawback is its questionable accuracy because ICP isn't being measured directly from a CSF-filled space.

For subdural monitoring, a fiber-optic transducer tipped catheter is tunneled through a burr hole, and its tip is placed on brain tissue under the dura mater. The main drawback to this method is its inability to drain CSF.

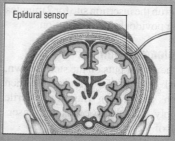

Epidural sensor

(continued)

Understanding ICP monitoring *(continued)*

Intraparenchymal monitoring

In this procedure, the doctor inserts a catheter through a small subarachnoid bolt and, after puncturing the dura, advances the catheter a few centimeters into the brain's white matter. There's no need to balance or calibrate the equipment after insertion.

Although this method doesn't provide direct access to CSF, measurements are accurate because brain tissue pressures correlate well with ventricular pressures. It may be used to obtain ICP measurements in patients with compressed or dislocated ventricles.

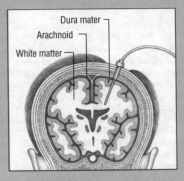

tection of decompensation during the procedure.

• Place the patient in the supine position, and elevate the head of the bed 30 degrees or as ordered. Document the number of bed crank rotations, or hang a yardstick on an I.V. pole and mark the exact elevation.

• Place linen-saver pads under the patient's head. Shave or clip his hair at the insertion site as indicated by the doctor, *to decrease the risk of infection.* Carefully fold and remove the linen-saver pads *to avoid spilling loose hair onto the bed.*

• Drape the patient with sterile drapes.

• Scrub the insertion site for 2 minutes with povidone-iodine solution.

Implementation

• The doctor puts on the sterile gown, mask, and sterile gloves. He then opens the interior wrap of the sterile supply tray and proceeds with insertion of the catheter or bolt.

• *To facilitate placement of the device,* hold the patient's head in your hands or attach a long strip of 4″ roller gauze to one side rail and bring it across the patient's forehead to the opposite rail. Reassure the conscious patient *to help ease his anxiety.* Talk to him frequently *to assess his level of consciousness (LOC) and detect signs of deterioration.* Watch for cardiac arrhythmias and abnormal respiratory patterns.

• After insertion, apply povidone-iodine ointment and a sterile dressing to the site. If not done by the doctor, connect the catheter to the appropriate monitoring device, depending on the system used. (See *Setting up an ICP monitoring system.*)

• If the doctor has set up a drainage system, attach the drip chamber to the headboard or bedside I.V. pole, as ordered.

Nursing alert: Positioning the drip chamber too high may raise ICP; positioning it too low may cause excessive CSF drainage.

Setting up an ICP monitoring system

To set up an intracranial pressure (ICP) monitoring system, follow these steps:

• Begin by opening a sterile towel. On the sterile field, place a 20-ml luer-lock syringe, an 18G needle, a 250-ml bag filled with normal saline solution (with outer wrapper removed), and a disposable transducer.
• Put on sterile gloves and gown and fill the 20 ml syringe with normal saline solution from the I.V. bag.
• Remove the injection cap from the patient line and attach the syringe. Turn the system stopcock off to the short end of the patient line, and flush through to the drip chamber, as shown below. Allow a few drops to flow through the flow chamber (the manometer), the tubing, and the one-way valve into the drainage bag. (Fill the tubing and the manometer slowly to minimize air bubbles. If any air bubbles surface, be sure to force them from the system.)

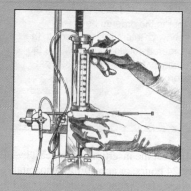

• Next, connect the transducer to the monitor. Put on a clean pair of sterile gloves. Keeping one hand sterile, turn the patient stopcock off to the patient.
• Align the zero point with the center line of the patient's head, level with the middle of the ear, as shown (below).

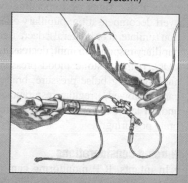

• Attach the manometer to the I.V. pole at the head of the bed (as shown above, next column). Slide the drip chamber onto the manometer, and align the chamber to the zero point, as shown.

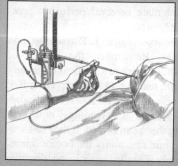

• Lower the flow chamber to zero, and turn the stopcock off to the dead-end cap. With a clean hand,
(continued)

Setting up an ICP monitoring system (continued)

balance the system according to monitor guidelines.
• Turn the system stopcock off to drainage, and raise the flow chamber to the ordered height, as shown. Return the stopcock to the ordered position, and observe the monitor for the return of ICP patterns.

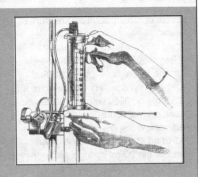

• Inspect the insertion site at least every 24 hours, or according to hospital policy, for redness, swelling, and drainage. Clean the site, reapply povidone-iodine ointment, and apply a fresh sterile dressing.
• Hourly, or as ordered, assess the patient's clinical status, and take routine and neurologic vital signs. Make sure you have obtained orders for waveforms and pressure parameters from the doctor.
• Calculate cerebral perfusion pressure hourly.
• Observe digital ICP readings and waves. Remember, the pattern of readings is more significant than any single reading. (See Interpreting ICP waveforms.) If you observe continually elevated ICP readings, note how long they're sustained. If they last several minutes, notify the doctor immediately. Finally, record and describe any CSF drainage.

Complications

• CNS infection, the most common hazard of ICP monitoring, can result from contamination of the equipment setup or of the insertion site.

Nursing alert. Excessive loss of CSF can result from faulty stopcock placement or a drip chamber that's positioned too low. Such loss can rapidly decompress the cranial contents and damage bridging cortical veins, leading to hematoma formation. Decompression can also lead to rupture of existing hematomas or aneurysms, causing hemorrhage.
• Watch for signs of impending or overt decompensation: pupillary dilation (unilateral or bilateral); decreased pupillary response to light; decreasing LOC; rising systolic blood pressure and widening pulse pressure; bradycardia; slowed, irregular respirations; and, in late decompensation, decerebrate posturing.

Nursing considerations

• In infants, ICP monitoring can be performed without penetrating the scalp. In this external method, a photoelectric transducer with a pressure-sensitive membrane is taped to the anterior fontanel. The transducer responds to pressure at the site and transmits readings to a bedside monitor and recording system. The external

Interpreting ICP waveforms

Three waveforms, A, B, and C, are used to monitor intracranial pressure (ICP). *A waves* are an ominous sign of intracranial decompensation and poor compliance. *B waves* correlate with changes in respiration, and *C waves* with changes in arterial pressure.

A normal ICP waveform typically shows a steep upward systolic slope followed by a downward diastolic slope with a dicrotic notch. In most cases, this waveform occurs continuously and

Normal waveform

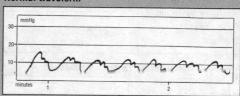

indicates an ICP between 0 and

15 mm Hg — normal pressure.

The most clinically significant ICP waveforms are A waves, which may reach elevations of 50 to 100 mm Hg, persist for 5 to 20 minutes, then drop sharply. A waves may come and go, spiking from temporary rises in thoracic pressure or from any condition

A waves

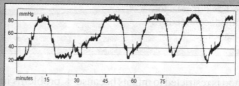

that increases ICP beyond the brain's compliance limits. Activities such as sustained coughing or straining

with bowel movements can cause temporary elevations in thoracic pressure.

B waves, which appear sharp and rhythmic, with a sawtooth pattern, occur every 1½ to 2 minutes and may reach elevations of 50 mm Hg. The clinical significance of B waves isn't clear, but they correlate with respiratory changes and may occur more

B waves

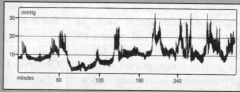

frequently with decreasing compensation. Because B waves sometimes precede A waves,

notify the doctor if B waves occur frequently.

(continued)

Interpreting ICP waveforms (continued)

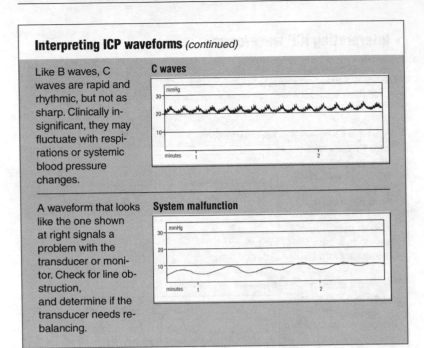

Like B waves, C waves are rapid and rhythmic, but not as sharp. Clinically insignificant, they may fluctuate with respirations or systemic blood pressure changes.

C waves

A waveform that looks like the one shown at right signals a problem with the transducer or monitor. Check for line obstruction, and determine if the transducer needs rebalancing.

System malfunction

method is restricted to infants because pressure readings can be obtained only at fontanels, the incompletely ossified areas of the skull.

• In some instances, a Doppler ultrasonic transducer may be used for noninvasive ICP monitoring. (See *Understanding transcranial Doppler ultrasonography*.)

• Osmotic diuretic agents such as mannitol reduce cerebral edema by shrinking intracranial contents. Given by I.V. drip or bolus, mannitol draws water from tissues into plasma; it does not cross the blood-brain barrier. Monitor serum electrolyte levels and osmolality readings closely because *the patient may become dehydrated very quickly*. Be aware that a rebound increase in ICP may occur. If your patient has congestive heart failure or severe renal dysfunction, monitor for problems in adapting to the increased intravascular volumes.

• Fluid restriction, usually 1,200 ml to 1,500 ml per day, avoids causing or increasing cerebral edema.

• Although steroid therapy is controversial, steroids may be used to lower elevated ICP by reducing sodium and water concentration in the brain. *Because they may also produce peptic ulcers,* they're usually given with antacids and cimetidine or ranitidine. Observe for possible GI bleeding. Also monitor urine glucose and acetone levels because *steroids may cause glycosuria in patients with borderline diabetes.*

Barbiturate-induced coma depresses the reticular activating system and reduces the brain's metabolic demand. Reduced demand for oxygen

TECHNOLOGY UPDATE

Understanding transcranial Doppler ultrasonography

A noninvasive procedure, Doppler ultrasonography monitors blood flow changes and emboli in the intracranial vessels, specifically the circle of Willis. The transcranial Doppler transducer is positioned at the temporal region of the patient's head (below, left). It transmits pulses of high-frequency ultrasound, which are reflected back to the transducer by the red blood cells moving in the vessel being monitored. The reflected pulses are electronically processed into an audible signal and a waveform display (below, right) that provides information about blood flow, emboli, and other diagnostic parameters.

Transducer placement
Once the Doppler transducer is positioned on the patient's head to provide the strongest, highest pitched signal and the best waveform, it's locked into place at the chosen angle with set screws and a headband.

Transcranial Doppler signal
The displayed waveform is actually a moving graph of blood flow velocities. The heart's contractions speed up blood cell movement during systole and slow it down during diastole, resulting in a waveform that varies in velocity over the cardiac cycle.

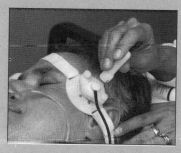

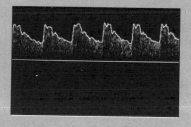

and energy reduces cerebral blood flow, thereby lowering ICP.

• Hyperventilation with oxygen from a handheld resuscitation bag or respirator helps rid the patient of excess carbon dioxide, thereby constricting cerebral vessels and reducing cerebral blood volume and ICP. However, only normal brain tissues respond because blood vessels in damaged areas have reduced vasoconstrictive ability.

• Before tracheal suctioning, hyperventilate the patient with 100% oxygen as ordered. Apply suction for a maximum of 15 seconds. Avoid inducing hypoxia *because it greatly increases cerebral blood flow.*

• Because fever raises brain metabolism, which increases cerebral blood flow, fever-reduction (achieved by administering acetaminophen, alcohol sponge baths, and a hypothermia blanket) also helps to reduce ICP. However, rebound increases in ICP and brain edema may occur if rapid rewarming takes place after hypothermia or if cooling measures induce shivering.

• Withdrawal of CSF through the drainage system reduces CSF volume, and thus reduces ICP. Although less commonly used, surgical removal of a skull-bone flap provides room for the swollen brain to expand. If this procedure is performed, keep the site clean and dry *to prevent infection* and maintain sterile technique when changing the dressing.

Documentation

• Record the time and date of the insertion procedure and the patient's response.

• Note the insertion site and the type of monitoring system used.

• Record ICP digital readings and waveforms at least once per shift, and record CPP hourly in your notes, on a flowchart, or directly on readout strips, depending on hospital policy.

• Document any factors that may affect ICP — for example, drug therapy, stressful procedures, or sleep.

• Record routine and neurologic vital signs hourly, and describe the patient's clinical status.

• Note the amount, character, and frequency of any CSF drainage (for example, "between 6 p.m. and 7 p.m., 15 ml of blood-tinged CSF").

Intradermal injection

Used primarily for diagnostic purposes, as in allergy or tuberculin testing, intradermal injections are administered in small amounts, usually 0.5 ml or less, into the outer layers of the skin. Because little systemic absorp-tion of intradermally injected agents takes place, this type of injection is used primarily to produce a local effect.

The ventral forearm is the most commonly used site for intradermal injection because of its easy accessibility and lack of hair. In extensive allergy testing, the outer aspect of the upper arms may be used, or the back, between the scapulae. (See *Intradermal injection sites.*)

≫ Key nursing diagnoses and patient outcomes

Use these nursing diagnoses as a guide when developing your plan of care for a patient receiving intradermal medications.

Knowledge deficit related to lack of exposure

Based on this nursing diagnosis, you'll establish the following patient outcomes. The patient will:

• state or demonstrate understanding of what has been taught.

• demonstrate ability to perform new health-related behaviors as they are taught.

High risk for injury related to performing procedure

Based on this nursing diagnosis, you'll establish the following patient outcomes. The patient will:

• identify factors that increase potential for injury.

• assist in identifying and applying safety measures to prevent injury.

Equipment

♦ patient's medication record and chart ♦ tuberculin syringe with a 26G or 27G ½″ to ⅝″ needle ♦ prescribed medication ♦ gloves ♦ alcohol sponges.

Patient preparation
• Verify the patient's identity by checking his name, room number, and bed number on his wristband against his medical record.
• Tell him where you will be giving the injection.
• Instruct the patient to sit up and to extend his arm and support it on a flat surface, with the ventral forearm exposed.

Implementation
• Put on gloves.
• With an alcohol sponge, clean the surface of the ventral forearm about two or three fingerbreadths distal to the antecubital space. Be sure the test site you have chosen is free of hair or blemishes. Allow the skin to dry completely before administering the injection.
• While holding the patient's forearm in your hand, stretch the skin taut with your thumb.
• With your free hand, hold the needle at a 15-degree angle to the patient's arm, with its bevel up.
• Insert the needle about $\frac{1}{8}$" (0.3 cm) below the epidermis at sites 2" (5 cm) apart. Stop when the needle's bevel tip is under the skin, and inject the antigen slowly. You should feel some resistance as you do this, and a wheal should form as you inject the antigen. (See *Giving an intradermal injection*, page 456.) If no wheal forms, you have injected the antigen too deeply; withdraw the needle and administer another test dose at least 2" (5 cm) from the first site.
• Withdraw the needle at the same angle at which it was inserted. Do not

Intradermal injection sites

The most common intradermal injection site is the ventral forearm. Other sites (indicated by dotted areas) include the upper chest, upper arm, and shoulder blades. Skin in these areas is usually lightly pigmented, thinly keratinized, and relatively hairless, facilitating detection of adverse reactions.

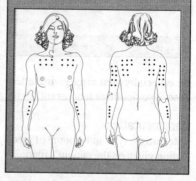

rub the site. *This could irritate the underlying tissue, which may affect test results.*
• Circle each test site with a marking pen, and label each site according to the recall antigen given. Instruct the patient to refrain from washing off the circles until the test is completed.
• Dispose of needles and syringes according to hospital policy.
• Remove and discard your gloves.
• Assess the patient's response to the skin testing in 24 to 48 hours.

Nursing considerations
• In patients hypersensitive to the test antigens, a severe anaphylactic response can result. This requires immediate epinephrine injection and other emergency resuscitation procedures.

Giving an intradermal injection

Secure the forearm. Insert the needle at a 10- to 15-degree angle so it just punctures skin surface. When injected, the drug should raise a small wheal.

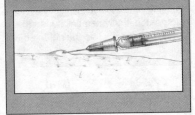

Be especially alert after giving a test dose of penicillin or tetanus antitoxin.

Documentation
• Record the type and amount of medication given on the patient's medication record.
• Record the time given and the location of the injection site. Note any skin reactions as well as any other adverse reactions.

Intramuscular injection

Intramuscular (I.M.) injections deposit medication deep into muscle tissue, which is well-vascularized and can absorb it quickly. This route of administration provides rapid systemic action and absorption of relatively large doses (up to 5 ml in appropriate sites). I.M. injections are recommended for patients who are uncooperative or can't take medication orally and for drugs that are altered by digestive juices. Because muscle tissue has few sensory nerves, I.M. injection allows less painful administration of irritating drugs.

The site for an I.M. injection must be chosen carefully, taking into account the patient's general physical status and the purpose of the injection. I.M. injections should not be administered at inflamed, edematous, or irritated sites, or at sites containing moles, birthmarks, scar tissue, or other lesions. I.M. injections may also be contraindicated in patients with impaired coagulation mechanisms and in patients with occlusive peripheral vascular disease, edema, and shock because these conditions impair peripheral absorption. I.M. injections require sterile technique to maintain the integrity of muscle tissue.

Oral or I.V. routes are preferred for administration of drugs that are poorly absorbed by muscle tissue, such as phenytoin, digoxin, chlordiazepoxide, diazepam, and haloperidol.

≫ Key nursing diagnoses and patient outcomes
Use these nursing diagnoses as a guide when developing your plan of care for a patient who's receiving I.M. injections.

Knowledge deficit related to lack of exposure
Based on this nursing diagnosis, you'll establish the following patient outcomes. The patient will:
• state or demonstrate understanding of what has been taught.
• demonstrate ability to perform new health-related behaviors as they are taught.

Risk for injury related to improper technique

Based on this nursing diagnosis, you'll establish the following patient outcomes. The patient will:
• identify factors that increase risk for injury.
• assist in identifying and applying safety measures to prevent injury.

Equipment

♦ patient's medication record and chart ♦ prescribed medication ♦ diluent or filter needle if needed ♦ 3- to 5-ml syringe ♦ 20G to 25G 1″ to 3″ needle ♦ gloves ♦ alcohol sponges.

The prescribed medication must be sterile. The needle may be packaged separately or already attached to the syringe. Needles used for I.M. injections are longer than subcutaneous needles *because they must reach deep into the muscle.* Needle length also depends on the injection site, the patient's size, and the amount of subcutaneous fat covering the muscle. The needle gauge for I.M. injections should be larger to accommodate viscous solutions and suspensions.

Equipment preparation

• Verify the order on the patient's medication record by checking it against the doctor's order. Also note if the patient has any allergies, especially before the first dose.
• Check the prescribed medication for color and clarity.
• Note the expiration date.
• Never use medication that's cloudy or discolored or that contains a precipitate unless the manufacturer's instructions allow it. Remember also that for some drugs (such as suspensions) the presence of drug particles

is normal. Observe for any abnormal changes. If in doubt, check with the pharmacist.
• Choose equipment appropriate to the prescribed medication and injection site, and make sure it works properly. The needle should be straight, smooth, and free of burrs.
• Wipe the stopper of the medication vial with an alcohol sponge, and then draw up the prescribed amount of medication using the three-label check system — read the label as you select the medication, as you draw up the medication, and after you have completed drawing up the medication *to verify the correct dosage.*
• Then draw about 0.2 cc of air into the syringe according to hospital policy. When the syringe is inverted during the injection, the air bubble rises to the plunger end of the syringe and follows the medication into the injection site. The air clears the needle of medication and helps prevent leakage into the subcutaneous tissue following injection by creating an air block that reduces reflux (tracking) along the needle path.
• Gather all necessary equipment, and proceed to the patient's room.

Implementation

• Confirm the patient's identity by asking his name and checking his wristband for name, room number, and bed number.
• Provide privacy and explain the procedure to the patient.
• Wash your hands.
• Select an appropriate injection site. The gluteal muscles (gluteus medius and minimus and the upper outer corner of the gluteus maximus) are used most commonly for healthy adults, al-

though the deltoid muscle may be used for a small-volume injection (2 ml or less). For infants and children, the vastus lateralis muscle of the thigh is used most often *because it's usually the best developed and contains no large nerves or blood vessels, minimizing the risk of serious injury.* The rectus femoris muscle may also be used in infants but is usually contraindicated in adults. Remember to always rotate injection sites for patients who require repeated injections.

• Position and drape the patient appropriately, making sure the site is well-exposed and that lighting is adequate.

• Loosen the protective needle sheath, but don't remove it.

• After selecting the injection site, gently tap it *to stimulate nerve endings and minimize pain when the needle is inserted.* (See *Locating intramuscular injection sites.*) Then clean the skin at the site with an alcohol sponge. Move the sponge outward in a circular motion to a circumference of about 2" (5 cm) from the injection site. Then allow the skin to dry *to avoid introducing alcohol into the needle puncture, which causes pain.* Keep the alcohol sponge for later use.

• Put on gloves. With the thumb and index finger of your nondominant hand, gently stretch the skin of the injection site taut.

• Holding the syringe in your dominant hand, remove the needle sheath by slipping it between the free fingers of your nondominant hand and then drawing back the syringe.

• Position the syringe at a 90-degree angle to the skin surface, with the needle a couple of inches from the skin. Tell the patient that he will feel a prick as you insert the needle. Then quickly

and firmly thrust the needle through the skin and subcutaneous tissue, deep into the muscle.

• Support the syringe with your nondominant hand, if desired. Pull back slightly on the plunger with your dominant hand to aspirate for blood. If no blood appears, place your thumb on the plunger rod and *slowly* inject the medication into the muscle. *A slow, steady injection rate allows the muscle to distend gradually and accept the medication under minimal pressure.* You should feel little or no resistance against the force of the injection. The air bubble in the syringe should follow the medication into the injection site.

Note. If blood appears in the syringe on aspiration, the needle is in a blood vessel. If this occurs, stop the injection, withdraw the needle, prepare another injection with new equipment, and inject another site. Don't inject the bloody solution.

• After the injection, gently but quickly remove the needle at a 90-degree angle.

• Using a gloved hand, cover the injection site immediately with the used alcohol sponge, apply gentle pressure, and unless contraindicated, massage the relaxed muscle *to help distribute the drug and promote absorption.*

• Remove the alcohol sponge and inspect the injection site for signs of active bleeding or bruising. If bleeding continues, apply pressure to the site; if bruising occurs, you may apply ice.

• Watch for adverse reactions at the site for 30 minutes after the injection.

• Discard all equipment according to universal precautions and your hospital's policy. Don't attempt to recap any needles; dispose of them in an

Locating intramuscular injection sites

Deltoid

First find the lower edge of the acromial process and the point on the lateral arm in line with the axilla. Insert the needle 1″ to 2″ (2.5 to 5 cm) below the acromial process, usually two to three fingerbreadths, at a 90-degree angle or angled slightly toward the process. Typical injection: 0.5 ml (range: 0.5 to 2 ml).

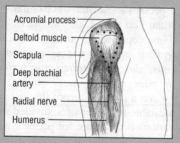

Acromial process
Deltoid muscle
Scapula
Deep brachial artery
Radial nerve
Humerus

Dorsogluteal

Inject above and outside a line drawn from the posterior superior iliac spine to the greater trochanter of the femur. Or divide the buttock into quadrants and inject in the upper outer quadrant, about 2″ to 3″ (5 to 7.6 cm) below the iliac crest. Insert the needle at a 90-degree angle. Typical injection: 1 to 4 ml (range: 1 to 5 ml).

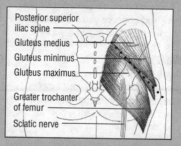

Posterior superior iliac spine
Gluteus medius
Gluteus minimus
Gluteus maximus
Greater trochanter of femur
Sciatic nerve

Ventrogluteal

First locate the greater trochanter of the femur with the heel of your hand. Then, spread your index and middle fingers from the anterior superior iliac spine to as far along the iliac crest as you can reach. Insert the needle between the two fingers at a 90-degree angle to the muscle. (Remove your hand before inserting the needle.) Typical injection: 1 to 4 ml (range: 1 to 5 ml).

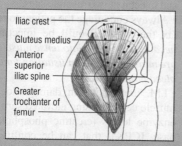

Iliac crest
Gluteus medius
Anterior superior iliac spine
Greater trochanter of femur

Vastus lateralis

Use the lateral muscle of the quadriceps group, from a handbreadth below the greater trochanter to a handbreadth above the knee. Insert the needle into the middle third of the muscle parallel to the surface on which the patient is lying. You may have to bunch the muscle before insertion. Typical injection: 1 to 4 ml (range: 1 to 5 ml; 1 to 3 ml for infants).

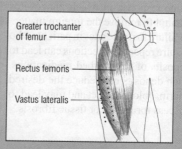

Greater trochanter of femur
Rectus femoris
Vastus lateralis

BETTER CHARTING

Documenting administration of narcotic drugs

Regulations require narcotic drugs to be counted after each nursing shift to ensure an accurate drug count. Before administering a narcotic, verify the amount of drug in the container, and sign out the medication on the appropriate form.

Another regulation requires that a second nurse document your activity and observe you if a narcotic of part of a dose must be wasted.

What to report

If you discover a discrepancy in the narcotic count, follow your employer's policy for reporting this. You'll need to file an incident report as well. An investigation will follow.

appropriate sharps container *to avoid needle-stick injuries.*

Complications

• Accidental injection of concentrated or irritating medications into subcutaneous tissue, or into other areas where it can't be fully absorbed, can cause sterile abscesses to develop. Such abscesses result from a natural immune response in which phagocytes attempt to remove the foreign matter.

• Failure to rotate sites in patients who require repeated injections can lead to deposits of unabsorbed medications. Such deposits can reduce the desired pharmacologic effect and may lead to abscess formation or tissue fibrosis.

Nursing considerations

• To slow absorption, some drugs for I.M. administration are dissolved in oil or other special solutions. Mix these preparations well before drawing them into the syringe.

• Never use the gluteal muscles (which develop from repeated walking) as the injection site for a child under age 3 or who has been walking for less than a year.

• Never inject into sensitive muscles, especially those that twitch or tremble when you assess site landmarks and tissue depth with your fingertips. *Injections in these trigger areas may cause sharp or referred pain such as the pain caused by nerve trauma.*

• Keep a rotation record that lists all available injection sites, divided into various body areas, for patients who require repeated injections. Rotate from a site in the first area to a site in each of the other areas. Then return to a site in the first area that is at least 1" (2.5 cm) away from the previous injection site in that area.

• If the patient has experienced pain or emotional trauma from repeated injections, consider numbing the area before cleaning it by holding ice on it for several seconds. If you must inject more than 5 ml of solution, divide the solution and inject it at two separate sites.

• Always encourage the patient to relax the muscle you'll be injecting *because injections into tense muscles are more painful than usual and may bleed more readily.*

• I.M. injections can damage local muscle cells, causing elevated serum enzyme levels (creatine phosphokinase, [CPK]) that can be confused with the elevated enzymes resulting from damage to cardiac muscle, as in myocardial infarction. To distinguish between skeletal and cardiac muscle damage, diagnostic tests for suspected myocardial infarction must identify the isoenzyme of CPK specific to cardiac muscle and include tests for lactate dehydrogenase and aspartate aminotransferase. If it's important to measure these enzyme levels, suggest that the doctor switch to I.V. administration, with dosages adjusted accordingly.

Documentation

• Chart the drug administered, dose, date, time, route of administration, and injection site.
• Note the patient's tolerance of injection and its effects, including any adverse effects.
• When you administer a narcotic, you must give the drug and document administration according to federal, state, and institutional regulations. (See *Documenting administration of narcotic drugs*.)

Intrapleural injection

An intrapleural drug is injected through the chest wall into the pleural space or instilled through a chest tube placed intrapleurally for drainage. Intrapleural administration provides superior chemotherapeutic effects, reduces drug toxicity, and maintains higher and longer-lasting pleural drug concentrations. Increasingly, doctors are using it to promote analgesia, treat spontaneous pneumothorax, resolve pleural effusions, and administer chemotherapy.

Intrapleurally administered drugs diffuse across the parietal pleura and innermost intercostal muscles to affect the intercostal nerves. During intrapleural injection of a drug, the needle passes through the intercostal muscles and parietal pleura on its way to the pleural space. The internal intercostal muscle is a key landmark for placement of the needle because it resists the advancing needle.

Drugs commonly given by intrapleural injection include tetracycline, streptokinase, anesthetics, and chemotherapeutic agents (to treat malignant pleural effusion or lung adenocarcinoma).

Contraindications for intrapleural administration include pleural fibrosis or adhesions, which interfere with diffusion of the drug to the intended site; pleural inflammation; sepsis; and infection at the puncture site. Patients with bullous emphysema and those receiving respiratory therapy using positive end-expiratory pressure also shouldn't have intrapleural injections because the injections may exacerbate an already compromised pulmonary condition.

≫ Key nursing diagnoses and patient outcomes

Use these nursing diagnoses as a guide when developing your plan of care for a patient who is being treated with intrapleural medication.

Knowledge deficit related to lack of exposure

Based on this nursing diagnosis, you'll establish the following patient outcomes. The patient will:
• state or demonstrate understanding of what has been taught.

• demonstrate ability to perform new health-related behaviors as they are taught.

Risk for injury related to improper technique

Based on this nursing diagnosis, you'll establish the following patient outcomes. The patient will:
• identify factors that increase risk for injury.
• assist in identifying and applying safety measures to prevent injury.

Equipment

An intrapleural drug is given through a #16 to #20 or #28 to #40 chest tube if the patient has empyema, pleural effusion, or pneumothorax. For any other patient, it is given through a 16G to 18G blunt-tipped intrapleural (epidural) needle and catheter. Accessory equipment depends on which type of access device the doctor uses. All equipment must be sterile.

For intrapleural catheter insertion: ♦ gloves ♦ gauze ♦ antiseptic solution such as povidone-iodine ♦ drape ♦ local anesthetic, such as 1% lidocaine ♦ 3-ml and 5-ml syringes with 22G 1″ and 25G ⅝″ needles ♦ 18G needle or scalpel ♦ 16G to 18G blunt-tipped intrapleural needle and catheter ♦ saline-lubricated glass syringe ♦ dressings ♦ sutures ♦ tape.

For chest tube insertion: ♦ towels ♦ gloves ♦ gauze ♦ antiseptic solution such as povidone-iodine ♦ 3- to 5-ml syringe ♦ anesthetic such as 1% lidocaine ♦ 18G needle or scalpel ♦ chest tube with or without trocar (#16 to #20 catheter for air or serous fluid, #28 to #40 for blood, pus, or thick fluid) ♦ two rubber-tipped clamps ♦ sutures ♦ drain dressings

♦ tape ♦ thoracic drainage system and tubing.

For drug administration: ♦ sterile gloves ♦ sterile gauze pads ♦ povidone-iodine solution ♦ ordered medication ♦ appropriate-sized needles and syringes ♦ 1% lidocaine if necessary ♦ dressings ♦ tape.

Patient preparation

• Explain the procedure to the patient *to allay his fears.*
• Encourage him to follow instructions.

Implementation

Go by the following steps to administer drugs intrapleurally.

Intrapleural catheter insertion

• The doctor inserts the intrapleural catheter at the patient's bedside, with the nurse assisting.
• Position the patient with the affected side up. The doctor will insert the catheter into the fourth to eighth intercostal space, 3″ to 4″ (7.5 to 10 cm) from the posterior midline. (See *Giving intrapleural drugs.*)
• The doctor puts on sterile gloves, cleans around the puncture site with antiseptic-soaked gauze, then covers the area with a sterile drape. Next, he fills the 3- to 5-ml syringe with local anesthetic and injects it into the patient's skin and deep tissues.
• The doctor punctures the skin with the 18G needle or scalpel, which helps the blunt-tipped intrapleural needle penetrate the skin over the superior edge of the lower rib in the chosen interspace. Keeping the bevel tilted upward, he directs the needle medially at a 30- to 40-degree angle to the skin. When the needle tip punctures the

Giving intrapleural drugs

In intrapleural administration, the doctor injects a drug into the pleural space using a catheter.

Help the patient lie on one side with the affected side up. The doctor inserts a needle into the fourth to eighth intercostal space, 3″ to 4″ (7.5 to 10 cm) from the posterior midline. He then advances the needle medially over the superior edge of the patient's rib through the intercostal muscles, until it tangentially penetrates the parietal pleura, as shown.

The catheter is advanced into the pleural space through the needle, which is then removed.

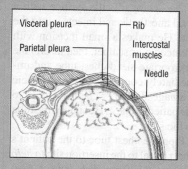

posterior intercostal membrane, he removes the stylet and attaches a saline-lubricated glass syringe containing 2 to 4 cc of air to the needle hub.

• During puncture, tell the patient to hold his breath (or momentarily disconnect him from mechanical ventilation) until the needle is removed. *This helps prevent the needle from injuring lung tissue.*

• The doctor advances the needle slowly, taking care not to apply pressure to the plunger. When the needle punctures the parietal pleura, negative intrapleural pressure moves the plunger outward. The doctor then removes the syringe from the needle and threads the intrapleural catheter through the needle until he has advanced it about 2″ (5 cm) into the pleural space. Without removing the catheter, he carefully withdraws the needle.

• Tell the patient he can breathe again (or reconnect mechanical ventilation).

• After inserting the catheter, the doctor coils it to prevent kinking, then sutures it securely to the patient's skin. He con-

firms placement by aspirating the catheter. Resistance indicates correct placement in the pleural space, aspirated blood means the catheter probably is misplaced in a blood vessel, and aspirated air means it's probably in a lung. The doctor will order a chest X-ray at this time to detect pneumothorax.

• Apply a sterile dressing over the insertion site to prevent catheter dislodgment. Take the patient's vital signs every 15 minutes for the first hour after the procedure, then as needed.

Chest tube insertion

• The doctor inserts the chest tube, assisted by the nurse.

• First, position the patient with the affected side up, and drape him with sterile towels.

• The doctor puts on gloves and cleans the appropriate site with gauze-soaked antiseptic solution. If the patient has a pneumothorax, the doctor uses the second intercostal space as the access site *because air rises to the top of the pleural space.* If the patient has a hemothorax or pleural effusion, the doctor uses the sixth to eighth intercostal space *because fluid settles to the bottom of the pleural space.*

• The doctor fills the syringe with a local anesthetic and injects it into the site. He makes a small incision with the needle or scalpel, then inserts the appropriate-sized chest tube and immediately connects it to the thoracic drainage system or clamps it close to the patient's chest. He sutures the tube to the skin.

• Tape the chest tube to the patient's chest distal to the insertion site *to help prevent accidental dislodgment.* Also tape the junction of the chest tube and drainage tube *to prevent their separation.* Apply sterile drain dressings, and tape them to the site.

• After insertion, the doctor checks tube placement with a chest X-ray. Take the patient's vital signs every 15 minutes for 1 hour, then as needed. Auscultate his lungs at least every 4 hours *to assess air exchange in the affected lung.* Diminished or absent breath sounds mean the lung hasn't reexpanded.

Drug administration

• The doctor injects medication through the intrapleural catheter or chest tube, with the nurse assisting.

• If the patient will receive chemotherapy, the doctor will probably ask you to give an antiemetic at least ½ hour beforehand.

• Position the patient with the affected side up. Help the doctor move the dressing away from the intrapleural catheter or chest tube and clamp the drainage tube if present.

• The doctor disinfects the access port of the catheter or chest tube with antiseptic-soaked gauze. Draw up the appropriate medication dose, and hand it to the doctor with the vial so he can verify the correct dose.

• The doctor injects the medication. If it's an anesthetic, he gives a bolus or loading dose initially, then changes to a continuous infusion. If it's tetracycline, he mixes it with an anesthetic such as lidocaine *to alleviate pain during injection.*

• Reapply the dressings around the catheter. Monitor the patient closely during and after drug administration *to gauge the effectiveness of drug therapy and to check for complications and adverse effects.*

Complications

• Pneumothorax or tension pneumothorax may occur if the doctor accidentally injects air into the pleural cavity. These complications are more likely in a patient who is on mechanical ventilation.

• Accidental catheter placement in the lung can lead to respiratory distress; catheter placement within a vessel can increase the medication's effects.

• With catheter fracture, lung puncture may occur.

• Laceration of intercostal vessels can cause bleeding.

• Local anesthetic toxicity can lead to tinnitus, metallic taste, light-headedness, somnolence, visual and auditory disturbances, restlessness, delirium, slurred speech, nystagmus, muscle tremor, seizures, arrhythmias, and cardiovascular collapse. A local anesthetic containing epinephrine can cause tachycardia and hypertension.

• Intrapleural chemotherapeutic drugs can irritate the pleura chemically and cause such systemic effects as neutropenia and thrombocytopenia. Administering intrapleural tetracycline without an anesthetic causes pain.
• The insertion site can become infected. However, meticulous skin preparation, strict aseptic technique, and sterile dressings usually prevent infection.

Nursing considerations

• Make sure the patient has signed a consent form.
• Before catheter insertion, ask the patient to urinate to reduce the risk of bladder perforation and promote comfort.
• If the patient is receiving a continuous infusion, label the solution bag clearly. Cover all injection ports so other drugs aren't injected into the pleural space accidentally.
• If the chest tube accidentally dislodges, cover the site at once with a sterile gauze pad, and tape it in place. Stay with the patient, monitor his vital signs, and observe carefully for signs and symptoms of tension pneumothorax: hypotension, distended neck veins, absent breath sounds, tracheal shift, hypoxemia, dyspnea, tachypnea, diaphoresis, chest pain, and weak, rapid pulse. Have another nurse call the doctor, and gather the equipment needed to reinsert the tube.
• Keep rubber-tipped clamps at the bedside. If a commercial chest-tube system cracks or a tube disconnects, use the clamps to clamp the chest tube close to the insertion site temporarily. However, be sure to observe the patient closely for signs of tension pneumothorax because no air can escape

from the pleural space while the tube is clamped.
• You can wrap a piece of petroleum gauze around the chest tube at the insertion site to make an airtight seal; then apply the sterile dressing. After the chest tube is removed, use the petroleum gauze to dress the wound; then cover it with a new piece of sterile gauze.
• After the catheter has been removed, inspect the skin at the entry site for signs of infection; then cover the wound with a sterile dressing.

Documentation

• Document the drug administered, drug dosage, the patient's response to the treatment, and the condition of the catheter insertion site.

Isolation precautions

The Guidelines for Isolation Precautions in Hospitals were developed by the Centers for Disease Control and Prevention (CDC) and the Hospital Infection Control Practices Advisory Committee (HICPAC). These guidelines contain two levels of precautions: Standard precautions and transmission-based precautions. Transmission-based precautions are divided into three types: airborne, droplet, and contact precautions.

Standard precautions are designed to decrease the risk of transmission of microorganisms from recognized and unrecognized sources of infection in hospitals. They should be followed at all times and with every patient.

Standard precautions combine the major features of the former "Universal Precautions," developed in response to the increasing incidence of immunodeficiency virus infections, hepatitis B virus infections, and other bloodborne diseases, as well as to "Body Substance Isolation," developed as a way of decreasing the risk of pathogen transmission from moist body surfaces. Because standard precautions reduce the risk of transmission of bloodborne and other pathogens, many patients with diseases or conditions that previously required category- or disease-specific isolation precautions now require only standard precautions.

Substances covered by standard precautions include blood and all other bodily fluids (even if blood is not visible), bodily secretions, and bodily excretions (excluding sweat). Standard precautions should also be followed in the presence of non-intact skin or exposed mucous membranes.

In addition to standard precautions, transmission-based precautions should be followed whenever a patient is known or suspected to be infected with a highly contagious and epidemiologically important pathogen transmitted by air or droplets or by contact with dry skin or other contaminated surfaces. Examples of such pathogens include those that cause measles (spread through the air), influenza, (spread through droplets) or GI, respiratory, skin, or wound infections (spread through contact).

Transmission-based precautions replace all older categories of isolation precautions including strict isolation, contact isolation, respiratory isolation, enteric precautions, drainage/secretion precautions, and most other disease-specific precautions. One or more types of transmission-based precau-

tions may be combined and followed when a patient has a disease that has multiple routes of transmission.

The CDC and HICPAC believe the foregoing precautions should end the confusion that often exists when implementing or interpreting the former guidelines.

≫ Key nursing diagnoses and patient outcomes

Use this nursing diagnosis as appropriate when developing plans of care.

Risk for infection related to hospital admission

Based on this nursing diagnosis, you'll establish the following patient outcomes. The patient will:
• remain free of all signs and symptoms of infection.
• state factors that put him at risk of infection.
• identify signs and symptoms of infection.

Equipment

♦ gloves ♦ masks ♦ face shields ♦ goggles ♦ glasses ♦ gowns ♦ resuscitation masks ♦ antimicrobial soap.

Patient preparation

• Explain the purpose of standard precautions, and, if applicable, transmission-based precautions to the patient and the family so they understand the need to prevent disease transmission. Also explain how these precautions are implemented.

Implementation

The following actions should be taken when implementing isolation precautions.

Standard precautions

• Wash your hands immediately if they become contaminated with blood or bodily fluids. Also wash your hands before and after patient care and after removing gloves.

• Wear gloves if you could come into contact with blood, tissues, bodily fluids, secretions, excretions, or contaminated surfaces or objects.

• Change your gloves between tasks and procedures on the same patient if you make contact with anything that might have a high concentration of microorganisms and between patient contacts, to avoid cross contamination.

• Wear a gown, eye protection (goggles, glasses), or face shield, and a mask during procedures likely to generate droplets of blood or body fluids, secretions, or excretions, such as surgery, endoscopic procedures, or dialysis.

• Carefully handle used patient care equipment soiled with blood, body fluids, secretions, or excretions to avoid exposure to skin and mucous membranes, clothing contaminations, and transfer of microorganisms to other patients and environments.

• Ensure that hospital procedures for routine care, cleaning, and disinfection of environmental surfaces, beds, bedrails, and bedside equipment are followed.

• Handle contaminated linens in a manner that prevents contamination and the transfer of microorganisms. Do not shake contaminated linens. Keep them away from your body. Place in properly labelled containers. Ensure that linens are transported and processed according to hospital policy.

• Handle used needles or other sharp implements carefully. Do not bend, break, reinsert them into their original sheaths, or unnecessarily handle them. Discard them intact immediately after use into an impervious disposal box. Those measures reduce the risk of accidental injury and infection.

• Use mouthpieces, resuscitation bags, or other ventilation devices in place of mouth-to-mouth resuscitation whenever possible.

• Place patients who cannot maintain appropriate hygiene or who contaminate the environment in a private room. Notify infection control personnel.

• If you have an exudative lesion, avoid all direct patient contact until the condition has resolved and you've been cleared by the employee health provider.

Airborne transmission-based precautions

In addition to standard precautions follow these precautions:

• Place the patient in a private room that has monitored negative air pressure in relation to surrounding areas. The room should have 6 to 12 air exchanges per hour and appropriate outdoor-air discharge or high-efficiency filtration of room-air. Keep the door closed and the patient in the room. If a private room is not available, place the patient in a room with a patient who has an active infection with the same microorganism. Consult with infection control personnel if a private room is not available.

• Wear respiratory protection (masks or face shields) when entering the room of a patient with a known or suspected respiratory infection. Persons immune to measles and varicella do not need to wear respiratory protection when entering the room of a patient with these illnesses.

• Limit patient transport and patient movement out of the room. If the patient must leave the room, have him wear a surgical mask, if possible.

Droplet transmission-based precautions

In addition to standard precautions, follow these precautions:
• Place the patient in a private room or, if one is not available, in a room with another patient who has an active infection with the same microorganisms. If this is not possible, consult infection control personnel. Special ventilation of the room is not necessary.
• Wear a mask when working within 3′ (1 m) of the patient.
• Keep visitors at least 3′ away from the infected patient.
• Limit movement of the patient from the room. If the patient needs to leave the room, have him wear a surgical mask, if possible.

Contact transmission-based precautions

In addition to standard precautions, follow these precautions:
• Place the patient in a private room or, if one is not available, in a room with another patient who has an active infection with the same microorganisms. If this is not possible, consult infection control personnel. Special ventilation of the room is not necessary.
• Wear gloves whenever you enter the room. Always change gloves after contact with infected material. Remove gloves before leaving the patient's room, and wash your hands immediately with an antimicrobial soap or a waterless antiseptic agent. Do not touch contaminated surfaces after washing your hands.
• Wear a gown when entering the patient's room if you think your clothing will have extensive contact with the patient, environmental surfaces, or items in the patient's room, or if the patient has diarrhea or is incontinent. Remove the gown before leaving the patient's room.
• Limit movement of the patient from the room.
• Avoid sharing patient-care equipment.

Complications

Failure to follow isolation precautions correctly may lead to exposure to disease and all of their attendant complications.

Nursing considerations

• Additional precautions, such as special respirators are necessary for preventing the transmission of tuberculosis.
• No special precautions are needed for dishes, glasses, or eating utensils because the hot water and detergents used in hospitals are able to decontaminate them.

Documentation

Record any special needs for standard or transmission-based precautions.

I.V. controller and pump use

Various types of controllers and pumps electronically regulate the flow of I.V. solutions or drugs with ex-

Regulating flow rate electronically

Controllers and infusion pumps, such as the two shown at right, electronically regulate the flow of I.V. solutions and drugs. You'll use them when a precise flow rate is required — for instance, when administering total parenteral nutrition solutions and chemotherapeutic or cardiovascular agents.

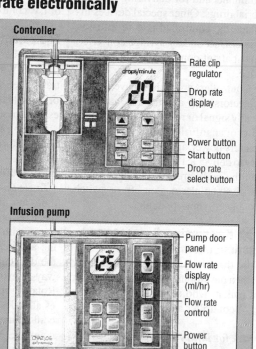

Controller

- Rate clip regulator
- Drop rate display
- Power button
- Start button
- Drop rate select button

Infusion pump

- Pump door panel
- Flow rate display (ml/hr)
- Flow rate control
- Power button

treme accuracy. (See *Regulating flow rate electronically*.)

Controllers regulate gravity flow by counting drops and achieve the desired infusion rate by compressing the I.V. tubing. However, because controllers simply count drops, which aren't always of equal size, these devices fail to achieve the accuracy of volumetric pumps, which measure flow rate in milliliters per hour.

• Volumetric pumps, used for high-pressure infusion of drugs or for highly accurate delivery of fluids or drugs, have mechanisms to propel the solution at the desired rate under pressure. (Pressure is brought to bear only when

gravity flow rates are insufficient to maintain preset infusion rates.) The peristaltic pump applies pressure to the I.V. tubing to force the solution through it. (Not all peristaltic pumps are volumetric; some count drops.) The piston-cylinder pump pushes the solution through special disposable cassettes. Most of these pumps operate at high pressures (up to 45 psi) and can deliver from 1 to 999 ml/hour with about 98% accuracy. (Some newer pumps operate at 10 to 25 psi.) The portable syringe pump, another type of volumetric pump, delivers very small amounts of fluid over a long period. It's used for administering fluids to infants and for delivering intra-arterial drugs. Other special devices include the controlled-release infusion system, secondary syringe converter, and patient-controlled analgesia device.

• Controllers and pumps have various detectors and alarms that automatically signal or respond to the completion of an infusion, air in the line, low battery power, and occlusion or inability to deliver at the set rate. Depending on the problem, these devices sound or flash an alarm, shut off, or switch to a keep-vein-open rate.

≫ Key nursing diagnoses and patient outcomes

Use these nursing diagnoses as a key when developing your plan of care for a patient who requires the use of an I.V. controller and pump.

Risk for injury related to I.V. therapy

Based on this nursing diagnosis, you'll establish these patient outcomes. The patient will:

• remain free from injury from I.V. therapy.

• show signs of fluid and electrolyte balance.

• show no signs of fluid volume excess or depletion from use of controllers and pumps.

• communicate the importance of not altering rates on controllers and pumps.

Knowledge deficit related to lack of exposure to I.V. control equipment

Based on this nursing diagnosis, you'll establish the following patient outcome. The patient will:

• communicate understanding of use of I.V. control equipment.

Equipment

♦ controller or peristaltic pump ♦ I.V. pole ♦ I.V. solution ♦ sterile administration set ♦ sterile peristaltic tubing or cassette if needed ♦ alcohol sponges ♦ adhesive tape.

Tubing and cassette vary with each manufacturer.

Equipment preparation

• *To set up a controller:* First, attach the controller to the I.V. pole. Then clean the port on the I.V. solution container with an alcohol sponge, insert the administration set spike, and fill the drip chamber no more than halfway to avoid miscounting the drops. Rotate the chamber so the fluid touches all sides to remove any vapor that could interfere with correct drop counting. Now, prime the tubing and close the clamp. Position the drop sensor above the fluid level in the drip chamber and below the drop port to ensure correct drop counting. Insert the peristaltic tubing into the controller, close the door, and open the flow clamp completely.

• *To set up a volumetric pump:* First, attach the pump to the I.V. pole. Then, swab the port on the I.V. container with alcohol, insert the administration set spike, and completely fill the drip chamber to prevent air bubbles from entering the tubing. Next, prime the tubing and close the clamp. Now, follow the manufacturer's instructions for placement of tubing.

Patient preparation

• Explain the need for controller or pump to the patient.

• Explain the importance of not tampering with equipment.

Implementation
• Position the controller or pump on the same side of the bed as the I.V. or anticipated venipuncture site *to avoid crisscrossing I.V. lines over the patient.* Perform the venipuncture, if necessary .
• Plug in the machine and attach its tubing to the needle or catheter hub. If you're using a controller, position the drip chamber 30″ (76.2 cm) above the infusion site *to ensure accurate gravity flow.*
• Depending on the machine, turn it on and press the start button. Set the appropriate dials on the front panel to the desired infusion rate and volume. Always set the volume dial at 50 ml less than the prescribed volume or 50 ml less than the volume in the container *so you can hang a new container before the old one empties completely.*
• Check the patency of the I.V. line, and watch for infiltration. If you're using a controller, monitor the accuracy of the infusion rate.
• Tape all connections and recheck the controller's drip rate because taping may alter it.
• Turn on the alarm switches. Then explain the alarm system to the patient *to prevent anxiety when a change in the infusion activates the alarm.*

Complications
• Complications associated with I.V. controllers and pumps are the same as those associated with peripheral lines.
• Keep in mind that infiltration can develop rapidly with infusion by a volumetric pump because the increased subcutaneous pressure won't slow the infusion rate until significant edema occurs.

Nursing considerations
• Monitor the pump or controller and the patient frequently to ensure the device's correct operation and flow rate and to detect infiltration and such complications as infection and air embolism.
• If electrical power fails, the pumps will automatically switch to battery power.
• Check the manufacturer's recommendations before administering opaque fluids such as blood because some pumps fail to detect opaque fluids and others may cause hemolysis of infused blood.
• Move the tubing in controllers every few hours *to prevent permanent compression or tubing damage.* Change the tubing and cassette every 48 hours or according to hospital policy.
• Remove I.V. solutions from the refrigerator 1 hour before infusing them to help release small gas bubbles from the solutions. Small bubbles in the solution can join to form larger bubbles, which can activate the pump's air-in-line alarm.

Home care
• Make sure the patient and his family understand the purpose of using the pump or controller.
• Demonstrate how the device works, if necessary.
• Demonstrate how to maintain the system (tubing, solution, and site assessment and care) until you're confident that the patient and family can proceed safely. Have the patient repeat the demonstration if time permits.
• Discuss which complications to watch for, such as infiltration, and re-

view what measures to take if complications occur.

• Schedule a teaching session with the patient or family so you can answer questions they may have about the procedure before the patient's discharge.

Documentation

• Besides routine documentation of the I.V. infusion, record the use of a controller or pump on the I.V. record and in your notes.

I.V. flow rate calculation and control

Calculated from a doctor's orders, flow rate is usually expressed as the total volume of I.V. solution infused over a prescribed interval or as the total volume given in milliliters per hour (ml/hr). Many devices can regulate the flow of I.V. solution, including clamps, controllers, the flow regulator (or rate minder), and the volumetric pump. (See *Using I.V. clamps.*)

When regulated by a clamp or controller, flow rate is usually measured in drops per minute, by a volumetric pump in milliliters per hour. The flow regulator can be set to deliver the desired amount of solution, also in milliliters per hour. Less accurate than infusion pumps or controllers, flow regulators are most reliable when used with inactive adult patients. With any device, flow rate can be easily monitored by using a time tape, which indicates the prescribed solution level at hourly intervals.

⟫ Key nursing diagnoses and patient outcomes

Use this nursing diagnosis as a guide when developing your plan of care for a patient who is receiving I.V. therapy.

Fluid volume deficit related to (specify)

Based on this nursing diagnosis, you'll establish the following patient outcomes. The patient will:
• maintain normal vital signs.
• maintain normal skin turgor and moist mucous membranes.
• maintain an adequate urine output.
• maintain normal electrolyte levels.

Equipment

♦ I.V. administration set with clamp ♦ 1″ paper or adhesive tape (or premarked time tape) ♦ infusion pump and controller (if infusing drugs) ♦ watch with second hand ♦ drip rate chart as necessary ♦ pen.

Standard macrodrip sets deliver 10 to 20 drops/ml, depending on the manufacturer; microdrip sets, 60 drops/ml; and blood transfusion sets, 10 drops/ml. A commercially available adapter can convert a macrodrip set to a microdrip system.

Patient preparation

• Observe the I.V. site for any signs of infiltration or phlebitis.

Implementation

• Flow rate requires close monitoring and correction because such factors as venous spasm, venous pressure changes, patient movement or manipulation of the clamp, and bent or kinked tubing can cause the rate to vary markedly.

To calculate and set the drip rate

• Follow the steps in *Calculating flow rates,* page 474, to determine the proper drip rate, or use your unit's chart.
• After calculating the desired drip rate, remove your watch and hold it next to the drip chamber of the I.V. administration set *to allow simultaneous observation of the watch and the drops.*
• Release the clamp to the approximate drip rate. Then count drops for 1 minute *to account for flow irregularities.*
• Adjust the clamp as necessary, and count drops for 1 minute. Continue to adjust the clamp and count drops until the correct rate is achieved.

To make a time tape

• Calculate the number of milliliters to be infused per hour. Place a piece of tape vertically on the container alongside the volume-increment markers.
• Starting at the current solution level, move down the number of milliliters to be infused in 1 hour, and mark the appropriate time and a horizontal line on the tape at this level. Then continue to mark 1 hour intervals until you reach the bottom of the container.
• Check the flow rate every 15 minutes until it's stable. Then recheck it every hour or according to hospital policy, and adjust as necessary.
• With each check, inspect the I.V. site for complications and assess the patient's response to therapy.

Complications

An excessively slow flow rate may cause insufficient intake of fluids, drugs, and nutrients. An excessively rapid rate of infusion may cause circulatory overload — possibly leading

Using I.V. clamps

With a roller clamp or screw clamp, you can increase or decrease flow through the I.V. line by turning a wheel or screw.

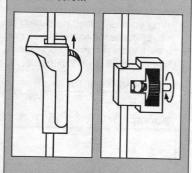

With a slide clamp, you can open or close the line by moving the clamp horizontally. However, you can't make fine adjustments to flow rate.

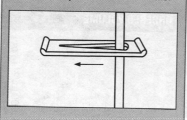

to congestive heart failure and pulmonary edema as well as drug side effects. (See *Managing I.V. flow rate deviations*, page 475.)

Nursing considerations

• If the infusion rate slows significantly, a slight rate increase may be necessary. If the rate must be increased by more than 30%, consult the doctor.
• When infusing drugs, use an I.V. pump or controller, if possible, to avoid flow rate inaccuracies.

(Text continues on page 476.)

Calculating flow rates

When calculating the flow rate of I.V. solutions, remember that the number of drops required to deliver 1 ml varies with the type and manufacturer of the administration set used. The illustration on the left shows a standard (macrodrip) set, which delivers from 10 to 20 drops/ml. The illustration in the center shows a pediatric (microdrip) set, which delivers about 60 drops/ml. The illustration on the right shows a blood transfusion set, which delivers about 10 drops/ml.

To calculate the flow rate, you must know the calibration of the drip rate for each manufacturer's product. As a quick guide, refer to the chart below. Use this formula to calculate specific drip rates:

$$\frac{\text{Volume of infusion (in ml)}}{\text{time of infusion (in minutes)}} \times \text{drip factor (in drops/ml)} = \text{drops/minute}$$

Macrodrip

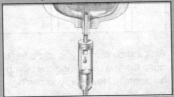

Microdrip

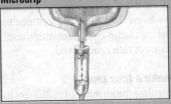

ORDERED VOLUME

ADMINISTRATION SET	DRIP FACTOR	DROPS/ MINUTE TO INFUSE					
		500 ml/24 hr or 21 ml/hr	1,000 ml/24 hr or 42 ml/hr	1,000 ml/20 hr or 50 ml/hr	1,000 ml/10 hr or 100 ml/hr	1,000 ml/8 hr or 125 ml/hr	1,000 ml 6 hr or 166 ml/hr
Macrodrip							
Abbott	15	5	10	12	25	31	42
Baxter Healthcare	10	3	7	8	17	21	28
Cutter	20	7	14	17	34	42	56
IVAC	20	7	14	17	34	42	56
McGaw	15	5	10	12	25	31	42
Microdrip							
Various manufacturers	60	21	42	50	100	125	166

PROBLEM SOLVER

Managing I.V. flow rate deviations

PROBLEM	CAUSE	INTERVENTION
Flow rate too fast	• Patient or visitor manipulates the clamp	• Instruct the patient not to touch the clamp, and place tape over it. Restrain the patient or administer the I.V. with an infusion pump or a controller if necessary.
	• Tubing disconnected from the catheter	• Wipe the distal end of the tubing with alcohol, reinsert firmly into the catheter hub, and tape at the connection site. Consider using tubing with luer connections.
	• Change in patient position	• Administer the I.V. with an infusion pump or a controller to ensure the correct flow rate.
	• Bevel against vein wall (positional cannulation)	• Manipulate the cannula, and place a $2'' \times 2''$ gauze pad under or over the catheter hub to change the angle. Reset the flow clamp at the desired rate. If necessary, remove the cannula and reinsert.
	• Flow clamp drifting as a result of patient movement	• Place tape below the clamp.
Flow rate too slow	• Venous spasm after insertion	• Apply warm soaks over site.
	• Venous obstruction from bending arm	• Secure with an arm board if necessary.
	• Pressure change (decreasing fluid in bottle causes solution to run slower due to decreasing pressure)	• Readjust the flow rate.
	• Elevated blood pressure	• Readjust the flow rate. Use an infusion pump or a controller to ensure correct flow rate.
	• Cold solution	• Allow the solution to warm to room temperature before hanging.
	• Change in solution viscosity from medication added	• Readjust the flow rate.

(continued)

Managing I.V. flow rate deviations (continued)

PROBLEM	CAUSE	INTERVENTION
Flow rate too slow (continued)	• I.V. container too low or patient's arm or leg too high	• Hang the container higher or remind the patient to keep his arm below heart level.
	• Bevel against vein wall (positional cannulation)	• Withdraw the needle slightly, or place a folded $2'' \times 2''$ gauze pad over or under the catheter hub to change the angle.
	• Excess tubing dangling below insertion site	• Replace the tubing with a shorter piece, or tape the excess tubing to the I.V. pole, below the flow clamp (make sure the tubing is not kinked).
	• Cannula too small	• Remove the cannula in use and insert a larger-bore cannula, or use an infusion pump.
	• Infiltration or clotted cannula	• Remove the cannula in use and reinsert a new cannula.
	• Kinked tubing	• Check the tubing over its entire length and unkink it.
	• Clogged filter	• Remove the filter and replace with a new one.
	• Tubing memory (tubing compressed at area clamped)	• Massage or milk the tubing by pinching and wrapping it around a pencil four or five times. Quickly pull the pencil out of the coiled tubing.

• Always use a pump or controller when infusing solutions through a central line.

• Large-volume solution containers have approximately 10% more fluid than the amount indicated on the bag *to allow for tubing purges.* Thus, a 1,000-ml bag or bottle will contain an additional 100 ml; similarly, a 500-ml container will hold an extra 50 ml and a 250-ml container, 25 ml.

Documentation

• Record the original flow rate when setting up a peripheral line.
• If you adjust the rate, record the change, the date and time, and your initials.

I.V. therapy preparation

Proper selection and preparation of equipment is essential to accurate delivery of an I.V. solution. Selection of an I.V. administration set depends on the rate and type of infusion desired and the type of I.V. solution container used. Two types of drip system are available: the macrodrip set and the microdrip set. The macrodrip set can deliver a solution in large quantities and at rapid rates because it delivers a larger amount of solution with each drop than the microdrip set. The microdrip set, used for pediatric and certain adult patients requiring small or closely regulated amounts of I.V. solution, delivers a smaller quantity of solution with each drop.

Administration tubing with a secondary injection port permits separate or simultaneous infusion of two solutions; tubing with a piggyback port and a back-check valve permits intermittent infusion of a secondary solution and, on its completion, a return to infusion of the primary solution. Vented I.V. tubing is selected for solutions in nonvented bottles, nonvented tubing for solutions in bags or vented bottles. Assembly of I.V. equipment requires aseptic technique to prevent contamination, which can cause local or systemic infection. (See *New dressing saves time*.)

≫ Key nursing diagnoses and patient outcomes

Use these nursing diagnoses as a guide when developing your plan of care for a patient who needs I.V. therapy.

Risk for infection related to I.V. therapy

Based on this nursing diagnosis, you'll establish the following patient outcomes. The patient will:
• maintain a normal body temperature.
• show no signs of infection at the I.V. site.
• take precautions to keep I.V. site dry.

Knowledge deficit related to lack of exposure to I.V. therapy

Based on this nursing diagnosis, you'll establish the following patient outcomes. The patient will:
• verbalize understanding of need for I.V. therapy.
• verbalize understanding of precautions and care of I.V. site.

TECHNOLOGY UPDATE

New dressing saves time

When you insert an I.V. line, you have multiple choices as you decide what dressing to use. Today, you may choose a dressing that not only covers the site but also aims to lower the chance of infection. The dressing includes a foam disk that sits around the catheter at the insertion site. It is able to absorb fluid and is also embedded with an antimicrobial agent. This is released continuously in order to reduce skin organisms.

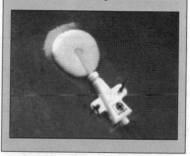

Equipment

♦ I.V. solution ♦ I.V. administration set ♦ in-line filter if needed ♦ I.V. pole ♦ alcohol sponges ♦ medication and label if necessary.

Equipment preparation

• Verify the type, volume, and expiration date of the I.V. solution.
• Discard any outdated solution.
• If the solution is contained in a glass bottle, inspect for chips or cracks; if it's in a plastic bag, squeeze to detect leaks.
• Examine the I.V. solution for particles, abnormal discoloration, and cloudiness. If present, discard the so-

lution and notify the pharmacy or dispensing department.
• If ordered, add medication to the solution, and place a completed medication-added label on the container.
• Remove the administration set from its box and observe for cracks, holes, and missing clamps.

Patient preparation
• Explain the need for I.V. therapy to the patient.

Implementation
• Wash your hands thoroughly *to prevent introducing contaminants during preparation.*
• Slide the flow clamp of the administration set tubing down to the drip chamber or injection port, and close the clamp.

Preparing a bag
• Place the bag on a flat, stable surface or hang it on an I.V. pole.
• Remove the protective cap or tear the tab from the tubing insertion port.
• Remove the protective cap from the administration set spike.
• Holding the port carefully and firmly with one hand, insert the spike with your other hand.

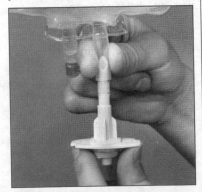

• Hang the bag on the I.V. pole if you haven't already, and squeeze the drip chamber until it's half full.

Preparing a nonvented bottle
• Remove the bottle's metal cap and inner disk if present.
• Place the bottle on a stable surface and wipe the rubber stopper with an alcohol sponge.
• Remove the protective cap from the administration set spike, and push the spike through the center of the bottle's rubber stopper. Avoid twisting or angling the spike *to prevent pieces of the stopper from breaking off and falling into the solution.*
• Invert the bottle. You'll hear a hissing sound and see air bubbles rise if its vacuum is intact (this may not occur if you've already added medication). If the vacuum isn't intact, discard the bottle and begin again.
• Hang the bottle on the I.V. pole and squeeze the drip chamber until it's half full.

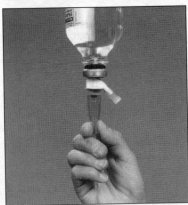

Preparing a vented bottle
• Remove the bottle's metal cap and latex diaphragm *to release the vacuum.* If the vacuum isn't intact (except

When to use an in-line filter

An in-line filter removes pathogens and particles from I.V. solutions, helping to reduce the risk of infusion phlebitis. But because in-line filters are expensive and their installation cumbersome and time-consuming, they're not routinely used. Many institutions require use of a filter only when administering an admixture. If you're unsure of whether to use a filter, check hospital policy or follow this list of do's and don'ts.

Do's

Use an in-line filter:
• when administering solutions to an immunodeficient patient.
• when administering total parenteral nutrition.
• when using additives comprising many separate particles such as antibiotics requiring reconstitution or when administering several additives.
• when using rubber injection sites or plastic diaphragms repeatedly.
• when phlebitis is likely to occur.

Be sure to change the in-line filter according to the manufacturer's recommendations (typically every 24 to 96 hours). *If you don't, bacteria trapped in the filter release endo-toxin, a pyrogen small enough to pass through the filter into the bloodstream.*

Use an add-on filter of larger pore size (1.2 microns) when infusing lipid emulsions and albumin mixed with nutritional solutions.

Don'ts

Don't use an in-line filter:
• when administering solutions with large particles *that will clog a filter and stop I.V. flow,* such as blood and its components, suspensions, lipid emulsions, and high-molecular-volume plasma expanders.
• when administering a drug dose of 5 mg or less *because the filter may absorb it.*

---

after medication has been added), discard the bottle and begin again.
• Place the bottle on a stable surface, and wipe the rubber stopper with an alcohol sponge.
• Remove the protective cap from the administration set spike, and push the spike through the insertion port next to the air vent tube opening.
• Hang the bottle on the I.V. pole, and squeeze the drip chamber until it's half full.

Priming the I.V. tubing

• If necessary, attach a filter to the opposite end of the I.V. tubing, and follow the manufacturer's instructions for filling and priming it. Purge the tubing before attaching the filter to avoid forcing air into the filter and possibly clogging some filter channels. Most filters are positioned with the distal end of the tubing facing upward so that the solution will completely wet the filter membrane and all air bubbles will be eliminated from the line. (See *When to use an in-line filter.*)
• If you're not using a filter, aim the distal end of the tubing over a wastebasket or sink and slowly open the flow clamp. (Most distal tube coverings allow the solution to flow without having to remove the protective cover.)

Teaching your patient about I.V. therapy

Many patients feel apprehensive about peripheral I.V. therapy; therefore, before you begin therapy, teach your patient what to expect before, during, and after the procedure. Thorough patient teaching can reduce anxiety, making therapy easier. Follow these guidelines.

Before insertion
• Describe the procedure. Tell him that "intravenous" means inside the vein and that a plastic catheter or needle will be placed in his vein. Explain that fluids containing certain nutrients or medications will flow from a bag or bottle, through a length of tubing, then through the plastic catheter or needle into his vein.

• Tell him approximately how long the catheter or needle will stay in place. Explain that the doctor will decide how much and what type of fluid the patient needs.

• If the patient will receive a local anesthetic at the insertion site, ask him if he's allergic to lidocaine. If in doubt, use another anesthetic. Tell him this will numb the site to reduce the pain of I.V. device insertion.

• If no anesthetic will be used, tell the patient that he may feel transient pain at the insertion site but that the discomfort will stop once the catheter or needle is in place.

• Tell him that I.V. fluid may feel cold at first but that this sensation should last only a few minutes.

During therapy
• Instruct the patient to report any discomfort after the catheter or needle has been inserted and the fluid has begun to flow.

• Explain any restrictions as ordered. As appropriate, tell the patient that he may be able to walk while receiving I.V. therapy and, depending on the insertion site and the device, he may also be able to shower or take a tub bath during therapy.

• Teach him how to care for the I.V. line. Tell him not to pull at the insertion site or tubing, not to remove the container from the I.V. pole, and not to kink the tubing or lie on it. Instruct him to call a nurse if the flow rate suddenly slows down or speeds up.

At removal
• Explain that removing a peripheral I.V. line is a simple procedure. Tell the patient that pressure will be applied to the site until the bleeding stops. Reassure him that once the device is out and the bleeding stops, he'll be able to use the affected arm or leg as before therapy.

• Leave the clamp open until I.V. solution flows through the entire length of tubing, forcing out all air.

• Invert all Y-injection sites and backcheck valves and tap them, if necessary, to fill them with solution.

• After priming the tubing, close the clamp. Then loop the tubing over the I.V. pole.

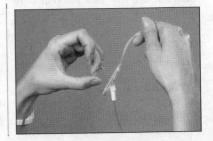

BETTER CHARTING

Documenting insertion of a venipuncture device

Once you establish an I.V. route, remember to document the date, time, and venipuncture site together with the equipment used, such as the type and gauge of catheter or needle. Record how the patient tolerated the procedure and any patient teaching that you performed with the patient and his family, such as explaining the purpose of I.V. therapy, describing the procedure itself, and discussing any possible complications.

You'll need to update your records each time you change the insertion site and change the venipuncture device or the I.V. tubing. Also document any reason for

1/6/97	0200	A #20 Fr. angiocath inserted in the anterior portion of the right hand. Good blood return noted. I.V. of 1000 ml D5½NSS with 20 mEq KCL running at 125 ml/hr. On Imed. I.V. tolerated well. Taught pt. about the need for I.V. therapy, its complications, and how to ambulate with I.V. Pt. stated that he understood. ———— Kathy Collins, RN

changing the I.V. site, such as extravasation, phlebitis, occlusion, patient removal, or routine change according to hospital policy.

• Label the container with the patient's name and room number, the date and time, the container number, the ordered rate and duration of infusion, and your initials.

Nursing considerations
• Before initiating I.V. therapy, the patient should be instructed in what to expect. (See *Teaching your patient about I.V. therapy.*)
• Always use aseptic technique when preparing I.V. solutions. If you contaminate the administration set or container, replace it with a new one to prevent introducing contaminants into the system.
• If necessary, you can use vented tubing with a vented bottle. To do this, don't remove the latex diaphragm. In-

stead, insert the spike into the larger indentation in the diaphragm.
• Change I.V. tubing every 48 or 72 hours according to hospital policy or more frequently if you suspect contamination. Change the filter according to manufacturer's recommendations or sooner if it becomes clogged.

Documentation
• Document the type of solution used and any additives to the solution. (See *Documenting insertion of a venipuncture device.*)

J

Jugular vein inspection

Inspecting the right jugular venous pulse can provide information about the dynamics of the right side of the heart. Distention of jugular veins can also be used to obtain a rough estimate of central venous pressure (CVP).

≫ Key nursing diagnoses and patient outcomes

Use these nursing diagnoses as a guide when developing your plan of care for a patient who needs jugular vein inspection.

Knowledge deficit related to lack of exposure to assessment techniques
Based on this nursing diagnosis, you'll establish the following patient outcomes. The patient will:
• communicate a need to know about techniques used to develop plan of care.
• verbalize an understanding of what is taught.

Anxiety related to techniques used during assessment
Based on this nursing diagnosis, you'll establish the following patient outcomes. The patient will:
• verbalize feelings of anxiety during assessment.
• remain calm during assessment.
• use relaxation techniques during assessment when appropriate.

Equipment

♦ stethoscope ♦ light source ♦ centimeter ruler ♦ warm, quiet, private setting with adequate lighting.

Patient preparation

• Explain the procedure.

Implementation

• Wash your hands.
• Begin by observing the jugular veins to detect distention. Assist the patient into semi-Fowler's position. Turn his head slightly away from the side you're examining. Angle the light source (a penlight, for example) to cast shadows along the neck. (The shadows will help you see pulse wave motion.) Measure the level of distention in fingerbreadths above the clavicle.
• With the patient in the same position, estimate central venous pressure. Begin by palpating the clavicles where they join the sternum (the suprasternal notch). Place your fingers here and slide them down the sternum until you feel a bony protuberance, known as the angle of Louis (or the sternal angle). Place a centimeter ruler vertically (perpendicular to the chest) at this angle. From the ruler, extend a sturdy square-cornered piece of paper horizontally along the highest level of venous pulsation. Normally, venous pressure is seen below the angle of Louis or less than 1.6″ (4 cm) above it. A total distance that exceeds 4″ (10 cm) may indicate elevated CVP and right-sided heart failure.

Nursing considerations

• You'll see jugular vein distention only if the patient has right-sided heart dysfunction.

• Focus on areas related to the patient's chief complaint.

• Use your eyes, ears, and sense of smell to observe the patient.

• Note any unusual findings as well as predictable ones.

Documentation

• Document normal and abnormal findings.

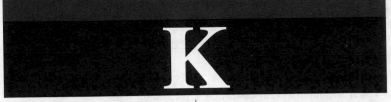

Kidney and bladder palpation

Palpation of the kidneys and bladder can help detect any lumps, masses, or tenderness. Abnormal kidney palpation findings may signify various problems. A lump, a mass, or tenderness may indicate a tumor or cyst. A soft kidney may reflect chronic renal disease; a tender kidney, acute infection. Unequal kidney size may reflect hydronephrosis, a cyst, a tumor, or another disorder. Bilateral enlargement suggests polycystic kidney disease.

Abnormal bladder palpation findings include a lump or a mass, possibly signaling a tumor or a cyst, or tenderness, which may stem from infection.

➤➤ Key nursing diagnoses and patient outcomes

Use these nursing diagnoses as a guide when developing your plan of care.

Knowledge deficit related to lack of exposure to assessment techniques

Based on this nursing diagnosis, you'll establish the following patient outcomes. The patient will:
• communicate a need to know about techniques used to develop plan of care.
• verbalize an understanding of what is taught.

Anxiety related to techniques used during assessment

Based on this nursing diagnosis, you'll establish the following patient outcomes. The patient will:

• verbalize feelings of anxiety during assessment.
• remain calm during assessment.
• utilize relaxation techniques during assessment when appropriate.

Equipment
♦ flashlight or gooseneck lamp.

Patient preparation
• Explain the procedure to the patient and assure his privacy.
• Have the patient lie in a supine position.
• Tell the patient what to expect such as occasional discomfort as pressure is applied.
• Encourage the patient to relax because muscle tension or guarding can interfere with performance and results of palpation.

Implementation
To achieve optimal results, have the patient relax his abdomen by taking deep breaths through his mouth. (See *Palpating the urinary organs*.)

Nursing considerations
• Avoid palpating an area known to be tender at the start of your examination. Instead, work around the area; then gently palpate it at the end of the examination. This progression will minimize your patient's discomfort and apprehension.

If you can't palpate because the patient fears pain, try distracting him with conversation.

Documentation
• Document any normal and abnormal findings.

Palpating the urinary organs

In the normal adult, the kidneys usually can't be palpated because of their location deep within the abdomen. However, they may be palpable in a thin patient or in one with reduced abdominal muscle mass. (Because the right kidney is slightly lower than the left, it may be easier to palpate.) Keep in mind that both kidneys descend with deep inhalation.

The bladder normally feels firm and relatively smooth. However, keep in mind that an adult's bladder may not be palpable.

Using bimanual palpation, begin on the patient's right side and proceed as follows.

Kidney palpation

1. Help the patient to a supine position, and expose the abdomen from the xiphoid process to the symphysis pubis. Standing at the right side, place your left hand under the back, midway between the lower costal margin and the iliac crest.

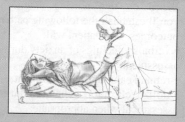

2. Next, place your right hand on the patient's abdomen, directly above your left hand. Angle this hand slightly toward the costal margin. To palpate the right lower edge of the right kidney, press your right fingertips about 1½″ (4 cm) above the right iliac crest at the midinguinal line; press your left fingertips upward into the right costovertebral angle.

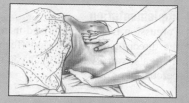

3. Instruct the patient to inhale deeply so that the lower portion of the right kidney can move down between your hands. If it does, note the shape and size of the kidney. Normally, it feels smooth, solid, and firm, yet elastic. Ask the patient if palpation causes tenderness. (*Note:* Avoid using excessive pressure to palpate the kidney because this may cause intense pain.)

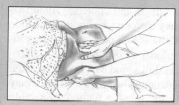

4. To assess the left kidney, move to the patient's left side and position your hands as described above, but with this change: Place your right hand 2″ (5 cm) above the left iliac crest. Then apply pressure with both hands as the patient inhales. If the left kidney can be palpated, compare it with the right kidney; it should be the same size.

Bladder palpation

Before palpating the bladder, make sure the patient has voided. Then locate the edge of the bladder by

(continued)

Palpating the urinary organs (continued)

pressing deeply in the midline about 1″ to 2″ (2.5 to 5 cm) above the symphysis pubis. As the bladder is palpated, note its size and location and check for lumps, masses, and tenderness. The bladder normally feels firm and relatively smooth. During deep palpation, the patient may report the urge to urinate — a normal response.

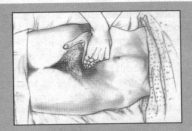

Kidney and bladder percussion

Percussion of the kidneys is done to detect any tenderness or pain. Percussion of the bladder is done to evaluate its position and contents. Abnormal kidney percussion findings include tenderness and pain, suggesting glomerulonephritis or glomerulonephrosis. A dull sound heard on percussion in a patient who has just urinated may indicate urine retention, reflecting bladder dysfunction or infection.

≫ Key nursing diagnoses and patient outcomes
Use these nursing diagnoses as a guide when developing your plan of care.

Knowledge deficit related to lack of exposure to assessment techniques
Based on this nursing diagnosis, you'll establish the following patient outcomes. The patient will:
• communicate a need to know about techniques used to develop plan of care.

• verbalize an understanding of what is taught.

Anxiety related to techniques used during assessment
Based on this nursing diagnosis, you'll establish the following patient outcomes. The patient will:
• verbalize feelings of anxiety during assessment.
• remain calm during assessment.
• utilize relaxation techniques during assessment when appropriate.

Equipment
♦ flashlight or gooseneck lamp.

Patient preparation
• Explain the procedure to the patient and tell him what to expect.
• Maintain patient privacy.
• Before percussing the bladder, have the patient urinate.

Implementation
Percussion may be performed using the direct or indirect method. Technique also varies with the organ you're percussing.

Percussing the urinary organs

Percuss the kidneys and bladder using these techniques.

Kidney percussion

With the patient sitting upright, percuss each costovertebral angle (the angle over each kidney whose borders are formed by the lateral and downward curve of the lowest rib and the vertebral column). To perform mediate percussion, place your left palm over the costovertebral angle, and gently strike it with your right fist. To perform immediate percussion, gently strike your fist over each costovertebral angle. Normally, the patient will feel a thudding sensation or pressure during percussion.

Bladder percussion

Using mediate percussion, percuss the area over the bladder, beginning 2″ (5 cm) above the symphysis pubis. To detect differences in sound, percuss toward the bladder's base. Percussion normally produces a tympanic sound. (Over a urine-filled bladder, it produces a dull sound.)

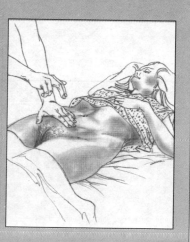

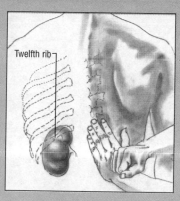

Twelfth rib

Indirect percussion

• To percuss the kidneys using the indirect fist method, have the patient sit up.

• Place the ball of one hand over the costovertebral angle, and strike it with the ulnar surface of your other fist.

• Use just enough force to cause a painless, but perceptible thud.

Direct percussion

• To use the direct method, strike the costovertebral angle directly with your fist, without putting your other hand down first.

• Be sure to percuss both sides of the body to assess both kidneys.

Percussing the bladder

• To percuss the bladder, tell the patient to lie in a supine position. Begin about 2″ (5 cm) above the symphysis pubis and percuss toward and over the bladder.

• You should hear tympany over the bladder. (See *Percussing the urinary organs,* page 487.)

Nursing considerations

• Avoid percussing kidneys or bladder known to be tender at the start of your examination. Instead, work around the area; then gently percuss it at the end of the examination.

Documentation

• Document normal and abnormal findings.

L

Lipid emulsion administration

Typically given as a separate solution in conjunction with total parenteral nutrition, lipid emulsions are a source of calories and essential fatty acids. A deficiency in essential fatty acids can hinder wound healing, adversely affect production of red blood cells, and impair prostaglandin synthesis.

Although lipid emulsions are usually given in conjunction with parenteral nutrition solution, they may also be given alone. You may administer them through either a peripheral or central venous line.

Lipid emulsions must be used cautiously in patients who have liver disease, pulmonary disease, anemia, or coagulation disorders and in those who are at risk for developing a fat embolism. Their use is contraindicated in patients who have a condition that disrupts normal fat metabolism (such as pathologic hyperlipidemia, lipid nephrosis, and acute pancreatitis).

≫ Key nursing diagnoses and patient outcomes

Use these nursing diagnoses as a guide when developing your plan of care for a patient who is receiving lipid emulsions.

Altered nutrition: less than body requirements related to (specify)

Based on this nursing diagnosis, you'll establish the following patient outcomes. The patient will:

- show no evidence of weight loss.
- gain (specify) lb (kg) weekly.
- tolerate lipid emulsion infusion without adverse effects.

Knowledge deficit related to lack of exposure to the administration of lipid emulsions

Based on this nursing diagnosis, you'll establish the following patient outcomes. The patient will:

- express an interest in learning treatment regimen.
- communicate understanding of special dietary needs.

Equipment

♦ I.V. administration set with vented spike (a separate adapter may be used if an administration set with vented spike isn't available) ♦ access pin with reflux valve ♦ tape ♦ time tape ♦ alcohol sponges.

If administering the lipid emulsion as part of a 3-in-1 solution, also obtain a filter that's 1.2 microns or greater because lipids will clog a smaller filter.

Equipment preparation

- Inspect the lipid emulsion for opacity and for consistency of color and texture. If the emulsion looks frothy or oily or contains particles, or if you think its stability or sterility is questionable, return the bottle to the pharmacy.
- To prevent aggregation of fat globules, don't shake the lipid container excessively.
- Protect the emulsion from freezing, and never add anything to it.

• Make sure you have the correct lipid emulsion, and verify the doctor's order and the patient's name.

Patient preparation

• Explain the procedure to the patient *to promote his cooperation.*

Implementation

Follow these steps to administer lipid emulsions.

To connect the tubing

• First, connect the I.V. tubing to the access pin. Access pins with reflux valves take the place of needles when connecting piggyback tubing to primary tubing.

• Close the flow clamp on the I.V. tubing. If the tubing doesn't contain luer-lock connections, tape all connections securely *to prevent accidental separation, which can lead to air embolism, exsanguination, or sepsis.*

• Using aseptic technique, remove the protective cap from the lipid emulsion bottle, and wipe the rubber stopper with an alcohol sponge.

• Hold the bottle upright and, using strict aseptic technique, insert the vented spike through the inner circle of the rubber stopper.

• Invert the bottle, and squeeze the drip chamber until it fills to the level indicated in the tubing package instructions.

• Open the flow clamp and prime the tubing. Gently tap the tubing *to dislodge air bubbles trapped in the Y-ports.* If necessary, attach a time tape to the lipid emulsion container *to allow accurate measurement of fluid intake.*

• Label the tubing, noting the date and time the tubing was hung.

To start the infusion

• If this is the patient's first lipid infusion, administer a test dose at the rate of 1 ml/minute for 30 minutes.

• Monitor the patient's vital signs, and watch for signs and symptoms of an adverse reaction, such as fever; flushing, sweating, or chills; a pressure sensation over the eyes; nausea; vomiting; headache; chest and back pain; tachycardia; dyspnea; and cyanosis. An allergic reaction is usually due either to the source of lipids or to eggs, which occur in the emulsion as egg phospholipids, an emulsifying agent.

• If the patient has no adverse reactions to the test dose, begin the infusion at the prescribed rate. Use an infusion pump if you'll be infusing the lipids at less than 20 ml/hour. The maximum infusion rate is 125 ml/hour for a 10% lipid emulsion and 60 ml/hour for a 20% lipid emulsion.

Complications

• Immediate or early adverse reactions to lipid emulsion therapy, which occur in fewer than 1% of patients, include fever, dyspnea, cyanosis, nausea and vomiting, headache, flushing, diaphoresis, lethargy, syncope, chest and back pain, slight pressure over the eyes, irritation at the infusion site, hyperlipidemia, hypercoagulability, and thrombocytopenia. Thrombocytopenia has been reported in infants receiving a 20% I.V. lipid emulsion.

• Delayed but uncommon complications associated with prolonged administration of lipid emulsion include hepatomegaly, splenomegaly, jaundice secondary to central lobular cholestasis, and blood dyscrasias (such as thrombocytopenia, leukopenia, and transient increases in liver function studies).

• Dry or scaly skin, thinning hair, abnormal liver function studies, and thrombocytopenia may indicate a deficiency of essential fatty acids.

• For unknown reasons, some patients develop brown pigmentation in the reticuloendothelial system.

• In premature or low-birth-weight infants, peripheral parenteral nutrition with a lipid emulsion may cause lipids to accumulate in the infants' lungs.

• Report any adverse reactions to the patient's doctor so that he can change the parenteral nutrition regimen as needed.

Nursing considerations

• Always maintain strict aseptic technique while preparing and handling equipment.

• Observe the patient's reaction to the lipid emulsion. Most patients report a feeling of satiety; some complain of an unpleasant metallic taste.

• Change the I.V. tubing and the lipid emulsion container every 24 hours.

• Monitor the patient for hair or skin changes. Also, closely monitor his lipid tolerance rate. Cloudy plasma in a centrifuged sample of citrated blood indicates that the lipids haven't been cleared from the patient's bloodstream.

• A lipid emulsion may clear from the blood at an accelerated rate in patients with full-thickness burns, multiple traumatic injuries, or a metabolic imbalance. This is because catecholamines, adrenocortical hormones, thyroxine, and growth hormone enhance lipolysis and embolization of fatty acids.

• Obtain weekly laboratory tests as ordered. Usual tests include liver function studies, prothrombin time, platelet count, and serum triglyceride levels. Whenever possible, draw blood for triglyceride levels at least 6 hours after the completion of the lipid emulsion infusion *to avoid false-high results.*

• A lipid emulsion is an excellent medium for bacterial growth. Therefore, never rehang a partially empty bottle of emulsion.

Documentation

• Record the times of all dressing changes and solution changes, the condition of the catheter insertion site, your observations of the patient's condition, and any complications and resulting treatments.

Liver biopsy, percutaneous

Percutaneous biopsy of the liver is the needle aspiration of a core of tissue for histologic analysis. This procedure is performed under a local or general anesthetic. Findings may help to identify hepatic disorders after ultrasonography, computerized tomography, and radionuclide studies have failed to detect them. The normal liver consists of sheets of hepatocytes supported by a reticulin framework.

Examination of the hepatic tissue may reveal diffuse hepatic disease, such as cirrhosis or hepatitis, or granulomatous infections such as tuberculosis. Primary malignant tumors include hepatocellular carcinoma, cholangiocellular carcinoma, and angiosarcoma, but hepatic metastasis is more common.

Nonmalignant findings with a known focal lesion require further studies, such as laparotomy or laparoscopy with biopsy.

» Key nursing diagnoses and patient outcomes

Use these nursing diagnoses as a guide when developing your plan of care for a patient who needs liver biopsy.

Fear related to unknown results
Based on this nursing diagnosis, you'll establish the following patient outcomes. The patient will:
• communicate his feelings of fear.
• use available support systems to help with coping.
• demonstrate relaxation techniques to help with fear and to cope better.

Knowledge deficit related to lack of exposure to procedure
Based on this nursing diagnosis, you'll establish the following patient outcomes. The patient will:
• communicate a need to know and become involved with care.
• verbalize reason for diagnostic test and what to expect during procedure.

Risk for injury related to invasive procedure
Based on this nursing diagnosis, you'll establish the following patient outcomes. The patient will:
• show no signs or symptoms of bleeding from biopsy.
• have normal vital signs during and after procedure.
• communicate reasons to notify nurse or doctor.

Equipment
♦ Local anesthetic (usually 1% or 2% lidocaine) ♦ Menghini needle ♦ 5-ml syringe ♦ sterile normal saline solution for injection ♦ sterile specimen container with 10% formalin solution ♦ labels ♦ sterile 4″ × 4″ gauze pads ♦ tape ♦ small pillow or sandbag.

Patient preparation
• Explain to the patient that this test is used to diagnose liver disorders.
• Describe the procedure to the patient, and answer any questions.
• Instruct the patient to restrict food and fluids for 4 to 8 hours before the test.
• Tell him who will perform the biopsy and where; that the biopsy needle remains in the liver about 1 second; that the entire procedure takes about 10 to 15 minutes; and that test results are usually available in 1 day.
• Make sure the patient or an appropriate family member has signed a consent form.
• Check patient history for hypersensitivity to the local anesthetic.
• Make sure prothrombin time and platelet count tests have been performed and that the results are recorded on the patient's chart.
• Just before the biopsy, tell the patient to void; then, record vital signs.
• Inform him that he will receive a local anesthetic but may experience pain similar to that of a punch in his right shoulder as the biopsy needle passes the phrenic nerve.

Implementation
• For aspiration biopsy using the Menghini needle, place the patient in a supine position, with his right hand under his head. Instruct him to main-

tain this position and remain as still as possible during the procedure.
• The liver is palpated, the biopsy site is selected and marked, and the anesthetic is then injected.
• The needle flange is set to control the depth of penetration, and 2 ml of sterile normal saline solution are drawn into the syringe.
• The syringe is attached to the biopsy needle, and the needle is introduced into the subcutaneous tissue, through the right eighth or ninth intercostal space, between the anterior and posterior axillary lines.
• Next, 1 ml of normal saline solution is injected to clear the needle and the plunger; then the plunger is drawn back to the 4-ml mark to create negative pressure.
• At this point in the procedure, ask the patient to take a deep breath, exhale, and hold his breath at the end of expiration to prevent any movement of the chest wall.
• As the patient holds his breath, the biopsy needle is quickly inserted into the liver and withdrawn in 1 second.
• After the needle is withdrawn, tell the patient to resume normal respirations.
• The tissue specimen is then placed in a properly labeled specimen cup containing 10% formalin solution.
• Again, 1 ml of normal saline solution is injected to clear the needle of the tissue specimen.
• Apply pressure to the biopsy site to stop bleeding.
• Position the patient on his right side for 2 hours, with a small pillow or sandbag under the costal margin to provide extra pressure. Advise bed rest for 24 hours.

• Check the patient's vital signs every 15 minutes for 1 hour, then every 30 minutes for 4 hours, and every 4 hours thereafter for 24 hours. Throughout, observe carefully for signs of shock.
• If the patient experiences pain, which may persist for several hours after the test, administer an analgesic.
• Inform the patient that he may resume his normal diet.

Complications
• Immediately report bleeding or signs of bile peritonitis: tenderness and rigidity around the biopsy site.
• Be alert for symptoms of pneumothorax: rising respiration rate, depressed breath sounds, dyspnea, persistent shoulder pain, and pleuritic chest pain. Report such complications promptly.

Nursing considerations
• Because many patients with hepatic disorders have clotting defects, testing for hemostasis should precede liver biopsy.
• Percutaneous liver biopsy is contraindicated in a patient with a platelet count below 100,000/mm³; prothrombin time longer than 15 seconds; empyema of the lungs, pleurae, peritoneum, biliary tract, or liver; vascular tumor; hepatic angiomas; hydatid cyst; or tense ascites. If extrahepatic obstruction is suspected, ultrasonography or subcutaneous transhepatic cholangiography should rule out this condition before the biopsy is considered.
• Send the specimen to the laboratory immediately.

Documentation
• Document the time, date, and the patient's tolerance of the procedure.
• Document the presence of any postprocedure complications and your nursing interventions.

Lumbar puncture

This procedure involves insertion of a sterile needle into the subarachnoid space of the spinal canal, usually between the third and fourth lumbar vertebrae. The procedure may be performed for several reasons: to detect increased intracranial pressure (ICP) or the presence of blood in cerebrospinal fluid (CSF), which indicates cerebral hemorrhage; to obtain CSF specimens for laboratory analysis; or to inject dyes or gases for contrast in radiologic studies of the brain and spinal cord. Lumbar puncture is also used therapeutically to administer drugs or anesthetics and to relieve ICP by removing CSF.

Performed by a doctor with a nurse assisting, lumbar puncture requires sterile technique and careful patient positioning. This procedure is contraindicated in patients with lumbar deformity or infection at the puncture site. It should be performed cautiously in patients with increased ICP because the rapid reduction in pressure that follows withdrawal of fluid can cause tonsillar herniation and medullary compression.

≫ Key nursing diagnoses and patient outcomes
Use these nursing diagnoses as a guide when developing your plan of care for a patient who needs lumbar puncture.

Anxiety related to lack of exposure to procedure
Based on this nursing diagnosis, you'll establish the following patient outcomes. The patient will:
• verbalize feelings of anxiety.
• use support systems to assist with coping.
• perform stress-reduction techniques to avoid anxiety symptoms.
• demonstrate abated physical symptoms of anxiety.

Pain related to adverse effect of procedure
Based on this nursing diagnosis, you'll establish the following patient outcomes. The patient will:
• maintain flat position for 8 to 12 hours after procedure.
• identify pain characteristics if present.
• express a feeling of comfort and relief from pain.

Equipment
♦ overbed table ♦ one or two pairs of sterile gloves for the doctor ♦ sterile gloves for the nurse ♦ povidone-iodine solution ♦ sterile gauze pads ♦ alcohol sponges ♦ sterile fenestrated drape ♦ 3-ml syringe for local anesthetic ♦ 25G ¾″ sterile needle for injecting anesthetic ♦ local anesthetic (usually 1% lidocaine) ♦ 18G or 20G 3 ½″ spinal needle with stylet (22G needle for children) ♦ three-way stopcock ♦ manometer ♦ small adhesive bandage ♦ three sterile collection tubes with stoppers ♦ laboratory request forms ♦ labels ♦ light source such as a gooseneck lamp.

Disposable lumbar puncture trays containing most of the needed sterile equipment are generally available.

Patient preparation

- Explain the procedure to the patient *to ease his anxiety and ensure cooperation.*
- Make sure a consent form has been signed.
- Inform the patient that he may experience headache after lumbar puncture, but reassure him that his cooperation during the procedure minimizes such an effect.
- Immediately before the procedure, provide privacy and instruct the patient to void.

Implementation

- Wash your hands thoroughly.
- Open the equipment tray on an overbed table, being careful not to contaminate the sterile field when you open the wrapper.
- Provide adequate lighting at the puncture site, and adjust the height of the patient's bed *to allow the doctor to perform the procedure comfortably.*
- Position the patient (see *Positioning for lumbar puncture*) and reemphasize the importance of remaining as still as possible *to minimize discomfort and trauma.*
- The doctor cleans the puncture site with sterile gauze pads soaked in povidone-iodine solution, wiping in a circular motion away from the puncture site; he uses three different pads *to prevent contamination of spinal tissues by the body's normal skin flora.* After allowing the skin to dry, he may wipe the area in a similar manner with alcohol sponges *to improve his view of the puncture site.* Next, he drapes the area with the fenestrated drape *to provide a sterile field.* (If the doctor uses povidone-iodine sponges instead of sterile gauze pads, he may remove

Positioning for lumbar puncture

Have the patient lie on his side at the edge of the bed, with his chin tucked to his chest and his knees drawn up to his abdomen. Make sure the patient's spine is curved and his back is at the edge of the bed, as shown here. This position widens the spaces between the vertebrae, easing insertion of the needle.

To help the patient maintain this position, place one of your hands behind his neck and the other hand behind his knees, and pull gently. Hold the patient firmly in this position throughout the procedure to prevent accidental needle displacement.

Patient positioning

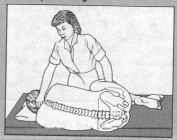

Typically, the doctor inserts the needle between the third and fourth lumbar vertebrae, as shown below.

Needle insertion

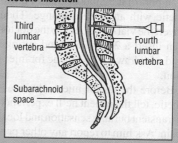

BETTER CHARTING

Documenting lumbar puncture

During lumbar puncture, observe the patient closely for signs such as a change in level of consciousness, dizziness, or changes in vital signs. Report these observations to the doctor, and document them carefully.

Also record the cerebrospinal fluid (CSF) pressure initially and during the procedure. Record obtaining the test tube specimens of CSF as they are obtained. Document the patient's tolerance of the procedure and any pertinent information about specimens in the chart.

Monitor the patient's condition, and keep him in a flat supine position for 6 to 12 hours. Encourage fluid intake, assess him for headache, and check the puncture site for leaking CSF. Document all your observations and interventions.

his sterile gloves and put on another pair *to avoid introducing povidone-iodine into the subarachnoid space with the lumbar puncture needle.*)

• If there is no ampule of anesthetic on the equipment tray, clean the injection port of a multidose vial of anesthetic with an alcohol sponge. Then invert the vial 45 degrees so the doctor can insert a 25G needle and syringe and withdraw the anesthetic for injection.

• Before the doctor injects the anesthetic, tell the patient he'll experience a transient burning sensation and local pain. Ask him to report any other persistent pain or sensations *because these may indicate irritation or puncture of a nerve root, requiring repositioning of the needle.*

• When the doctor inserts the sterile spinal needle into the subarachnoid space between the third and fourth lumbar vertebrae, instruct the patient to remain still and breathe normally. If necessary, hold the patient firmly in position *to prevent sudden movement that may displace the needle.*

• If a lumbar puncture is being performed to administer contrast media for radiologic studies or spinal anesthetic, the doctor injects the dye or anesthetic at this time.

• When the needle is in place, the doctor attaches a manometer with a three-way stopcock to the needle hub *to read CSF pressure.* If ordered, help the patient extend his legs *to provide a more accurate pressure reading.*

• The doctor then detaches the manometer and allows fluid to drain from the needle hub into the collection tubes. When he has collected approximately 2 or 3 ml in each tube, mark the tubes in sequence, stopper them securely, and label them properly.

• If the doctor suspects an obstruction in the spinal subarachnoid space, he may check for Queckenstedt's sign. He first takes an initial CSF pressure reading. Then compress the patient's jugular vein for 10 seconds, as ordered. *This temporarily obstructs blood flow from the cranium, increasing ICP* and — if no subarachnoid block exists — *causes CSF pressure to rise as well.* The doctor then takes pressure readings every 10 seconds until the pressure stabilizes.

• After the doctor collects the specimens and removes the spinal needle, clean the puncture site with povidone-

iodine and apply a small adhesive bandage.
• Send the CSF specimens to the laboratory immediately, with properly completed laboratory request forms.

Complications
• Headache is the most common adverse effect of lumbar puncture.
• Other adverse effects may include a reaction to the anesthetic, meningitis, epidural or subdural abscess, bleeding into the spinal canal, CSF leakage through the dural defect remaining after needle withdrawal, local pain caused by nerve root irritation, edema or hematoma at the puncture site, transient difficulty in voiding, and fever.
• The most serious complications of lumbar puncture, although rare, are tonsillar herniation and medullary compression.

Nursing considerations
• Sedatives and analgesics are usually withheld before this test if there is evidence of a central nervous system disorder *because they may mask important symptoms.*
• During lumbar puncture, watch closely for signs of adverse reaction: elevated pulse rate, pallor, or clammy skin. Alert the doctor immediately to any significant changes.
• The patient may be ordered to lie flat for 8 to 12 hours after the procedure. If necessary, place a patient care reminder on his bed to this effect.
• Collected CSF specimens must be sent to the laboratory immediately; they cannot be refrigerated for later transport.

Documentation
• Record the initiation and completion times of the procedure, the patient's response, the administration of drugs, the number of specimen tubes collected, the time of transport to the laboratory, and the color, consistency, and any other characteristics of the collected specimens. (See *Documenting lumbar puncture.*)

Lung perfusion scan

A lung perfusion scan produces an image of pulmonary blood flow after I.V. injection of a radiopharmaceutical, either human serum albumin microspheres or macroaggregated albumin bonded to technetium. The purpose of this diagnositic procedure is to assess arterial perfusion of the lungs, detect pulmonary emboli, aid preoperative evaluation of pulmonary function in a patient with marginal lung reserves, help confirm pulmonary vascular obstruction such as pulmonary emboli, and help determine ventilation-perfusion ratios (when performed in conjunction with a lung ventilation scan).

Hot spots are areas showing high uptake of the radioactive substance with normal blood perfusion; a normal lung shows a uniform uptake.

Cold spots are areas showing low radioactive uptake indicating poor perfusion and suggesting embolism, but a ventilation scan is necessary to confirm diagnosis. Decreased regional blood flow without vessel obstruction may indicate pneumonitis.

≫ Key nursing diagnoses and patient outcomes

Use these nursing diagnoses as a guide when developing your plan of care.

Impaired gas exchange related to (specify)

Based on this nursing diagnosis, you'll establish the following patient outcomes. The patient will:
• maintain respiratory rate within +/- 5 of baseline.
• express feeling of comfort in maintaining air exchange.
• have normal breath sounds.
• perform activities of daily living to level of tolerance.

Knowledge deficit related to lack of exposure to diagnositic procedure

Based on this nursing diagnosis, you'll establish the following patient outcomes. The patient will:
• communicate an understanding of purpose of procedure.
• communicate a desire to know his role during the procedure.

Patient preparation

• Tell the patient that the test helps evaluate respiratory function.
• Explain that there are no food or fluid restrictions before the test.
• Describe the test, including who will perform it, where it will take place, and how long it will take (15 to 30 minutes).
• Tell the patient that a radiopharmaceutical will be injected into a vein in his arm and that he'll then sit in front of or lie under a camera.
• Explain that neither the camera nor the uptake probe emits radiation and that the amount of radioactivity in the radiopharmaceutical is minimal.

• Assure the patient that he'll be comfortable during the test and that he doesn't have to remain perfectly still.
• On the test request slip, note whether the patient has conditions such as chronic obstructive pulmonary disease, vasculitis, pulmonary edema, tumor, sickle cell disease, or parasitic disease.

Implementation

• Half of the radiopharmaceutical is injected I.V. while the patient is in a supine position; the remaining half is injected while the patient is in a prone position.
• After the injection, the gamma camera takes a series of single stationary images in the anterior, posterior, oblique, and both lateral chest views.
• Images, which are projected on an oscilloscope screen, show the distribution of radioactive particles.
• If a hematoma develops at the injection site after the test, apply warm soaks.

Nursing considerations

• A lung scan is contraindicated in patients hypersensitive to the radiopharmaceutical.

Documentation

• Document the time, date, and the patient's tolerance of the procedure.

Lung ventilation scan

This nuclear diagnostic scan is performed after the patient inhales a mixture of air and radioactive gas that delineates areas of the lung ventilated during respiration. The scan records the distribution of the gas during three phases: the buildup of radioactive gas (wash-in phase); the time after rebreathing when radioactivity reaches a steady level (equilibrium phase); and after removal of the radioactive gas from the lungs (wash-out phase).

This scan helps diagnose pulmonary emboli, identify areas of the lung capable of ventilation, evaluate regional respiratory function, and locate regional hypoventilation (usually caused by smoking or chronic obstructive pulmonary disease). It also helps distinguish between parenchymal disease, such as emphysema, sarcoidosis, bronchogenic carcinoma, and tuberculosis, and conditions from vascular abnormalities such as pulmonary emboli (performed with a lung perfusion scan). Normal findings include an equal distribution of gas in both lungs and normal wash-in and wash-out phases.

Unequal gas distribution in both lungs indicates poor ventilation or airway obstruction in areas with low radioactivity.

When compared with a lung scan (perfusion scan) of such vascular obstructions as pulmonary embolism, the perfusion to the embolized area is decreased, but the ventilation to this area is maintained; in parenchymal disease such as pneumonia, ventilation is abnormal within the areas of consolidation.

≫ Key nursing diagnoses and patient outcomes

Use these nursing diagnoses as a guide when developing your plan of care.

Impaired gas exchange related to (specify)
Based on this nursing diagnosis, you'll establish the following patient outcomes. The patient will:
• maintain respiratory rate within +/- 5 of baseline.
• express feeling of comfort in maintaining air exchange.
• have normal breath sounds.
• perform activities of daily living to level of tolerance.

Knowledge deficit related to lack of exposure to diagnostic procedure
Based on this nursing diagnosis, you'll establish the following patient outcomes. The patient will:
• communicate an understanding of purpose of procedure.
• communicate a desire to know his role during the procedure.

Equipment
♦ breathing mask that fits tightly over patient's nose and mouth ♦ radioactive gas (xenon 133 or krypton 85) nuclear scanner.

Patient preparation
• Describe the procedure and explain the test.
• Tell the patient there are no food or fluid restrictions.
• Tell him who will perform the test, where it will take place, and that it will take 15 to 30 minutes.
• Ask the patient to remove all jewelry or metal from the scanning field.
• Explain that he'll be asked to hold his breath for a short time after inhaling a gas and that he must remain still while a machine scans his chest.
• Reassure him that a minimal amount of radioactive gas is used.

Implementation
• After the patient inhales air mixed with a small amount of radioactive gas, a nuclear scanner monitors the distribution of the gas in the patient's lungs.
• The patient's chest is scanned as he exhales.

Nursing considerations
• Watch for leaks in the closed radioactive-gas system that may contaminate the surrounding atmosphere.
• In a patient on mechanical ventilation, krypton gas must be used instead of xenon gas.

Documentation
• Document the time, date, and the patient's tolerance of the procedure.

Lymph node palpation

Lymph usually travels through more than one lymph node because numerous nodes line the lymphatic channels that drain a particular region. For example, axillary nodes filter drainage from the arms and femoral nodes filter drainage from the legs. This pattern prevents organisms that enter peripheral body areas from migrating unchallenged to central body locations. Lymph nodes are also a principal source of circulating lymphocytes, which provide specific immune responses.

≫ Key nursing diagnoses and patient outcomes
Use these nursing diagnoses as a guide when developing your plan of care.

Knowledge deficit related to lack of exposure to assessment techniques
Based on this nursing diagnosis, you'll establish the following patient outcomes. The patient will:
• communicate a need to know about techniques used to develop plan of care.
• verbalize an understanding of what is taught.

Anxiety related to techniques used during assessment
Based on this nursing diagnosis, you'll establish the following patient outcomes. The patient will:
• verbalize feelings of anxiety during assessment.
• remain calm during assessment.
• use relaxation techniques during assessment, when appropriate.

Equipment
♦ flashlight or gooseneck lamp.

Patient preparation
• Explain the procedure.
• Provide privacy.

Implementation
• Use the pads of your index and middle fingers to palpate the patient's superficial lymph nodes in the head and neck, and in the axillary, epitrochlear, inguinal, and popliteal areas.
• Apply gentle pressure and rotary motion to feel the underlying nodes without obscuring them by pressing them into deeper soft tissues. (See *Palpating the lymph nodes*.)
• Lymph nodes usually can't be felt in a healthy patient. If palpation reveals nodal enlargement or other abnormalities, note size, shape, surface, con-
(Text continues on page 504.)

Palpating the lymph nodes

When assessing a patient for signs of an immune disorder, you'll need to palpate the superficial lymph nodes of the head and neck, and the axillary, epitrochlear, inguinal, and popliteal nodes with the pads of the index and middle fingers. Always palpate gently, beginning with light pressure and gradually increasing pressure.

Head and neck nodes

Head and neck nodes are best palpated with the patient in a sitting position.

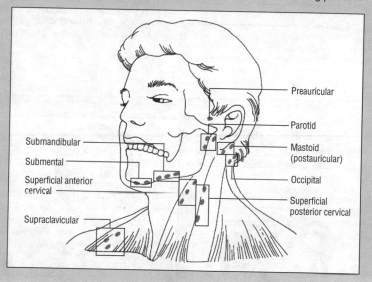

Preauricular

Parotid

Submandibular

Mastoid (postauricular)

Submental

Superficial anterior cervical

Occipital

Superficial posterior cervical

Supraclavicular

To palpate the submandibular, submental, anterior cervical, and occipital nodes, position your fingers as shown. Palpate over the mandibular surface, and continue moving up and down the entire neck. Flex the head forward or to the side being examined. This relaxes the tissues and makes enlarged nodes more palpable. Reverse your hand position to palpate the opposite side.

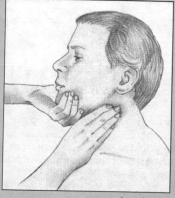

(continued)

Palpating the lymph nodes *(continued)*

Axillary and epitrochlear nodes

Palpate the axillary and epitrochlear nodes with the patient sitting. You can also palpate the axillary nodes with the patient lying in a supine position.

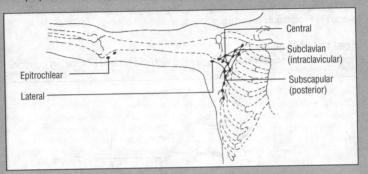

To palpate the preauricular, parotid, and mastoid nodes, position your fingers as shown.

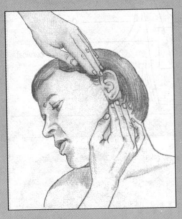

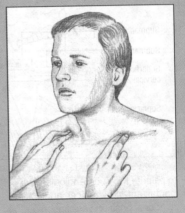

To palpate the posterior cervical nodes and spinal nerve chain, place your fingertip pads along the anterior surface of the trapezius muscle. Then move your fingertips toward the posterior surface of the sternocleidomastoid muscle.

To palpate the supraclavicular nodes, encourage the patient to relax so that the clavicles drop. To relax the soft tissues of the anterior neck, flex his head slightly forward with your free hand. Then hook your left index finger over the clavicle lateral to the sternocleidomastoid muscle. Rotate your fingers deeply into this area to feel these nodes.

Palpating the lymph nodes (continued)

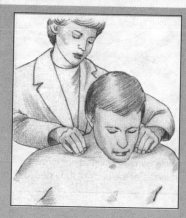

To palpate the axillary nodes, use your nondominant hand to support the patient's relaxed right arm and put your other hand as high in his right axilla as possible. Then palpate the axillary nodes, gently pressing the soft tissues against the chest wall and the muscles surrounding the axilla (the pectorals, latissimus dorsi, subscapular, and anterior serratus). Repeat this procedure for the left axilla.

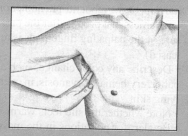

To palpate the epitrochlear lymph nodes, place your fingertips in the depression above and posterior to the medial area of the elbow and palpate gently.

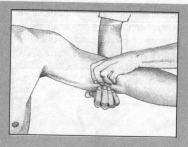

Inguinal and popliteal nodes

Palpate the inguinal and popliteal nodes with the patient lying in a supine position. You can also palpate the popliteal nodes with the patient sitting or standing.

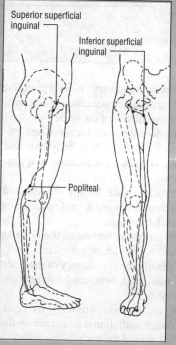

Superior superficial inguinal

Inferior superficial inguinal

Popliteal

(continued)

Palpating the lymph nodes *(continued)*

To palpate the inferior superficial inguinal lymph nodes (femoral), gently press below the junction of the saphenous and femoral veins.

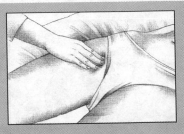

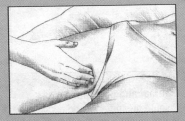

To palpate the superior superficial inguinal lymph nodes, press along the course of the saphenous veins from the inguinal area to the abdomen.

To palpate the popliteal nodes, press gently along the posterior muscles at the back of the knee.

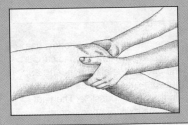

sistency, symmetry, mobility, color, tenderness, temperature, pulsations, and vascularity of the node.

• To describe node location, use reference points, such as body axis and lines, or sketch the location if appropriate.

• Indicate node length, width, and depth in centimeters, and describe or sketch the shape.

• Describe the surface of the node as smooth, nodular, or irregular.

• Identify the consistency of the node as hard, soft, firm, resilient, spongy, or cystic.

• Evaluate node symmetry by comparing it with similar structures on the other side of the body.

• Describe the node's mobility. If it's immobile, indicate whether it's fixed to overlying tissue, underlying tissue, or both.

• During palpation, note whether any tenderness is elicited by palpation, movement, or rebound phenomenon (tenderness that occurs after the pressure of the palpating fingerpads is released).

• Describe any color change, such as pallor, erythema, or cyanosis, in overlying skin.

• Note whether the site feels warm.

• Be alert for pulsations in the mass; plan to auscultate a pulsating mass for a bruit.

• If the node exhibits increased vascularity, describe any changes in overlying blood vessels.

• Use a flashlight to assess further an abnormal lump in an area that can be transilluminated such as the scrotum.

• Describe the results of transillumination along with the other characteristics.

• A lump that allows light to pass through means it's filled with fluid, which usually indicates a cyst rather than a node.

Nursing considerations

• Enlarged lymph nodes may result from enlarged or more numerous lymphocytes and reticuloendothelial cells that normally line the node or from infiltration by foreign cells such as metastatic cancer cells. The clinical significance of a palpated node depends on its location and the patient's age. In a child, swollen nodes may indicate a mild infection; in an adult, they're usually more significant.

• Red streaks in the skin, palpable nodes, and lymphedema may indicate a lymphatic disorder.

• Enlarged nodes suggest current or recent inflammation.

• Tender nodes usually denote infection.

• In acute infection, nodes are large, tender, and discrete; in chronic infection, they become confluent.

• Metastasized cancer usually affects nodes unilaterally, causing them to become discrete, nontender, firm or hard, and fixed.

• Generalized lymphadenopathy (involving three or more node groups) can indicate an autoimmune disorder such as SLE or an infectious or neoplastic disorder. In SLE, nodal enlargement may be local or general.

Documentation

• Document any normal and abnormal findings.

M

Magnetic resonance imaging (MRI)

This noninvasive diagnostic technique, also called nuclear magnetic resonance, may be superior to computed tomography scanning in detecting cerebellar lesions and metastatic bone marrow disease and in identifying soft-tissue masses. Because MRI uses a strong magnetic field rather than ionizing radiation, it may allow safe serial studies of children and pregnant women. MRI cannot, however, be used in patients with pacemakers or metal surgical clips in such vital areas as the brain because the magnetic force affects metal.

≫ Key nursing diagnoses and patient outcomes

Use these nursing diagnoses as a guide when developing your plan of care.

Knowledge deficit related to diagnostic procedure
Based on this nursing diagnosis, you'll establish the following patient outcome. The patient will:
• verbalize purpose for the diagnostic procedure.

Fear related to potential outcome of procedure
Based on this nursing diagnosis, you'll establish the following patient outcomes. The patient will:
• communicate feelings about potential outcome of procedure.
• use available support systems, such as family and significant others.

Anxiety related to claustrophobia during procedure
Based on this nursing diagnosis, you'll establish the following patient outcome. The patient will:
• verbalize feelings of claustrophobia during procedure.

Equipment
♦ MRI scanner and computer ♦ display screen ♦ recorder (film or magnetic tape).

Patient preparation
• Explain to the patient that this test assesses bone and soft tissue.
• Tell him who will perform the test, where it will be done, and that it will take up to 90 minutes.
• Explain that although MRI is painless and involves no exposure to radiation from the scanner, a radioactive contrast dye may be used, depending on the type of tissue being studied.
• Emphasize that the opening for the patient's head and body in the MRI scanner is quite small and deep. Ask if claustrophobia has ever been a problem; if it has, the patient might not be able to tolerate the scan and may need sedation.
• Tell him that he'll hear the scanner clicking, whirring, and thumping as it moves inside its housing.
• Reassure him that he'll be able to communicate with the technician at all times.
• Instruct him to remove all metallic objects, including jewelry, hair pins, or watch. Ask whether he has any surgically implanted joints, pins, clips, valves, pumps, or pacemakers containing metal that could be affected by

the strong MRI magnet; he won't be able to undergo the test if he does.
• If the test involves contrast medium, ask the patient about allergies.
• Make sure that an appropriate consent form has been signed by the patient or a responsible family member.
• Tell him he must remain still during the procedure.
• Tell the patient that he may resume normal activity after the test.
• Provide emotional support to the patient with anxiety about claustrophobia or anxiety over his diagnosis.

Implementation

• At the scanner-room door, check the patient one last time for metal objects.
• The patient is placed on a narrow, padded, nonmetallic table that moves into the scanner tunnel.
• While the patient lies in the strong magnetic field, the area to be studied is stimulated with radiofrequency waves.
• The resulting images are displayed on a monitor and recorded on film or magnetic tape for permanent storage.
• Observe the patient for postural hypotension if the test took a long time.

Complications

• Postural hypotension may occur if the test takes longer than 90 minutes.

Nursing considerations

• If the patient has an I.V. line, make sure the indwelling catheter is nonmetallic.

Documentation

• Chart the time, date, and the patient's tolerance of the procedure.

Manual ventilation

A hand-held resuscitation bag is an inflatable device that can be attached to a face mask or directly to an endotracheal or tracheostomy tube to allow manual delivery of oxygen or room air to the lungs of a patient who can't breathe on her own. Usually used in an emergency, manual ventilation also can be performed while the patient is disconnected temporarily from a mechanical ventilator, such as during a tubing change, during transport, or before suctioning. In such instances, use of the hand-held resuscitation bag maintains ventilation. Oxygen administration with a resuscitation bag can help improve a compromised cardiorespiratory system.

≫ Key nursing diagnoses and patient outcomes

Use these nursing diagnoses as a guide when developing your plan of care for a patient requiring manual ventilation.

Ineffective breathing pattern related to decreased energy

Based on this nursing diagnosis, you'll establish the following patient outcomes. The patient will:
• achieve maximum lung expansion with adequate ventilation.
• report feeling comfortable with breathing.

Gas exchange impairment related to altered oxygen supply

Based on this nursing diagnosis, you'll establish the following patient outcomes. The patient will:
• cough effectively.

• expectorate sputum.

Equipment

♦ hand-held resuscitation bag ♦ mask ♦ oxygen source (wall unit or tank) ♦ oxygen tubing ♦ nipple adapter attached to oxygen flowmeter ♦ optional: positive end-expiratory pressure (PEEP) valve, oxygen accumulator.

Equipment preparation

• Unless the patient is intubated or has a tracheostomy, select a mask that fits snugly over the mouth and nose. Attach the mask to the resuscitation bag.
• If oxygen is readily available, connect the hand-held resuscitation bag to the oxygen. Attach one end of the tubing to the bottom of the bag and the other end to the nipple adapter on the flowmeter of the oxygen source.
• Turn on the oxygen and adjust the flow rate according to the patient's condition. For example, if the patient has a low partial pressure of oxygen in arterial blood, he'll need a higher fraction of inspired oxygen (FIO_2). To increase the concentration of inspired oxygen, you can add an oxygen accumulator (also called an oxygen reservoir). This device, which attaches to an adapter on the bottom of the bag, permits an FIO_2 of up to 100%. Then, if time allows, set up suction equipment.

Patient preparation

• Before using the hand-held resuscitation bag, check the patient's upper airway for foreign objects. If present, remove them because this alone may restore spontaneous respirations in some instances. Also, foreign matter or secretions can obstruct the airway and impede resuscitation efforts. Suction the patient *to remove any secretions that may obstruct the airway.* If necessary, insert an oropharyngeal or nasopharyngeal airway *to maintain airway patency.* If the patient has a tracheostomy or endotracheal tube in place, suction the tube.
• If appropriate, remove the bed's headboard and stand at the head of the bed *to help keep the patient's neck extended and to free space at the side of the bed for other activities, such as cardiopulmonary resuscitation.*

Implementation

• Tilt the patient's head backward, if not contraindicated, and pull his jaw forward *to move the tongue away from the base of the pharynx and prevent obstruction of the airway.* (See *How to apply a hand-held resuscitation bag and mask.*)
• Keeping your nondominant hand on the patient's mask, exert downward pressure *to seal the mask against his face.* For the adult patient, use your dominant hand to compress the bag every 5 seconds *to deliver about 1 liter of air.* For a child, deliver 15 breaths/minute, or one compression of the bag every 4 seconds; for the infant, 20 breaths/minute, or one compression every 3 seconds. Infants and children should receive 250 to 500 cc of air with each bag compression.
• Deliver breaths with the patient's own inspiratory effort, if any is present. Don't attempt to deliver a breath as the patient exhales.
• Observe the patient's chest *to ensure that it rises and falls with each compression.* If ventilation fails to occur, check the fit of the mask and the patency of the patient's airway; if neces-

sary, reposition the patient's head and ensure patency with an oral airway.

Complications

• Aspiration of vomitus can result in pneumonia, and gastric distention may result from air forced into the patient's stomach.

Nursing considerations

• Avoid neck hyperextension if the patient has a possible cervical injury; instead, use the jaw-thrust technique to open the airway. If you need both hands to keep the patient's mask in place and maintain hyperextension, use the lower part of your arm to compress the bag against your side.

• Observe for vomiting through the clear part of the mask. If vomiting occurs, stop the procedure immediately, lift the mask, wipe and suction vomitus, and resume resuscitation.

• Underventilation commonly occurs because the hand-held resuscitation bag is difficult to keep positioned tightly on the patient's face while ensuring an open airway. What's more, the volume of air delivered to the patient varies with the type of bag used and the hand size of the person compressing the bag. An adult with a small or medium-sized hand may not consistently deliver 1 liter of air. For these reasons, have someone assist with the procedure, if possible. (See *Using a PEEP valve*, page 510.)

Documentation

• In an emergency, record the date and time of the procedure; manual ventilation efforts; any complications and the nursing action taken; and the patient's response to treatment, accord-

How to apply a hand-held resuscitation bag and mask

Place the mask over the patient's face so that the apex of the triangle covers the bridge of his nose and the base lies between his lower lip and chin.

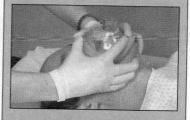

Make sure that the patient's mouth remains open underneath the mask. Attach the bag to the mask and to the tubing leading to the oxygen source.

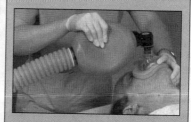

Or, if the patient has a tracheostomy or an endotracheal tube in place, remove the mask from the bag and attach the hand-held resuscitation bag directly to the tube.

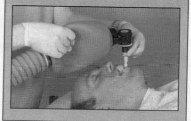

Using a PEEP valve

Add positive end-expiratory pressure (PEEP) to manual ventilation by attaching a PEEP valve to the resuscitation bag. This may improve oxygenation if the patient hasn't responded to increased fraction of inspired oxygen levels. Always use a PEEP valve to manually ventilate a patient who has been receiving PEEP on the ventilator.

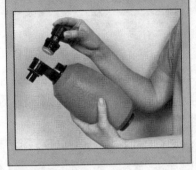

ing to your hospital's protocol for respiratory arrest.

• In a nonemergency situation, record the date and time of the procedure, reason and length of time the patient was disconnected from mechanical ventilation and received manual ventilation, any complications and the nursing action taken, and the patient's tolerance for the procedure.

Mechanical traction

Mechanical traction exerts a pulling force on a part of the body—usually the spine, pelvis, or long bones of the arms and legs. It can be used to reduce fractures, treat dislocations, correct or prevent deformities, improve or correct contractures, or decrease muscle spasms. Depending on the injury or condition, an orthopedist may order either skin or skeletal traction.

Applied directly to the skin and thus indirectly to the bone, skin traction is ordered when a light, temporary, or noncontinuous pulling force is required. Contraindications for skin traction include a severe injury with open wounds, an allergy to tape or other skin traction equipment, circulatory disturbances, dermatitis, and varicose veins.

In skeletal traction, an orthopedist inserts a pin or wire through the bone and attaches the traction equipment to the pin or wire to exert a direct, constant, longitudinal pulling force. Indications for skeletal traction include fractures of the tibia, femur, and humerus. Infections such as osteomyelitis contraindicate skeletal traction.

Nursing responsibilities for this procedure include setting up the traction frame. (See *Traction frames*.) The design of the patient's bed usually dictates whether to use a claw clamp or I.V.-post-type frame.(However, the claw-type Balkan frame is rarely used.) Setup of the specific traction can be done by a nurse with special skills, an orthopedic technician, or by the doctor. Instructions for setting up these traction units usually accompany the equipment. (See *Comparing traction types*, page 512). After the patient is placed in the specific type of traction ordered by the orthopedist, the nurse is responsible for preventing complications from immobility; for routinely inspecting the equipment; for adding traction weights, as ordered; and, in patients with skeletal traction, for *monitoring the pin insertion sites for signs of infection.*

Traction frames

You may encounter three types of fraction frames, as described below.

Claw-type basic frame
With this frame, claw attachments secure the uprights to the footboard and headboard.

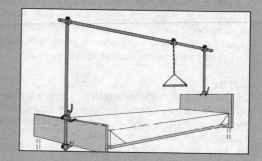

I.V.-type basic frame
With this frame, I.V. posts placed in I.V. holders support the horizontal bars across the foot and head of the bed. These horizontal bars then support the two uprights.

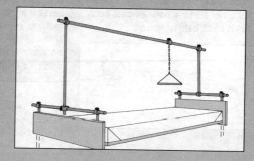

I.V.-type Balkan frame
This frame features I.V. posts and horizontal bars (secured in the same manner as those for the I.V.-type basic frame) that support four uprights.

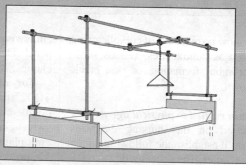

≫ Key nursing diagnoses and patient outcomes
Use these nursing diagnoses as a guide when developing your plan of care for a patient who is being treated with mechanical traction.

Mobility impairment related to neuromuscular impairment
Based on this nursing diagnosis, you'll establish the following patient outcomes. The patient will:
• maintain muscle strength and joint range of motion.

Comparing traction types

Traction therapy restricts movement of a patient's affected limb or body part and may confine the patient to bed rest for an extended period. The limb is immobilized by pulling with equal force on each end of the injured area — an equal mix of traction and countertraction. Weights provide the pulling force. Countertraction is produced by using other weights or by positioning the patient's body weight against the traction pull.

Skin traction
This procedure immobilizes a body part intermittently over an extended period through direct application of a pulling force on the patient's skin. The force may be applied using adhesive or nonadhesive traction tape or other skin traction devices, such as a boot, belt, or halter.

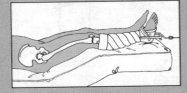

Adhesive attachment allows more continuous traction, whereas nonadhesive attachment allows easier removal for daily skin care.

Skeletal traction
This procedure immobilizes a body part for prolonged periods by attaching weighted equipment directly to the patient's bones. This may be accomplished with pins, screws, wires, or tongs.

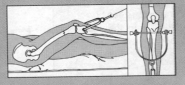

• show no evidence of complications, such as contractures, venous stasis, thrombus formation, or skin breakdown.

Pain related to physical agents
Based on this nursing diagnosis, you'll establish the following patient outcomes. The patient will:
• express a feeling of comfort and relief from pain.
• state and carry out appropriate interventions for pain relief.

Equipment
For a claw-type basic frame: ♦ 102″ (259-cm) plain bar ♦ two 66″ (168-cm) swivel-clamp bars ♦ two upper-panel clamps ♦ two lower-panel clamps.
For an I.V.-type basic frame: ♦ 102″ plain bar ♦ 27″ (68.6-cm) double-clamp bar ♦ 48″ (122-cm) swivel-clamp bar ♦ two 36″ (91.4-cm) plain bars ♦ four 4″ (10-cm) I.V. posts with clamps ♦ cross clamp.
For an I.V.-type Balkan frame: ♦ two 102″ plain bars ♦ two 48″ swivel-clamp bars ♦ five 36″ plain bars ♦ two 27″ double-clamp bars ♦ four 4″ I.V. posts with clamps ♦ eight cross clamps.
For all frame types: ♦ trapeze with clamp ♦ wall bumper or roller.

For skeletal traction care: ♦ sterile cotton-tipped applicators ♦ prescribed antiseptic solution ♦ sterile gauze pads ♦ povidone-iodine solution ♦ optional: antimicrobial ointment.

Equipment preparation

• Arrange with central supply or the appropriate department to have the traction equipment transported to the patient's room on a traction cart. If appropriate, gather the equipment for pin-site care at the patient's bedside. Pin-site care protocols may vary with each hospital or doctor.

Patient preparation

• Explain the purpose of traction to the patient. Emphasize the importance of maintaining proper body alignment after the traction equipment is set up.

Implementation

Here are the steps involved in mechanical traction.

To set up a claw-type basic frame

• Attach one lower panel and one upper panel clamp to each 66" swivel-clamp bar.

• Fasten one bar to the footboard and one to the headboard by turning the clamp knobs clockwise until they are tight and then pulling back on the upper clamp's rubberized bar until it is tight.

• Secure the 102" horizontal plain bar atop the two vertical bars, making sure the clamp knobs point up.

• Using the appropriate clamp, attach the trapeze to the horizontal bar about 2' (0.6 m) from the head of the bed.

To set up an I.V.-type basic frame

• Attach one 4" I.V. post with clamp to each end of both 36" horizontal plain bars.

• Secure an I.V. post in each I.V. holder at the bed corners. Using a cross clamp, fasten the 48" vertical swivel-clamp bar to the middle of the horizontal plain bar at the foot of the bed.

• Fasten the 27" vertical double-clamp bar to the middle of the horizontal plain bar at the head of the bed.

• Attach the 102" horizontal plain bar to the tops of the two vertical bars, making sure the clamp knobs point up.

• Using the appropriate clamp, attach the trapeze to the horizontal bar about 2' from the head of the bed.

To set up an I.V.-type Balkan frame

• Attach one 4" I.V. post with clamp to each end of two 36" horizontal plain bars.

• Secure an I.V. post in each I.V. holder at the bed corners.

• Attach a 48" vertical swivel-clamp bar, using a cross clamp, to each I.V. post clamp on the horizontal plain bar at the foot of the bed.

• Fasten one 36" horizontal plain bar across the midpoints of the two 48" swivel-clamp bars, using two cross clamps.

• Attach a 27" vertical double-clamp bar to each I.V. post clamp on the horizontal bar at the head of the bed.

• Using two cross clamps, fasten a 36" horizontal plain bar across the midpoints of two 27" double-clamp bars.

• Clamp a 102" horizontal plain bar onto the vertical bars on each side of the bed, making sure the clamp knobs point up.

• Use two cross clamps to attach a 36" horizontal plain bar across the two

overhead bars, about 2' from the head of the bed.
• Attach the trapeze to this 36" horizontal bar.

After setting up any frame

• Attach a wall bumper or roller to the vertical bar or bars at the head of the bed. *This protects the walls from damage caused by the bed or equipment.*

Caring for the traction patient

• Show the patient how much movement he's allowed and instruct him not to readjust the equipment. Also tell him to report any pain or pressure from the traction equipment.
• At least once a shift, make sure that the traction equipment connections are tight and that no parts touch the bedding, the patient, or other inappropriate portions of the apparatus. Check for impingements, such as ropes rubbing on the footboard or getting caught between pulleys. *Friction and impingement reduce the effectiveness of traction.*
• Inspect the traction equipment *to ensure the correct alignment.*
• Inspect the ropes for fraying, which can eventually cause a rope to break.
• Make sure the ropes are positioned properly in the pulley track. An improperly positioned rope changes the degree of traction.
• To prevent tampering and aid stability and security, make sure that all rope ends are taped above the knot.
• Inspect the equipment regularly to make sure that the traction weights hang freely. Weights that touch the floor, bed, or each other reduce the amount of traction.
• About every 2 hours, check the patient for proper body alignment and

reposition the patient as necessary. *Misalignment causes ineffective traction and may keep the fracture from healing properly.*
• *To prevent complications from immobility,* assess neurovascular integrity routinely. The patient's condition, the hospital routine, and the doctor's orders determine the frequency of neurovascular assessments.
• Provide skin care, encourage coughing and deep breathing exercises, and assist with ordered range-of-motion exercises for unaffected extremities. Typically, an order for elastic support stockings is written. Check elimination patterns and provide laxatives, as ordered.
• For the patient with skeletal traction, make sure that the protruding pin or wire ends are covered with cork *to prevent them from tearing the bedding or injuring the patient and staff.*
• Check the pin site and surrounding skin regularly for signs of infection.
• If ordered, clean the pin site and surrounding skin. Pin-site care varies, but you'll usually follow guidelines like these: Use sterile technique; avoid digging at pin sites with the cotton-tipped applicator; if ordered, clean the pin site and surrounding skin with a cotton-tipped applicator dipped in ordered antiseptic; if ordered, apply antimicrobial ointment to the pin sites; apply a loose sterile dressing, or dress with sterile gauze pads soaked in povidone-iodine solution. Perform pin-site care as often as necessary, depending on the amount of drainage.

Complications

• Immobility during traction may result in pressure ulcers; muscle atro-

phy, weakness, or contractures; and osteoporosis.
• Immobility can also cause GI disturbances, such as constipation; urinary problems, including stasis and calculi; respiratory problems, such as stasis of secretions and hypostatic pneumonia; and circulatory disturbances, including stasis and thrombophlebitis.
• Prolonged immobility, especially after traumatic injury, may promote depression or other emotional disturbances.
• Skeletal traction may cause osteomyelitis originating at the pin or wire sites.

Nursing considerations

• When using skin traction, apply ordered weights slowly and carefully *to avoid jerking the affected extremity. To avoid injury in case the ropes break*, arrange the weights so they don't hang over the patient.

Documentation

• In the patient record, document the amount of traction weight used daily, noting the application of additional weights and the patient's tolerance.
• Document equipment inspections and patient care, including routine checks of neurovascular integrity, skin condition, respiratory status, and elimination patterns. If applicable, note the condition of the pin site and any care given.

Mechanical ventilation

A mechanical ventilator moves air in and out of a patient's lungs, but doesn't ensure adequate gas ex-

change. Mechanical ventilators use positive or negative pressure to ventilate patients.

Positive-pressure ventilators exert a positive pressure on the airway, which causes inspiration while increasing tidal volume (VT). The inspiratory cycles of these ventilators may vary in volume, pressure, or time. For example, a volume-cycled ventilator (the type used most commonly) delivers a preset volume of air each time, regardless of the amount of lung resistance. A pressure-cycled ventilator generates flow until the machine reaches a preset pressure, regardless of the volume delivered or the time required to achieve the pressure. A time-cycled ventilator generates flow for a preset amount of time. A high-frequency ventilator uses high respiratory rates and low VT to maintain alveolar ventilation.

Negative-pressure ventilators act by creating negative pressure, which pulls the thorax outward and allows air to flow into the lungs. Examples of such ventilators are the iron lung, the cuirass (chest shell), and the body wrap. Negative-pressure ventilators are used mainly to treat neuromuscular disorders, such as Guillain-Barré syndrome, myasthenia gravis, and poliomyelitis.

Other indications for ventilator use include central nervous system disorders, such as cerebral hemorrhage and spinal cord transsection, adult respiratory distress syndrome, pulmonary edema, chronic obstructive pulmonary disease, flail chest, and acute hypoventilation.

≫ Key nursing diagnoses and patient outcomes

Use these nursing diagnoses as a guide when developing your plan of care for a patient requiring mechanical ventilation.

Ineffective breathing pattern related to decreased energy

Based on this nursing diagnosis, you'll establish the following patient outcomes. The patient will:
• achieve maximum lung expansion with adequate ventilation.
• report feeling comfortable with breathing.

Gas exchange impairment related to altered oxygen supply

Based on this nursing diagnosis, you'll establish the following patient outcomes. The patient will:
• cough effectively.
• expectorate sputum.

Equipment

♦ oxygen source ♦ air source that can supply 50 psi ♦ mechanical ventilator ♦ humidifier ♦ ventilator circuit tubing, connectors, and adapters ♦ condensation collection trap ♦ spirometer, respirometer, or electronic device to measure flow and volume ♦ in-line thermometer ♦ probe for gas sampling and measuring airway pressure ♦ bacterial filter ♦ gloves ♦ hand-held resuscitation bag with reservoir ♦ suction equipment ♦ sterile distilled water ♦ equipment for arterial blood gas (ABG) analysis ♦ soft restraints, if indicated. ♦ optional: oximeter.

Equipment preparation

• In most hospitals, respiratory therapists assume responsibility for setting up the ventilator.
• If necessary, check the manufacturer's instructions for setting it up.
• In most cases, you'll need to add sterile distilled water to the humidifier and connect the ventilator to the appropriate gas source.

Patient preparation

• Verify the doctor's order for ventilator support. If the patient is not already intubated, prepare him for intubation.
• When possible, explain the procedure to the patient and his family *to help reduce anxiety and fear.* Assure the patient and his family that staff members are nearby to provide care.
• Perform a complete physical assessment and draw blood for ABG analysis *to establish a baseline.*
• Suction the patient if necessary.

Implementation

• Plug the ventilator into the electrical outlet and turn it on. Adjust the settings on the ventilator as ordered.
• Make sure that the ventilator's alarms are set, as ordered, and that the humidifier is filled with sterile distilled water.
• Put on gloves if you haven't already.
• Connect the endotracheal tube to the ventilator.
• Observe for chest expansion and auscultate for bilateral breath sounds *to verify that the patient is being ventilated.*
• Monitor the patient's ABG values after the initial ventilator setup (usually 20 to 30 minutes), after any changes in ventilator settings, and as the patient's clinical condition indi-

cates *to determine whether the patient is being adequately ventilated and to avoid oxygen toxicity.* Be prepared to adjust ventilator settings depending on ABG analysis.

• Check the ventilator tubing frequently for condensation, *which can cause resistance to airflow and which may also be aspirated by the patient.* As needed, drain the condensate into a collection trap or briefly disconnect the patient from the ventilator (ventilating him with a hand-held resuscitation bag if necessary), and empty the water into a receptacle. Do not drain the condensate into the humidifier *because the condensation may be contaminated with the patient's secretions.*

• Check the in-line thermometer to make sure that the temperature of the air delivered to the patient is close to body temperature.

• When monitoring the patient's vital signs, count spontaneous breaths as well as ventilator-delivered breaths.

• Change, clean, or dispose of the ventilator tubing and equipment, according to hospital policy, *to reduce the risk of bacterial contamination.* Typically, ventilator tubing should be changed every 48 to 72 hours, and sometimes more often.

• When ordered, begin to wean the patient from the ventilator. (See *Weaning the patient from the ventilator,* page 518.)

Complications

• Mechanical ventilation can cause tension pneumothorax, decreased cardiac output, oxygen toxicity, fluid volume excess caused by humidification, infection, and such GI complications as distention or bleeding from stress ulcers.

Nursing considerations

• Be sure that the ventilator alarms are on at all times. *These alarms alert the nursing staff to potentially hazardous conditions and changes in patient status.* If an alarm sounds and the problem can't be identified easily, disconnect the patient from the ventilator and use a hand-held resuscitation bag to ventilate him. (See *Responding to ventilator alarms, pages 520 and 521.*)

• Provide emotional support to the patient during all phases of mechanical ventilation *to reduce anxiety and promote successful treatment.* Even if the patient is unresponsive, continue to explain all procedures and treatments to him.

• Unless contraindicated, turn the patient from side to side every 1 to 2 hours *to facilitate lung expansion and removal of secretions.* Perform active or passive range-of-motion exercises for all extremities *to reduce the hazards of immobility.* If the patient's condition permits, position him upright at regular intervals *to increase lung expansion.* When moving the patient or the ventilator tubing, be careful to prevent condensation in the tubing from flowing into the lungs *because aspiration of this contaminated moisture can cause infection.* Provide care for the patient's artificial airway as needed.

• Assess the patient's peripheral circulation, and monitor his urine output for signs of decreased cardiac output. Watch for signs and symptoms of fluid volume excess or dehydration.

• Place the call light within the patient's reach, and establish a method of communication such as a commu-

Weaning the patient from the ventilator

Successful weaning depends on the patient's ability to breathe on his own. That means he must have a spontaneous respiratory effort that can keep him ventilated, a stable cardiovascular system, and sufficient respiratory muscle strength and level of consciousness to sustain spontaneous breathing. He also should meet some or all of the following criteria.

Criteria
- PaO_2 of 60 mm Hg (50 mm Hg or the ability to maintain baseline levels if he has chronic lung disease) or a fraction of inspired oxygen (FIO_2) at or below 0.4
- $PaCO_2$ of less than 40 mm Hg (or normal for the patient), or an FIO_2 of 0.4 or less if his $PaCO_2$ is 60 mm Hg or more
- Vital capacity of more than 10 ml/kg of body weight
- Maximum inspiratory pressure over -20 cm H_2O
- Minute ventilation under 10 liters/minute with a respiratory frequency of less than 28 to 30 breaths/minute
- Forced expiratory volume in the first second of more than 10 ml/kg of body weight
- Ability to double his spontaneous resting minute ventilation
- Adequate natural airway or a functioning tracheostomy
- Ability to cough and mobilize secretions
- Successful withdrawal of any neuromuscular blocker, such as pancuronium
- Clear or clearing chest X-ray
- Absence of infection, acid-base or electrolyte imbalance, hyperglycemia, arrhythmias, renal failure, anemia, fever, or excessive fatigue

Short-term ventilation
If the patient has received mechanical ventilation for a short time,

weaning may be accomplished by progressively decreasing the frequency and tidal volume of the ventilated breaths. Then the patient's endotracheal tube can be converted to a T tube to assess whether his spontaneous respirations are adequate before extubation. If the patient has been mechanically ventilated with 5 cm H_2O or less of PEEP, the adequacy of his spontaneous breathing can be assessed by using a trial of CPAP on the ventilator.

Long-term ventilation
If the patient has received mechanical ventilation for a long time, weaning is usually accomplished by switching the ventilator to pressure support ventilation (PSV), with or without intermittent mandatory ventilation (IMV). This way, each of the patient's spontaneous breaths is augmented by the ventilator. As the patient's own respirations improve, the IMV and the PSV can be decreased.

If the patient doesn't progress satisfactorily using one of these methods, an alternative method of weaning is to disconnect the patient from the ventilator and place him on a T tube or tracheostomy collar for the ordered amount of time before reconnecting him to the ventilator. The patient then alternates between being on and off the ventilator, with the time off the venti-

Weaning the patient from the ventilator *(continued)*

lator increasing with each trial. Eventually, the patient will be able to breathe on his own all day. But, even then, he should be reconnect-ed to the ventilator for a few nights so that he can obtain adequate rest and conserve the energy required to breathe on his own the next day.

nication board because intubation and mechanical ventilation impair the patient's ability to speak. An artificial airway may help the patient to speak by allowing air to pass through his vocal cords.

• Administer a sedative or neuromuscular blocking agent, as ordered, *to relax the patient or eliminate spontaneous breathing efforts that can interfere with the ventilator's action.* Remember that the patient receiving a neuromuscular blocking drug requires close observation *because of his inability to breathe or communicate.*

• If the patient is receiving a neuromuscular blocking agent, make sure that he also receives a sedative. *Neuromuscular blocking agents cause paralysis without altering the patient's level of consciousness.* Reassure the patient and his family that the paralysis is temporary. Also make sure that emergency equipment is readily available in case the ventilator malfunctions or the patient is extubated accidentally. Continue to explain all procedures to the patient, and take extra steps to ensure his safety, such as raising the side rails during turning and covering and lubricating his eyes.

• Ensure that the patient gets adequate rest and sleep *because fatigue can delay weaning from the ventilator.* Provide subdued lighting, safely muffle equipment noises, and restrict staff ac-cess to the area *to promote quiet during rest periods.*

• When weaning the patient, continue to observe for signs of hypoxia. Schedule weaning to fit comfortably and realistically with the patient's daily regimen. Avoid scheduling sessions after meals, baths, or lengthy therapeutic or diagnostic procedures. Have the patient help you set up the schedule *to give him some sense of control over a frightening procedure.* As the patient's tolerance for weaning increases, help him sit up out of bed *to improve his breathing and sense of well-being.* Suggest diversionary activities *to take his mind off breathing.*

Home care

• If the patient will be discharged on a ventilator, evaluate the family's or the caregiver's ability and motivation to provide such care. Well before discharge, develop a teaching plan that will address the patient's needs. For example, teaching should include information about ventilator care and settings, artificial airway care, suctioning, respiratory therapy, communication, nutrition, therapeutic exercise, the signs and symptoms of infection, and ways to troubleshoot minor equipment malfunctions.

• Also evaluate the patient's need for adaptive equipment, such as a hospital bed, wheelchair or walker with a ventilator tray, patient lift, and bedside

PROBLEM SOLVER

Responding to ventilator alarms

SIGNAL	POSSIBLE CAUSE	INTERVENTIONS
Low-pressure alarm	• Tube disconnected from ventilator	• Reconnect the tube to the ventilator.
	• Endotracheal tube displaced above vocal cords or tracheostomy tube extubated	• Check tube placement and reposition if needed. If extubation or displacement has occurred, ventilate the patient manually and call the doctor immediately.
	• Leaking tidal volume from low cuff pressure (from an underinflated or ruptured cuff or a leak in the cuff or one-way valve)	• Listen for a whooshing sound around the tube, indicating an air leak. If you hear one, check cuff pressure. If you can't maintain pressure, call the doctor; he may need to insert a new tube.
	• Ventilator malfunction	• Disconnect the patient from the ventilator and ventilate him manually if necessary. Obtain another ventilator.
	• Leak in ventilator circuitry (from loose connection or hole in tubing, loss of temperature-sensitive device, or cracked humidification jar)	• Make sure all connections are intact. Check for holes or leaks in the tubing and replace if necessary. Check the humidification jar and replace if cracked.
High-pressure alarm	• Increased airway pressure or decreased lung compliance caused by worsening disease	• Auscultate the lungs for evidence of increasing lung consolidation, barotrauma, or wheezing. Call the doctor if indicated.
	• Patient is biting on oral endotracheal tube	• Insert a bite block if needed.
	• Secretions in airway	• Look for secretions in the airway. To remove them, suction the patient or have him cough.
	• Condensate in large-bore tubing	• Check tubing for condensate and remove any fluid.

Responding to ventilator alarms (continued)

SIGNAL	POSSIBLE CAUSE	INTERVENTIONS
High-pressure alarm (continued)	• Intubation of right mainstem bronchus	• Check tube position. If it has slipped, call the doctor; he may need to reposition it.
	• Patient coughing, gagging, or attempting to talk	• If the patient fights the ventilator, the doctor may order a sedative or neuromuscular blocking agent.
	• Chest wall resistance	• Reposition the patient if it improves chest expansion. If repositioning doesn't help, administer the prescribed analgesic.
	• Failure of high-pressure relief valve	• Have the faulty equipment replaced.
	• Bronchospasm	• Assess the patient for the cause. Report to the doctor and treat as ordered.

commode. Determine whether the patient needs to travel; if so, select appropriate portable and backup equipment.
• Before discharge, have the patient's caregiver demonstrate his ability to use the equipment. At discharge, contact a durable medical equipment vendor and a home health nurse to follow up with the patient. Also refer the patient to community resources, if available.

Documentation
• Document the date and time of initiation of mechanical ventilation.
• Name the type of ventilator used for the patient and note its settings.
• Describe the patient's subjective and objective response to mechanical ventilation (including vital signs, breath sounds, use of accessory muscles, intake and output, and weight).

• List any complications and nursing actions taken.
• Record all pertinent laboratory data, including ABG analysis results and oxygen saturation levels.
• During weaning, record the date and time of each session; the weaning method; and baseline and subsequent vital signs, oxygen saturation levels, and ABG values. Again describe the patient's subjective and objective responses (including level of consciousness, respiratory effort, arrhythmias, skin color, and need for suctioning).
• List all complications and nursing actions taken. If the patient was receiving pressure support ventilation (PSV) or using a T-piece or tracheostomy collar, note the duration of spontaneous breathing and the patient's ability to maintain the weaning sched-

ule. If using intermittent mandatory ventilation, with or without PSV, record the control breath rate, the time of each breath reduction, and the rate of spontaneous respirations.

Mixed venous oxygen saturation

Monitoring mixed venous oxygen saturation ($S\bar{v}O_2$) allows rapid detection of impaired oxygen delivery, such as from decreased cardiac output, hemoglobin level, or arterial oxygen saturation. It's also used to aid evaluation of a patient's response to drug administration, endotracheal tube suctioning, ventilator setting changes, positive end-expiratory pressure, and fraction of inspired oxygen.

Monitoring is done with a fiber-optic thermodilution pulmonary artery catheter. $S\bar{v}O_2$ saturation usually ranges from 60% to 80%, with the normal value being 75%.

≫ Key nursing diagnoses and patient outcomes

Use these nursing diagnoses as a guide when developing your plan of care.

Impaired gas exchange related to altered oxygen supply

Based on this nursing diagnosis, establish the following patient outcomes. The patient will:
• maintain respiratory rate within +/- 5 of baseline.
• express feeling of comfort while maintaining air exchange.
• have normal breath sounds.

• have ABG levels that return to baseline: (specify) pH; (specify) PaO_2; (specify) $PaCO_2$.

Altered cardiopulmonary tissue perfusion related to decreased cellular exchange

Based on this nursing diagnosis, establish the following patient outcomes. The patient will:
• attain hemodynamic stability as evidenced by: pulse not less than __ beats/minute and not greater than __ beats/minute, blood pressure not less than __mm Hg and not greater than __mm Hg, respirations +/- 5 breaths/minute of baseline rate.
• have warm and dry skin.
• maintain adequate cardiac output.
• not experience arrythmias.
• have an $S\bar{v}O_2$ saturation ranging from 60% to 80%.

Equipment

♦ fiber-optic pulmonary artery (PA) catheter ♦ CO-oximeter monitor ♦ optical module and cable ♦ gloves.

Equipment preparation

• Review the manufacturer's instructions for assembly and use of the fiber-optic PA catheter.
• Connect the optical module and cable to the monitor.
• Peel back the wrapping covering the catheter just enough to uncover the fiber-optic connector. Attach the fiber-optic connector to the optical module; keep the rest of the catheter in its sterile wrapping.
• Calibrate the fiber-optic catheter by following the manufacturer's instructions. (See *$S\bar{v}O_2$ monitoring equipment.*)

S$\overline{v}$O$_2$ monitoring equipment

The S$\overline{v}$O$_2$ monitoring system consists of a flow-directed pulmonary artery (PA) catheter with fiber-optic filaments, an optical module, and a CO-oximeter. The CO-oximeter displays a continuous digital S$\overline{v}$O$_2$ value; the strip recorder prints a permanent record.

Catheter insertion follows the same technique as with any thermodilution flow-directed PA catheter. The distal lumen connects to an external PA pressure monitoring system; the proximal or central venous pressure (CVP) lumen connects to another monitoring system or to a continuous flow administration unit; and the optical module connects to the CO-oximeter unit.

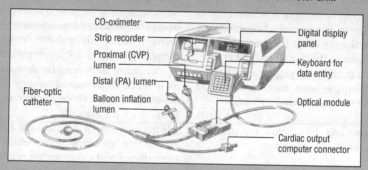

CO-oximeter
Strip recorder
Proximal (CVP) lumen
Distal (PA) lumen
Fiber-optic catheter
Balloon inflation lumen
Digital display panel
Keyboard for data entry
Optical module
Cardiac output computer connector

Normal SvO$_2$ waveform

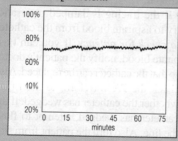

S$\overline{v}$O$_2$ with patient activities

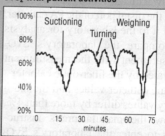

S$\overline{v}$O$_2$ with PEEP and F$_{IO_2}$ changes

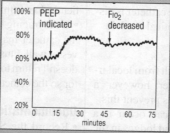

Patient preparation

• Explain the procedure to the patient to allay fears and promote the patient's cooperation.

Implementation

• Wash your hands and put on gloves.
• Assist with insertion of the fiber-optic catheter as you would for a PA catheter.
• Once the catheter is inserted, confirm that the light intensity tracing on the graphic printout is within normal range to ensure correct position and functioning of the catheter.
• Observe the digital readout and record the $S\overline{v}O_2$ on graph paper. Repeat readings at least once each hour *to monitor and document trends*.
• Set the machine alarms at 10% above and 10% below the patient's current $S\overline{v}O_2$ reading.

To recalibrate the monitor

• Draw a mixed venous blood sample from the distal port of the PA catheter. Send it to the laboratory for analysis to compare the laboratory's $S\overline{v}O_2$ measurement with the measurement indicated by the fiber-optic catheter.
• If the catheter values and the laboratory values differ by more than 4%, follow the manufacturer's instructions to enter the laboratory's $S\overline{v}O_2$ value into the oximeter.
• Recalibrate the monitor every 24 hours, or whenever the catheter is disconnected from the optical module.

Complications

• Thrombosis can result from local irritation by the catheter; however, a heparinized flush helps prevent this.
• Thromboembolism can occur if a thrombus breaks off and lodges in the circulatory system.

• Monitor the patient for signs and symptoms of infection — such as redness or drainage — at the catheter site.

Nursing considerations

• If the patient's $S\overline{v}O_2$ drops below 60%, or if it varies by more than 10% for 3 minutes or longer, reassess the patient. If the $S\overline{v}O_2$ does not return to the baseline value after appropriate nursing interventions, notify the doctor. *A decreasing $S\overline{v}O_2$, or a value less than 60%, indicates impaired oxygen delivery, which may be due to hemorrhage, hypoxia, shock, arrhythmias, or suctioning. $S\overline{v}O_2$ can also decrease as a result of increased oxygen demand due to hyperthermia, shivering, or seizures, for example.*
• If the intensity of the tracing is low, ensure that all connections between the catheter and oximeter are secure and that the catheter is patent and not kinked.
• If the tracing is damped or erratic, try to aspirate blood from the catheter *to check for patency*. If you can't aspirate blood, notify the patient's doctor so that the catheter can be replaced. Also check the PA waveform to determine whether the catheter has wedged. If the catheter has wedged, attempt to flush the line. Also turn the patient from side to side and instruct him to cough. If the catheter remains wedged, notify the patient's doctor immediately.
• If the tracing shows a high intensity, the catheter may be pressing against a vessel wall. Flush the line. If the tracing doesn't return to normal, notify the doctor so the catheter can be repositioned.

Documentation

• Record the $S\overline{v}O_2$ value on a flowchart and attach a tracing, as ordered.

At the same time, note any significant changes in the patient's status and the results of any medical or nursing interventions. For comparison, note the $S\bar{v}O_2$ as measured by the fiber-optic catheter whenever a blood sample is obtained for laboratory analysis of mixed venous oxygen saturation.

Mouth care

Given in the morning, at bedtime, or after meals, mouth care entails brushing and flossing the teeth and inspecting the mouth. It removes soft plaque deposits and calculus from the teeth, cleans and massages the gums, reduces mouth odor, and helps prevent infection. By freshening the patient's mouth, mouth care also enhances appreciation of food, thereby aiding appetite and nutrition.

Although the ambulatory patient can usually perform mouth care alone, the bedridden patient may require partial or full assistance. The comatose patient requires use of suction equipment to prevent aspiration during oral care.

≫ Key nursing diagnoses and patient outcomes

Use these nursing diagnoses as a guide when developing your plan of care for a patient who requires mouth care.

Altered oral mucous membrane related to (specify)

Based on this nursing diagnosis, you'll establish the following patient outcomes. The patient will:
• state increased comfort.
• maintain pink and moist oral mucous membranes.

• explain oral care routine.

Bathing/hygiene self-care deficit related to (specify)

Based on this nursing diagnosis, you'll establish the following patient outcomes. The patient will:
• communicate feelings about limitations.
• have self-care needs met.
• achieve highest functional level.

Equipment

♦ towel or facial tissues ♦ emesis basin ♦ trash bag ♦ mouthwash ♦ toothbrush and toothpaste ♦ pitcher and glass ♦ drinking straw ♦ dental floss ♦ gloves ♦ dental floss holder if available ♦ small mirror if necessary ♦ optional: oral irrigating device.

For the comatose or debilitated patient as needed: ♦ linen-saver pad ♦ bite-block ♦ petroleum jelly ♦ hydrogen peroxide ♦ mineral oil ♦ cotton-tipped mouth swab ♦ oral suction equipment or gauze pads ♦ optional: lemon-glycerin swabs or mouth care kit, tongue blade, $4'' \times 4''$ gauze pads, adhesive tape.

Equipment preparation

• Fill a pitcher with water, and bring it and other equipment to the patient's bedside.
• If you'll be using oral suction equipment, connect the tubing to the suction bottle and suction catheter, insert the plug into an outlet, and check for correct operation.
• If necessary, devise a bite-block to protect yourself from being bitten during the procedure. Wrap a gauze pad over the end of a tongue blade, fold

the edge in, and secure it with adhesive tape.

Patient preparation
- Explain the procedure to the patient.
- Provide privacy.

Implementation
- Wash your hands.
- Put on gloves.

Supervising mouth care
- For the bedridden patient capable of self-care, encourage him to perform his own mouth care.
- If allowed, place the patient in Fowler's position. Place the overbed table in front of the patient, and arrange the equipment on it. Open the table and set up the built-in mirror if available, or position a small mirror on the table.
- Drape a towel over the patient's chest to protect his gown. Instruct him to floss his teeth while looking into the mirror.
- Observe the patient *to be sure he's flossing correctly,* and correct him if necessary. Tell him to wrap the floss around the second or third fingers of both hands. Starting with his back teeth and without injuring the gums, he should insert the floss as far as possible into the space between each pair of teeth. Then he should clean the surfaces of adjacent teeth by pulling the floss up and down against the side of each tooth. After the patient flosses a pair of teeth, remind him to use a clean 1″ (2.5-cm) section of floss for the next pair.
- After the patient flosses, mix mouthwash and water in a glass, place a straw in the glass, and position the emesis basin nearby. Then instruct the patient to brush his teeth and gums while looking into the mirror. Encourage

him to rinse frequently during brushing, and provide facial tissues for him to wipe his mouth.

Performing mouth care
- For the comatose patient or the conscious patient incapable of self-care, you'll perform mouth care. If the patient wears dentures, clean them thoroughly. (See *Dealing with dentures.*)

Some patients may benefit from using an oral irrigating device, such as a Water Pik. (See *Using an oral irrigating device,* page 528.)
- Raise the bed to a comfortable working height *to prevent back strain.* Then lower the head of the bed, and position the patient on his side, with his face extended over the edge of the pillow *to facilitate drainage and prevent fluid aspiration.*
- Arrange the equipment on the overbed table or bedside stand, including the oral suction equipment, if necessary. Turn on the machine. If a suction machine isn't available, wipe the inside of the patient's mouth frequently with a gauze pad.
- Place a linen-saver pad under the patient's chin and an emesis basin near his cheek *to absorb or catch drainage.*
- Lubricate the patient's lips with petroleum jelly *to prevent dryness and cracking.* Reapply lubricant as needed during oral care.
- If necessary, insert the bite-block *to hold the patient's mouth open during oral care.*
- Using a dental floss holder, hold the floss against each tooth and direct it as close to the gum as possible without injuring the sensitive tissues around the tooth.

Dealing with dentures

Prostheses made of acrylic resins, vinyl composites, or both, dentures replace some or all of the patient's natural teeth. Dentures require proper care to remove soft plaque deposits and calculus and to reduce mouth odor. Dentures must be removed from the comatose or presurgical patient to prevent possible airway obstruction.

Preparation

Start by assembling the following equipment: emesis basin ♦ labeled denture cup ♦ toothbrush or denture brush ♦ gloves ♦ toothpaste ♦ denture cleaner ♦ paper towel ♦ cotton-tipped ♦ mouthwash ♦ gauze ♦ optional: adhesive denture liner. Wash your hands and put on gloves.

Removing dentures

• To remove a full upper denture, grasp the front and palatal surfaces of the denture with your thumb and forefinger. Position the index finger of your opposite hand over the upper border of the denture, and press *to break the seal between denture and palate.* Grasp the denture with gauze *because saliva can make it slippery.*

• To remove a full lower denture, grasp the front and lingual surfaces of the denture with your thumb and index finger, and gently lift up.

• To remove partial dentures, first ask the patient or a caregiver how the prothesis is retained and how to remove it. If the partial denture is held in place with clips or snaps, then exert equal pressure on the border of each side of the denture. Avoid lifting the clasps, *which easily bend or break.*

Oral and denture care

• After removing dentures, place them in a properly labeled denture cup. Add warm water and a commercial denture cleaner *to remove stains and hardened deposits.* Follow package directions. Avoid soaking dentures in mouthwash containing alcohol *because it may damage a soft liner.*

• Instruct the patient to rinse his mouth with mouthwash. Then stroke the palate, buccal surfaces, gums, and tongue with a soft toothbrush or cotton-tipped mouth swab. Inspect for irritated areas or sores *because they may indicate a poorly fitting denture.*

• Line the sink basin with a paper towel and fill it with water *to cushion the dentures in case you drop them.* Hold the dentures over the basin, wet them with warm water, and apply toothpaste to a denture brush or long-bristled toothbrush. Clean the dentures using only moderate pressure and warm water.

• Clean the denture cup, and place the dentures in it. Rinse the brush, and clean and dry the emesis basin. Return all equipment to the patient's bedside stand.

Inserting dentures

• If the patient desires, apply adhesive liner to the dentures. Moisten them with water, if necessary, *to reduce friction and ease insertion.*

• Encourage the patient to wear his dentures *to enhance his appearance, facilitate eating and speaking, and prevent changes in the gum line that may affect denture fit.*

Using an oral irrigating device

An oral irrigating device such as the Water Pik directs a pulsating jet of water around the teeth to massage gums and remove debris and food particles. It's especially useful for cleaning areas missed by brushing, such as around bridgework, crowns, and dental wires. Because this device enhances oral hygiene, it benefits patients undergoing head and neck irradiation, which can damage teeth and cause severe caries. The device also maintains oral hygiene in a patient with a fractured jaw or with mouth injuries that limit standard mouth care.

Equipment
To use the device, first assemble the following equipment: ◆ oral irrigating device ◆ towel ◆ emesis basin ◆ pharyngeal suction apparatus ◆ salt solution or mouthwash if ordered ◆ soap.

Implementation
• Turn the patient to his side *to prevent aspiration of water.* Then, place a towel under his chin and an emesis basin next to his cheek *to absorb or catch drainage.*
• Insert the oral irrigating device's plug into a nearby electrical outlet. Remove the device's cover, turn it upside down, and fill it with lukewarm water, mouthwash, or salt solution as ordered. When using a salt solution, dissolve the salt beforehand in a separate container. Then pour the solution into the cover.
• Secure the cover to the base of the device. Remove the water hose handle from the base, and snap the jet tip into place. If necessary, wet the grooved end of the tip *to ease insertion.* Adjust the pressure dial to the setting most comfortable for the patient. If his gums are tender and prone to bleed, choose a low setting.
• Adjust the knurled knob on the handle *to direct the water jet,* place the jet tip in the patient's mouth,

and turn on the device. Instruct the alert patient to keep his lips partially closed *to avoid spraying water.*
• Direct the water at a right angle to the gum line of each tooth and between teeth. Avoid directing water under the patient's tongue *because this may injure sensitive tissue.*

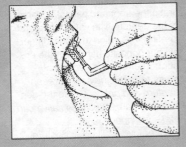

After irrigating each tooth, pause briefly and instruct the patient to expectorate the water or solution into the emesis basin. If he's unable to do so, suction it from the sides of the mouth with the pharyngeal suction apparatus. After irrigating all teeth, turn off the device, and remove the jet tip from the patient's mouth.
• Empty the remaining water or solution from the cover, remove the jet tip from the handle, and return the handle to the base. Clean the jet tip with soap and water, rinse the cover, and dry them both and return them to storage.

• After flossing the patient's teeth, mix mouthwash and water in a glass and place the straw in it.
• Wet the toothbrush with water. If necessary, use hot water *to soften the bristles.* Apply toothpaste.
• Brush the patient's lower teeth from the gum line up, the upper teeth from the gum line down. Place the brush at a 45-degree angle to the gum line, and press the bristles gently into the gingival sulcus. Using short, gentle strokes *to prevent gum damage, brush* the facial surfaces (toward the cheek) and the lingual surfaces (toward the tongue) of the bottom teeth. Use just the tip of the brush for the lingual surfaces of the front teeth. Then, using the same technique, brush the facial and lingual surfaces of the top teeth. Next, brush the biting surfaces of the bottom and top teeth, using a back and forth motion. If possible, ask the patient to rinse frequently during brushing by taking the mouthwash solution through the straw. Hold the emesis basin steady under the patient's cheek, and wipe his mouth and cheeks with facial tissues as needed.
• After brushing the patient's teeth, dip a cotton-tipped mouth swab into the mouthwash solution. Press the swab against the side of the glass to remove excess moisture. Gently stroke the gums, buccal surfaces, palate, and tongue *to clean the mucosa and stimulate circulation.* Replace the swab as necessary for thorough cleaning. Avoid inserting the swab too deeply *to prevent gagging and vomiting.*

After mouth care
• Assess the patient's mouth for cleanliness and tooth and tissue condition. Then remove your gloves, rinse the

toothbrush, and clean the emesis basin and glass. Empty and clean the suction bottle if used, and place a clean suction catheter on the tubing. Return reusable equipment to the appropriate storage location, and properly discard disposable equipment in the trash bag.

Nursing considerations
• Use cotton-tipped mouth swabs to clean the teeth of a patient with sensitive gums. *These swabs produce less friction than a toothbrush but don't clean as well.*
• Clean the mouth of a toothless comatose patient by wrapping a gauze pad around your index finger, moistening it with mouthwash, and gently swabbing the oral tissues. If necessary, moisten gauze pads in an equal mixture of hydrogen peroxide and water *to remove tenacious mucus.*
• Remember that mucous membranes dry quickly in the patient breathing through his mouth or receiving oxygen therapy. Moisten his mouth and lips regularly with mineral oil, lemon-glycerin swabs, or water. If you use water as the lubricant, place a short straw in a glass of water and stop the open end with your finger. Remove the straw from the water and, with your finger in place, position it in the patient's mouth. Release your finger slightly to let the water flow out gradually. If the patient is comatose, suction excess water *to prevent aspiration.*

Documentation
• Record the date and time of mouth care in your notes.
• Document any unusual conditions, such as bleeding, edema, mouth odor, excessive secretions, or plaque on the tongue.

N

Nasal irrigation

Irrigation of the nasal passages soothes irritated mucous membranes and washes away crusted mucus, secretions, and foreign matter. Left unattended, these deposits may impede sinus drainage and nasal airflow and cause headaches, infections, and unpleasant odors. Irrigation may be done with a bulb syringe or an electronic oral irrigating device.

Nasal irrigation benefits patients with either acute or chronic nasal conditions, including sinusitis, rhinitis, Wegener's granulomatosis, and Sjögren's syndrome. In addition, the procedure may help people who regularly inhale toxins or allergens — paint fumes, sawdust, pesticides, or coal dust, for example. Nasal irrigation is routinely recommended after some nasal surgeries *to enhance healing by removal of postoperative eschar and to aid remucosolization of the sinus cavities and ostia.*

Contraindications for nasal irrigation may include advanced destruction of the sinuses, frequent nosebleeds, and foreign bodies in the nasal passages (which could be driven farther into the passages by the irrigant). However, some patients with these conditions may benefit from irrigation.

❯❯ Key nursing diagnoses and patient outcomes

Use these nursing diagnoses as a guide when developing your plan of care for a patient who is receiving nasal irrigation.

Risk for infection related to (specify)

Based on this nursing diagnosis, you'll establish the following patient outcomes. The patient will:
• maintain a normal body temperature.
• show no signs and symptoms of infection.
• communicate understanding of signs and symptoms to report to nurse or doctor.

Knowledge deficit related to lack of exposure to procedure

Based on this nursing diagnosis, you'll establish the following patient outcomes. The patient will:
• communicate a desire to become informed about procedure.
• correctly return demonstrate procedure if to be performed independently in home.

Equipment

♦ bulb syringe or an oral irrigating device (such as a Water Pik) ♦ rigid or flexible disposable irrigation tips (for one-patient use) ♦ hypertonic saline solution ♦ plastic sheet ♦ apron or towels ♦ facial tissues ♦ bath basin ♦ gloves.

Equipment preparation

• Warm the saline solution to about 105° F (40.5° C).
• If you'll be irrigating with a bulb syringe, draw some irrigant into the bulb and then expel it. *This will rinse any*

residual solution from the previous irrigation and warm the bulb.

• If you're using an oral irrigating device, plug it into an electrical outlet in an area near the patient. Then run about 1 cup (240 ml) of saline solution through the tubing *to rinse residual solution from the lines and warm the tubing.* Next, fill the reservoir of the device with warm saline solution.

Patient preparation

• Explain the procedure to the patient.
• Have the patient sit comfortably near the equipment in a position that allows the bulb or catheter tip to enter his nose and the returning irrigant to flow into the bath basin or sink. (See *Positioning the patient for nasal irrigation.*)
• Remind the patient to keep his mouth open and to breathe rhythmically during irrigation. This causes the soft palate to seal the throat, allowing the irrigant to stream out the opposite nostril and carry discharge with it.
• Instruct the patient not to speak or swallow during the irrigation *to avoid forcing infectious material into the sinuses or eustachian tubes.*
• *To avoid injuring the nasal mucosa,* remove the irrigating tip from the patient's nostril if he reports the need to sneeze or cough.

Implementation

• Wash your hands and put on gloves.

To use a bulb syringe

• Fill the bulb syringe with saline solution and insert the tip about ½" (1.3 cm) into the patient's nostril.
• Squeeze the bulb until a gentle stream of warm irrigant washes through the nose. Avoid forceful

Positioning the patient for nasal irrigation

Whether you're teaching a patient to perform nasal irrigation with a bulb syringe or an oral irrigating device, the irrigation will progress more easily once the patient learns how to hold her head for safety, comfort, and effectiveness.

Help the patient to sit upright with her head bent forward over the basin or sink and well-flexed on her chest. Her nose and ear should be on the same vertical plane.

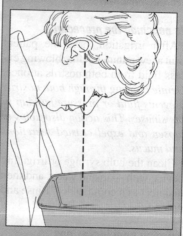

Explain that she's less likely to breathe in the irrigant when holding her head in this position. Additionally, this position should keep the irrigant from entering the eustachian tubes, which will now lie above the level of the irrigation stream.

squeezing, *which may drive debris from the nasal passages into the sinuses or eustachian tubes and introduce infection.* Alternate the nostrils until the return irrigant runs clear.

To use an oral irrigation device

• Insert the irrigation tip into the nostril about ½" to 1" (1.3 to 2.5 cm), and turn on the irrigating device. Begin with a low pressure setting (increasing the pressure as needed) *to obtain a gentle stream of irrigant.* Again, be careful not to drive material from the nose into the sinuses or eustachian tubes. Irrigate both nostrils.
• Inspect returning irrigant. Changes in color, viscosity, or volume may signal an infection and should be reported to the doctor. Also report blood or necrotic material.

To conclude the procedure

• After irrigation, have the patient wait a few minutes before blowing excess fluid from both nostrils at once. *Gentle blowing through both nostrils prevents fluid or pressure buildup in the sinuses. This action also helps to loosen and expel crusted secretions and mucus.*
• Clean the bulb syringe or irrigating device with soap and water, and then disinfect as recommended. Rinse and dry.

Nursing considerations

• Expect fluid to drain from the patient's nose for a brief time after the irrigation and before he blows his nose.
• Be sure to insert the irrigation tip far enough to ensure that the irrigant cleans the nasal membranes before draining out. A typical amount of irrigant ranges from 500 to 1,000 ml.

Home care

• To continue nasal irrigations at home, teach the patient how to prepare saline solution.

• Tell him to fill a clean 1 qt (1 L) plastic bottle with bottled or distilled water, add 1½ tsp of canning salt, and shake the solution until the salt dissolves.
• Teach him how to disinfect used irrigation devices.

Documentation

• Write down the time and duration of the procedure and the amount of irrigant used.
• Describe the appearance of the returned solution.
• Record your assessment of the patient's comfort level and breathing ease before and after the procedure.
• Document patient-teaching content.

Nasal medication instillation

Nasal medications are instilled by means of drops, a spray (using an atomizer), or an aerosol (using a nebulizer). Most drugs instilled by these methods produce local rather than systemic effects. Drops can be directed at a specific area; sprays and aerosols diffuse medication throughout the nasal passages.

Most nasal medications such as phenylephrine are vasoconstrictors, which relieve nasal congestion by coating and shrinking swollen mucous membranes. Because vasoconstrictors may be absorbed systemically, they are usually contraindicated in hypertensive patients. Other types of nasal medications include antiseptics, anesthetics, and corticosteroids. Local anesthetics may be administered to promote patient comfort during rhinolaryngologic examination, laryngoscopy, bronchoscopy, and endotracheal intubation. Corticosteroids reduce inflammation in allergic or inflammatory conditions and in nasal polyps.

≫ Key nursing diagnoses and patient outcomes

Use these nursing diagnoses as a guide when developing your plan of care for a patient receiving nasal medications.

Knowledge deficit related to lack of exposure

Based on this nursing diagnosis, you'll establish these patient outcomes. The patient will:
• state or demonstrate understanding of what has been taught.
• demonstrate ability to perform new health-related behaviors as they are taught.

High risk for injury related to improper technique

Based on this nursing diagnosis, you'll establish the following patient outcomes. The patient will:
• identify factors that increase risk for injury.
• assist in identifying and applying safety measures to prevent injury.

Equipment

♦ prescribed medication ♦ patient's medication record and chart ♦ emesis basin (with nose drops only) ♦ facial tissues ♦ optional: pillow, small piece of soft rubber or plastic tubing, gloves.

Patient preparation

• Explain the procedure to the patient and provide privacy.

Implementation

• Verify the order on the patient's medication record by checking it against the doctor's order. Note the concentration of the medication. Phenylephrine, for example, is available in various concentrations from 0.125% to 1%.
• Confirm the patient's identity by asking his name and checking the name, room number, and bed number on his wristband.
• Wash your hands. Don gloves if you notice any drainage from the nares.

Instilling nose drops

• When possible, position the patient so the drops flow back into the nostrils, toward the affected area. (See *Positioning the patient for nose drop instillation,* page 534.)
• Draw up some medication into the dropper.
• Push up the tip of the patient's nose slightly. Position the dropper just above the nostril, and direct its tip toward the midline of the nose *so the drops flow toward the back of the nasal cavity rather than down the throat.*
• Insert the dropper about ⅜" (1 cm) into the nostril. Make sure the dropper doesn't touch the sides of the nostril *because this would contaminate the dropper or could cause the patient to sneeze.*
• Instill the prescribed number of drops, observing the patient carefully for any signs of discomfort.
• *To prevent the drops from leaking out of the nostrils,* ask the patient to keep his head tilted back for at least 5 minutes and to breathe through his mouth. *This also allows sufficient time for the medication to constrict mucous membranes.*

Positioning the patient for nose drop instillation

To reach the ethmoidal and sphenoidal sinuses, have the patient lie on his back with his neck hyperextended and his head tilted back over the edge of the bed. Support his head with one hand to prevent neck strain.

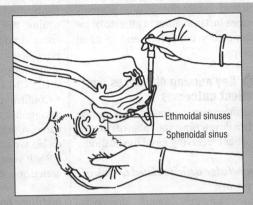

Ethmoidal sinuses
Sphenoidal sinus

To reach the maxillary and frontal sinuses, have the patient lie on his back with his head toward the affected side and hanging slightly over the edge of the bed. Ask him to rotate his head laterally after hyperextension, and support his head with one hand to prevent neck strain.

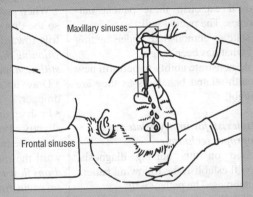

Maxillary sinuses
Frontal sinuses

To administer drops to relieve ordinary nasal congestion, help the patient to a reclining or supine position with his head tilted slightly toward the affected side. Aim the dropper upward, toward the patient's eye, rather than downward toward his ear.

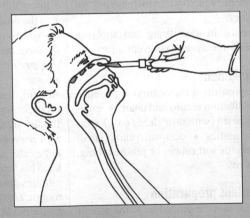

• Keep an emesis basin handy *so the patient can expectorate any medication that flows into the oropharynx and mouth.* Use a facial tissue to wipe any excess medication from the patient's nostrils and face.

• Clean the dropper by separating the plunger and pipette and flushing them with warm water. Allow them to air-dry.

Using a nasal spray

• Have the patient sit upright with his head tilted back slightly. If this position is uncomfortable, have the patient lie on his back with his shoulders elevated, neck hyperextended, and head tilted back over the edge of the bed. Support his head with one hand *to prevent neck strain.*

• Remove the protective cap from the atomizer.

• *To prevent air from entering the nasal cavity and to allow the medication to flow in properly,* occlude one of the patient's nostrils with your finger. Insert the atomizer tip into the open nostril.

• Instruct the patient to inhale, and as he does so, squeeze the atomizer once, quickly and firmly. Use just enough force to coat the inside of the patient's nose with medication. Then tell the patient to exhale through his mouth.

• If ordered, spray the nostril again. Then repeat the procedure in the other nostril.

• Instruct the patient to keep his head tilted back for several minutes and to breathe slowly through his nose *so the medication has time to work.* Tell him not to blow his nose for several minutes.

Using a nasal aerosol

• Instruct the patient to blow his nose gently *to clear his nostrils.*

• Insert the medication cartridge according to the manufacturer's directions. With some models, you'll fit the medication cartridge over a small hole in the adapter. When inserting a refill cartridge, first remove the protective cap from the stem. Spacer inhalers may be recommended.

• Shake the aerosol well immediately before each use, and remove the protective cap from the adapter tip.

• Hold the aerosol between your thumb and index finger with your index finger positioned on top of the medication cartridge.

• Tilt the patient's head back, and carefully insert the adapter tip in one nostril while sealing the other nostril with your finger.

• Press the adapter and cartridge together firmly *to release one measured dose of medication.*

• Shake the aerosol and repeat the procedure to instill medication into the other nostril.

• Remove the medication cartridge and wash the nasal adapter in lukewarm water daily. Allow the adapter to dry thoroughly before reinserting the cartridge.

Complications

Some nasal medications may cause:
• restlessness
• palpitations
• nervousness
• other systemic effects.

As for systemic effects, excessive use of corticosteroid aerosols, for instance, may cause hyperadrenocorticism and adrenal suppression.

Nursing considerations

- Before instilling nose drops in a young child or an uncooperative patient, attach a small piece of tubing to the end of the dropper *to avoid damaging mucous membranes.*
- When using an aerosol, be careful not to puncture or incinerate the pressurized cartridge. Store it at temperatures below 120° F (48.9° C).
- *To prevent the spread of infection,* label the medication bottle so that it will be used only for that patient.

Home care

- Ideally, a nasal spray should be self-administered by the patient. Teach the patient how to instill nasal medications correctly *so he can continue treatment after discharge* if necessary.
- Caution him against using nasal medications longer than prescribed *because they may cause a rebound effect that worsens the condition.* A rebound effect occurs when the medication loses its effectiveness and relaxes the vessels in the nasal turbinates, producing a stuffiness that can be relieved only by discontinuing the medication.
- Inform the patient of possible adverse reactions. For example, explain that when receiving corticosteroids by aerosol therapy, therapeutic effects may not appear for 2 days to 2 weeks.

Documentation

- Record the medication instilled and its concentration, the number of drops or instillations administered, and whether the medication was instilled in one or both nostrils.
- Note the time, date, and any resulting adverse effects.

Nasal packing

In the highly vascular nasal mucosa, even seemingly minor injuries can cause major bleeding and blood loss. When such routine therapeutic measures as direct pressure, cautery, or vasoconstrictive medications fail to control epistaxis (nosebleed), the patient's nose may have to be packed to stop anterior bleeding (which runs out of the nose) or posterior bleeding (which runs down the throat). If blood drains into the nasopharyngeal area or the lacrimal ducts, the patient may appear to bleed from the mouth and eyes as well.

Most nasal bleeding originates at a plexus of arterioles and venules in the anteroinferior septum. Only about 1 in 10 nosebleeds occurs in the more vascular posterior nose, which usually bleeds more heavily than the anterior location.

A nurse typically assists a doctor with anterior or posterior nasal packing, depending on the bleeding site (see *Types of nasal packing*) or assists with nasal balloon catheterization, a procedure that applies pressure to a posterior bleeding site (see *Nasal balloon catheters,* page 539).

Whichever procedure the patient undergoes, the nurse should provide ongoing encouragement and support to reduce his discomfort and anxiety. In addition, the nurse should perform ongoing assessment to determine the procedure's success and detect possible complications.

Types of nasal packing

Depending on its source, your patient's nosebleed may be controlled with anterior or posterior nasal packing.

Anterior nasal packing

The doctor may treat an anterior nosebleed by packing the anterior nasal cavity with a 3′ to 4′ (0.9- to 1.2-m) strip of antibiotic-impregnated petroleum gauze or with a nasal tampon.

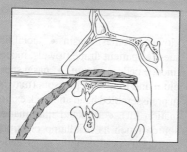

A nasal tampon is made of tightly compressed absorbent material with or without a central breathing tube. The doctor inserts a lubricated tampon along the floor of the nose and, with the patient's head tilted backward, instills 5 to 10 ml of antibiotic or normal saline solution. The tampon expands as a result, stopping the bleeding. It should be moistened periodically, and the central breathing tube should be suctioned regularly.

In a child or a patient with blood dyscrasia, the doctor may fashion an absorbable pack by moistening a gauzelike, regenerated cellulose material with a vasoconstrictor. Applied to a visible bleeding point, this substance will swell to form a clot. Because it's absorbable, the packing doesn't need removal.

Posterior nasal packing

Posterior packing consists of a gauze roll shaped and secured by three sutures (one suture at each end and one in the middle) or a balloon-type catheter. To insert the packing, the doctor advances one or two soft catheters into the patient's nostrils. When the catheter tips appear in the nasopharynx, the doctor grasps them with a Kelly clamp or bayonet forceps and pulls them forward through the patient's mouth. He secures the two end sutures to the catheter tip and draws the catheter back through the patient's nostrils.

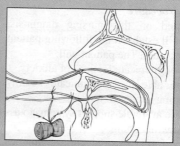

This step brings the packing into place with the end sutures hanging from the patient's nostril. (The middle suture emerges from the patient's mouth to free the packing, when needed.)

The doctor may weight the nose sutures with a clamp. Then he will pull the packing securely into place behind the soft palate and against the posterior end of the septum (nasal choana).

(continued)

Types of nasal packing (continued)

Finally, after he examines the patient's throat (to ensure that the uvula hasn't been forced under the packing), he will insert anterior packing and secure the whole apparatus by tying the posterior pack strings around rolled gauze or a dental roll at the nostrils.

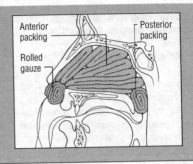

>> Key nursing diagnoses and patient outcomes

Use these nursing diagnoses as a guide when developing your plan of care for a patient who needs nasal packing.

Anxiety related to lack of exposure to procedure

Based on this nursing diagnosis, you'll establish the following patient outcomes. The patient will:
• communicate feelings of anxiety.
• be able to communicate healthy coping strategies.
• use available support systems to assist with coping.
• perform stress-reduction techniques to avoid anxiety symptoms.

Risk for aspiration related to nasal packing

Based on this nursing diagnosis, you'll establish the following patient outcomes. The patient will:
• show no signs of aspiration.
• maintain a patent airway.
• exhibit normal skin color.

Equipment

For anterior and posterior packing:
♦ gowns ♦ goggles ♦ masks ♦ sterile gloves ♦ emesis basin ♦ facial tissues ♦ patient drape (towels, incontinence pads, or gown) ♦ nasal speculum and tongue depressors (may be in preassembled head and neck examination kit) ♦ directed illumination source (such as headlamp or strong flashlight) or fiberoptic nasal endoscopes, light cables, and light source ♦ suction apparatus with sterile suction-connecting tubing and sterile nasal aspirator tip ♦ sterile bowl and sterile saline solution for flushing out suction apparatus ♦ sterile tray or sterile towels ♦ sterile cotton-tipped applicators ♦ local anesthetic spray (topical 4% lidocaine) or vial of local anesthetic solution (such as 2% lidocaine or 1% to 2% lidocaine with epinephrine 1:100,000) ♦ sterile cotton balls or cotton pledgets ♦ 10-ml syringe with 22G 1 ½″ needle ♦ silver nitrate sticks ♦ electrocautery device with grounding plate and small tip ♦ topical nasal decongestant (such as 1½% to 2% phenylephrine or 4% cocaine) ♦ absorbable hemostatic (such as Gelfoam, Avitene, Surgicel, or thrombin) ♦ sterile normal saline solution (1-g container and 60-ml syringe with luer-lock tip, or 5-ml

Nasal balloon catheters

To control epistaxis, the doctor may use a balloon catheter instead of nasal packing. Self-retaining and disposable, the catheter may have a single balloon or a double balloon to apply pressure to bleeding nasal tissues. If bleeding is still uncontrolled, the doctor may choose to use arterial ligation, cryotherapy, or arterial embolization.

Once inserted and inflated, the single-balloon catheter (shown below) compresses the blood vessels while a soft, collapsible external bulb prevents the catheter from dislodging posteriorly.

Anterior nasal balloon catheter

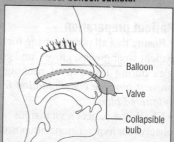

Balloon
Valve
Collapsible bulb

The double-balloon catheter (shown in the next column) is used for simultaneous anterior and posterior nasal packing. It compresses the posterior vessels serving the nose and the posterior bleeding vessels; the anterior balloon compresses bleeding intranasal vessels. This catheter contains a central airway for breathing comfort.

Double nasal balloon for simultaneous anterior and posterior packing

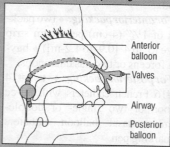

Anterior balloon
Valves
Airway
Posterior balloon

Providing routine care

The tip of the single-balloon catheter will be inserted in the nostrils until it reaches the posterior pharynx. Then, the balloon will be inflated with normal saline solution, pulled gently into the posterior nasopharynx, and secured at the nostrils with the collapsible bulb. With a double-balloon catheter, the posterior balloon is inflated with normal saline solution; then the anterior balloon is inflated.

To check catheter placement, mark the catheter at the nasal vestibule; then inspect for that mark and observe the oropharynx for the posteriorly placed balloon. Assess the nostrils for irritation or erosion. Remove secretions by gently suctioning the airway of a double-balloon catheter or by dabbing away crusted external secretions if the patient has a catheter with no airway.

To prevent damage to nasal tissue, the doctor may order the balloon deflated for 10 minutes every 24 hours. If bleeding recurs or remains uncontrolled, reinflate the balloon and contact the doctor, who may add packing.

bullets for moistening nasal tampons) ♦ hypoallergenic tape ♦ antibiotic ointment ♦ equipment for measuring vital signs ♦ equipment for drawing blood.

For anterior packing: ♦ two packages of $1\frac{1}{2}''$ (4-cm) petroleum strip gauze (3' to 4' [0.9- to 1.2-m]) ♦ bayonet forceps or two nasal tampons.

For posterior packing: ♦ two #14 or #16 French catheters with 30-cc balloon or two single- or double-chamber nasal balloon catheters ♦ marking pen.

For assessment and bedside use: ♦ tongue depressors ♦ flashlight ♦ long hemostats or sponge forceps ♦ 60-ml syringe for deflating balloons (if applicable) ♦ if nasal tampons are in place: saline bullets for applying moisture, small flexible catheters for suctioning central breathing tube ♦ drip pad or moustache dressing supplies ♦ mouth care supplies ♦ water or artificial saliva ♦ external humidification.

Equipment preparation

• Assemble all equipment at the patient's bedside.

• Make sure the headlamp works.

• Plug in the suction apparatus, and connect the tubing from the collection bottle to the suction source.

• Test the suction equipment to make sure it works properly. At the bedside, create a sterile field. (Use the sterile towels or the sterile tray.)

• Using sterile technique, place all sterile equipment on the sterile field.

• If the doctor will inject a local anesthetic rather than spray it into the nose, place the 22G $1\frac{1}{2}''$ needle attached to the 10-ml syringe on the sterile field. When the doctor readies the syringe,

clean the stopper on the anesthetic vial and hold the vial so he can withdraw the anesthetic. This practice allows the doctor to avoid touching his sterile gloves to the nonsterile vial.

• Open the packages containing the sterile suction-connecting tubing and aspirating tip, and place them on the sterile field. Fill the sterile bowl with normal saline solution *so the suction tubing can be flushed as necessary.* Thoroughly lubricate the anterior or posterior packing with antibiotic ointment.

• If the patient needs a nasal balloon catheter, test the balloon for leaks by inflating the catheter with normal saline solution. Remove the solution before insertion.

Patient preparation

• Ensure that all people caring for the patient wear gowns, gloves, and goggles during insertion of packing *to prevent possible contamination from splattered blood.*

• Check the patient's vital signs, and observe for hypotension with postural changes. *Hypotension suggests significant blood loss.* Also monitor airway patency because the patient will be at risk for aspirating or vomiting swallowed blood.

• Explain the procedure to the patient and offer reassurance *to reduce his anxiety and promote cooperation.*

• Administer a sedative or tranquilizer, if ordered, *to reduce the patient's anxiety and decrease sympathetic stimulation, which can exacerbate a nosebleed.*

• Assist the patient to sit with his head tilted forward *to minimize blood drainage into the throat and prevent aspiration.*

Implementation

- Wash your hands.
- Don protective gear.
- Turn on the suction apparatus and attach the connecting tubing *so the doctor can aspirate the nasal cavity to remove clots before locating the bleeding source.*
- To inspect the nasal cavity, the doctor will use a nasal speculum and an external light source, or a fiber-optic nasal endoscope. To remove collected blood and help visualize the bleeding vessel, he will use suction or cotton-tipped applicators. The nose may be treated early with topical vasoconstrictors such as phenylephrine *to slow bleeding and aid visualization.*

For anterior nasal packing

- Help the doctor to apply topical vasoconstricting agents to control bleeding or to use chemical cautery with silver nitrate sticks.
- *To enhance the vasoconstrictor's action,* apply manual pressure to the nose for about 10 minutes.
- If bleeding persists, you may assist with insertion of an absorbable nasal pack directly on the bleeding site. The material will swell, forming an artificial clot.
- Prepare to assist with electrocautery or insertion of anterior nasal packing if these methods fail. (Even if only one side is bleeding, both sides may require packing to apply sufficient pressure to the bleeding site.)
- While the patient has the anterior pack in place, use the cotton-tipped applicators to apply petroleum jelly to his lips and nostrils *to prevent drying and cracking.*

For posterior nasal packing

- Wash your hands and put on sterile gloves.
- If the doctor identifies the bleeding source in the posterior nasal cavity, lubricate the soft catheters *to ease insertion.*
- Instruct the patient to open his mouth and to breathe normally through his mouth during catheter insertion *to minimize gagging as the catheters pass through the nostrils.*
- Assist the doctor, as directed, to insert the packing.
- Help the patient assume a comfortable position with his head elevated 45 to 90 degrees. Assess him for airway obstruction or any respiratory changes.
- Monitor the patient's vital signs regularly *to detect changes that may indicate hypovolemia or hypoxemia.*

Complications

- The pressure of a posterior pack on the soft palate may lead to hypoxemia from stimulation of the sinobronchial reflex.
- Patients with posterior nosebleeds are at special risk for aspiration of blood because posterior packing partially obstructs the upper airway.
- Patients with underlying pulmonary conditions, such as chronic obstructive pulmonary disease or asthma, are at special risk for exacerbation of the condition or for hypoxemia while nasal packing is in place. Hypoxemia can be detected with pulse oximetry. Signs and symptoms include tachycardia, confusion, cyanosis, and restlessness.
- Airway obstruction may occur if a posterior or anterior nasal pack slips backward. The patient may complain

Preventing recurrent nosebleeds

Review the following self-care guidelines to reduce your patient's chances for recurrent nosebleeds:
• Because nosebleeds can result from dry mucous membranes, suggest that the patient use a cool-mist room vaporizer or humidifier as needed, especially in dry environments.
• Teach the patient how to minimize pressure on nasal passages. Advise him, for instance, to avoid constipation and consequent straining during defecation. Recommend a fiber-rich diet and adequate fluid intake, and warn him to forgo extreme physical exertion for 24 hours after the nosebleed stops. Also caution him to avoid aspirin (which has anticoagulant properties), alcoholic beverages, and tobacco for at least 5 days.
• If the patient gets a nosebleed despite these precautions, tell him to keep his head higher than his heart and, using his thumb and forefinger, to press the soft portion of the nostrils together and against the facial bones. (Recommend against direct pressure if he has a facial injury or nasal fracture.) Tell him to maintain pressure for up to 10 minutes and then reassess bleeding. If it's uncontrolled, he should reapply pressure for another 10 minutes with ice between the thumb and forefinger.
• After a nosebleed or after nasal packing is removed, caution the patient to avoid rubbing or picking his nose, putting a handkerchief or tissue in his nose, or blowing his nose forcefully for at least 48 hours. After this time, he may blow his nose gently and use salt-water nasal spray to clear nasal clots.

of difficulty swallowing and pain or discomfort. In patients with posterior packs, otitis media may develop because the pack blocks the eustachian tube openings. Other possible complications include hematotympanum and pressure necrosis of nasal structures, especially the septum.
• Sedation may cause hypotension in a patient with significant blood loss and may also increase the patient's risk of aspiration and hypoxemia

Nursing considerations
• Patients with posterior packing usually are hospitalized for monitoring. If mucosal oozing persists, apply a moustache dressing by securing a folded gauze pad over the nasal vestibules with tape or a commercial nasal dressing holder. Change the pad when soiled.
• Test the patient's call bell to make sure he can summon help if needed. Also keep emergency equipment (flashlight, tongue depressor, syringe, and hemostats) at the patient's bedside *to speed packing removal if it becomes displaced and occludes the airway.*
• Once the packing is in place, compile assessment data carefully to help detect the underlying cause of nosebleeds. Mechanical factors include a deviated septum, injury, and a foreign body. Environmental factors include drying and erosion of the nasal mucosa. Other possible causes are upper respiratory tract infection, anticoagulant or salicylate therapy, blood dyscrasia, cardiovascular or hepatic disorders, tumors of the nasal cavity or paranasal sinuses, chronic nephritis, and familial hemorrhagic telangiectasia.

• If significant blood loss occurs or if the underlying cause remains unknown, expect the doctor to order a complete blood count and coagulation profile as soon as possible. Blood transfusion may be necessary. After the procedure, the doctor may order arterial blood gas analysis to detect any pulmonary complications and arterial oxygen saturation monitoring to assess for hypoxemia. If necessary, prepare to administer supplemental humidified oxygen with a face mask, and give antibiotics and decongestants as ordered.

• Because a patient with nasal packing must breathe through his mouth, provide thorough mouth care often. Artificial saliva, room humidification, and ample fluid intake also relieve dryness caused by mouth breathing.

• Until the pack is removed, the patient should be on modified bed rest. As ordered, administer moderate doses of nonaspirin analgesics and sedatives along with prophylactic antibiotics *to prevent sinusitis or related infections.*

• Nasal packing is usually removed in 2 to 5 days. After an anterior pack is removed, instruct the patient to avoid rubbing or picking his nose, inserting any object (such as a handkerchief or tissue) into his nose, and blowing his nose forcefully for 48 hours or as ordered.

Home care
• Tell the patient to expect reduced smell and taste ability.

• Make sure he has a working smoke detector at home.

• Advise him to eat soft foods because his eating and swallowing abilities will be impaired.

• Instruct him to drink fluids often or to use artificial saliva to cope with dry mouth.

• Teach him measures to prevent nosebleeds and tell him to seek medical help if these measures fail to stop bleeding. (See *Preventing recurrent nosebleeds.*)

Documentation
• Record the type of pack used to ensure its removal at the appropriate time.

• On the intake and output record, document the estimated blood loss and all fluid administered.

• Note the patient's vital signs, his response to sedation or position changes, the results of any laboratory tests, and any drugs administered, including topical agents.

• Record any unusual findings or complications.

• Document charge instructions and clinical follow-up plans.

Nasoenteric-decompression tube care

The patient with a nasoenteric-decompression tube needs special care and continuous monitoring to ensure tube patency, to maintain suction and bowel decompression, and to detect such complications as fluid-electrolyte imbalances related to aspiration of intestinal contents. Precise intake and output records form an integral part of the patient's care. Frequent mouth and nose care is also essential to provide comfort and to prevent skin breakdown. Finally, a patient with a nasoenteric-decompression tube will need encouragement and support during insertion and removal of the tube and while the tube is in place.

>> Key nursing diagnoses and patient outcomes

Use these nursing diagnoses as a guide when developing your plan of care for a patient who needs nasoenteric decompression.

Risk for fluid volume deficit related to enteric decompression

Based on this nursing diagnosis, you'll establish the following patient outcomes. The patient will:
• maintain normal vital signs and skin color and turgor.
• maintain urine output of at least (specify) ml/hr.
• have an output equal to or more than intake.
• maintain normal electrolyte levels.

Risk for impaired skin integrity related to presence of nasoenteric tube

Based on this nursing diagnosis, you'll establish the following patient outcomes. The patient will:
• show no signs of skin breakdown in nares.
• maintain adequate circulation to nares.
• report no signs of discomfort at nares.

Anxiety related to presence of nasoenteric-decompression tube

Based on this nursing diagnosis, you'll establish the following patient outcomes. The patient will:
• verbalize feelings of anxiety.

• ask questions related to plan of care in an attempt to decrease anxiety.
• use available support systems to assist with coping.
• perform stress-reduction techniques to avoid anxiety symptoms.

Equipment

♦ suction apparatus with intermittent suction capability (stationary or portable unit) ♦ container of water ♦ intake and output record sheets ♦ mouthwash and water mixture ♦ lemon-glycerin swabs ♦ petroleum jelly or water-soluble lubricant ♦ cotton-tipped applicators ♦ safety pin ♦ tape or rubber band ♦ disposable irrigation set ♦ irrigant ♦ labels for tube lumens ♦ optional: throat comfort measures such as gargle, viscous lidocaine, sour hard candy, throat lozenges, ice collar, or chewing gum.

Equipment preparation

• Assemble the suction apparatus and set up the suction unit.
• If indicated, test the unit by turning it on and placing the end of the suction tubing in a container of water. If the tubing draws in water, the unit works.

Patient preparation

• Explain to the patient and his family the purpose of the procedure.
• Answer questions clearly and thoroughly *to ease anxiety and enhance cooperation.*

Implementation

• After inserting the tube, have the patient lie quietly on his right side for about 2 hours *to promote the tube's passage.* After the tube advances past the pylorus, the patient's activity level may increase as ordered.

• After the tube advances to the desired position, coil the excess external tubing and secure it to the patient's gown or bed linens with a safety pin attached to tape or a rubber band looped around the tubing. *This may prevent kinks in the tubing, which would interrupt suction.* And once in the desired location, the tube may be taped to the patient's face.

• Maintain slack in the tubing *so the patient can move comfortably and safely in bed.* Show him how far he can move without dislodging the tube.

• After securing the tube, connect it to the tubing on the suction machine *to begin decompression.*

• Check the suction machine at least every 2 hours *to confirm proper functioning and to ensure continued tube patency and bowel decompression.* Excessive negative pressure may draw the mucosa into the tube openings, impair the suction's effectiveness, and injure the mucosa. By using intermittent suction, you may circumvent these problems. To check functioning in an intermittent suction unit, look for drainage in the connecting tube and for drainage dripping into the collecting container. Empty the container every 8 hours and measure the contents.

• After decompression and before extubation, as ordered, provide a clear-to-full liquid diet *to assess bowel function.*

• Record intake and output accurately *to monitor the patient's fluid balance.* If you irrigate the tube, its length may prohibit aspiration of the irrigant, so record the amount of instilled irrigant as "intake." Typically, normal saline solution supersedes water as the preferred irrigant because water, which is hypotonic, may increase electrolyte loss through osmotic action, especially if you irrigate the tube often.

• Observe the patient for signs and symptoms of disorders related to suctioning and intubation. These signs and symptoms may suggest dehydration, a fluid-volume deficit, or a fluid-electrolyte imbalance: dry skin and mucous membranes, decreased urine output, lethargy, exhaustion, and fever.

• Watch for signs and symptoms of pneumonia related to the patient's inability to clear his pharynx or cough effectively with a tube in place. Be alert for fever, chest pain, tachypnea or labored breathing, and diminished breath sounds over the affected area.

• Observe drainage characteristics, including amount, color, consistency, odor, and any unusual changes.

• Provide mouth care frequently (at least every 4 hours). *This increases patient comfort and promotes a healthy oral cavity. If the tube remains in place for several days, mouth-breathing will leave the patient's lips, tongue, and other tissues dry and cracked.*

• Encourage the patient to brush his teeth or rinse his mouth with the mouthwash and water mixture.

• Lubricate the patient's lips with either lemon-glycerin swabs or petroleum jelly applied with a cotton-tipped applicator.

• At least every 4 hours, gently clean and lubricate the patient's external nostrils with either petroleum jelly or water-soluble lubricant on a cotton-tipped applicator *to prevent skin breakdown.*

• Watch for peristalsis to resume, signaled by bowel sounds, passage of fla-

PROBLEM SOLVER

Clearing a nasoenteric-decompression tube obstruction

If your patient's nasoenteric-decompression tube appears to be obstructed, notify the doctor right away. He may order measures, such as these, to restore patency quickly and efficiently.

First, disconnect the tube from the suction source and irrigate with normal saline solution. Use gravity flow to help clear the obstruction unless ordered otherwise.

If irrigation doesn't reestablish patency, the tube may be obstructed by its position against the gastric mucosa. To rectify this, tug slightly on the tube to move it away from the mucosa.

If gentle tugging doesn't restore patency, the tube may be kinked and may need additional manipulation. Before proceeding, though, take these precautions:
• Never reposition or irrigate a nasoenteric-decompression tube (without a doctor's order) in a patient who has had GI surgery.
• Avoid manipulating a tube in a patient who had the tube inserted during surgery. To do so may disturb new sutures.
• Don't try to reposition the tube in a patient who was difficult to intubate (because of an esophageal stricture, for example).

tus, decreased abdominal distention, and possibly, a spontaneous bowel movement. *These signs may require tube removal.*

Complications
• Besides fluid-volume deficit, electrolyte imbalance, and pneumonia, potential complications include mercury poisoning (from a ruptured mercury-filled balloon) and intussusception of the bowel (from the weight of the mercury in the balloon).

Nursing considerations
• For a Miller-Abbott tube, clamp the lumen leading to the mercury balloon and label it DO NOT TOUCH. Label the other lumen SUCTION. *Marking the tube in this way may prevent accidentally instilling irrigant into the wrong lumen and possibly rupturing the mercury balloon.*
• If the suction machine works improperly, replace it immediately. If the machine works properly but no drainage accumulates in the collection container, suspect an obstruction in the tube.
• As ordered, irrigate the tube with the irrigation set *to clear the obstruction.* (See *Clearing a nasoenteric-decompression tube obstruction.*)
• If your patient is ambulatory and his tube connects to a portable suction unit, he may move short distances while connected to the unit. Or, if feasible and ordered, the tube can be disconnected and clamped for a brief time while he moves about.
• If the tubing irritates the patient's throat or makes him hoarse, offer relief with mouthwash, gargles, viscous lidocaine, sour hard candy, throat lozenges, an ice collar, or chewing gum as appropriate.
• If the tip of the balloon falls below the ileocecal valve (confirmed by X-ray), the tube can't be removed na-

sally. It has to be advanced and removed through the anus.

• If the balloon at the end of the tube protrudes from the anus, notify the doctor. Most likely, the tube can be disconnected from suction, the proximal end severed, and the remaining tube removed gradually through the anus either manually or by peristalsis.

Documentation

• Record the frequency and type of mouth and nose care given.

• Describe the therapeutic effect, if any.

• Document in your notes the amount, color, consistency, and odor of the drainage obtained each time you empty the collection container.

• Record the amount of drainage on the intake and output sheet. Always write down the amount of any irrigant or other fluid introduced through the tube or taken orally by the patient.

• If the suction machine malfunctions, note the length of time it didn't appear to be functioning and the nursing action taken. Document the amount and character of any vomitus. Also note the patient's tolerance of the tube's insertion and removal.

Nasoenteric-decompression tube insertion and removal

The nasoenteric-decompression tube is inserted nasally and advanced beyond the stomach into the intestinal tract. It's used to aspirate intestinal contents for analysis and to treat intestinal obstruction. The tube may also help to prevent nausea, vomiting, and abdominal distention after GI surgery. A doctor will usually insert or remove a nasoenteric-decompression tube, but sometimes, a nurse will remove it.

A balloon or rubber bag at one end of the tube holds mercury (or air or water) to stimulate peristalsis and facilitate the tube's passage through the pylorus and into the intestinal tract. (See *Common types of nasoenteric-decompression tubes*, page 548.)

≫ Key nursing diagnoses and patient outcomes

Use these nursing diagnoses as a guide when developing your plan of care for a patient who needs nasoenteric decompression.

Risk for fluid volume deficit related to enteric decompression

Based on this nursing diagnosis, you'll establish the following patient outcomes. The patient will:

• maintain normal vital signs and skin color and turgor.

• maintain urine output of at least (specify) ml/hr.

• have an output equal to or more than intake.

• maintain normal electrolyte levels.

Risk for impaired skin integrity related to presence of nasoenteric tube

Based on this nursing diagnosis, you'll establish the following patient outcomes. The patient will:

• show no signs of skin breakdown in nares.

• maintain adequate circulation to nares.

• report no signs of discomfort at nares.

Common types of nasoenteric-decompression tubes

The type of nasoenteric-decompression tube chosen for your patient will depend on the size of the patient and his nostrils, the estimated duration of intubation, and the reason for the procedure. For example, to remove viscous material from the patient's intestinal tract, the doctor may select a tube with a wide bore and a single lumen.

Whichever tube you use, you'll need to provide good mouth care and check the patient's nostrils often for signs of irritation. If you see any signs of irritation, retape the tube so it doesn't cause tension. Then, lubricate the nostril. Or check with the doctor to see if the tube can be inserted through the other nostril.

Most tubes are impregnated with a radiopaque mark so that placement can be confirmed easily by X-ray or other imaging technique. The following are among the most commonly used types of nasoenteric-decompression tubes.

Cantor tube

This single-lumen, 10' (3 m) long tube has a balloon that can hold mercury at its distal tip. The Cantor tube may be used to relieve bowel obstructions and to aspirate intestinal contents.

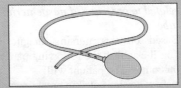

Harris tube

Measuring only 6' (1.8 m) long, this single-lumen tube (top right) also ends with a balloon that holds mercury. Used chiefly for treating a bowel obstruction, the Harris tube allows lavage of the intestinal tract — usually with a Y-tube attached.

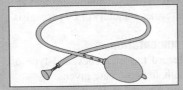

Miller-Abbott tube

This 10' tube has two lumens: one for inflating the distal balloon with air and one for instilling mercury or water. Also used for bowel obstruction, the tube allows aspiration of intestinal contents.

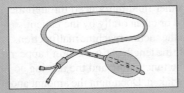

Dennis tube

This three-lumen sump tube is used to decompress the intestinal tract before or after GI surgery. Each lumen is marked to denote its use: irrigation, drainage, and balloon inflation.

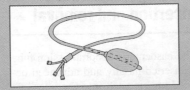

Anxiety related to presence of nasoenteric-decompression tube
Based on this nursing diagnosis, you'll establish the following patient outcomes. The patient will:
• verbalize feelings of anxiety.
• ask questions related to plan of care in an attempt to decrease anxiety.
• use available support systems to assist with coping.
• perform stress-reduction techniques to avoid anxiety symptoms.

Equipment

♦ sterile 10-cc syringe ♦ 21G needle ♦ nasoenteric-decompression tube ♦ container of water ♦ 5 to 10 ml of mercury or water as ordered ♦ suction-decompression equipment ♦ gloves ♦ towel or linen-saver pad ♦ water-soluble lubricant ♦ $4'' \times 4''$ gauze pad ♦ ½" hypoallergenic tape ♦ bulb syringe or 60-ml catheter-tip syringe ♦ stethoscope ♦ cotton-tipped applicators ♦ rubber band ♦ safety pin ♦ clamp ♦ specimen container ♦ basin of ice or warm water ♦ penlight ♦ waterproof marking pen ♦ glass of water with straw ♦ optional: ice chips, local anesthetic.

Equipment preparation

• Stiffen a flaccid tube by chilling it in a basin of ice *to facilitate insertion.* To make a stiff tube flexible, dip it into warm water.
• Check the tube's balloon for leaks. If you're using a Cantor or Harris tube, inject 10 cc of air into the balloon with a 10-cc syringe and 21G needle. If you're using a Miller-Abbott or Dennis tube, attach a 10-cc syringe to the distal balloon port. Immerse the balloon in a container of water and watch for air bubbles. Bubble-free water

means a leak-free balloon. Then remove the balloon from the water. Mercury, air, or water is added to the balloon either before or after insertion of the tube, depending on the type of tube used. Follow the manufacturer's recommendations.
• Set up suction-decompression equipment if ordered, and make sure it works properly.

Patient preparation

• Explain the procedure to the patient, forewarning him that he may experience some discomfort.
• Provide privacy and adequate lighting. Wash your hands and put on gloves.
• Position the patient as the doctor specifies. The most common positions to facilitate tube insertion are semi-Fowler's or high Fowler's positions. You may also need to help the patient hold his neck in a hyperextended position.
• Protect the patient's chest with a linen-saver pad or towel.
• Agree with the patient on a signal that can be used to stop the insertion briefly if necessary.

Implementation
To assist with insertion

• The doctor assesses the patency of the patient's nostrils. To evaluate which nostril has better airflow in a conscious patient, he holds one nostril closed and then the other as the patient breathes. In an unconscious patient, he examines each nostril with a penlight *to check for polyps, a deviated septum, or other obstruction.*
• *To decide how far the tube must be inserted to reach the stomach,* the doctor places the tube's distal end at the

tip of the patient's nose and then extends the tube to the earlobe and down to the xiphoid process. He either marks the tube with a waterproof marking pen or holds it at this point.

• The doctor applies water-soluble lubricant to the first few inches of the tube *to reduce friction and tissue trauma and to facilitate insertion.*

• If the balloon already contains mercury or water, the doctor holds it so the fluid runs to the bottom. Then he pinches the balloon closed *to retain the fluid as the insertion begins.*

• Direct the patient to breathe through his mouth or to pant as the balloon enters his nostril. After the balloon begins its descent, the doctor releases his grip on it, *allowing the weight of the fluid to pull the tube into the nasopharynx.* When the tube reaches the nasopharynx, the doctor instructs the patient to lower his chin and to swallow. In some cases, the patient may sip water through a straw *to facilitate swallowing as the tube advances.* After the tube reaches the trachea, however, the patient won't be offered water. This prevents injury from aspiration. The doctor continues to advance the tube slowly *to prevent it from curling or kinking in the stomach.*

• *To confirm the tube's passage into the stomach,* the doctor aspirates stomach contents with a bulb syringe.

• When the doctor confirms proper placement of a Miller-Abbott tube, he injects the appropriate amount of mercury (commonly between 2 and 5 ml) into the balloon lumen.

• *To keep the tube out of the patient's eyes and to help avoid undue skin irritation,* fold a 4″ × 4″ gauze pad in half and tape it to the patient's fore-

head with the fold directed toward the patient's nose. The doctor can slide the tube through this sling, leaving enough slack for the tube to advance.

• Position the patient, as directed, *to help advance the tube.* Commonly, the patient will lie on his right side until the tube clears the pylorus (about 2 hours). The doctor confirms passage by X-ray.

• After the tube clears the pylorus, the doctor may direct you to advance it 2″ to 3″ (5 to 7.6 cm) every hour and to reposition the patient until the premeasured mark reaches the patient's nostril. Gravity and peristalsis will help to advance the tube. (Notify the doctor if you cannot advance the tube.)

• Be sure to keep the remaining premeasured length of tube well lubricated *to ease passage and prevent irritation.*

• Avoid taping the tube while it advances to the premeasured mark, unless the doctor directs you to do so.

• After the tube progresses the necessary distance, the doctor will order an X-ray *to confirm tube positioning.* Once the tube's in place, secure the external tubing with tape *to prevent further progression.*

• Loop a rubber band around the tube and pin the rubber band to the patient's gown with a safety pin.

• If ordered, attach the tube to intermittent suction.

To remove the tube

• Assist the patient into semi-Fowler's or high Fowler's position. Drape a linen-saver pad or towel across the patient's chest.

• Put on gloves.

• Clamp the tube and disconnect it from the suction. *This prevents the patient from aspirating any gastric contents that leak from the tube during withdrawal.*

• If your patient has a double-lumen Miller-Abbott tube or a triple-lumen Dennis tube, attach a 10-ml syringe to the balloon port and withdraw the mercury. Place the mercury in a specimen container and follow your hospital's protocol for safe disposal. (If you're working with a single-lumen Cantor or Harris tube, you'll withdraw the mercury after you remove the tube.)

• Slowly withdraw between 6″ and 8″ (15 cm and 20 cm) of the tube. Wait 10 minutes and withdraw another 6″ to 8″. Wait another 10 minutes. Continue this procedure until the tube reaches the patient's esophagus (with about 18″ [46 cm] of the tube remaining inside the patient). At this point, you can gently withdraw the tube completely with the mercury in the balloon.

Complications

Nasoenteric-decompression tubes may cause:

• reflux esophagitis
• nasal or oral inflammation
• nasal, laryngeal, or esophageal ulceration.

Nursing considerations

• For a double- or triple-lumen tube, note which lumen accommodates balloon inflation and which accommodates drainage.

• An alternate method for removing a single-lumen tube is to withdraw it gently into the pharynx. Ask the patient to open his mouth. Then grasp

the tube and mercury balloon and gently pull them outside of the patient's mouth. Remove mercury from the bag with a needle and syringe. Then pull the tube and empty balloon through the patient's nose. Never forcibly remove a tube if you meet resistance. Notify the doctor.

• Apply a local anesthetic, if ordered, to the nostril or the back of the throat *to dull sensations and the gag reflex for intubation.* Letting the patient gargle with a liquid anesthetic or hold ice chips in his mouth for a few minutes serves the same purpose.

• Mercury can be disposed of only by a licensed hazardous-waste disposal company. Put the container of mercury into a plastic bag, and send it to the appropriate department for disposal.

Documentation

• Record the date and time the nasoenteric-decompression tube was inserted and by whom.

• Note the patient's tolerance of the procedure; the type of tube used; the suction type and amount; and the color, amount, and consistency of drainage.

• Note the date, time, and name of the person removing the tube and the patient's tolerance of the removal procedure.

Nasogastric tube care

Providing effective nasogastric (NG) tube care requires meticulous monitoring of the patient and the equipment. Monitoring the patient involves checking drainage from the NG tube and assessing GI function. Monitoring the equipment involves verifying correct tube placement and irrigating the tube to ensure patency and to prevent mucosal damage.

Specific care varies only slightly for the most commonly used NG tubes: the single-lumen Levin tube and the double-lumen Salem sump tube.

≫ Key nursing diagnoses and patient outcomes

Use these nursing diagnoses as a guide when developing your plan of care for a patient who needs an NG tube.

Risk for fluid volume deficit related to NG tube

Based on this nursing diagnosis, you'll establish the following patient outcomes. The patient will:
• maintain normal vital signs and skin color and turgor.
• maintain urine output of at least (specify) ml/hr.
• have an output equal to or more than intake.
• maintain normal electrolyte levels.

Risk for impaired skin integrity related to presence of NG tube

Based on this nursing diagnosis, you'll establish the following patient outcomes. The patient will:
• show no signs of skin breakdown in nares.
• maintain adequate circulation to nares.
• report no signs of discomfort at nares.

Anxiety related to presence of NG tube

Based on this nursing diagnosis, you'll establish the following patient outcomes. The patient will:

• verbalize feelings of anxiety.
• ask questions related to plan of care in an attempt to decrease anxiety.
• use available support systems to assist with coping.
• perform stress-reduction techniques to avoid anxiety symptoms.

Equipment

♦ irrigant (usually normal saline solution) ♦ irrigant container ♦ 60-ml catheter-tip syringe ♦ bulb syringe ♦ suction equipment ♦ lemon-glycerin swabs or toothbrush and toothpaste ♦ petroleum jelly ♦ 1½″ or 1″ hypoallergenic tape ♦ water-soluble lubricant ♦ gloves ♦ stethoscope ♦ linen-saver pad ♦ optional: emesis basin.

Equipment preparation

• Make sure the suction equipment works properly. (See *Common gastric suction devices.*)
• When using a Salem sump tube with suction, connect the larger, primary lumen (for drainage and suction) to the suction equipment and select the appropriate setting as ordered (usually low constant suction). If the doctor doesn't specify the setting, follow the manufacturer's directions.
• A Levin tube usually calls for intermittent low suction.

Patient preparation

• Explain the procedure to the patient and provide privacy.

Implementation

• Wash your hands and put on gloves.

To irrigate the NG tube

• Review the irrigation schedule (usually every 4 hours), if the doctor orders this procedure.

Common gastric suction devices

A variety of portable or wall-mounted suction devices are available for applying negative pressure to nasogastric (NG) and other drainage tubes. Two common types are shown here.

Portable suction machine

In the portable suction machine, a vacuum created intermittently by an electric pump draws gastric contents up the NG tube and into the collecting bottle.

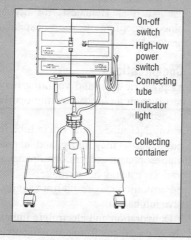

Stationary suction machine

A stationary wall-unit apparatus can provide intermittent or continuous suction. On-off switches and variable power settings let you set and adjust the suction force on either machine.

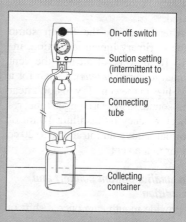

• Inject 10 cc of air and auscultate the epigastric area with a stethoscope and aspirate stomach contents to check correct positioning in the stomach and to prevent the patient from aspirating the irrigant.

• Measure the amount of irrigant in the bulb syringe or in the 60-ml catheter-tip syringe (usually 30 ml) *to maintain an accurate intake and output record.*

• When using suction with a Salem sump tube or a Levin tube, unclamp and disconnect the tube from the suction equipment while holding it over a linen-saver pad or an emesis basin *to collect any drainage.*

• Slowly instill the irrigant into the NG tube. (When irrigating the Salem sump tube, you may instill small amounts of solution into the vent lumen without interrupting suction; however, you should instill greater amounts into the larger, primary lumen.)

• Gently aspirate the solution with the bulb syringe or 60-ml catheter-tip syringe or connect the tube to the suction equipment, as ordered. *Gentle aspiration prevents excessive pressure on a suture line and on delicate gastric mucosa.*

• Reconnect the tube to suction after completing irrigation.

To instill a solution through the NG tube

• If the doctor orders *instillation,* inject the solution, but do not aspirate it. Note the amount of instilled solution as "intake" on the intake and output record.

• Reattach the tube to suction as ordered.

• After attaching the Salem sump tube's primary lumen to suction, instill 10 to 20 cc of air into the vent lumen *to verify patency.* Listen for a soft hiss in the vent. If you don't hear this sound, suspect a clogged tube; recheck patency by instilling 10 ml of normal saline solution and 10 to 20 cc of air in the vent.

To monitor patient comfort and condition

• Provide mouth care once a shift or as needed. Depending on the patient's condition, use lemon-glycerin swabs to clean his teeth or assist him to brush them with toothbrush and toothpaste. Coat the patient's lips with petroleum jelly *to prevent dryness from mouth breathing.*

• Change the tape securing the tube as needed or at least daily. Clean the skin, apply fresh tape, and dab water-soluble lubricant on the nostrils as needed.

• Regularly check the tape that secures the tube *because sweat and nasal secretions may loosen the tape.*

• Assess bowel sounds regularly (every 4 to 8 hours) *to verify GI function.*

• Measure the drainage amount and update the intake and output record every 8 hours. Be alert for electrolyte imbalances with excessive gastric output.

• Inspect gastric drainage. Note color, consistency, odor, and amount. Normal gastric secretions have no color or appear yellow-green from bile and have a mucoid consistency. Immediately report any drainage with a coffee-bean color. *This may indicate bleeding.* If you suspect that the drainage contains blood, use a screening test (such as Hematest) for occult blood according to your hospital's protocol.

Complications

• Epigastric pain and vomiting may result from a clogged or improperly placed tube.

• Any NG tube — the Levin tube in particular — may move and aggravate esophagitis, ulcers, or esophageal varices, causing hemorrhage.

• Perforation may result from aggressive intubation.

• Dehydration and electrolyte imbalances may result from removing body fluids and electrolytes by suctioning.

• Pain, swelling, and salivary dysfunction may signal parotitis, which occurs in dehydrated, debilitated patients.

• Intubation can cause nasal skin breakdown and discomfort and increased mucous secretions.

• Aspiration pneumonia may result from gastric reflux.

• Vigorous suction may damage the gastric mucosa and cause significant bleeding, possibly interfering with endoscopic assessment and diagnosis.

Nursing considerations

• Irrigate the NG tube with 30 ml of irrigant before and after instilling medication. (See "Nasogastric tube drug administration".) Wait about 30 minutes, or as ordered, after instillation before reconnecting the suction equipment *to allow sufficient time for the medication to be absorbed.*

• When no drainage appears, check the suction equipment for proper function. Then, holding the NG tube over a linen-saver pad or an emesis basin, separate the tube and the suction source. Check the suction equipment by placing the suction tubing in an irrigant container. If the apparatus draws the water, check the NG tube for proper function. Be sure to note the amount of water drawn into the suction container on the intake and output record.

• A dysfunctional NG tube may be clogged or incorrectly positioned. Attempt to irrigate the tube, reposition the patient, or rotate and reposition the tube. However, if the tube was inserted during surgery, avoid this maneuver *to ensure that the movement doesn't interfere with gastric or esophageal sutures.* Notify the doctor.

• If you can ambulate the patient and interrupt suction, disconnect the NG tube from the suction equipment. Clamp the tube *to prevent stomach contents from draining out of the tube.*

• If the patient has a Salem sump tube, watch for gastric reflux in the vent lumen when pressure in the stomach exceeds atmospheric pressure. This problem may result from a clogged primary lumen or from a suction system that's set up improperly. Assess the suction equipment for proper functioning. Then, irrigate the NG tube and instill 30 cc of air into the vent tube *to maintain patency.* Don't attempt to stop reflux by clamping the vent tube. Unless contraindicated, elevate the patient's torso more than 30 degrees, and keep the vent tube above his midline *to prevent a siphoning effect.*

Documentation

• Regularly record tube placement confirmation (usually every 4 to 8 hours).

• Keep a precise record of fluid intake and output, including the instilled irrigant in fluid input.

• Track the irrigation schedule and note the actual time of each irrigation.

• Describe drainage color, consistency, odor, and amount. Also note tape change times and condition of the nares.

Nasogastric tube drug administration

Besides providing an alternate means of nourishment, the nasogastric (NG) tube allows direct instillation of medication into the GI system of patients who can't ingest it orally. Before instillation, the patency and positioning of the tube must be carefully checked because this procedure is contraindicated if the tube is obstructed or improperly positioned or if the patient is vomiting around the tube or his bowel sounds are absent.

Oily medications and enteric-coated or sustained-release tablets should not be given through an NG tube. Oily medications cling to the sides of the tube and resist mixing with the irrigating solution. And crushing enteric-coated or sustained-release tablets to facilitate transport through the tube destroys their intended effect.

>> Key nursing diagnoses and patient outcomes

Use these nursing diagnoses as a guide when developing your plan of care for a patient who is receiving medications through an NG tube.

Knowledge deficit related to lack of exposure

Based on this nursing diagnosis, you'll establish the following patient outcomes. The patient will:
• state or demonstrate understanding of what has been taught.
• demonstrate ability to perform new health-related behaviors as they are taught.

Risk for injury related to improper technique

Based on this nursing diagnosis, you'll establish these patient outcomes. The patient will:
• identify factors that increase risk for injury.
• assist in identifying and applying safety measures to prevent injury.

Equipment

◆ patient's medication record and chart ◆ prescribed medication ◆ towel or linen-saver pad ◆ 50- or 60-ml piston type catheter-tip syringe ◆ feeding tubing ◆ two $4'' \times 4''$ gauze pads ◆ stethoscope ◆ gloves ◆ diluent ◆ cup for mixing medication and fluid ◆ spoon ◆ 50 ml of water ◆ rubber band ◆ gastrostomy tube and funnel if needed ◆ optional: pill-crushing equipment (mortar and pestle, for ex-

ample), clamp (if not already attached to tube).

For maximum control of suction, use a piston syringe instead of a bulb syringe. The liquid for diluting the medication can be juice, water, or a nutritional supplement.

Equipment preparation

• Gather necessary equipment for use at the patient's bedside. Liquids should be at room temperature. Administering cold liquid through the NG tube can cause abdominal cramping. Although this is not a sterile procedure, make sure the cup, syringe, spoon, and gauze are clean.

Implementation

• Verify the order on the patient's medication record by checking it against the doctor's order.
• Wash your hands and don gloves.
• Check the label on the medication three times before preparing it for administration to make sure you'll be giving the medication correctly.
• If the prescribed medication is in tablet form, crush the tablets to ready them for mixing in a cup with the diluting liquid. Bring the medication and equipment to the patient's bedside.
• Explain the procedure to the patient, if necessary, and provide privacy.
• Confirm the patient's identity by asking his name and checking the name, room number, and bed number on his wristband.
• Unpin the tube from the patient's gown. To avoid soiling the sheets during the procedure, fold back the bed linens to the patient's waist and drape his chest with a towel or linen-saver pad.

• Elevate the head of the bed so the patient is in Fowler's position, as tolerated.

• After unclamping the tube, take the 50- or 60-ml syringe and create a 10-cc air space in its chamber. Then attach the syringe to the end of the tube.

• Auscultate the patient's abdomen about 3″ (7.5 cm) below the sternum with the stethoscope. Then, gently insert the 10 cc of air into the tube. You should hear the air bubble entering the stomach. If you hear this sound, gently draw back on the piston of the syringe. The appearance of gastric contents implies that the tube is patent and in the stomach. (However, only an X-ray positively confirms the tube's position.) If no gastric contents appear when you draw back on the piston of the syringe, the tube may have risen into the patient's esophagus, in which case you'll have to advance it before proceeding.

• If you meet resistance when aspirating for stomach contents, stop the procedure. Resistance may indicate a nonpatent tube or improper tube placement. (Keep in mind that some smaller NG tubes may collapse when aspiration is tried.) If the tube seems to be in the stomach, resistance probably means the tube is lying against the stomach wall. To relieve resistance, withdraw the tube slightly or turn the patient.

• After you have established that the tube is patent and in the correct position, clamp the tube, detach the syringe, and lay the end of the tube on the 4″ × 4″ gauze pad.

• Mix the crushed tablets with the diluent. If the medication is in capsule form, open the capsules and empty their contents into the liquid. Pour liquid medications directly into the diluting liquid. Stir well with the spoon. (If the medication was in tablet form, make sure the particles are small enough to pass through the eyes at the distal end of the tube.)

• Reattach the syringe, without the piston, to the end of the tube and open the clamp.

• Deliver the medication slowly and steadily. (See *Giving medications through an NG tube, page 558.*)

• If the medication flows smoothly, slowly add more until the entire dose has been given. If the medication doesn't flow properly, don't force it. It may be too thick to flow through the tube. If so, dilute it with water. If you suspect tube placement is inhibiting flow, stop the procedure and reevaluate the placement.

• Watch the patient's reaction throughout the instillation. If he shows any sign of discomfort, stop the procedure immediately.

• As the last of the medication flows out of the syringe, start to irrigate the tube by adding 30 to 50 ml of water. (If your patient is a child, use only 15 to 30 ml of water.) Irrigation clears medication from the sides of the tube and from the distal end, reducing the risk of clogging.

• When the water stops flowing, quickly clamp the tube. Detach the syringe and dispose of it properly.

• Fasten the NG tube to the patient's gown.

• Remove the towel or linen-saver pad and replace bed linens.

• Leave the patient in Fowler's position, or have him lie on his right side with the head of the bed partially elevated. Have him maintain this position for at least 30 minutes after the

Giving medications through an NG tube

Introducing air into the stomach

Holding the nasogastric (NG) tube at a level somewhat above the patient's nose, pour up to 30 ml of diluted medication into the syringe barrel. *To prevent air from entering the patient's stomach,* hold the tube at a slight angle and add more medication before the syringe empties. If necessary, raise the tube slightly higher to increase the flow rate.

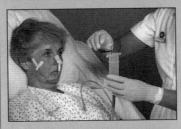

Esophageal reflux

After you've delivered the whole dose, position the patient on her right side, head slightly elevated, *to minimize esophageal reflux.*

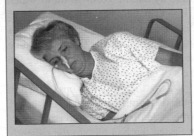

procedure to facilitate the downward flow of medication into his stomach and prevent esophageal reflux.
• You may be asked to deliver medications through a gastrostomy tube. (See *Giving medications through a gastrostomy tube.*)

If medication is prescribed for a patient with a gastrostomy feeding button, ask the doctor to order the liquid form of the drug, if possible. If not, you may administer a tablet or capsule if it is dissolved in 30 to 50 ml of warm water (15 to 30 ml for children). To administer medication this way, use the same procedure as for feeding patient through the button (See "Feeding button care," pages 342 to 345.). Then draw up the dissolved medication into a syringe and inject it into the feeding tube.
• Next, withdraw the medication syringe and flush the tube with 50 ml of warm water. (For children, flush the tube with 30 ml.)
• Then replace the safety plug, and keep the patient upright at a 30-degree angle for 30 minutes after giving the medication.

Nursing considerations

• To prevent instillation of too much fluid (more than 400 ml of liquid at one time for an adult), plan the drug instillation so that it doesn't coincide with the patient's regular tube feeding, if possible.
• When you must schedule a tube feeding and medication instillation simultaneously, administer the medication first *to ensure that the patient receives the prescribed drug therapy even if he can't tolerate an entire feeding.* Remember to avoid giving the patient foods that interact adversely with the medication.
• If the patient receives continuous tube feedings, stop the feeding and check the quantity of residual stomach contents. If it's greater than 150 ml, withhold the medication and feeding and notify the doctor. *An excessive*

Giving medications through a gastrostomy tube

Surgically inserted into the stomach, a gastrostomy tube reduces the risk of fluid aspiration into the lungs, a constant danger with a nasogastric (NG) tube.

To administer medication by this route, prepare the patient and medication as you would for an NG tube. Then, gently lift the dressing around the tube *to assess the skin for irritation caused by gastric secretions.* Report any redness or irritation to the doctor. If no irritation appears, follow these steps:

• Remove the dressing that covers the tube. Then remove the dressing or plug at the tip of the tube and attach the syringe or funnel to the tip.

• Release the clamp and instill about 10 ml of water into the tube through the syringe *to check for patency.* If the water flows in easily, the tube is patent. If it flows in slowly, raise the funnel to increase pressure. If the water still doesn't flow properly, stop the procedure and notify the doctor.

• Pour up to 30 ml of medication into the syringe or funnel. Tilt the tube *to allow air to escape as the fluid flows downward.* Just before the syringe empties, add medication as needed.

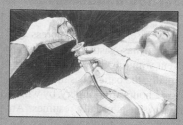

• After giving the medication, pour in about 30 ml of water *to irrigate the tube.*

• Tighten the clamp; then place a 4″ × 4″ gauze pad on the end of the tube, and secure it with a rubber band.

• Cover the tube with two more 4″ × 4″ gauze pads, and secure them firmly with tape.

• Keep the head of the bed elevated for at least 30 minutes after the procedure *to aid digestion.*

---

amount of residual contents may indicate intestinal obstruction or paralytic ileus.

• If the NG tube is attached to suction, be sure to turn off the suction for 20 to 30 minutes after administering medication.

• If possible, teach the patient who requires long-term treatment to instill his medication himself through the NG tube. Have him observe you as you perform the procedure several times before you allow him to try it himself.

• Be sure to remain with the patient when he performs the procedure for the first few times so you can provide assistance and answer any questions. As the patient performs the procedure, give him positive reinforcement and correct any errors in his technique, as necessary.

Documentation

• Record the instillation of medication, the date and time of instillation, the dose, and the patient's tolerance of the procedure.

• On his intake and output sheet, note the amount of fluid instilled.

Nasogastric tube insertion and removal

Usually inserted to decompress the stomach, a nasogastric (NG) tube can prevent vomiting after major surgery. Normally, the patient has the tube for 48 to 72 hours after surgery, by which time peristalsis usually resumes. An NG tube may remain in place for shorter or longer periods, however, depending on its use.

The NG tube has other diagnostic and therapeutic applications, especially in assessing and treating upper GI bleeding, collecting gastric contents for analysis, performing gastric lavage, aspirating gastric secretions, and administering medications and nutrients.

Inserting an NG tube requires close observation of the patient and verification of proper placement. Removing the tube requires careful handling to prevent injury or aspiration. The tube must be inserted with extra care in pregnant patients and in those with an increased risk of complications. For example, the doctor will order an NG tube for a patient with aortic aneurysm, myocardial infarction, gastric hemorrhage, or esophageal varices only if he believes that the benefits outweigh the risks of intubation.

• Most NG tubes have a radiopaque marker or strip at the distal end so that the tube's position can be verified by X-ray studies. If the position can't be confirmed, the doctor may order fluoroscopy to verify placement.

The most common NG tubes are the Levin tube, which has one lumen, and the Salem sump tube, which has two lumens, one for suction and drainage and a smaller one for ventilation. Air flows through the vent lumen continuously. This protects the delicate gastric mucosa by preventing a vacuum from forming should the tube adhere to the stomach lining. The Moss tube, which has a triple lumen, is usually inserted during surgery. (See *Types of NG tubes.*)

≫ Key nursing diagnoses and patient outcomes

Use these nursing diagnoses as a guide when developing your plan of care for a patient who needs an NG tube.

Risk for fluid volume deficit related to NG tube

Based on this nursing diagnosis, you'll establish the following patient outcomes. The patient will:
• maintain normal vital signs and skin color and turgor.
• maintain urine output of at least (specify) ml/hr.
• have an output equal to or more than intake.
• maintain normal electrolyte levels.

Risk for impaired skin integrity related to presence of NG tube

Based on this nursing diagnosis, you'll establish the following patient outcomes. The patient will:
• show no signs of skin breakdown in nares.
• maintain adequate circulation to nares.
• report no signs of discomfort at the nares.

Types of NG tubes

The doctor will choose the type and diameter of nasogastric (NG) tube that best suits the patient's needs, including lavage, aspiration, enteral therapy, or stomach decompression. Choices may include the Levin, Salem sump, and Moss tubes.

Levin tube

This rubber or plastic tube has a single lumen that's 42″ to 50″ (107 to 127 cm) long and has holes at the tip and along the side.

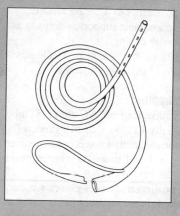

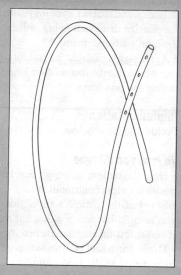

Moss tube

This tube has a radiopaque tip and three lumens. The first, positioned and inflated at the cardia, serves as a balloon inflation port. The second is an esophageal aspiration port. The third is a duodenal feeding port.

Salem sump tube

This double-lumen tube (above right) is made of clear plastic and has a blue sump port (pigtail) that allows atmospheric air to enter the patient's stomach. Thus, the tube floats freely and doesn't adhere to or damage gastric mucosa. The larger port of this 48″ (122-cm) tube serves as the main suction conduit. The tube has openings at the sides and the tip; markings at 45, 55, 65, and 75 cm; and a radiopaque line to verify placement.

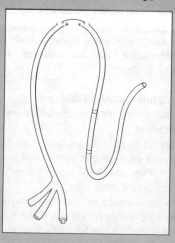

Anxiety related to presence of NG tube

Based on this nursing diagnosis, you'll establish the following patient outcomes. The patient will:
• verbalize feelings of anxiety.
• ask questions related to plan of care in an attempt to decrease anxiety.
• use available support systems to assist with coping.
• perform stress-reduction techniques to avoid anxiety symptoms.

Equipment

For inserting an NG tube: ◆ tube (usually #14, #16, or #18 French for a normal adult) ◆ towel or linen-saver pad ◆ facial tissues ◆ emesis basin ◆ penlight ◆ 18MÆ or 2″ hypoallergenic tape ◆ gloves ◆ water-soluble lubricant ◆ cup or glass of water with straw (if appropriate) ◆ stethoscope ◆ tongue blade ◆ catheter-tip or bulb syringe or irrigation set ◆ safety pin ◆ ordered suction equipment ◆ optional: metal clamp, ice, warm water, large basin or plastic container, rubber band.

For removing an NG tube: ◆ stethoscope ◆ catheter-tip syringe ◆ normal saline solution ◆ towel or linen-saver pad ◆ adhesive remover ◆ optional: clamp.

Equipment preparation

• Gather and prepare all necessary equipment.
• Inspect the NG tube for defects, such as rough edges or partially closed lumens. Then, check the tube's patency by flushing it with water.
• *To ease insertion,* increase a stiff tube's flexibility by coiling it around your gloved fingers for a few seconds or by dipping it into warm water. Stiff-en a limp tube by briefly chilling it in ice.

Patient preparation

• Whether you're inserting or removing an NG tube, be sure to provide privacy and wash and glove your hands before inserting the tube.
• Explain the procedure to the patient *to ease anxiety and promote cooperation.* Inform her that she may experience some nasal discomfort, that she may gag, and that her eyes may water. Emphasize that swallowing will ease the tube's advancement.
• Agree on a signal that the patient can use if she wants you to stop briefly during the procedure.

Implementation

Follow the steps below.

To insert an NG tube

• Help the patient into high Fowler's position unless contraindicated.
• Stand at the patient's right side if you're right-handed or at her left side if you're left-handed *to ease insertion.*
• Drape the towel or linen-saver pad over the patient's chest *to protect her gown and bed linens from spills.*
• Have the patient gently blow her nose *to clear her nostrils.*
• Place the facial tissues and emesis basin well within the patient's reach.
• Help the patient face forward with her neck in a neutral position.
• To determine how long the NG tube must be to reach the stomach, hold the end of the tube at the tip of the patient's nose. Extend the tube to the patient's earlobe and then down to the xiphoid process.
• Mark this distance on the tubing with the tape. (Average measurements

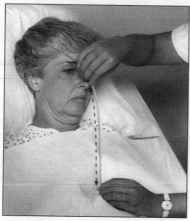

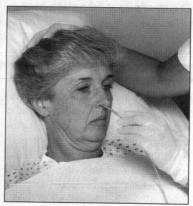

for an adult range from 22″ to 26″ [56 to 66 cm].)

• To determine which nostril will allow easier access, use a penlight and inspect for a deviated septum or other abnormalities. Ask the patient if she ever had nasal surgery or a nasal injury. Assess airflow in both nostrils by occluding one nostril at a time while the patient breathes through her nose. Choose the nostril with the better airflow.

• Lubricate the first 3″ (7.6 cm) of the tube with a water-soluble gel to minimize injury to the nasal passages. Using a water-soluble lubricant prevents lipoid pneumonia that may result from aspirating an oil-based lubricant or from accidental slippage of the tube into the trachea.

• Instruct the patient to hold her head straight and upright.

• Grasp the tube with the end pointing downward, curve it if necessary, and carefully insert it into the more patent nostril.

• Aim the tube downward and toward the ear closer to the chosen nostril. Advance it slowly *to avoid pressure on*

the turbinates and resultant pain and bleeding.

• When the tube reaches the nasopharynx, you'll feel resistance. Instruct the patient to lower her head slightly *to close the trachea and open the esophagus.* Then rotate the tube 180 degrees toward the opposite nostril *to redirect it so that the tube won't enter the patient's mouth.*

• Unless contraindicated, offer the patient a cup or glass of water with a straw. Direct her to sip and swallow as you slowly advance the tube. This helps the tube pass to the esophagus. (If you aren't using water, ask the patient to swallow.)

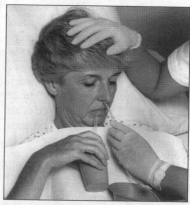

To ensure proper tube placement

• Use a tongue blade and penlight to examine the patient's mouth and throat for signs of a coiled section of tubing (especially in an unconscious patient).

• Keep an emesis basin and facial tissues readily available for the patient.

• As you carefully advance the tube and the patient swallows, watch for respiratory distress signs, *which may mean the tube is in the bronchus and must be removed immediately.*

• Stop advancing the tube when the tape mark reaches the patient's nostril.

• Attach a catheter-tip or bulb syringe to the tube as shown below and try to aspirate stomach contents. If you do not obtain stomach contents, position the patient on her left side *to move the contents into the stomach's greater curvature,* and aspirate again.

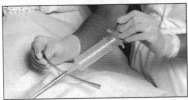

• When confirming tube placement, never place the tube's end in a container of water. *If the tube should be mispositioned in the trachea, the patient may aspirate water.* Besides, water without bubbles does not confirm proper placement. *Instead, the tube may be coiled in the trachea or the esophagus.*

• If you still can't aspirate stomach contents, advance the tube 1″ to 2″ (2.5 to 5 cm). Then inject 10 cc of air into the tube. At the same time, auscultate for air sounds with your stethoscope placed over the epigastric region. *You should hear a whooshing sound if the tube is patent and properly positioned in the stomach.*

• If these tests don't confirm proper tube placement, you'll need X-ray verification.

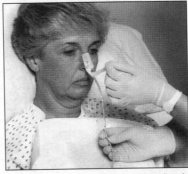

• Secure the NG tube to the patient's nose with hypoallergenic tape (or other designated tube holder). You will need about 4″ (10 cm) of 1″ tape. Split one end of the tape up the center about 1½″ (4 cm). Make tabs on the split ends (by folding sticky sides together). Stick the uncut tape end on the patient's nose so that the split in the tape starts about ½″ (1 cm) to 1½″ from the tip of her nose. Crisscross the tabbed ends around the tube. Then apply another piece of tape over the bridge of the nose to secure the tube.

• Alternatively, stabilize the tube with a prepackaged product that secures and cushions it at the nose.

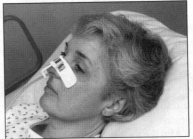

• *To reduce discomfort from the weight of the tube,* tie a slip knot around the tube with a rubber band,

and then secure the rubber band to the patient's gown with a safety pin, or wrap another piece of tape around the end of the tube and leave a tab. Then fasten the tape tab to the patient's gown with a safety pin.

• Attach the tube to suction equipment, if ordered, and set the designated suction pressure.

To remove an NG tube

• Explain the procedure to the patient, informing her that it may cause some nasal discomfort and sneezing or gagging.

• Assess bowel function by auscultating for peristalsis or flatus.

• Help the patient into semi-Fowler's position. Then drape a towel or linensaver pad across her chest to protect her gown and bed linens from spills.

• Using a catheter-tip syringe, flush the tube with 10 ml of normal saline solution *to ensure that the tube doesn't contain stomach contents that could irritate tissues during tube removal.*

• Untape the tube from the patient's nose, and then unpin it from her gown.

• Clamp the tube by folding it in your hand.

• Ask the patient to hold her breath *to close the epiglottis.* Then withdraw the tube gently and steadily.(When the distal end of the tube reaches the nasopharynx, you can pull it quickly.)

• When possible, immediately cover and remove the tube *because its sight and odor may nauseate the patient.*

• Assist the patient with thorough mouth care, and clean the tape residue from her nose with adhesive remover.

• For the next 48 hours, monitor the patient for signs of GI dysfunction, including nausea, vomiting, abdominal distention, and food intolerance. GI

Using an NG tube at home

If your patient will need to have a nasogastric (NG) tube in place at home (for short-term feeding or gastric decompression, for example), find out who will insert the tube. If the patient will have a home care nurse, identify her and, if possible, tell the patient when to expect her.

If the patient or a family member will perform the procedure, you'll need to provide additional instruction and supervision. Use this checklist to assemble your teaching topics:

☐ how and where to obtain equipment needed for home intubation
☐ how to insert the tube
☐ verifying tube placement by aspirating stomach contents
☐ correcting tube misplacement
☐ preparing formula for tube feeding
☐ how to store formula if appropriate
☐ administering formula through the tube
☐ how to remove and dispose of an NG tube
☐ how to clean and store a reusable NG tube
☐ how to use the NG tube for gastric decompression if appropriate
☐ how to set up and operate suctioning equipment
☐ troubleshooting suctioning equipment
☐ how to perform mouth care and other hygienic procedures.

dysfunction may necessitate reinsertion of the tube.

Complications

Potential complications of prolonged intubation with an NG tube include:

BETTER CHARTING

Documenting NG tube insertion and removal

Document the date, time, and route of nasogastric (NG) tube insertion and removal.

Also note how the patient tolerated the procedures.

Include in your notes any signs and symptoms signaling complications, such as nausea, vomiting, and abdominal distention. Document any subsequent irrigation procedures and continuing problems after irrigation.

Note any unusual events following NG removal, such as nausea, vomiting, abdominal distention, and food intolerance.

1/15/97	1605	#12 Fr. NG tube placed in ①
		nostril. Placement verified and
		attached to low intermittent
		suction as ordered. Drainage
		pale green; heme –. Irrigated
		with 30 ml NSS q 2 hr. Pt. tol–
		erated procedure. Hypoactive
		b.s. in all 4 quadrants. ——
		—— Mark Porter, RN

- skin erosion at the nostril
- sinusitis
- esophagitis
- esophagotracheal fistula
- gastric ulceration
- pulmonary and oral infection
- electrolyte imbalances and dehydration (from suctioning).

Nursing considerations

- A helpful device for calculating the correct tube length is Ross-Hanson tape. Place the narrow end of this measuring tape at the tip of the patient's nose. Again, extend the tape to the patient's earlobe and down to the tip of the xiphoid process. Mark this distance on the edge of the tape labeled "nose to ear to xiphoid." The corresponding measurement on the opposite edge of the tape is the proper insertion length.
- If the patient has a deviated septum or other nasal condition that prevents nasal insertion, pass the tube orally after removing any dentures, if necessary. Sliding the tube over the tongue, proceed as you would for nasal insertion.
- When using the oral route, remember to coil the end of the tube around your hand. *This helps curve and direct the tube downward at the pharynx.*
- If your patient lies unconscious, tilt her chin toward her chest *to close the trachea.* Then advance the tube between respirations *to ensure that it doesn't enter the trachea.*
- While advancing the tube in an unconscious patient (or in a patient who can't swallow), stroke the patient's neck *to encourage the swallowing reflex and to facilitate passage down the esophagus.*
- While advancing the tube, observe for signs that it has entered the trachea, such as choking or breathing difficulties in a conscious patient and cyanosis in an unconscious patient or a patient without a cough reflex. If these signs occur, remove the tube immediately. Allow the patient time to rest; then try to reinsert the tube.
- After tube placement, vomiting suggests tubal obstruction or incorrect position. Assess immediately to determine the cause.

Home care
• An NG tube may be inserted or removed at home.
• Indications for insertion include gastric decompression and short-term feeding.
• A home care nurse or the patient may insert the tube, deliver the feeding, and remove the tube. (See *Using an NG tube at home*, page 565.)

Documentation
• Record the type and size of the NG tube and the date, time, and route of insertion.
• Note the type and amount of suction, if used, and describe the drainage, including amount, color, character, consistency, and odor.
• Note the patient's tolerance of the procedure. (See *Documenting NG tube insertion and removal.*)
• When you remove the tube, make sure to record the date and time.
• Describe the color, consistency, and amount of gastric drainage.
• Note the patient's tolerance of the procedure.

Neonatal vital signs measurement

Measuring vital signs establishes the baseline of any neonatal assessment. Typically, the nurse visually assesses the respiratory rate by watching and counting the neonate's breaths, although she may auscultate the lungs with a pediatric stethoscope and watch for labored or abnormal breathing. She measures the heart rate apically — also with a pediatric stethoscope — and takes the first neonatal temperature rectally to verify rectal patency. Subsequent temperature readings are axillary to avoid injuring the rectal mucosa. Blood pressure may be assessed by sphygmomanometer or by palpation or auscultation. An electronic vital signs monitor may also be used.

When the neonate arrives in the nursery, additional procedures may be required to ensure the neonate's safety and progress in the nursery. Depending on hospital protocol, these may include an identification and weight check, placement in radiant warming equipment, a vitamin K_1 injection to stimulate neonatal clotting mechanisms, and eye treatments with an antibiotic or silver nitrate to guard against infections.

⟫ Key nursing diagnoses and patient outcomes
Use these nursing diagnoses as a guide when developing your plan of care.

Anxiety related to parental concern about proper procedure and vital sign interpretation
Based on this nursing diagnosis, you'll establish the following outcomes. The parent will:
• develop effective coping behaviors.
• maintain autonomy without fears of being handicapped.

Knowledge deficit related to parental understanding of precedures and interpretation of results
Based on this nursing diagnosis, you'll establish the following outcomes. The parent will:
• communicate a need to know.

Normal vital signs in full-term neonates

Use these ranges (or those established by your hospital) to guide assessment of neonatal status.

Respiratory rate
30 to 50 breaths/minute

Heart rate (apical)
110 to 160 beats/minute

Temperature
Axillary: 97.5° to 99° F (36.4° to 37.2° C)
Rectal: one degree higher than axillary

Blood pressure
Systolic: 60 to 80 mm Hg
Diastolic: 40 to 50 mm Hg

• demonstrate ability to perform new health-related behaviors as they are taught.

Equipment
♦ pediatric stethoscope ♦ watch with second hand ♦ thermometer (mercury or electronic with rectal probe and cover) ♦ water-soluble lubricant ♦ sphygmomanometer with 1″ (2.5-cm) cuff ♦ gloves ♦ optional: Doppler ultrasound device with conduction gel or an electronic vital signs monitor.

Equipment preparation
• Assemble the equipment beside the patient.
• If you're using a mercury thermometer, shake it until the mercury drops under 96° F (35.5° C).

• If you have an electronic thermometer, apply the cover to the rectal probe.
• Using water-soluble lubricant, coat the thermometer or probe cover before taking a rectal temperature.

Implementation
• Wash your hands.

To determine respiratory rate
• Observe respirations first, before the neonate becomes agitated or too active. Watch and count respiratory movements for 1 minute. Then record the result.
• Expect to see mostly diaphragmatic respirations. Also expect an irregular respiratory rate and pattern, varying from slow and shallow to rapid and deep. (See *Normal vital signs in full-term neonates.*)
• Abnormally fast breathing (tachypnea) may signal a perinatal problem. A lapse of 15 seconds or more after a complete respiratory cycle (one expiration and one inspiration) indicates apnea.
• Check for labored breathing (sometimes resulting from blocked nasal passages). Observe for uneven chest expansion, nasal flaring, visible chest retractions, expiratory grunts, and inspiratory stridor (a high-pitched sound audible without a stethoscope).
• *To evaluate breath sounds,* auscultate the anterior and posterior lung fields, placing the stethoscope over each lung lobe for at least 5 seconds for a total time of 1 minute. Normal breath sounds are clear and the same bilaterally. However, immediately after birth, you may hear crackles resulting from retained fetal lung fluid.

• Observe the chest as it rises and falls; normal movement should be symmetrical. Also, determine any difference between the anterior and posterior diameters of the chest, which normally should be equal. *Unequal diameters suggest hyperinflated lungs or respiratory distress.*

To assess heart rate

• Place the stethoscope over the apical impulse on the fourth or fifth intercostal space at the left midclavicular line over the cardiac apex. Listen to and count the heartbeats for 1 minute *to learn the heart rate and to detect any abnormalities in quality or rhythm.*

• If you hear an unorthodox rhythm, assess whether the irregularity follows a definite or random pattern. *This evaluation helps to identify the type of abnormality.* For example, atrial fibrillation is an irregular rhythm with an irregular pattern.

• Auscultate for variations from the normal *lub-dub* systole-diastole sounds. Determine whether the first and second heart sounds are separate and distinct or split into two sounds. Assess for extra heartbeats and sounds that stretch into the next sound. *Such abnormal sounds may indicate a heart murmur — from patent ductus arteriosus, for example, as blood rushes through the abnormal opening.*

To take temperature rectally

• Wash your hands and put on gloves.

• With the neonate lying in a supine position, firmly grasp his ankles with your index finger between them *to prevent skin trauma.* Place a diaper over the penis of a male neonate *to absorb urine if he urinates.*

• Still holding the neonate's ankles, insert the lubricated thermometer no more than 2″ (1.3 cm) — *any farther could cause rectal injury.* Place the palm of your hand on his buttocks, and hold the thermometer between your index and middle fingers. *This stabilizes the thermometer and prevents breakage if the neonate moves suddenly. To inhibit the defecation response induced by inserting a rectal thermometer,* press the buttocks together. If you meet resistance during insertion, withdraw the thermometer and notify the doctor.

• Hold a mercury thermometer in place for 3 minutes and an electronic thermometer until the temperature registers. Remove the thermometer and read the number on the scale where the mercury stops or on the digital display panel. Record the result.

To take an axillary temperature

• Dry the axillary skin. Then place the thermometer in the axilla and hold it along the outer aspect of the neonate's chest between the axillary line and the arm for at least 3 minutes *because axillary temperature takes this long to register.* Hold an electronic thermometer in place until the temperature registers.

• Reassess axillary temperature in 15 to 30 minutes if it registers outside the normal range. If the temperature remains abnormal, notify the doctor. *A subnormal temperature may result from infection, and an elevated temperature may result from dehydration or reflect the environment, such as a malfunctioning overhead warmer.*

• Document the temperature.

Alternative methods for assessing neonatal blood pressure

Besides using a standard sphygmomanometer for assessing neonatal blood pressure, you may use palpation or auscultation.

Palpation
Feel for the neonate's radial or brachial pulse, which is the systolic blood pressure.

Auscultation
If you're using a pediatric stethoscope with amplification, listen for diastolic and systolic sounds at the brachial artery.
If you're using a Doppler blood pressure monitor, place the cuff directly over the brachial or popliteal artery *to ensure an accurate reading.* The device automatically inflates the cuff. *For greatest accuracy,* keep the cuffed arm or leg extended during cuff inflation. (Also observe the extremity's color. *Duskiness signifies reduced blood flow.*)

To determine blood pressure
• Measure blood pressure in a quiet neonate.
• Make sure that the blood pressure cuff is small enough for the patient (cuff width should be about half the circumference of the neonate's arm) because *the cuff size affects the accuracy of readings.*
• Wrap the cuff one or two fingerbreadths above the antecubital or popliteal area. With the stethoscope held directly over the chosen artery, hold the cuffed extremity firmly *to keep it extended* and inflate the cuff no faster

than 5 mm Hg/second. (See *Alternative methods for assessing neonatal blood pressure.*)
• *To determine whether subsequent blood pressure readings are within the neonate's normal range,* compare the readings to baseline values. Report any significant deviation.

Nursing considerations
• If desired, count respirations while auscultating the heart rate.
• When listening to neonatal heart tones immediately after birth, you may hear murmurs. These may result from a delayed closing of fetal blood shunts.
• Excessive neonatal activity — such as restlessness and crying — during a vital signs assessment may elevate the heart rate above normal. For this reason, describe the neonate's activity along with measured findings.

Documentation
• Record vital signs and related measurements in your notes, a special neonatal appraisal form, or a flowchart. Include any observations about the neonate's condition, such as abnormal breath sounds.

Nephrostomy and cystostomy tube care

Two urinary diversion techniques — nephrostomy and cystostomy — are used to ensure adequate drainage from the kidneys (nephrostomy) or bladder (cystostomy) and help prevent urinary tract infection or kidney failure. (See *Urinary diversion techniques.*)

Urinary diversion techniques

Nephrostomy and cystostomy are used to create permanent diversion, relieve obstruction from an inoperable tumor, or provide an outlet for urine after cystectomy. Temporary diversion can relieve obstruction from a calculus or ureteral edema. In *nephrostomy,* a catheter is inserted percutaneously through the flank into the renal pelvis. In *cystostomy,* a catheter is inserted percutaneously through the suprapubic area into the bladder.

Nephrostomy

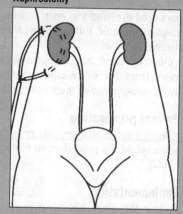

Cystostomy

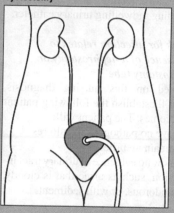

A nephrostomy tube is used to drain urine directly from a kidney when the normal flow of urine is obstructed. It is usually placed percutaneously, although it may be surgically inserted through the renal cortex and medulla into the renal pelvis from a lateral incision in the flank. The usual indication for nephrostomy is a disease that causes urinary obstruction, such as calculi in the ureter or ureteropelvic junction, or an obstructing tumor. Draining urine with a nephrostomy tube also promotes healing of kidney tissue damaged by obstructive disease.

A cystostomy tube is used to drain urine from the bladder, diverting it from the urethra. It is inserted about

2″ (5 cm) above the symphysis pubis. A cystostomy tube may be used alone or with an indwelling urethral catheter. Cystostomy is indicated after some gynecologic procedures, bladder surgery, and prostatectomy, and for patients with severe urethral stricture or traumatic injury.

❯❯ Key nursing diagnoses and patient outcomes

Use these nursing diagnoses as a guide when developing your plan of care for the patient with a nephrostomy or cystostomy tube.

Altered urinary elimination due to presence of a urinary diversion device

Based on this nursing diagnosis, you'll establish the following patient outcomes. The patient will:
• maintain fluid balance (intake equals output).
• experience minimal complications.
• describe feelings and concerns regarding indwelling urinary catheter.

Risk for infection related to presence of a nephrostomy or cystostomy tube

Based on this nursing diagnosis, you'll establish the following patient outcomes. The patient will:
• have no pathogens in cultures.
• remain afebrile.
• show no evidence of urinary tract infection, such as urine that is cloudy, malodorous, or with sediment.

Equipment

For dressing changes: ♦ $4'' \times 4''$ gauze pads ♦ povidone-iodine solution or povidone-iodine sponges ♦ sterile cup or emesis basin paper bag ♦ linen-saver pad ♦ clean gloves (for dressing removal) ♦ sterile gloves (for new dressing) ♦ forceps ♦ precut $4'' \times 4''$ drain dressings or transparent semipermeable dressings ♦ adhesive tape (preferably hypoallergenic).

For nephrostomy-tube irrigation: ♦ 3-ml syringe ♦ alcohol sponge or povidone-iodine sponge ♦ normal saline solution ♦ optional: hemostat.

Commercially prepared sterile dressing kits and povidone-iodine sponges may be available.

Equipment preparation

• Wash your hands and assemble all equipment at the patient's bedside.
• Open several packages of gauze pads, place them in the sterile cup or emesis basin, and pour the povidone-iodine solution over them. Or, open several packages of povidone-iodine sponges.
• If you're using a commercially packaged dressing kit, open it, using aseptic technique. Fill the cup with antiseptic solution.
• Open the paper bag, and position it away from the other equipment *to avoid contaminating the sterile field.*

Patient preparation

• Wash your hands, provide privacy, and explain the procedure to the patient.

Implementation

Follow the steps below to provide nephrostomy and cystostomy tube care.

To change a dressing

• Help the patient to lie on his back (for a cystostomy tube) or the side opposite the tube (for a nephrostomy tube) *so you can see the tube clearly and change the dressing more easily.*
• Place the linen-saver pad under the patient *to absorb excess drainage and keep the patient dry.*
• Put on the clean gloves. Carefully remove the tape from around the tube, and then remove the wet or soiled dressing. Discard the tape and dressing in the paper bag. Remove the gloves and discard them in the bag.
• Put on the sterile gloves. Pick up a saturated pad or dip a dry one into the cup of antiseptic solution.

• To clean the wound, wipe only once with each pad or sponge, moving from the insertion site outward. Discard the used pad or sponge in the paper bag. Don't touch the bag *to avoid contaminating your gloves.*

• Pick up a sterile 4″ × 4 ″ drain dressing and place it around the tube. If necessary, overlap two drain dressings to provide maximum absorption. Or, depending on your hospital's policy, apply a transparent semipermeable dressing over the site and tubing *to allow observation of the site without removing the dressing.*

• Use hypoallergenic tape to secure the dressing. Then tape the tube to the patient's lateral abdomen *to prevent tension on the tube.* (See *Taping a nephrostomy tube*, page 574.)

• Dispose of all equipment appropriately. Clean the patient as necessary.

To irrigate a nephrostomy tube

• Fill the 3-ml syringe with the normal saline solution.

• Clean the junction of the nephrostomy tube and drainage tube with the alcohol sponge or povidone-iodine sponge, and disconnect the tubes.

• Insert the syringe into the nephrostomy tube opening, and instill 2 to 3 ml of saline solution into the tube.

• Slowly aspirate the solution back into the syringe. *To avoid damaging the patient's renal pelvis tissue,* never pull back forcefully on the plunger.

• If the solution doesn't return, remove the syringe from the tube and reattach the drainage tubing *to allow the solution to drain by gravity.*

• Dispose of all equipment appropriately.

Complications

• The patient has an increased risk of infection because nephrostomy and cystostomy tubes provide direct openings to the kidneys or bladder.

Nursing considerations

• Change dressings once a day or more often if needed.

• When necessary, irrigate a cystostomy tube as you would an indwelling catheter. Be sure to perform the irrigation gently *to avoid damaging any suture lines.*

   Note. Never irrigate a nephrostomy tube with more than 5 ml of solution *because the capacity of the renal pelvis is usually between 4 and 8 ml.* (Remember that the purpose of irrigation is to keep the tube patent, not to lavage the renal pelvis.)

• Check a nephrostomy tube frequently for kinks or obstructions. Kinks are likely to occur if the patient lies on the insertion site. Suspect an obstruction when the amount of urine in the drainage bag decreases or the amount of urine around the insertion site increases. Pressure created by urine backing up in the tube can damage nephrons. Gently curve a cystostomy tube *to prevent kinks.*

• If a blood clot or mucus plug obstructs a nephrostomy or cystostomy tube, try milking the tube *to restore its patency.* With your nondominant hand, hold the tube securely above the obstruction *to avoid pulling the tube out of the incision.* Then place the flat side of a closed hemostat under the tube, just above the obstruction. Pinch the tube against the hemostat, and slide both your finger and the hemostat toward you, away from the patient.

Taping a nephrostomy tube

To tape a nephrostomy tube directly to the skin, cut a wide piece of hypoallergenic adhesive tape twice lengthwise to its midpoint.

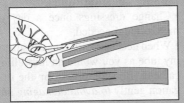

Apply the uncut end of the tape to the skin so that the midpoint meets the tube. Wrap the middle strip around the tube in spiral fashion. Tape the other two strips to the patient's skin on both sides of the tube.

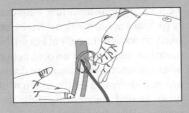

For greater security, repeat this step with a second piece of tape, applying it in the reverse direction. You may also apply two more strips of tape perpendicular to and over the first two pieces.

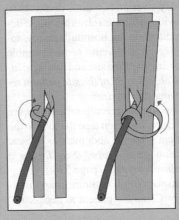

Always apply another strip of tape lower down on the tube in the direction of the drainage tube to further anchor the tube. Don't put tension on any sutures that prevent tube dislocation.

• Typically, cystostomy tubes for postoperative urologic patients are checked hourly for the first 24 hours *to ensure adequate drainage and tube patency.* To check tube patency, note the amount of urine in the drainage bag and check the patient's bladder for distention.

Home care
• Tell the home care patient how to clean the insertion site with soap and water, check for skin breakdown, and change the dressing daily. Demonstrate the procedure.
• Teach the patient how to change the leg bag and drainage bag. A leg bag can be used during the day and a larger drainage bag can be used overnight.
• Stress the importance of reporting to the doctor signs of infection (red skin or white, yellow, or green drainage at the insertion site) or tube displacement (drainage that smells like urine).
• Whether the patient uses a drainage bag or larger container, explain how to wash the device daily with a 1:3

vinegar and water solution, rinse it with plain water, and dry it on a clothes hanger or over a towel rack. *This prevents crystalline buildup.*

Documentation

• Describe the color and amount of drainage from the nephrostomy or cystostomy tube, and record any color changes as they occur.

• If the patient has more than one tube, describe the drainage (color, amount, and character) from each tube separately.

• If irrigation is necessary, record the amount and type of irrigant used and whether or not you obtained a complete return.

Neurologic vital signs measurement

Neurologic vital signs supplement the routine measurement of temperature, pulse rate, and respirations by evaluating the patient's level of consciousness (LOC), pupillary activity, and orientation to place, time, date, situation, and person. They provide a simple, indispensable tool for quickly checking the patient's neurologic status.

LOC — a measure of environmental and self-awareness — reflects cortical function and usually provides the first sign of central nervous system (CNS) deterioration. Changes in *pupillary activity* — pupil size, shape, equality, and response to light — may signal increased intracranial pressure (ICP), which is associated with a space-occupying lesion.

Evaluating muscle strength and tone, reflexes, and posture also may help identify CNS damage. Finally, changes in vital signs alone rarely indicate neurologic compromise, and any changes should be related to a complete neurologic assessment. Because vital signs are controlled at the medullary level, changes related to neurologic compromise are ominous.

⟫ Key nursing diagnoses and patient outcomes

Use these nursing diagnoses as a guide when developing your plan of care.

Anxiety related to environmental conflict

Based on this nursing diagnosis, you'll establish the following patient outcomes. The patient will:

• develop effective coping behaviors.

• maintain autonomy and independence without handicapping fears.

Knowledge deficit related to lack of exposure

Based on this nursing diagnosis, you'll establish the following patient outcomes. The patient will:

• communicate a need to know.

• demonstrate ability to perform new health-related behaviors as they are taught.

Equipment

◆ penlight ◆ thermometer ◆ sterile cotton ball or cotton-tipped applicator ◆ stethoscope ◆ sphygmomanometer ◆ pupil size chart ◆ optional: pencil or pen.

Patient preparation

- Explain the procedure, even if the patient is unresponsive.
- Provide privacy.

Implementation

- Wash your hands.

Assessing LOC and orientation

- Assess the patient's LOC by evaluating his responses. Use standard guidelines, such as the Glasgow coma scale. (See *Using the Glasgow coma scale.*)

Begin by measuring the patient's response to verbal, light tactile (touch), or painful (nail bed pressure) stimuli. First, ask the patient his full name. If he responds appropriately, assess his orientation to place, time, date, and situation. Ask the patient where he is and then what day, season, and year it is. (Expect disorientation to affect the sense of date first, then time, place, caregivers, and finally self.) When the patient responds verbally, assess the quality of replies. For example, garbled words indicate difficulty with the motor nerves that govern speech muscles. Rambling responses indicate difficulty with thought processing and organization.

- Assess the patient's ability to understand and follow one-step commands that require a motor response. For example, ask him to open and close his eyes or stick out his tongue. Note whether he can maintain his LOC. If you must gently shake him to keep him focused on your verbal commands, he may be neurologically compromised.
- If the patient doesn't respond to commands, apply a painful stimulus. With moderate pressure, squeeze the nail beds on fingers and toes, and note his response. Check motor responses bilaterally *to rule out monoplegia (paralysis of a single area) and hemiplegia (paralysis of one side of the body).*

Examining pupils and eye movement

- Ask the patient to open his eyes. If he doesn't respond, gently lift his upper eyelids. Inspect each pupil for size and shape, and compare the two for equality. *To evaluate pupil size more precisely,* use a chart showing the various pupil sizes (given in increments of 1 mm, with the normal diameter ranging from 2 to 6 mm). Remember, pupil size varies considerably, and some patients have normally unequal pupils (anisocoria). Also see if the pupils are positioned in, or deviated from, the midline.
- Test the patient's direct light response. First, darken the room. Then hold each eyelid open in turn, keeping the other eye covered. Swing the penlight from the patient's ear toward the midline of the face. Shine the light directly into the eye. Normally, the pupil constricts immediately. When you remove the penlight, the pupil should dilate immediately. Wait about 20 seconds before testing the other pupil *to allow it to recover from reflex stimulation.*
- Now test consensual light response. Hold both eyelids open, but shine the light into one eye only. Watch for constriction in the other pupil, *which indicates proper nerve function at the optic chiasm.*
- Brighten the room and have the conscious patient open his eyes. Observe the eyelids for ptosis, or drooping. Then check extraocular movements.

Using the Glasgow coma scale

The Glasgow coma scale provides a standard reference for assessing or monitoring a patient with suspected or confirmed brain injury. You measure three responses to stimuli — eye opening, motor response, and verbal response — and assign a number to each of the possible responses within these categories. A score of 3 is the lowest and 15 is the highest. A score of 7 or less indicates coma. This scale is commonly used in the emergency department, at the scene of an accident, and for periodic evaluation of the hospitalized patient.

CHARACTERISTIC	RESPONSE	SCORE
Eye opening	• Spontaneous	4
	• To verbal command	3
	• To pain	2
	• No response	1
Best motor response	• Obeys commands	6
	• To painful stimuli	
	Localizes pain; pushes stimulus away	5
	Flexes and withdraws	4
	Abnormal flexion	3
	Extension	2
	No response	1
Best verbal response (Arouse patient with painful stimuli, if necessary)	• Oriented and converses	5
	• Disoriented and converses	4
	• Uses inappropriate words	3
	• Makes incomprehensible sounds	2
	• No response	1
	Total:	3 to 15

Hold up one finger and ask the patient to follow it with his eyes alone. As you move the finger up, down, laterally, and obliquely, see if the patient's eyes track together to follow your finger (conjugate gaze). Watch for involuntary jerking or oscillating eye movements (nystagmus).

• Check accommodation. Hold up one finger midline to the patient's face and several feet away. Have the patient focus on your finger. Then gradually move your finger toward his nose while he still focuses on your finger. This should cause his eyes to converge and both pupils to constrict equally.

• Test the corneal reflex by touching a wisp of cotton ball to the cornea. This normally causes an immediate blink reflex. Repeat for the other eye.

• If the patient is unconscious, test the oculocephalic (doll's eye) reflex. Hold the patient's eyelids open. Then quickly, but gently, turn his head to one side, then the other. If his eyes move in the opposite direction from

Identifying warning postures

Decorticate and decerebrate posturing are ominous signs of central nervous system deterioration.

Decorticate (abnormal flexion)
In decorticate posturing, the patient's arms are adducted and flexed, with the wrists and fingers flexed on the chest. The legs may be stiffly extended and internally rotated, with plantar flexion of the feet.

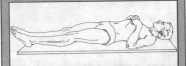

The decorticate posture may indicate a lesion of the frontal lobe, internal capsule, or cerebral peduncles.

Decerebrate (extension)
In decerebrate posturing, the patient's arms are adducted and extended with the wrists pronated and the fingers flexed. One or both of the legs may be stiffly extended, with plantar flexion of the feet.

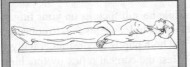

The decerebrate posture may indicate lesions of the upper brain stem.

the side to which you turn the head — eyes move right when the head moves left — the reflex is intact.

Note: Never test the doll's eye reflex if you know or suspect that the patient has a cervical spine injury.

Evaluating motor function
• If the patient is conscious, test his grip strength in both hands at the same time. Extend your hands, ask the patient to squeeze your fingers as hard as he can, and compare the strength of each hand. Grip strength is usually slightly stronger in the dominant hand.
• Test arm strength by having the patient close his eyes and hold his arms straight out in front of him with the palms up. See if either arm drifts downward or pronates *to indicate muscle weakness.*
• Test leg strength by having the patient raise his legs, one at a time, against gentle downward pressure from your hand. Gently push down on each leg at the midpoint of the thigh *to evaluate muscle strength.*

  Note. If decorticate or decerebrate posturing develops in response to stimuli, notify the doctor immediately. (See *Identifying warning postures.*)
• Flex and extend the extremities on both sides to evaluate muscle tone.
• Test the plantar reflex in all patients. Stroke the lateral aspect of the sole of the patient's foot with your thumbnail or another moderately sharp object. Normally, this elicits flexion of all toes. Watch for a positive Babinski's sign — dorsiflexion of the great toe with fanning of the other toes — *which indicates an upper motor neuron lesion.*
• Test for Brudzinski's and Kernig's signs in patients suspected of having meningitis.

Completing the examination

• Take the patient's temperature, pulse and respiratory rates, and blood pressure. Especially note his pulse pressure — which is the difference between systolic pressure and diastolic pressure — *because widening pulse pressure can indicate increasing ICP.*

Nursing considerations

Note. If a previously stable patient suddenly develops a change in neurologic or routine vital signs, assess his condition further, and notify the doctor immediately.

Documentation

• Baseline data require detailed documentation; subsequent notes can be brief unless the patient's condition changes.

• Record the patient's LOC and orientation, pupillary activity, motor function, and routine vital signs, as hospital policy directs. To save time while keeping complete records, the hospital may let you use abbreviations. Use only commonly understood abbreviations and terms to avoid misinterpretation of the patient's status. Examples include the following: $A + O \times 4$, alert and oriented to person, place, time, and date; *PERRLA,* pupils equal, round, reactive to light and accommodation; *PERL,* pupils equal, reactive to light; and *EOM,* extraocular movements.

• Describe the patient's behavior — for example, difficult to arouse by gentle shaking, sleepy, unresponsive to painful stimuli.

Nose, mouth, and throat inspection

To examine the nose, use direct inspection and olfactory function tests. Depending on the purpose of your assessment, you may also inspect the patient's mouth and throat and palpate the thyroid gland.

⟫ Key nursing diagnoses and patient outcomes

Use these nursing diagnoses as a guide when developing your plan of care.

Altered oral mucous membrane related to (specify)

Based on this nursing diagnosis, you'll establish the following patient outcomes. The patient will:

• have moist and pink oral mucous membranes.

• express feelings of increased comfort.

• correlate precipitating factors with appropriate oral care.

• demonstrate correct oral hygiene practices.

Impaired swallowing related to neuromuscular impairment

Based on this nursing diagnosis, you'll establish the following patient outcomes. The patient will:

• show no evidence of aspiration pneumonia.

• achieve adequate nutritional intake.

• maintain acceptable weight.

• demonstrate correct eating or feeding techniques to maximize swallowing.

Equipment

♦ penlight ♦ nasal speculum ♦ tongue blade ♦ sterile gauze ♦ clean gloves.

Patient preparation

• Wash your hands, provide privacy, and explain the procedure to the patient.

• When you're ready to inspect the nasal cavities, ask the patient to tilt his head back slightly.

Implementation

Here's how to inspect the nose, mouth, and throat.

Inspecting the nose

• Put on clean gloves *to protect you from contact with mucus or other body fluids.*

• Observe the nose for deviations in its shape, size, or color. The skin should be smooth and lesion-free, and the columella and the tip of the nose should lie midline without deviation. Expect the nostrils to be oval and symmetrical. Watch for nasal flaring or narrowing with respirations — signs of possible airway obstruction. Look for a transverse crease just above the tip of the nose, a sign of chronic nasal pruritus and allergies.

• Assess the ridge and the soft tissues of the nose by placing one finger on each side of the nasal arch. Gently palpate, moving the fingers from the nasal bridge to the tip.

• *To test both nasal patency and olfactory nerve (cranial nerve I) function,* have the patient block one nostril and inhale fumes from a familiar aromatic substance — such as soap, coffee, tobacco, or nutmeg — through the open nostril. Some examiners use 70% isopropyl alcohol for this test, but it can irritate the nasal mucosa, and many patients don't recognize its scent.

• Ask the patient to identify the aroma. Then have him block the other nostril and repeat the test, using a different aroma.

• *To evaluate patency,* occlude one nostril by pressing your finger on the side of the patient's nose. Then ask the patient to breathe in with his mouth closed. Breathing should be easy and noiseless. Similarly, check patency on the other side.

• Inspect the interior nasal cavity next. Hold the speculum in the palm of one hand and the penlight in the other hand. Have the patient tilt his head toward the light source.(See *Performing direct nasal inspection.*)

• Insert the speculum into the nostril, using your index finger for stability. Cautiously open the speculum, being careful not to overdilate the nostril or touch the nasal septum. Inspect the nasal mucosa, which should be deep pink. Note any discharge, masses, lesions, or mucosal swelling. Also check the nasal septum for perforation, bleeding, or crusting. Bluish turbinates suggest allergies. A rounded, elongated projection suggests a polyp. Next, inspect the opposite nostril.

Inspecting the mouth and throat

• Start by inspecting the lips. With the patient's mouth closed, observe the lips for symmetry and color. Pale lips may reflect anemia; a bluish hue suggests poor oxygenation.

• Note any edema or alterations in skin integrity. Then palpate the lips for lumps and surface abnormalities. Edema may result from allergies; dry, split lips may result from dehydration (from wind or heat). Cracks at the cor-

Performing direct nasal inspection

This illustration shows the proper placement of the nasal speculum during direct inspection of the nose. The inset shows the structures you should be able to see during this examination.

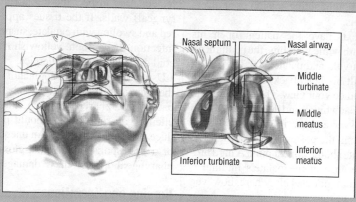

ners of the lips may indicate a vitamin deficiency. Lumps and skin changes may indicate irritation, infection, or cancer.

• Using the tongue blade and bright light, inspect the oral mucosa of the patient's open mouth. Place the tongue blade on top of the patient's tongue. Inspect the buccal surface of the mouth and lips. Normal mucosa appears moist, pinkish red, and smooth. The gums should appear pink with clearly defined margins at each tooth. Ulcerations, swelling, or bleeding may signal periodontal disease.

• *To inspect the dorsum of the tongue,* have your patient stick out the tongue as far as possible. A normal tongue appears dull red, moist, and glistening. The anterior surface should be slightly rough with papillae and small fissures. The posterior surface appears smooth and slightly uneven. Look for swelling, color deviations, a coating, or ul-

cerations. Normally, the tongue moves easily. At rest, it should lie straight to the front. Deviation to either side may indicate damage to the hypoglossal nerve.

• Have the patient place the tip of the tongue on the palate directly behind the front teeth. Inspect the tongue's ventral surface and the floor of the mouth. The ventral surface should be pink and smooth, with large veins between the frenulum and fimbriated folds. Note any swelling and varicosities.

Note. To assess for cyanosis in dark-skinned patients, look for a bluish discoloration of the mucous membranes in the mouth and under the tongue (or on the inner eyelids).

• Wrap the tip of the tongue with a piece of gauze. This will help you grasp the tongue and direct it to one side so you can inspect the lateral borders. Repeat the procedure, and inspect the other side. Both sides of the tongue should have a smooth, even texture. Note any nodules, ulcerations, or white patches.

• Palpate the tongue and the floor of the mouth, noting any lumps or ulcerations.

• Next, have the patient open his mouth while you shine the penlight on the uvula and palate. Ask the patient to tilt his head back, if necessary, to enhance your view. The palate should appear whitish and dome-shaped with transverse rugae in the anterior portion; in the posterior, soft portion, the palate should appear pink. A hard protuberance at the palate's midline is normal; nodules elsewhere, however, may be tumors.

• Using a tongue blade, depress the tongue and have the patient say ah. Observe the movement of the soft palate and the uvula (lying midline at the back of the soft palate). The soft palate should rise symmetrically with the uvula remaining midline. Deviation to one side may denote paralysis of the vagus nerve.

• Ask the patient to clench his teeth and smile as widely as possible. The upper teeth should rest evenly on the lower teeth. Note any protrusion of the upper teeth, failure of the upper teeth to overlap the lower teeth, or failure of the upper back teeth to meet the lower teeth (indicating malocclusion). Inability to adequately clench the teeth may indicate a damaged facial nerve.

• *To assess the teeth,* have the patient open his mouth wide. Teeth usually appear ivory or slightly yellow (although tea, coffee, and tobacco can darken them). Inspect for caries, missing teeth, and loose teeth.

• Using a tongue blade, depress the tongue and inspect the pharynx. Note the tonsils on both sides of the pharynx; if they're reddened, swollen, or covered with exudate, they may be infected. Also inspect the throat (pharyngeal) walls. If the tissues appear red and swollen with exudate, suspect infection. If you note yellowish mucoid drainage, suspect allergies.

• Using a cotton-tipped applicator (or the tongue blade), gently touch the back of the pharynx on each side to elicit a gag reflex. This should produce a bilateral response. An unequal or poor response may signal glossopharyngeal or vagal nerve damage.

Nursing considerations

• During your assessment of a patient's nose and throat, you may detect certain abnormalities. Some of the most common include nasal flaring, nasal drainage, paranasal sinus tenderness, pharyngitis, and peritonsillar abscess.

• In adults, some nasal flaring is normal during quiet breathing. Nasal flaring is also normal in children. But marked, regular flaring in an adult may be a sign of respiratory distress.

• The appearance of nasal drainage may help you determine its cause. Bloody drainage may result from frequent nose blowing or from spontaneous, traumatic epistaxis. Thick white or yellow drainage usually occurs with infection. Clear, thin drainage may simply indicate rhinitis. Or it may suggest cerebrospinal fluid leakage from a basilar skull fracture.

• A patient with viral pharyngitis will typically have slight swelling and inflammation of the pharynx. Streptococcal pharyngitis produces severe swelling and inflammation of the pharynx and exudate from the tonsils. With infectious mononucleosis, the patient may have enlargement or tenderness of the auricular, inguinal, and axillary lymph nodes as well as exudative pharyngitis.

• A peritonsillar abscess — also called quinsy — usually results from acute tonsillitis and causes painful swallowing and potential airway obstruction. In this condition, the streptococcal infection spreads from the tonsils to the surrounding soft tissue.

Documentation

• Note and document any tenderness or masses.
• Note any discharge and document its character and amount.
• Note any disparity in nostril sizes; such disparity may result from a deviated septum.
• Observe the lips for symmetry and color, and document any deviations.
• Note any edema and alterations in skin integrity.
• Note any nodules, ulcerations, or white patches on the tongue.
• Document the presence of caries and missing or loose teeth.

Nutritional assessment

A nutritional assessment includes a dietary history, an intake record, and a psychosocial assessment. (See *Dietary recall methods*, page 584.) This will help you confirm good nutrition or detect an alteration in nutritional status and the need for in-depth assessment and follow-up. It will also help you identify potential nutrition-related health problems, determine educational needs, and plan realistic patient outcomes.

≫ Key nursing diagnoses and patient outcomes

Use these nursing diagnoses as a guide when developing your plan of care.

Impaired swallowing related to neuromuscular impairment

Based on this nursing diagnosis, you'll establish the following patient outcomes. The patient will:
• show no evidence of aspiration pneumonia.
• achieve adequate nutritional intake.
• maintain weight.
• demonstrate correct eating or feeding techniques to maximize swallowing.

Altered nutrition: Less than body requirements

Based on this nursing diagnosis, you'll establish the following patient outcomes. The patient will:
• show no evidence of further weight loss.
• tolerate oral, tube, or I.V. feedings without adverse effects.
• take in a specified number of calories daily.
• gain a specified number of pounds weekly.
• demonstrate the ability to plan a diet after discharge.

Equipment

♦ calipers for measuring the triceps muscle's skin-fold thickness ♦ a tape measure ♦ a bedside or bed scale.

Dietary recall methods

Choose one of the dietary recall methods described below to assess a patient's dietary patterns.

24-hour dietary recall
Ask the patient to recall everything he ate or drank within the past 24 hours (or yesterday), when he consumed it, the amount, and how he prepared it. If assessing an infant or small child, determine the feeding schedule, the types and amounts of food and drink, and whether intake is adequate. Ask hospitalized patients to write down 24-hour food intake on a typical day.

Dietary inventory
Have the patient complete a 3-, 7-, or 14-day diary, recording everything he ate or drank, the time he ate it, the amount, and how he prepared it. Also have him record the place where he ate, whether he ate alone or with others, and whether he ate because of hunger or thirst, or for some other reason. Keep in mind that a patient may consciously or unconsciously modify his diet during the recorded time.

Food frequency form
This form provides an overview of the quality and variety of a patient's diet. The patient indicates how often he eats each food item listed.

Agency dietary history questionnaires
These usually combine dietary intake inventory with questions about factors that affect food intake. When using dietary recall intake forms, ask the patient to indicate the addition of any seasoning to the food.

Implementation
• Obtain and record the patient's weight at the same time each day *to ensure the most accurate reading.*

• Unless your patient has an urgent complaint, take the time to perform anthropometric arm measurements. *These measurements provide information about the caloric reserves in subcutaneous fat and indicate skeletal muscle mass.* First, locate and mark the midpoint of the patient's upper arm. Then, measure the skin-fold thickness with the calipers, measure the midarm circumference with a tape measure, and calculate the midarm muscle circumference. (See *Taking anthropometric arm measurements.*)

• Monitor fluid intake and output *to determine whether an imbalance exists and because body weight may increase as a result of fluid retention.*

• Monitor frequency, consistency, amount, and color of stool *to detect changes.*

• Auscultate for bowel sounds once per shift *to identify increased or decreased sounds.*

• Provide foods appropriate to the patient's prescribed diet *to avoid altering stool consistency.*

• Assess the patient's skin for dryness or lesions, which may occur with nutritional deficiencies. These skin changes should improve with nutrient replenishment.

• Monitor and document the status of any wounds, including size, color, and presence of drainage or odor, *to assess changes.*

• Assess physical limitations *to determine the patient's need for assistance.*

• Reassure the malnourished patient that proper limb functioning will re-

Taking anthropometric arm measurements

Follow these steps to determine triceps skin-fold thickness, midarm circumference, and midarm muscle circumference.

Triceps skin-fold thickness
Determine the triceps skin-fold thickness by grasping the patient's skin between the thumb and forefinger about 1 cm above the midpoint, as shown below. Hold the calipers at the midpoint and squeeze for about 3 seconds. Record the measurement registered on the handle gauge to the nearest 0.5 mm. Take two more readings; then average all three to compensate for any error.

Midarm circumference and midarm muscle circumference
At the midpoint, measure the midarm circumference, as shown here. Then calculate midarm muscle circumference by multiplying the triceps skin-fold thickness (in centimeters) by 3.143 and subtracting the result from the midarm circumference.

Record all three measurements as percentages of the standard measurements by using the following formula:

$$\frac{\text{Actual measurement}}{\text{Standard measurement}} \times 100$$

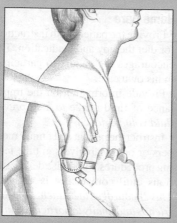

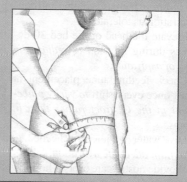

Compare the patient's percentage measurement with the standard. A measurement less than 90% of the standard indicates caloric deprivation, over 90% adequate or more than adequate energy reserves.

MEASUREMENT	STANDARD	90%
Triceps skin-fold thickness	Men: 12.5 mm Women: 16.5 mm	Men: 11.3 mm Women: 14.9 mm
Midarm circumference	Men: 29.3 cm Women: 28.5 cm	Men: 26.4 cm Women: 25.7 cm
Midarm muscle circumference	Men: 25.3 cm Women: 23.2 cm	Men: 22.8 cm Women: 20.9 cm

turn with nutritional repletion. *Reassurance will allay his anxiety.*
• Assess for signs of dehydration, including low urine output, dry skin, and sunken eyes. These may occur with fluid imbalance.
• Administer fluids, as prescribed, *to meet the patient's fluid requirements.*
• Carefully monitor the patient's response to fluid intake *to prevent complications of fluid overload,* including respiratory distress and edema.
• For patients receiving tube feedings, administer the prescribed amount of tube feeding *to provide needed nutrition.*
• Begin the tube feeding regimen with a small amount and diluted concentration *to decrease diarrhea and improve absorption.* Increase volume and concentration as tolerated.
• Elevate the head of the bed 30 degrees during infusion *to reduce the risk of aspiration.*
• Check feeding tube placement at least once every shift *to verify placement in the GI tract rather than in lungs.*
• Give water and juices, as needed, *to maintain adequate hydration.*
• Provide nostril care every 4 hours *to prevent ulceration and skin breakdown.* Tape the nasogastric tube *to prevent tube displacement.*
• Ensure proper temperature of food (room temperature), and change feeding tube bags and tubing at least every 24 hours or according to facility policy *to encourage optimal food intake.*

• Auscultate and record breath sounds every 4 hours *to monitor for aspiration.* Report wheezes, rhonchi, crackles, or decreased breath sounds. If aspiration is suspected, stop tube feeding. Keep suction apparatus at the patient's bedside and suction as needed. Turn the patient on his side *to avoid further aspiration.*

Nursing considerations
• If possible, use continuous infusion pump when giving tube feedings *to avoid diarrhea.*
• Put food coloring in tube feeding *to monitor for aspiration.*

Home care
• Provide the patient with instructions for diet therapy and medication. This encourages the patient to participate in his own care.
• Provide information on the importance of fluid intake *to help prevent fluid volume deficit.*
• Instruct the patient and family members or other caregivers in tube feeding procedures. Supervise demonstrations until competence is achieved. *This encourages the patient as well as friends and family to participate in the patient's care.*

Documentation
• Document the patient's daily weight, anthropometric arm measurements, intake and output, and abnormalities noted during daily assessments.

O

Ommaya reservoir drug infusion

Also known as the subcutaneous cerebrospinal fluid (CSF) reservoir, the Ommaya reservoir allows delivery of long-term drug therapy to the CSF via the brain's ventricles. The reservoir spares the patient repeated lumbar punctures to administer chemotherapeutic drugs, analgesics, antibiotics, and antifungals. It's most commonly used for chemotherapy and pain management, specifically for treating central nervous system (CNS) leukemia, malignant CNS disease, or meningeal carcinomatosis.

The reservoir is a mushroom-shaped silicone apparatus with an attached catheter. It's surgically implanted beneath the patient's scalp in the nondominant lobe, and the catheter is threaded into the ventricle through a burr hole in the skull. (See *How the Ommaya reservoir works,* page 588.) Besides providing convenient, comparatively painless access to CSF, the Ommaya reservoir permits consistent and predictable drug distribution throughout the subarachnoid space and CNS. It also allows measurement of intracranial pressure (ICP).

Before the reservoir is inserted, the patient may receive a local or general anesthetic, depending on his condition and the doctor's preference. After an X ray confirms placement of the reservoir, a pressure dressing is applied for 24 hours, followed by a gauze dressing for another day or two.

The sutures may be removed in about 10 days. However, the reservoir can be used within 48 hours to deliver drugs, obtain CSF pressure measurements, drain CSF, and withdraw CSF specimens.

The doctor usually injects drugs into the Ommaya reservoir, but a specially trained nurse may perform this procedure if allowed by hospital policy and the state's nurse practice act. This sterile procedure usually takes 15 to 30 minutes.

≫ Key nursing diagnoses and patient outcomes

Use these nursing diagnoses as a guide when developing your plan of care for a patient who is receiving medications through an Ommaya reservoir.

Knowledge deficit related to lack of exposure

Based on this nursing diagnosis, you'll establish the following patient outcomes. The patient will:
• state or demonstrate understanding of what has been taught.
• demonstrate ability to perform new health-related behaviors as they are taught.

High risk for injury related to improper technique

Based on this nursing diagnosis, you'll establish the following patient outcomes. The patient will:
• identify factors that increase his risk of injury.
• assist in identifying and applying safety measures to prevent injury.

How the Ommaya reservoir works

To insert an Ommaya reservoir, the doctor drills a burr hole and inserts the device's catheter through the patient's nondominant frontal lobe into the lateral ventricle. The reservoir, which has a self-sealing silicone injection dome, rests over the burr hole under a scalp flap. This creates a slight, soft bulge on the scalp, approximately the size of a quarter. Usually, drugs are injected into the dome with a syringe.

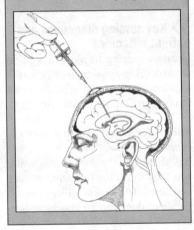

Equipment

♦ preservative-free prescribed drug ♦ gloves ♦ povidone-iodine solution ♦ sterile towel ♦ two 3-ml syringes ♦ 25G needle or 22G Huber needle ♦ sterile gauze pad ♦ collection tubes for CSF, if ordered ♦ vial of bacteriostatic normal saline solution.

Patient preparation

• Using the sterile towel, establish a sterile field near the patient. Prepare a syringe with the preservative-free drug to be instilled and place it, the CSF collection tubes, and the normal saline solution on the sterile field.

• Explain the procedure before reservoir insertion. Make sure the patient and his family understand the potential complications, and answer any questions they may have.

• Reassure the patient that any hair shaved for the implant will grow back and that only a coin-sized patch must remain shaved for injections. (Hair regrowth will be slower if the patient is receiving chemotherapy.)

Implementation

• Obtain baseline vital signs.

• Position the patient so he's either sitting or reclining.

• Put on gloves and prepare the patient's scalp with the povidone-iodine solution, working in a circular motion from the center outward.

• Placing the 25G needle at a 45-degree angle, insert it into the reservoir and aspirate 3 ml of clear CSF into the syringe. (If the aspirate isn't clear, check with the doctor before continuing.)

• Continue to aspirate as many millimeters of CSF as you will instill of the drug. Then detach the syringe from the needle hub, attach the drug syringe, and instill the medication slowly, monitoring the patient for headache, nausea, and dizziness. (Some hospitals use the CSF to deliver the drug, instead of a preservative-free diluent.)

• Instruct the patient to lie quietly for about 15 to 30 minutes after the procedure. *This may prevent meningeal irritation, which can cause nausea and vomiting.*

• Cover the site with a sterile gauze pad, and apply gentle pressure for a moment or two until superficial bleeding stops.

• Monitor the patient for adverse drug reactions and signs of increased ICP, such as nausea, vomiting, pain, or dizziness. Assess for adverse reactions every 30 minutes for 2 hours, then every hour for 2 hours, and finally every 4 hours.

Complications

• Infection may develop but can usually be treated successfully by injection of antibiotics directly into the reservoir. Persistent infection may require removal of the reservoir.

• Catheter migration or blockage may cause symptoms of increased ICP, such as headache and nausea. If the doctor suspects this problem, he may gently push and release the reservoir several times (a technique called pumping). With his finger on the patient's scalp, the doctor can feel the reservoir refill. Slow filling suggests catheter migration or blockage, which must be confirmed by computed tomography scan. Surgical correction is required.

Nursing considerations

• Occasionally, the doctor may wish to prescribe an antiemetic to be administered 30 minutes before the procedure to control nausea and vomiting.

• After the reservoir is implanted, the patient may resume normal activities. Instruct him to protect the site from bumps and traumatic injury while the incision heals.

• Tell him that, unless complications develop, the reservoir may function for years.

• Instruct the patient and his family to notify the doctor if any signs of infection develop at the insertion site (for example, redness, swelling, tenderness, or drainage) or if the patient develops a headache, a stiff neck, or a fever, which may indicate a systemic infection.

Documentation

• Record the appearance of the reservoir insertion site before and after access, the patient's tolerance of the procedure, the amount of CSF withdrawn, its appearance, and the name and dosage of the drug instilled.

Ophthalmoscopic examination

An ophthalmoscopic examination provides magnified views of the vascular and nerve tissue of the fundus of the eye, including the optic disk, retinal vessels, macula, and retina. The instrument used in this test — either the direct or the indirect ophthalmoscope — is considered one of the most important diagnostic tools in ophthalmology. Most examiners use the direct ophthalmoscope — a small, handheld instrument consisting of a light source, viewing device, reflecting device to channel light into a patient's eyes, and spherical lenses (to correct any refractive errors of either the patient or the examiner). The direct model is easier to use than the indirect.

Normal ophthalmoscopic findings include the following:

• red reflex — an orange glow reflected by the retina — that's visible through the aperture when the beam of light from the ophthalmoscope is directed into the pupil

• optic disk, which lies to the nasal side of the fundus center and is typically pink, with darker edges at its nasal border (however, its color varies widely)

• physiologic cup, a pale depression in the center of the optic disk, which varies widely in size (it tends to be larger in a patient with myopia and smaller in one with hyperopia)

• semitransparent retina surrounding the optic disk, with retinal vessels branching out from the disk

• macula, a darkly pigmented area of the retina, with a small, even darker spot called the fovea in the center

• tiny light reflex at the center of the fovea, caused by reflection of the ophthalmoscopic light from the concave inner surface of the area.

Abnormal ophthalmoscopic findings may include the following:

• an absent or diminished red reflex, which may result from gross corneal lesions, dense opacities of the aqueous or vitreous, cataracts, or detached retina

• a cloudy vitreous that obscures the fundus, possibly caused by inflammatory disease of the optic disk, retina, or uvea

• optic neuritis, which causes the optic disk to become elevated and more vascular and may produce small hemorrhages

• optic nerve atrophy, which makes the disk appear white

• papilledema, such as from increased intracranial pressure, which causes abnormal elevation of the disk, blurring of disk margins, engorged vessels, and hemorrhages

• physiologic cup that appears enlarged and gray, with white edges, reflecting glaucoma

• a milky-white retina, which signals the acute phase of central retinal artery occlusion; the fovea, in contrast to the ischemic macula, appears as a bright red spot

• widespread retinal hemorrhaging, patches of white exudate, and disk elevation, indicating central retinal vein occlusion

• gray elevated areas, possibly with areas of red vascular choroid exposed by retinal tears, signalling retinal detachments

• a dark lesion, which may indicate a choroidal tumor.

Interpretation of ophthalmoscopic findings depends largely on the examiner's knowledge and experience, because an abnormality can arise from several sources. After an ophthalmoscopic evaluation, referral for complete medical evaluation may be necessary.

≫ Key nursing diagnoses and patient outcomes

Use these nursing diagnoses as a guide when developing your plan of care.

Sensory or perceptual alteration (visual) related to altered sensory reception, transmission, or integration

Based on this nursing diagnosis, you'll establish the following patient outcomes. The patient will:

• discuss impact of vision loss on lifestyle.

• express feelings of safety, comfort, and security.

• show interest in surroundings.

• use appropriate resources when needed.

Risk for injury related to sensory deficits

Based on this nursing diagnosis, you'll establish the following patient outcomes. The patient will:
• identify factors that increase risk of injury.
• identify and apply safety measures to prevent injury.
• perform activities of daily living optimally within sensorimotor limitations.

Equipment

♦ ophthalmoscope ♦ mydriatic (dilating) eyedrops.

Patient preparation

• Explain to the patient that this test permits examination of the interior back of the eye.
• Describe the test, including who will perform it, where it will take place, and how long it takes to perform (usually less than 5 minutes).
• Advise the patient that eyedrops may be instilled *to dilate the pupils for a clearer examination.* Reassure him that he'll feel no discomfort during the test.
• Have the patient sit upright in the examination chair. Dim the room lights *to keep their reflections from interfering with the examination.*

Implementation

• Turn on the ophthalmoscope by pressing the ON/OFF switch and rotating the rheostat clockwise until the desired light intensity is reached. Shine the light onto the palm of your hand, and rotate the aperture selector until a large, round beam of white light appears. (See *Parts of an ophthalmoscope,* page 592.)

• Next, select the proper lens. Choose a lens setting of zero diopter (a measurement of refractive power) if both you and the patient have normal vision.
• If either you or the patient has myopia (nearsightedness), adjust the lens for a longer focus. Turn the lens selector counterclockwise to the red numbers (negative diopters) until you can see the retina clearly.
• *To focus the lens for hyperopia (farsightedness),* turn the lens selector clockwise to the black numbers (positive diopters) until you can see the retina clearly.
• Adjust the lens to a positive setting if the patient has had a cataract removed. If the patient wears a contact lens, however, you may be able to see the retina with the lens set at 0.
• Dim the room lights *to keep reflections from interfering with the examination. This also helps to dilate the patient's pupils,* but you may need to administer mydriatic eyedrops to dilate them sufficiently.
• *To examine the patient's right eye,* hold the ophthalmoscope in your right hand with your index finger on the lens selector *so that you can focus during the examination.*
• Place the ophthalmoscope over your eye, bracing it near your eyebrow. Make sure you can see through the aperture.
• *To steady yourself and the patient,* place your free hand on the patient's shoulder.
• Direct the patient to look slightly up and over your shoulder and to gaze at a specific point on the wall. With the ophthalmoscope about 12″ to 15″ (30 to 38 cm) away from the patient, shine the light through the patient's pupil.

Parts of an ophthalmoscope

Made of mirrors, a light, and several lenses, this battery-operated instruments allows you to see such structures as the retina, optic disk, macula, fovea centralis, and arteries and veins.

Front view

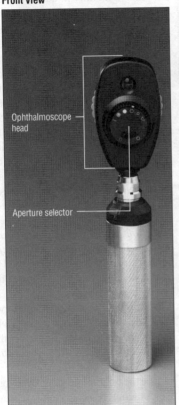

Ophthalmoscope head

Aperture selector

Back view

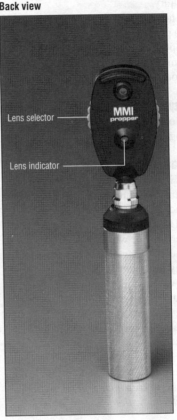

MMI propper

Lens selector

Lens indicator

Apertures

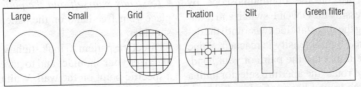

Large	Small	Grid	Fixation	Slit	Green filter

You'll see the red reflex, an orange glow reflected by the retina. Keeping the light beam focused, move toward the patient until the ophthalmoscope almost touches the patient's eyelashes.

• As you approach the patient, retinal details become sharper, although you may need to readjust the lens to keep the retina in focus. If the light shines too brightly, dim it slightly by adjusting the rheostat. Now, look for the optic disk, a yellowish orange to creamy pink oval or round structure located on the nasal side of the retina. If you don't see it, locate a blood vessel and follow it toward the center of the retina until the optic disk appears.

• Next, assess the eye's vascular supply by following the vessels in each of four directions. Note the size ratio of arterioles to veins (normally 2:3 or 4:5), and evaluate the character and distribution of the vessels (normally free of exudate) and arteriovenous crossings (normally smooth).

• As you observe, be alert for lesions. Sketch or photograph fundal lesions for further study.

• Finally, inspect the macula, located temporally to the optic disk. A normal macula appears as a yellow dot surrounded by a deep-pink periphery without blood vessels.

• Repeat the examination on the other eye.

Complications
• The patient may have a hypersensitivity reaction to the mydriatic eyedrops.

• A corneal laceration could occur with an uncooperative or violent patient.

Nursing considerations
• Before instilling eyedrops, check the patient's history for previous use of dilating eyedrops, indications of possible hypersensitivity, and narrow-angle glaucoma.

• Mydriatic drops are contraindicated for patients with head injury or coma who require regular pupillary monitoring.

• Make sure the patient maintains fixed vision throughout the procedure.

Home care
• Warn the patient that mydriatic drops cause temporarily blurred vision.

• Tell the patient not to drive or operate heavy machinery until the temporary blurred vision has worn off.

• Tell the patient that he may wear dark glasses to ease the discomfort of photophobia.

Documentation
• Document the time and place of the ophthalmoscopic examination, name of the mydriatic eyedrops used, normal and abnormal findings of each eye structure examined, and the patient's tolerance of the procedure.

Oral drug administration

Because oral administration of drugs is usually the safest, most convenient, and least expensive method, most drugs are administered by this route. Drugs for oral administration are available in many forms: capsules, tablets, enteric-coated tablets, syrups, elixirs, oils, liquids, suspensions, powders, and granules. Some require special preparation before administration, such as mixing with juice to make them more palatable; oils, powders, and granules most often require such preparation.

Oral drugs are sometimes prescribed in higher dosages than their parenteral equivalents because, after absorption through the GI system, they are immediately broken down by the liver, before they reach the systemic circulation. Oral administration is contraindicated for unconscious patients; it may also be contraindicated in patients with nausea and vomiting and in those unable to swallow.

≫ Key nursing diagnoses and patient outcomes

Use these nursing diagnoses as a guide when developing your plan of care for a patient receiving oral medication.

Knowledge deficit related to lack of exposure to information on oral drug administration

Based on this nursing diagnosis, you'll establish the following patient outcomes. The patient will:
• state or demonstrate understanding of what has been taught.
• demonstrate ability to perform new health-related behaviors as they are taught.

Risk for injury related to improper technique

Based on this nursing diagnosis, you'll establish the following patient outcomes. The patient will:
• identify factors that increase risk for injury.
• assist in identifying and applying safety measures to prevent injury.

Equipment

♦ patient's medication record and chart ♦ prescribed medication ♦ medication cup ♦ optional: appropriate vehicle, such as jelly or applesauce, for crushed pills commonly used with children or elderly patients and juice, water, or milk for liquid medications; drinking straw; mortar and pestle for crushing pills.

Implementation

• Verify the order on the patient's medication record by checking it against the doctor's order.
• Wash your hands.
• Check the label on the medication three times before administering it *to make sure you'll be giving the prescribed medication.* Check when you take the container from the shelf or drawer, again before you pour the medication into the medication cup, and again before returning the container to the shelf or drawer. If you're administering a unit-dose medication, check the label for the final time at the patient's bedside immediately after pouring the medication and before discarding the wrapper.
• Confirm the patient's identity by asking his name and checking the name, room number, and bed number on his wristband.
• Assess the patient's condition, including level of consciousness and vital signs, as needed. *Changes in the patient's condition may warrant withholding medication.* For example, you may need to withhold a medication that will slow the patient's heart rate if his apical pulse rate is below 60.
• Give the patient his medication and, as needed, an appropriate vehicle or liquid *to aid swallowing, minimize ad-*

verse effects, or promote absorption. For example, cyclophosphamide is given with fluids *to minimize adverse effects;* antitussive cough syrup is given without a fluid *to avoid diluting its soothing effect on the throat.* If appropriate, crush the medication *to facilitate swallowing.*

• Stay with the patient until he has swallowed the drug. If he seems confused or disoriented, check his mouth *to make sure he has swallowed it.* Return and reassess the patient's response within 1 hour after giving the medication.

Nursing considerations

• Make sure you have a written order for every medication given. Verbal orders should be signed by the doctor within the specified time period. (Hospitals usually require a signature within 24 hours; long-term care facilities, within 48 hours.)

• Use care in measuring out the prescribed dose of liquid oral medication. (See *Measuring liquid medications.*)

• Don't give medication from a poorly labeled or unlabeled container. Don't attempt to label or reinforce drug labels yourself. This must be done by a pharmacist.

• Never give a medication poured by someone else. Never allow your medication cart or tray out of your sight. This prevents anyone from rearranging the medications or taking one without your knowledge. Never return unwrapped or prepared medications to stock containers. Instead, dispose of them and notify the pharmacy. Keep in mind that the disposal of any narcotic drug must be co-signed by another nurse, as mandated by law.

Measuring liquid medications

To pour liquids, hold the medication cup at eye level. Use your thumb to mark off the correct level on the cup.

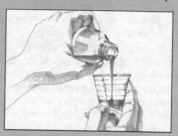

Then set the cup down and read the bottom of the meniscus at eye level *to ensure accuracy.* If you've poured too much medication into the cup, discard the excess. Don't return it to the bottle. Here are some additional tips:

• Hold the container so that the medication flows from the side opposite the label *so it won't run down the container and stain or obscure the label.* Remove drips from the lip of the bottle first, then from the sides, using a clean, damp paper towel.

• For a liquid measured in drops, use only the dropper supplied with the medication.

• If the patient questions you about his medication or the dosage, check his medication record again. If the medication is correct, reassure him. Make sure you tell him about any changes in his medication or dosage. Instruct him, as appropriate, about possible adverse effects. Ask him to report anything that he feels may be an adverse effect.

BETTER CHARTING

Documenting drugs given p.r.n.

Chart all drugs administered as needed (p.r.n.). For eye, ear, or nose drops, for example, chart the number of drops and where they were inserted. For suppositories, chart the type (rectal, vaginal, or urethral) and how it was tolerated. For dermal drugs, chart the size and location of the area to which you applied the drug. Also describe the condition of the skin or wound. For dermal patch, chart the location of the patch.

If you administer all drugs according to the accepted standards, you don't need to include more specific information in the chart. However if the medication administration record doesn't include space to document exceptional data (such as the patient's response to drugs given p.r.n. or any deviations from the drug order, such as patient refusal), document the information as a narrative in the chart.

12/8/97	0900	Pt. refused KCL elixir, stating that it makes her feel nauseated and she can't stand the taste. Dr. Miller notified. K-Dur tabs ordered and given. Pt. tolerated K-Dur well. — Betty Shiffer, RN

• *To avoid damaging or staining the patient's teeth,* give acid or iron preparations through a straw. Unpleasant-tasting liquids are usually more palatable if taken through a straw *because the liquid contacts fewer taste buds.*
• Oral medications are relatively easy to give to infants *because of their nat-*

ural *sucking instinct and, in infants under 4 months, their undeveloped sense of taste.*
• If the patient can't swallow a whole tablet or capsule, ask the pharmacist if the drug is available in liquid form or if it can be administered by another route. If not, ask him if you can crush the tablet or open the capsule and mix it with food. Keep in mind that many enteric-coated or timed-release medications and gelatin capsules should not be crushed. Remember to contact the doctor for an order to change the route of administration when necessary.

Documentation

• Note the drug administered, the dose, the date and time, and the patient's reaction, if any.
• If the patient refuses a drug, document the refusal and notify the charge nurse and the patient's doctor, as needed.
• Note whether a drug was omitted or withheld for other reasons, such as radiology or laboratory tests, or if, in your judgment, the drug was contraindicated at the ordered time.
• Sign out all narcotics given on the appropriate narcotics record. Also chart drugs administered as needed (p.r.n.). (See *Documenting drugs given p.r.n.*)

Oronasopharyngeal suction

Oronasopharyngeal suction removes secretions from the pharynx by means of a suction catheter inserted through the mouth or nostril. Used to maintain a patent airway, this procedure is indicated for a patient who's unable to clear his airway effectively with coughing and expectoration — for example, an unconscious or severely debilitated patient or an intubated patient who has secretions pooled above the cuff of the artificial airway. The procedure should be done as often as necessary, depending on the patient's condition.

Because the catheter may inadvertently slip into the lower airway or esophagus, oronasopharyngeal suction is an aseptic procedure that requires sterile equipment. However, clean technique may be used for a tonsil tip suction device. In fact, an alert patient can use a tonsil tip suction device himself to remove secretions.

Nasopharyngeal suctioning should be performed with caution in patients who have nasopharyngeal bleeding or spinal fluid leakage into the nasopharyngeal area. Also be alert when performing this procedure on patients who are receiving anticoagulant therapy or who have blood dyscrasias because these conditions increase the risk of bleeding.

>> Key nursing diagnoses and patient outcomes

Use these nursing diagnoses as a guide when developing your plan of care for a patient requiring oronasopharyngeal suctioning.

Ineffective breathing pattern related to decreased energy

Based on this nursing diagnosis, you'll establish the following patient outcomes. The patient will:
• achieve maximum lung expansion with adequate ventilation.

• report feeling comfortable with breathing.

Impaired gas exchange related to altered oxygen supply

Based on this nursing diagnosis, you'll establish the following patient outcomes. The patient will:
• cough effectively.
• expectorate sputum.

Equipment

♦ wall suction or portable suction apparatus ♦ collection bottle ♦ connecting tubing ♦ water-soluble lubricant ♦ normal saline solution or sterile water ♦ disposable sterile container ♦ sterile suction catheter (a #12 or #14 French for an adult, #8 or #10 French for a child, or pediatric feeding tube for an infant) ♦ sterile gloves ♦ tonsil tip suction device ♦ clean gloves ♦ nasopharyngeal or oropharyngeal airway (optional for frequent suctioning) ♦ overbed table ♦ waterproof trash bag ♦ soap, water, and 70% alcohol for cleaning catheters.

A sterile catheter, disposable container, and sterile gloves are available in a commercially prepared kit.

Equipment preparation

• Check your hospital's policy to determine whether a doctor's order is required for oronasopharyngeal suctioning.
• Review the patient's arterial blood gas or oxygen saturation values, and check vital signs.
• Evaluate the patient's ability to cough and deep-breathe to determine his ability to move secretions up the tracheobronchial tree.
• Check the patient's history for a deviated septum, nasal polyps, nasal

obstruction, traumatic injury, epistaxis, or mucosal swelling.
• If no contraindications exist, gather and place the suction equipment on the patient's overbed table or bedside stand.
• Position the table or stand on your preferred side of the bed *to facilitate suctioning.*
• Attach the collection bottle to the suctioning unit, and attach the connecting tubing to it.
• Date and then open the bottle of normal saline solution or sterile water.
• Open the waterproof trash bag.

Implementation

• Explain the procedure to the patient, even if he's unresponsive. Inform him that suctioning may stimulate transient coughing or gagging but that it helps to loosen secretions. If the patient has been suctioned previously, simply summarize the reasons for the procedure. Continue to reassure the patient throughout the procedure *to minimize anxiety and fear, which can increase oxygen consumption.* Also, ask the patient which nostril is more patent.
• Wash your hands.
• Place the patient in semi-Fowler's or high Fowler's position, if tolerated, *to promote lung expansion and effective coughing.*
• Turn on the suction from the wall or portable unit, and set the pressure according to hospital policy. Usually, the pressure is set between 80 and 120 mm Hg; higher pressure can cause excessive trauma without enhancing secretion removal. Occlude the end of the connecting tubing *to check suction pressure.*

• Using strict aseptic technique, open the suction catheter kit or the sterile catheter, container, and gloves. Put on the gloves and consider your dominant hand sterile and your nondominant hand nonsterile. Using your nondominant (nonsterile) hand, pour the sterile water or saline into the sterile container.
• With your nondominant hand, place a small amount of water-soluble lubricant on the sterile area. The lubricant is used *to facilitate passage of the catheter during nasopharyngeal suctioning.*
• Pick up the catheter with your dominant (sterile) hand and attach it to the connecting tubing. Use your nondominant hand to control the suction valve while your dominant hand manipulates the catheter.
• Instruct the patient to cough and breathe slowly and deeply several times before beginning suction. *Coughing helps loosen secretions and may decrease the amount of suctioning necessary, while deep-breathing helps minimize or prevent hypoxia.* (See *Tips on airway clearance.*)

For nasal insertion

• Raise the tip of the patient's nose with your nondominant hand *to straighten the passageway and facilitate insertion of the catheter.* Without applying suction, gently insert the suction catheter into the patient's nares. Roll the catheter between your fingers *to help it advance through the turbinates.* Continue to advance the catheter approximately 5″ to 6″ (12.7 to 15 cm) until you reach the pool of secretions or the patient begins to cough.

Tips on airway clearance

Deep breathing and coughing are vital for removing secretions from the lungs. Additional methods to help clear the airway include diaphragmatic breathing and forced expiration. Here's how to teach these methods to your patients.

Diaphragmatic breathing

First, tell the patient to lie in a supine position, with his head elevated 15 to 20 degrees on a pillow. Tell him to place one hand on his abdomen, and then to inhale so that he can feel his abdomen rise. Explain that this is what's known as breathing with the diaphragm.

Next, instruct the patient to exhale slowly through his nose — or, even better, through pursed lips — while letting his abdomen collapse. Explain that this action decreases his respiratory rate and increases his tidal volume.

Suggest that the patient perform this exercise for 30 minutes several times a day. After he becomes accustomed to the position, and after he's learned to breathe using his diaphragm, he may apply abdominal weights of 4 to 5 kg. The weights enhance the movement of the diaphragm toward the head during expiration.

To enhance the effectiveness of exercise, the patient may also manually compress the lower costal margins, perform straight leg lifts, and coordinate the breathing technique with a physical activity, such as walking.

Forced expiration

Another technique you should teach the patient is forced expiration. First, explain that forced expiration helps clear secretions while causing less traumatic injury than does a cough.

To perform the technique, tell the patient to forcefully expire without closing his glottis, starting with a mid- to low-lung volume. Tell him to follow this expiration with a period of diaphragmatic breathing and relaxation.

Advise the patient that if his secretions are in the central airways, he may have to use a more forceful expiration or a cough to clear them.

For oral insertion

• Without applying suction, gently insert the catheter into the patient's mouth. Advance the catheter approximately 3″ to 4″ (7.6 to 10 cm) along the side of the patient's mouth until you reach the pool of secretions or the patient begins to cough. Suction both sides of the patient's mouth and pharyngeal area.

• Using intermittent suction, withdraw the catheter from either the mouth or the nose with a continuous rotating motion *to minimize invagination of the mucosa into the catheter's tip and side ports.* Apply suction for only 10 to 15 seconds at a time *to minimize tissue trauma.*

• Between passes, wrap the catheter around your dominant hand *to prevent contamination.*

• If secretions are thick, clear the lumen of the catheter by dipping it in water and applying suction.

• Repeat the procedure until gurgling or bubbling sounds stop and respirations are quiet.

• After completing suctioning, pull your sterile glove off over the coiled catheter and discard it and the nonsterile glove along with the container of water.

• Flush the connecting tubing with normal saline solution or water.

• Replace the used items *so they're ready for the next suctioning,* and wash your hands.

Complications

• Increased dyspnea caused by hypoxia and anxiety may result from this procedure.

• Hypoxia can result because oxygen from the oronasopharynx is removed with the secretions. The amount of oxygen removed varies, depending upon the duration of the suctioning, suction flow and pressure, the size of the catheter in relation to the size of the patient's airway, and the patient's physical condition.

• Bloody aspirate can also result from prolonged or traumatic suctioning. Water-soluble lubricant can help to minimize traumatic injury.

Nursing considerations

• If the patient has no history of nasal problems, alternate suctioning between nostrils *to minimize traumatic injury.* If repeated oronasopharyngeal suctioning is required, the use of a nasopharyngeal or oropharyngeal airway will help with catheter insertion, reduce traumatic injury, and promote a patent airway. To facilitate catheter insertion for oropharyngeal suctioning, depress the patient's tongue with a tongue blade, or ask another nurse

to do so. *This helps you to visualize the back of the throat and also prevents the patient from biting the catheter.*

• If the patient has excessive oral secretions, consider using a tonsil tip catheter *because this allows the patient to remove oral secretions independently, as needed.*

• Let the patient rest after suctioning while you continue to observe him. The frequency and duration of suctioning depends on the patient's tolerance of the procedure and on any complications.

Home care

• Oronasopharyngeal suctioning may be performed in the home using a portable suction machine. Under these circumstances, suctioning is a clean rather than a sterile procedure. Properly cleaned catheters can be reused, putting less financial strain on patients.

Catheters should be cleaned by first washing them in soapy water and then boiling them for 10 minutes or soaking them in 70% alcohol for 3 to 5 minutes. The catheters should then be rinsed with normal saline solution or tap water.

• Whether the patient requires disposable or reusable suction equipment, you should make sure that he and his caregivers have received proper teaching and support.

Documentation

• Record the date, time, reason for suctioning, and technique used; amount, color, consistency, and odor (if any) of the secretions; the patient's respiratory status before and after the procedure; any complications and the nursing action taken; and the patient's tolerance of the procedure.

Oropharyngeal airway insertion

An oropharyngeal airway, a curved rubber or plastic device, is inserted into the mouth to the posterior pharynx to establish or maintain a patent airway. In an unconscious patient, the tongue usually obstructs the posterior pharynx. The oropharyngeal airway conforms to the curvature of the palate, removing the obstruction and allowing air to pass around and through the tube. It also facilitates oropharyngeal suctioning. The oropharyngeal airway is intended for short-term use, as in the postanesthesia or postictal stage. It may be left in place longer as an airway adjunct to prevent the orally intubated patient from biting the endotracheal tube.

The oropharyngeal airway is not the airway of choice for the patient with loose or avulsed teeth or recent oral surgery. Inserting this airway in the conscious or semiconscious patient may stimulate vomiting and laryngospasm; therefore, you'll usually insert the airway only in unconscious patients.

≫ Key nursing diagnoses and patient outcomes
Use these nursing diagnoses as a guide when developing your plan of care for a patient who requires oropharyngeal airway insertion.

Ineffective breathing pattern related to alterations in normal gas exchange
Based on this nursing diagnosis, you'll establish the following patient outcomes. The patient will:
• regain and maintain arterial blood gas (ABG) values within normal limits.
• regain his baseline respiratory rate and maintain stable respiration.

Inability to sustain spontaneous ventilation related to (specify)
Based on this nursing diagnosis, you'll establish the following patient outcomes. The patient will:
• show no signs of dyspnea at rest within 24 hours.
• have a chest X-ray that will indicate full lung expansion within 24 hours.

Anxiety related to inability to sustain spontaneous ventilation
Based on this nursing diagnosis, you'll establish the following patient outcomes. The patient will:
• verbally or nonverbally indicate that he feels less anxious.
• cope with this situation without demonstrating signs of severe anxiety (specify for individual).

Equipment
♦ oral airway of appropriate size ♦ tongue blade ♦ padded tongue blade ♦ gloves ♦ optional: suction equipment, handheld resuscitation bag or oxygen-powered breathing device.

Patient preparation
• Provide privacy.
• Select an airway of appropriate size for your patient; an oversized airway

Inserting an oral airway

Unless this position is contraindicated, hyperextend the patient's head as shown below before using either the cross-finger or tongue blade insertion method.

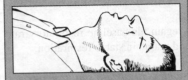

To insert an oral airway using the cross-finger method, place your thumb on the patient's lower teeth and your index finger on his upper teeth. Gently open his mouth by pushing his teeth apart.

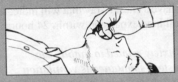

Insert the airway upside down to avoid pushing the tongue towards the pharynx, and slide it over the tongue toward the back of the mouth. Rotate the airway as it approaches the posterior wall of the pharynx so that it points downward, as shown below.

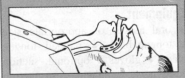

To use the tongue blade technique, open the patient's mouth and depress his tongue with the blade. Guide the airway over the back of the tongue as you did for the cross-finger technique.

can obstruct breathing by depressing the epiglottis into the laryngeal opening. Usually, you'll select a small size (#1 or 2) for an infant or child, a medium size (#4 or 5) for the average adult, and a large size (#6) for the large adult.

• If the patient is wearing dentures, remove them so they don't cause further airway obstruction.

• Be sure to confirm the correct size of the airway by placing the airway flange beside the patient's cheek, parallel to his front teeth. If the airway is the right size, the airway curve should reach to the angle of the jaw.

Implementation

• Explain the procedure to the patient even though he may not appear to be alert.

• Put on gloves *to prevent contact with body fluids.*

• If necessary, suction the patient.

• Place the patient in the supine position with his neck hyperextended, if this is not contraindicated.

• Insert the airway using the cross-finger or the tongue blade technique. (See *Inserting an oral airway.*)

• Auscultate the lungs *to ensure adequate ventilation.*

• After the airway is inserted, position the patient on his side *to decrease the risk of aspiration of vomitus.*

• Perform mouth care every 2 to 4 hours, as needed. Begin by holding the patient's jaws open with a padded tongue blade and gently removing the airway. Place the airway in a basin and rinse it with hydrogen peroxide followed by water. If secretions remain, use a pipe cleaner to remove them. Complete standard mouth care and reinsert the airway.

• While the airway is removed for mouth care, observe the mouth's mucous membranes *because tissue irritation or ulceration can result from prolonged airway use.*
• Frequently check the position of the airway *to ensure correct placement.*
• When the patient regains consciousness and is able to swallow, remove the airway by pulling it outward and downward, following the mouth's natural curvature. After the airway is removed, test the patient's cough and gag reflexes *to ensure that removal of the airway wasn't premature and that the patient can maintain his own airway.*
• *To test for the gag reflex,* use a cotton-tipped applicator to touch both sides of the posterior pharynx. *To test for the cough reflex,* gently touch the posterior oropharynx with the cotton-tipped applicator.

Complications
• Tooth damage or loss, tissue damage, and bleeding may result from insertion.
• If the airway is too long, it may press the epiglottis against the entrance of the larynx, producing complete airway obstruction. If the airway is not inserted properly, it may push the tongue posteriorly, aggravating the problem of upper airway obstruction.

Nursing considerations
• Clear breath sounds on auscultation indicate that the airway is the proper size and that it's in the correct position.
• Evaluate the patient's behavior *to provide the cue for airway removal.* The patient is likely to gag or cough

as he becomes more alert, indicating that he no longer needs the airway.
• Avoid taping the airway in place *because untaping it could delay airway removal, thus increasing the risk of aspiration.*

Documentation
• Record the date and time of the airway's insertion; size of the airway; removal and cleaning of the airway; condition of mucous membranes; any suctioning; any adverse reactions and the nursing action taken; and the patient's tolerance of the procedure.

Oropharyngeal handheld inhalers

Oropharyngeal handheld inhalers deliver topical medications to the respiratory tract, producing local and systemic effects. The mucosal lining of the respiratory tract absorbs the inhalant almost immediately. Examples of common inhalants are bronchodilators, used to improve airway patency and facilitate mucous drainage, and *mucolytics,* which attain a high local concentration to liquefy tenacious bronchial secretions. Types of handheld oropharyngeal inhalers include the metered-dose inhaler or nebulizer, the turbo-inhaler, and the nasal inhaler. (See *Types of handheld inhalers,* page 604.)

Inhalers may be contraindicated in patients who can't form an airtight seal around the device and in patients who lack the coordination or clear vision necessary to assemble a turbo-inhaler. Contraindications for specific inhalant drugs are also possible. For

Types of handheld inhalers

These devices use air under pressure to produce a mist containing tiny droplets of medication. Drugs delivered in this form (such as mucolytics or bronchodilators) can travel deep into the lungs.

Nasal inhaler

Metered-dose inhaler

Turbo-inhaler with capsules

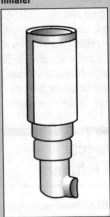
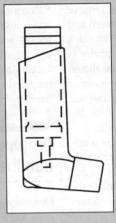
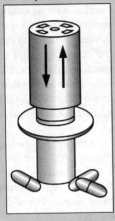

example, bronchodilators are contraindicated if the patient has tachycardia or a history of cardiac arrhythmias associated with tachycardia.

≫ Key nursing diagnoses and patient outcomes

Use these nursing diagnoses as a guide when developing your plan of care for a patient using a handheld oropharyngeal inhaler.

Ineffective breathing pattern related to (specify)

Based on this nursing diagnosis, you'll establish the following patient outcomes. The patient will:
• maintain respiratory rate within ± 5 breaths/minute of baseline.
• have normal arterial blood gas levels.

• demonstrate correct use of the inhaler.
• report ability to breathe comfortably.

Knowledge deficit related to use of handheld oropharyngeal inhaler

Based on this nursing diagnosis, you'll establish the following patient outcomes. The patient will:
• indicate need to know how to use inhaler.
• set realistic learning goals.
• state and demonstrate understanding of what has been taught.

Equipment

♦ patient's medication record and chart ♦ metered-dose inhaler ♦ turbo-inhaler or nasal inhaler ♦ prescribed medication ♦ normal saline solution (or another appropriate solution) for gargling ♦ optional: emesis basin.

Patient preparation

• Confirm the patient's identity by asking his name and by checking the name, room number, and bed number on his wristband.

• Explain the procedure to the patient.

Implementation

• Verify the order on the patient's medication record by checking it against the doctor's order.

• Check the label on the inhaler against the order on the medication record.

• Wash your hands.

Using a metered-dose inhaler

• Shake the inhaler bottle *to mix the medication and aerosol propellant.*

• Remove the mouthpiece and cap from the bottle.

• Insert the metal stem on the bottle into the small hole on the flattened portion of the mouthpiece. Then turn the bottle upside down.

• Have the patient exhale; then place the mouthpiece in his mouth and have him close his lips around it.

• As you firmly push the bottle down against the mouthpiece, instruct the patient to inhale slowly until his lungs feel full. *This action draws the medication into his lungs.* Compress the bottle against the mouthpiece only once.

• Remove the mouthpiece from the patient's mouth, and tell him to hold his breath for several seconds to allow the medication to reach the alveoli. Then instruct him to exhale slowly through pursed lips *to keep the distal bronchioles open, allowing increased absorption and diffusion of the drug and better gas exchange.*

• Have the patient gargle with normal saline solution, if desired, *to remove medication from the mouth and back of the throat.* (The lungs retain only about 10% of the inhalant; most of the remainder is exhaled, but substantial amounts may remain in the oropharynx.) Provide an emesis basin if the patient needs one.

• Rinse the mouthpiece thoroughly with warm water *to prevent accumulation of residue.*

Using a turbo-inhaler

• Hold the mouthpiece in one hand and, with the other hand, slide the sleeve away from the mouthpiece as far as possible.

• Unscrew the tip of the mouthpiece by turning it counterclockwise.

• Firmly press the colored portion of the medication capsule into the propeller stem of the mouthpiece.

• Screw the inhaler securely back together.

• Holding the inhaler with the mouthpiece at the bottom, slide the sleeve all the way down and then up again *to puncture the capsule and release the medication.* Do this only once.

• Have the patient exhale completely and tilt his head back. Then instruct him to place the mouthpiece in his mouth, close his lips around it, and inhale once — quickly and deeply — through the mouthpiece.

• Tell the patient to hold his breath for several seconds *to allow the medication to reach the alveoli. (Instruct him not to exhale through the mouthpiece.)*

• Remove the inhaler from the patient's mouth, and tell him to exhale as much air as possible.

• Repeat the procedure until all the medication in the device is inhaled.
• Have the patient gargle with normal saline solution, if desired, *to remove medication from the mouth and back of the throat.* Be sure to provide an emesis basin if the patient needs one.
• Discard the empty medication capsule, put the inhaler in its can, and secure the lid. Rinse the inhaler with warm water at least once a week.

Using a nasal inhaler

• Have the patient blow his nose *to clear his nostrils.*
• Shake the medication cartridge, and then insert it in the adapter. (When inserting a refill cartridge, first remove the protective cap from the stem.)
• Remove the protective cap from the adapter tip.
• Hold the inhaler with your index finger on top of the cartridge and your thumb under the nasal adapter. The adapter tip should be pointing toward the patient.
• Have the patient tilt his head back. Then tell him to place the adapter tip into one nostril while occluding the other nostril with his finger.
• Instruct the patient to inhale gently as he presses the adapter and the cartridge together firmly *to release a measured dose of medication.* Be sure to follow the manufacturer's instructions. With some medications, such as dexamethasone sodium phosphate (Turbinaire), inhaling during administration is not desirable.
• Tell the patient to remove the inhaler from his nostril and to exhale through his mouth.
• Shake the inhaler, and have the patient repeat the procedure in the other nostril.

• Have the patient gargle with normal saline solution *to remove medication from the mouth and throat.* Provide an emesis basin if he needs one.
• Remove the medication cartridge from the nasal inhaler, and wash the nasal adapter in lukewarm water. Let the adapter dry thoroughly before reinserting the cartridge.

Complications

• Overdosage is common.
• The patient may also have an adverse reaction to the inhalant drug.

Nursing considerations

• When using a turbo-inhaler or a nasal inhaler, make sure the pressurized cartridge isn't punctured or incinerated. Store the medication cartridge below 120° F (48.9° C).
• Spacer inhalers may be recommended *to provide greater therapeutic benefit for children or patients who have difficulty with coordination.* A spacer attachment is an extension to the inhaler's mouthpiece that provides more dead-air space for mixing the medication. Some inhalers have built-in spacers.
• If you're using a turbo-inhaler, keep the medication capsules wrapped until needed *to keep them from deteriorating.*
• Teach the patient how to use the inhaler *so that he can continue treatments after discharge, if necessary.* Explain that overdosage — which is common — can cause the medication to lose its effectiveness. Tell the patient to record the date and time of each inhalation and his response *to prevent overdosage and to help the doctor determine the drug's effectiveness.* Also, note if the patient uses an

unusual amount of medication — for example, more than one cartridge for a metered-dose nebulizer every 3 weeks.
• Inform the patient of possible adverse effects.

Documentation

• Record the inhalant administered, the dose, and the time.
• Note any significant change in the patient's heart rate after bronchodilation, and any other adverse reactions.

Otoscopic examination

Otoscopy is the direct visualization through an otoscope of the external auditory canal and the tympanic membrane. (See *Parts of an otoscope*, page 608.) It's a basic part of any physical examination of the ear and should be performed before other auditory or vestibular tests. Otoscopy indirectly provides information about the eustachian tube and the middle ear cavity.

≫ Key nursing diagnoses and patient outcomes

Use these nursing diagnoses as a guide when developing your plan of care.

Risk for injury related to sensory deficits

Based on this nursing diagnosis, you'll establish the following patient outcomes. The patient will:
• identify factors that increase risk of injury.
• identify and apply safety measures to prevent injury.
• perform activities of daily living optimally within sensorimotor limitations.

Sensory or perceptual alteration (auditory) related to altered sensory reception, transmission, or integration

Based on this nursing diagnosis, you'll establish the following patient outcomes. The patient will:
• discuss impact of auditory loss on lifestyle.
• express feelings of comfort and security.
• show interest in surroundings.
• state a plan to use community resources to assist with auditory deficit.

Equipment

♦ otoscope ♦ optional: gloves.

Equipment preparation

• Assemble the otoscope, if necessary.
• Attach the handle that houses the battery pack to the otoscope's head, which contains a light source and magnifying lens.
• Select and attach a speculum large enough to fit the patient's ear canal comfortably. (Speculum sizes typically range from 2 to 9 mm.)
• Press the light switch on the handle and adjust the beam by turning the rheostat located between the head and the handle.
• If desired, put on gloves.

Patient preparation

• Describe the procedure to the patient, and explain that this test permits examination of the ear canal and eardrum.
• Reassure the patient that the examination is usually painless and takes less than 5 minutes to perform.
• Have the patient sit in a comfortable position or lie down on the side opposite the ear you wish to examine.

Parts of an otoscope

An otoscope enables the visualization of the external ear canal and the tympanic membrane. Use this as a guide when assembling one.

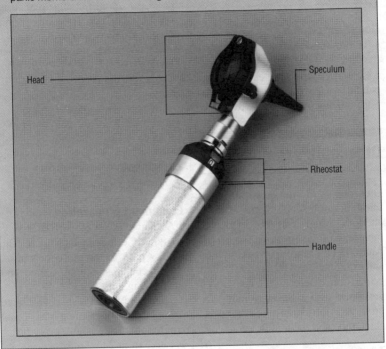

Implementation

• Have the patient tilt his head toward the shoulder opposite the ear you're examining. Keeping in mind how the ear canal curves in an adult, gently grasp the auricle and pull it up and back *to straighten the ear canal before inserting the speculum.*

• When examining a child's ear, gently pull the auricle downward *to straighten the ear canal before inserting the speculum.*

• Gently insert the otoscope into the ear canal using one of two techniques: either hold the handle of the otoscope facing down or facing up. Holding the otoscope with the handle facing up allows you to brace your hand against the patient's head *to stabilize the instrument.* This helps *to prevent injury if the patient moves suddenly.* If insertion is difficult, replace the speculum with a smaller one.

• Look through the lens, and gently advance the speculum until you see the eardrum. Obtain as full a view as possible, and note redness, swelling, lesions, discharge, foreign bodies, or scaling in the canal. Check the eardrum for color, contours, and perforation. Hairs and cerumen are seen in the distal two-thirds of the ear canal.

Landmarks of the tympanic membrane

Landmarks of the tympanic membrane include the umbo, handle of maleus, and cone of light.

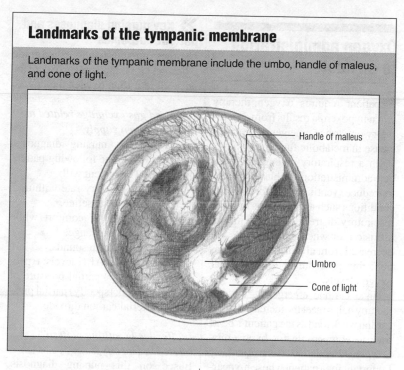

Note excessive cerumen that may obstruct your view; you may need to remove it to complete your inspection.
• Inspect the tympanic membrane. Typically, middle ear problems are evidenced by the tympanic membrane's appearance. Focus on the membrane's color and contour. It should be pearly gray and appear concave at the umbo. Then move the otoscope to identify landmarks on the tympanic membrane (See *Landmarks of the tympanic membrane*.) Be alert for perforations, bulging, missing landmarks, or a distorted cone of light.

Complications

Irritation of the canal lining can occur, especially with infection. Also, continuing to insert an otoscope against resistance may cause perforation or damage.

Nursing considerations

• Keep in mind the sensitivity of the ear canal's skin. *Improper technique can cause the patient considerable discomfort or pain.*
• Scarring, discoloration, or retraction or bulging of the tympanic membrane indicates a pathologic process.
• Movement of the tympanic membrane in tandem with respiration suggests abnormal patency of the eustachian tube.

Documentation

• Document the normal and abnormal findings of the canal, landmarks of the tympanic membrane, and the patient's tolerance of the procedure.

Oxygen administration to an adult

A patient requires oxygen therapy when hypoxemia results from a respiratory or cardiac emergency or an increase in metabolic function.

In a respiratory emergency, oxygen administration enables a patient to reduce ventilatory effort. When conditions such as atelectasis or adult respiratory distress syndrome impair diffusion, or when lung volumes are decreased from alveolar hypoventilation, this procedure boosts alveolar oxygen levels.

In a cardiac emergency, oxygen therapy helps meet the increased myocardial work load as the patient's heart tries to compensate for hypoxemia. Oxygen administration is particularly important for a patient whose myocardium is already compromised from myocardial infarction or cardiac arrhythmia, for example.

When metabolic demand is high, in cases of massive trauma, burns, or high fever, for instance, administering oxygen supplies the body with enough oxygen to meet cellular needs. This procedure also increases oxygenation when the blood's oxygen-carrying capacity is reduced, as with carbon monoxide poisoning or sickle cell crisis.

The adequacy of oxygen therapy is determined by arterial blood gas (ABG) analysis, oximetry monitoring, and clinical examinations. The patient's disease, physical condition, and age are considered when determining the most appropriate administration method.

≫ Key nursing diagnoses and patient outcomes

Use these nursing diagnoses as a guide when developing your plan of care for an adult requiring oxygen therapy.

Impaired gas exchange related to altered oxygen supply

Based on this nursing diagnosis, you'll establish the following patient outcomes. The patient will:
• maintain respiratory rate within 5 breaths/minute of baseline.
• express feeling of comfort while maintaining air exchange.
• have normal breath sounds.
• restore baseline ABG levels: (specify) pH; (specify) partial pressure of arterial oxygen; (specify) partial pressure of arterial carbon dioxide.

Ineffective breathing pattern related to (specify)

Based on this nursing diagnosis, you'll establish the following patient outcomes. The patient will:
• achieve maximum lung expansion with adequate ventilation.

Equipment

The equipment needed for this procedure depends on the type of delivery system ordered and may include some of the following items (see *Guide to oxygen delivery systems*): ◆ oxygen source (wall unit, cylinder, liquid tank, or concentrator) ◆ flowmeter ◆ adapter, if using a wall unit, or a pressure-reduction gauge, if using a cylinder ◆ sterile humidity bottle and adapters ◆ sterile distilled water OXYGEN PRECAUTION sign ◆ appropriate oxygen delivery system (a nasal cannula, simple mask, partial rebreather

(Text continues on page 615.)

Guide to oxygen delivery systems

Patients may receive oxygen through one of several administration systems. Each has its own benefits, drawbacks, and indications for use. Advantages and disadvantages of each system are compared below and on the following pages.

Nasal cannula

Oxygen is delivered through plastic cannulas in the patient's nostrils.

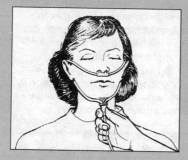

Advantages: safe and simple; comfortable and easily tolerated; nasal prongs can be shaped to fit any face; effective for low oxygen concentrations; allows movement, eating, and talking; inexpensive and disposable.

Disadvantages: can't deliver concentrations higher than 40%; can't be used in complete nasal obstruction; may cause headaches or dry mucous membranes if flow rate exceeds 6 liters/minute; can dislodge easily.

Administration guidelines: Ensure patency of the patient's nostrils with a flashlight. If patent, hook the cannula tubing behind the patient's ears and under the chin. Slide the adjuster upward under the chin to secure the tubing. If using an elastic strap to secure the cannula, position it over the ears and around the back of the head. Avoid applying too tightly, which can cause excess pressure on facial structures and cannula occlusion. With a nasal cannula, oral breathers achieve the same oxygen delivery as nasal breathers.

Simple mask

Oxygen flows through an entry port at the bottom of the mask and exits through large holes on the sides of the mask.

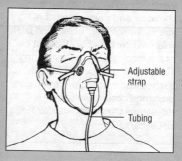

Adjustable strap

Tubing

Advantages: can deliver concentrations of 40% to 60%.

Disadvantages: hot and confining; may irritate patient's skin; tight seal that may cause discomfort is required for higher oxygen concentration; interferes with talking and eating; impractical for long-term therapy because of imprecision.

Administration guidelines: Select the mask size that offers the best fit. Place the mask over the patient's nose, mouth, and chin, and mold the flexible metal edge to the bridge of the nose. Adjust the elastic band around the head to hold

(continued)

Guide to oxygen delivery systems *(continued)*

the mask firmly but comfortably over the cheeks, chin, and bridge of the nose. For elderly or cachectic patients with sunken cheeks, tape gauze pads to the mask over the cheek area to try to create an airtight seal. Without this seal, room air dilutes the oxygen, preventing delivery of the prescribed concentration. A minimum of 5 liters/minute is required in all masks to flush expired carbon dioxide from the mask so the patient doesn't rebreathe it.

Partial rebreather mask

The patient inspires oxygen from a reservoir bag along with atmospheric air and oxygen from the mask. The first third of exhaled tidal volume enters the bag; the rest exits the mask. Because air entering the reservoir bag comes from the trachea and bronchi, where no gas exchange occurs, the patient rebreathes the oxygenated air he just exhaled.

feres with eating and talking; hot and confining; may irritate skin; bag may twist or kink; impractical for long-term therapy.

Administration guidelines: Follow procedures listed for the simple mask. If the reservoir bag collapses more than slightly during inspiration, raise the flow rate until you see only a slight deflation. Marked or complete deflation indicates insufficient oxygen flow; carbon dioxide will accumulate in the mask and bag. Keep the reservoir bag from twisting or kinking. Ensure free expansion by making sure it lies outside the patient's gown and bedcovers.

Nonrebreather mask

On inhalation, a one-way valve opens, directing oxygen from a reservoir bag into the mask. On exhalation, gas exits the mask through the one-way valve and enters the atmosphere. The patient only breathes air from the bag.

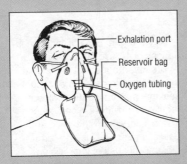

Exhalation port
Reservoir bag
Oxygen tubing

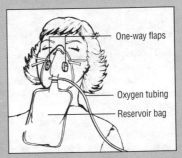

One-way flaps
Oxygen tubing
Reservoir bag

Advantages: effectively delivers concentrations of 40% to 60%; openings in mask allow patient to inhale room air if oxygen source fails.

Disadvantages: tight seal required for accurate oxygen concentration may cause discomfort; inter-

Advantages: delivers the highest possible oxygen concentration (60% to 90%) short of intubation and mechanical ventilation; effective for short-term therapy; doesn't dry mucous membranes; can be converted to a partial rebreather

Guide to oxygen delivery systems (continued)

mask, if necessary, by removing the one-way flap.

Disadvantages: requires a tight seal, which may be difficult to maintain and may cause discomfort; may irritate the patient's skin; impractical for long-term therapy.

Administration guidelines: Follow procedures listed for the simple mask. Make sure the mask fits very snugly. Make sure the one-way valves or flaps are secure and functioning. Because the mask excludes room air, valve malfunction can cause carbon dioxide buildup and suffocate an unconscious patient. If the reservoir bag collapses more than slightly during inspiration, raise the flow rate until you see only a slight deflation. Marked or complete deflation indicates an insufficient flow rate. Keep the reservoir bag from twisting or kinking. Ensure free expansion by making sure it lies outside the patient's gown and bedcovers.

Venturi mask

The mask is connected to a Venturi device that mixes a specific volume of air and oxygen.

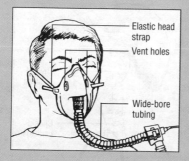

- Elastic head strap
- Vent holes
- Wide-bore tubing

Advantages: delivers highly accurate oxygen concentration de-

spite patient's respiratory pattern because the same amount of air is always entrained; dilute jets can be changed or dial turned to change oxygen concentration; doesn't dry mucous membranes; humidity or aerosol can be added.

Disadvantages: confining and may irritate skin; oxygen concentration may be altered if mask fits loosely, tubing kinks, oxygen intake ports become blocked, flow is insufficient, or patient is hyperpneic; interferes with eating and talking; condensate may collect and drip on the patient if humidification is used.

Administration guidelines: Make sure that the oxygen flow rate is set at the amount specified on each mask and that the Venturi valve is set for the desired fraction of inspired oxygen.

Aerosols

A face mask, hood, tent, or tracheostomy tube or collar is connected to wide-bore tubing that receives aerosolized oxygen from a jet nebulizer. The jet nebulizer, which is attached near the oxygen source, adjusts air entrainment in a manner similar to the Venturi device.

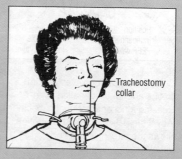

- Tracheostomy collar

(continued)

Guide to oxygen delivery systems *(continued)*

Advantages: administers high humidity; gas can be heated (when delivered through artificial airway) or cooled (when delivered through a tent).

Disadvantages: condensate collected in the tracheostomy collar or T tube may drain into the tracheostomy; the weight of the T tube can put stress on the tracheostomy tube.

Administration guidelines: Guidelines vary with the type of nebulizer used, including the ultrasonic, large volume, small volume, and in-line. When using a high-output nebulizer, watch for signs of overhydration, pulmonary edema, crackles, and electrolyte imbalance.

CPAP mask

This system allows the spontaneously breathing patient to receive continuous positive airway pressure (CPAP) with or without an artificial airway.

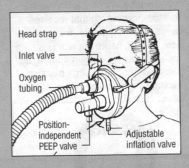

Head strap — Inlet valve — Oxygen tubing — Position-independent PEEP valve — Adjustable inflation valve

Advantages: noninvasively improves arterial oxygenation by increasing functional residual capacity; allows the patient to avoid intubation; allows the patient to talk and cough without interrupting positive pressure.

Disadvantages: requires a tight fit, which may cause discomfort;

heightened risk of aspiration if the patient vomits; increased risk of pneumothorax, diminished cardiac output, and gastric distention; contraindicated in patients with chronic obstructive pulmonary disease, bullous lung disease, low cardiac output, or tension pneumothorax.

Administration guidelines: Place one strap behind the patient's head and the other strap over his head to ensure a snug fit. Attach one latex strap to the connector prong on one side of the mask. Then, use one hand to position the mask on the patient's face while using the other hand to connect the strap to the other side of the mask. After the mask is applied, assess the patient's respiratory, circulatory, and GI function every hour. Watch for signs of pneumothorax, decreased cardiac output, a drop in blood pressure, and gastric distention.

Transtracheal oxygen

The patient receives oxygen through a catheter inserted into the base of his neck in a simple outpatient procedure.

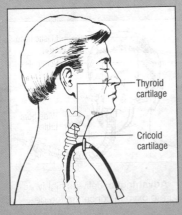

Thyroid cartilage

Cricoid cartilage

Guide to oxygen delivery systems *(continued)*

Advantages: supplies oxygen to the lungs throughout the respiratory cycle; provides continuous oxygen without hindering mobility; doesn't interfere with eating or talking; doesn't dry mucous membranes; catheter can easily be concealed by a shirt or scarf.

Disadvantages: not suitable for use in patients at risk for bleeding or those with severe bronchospasm, uncompensated respiratory acidosis, pleural herniation into the base of the neck, or high corticosteroid dosages.

Administration guidelines: After insertion, obtain a chest X-ray to confirm placement. Monitor the patient for bleeding, respiratory distress, pneumothorax, pain, coughing, or hoarseness. Don't use the catheter for about 1 week following insertion to decrease the risk of subcutaneous emphysema.

mask, or nonrebreather mask for low-flow and variable oxygen concentrations; Venturi mask, aerosol mask, tracheostomy collar, T tube, tent, or oxyhood for high-flow and specific oxygen concentrations) ♦ small-diameter and large-diameter connection tubing ♦ flashlight (for nasal cannula) ♦ water-soluble lubricant ♦ gauze pads and tape (for oxygen masks) ♦ jet adapter for Venturi mask (if adding humidity) ♦ optional: oxygen analyzer.

Equipment preparation

• Although a respiratory therapist typically is responsible for setting up, maintaining, and managing the equipment, you need working knowledge of the oxygen system used.

• Check the oxygen outlet port to verify flow. Pinch the tubing near the prongs to ensure that an audible alarm sounds if oxygen flow stops.

Patient preparation

• Assess the patient's condition. In an emergency, verify that the patient's airway is open before administering oxygen.

• Describe the procedure to the patient, and explain why oxygen is needed to ensure the patient's cooperation.

Implementation

• Check the patient's room to make sure it's safe for oxygen administration. Whenever possible, replace electrical devices with nonelectric ones and post a NO SMOKING sign in the patient's room. *Oxygen supports combustion and the smallest spark can cause a fire.*

• Place an OXYGEN PRECAUTION sign over the patient's bed and on the door to the room.

• Assist in placing the oxygen delivery device on the patient. Make sure it fits properly and is stable.

• Monitor the patient's response to oxygen therapy. Check the patient's ABG values during initial adjustments of oxygen flow. Once the patient is stabilized, pulse oximetry may be used instead. Check the patient frequently for signs of hypoxia, such as decreased level of consciousness,

Types of home oxygen therapy

Home oxygen therapy can be administered using an oxygen tank, an oxygen concentrator, or liquid oxygen.

Oxygen tank
Commonly used for patients who need oxygen on a standby basis or who need a ventilator at home, the oxygen tank has several disadvantages, including its cumbersome design and the need for frequent refills. Because oxygen is stored under high pressure, the oxygen tank also poses a potential hazard.

Oxygen concentrator
The oxygen concentrator extracts oxygen molecules from room air. It can be used for low oxygen flow (less than 4 liters/minute) and doesn't need to be refilled with oxygen. However, because the oxygen concentrator runs on electricity, it won't function during a power failure.

Liquid oxygen
This option is used commonly by patients who are oxygen-dependent but still mobile. The system includes a large liquid reservoir for home use. When the patient wants to leave the house, a portable unit is filled and worn over the shoulder; this supplies oxygen for up to several hours, depending on the liter flow.

increased heart rate, arrhythmias, restlessness, perspiration, dyspnea, use of accessory muscles, yawning or flared nostrils, cyanosis, and cool, clammy skin.

• Observe the patient's skin integrity *to prevent skin breakdown on pressure points from the oxygen delivery device.* Wipe moisture and perspiration from the patient's face and from the mask as needed.

• Remind the patient frequently to cough and practice deep breathing *to prevent atelectasis.*

• To prevent the development of serious lung damage, measure ABG values repeatedly *to determine whether high oxygen concentrations are still necessary.*

Complications
Complications may include oxygen toxicity leading to lung damage if the patient receives oxygen at a concentration greater than 60% for longer than 24 hours.

Nursing considerations
• Never administer oxygen at more than 2 liters/minute by nasal cannula to a patient with chronic lung disease unless you have a specific order to do so. *This is because some patients with chronic lung disease become dependent on a state of hypercapnia and hypoxia to stimulate their respirations; therefore, supplemental oxygen could cause them to stop breathing.* However, long-term oxygen therapy for 12 to 17 hours daily may help patients with chronic lung disease to sleep better, survive longer, and have reduced pulmonary hypertension.

• When monitoring the patient's response to a change in oxygen flow, check the pulse oximetry monitor or measure ABG values 20 to 30 minutes after adjusting the flow. Meanwhile, monitor the patient closely for any ad-

Transtracheal catheter care

Teach the patient with a transtracheal catheter how to care for the catheter as well as the skin surrounding the catheter. If the patient has a Heimlich Micro-Trach, tell him to clean around the catheter twice a day using a soapy cotton-tipped applicator and water. He also needs to irrigate the catheter while it's in place, two to three times a day, using normal saline solution. Tell him that this serves to loosen secretions and stimulate coughing. Instruct the patient to change the catheter once a month.

SCOOP catheter

If the patient has a SCOOP catheter, tell him to clean it two to three times a day to keep it free of mucus. Tell him that, before he begins cleaning, he should put on a nasal cannula, disconnect the oxygen tubing from the catheter, and then connect it to the cannula. Instruct the patient to irrigate the catheter by instilling 1.5 ml of normal saline solution into the catheter, as shown in the illustration below. Forewarn him that this may make him cough.

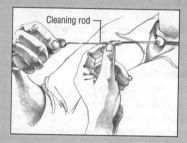

Cleaning rod

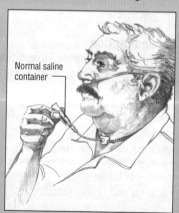

Normal saline container

Next, tell him to insert a cleaning rod (which he's cleaned beforehand) through the catheter as far as possible and then to pull it back.

After he has removed and reinserted the rod three times, tell him to remove the rod, instill 1.5 ml of normal saline solution into the catheter, and then reconnect the oxygen tubing to the catheter. As a final step, instruct him to clean the rod with antimicrobial soap and to store it in a dry place.

In addition to cleaning the catheter while it remains in place, the patient with a SCOOP 1 catheter needs to remove the catheter at least once weekly, the patient with a SCOOP 2 catheter at least once daily, for a more thorough cleaning. (The SCOOP 2 catheter has extra side holes to facilitate oxygen distribution.) After the catheter is removed, tell the patient to use antimicrobial soap, a cleaning rod, and lukewarm tap water to clean the catheter.

(continued)

Transtracheal catheter care (continued)

Reminders
Remind the patient never to remove or insert a SCOOP catheter while oxygen is flowing through it. Rather, he should put on a nasal cannula, disconnect the catheter from the oxygen source, and then remove the catheter. Next, he should insert a second SCOOP catheter, coated with water-soluble lubricant. Once the second catheter is secured, he can resume oxygen delivery through the catheter.

verse response to the change in oxygen flow.

Home care
• Before discharging a patient who will receive home oxygen therapy, make sure you know the types of oxygen therapy, the kinds of services that are available, and the service schedules offered by local home suppliers. Together with the doctor and the patient, choose the device best-suited to the patient. (See *Types of home oxygen therapy,* page 616.)
• If transtracheal oxygen therapy is to be given, teach the patient how to properly clean and care for the catheter. (See *Transtracheal catheter care,* page 617.) Tell the patient to keep the skin surrounding the insertion site clean and dry to prevent infection.
• Evaluate the patient and family members' ability and motivation to administer oxygen therapy at home. Make sure they understand the reason the patient is receiving oxygen and the safety issues for administering oxygen. Teach them how to properly use and clean the equipment and supplies.
• If your patient is to be discharged and will be using oxygen therapy at home for the first time, make sure his health insurance covers home oxygen therapy. If it doesn't, find out what criteria he must meet to obtain coverage. Without a third-party payer, the patient may not be able to afford home oxygen therapy.

Documentation
Document the following information:
• date and time of oxygen administration
• type of delivery device
• oxygen flow rate
• patient's vital signs, skin color, respiratory effort, and lung sounds
• patient response before and after therapy is initiated
• patient and family teaching.

P_Q

Pacemaker (permanent) insertion and care

A permanent pacemaker is a self-contained unit that's designed to operate for 3 to 20 years. A surgeon implants the device in a pocket under the patient's skin. This is usually done in an operating room or cardiac catheterization laboratory. Nursing responsibilities involve monitoring the electrocardiogram (ECG) and maintaining sterile technique.

A permanent pacemaker allows the patient's heart to beat on its own but prevents it from falling below a preset rate. Pacing electrodes can be placed in the atria, in the ventricles, or in both chambers (atrioventricular sequential and dual chamber). The most common pacing modes are VVI for single-chamber pacing and DDD for dual chamber pacing. (See *Understanding pacemaker codes,* page 620.)

Candidates for permanent pacemakers include patients with a myocardial infarction and persistent bradyarrhythmia and patients with complete heart block or slow ventricular rates stemming from congenital or degenerative heart disease or cardiac surgery. Patients who suffer Stokes-Adams attacks and those with Wolff-Parkinson-White syndrome or sick sinus syndrome also may benefit from a permanent pacemaker.

≫ Key nursing diagnoses and patient outcomes

Use these nursing diagnoses as a guide when developing your plan of care for a patient having a permanent pacemaker inserted.

Decreased cardiac output related to decreased stroke volume

Based on this nursing diagnosis, you'll establish the following patient outcomes. The patient will:
• attain hemodynamic stability as evidenced by pulse not less than __ beats/minute and not greater than __ beats/minute and blood pressure not less than __ mm Hg and not greater than __ mm Hg.
• have warm and dry skin.
• perform specified activities with proper pacemaker functioning.
• have a diminished heart workload.
• maintain adequate cardiac output.

Body image disturbance related to presence of pacemaker

Based on this nursing diagnosis, you'll establish the following patient outcomes. The patient will:
• acknowledge change in body image.
• participate in decision making about the pacemaker.
• express positive feelings about self.

Equipment

♦ sphygmomanometer ♦ stethoscope ♦ ECG monitor with oscilloscope and strip-chart recorder ♦ sterile dressing tray ♦ povidone-iodine ointment ♦ shaving supplies ♦ gauze dressing ♦ hypoallergenic tape ♦ antibiotics ♦ analgesics ♦ sedatives ♦ alcohol sponges ♦ emergency resuscitation equipment ♦ sterile gown and mask ♦ optional: I.V. line for emergency medications.

Understanding pacemaker codes

A permanent pacemaker's three-letter (or sometimes five-letter) code simply refers to how the pacemaker is programmed.

First letter (chamber that's paced)	Second letter (chamber that's sensed)	Third letter (how pulse generator responds)
A = atrium	A = atrium	I = inhibited
V = ventricle	V = ventricle	T = triggered
D = dual (both chambers)	D = dual (both chambers)	D = dual (inhibited and triggered)
O = not applicable	O = not applicable	O = not applicable

Examples of two common programming codes

DDD	**VVI**
Paces: atrium and ventricle	Paces: ventricle
Senses: atrium and ventricle	Senses: ventricle
Response: inhibited and triggered	Response: inhibited
This is a fully automatic, or universal, pacemaker.	This is a demand pacemaker.

Patient preparation

• Explain the procedure to the patient. Provide and review literature from the manufacturer or the American Heart Association so the patient can learn about the pacemaker and how it works. Emphasize that the pacemaker augments the patient's natural heart rate.

• Ensure that the patient or a responsible family member signs a consent form, and ask the patient about past allergic reactions to anesthetics or iodine.

Implementation
Preoperative care

• For pacemaker insertion, shave the patient's chest from the axilla to the midline and from the clavicle to the nipple line on the side selected by the doctor.

• Establish an I.V. line at a keep-vein-open rate *so that drugs can be administered promptly if the patient experiences a ventricular arrhythmia.*

• Obtain baseline vital signs and a baseline ECG.

• Administer a sedative, as ordered.

In the operating room

• If you'll be monitoring arrhythmias during the procedure, put on a gown and mask.

• Connect the ECG monitor to the patient, and run a baseline rhythm strip. Make sure the machine has enough paper to run additional rhythm strips during the procedure. Leave the monitor screen on throughout the procedure.

• During transvenous placement, the doctor, guided by a fluoroscope, passes the electrode catheter through the

Teaching the patient who has a permanent pacemaker

If your patient has a permanent pacemaker, make sure to teach him about daily care, safety and activity guidelines, and special precautions.

Daily care
- Clean your pacemaker site gently with soap and water when you take a shower or a bath. Leave the incision exposed to the air.
- Inspect your skin around the incision. A slight bulge is normal, but call your doctor if you feel discomfort or notice swelling, redness, a discharge, or other problems.
- Check your pulse for 1 minute as your nurse or doctor showed you — on the side of your neck, inside your elbow, or on the thumb side of your wrist. Your pulse rate should be the same as your pacemaker rate or faster. Contact your doctor if you think your heart is beating too fast or too slow.
- Take your medications, including those for pain, as prescribed. Even with a pacemaker, you still need the medication your doctor ordered.

Safety and activity
- Keep your pacemaker instruction booklet handy, and carry your pacemaker identification card at all times. This card has your pacemaker model number and other information needed by health care personnel who treat you.
- You can resume most of your usual activities when you feel comfortable doing so, but don't drive until the doctor gives you permission. Also avoid heavy lifting and stretching exercises for at least 4 weeks or as directed by your doctor.
- Try to use both arms equally to prevent muscle stiffness. And check

with your doctor before you golf, swim, play tennis, or perform other strenuous activities.

Electromagnetic interference
- Fortunately, today's pacemakers are designed and insulated to eliminate most electrical interference. You can safely operate common household electrical devices, including kitchen appliances, microwave ovens, razors, and sewing machines. And you can ride in or operate a motor vehicle without it affecting your pacemaker.
- Take care, however, to avoid direct contact with large running motors, high-powered CB radios and other similar equipment, welding machinery, and radar devices.
- If your pacemaker activates the metal detector in an airport, show your pacemaker identification card to the security official.
- Because the metal in your pacemaker makes you ineligible for certain diagnostic studies, such as magnetic resonance imaging, be sure to inform your doctors, dentist, and other health care personnel that you have a pacemaker.

Special precautions
- If you feel light-headed or dizzy when you're near any electrical equipment, moving away from the device should restore normal pacemaker function. Check with your doctor if you have questions about particular electrical devices.

(continued)

Teaching the patient who has a permanent pacemaker *(continued)*

• Notify your doctor if you experience any signs of pacemaker failure, such as palpitations, a fast heart rate, a slow heart rate (5 to 10 beats less than the pacemaker's setting), dizziness, fainting, shortness of breath, swollen ankles or feet, anxiety, forgetfulness, or confusion.

Checkups
• Be sure to schedule and keep regular checkup appointments with your doctor.
• If your doctor checks your pacemaker status by telephone, keep your transmission schedule and instructions in a handy place.

cephalic or external jugular vein and positions it under the trabeculae in the apex of the right ventricle. The surgeon then attaches the catheter to the pulse generator, inserts this into a pocket of subcutaneous tissue in the patient's chest wall, and sutures it closed, leaving a small outlet for a drainage tube.

Postoperative care
• Monitor the patient's ECG *to check for arrhythmias and to ensure correct pacemaker functioning.*
• Monitor the I.V. flow rate; the I.V. line is usually kept in place for 24 to 48 hours postoperatively *to allow for possible emergency treatment of arrhythmias.*
• Check the patient's sutures for signs of bleeding and infection (swelling, redness, or exudate). The doctor may order prophylactic antibiotics for up to 7 days after the implantation.
• Change the dressing and apply povidone-iodine ointment at least once every 24 to 48 hours or according to doctor's orders and hospital policy. If the dressing becomes soiled or the site is exposed to air, change the dressing immediately, regardless of when it was last changed.

• Check the patient's vital signs and level of consciousness (LOC) every 15 minutes for the first hour, every hour for the next 4 hours, every 4 hours for the next 48 hours, and then once every shift. (Confused, elderly patients with second-degree heart block won't show immediate improvement in LOC.)

Nursing alert. Watch for these signs and symptoms of a perforated ventricle, with resultant cardiac tamponade: persistent hiccups, distant heart sounds, pulsus paradoxus, hypotension with narrow pulse pressure, increased venous pressure, cyanosis, distended neck veins, decreased urine output, restlessness, or complaints of fullness in the chest. If any of these develops, notify the doctor immediately.

Complications
Insertion of a permanent pacemaker places the patient at risk for certain complications, such as:
• infection
• lead displacement
• perforated ventricle
• cardiac tamponade
• lead fracture and disconnection

TECHNOLOGY UPDATE

Transmitting pacemaker data by phone

The CarryAll pacemaker monitor by *Instromedix* lets people with pacemakers send information about their devices from their home to their health care facility. It's compatible with single chamber, dual chamber, and rate-responsive pacemakers in unipolar and bipolar pacing modes and transmits pacemaker pulse widths.

Patients attach the built-in wrist electrodes and follow the instructions printed on the inside of the unit. The unit contains a built-in modem, and the data is transmitted when the phone is placed in the CarryAll's cradle. It's equipped with an audible and visible alarm initiated by the clinician when more information is needed from the user during transmission.

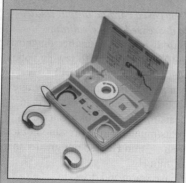

Photo courtesy of Instromedix, Inc., Hillsboro, Ore.

• twiddler's syndrome (which occurs if a pulse generator is too mobile within the subcutaneous pocket and the patient twists and turns it).

Nursing considerations
• If the patient wears a hearing aid, the pacemaker battery is placed on the opposite side.
• Watch for signs of pacemaker malfunction.

Home care
• Give the patient an identification card that lists the pacemaker type and manufacturer, serial number, pacemaker rate setting, date implanted, and the doctor's name. (See *Teaching the patient who has a permanent pacemaker*, pages 621 and 622.)
• Also provide the patient with information about telephone monitoring at home, if appropriate. (See *Transmitting pacemaker data by phone*.)

Documentation
• Document the type of pacemaker used, the serial number and the manufacturer's name, the pacing rate, the date of implantation, and the doctor's name.
• Note whether the pacemaker reduces or eliminates the patient's arrhythmias, and include other pertinent observations, such as the condition of the incision site.

Pacemaker (temporary) placement and care

A temporary pacemaker is usually inserted in an emergency. It consists of an external, battery-powered pulse generator and a lead or electrode system. There are four types of temporary pacemakers: transcutaneous, transvenous, transthoracic, and epicardial.

In a life-threatening situation, when time is critical, a transcutaneous pacemaker is the best choice. This device works by sending an electrical impulse from the pulse generator to the patient's heart by way of two electrodes, which are placed on the front and back of the patient's chest. Transcutaneous pacing is quick and effective, but it's used only until a doctor can establish transvenous pacing.

A transvenous pacemaker is more reliable and more comfortable than a transcutaneous pacemaker. Transvenous pacing involves threading an electrode catheter through a vein into the patient's right atrium or right ventricle. The electrode is then attached to an external pulse generator. As a result, the pulse generator can provide an electrical stimulus directly to the endocardium. This is the most common type of pacemaker.

A doctor may choose to insert a transthoracic pacemaker in an elective surgical procedure or as an emergency measure during cardiopulmonary resuscitation (CPR). To insert this type of pacemaker, the doctor performs a procedure similar to pericardiocentesis, in which a cardiac needle is used to pass an electrode through the chest wall and into the right ventricle. This procedure imposes a significant risk of coronary artery laceration and cardiac tamponade.

During cardiac surgery, the surgeon may insert electrodes through the epicardium of the right ventricle and — to institute atrioventricular sequential pacing — possibly the right atrium. From there, the electrodes pass through the chest wall, where they remain available if temporary pacing becomes necessary. This is called epicardial pacing.

Besides helping to correct conduction disturbances, a temporary pacemaker may aid in diagnosing conduction abnormalities. For example, during cardiac catheterization or an electrophysiology study, a temporary pacemaker may be used to locate conduction defects. In the process, the doctor might also learn whether the patient is at risk for developing an arrhythmia.

Among the contraindications to pacemaker therapy are electromechanical dissociation and ventricular fibrillation.

≫ Key nursing diagnoses and patient outcomes

Use these nursing diagnoses as a guide when developing your plan of care for a patient receiving a temporary pacemaker.

Decreased cardiac output related to decreased stroke volume

Based on this nursing diagnosis, you'll establish the following patient outcomes. The patient will:
• attain hemodynamic stability, as evidenced by: pulse not less than __ beats/minute and not greater than __ beats/minute, blood pressure not less than __ mm Hg and not greater than __ mm Hg
• have warm and dry skin.
• perform specific activities with proper pacemaker functioning.
• have a diminished heart workload.
• maintain adequate cardiac output.

Body image disturbance related to presence of pacemaker
Based on this nursing diagnosis, you'll establish the following patient outcomes. The patient will:
• acknowledge change in body image.
• participate in decision making about the pacemaker.
• express positive feelings about self.

Equipment
For transcutaneous pacing: ◆ transcutaneous pacing generator ◆ transcutaneous pacing electrodes ◆ cardiac monitor.

For all other types of temporary pacing: ◆ temporary pacemaker generator with new battery ◆ guide wire or introducer ◆ electrode catheter ◆ sterile gloves ◆ sterile dressings ◆ adhesive tape ◆ povidone-iodine solution ◆ nonconducting tape or rubber surgical glove ◆ pouch for external pulse generator ◆ emergency cardiac drugs ◆ intubation equipment ◆ defibrillator ◆ cardiac monitor with strip-chart recorder ◆ equipment to start a peripheral I.V. line, if appropriate ◆ I.V. fluids ◆ sedative ◆ optional: elastic bandage or gauze strips, restraints.

For transvenous pacing: ◆ all equipment listed for temporary pacing ◆ bridging cable ◆ percutaneous introducer tray or venous cutdown tray ◆ sterile gowns ◆ linen-saver pad ◆ antimicrobial soap ◆ alcohol sponges ◆ vial of 1% lidocaine ◆ 5-ml syringe ◆ fluoroscopy equipment, if necessary ◆ fenestrated drape ◆ prepackaged cutdown tray (for antecubital vein placement only) ◆ sutures ◆ receptacle for infectious wastes.

For transthoracic pacing: ◆ all equipment listed for temporary pacemaker ◆ transthoracic or cardiac needle.

For epicardial pacing: ◆ all equipment listed for temporary pacemakers ◆ atrial epicardial wires ◆ ventricular epicardial wires ◆ sterile rubber finger cot ◆ sterile dressing materials (if the wires won't be connected to a pulse generator).

Patient preparation
• Explain the procedure to the patient, if applicable.

Implementation
Follow the steps below for various types of pacing.

For transcutaneous pacing
• If necessary, clip the hair over the areas of electrode placement. However, don't shave the area. *(If you nick the skin, the current from the pulse generator could cause discomfort. Also, the nicks could become irritated or infected after the electrodes are applied.)*
• Attach monitoring electrodes to the patient in lead I, II, or III position. Do this even if the patient is already on telemetry monitoring *because you'll need to connect the electrodes to the pacemaker.* If you select the lead II position, adjust the LL electrode placement to accommodate the anterior pacing electrode and the patient's anatomy.
• Plug the patient cable into the electrocardiogram (ECG) input connection on the front of the pacing generator. Set the selector switch to the MONITOR ON position.
• You should now be able to see the ECG waveform on the monitor. Adjust the R-wave beeper volume to a

Proper electrode placement

Place the electrodes for a noninvasive temporary pacemaker at heart level, with the heart lying between the two electrodes. This placement ensures the shortest distance the electrical stimulus must travel to the heart.

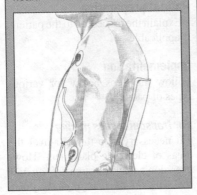

suitable level, and activate the alarm by pressing the ALARM ON button. Set the alarm for 10 to 20 beats lower and 20 to 30 beats higher than the intrinsic rate.

• Press the START/STOP button for a printout of the waveform.

• Next, apply the two pacing electrodes. Make sure the patient's skin is clean and dry *to ensure good skin contact.*

• Pull off the protective strip from the posterior electrode (marked BACK), and apply the electrode on the left side of the back, just below the scapula and to the left of the spine.

• The anterior pacing electrode (marked FRONT) has two protective strips: one covering the jellied area and one covering the outer rim. Expose the jellied area and apply it to the skin on the left side of the precordium in the usual V2 to V5 position. Move this electrode around *to get the best waveform.* Then, expose the electrode's outer rim and firmly press it to the skin. (See *Proper electrode placement.*)

• Now you're ready to pace the heart. After making sure the energy output in milliamperes (mA) is on 0, connect the electrode cable to the monitor output cable.

• Check the waveform, looking for a tall QRS complex in lead II.

• Next, turn the selector switch to PACER ON. Tell the patient that he might feel a thumping or twitching sensation and that you'll provide medication if the discomfort is intolerable.

• Now set the rate dial to 10 to 20 beats higher than the patient's intrinsic rhythm. Look for pacer artifact or spikes, which will appear as you increase the rate. If the patient doesn't have an intrinsic rhythm, set the rate at 60.

• Slowly increase the amount of energy delivered to the heart by adjusting the OUTPUT MA dial. Do this until capture is achieved (you'll see a pacer spike followed by a widened QRS complex that resembles a premature ventricular contraction). This is the pacing threshold. *To ensure consistent capture,* increase output by 10%. But don't go any higher *because you could cause the patient needless discomfort.*

• With full capture, the patient's heart rate should be approximately the same as the pacemaker rate set on the machine. The usual pacing threshold is between 40 and 80 mA.

For transvenous pacing

• Check the patient's history for hypersensitivity to local anesthetics.

Then attach the cardiac monitor to the patient and obtain a baseline assessment, including the patient's vital signs, skin color, level of consciousness (LOC), heart rate and rhythm, and emotional state. Next, insert a peripheral I.V. line if the patient doesn't already have one. Then begin an I.V. infusion of dextrose 5% in water at a keep-vein-open rate.

• Insert a new battery into the external pacemaker generator and then test it *to make sure it has a strong charge.* Connect the bridging cable to the generator, and align the positive and negative poles. *This cable allows slack between the electrode catheter and the generator, reducing the risk of accidental catheter displacement.*

• Place the patient in the supine position. If necessary, clip the hair around the insertion site. Next, open the supply tray while maintaining a sterile field. Using sterile technique, clean the insertion site with antimicrobial soap and then wipe the area with povidone-iodine solution. Cover the insertion site with a fenestrated drape. *Because fluoroscopy may be used during the placement of leadwires,* put on a protective apron.

• Provide the doctor with the local anesthetic.

• After anesthetizing the insertion site, the doctor will puncture the brachial, femoral, subclavian, or jugular vein and insert a guide wire or an introducer to advance the electrode catheter.

• As the catheter is advanced, watch the cardiac monitor. When the electrode catheter reaches the right atrium, you'll notice large P waves and small QRS complexes. As the catheter reaches the right ventricle, the P waves will become smaller while the QRS complexes enlarge. When the catheter touches the right ventricular endocardium, expect to see elevated ST segments, premature ventricular contractions, or both.

• Once in the right ventricle, the electrode catheter will send an impulse to the myocardium, causing depolarization. If the patient needs atrial pacing, either alone or with ventricular pacing, the doctor may place an electrode in the right atrium.

• Meanwhile, continuously monitor the patient's cardiac status and treat any arrhythmias, as appropriate. Also assess the patient for jaw pain and earache; *these symptoms indicate that the electrode catheter has missed the superior vena cava and has moved into the neck instead.*

• Once the electrode catheter is in place, attach the catheter leads to the bridging cable, lining up the positive and negative poles.

• Check the battery's charge by pressing the BATTERY TEST button.

• Set the pacemaker as ordered.

• The doctor will then suture the catheter to the insertion site. Afterward, put on sterile gloves and apply a sterile dressing to the site. Label the dressing with the date and time of application.

For transthoracic pacing

• Clean the skin to the left of the xiphoid process with povidone-iodine solution. Work quickly *because CPR must be interrupted for the procedure.*

• After interrupting CPR, the doctor will insert a transthoracic needle — and then the electrode catheter — through the patient's chest wall to the left of the xiphoid process into the right ventricle.

• Connect the electrode catheter to the generator, lining up the positive and negative poles. Watch the cardiac monitor for signs of ventricular pacing and capture.
• After the doctor sutures the electrode catheter into place, use sterile technique to apply a sterile $4'' \times 4''$ gauze dressing to the site. Tape the dressing securely, and label it with the date and time of application.
• Check the patient's peripheral pulses and vital signs to assess cardiac output. If you can't palpate a pulse, continue performing CPR.
• If the patient has a palpable pulse, assess his vital signs, ECG, and LOC.

For epicardial pacing

• Because epicardial pacemaker wires may be placed during cardiac surgery, inform the patient about this possibility during your preoperative teaching.
• During cardiac surgery, the doctor will hook epicardial wires into the epicardium just before the end of the surgery. Depending on the patient's condition, the doctor may insert either atrial or ventricular wires, or both.
• If indicated, connect the electrode catheter to the generator, lining up the positive and negative poles. Set the pacemaker as ordered.
• If the wires won't be connected to an external pulse generator, place them in a sterile rubber finger cot. Then cover both the wires and the insertion site with a sterile, occlusive dressing. *This will help protect the patient from microshock as well as infection.*

Complications

• Complications associated with pacemaker therapy include microshock, equipment failure, and competitive or fatal arrhythmias.
• Transcutaneous pacemakers can cause skin breakdown and muscle pain and twitching when the pacemaker fires.
• Transvenous pacemaker insertion can lead to pneumothorax or hemothorax, cardiac perforation and tamponade, diaphragmatic stimulation, pulmonary embolism, thrombophlebitis, and infection.
• If the doctor threads the electrode through the antecubital or femoral vein, venous spasm, thrombophlebitis, or lead displacement may result.
• Transthoracic pacemaker insertion can lead to pneumothorax, cardiac tamponade, emboli, sepsis, lacerations of the myocardium or coronary artery, and perforations of a cardiac chamber.
• Epicardial pacemakers impose a risk of infection, cardiac arrest, and diaphragmatic stimulation.

Nursing considerations

• Take steps to prevent microshock. This includes warning the patient not to use any electrical equipment that isn't grounded, such as telephones, electric shavers, TVs, or lamps.
• Other safety measures include placing a plastic cover supplied by the manufacturer over the pacemaker controls *to avoid an accidental setting change.* Also, insulate the pacemaker by covering all exposed metal parts, such as electrode connections and pacemaker terminals, with nonconducting tape, or place the pacing unit in a dry, rubber surgical glove.
• If the patient is disoriented or uncooperative, use restraints *to prevent accidental removal of pacemaker wires.*

PROBLEM SOLVER

When a temporary pacemaker malfunctions

Occasionally, a temporary pacemaker may fail to function appropriately. When this occurs, you'll need to take immediate action to correct the problem. Study the following chart to learn which steps to take when your patient's pacemaker fails to pace or capture.

Failure to pace
This happens when the pacemaker either doesn't fire or fires too often. The pulse generator may not be working properly, or it may not be conducting the impulse to the patient.

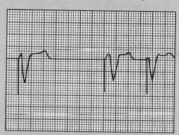

Nursing interventions
• If the pacing or sensing indicator flashes, check the connections to the cable and the position of the pacing electrode in the patient (by X-ray). The cable may have come loose, or the electrode may have been dislodged, pulled out, or broken.
• If the pulse generator is turned on but the indicators still aren't flashing, change the battery. If that doesn't help, use a different pulse generator.
• Check the settings if the pacemaker is firing too rapidly. If they're correct, or if altering them (according to hospital policy or the doctor's order) doesn't help, change the pulse generator.

Failure to capture
Here, you see pacemaker spikes but the heart isn't responding. This may be caused by changes in the pacing threshold from ischemia, an electrolyte imbalance (high or low potassium or magnesium levels), acidosis, an adverse reaction to a medication, a perforated ventricle, fibrosis, or the position of the electrode.

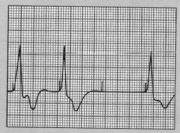

Nursing interventions
• If the patient's condition has changed, notify the doctor and ask him for new settings.
• If pacemaker settings are altered by the patient or others, return them to their correct positions. Then make sure the face of the pacemaker is covered with a plastic shield. Also, tell the patient or others not to touch the dials.
• If the heart isn't responding, try any or all of these suggestions: Carefully check all connections; increase the milliamperes slowly (according to
(continued)

When a temporary pacemaker malfunctions *(continued)*

hospital policy or the doctor's order); turn the patient on his left side, then on his right (if turning him to the left didn't help); reverse the cable in the pulse generator so the positive electrode wire is in the negative terminal and the negative electrode wire is in the positive terminal; schedule an anteroposterior or lateral chest X-ray to determine the position of the electrode.

Failure to sense intrinsic beats

This could cause ventricular tachycardia or ventricular fibrillation if the pacemaker fires on the vulnerable T wave. That could be caused by the pacemaker sensing an external stimulus as a QRS complex, which could lead to asystole, or by the pacemaker not being sensitive enough, which means it could fire anywhere within the cardiac cycle.

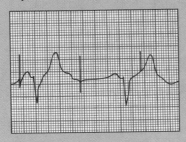

Nursing interventions

• If the pacing is undersensing, turn the sensitivity control completely to the right. If it's oversensing, turn it slightly to the left.
• If the pacemaker isn't functioning correctly, change the battery or the pulse generator.
• Remove items in the room causing electromechanical interference (razors, radios, cautery devices, and so on). Check the ground wires on the bed and other equipment for obvious damage. Unplug each piece and see if the interference stops. When you locate the cause, notify the hospital engineer and ask him to check it.
• If the pacemaker is still firing on the T wave and all else has failed, turn off the pacemaker. Make sure atropine is available in case the patient's heart rate drops. Be prepared to call a code and institute cardiopulmonary resuscitation if necessary.

• If the patient needs emergency defibrillation, make sure the pacemaker can withstand the procedure. If unsure, disconnect the pulse generator *to avoid damage.*
• When using a transcutaneous pacemaker, don't place the electrodes over a bony area *because bone conducts current poorly.* With female patients, place the anterior electrode under the patient's breast but not over the diaphragm.
• If the doctor inserts the electrode through the brachial or femoral vein, immobilize the patient's arm or leg *to avoid putting stress on the pacing wires.*
• After insertion of any temporary pacemaker, assess the patient's vital signs, skin color, LOC, and peripheral

pulses *to determine the effectiveness of the paced rhythm.* Perform a 12-lead ECG to serve as a baseline, and then perform additional ECGs daily or whenever clinical changes occur.

• If possible, obtain a rhythm strip before, during, and after pacemaker placement; any time the pacemaker settings are changed; and whenever the patient receives treatment for a complication due to the pacemaker.

• Continuously monitor the ECG reading, noting capture, sensing, rate, intrinsic beats, and competition of paced and intrinsic rhythms. If the pacemaker is sensing correctly, the sense indicator on the pulse generator should flash with each beat. (See *When a temporary pacemaker malfunctions,* pages 629 and 630.)

• Record the date and the time of pacemaker insertion, the type of pacemaker, the reason for insertion, and the patient's response. Note the pacemaker settings. Document any complications and the interventions taken.

• If the patient has epicardial pacing wires in place, clean the insertion site with povidone-iodine solution, and change the dressing daily. At the same time, monitor the site for signs of infection. Always keep the pulse generator nearby *in case pacing becomes necessary.*

Documentation

• Record the reason for pacing, the time it started, and the locations of the electrodes.

• For a transvenous or transthoracic pacemaker, note the date, the time, and reason for the temporary pacemaker.

• For any temporary pacemaker, record the pacemaker settings. Note the

---

BETTER CHARTING

Documenting pacemaker care

Record the date and time of temporary pacemaker placement, the reason for placement, the pacemaker settings, and the patient's response. Document the patient's level of consciousness and vital signs, noting which arm you used to obtain the blood pressure. As ECG monitoring continues, note capture, sensing rate, intrinsic beats, and competition of paced and intrinsic rhythms.

1/9/97	0920	Pt. c̄ temporary transvenous
		pacer in Ⓛ subclavian vein.
		Rate 70, mA2, mV full
		demand. 100% ventricular
		paced rhythm noted on moni-
		tor. ECG obtained. Pacer sens-
		ing & capturing correctly. Site
		w/o redness or swelling.
		Dressing D&I.——————
		————— John Mora, RN

patient's response to the procedure, along with any complications and the interventions taken.

• If possible, obtain rhythm strips before, during, and after pacemaker placement, and whenever pacemaker settings are changed or when the patient receives treatment for a complication caused by the pacemaker.

• As you monitor the patient, record his response to temporary pacing and note any changes in his condition. (See *Documenting pacemaker care.*)

Pain management

A patient with severe pain often seeks medical help not only for pain relief but also because he believes the pain signals a serious problem. This perception produces anxiety, which in turn increases the pain. To assess and manage pain properly, a nurse depends on the patient's subjective description in addition to objective tools.

Interventions to manage pain include analgesics as well as emotional support, comfort measures, and cognitive techniques to distract the patient. Severe pain usually requires a narcotic analgesic. Invasive measures such as epidural analgesia or patient-controlled analgesia may also be required.

>> Key nursing diagnoses and patient outcomes

Use the following nursing diagnoses as a guide when developing your plan of care for a patient requiring pain management. (In addition to the diagnoses below, other appropriate nursing diagnoses may include anxiety, activity intolerance, fear, risk for injury, knowledge deficit, powerlessness, and self-care deficit.)

Pain related to (specify)
Based on this nursing diagnosis, you'll establish the following patient outcomes. The patient will:
• identify pain characteristics.
• articulate factors that intensify pain and modify behavior accordingly.
• express a feeling of comfort and relief from pain.

• state and carry out appropriate interventions for pain relief.

Ineffective individual coping related to pain
Based on this nursing diagnosis, you'll establish the following patient outcomes. The patient will:
• communicate feelings about the present situation.
• become involved in planning own care.
• express feeling of having greater control over present situation.

Equipment
♦ pain assessment tool or scale ♦ oral hygiene supplies ♦ water ♦ nonnarcotic analgesic (such as aspirin or acetaminophen) ♦ optional: patient-controlled analgesia (PCA) device; mild narcotic (such as oxycodone or codeine); strong narcotic (such as methadone, levorphanol, morphine, or hydromorphone).

Patient preparation
• Explain to the patient how pain medications work together with other pain management therapies to provide relief.
• Explain that the goal of management is to keep pain at a low level to permit optimal bodily function.
• Work with the patient to develop a nursing plan of care that fits the patient's lifestyle.
• Suggest plans regarding prescribed medications, emotional support, comfort measures, cognitive techniques, and education about pain and pain management.
• Emphasize the importance of maintaining good bowel habits, respiratory function, and mobility *because pain*

How to assess pain

To assess pain properly, you'll need to consider the patient's description and your observations of the patient's physical and behavioral responses. Start by asking the following series of key questions (bearing in mind that the patient's responses will be shaped by his prior experiences, self-image, and beliefs about his condition):

- Where is the pain located? How long does it last? How often does it occur?
- What does the pain feel like? (Have the patient describe it.)
- What relieves the pain or makes it worse?
- How do you usually get relief from it?

Ask the patient to rank his pain on a scale of 0 to 10, with 0 denoting lack of pain and 10 denoting the worst pain level. This helps the patient verbally evaluate pain therapies.

Observe the patient's behavioral and physiologic responses to pain. Physiologic responses may be sympathetic or parasympathetic.

Behavioral responses
These include altered body position, moaning, sighing, grimacing, withdrawal, crying, restlessness, muscle twitching, and immobility.

Sympathetic responses
These are commonly associated with mild to moderate pain and include pallor, elevated blood pressure, dilated pupils, skeletal muscle tension, dyspnea, tachycardia, and diaphoresis.

Parasympathetic responses
These are commonly associated with severe, deep pain and include pallor, decreased blood pressure, bradycardia, nausea and vomiting, weakness, dizziness, and loss of consciousness.

may exacerbate any problems in these areas.

Implementation

- Assess the patient's pain by asking key questions. For instance, ask the patient to describe the duration, severity, and source of the pain. Also, note the patient's response to pain; look for physiologic or behavioral clues *to assess the severity of the pain.* (See *How to assess pain.*)
- Implement your plan of care. *Because individuals respond differently to pain,* you'll find that what works for one person may not work for another.

- If the patient is allowed oral intake, administer a nonnarcotic analgesic, such as acetaminophen or aspirin, every 4 to 6 hours as ordered.
- If the patient needs more relief than a nonnarcotic analgesic provides, administer a mild narcotic (such as oxycodone or codeine) as ordered.
- Administer a strong narcotic (such as methadone, levorphanol, morphine, or hydromorphone), as prescribed, if necessary. Give oral medications if possible. Check the appropriate drug information for each medication you administer.
- If ordered, provide instructions for using a PCA device. *This allows the*

Understanding patient-controlled analgesia

In patient-controlled analgesia (PCA), the patient controls I.V. delivery of an analgesic (usually morphine) by pressing a button on the delivery device so that he receives the amount of analgesia he needs when he needs it. The device prevents the patient from accidentally overdosing by imposing a lock-out time between doses, usually 6 to 10 minutes. During this interval, the patient will not receive the analgesic, even if he pushes the button. The accompanying illustrations show two of the more commonly used PCA devices.

The first device, shown below, is a reusable, battery-operated pump that delivers a drug dose when the patient presses a call button at the end of a cord.

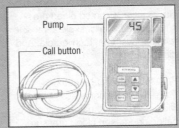

The other device, shown below, is disposable and mechanically operated. It contains an infuser and a unit that's worn like a wristwatch. The patient pushes a button on the device to receive the analgesic from a collapsible chamber.

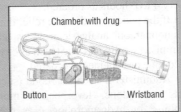

Indications and advantages

For patients who need parenteral analgesia, PCA therapy is typically given to trauma patients postopera-

tively and to terminal cancer and other patients with chronic diseases. To receive PCA therapy, a patient must be mentally alert, able to understand and comply with instructions and procedures, and have no history of allergy to the analgesic. Patients ineligible for PCA therapy include those with limited respiratory reserve, a history of drug abuse or chronic sedative or tranquilizer use, or a psychiatric disorder. Advantages are that PCA therapy ensures:
• no need for I.M. analgesics
• pain relief tailored to each patient's size and pain tolerance
• a sense of control over pain
• ability to sleep at night with minimal daytime drowsiness
• lower narcotic use compared with patients not on PCA
• improved postoperative deep-breathing, coughing, and ambulation.

PCA setup

To set up a PCA system, the doctor's order should include the:
• loading dose, given by I.V. push at the start of PCA therapy (typically 25 mg meperidine or 2 mg morphine)
• appropriate lock-out interval
• maintenance dose (also called the basal dose)

(continued)

Understanding patient-controlled analgesia *(continued)*

- amount the patient receives when he activates the device (typically 10 mg meperidine or 1 mg morphine)
- maximum amount the patient can receive within a specified time (if an adjustable device is used).

Nursing considerations
- Before your patient starts using the PCA device, teach him how it works.
- Have the patient practice with a sample device.
- Explain that he should take enough analgesic to relieve acute pain but not enough to induce drowsiness.

- Because the primary adverse effect of analgesics is respiratory depression, you must monitor your patient's respiratory rate routinely.
- Check for infiltration into the subcutaneous tissues and for catheter occlusion, which may cause the drug to back up in the primary I.V. tubing.
- If the analgesic makes your patient nauseous, you may need to administer an antiemetic drug.
- Monitor the patient's assessment of pain relief.
- If the patient reports insufficient pain relief, notify the doctor.

patient to personally control pain management and thereby decreases his anxiety. (See *Understanding patient-controlled analgesia.*)
- Provide emotional support by spending time talking with the patient. *This helps reduce feelings of anxiety and frustration, which can worsen pain.*
- Perform comfort measures, such as periodic repositioning, *to reduce muscle spasms and tension and to relieve pressure on bony prominences.* Changing the angle of the bed can reduce the pull on an abdominal incision, also diminishing pain. If appropriate, elevate a limb *to reduce swelling, inflammation, and pain.*
- Give the patient a back massage *to help relax tense muscles.*
- Perform passive range-of-motion exercises *to prevent stiffness and further loss of mobility, to relax tense muscles, and to provide comfort.*
- Take appropriate steps to maintain the patient's oral hygiene, such as

keeping a fresh water glass or cup at the bedside; *many medications tend to dry the mouth.*
- Wash the patient's face and hands.
- Use cognitive therapy to enhance the effect of analgesics. Implement techniques such as distraction, guided imagery, deep breathing, and relaxation. Use whichever method the patient feels most comfortable with. If possible, start these techniques when he feels little or no pain. If the patient feels persistent pain, begin with short, simple exercises. Before beginning, dim the lights, make sure the patient is not wearing restrictive clothing, and eliminate noise from the environment.
- *To distract the patient,* have him recall an interesting or pleasant experience or focus his attention on an enjoyable activity. For instance, he might use music as a distraction by turning on the radio when the pain begins. Have the patient close his eyes and concentrate on listening, raising

or lowering the volume as pain increases or subsides. Note, however, that distraction is usually effective only against brief pain episodes lasting less than 5 minutes.

• For guided imagery, help the patient concentrate on a peaceful, pleasant image. Encourage concentration on details of the image by asking about its sight, sound, smell, taste, and touch. *The positive emotions evoked by this exercise minimize pain.*

• For deep breathing, have the patient stare at an object, then slowly inhale and exhale while counting out loud at a comfortable rate and rhythm. Have him concentrate on the rise and fall of his abdomen or on a restful image. Encourage him to feel more and more weightless with each breath.

• For muscle relaxation, have the patient focus on a particular muscle group, then tense the muscles for 5 to 7 seconds and note the sensation. Next, have him relax the muscles and concentrate on the relaxed state. Ask him to note the difference between the tense and relaxed states. Proceed from one muscle group to another, covering the entire body.

Complications

• The most common adverse effects of analgesics include respiratory depression (the most serious), sedation, constipation, nausea, and vomiting.

Nursing considerations

• Evaluate your patient's response to pain management; reassess his condition and alter the plan of care as needed.

• Remind the patient that results of cognitive therapy techniques improve with practice. Help him through the initial sessions.

• Patients receiving narcotic analgesics are at risk for developing tolerance, dependence, or addiction. A patient with acute pain may have a smaller risk of dependence or addiction than one with chronic pain.

• If a patient receiving an opioid analgesic experiences abstinence syndrome when the drug is withdrawn abruptly, suspect physical dependence. The signs and symptoms include anxiety, irritability, chills and hot flashes, excessive salivation and tearing, rhinorrhea, sweating, nausea, vomiting, and seizures. Signs and symptoms are likely to begin in 6 to 12 hours and peak in 24 to 72 hours. *To reduce the risk of dependence,* discontinue a narcotic by decreasing the dose gradually each day. Or switch to an oral narcotic and decrease the patient's dose gradually.

• An addicted patient's behavior is characterized by compulsive drug use and a craving for the drug to experience effects other than pain relief. A patient demonstrating such behavior usually has a preexisting problem that's exacerbated by the narcotic use. Discuss the addicted patient's problem with support personnel, and make appropriate referrals to experts.

• During periods of intense pain, the patient's ability to concentrate diminishes. In such cases, help the patient select a cognitive technique that's simple to use, and encourage consistent practice.

Documentation

• Document each step of the nursing process.

• Record the subjective information you elicit, using the patient's words. Note the location, quality, and duration of the pain, and precipitating factors.

• Record your nursing diagnoses and the pain relief method selected. Summarize your actions and the patient's response.

• If the patient's pain wasn't relieved, note alternate treatments to consider the next time pain occurs.

• Record any complications of drug therapy.

Pap test

The Papanicolaou (Pap) test — also called a Pap smear — allows early detection of cervical cancer. The test involves scraping secretions from the cervix, spreading them on a slide, and immediately coating the slide with fixative spray or a solution to preserve specimen cells for nuclear staining. Cytologic evaluation is then used to determine cell maturity, morphology, and metabolic activity. Less commonly, the Pap test is used to evaluate the vaginal pool (an area that collects cells from the endometrium, vagina, and cervix), prostatic secretions, urine, gastric secretions, cavity fluids, bronchial aspirations, and sputum.

≫ Key nursing diagnoses and patient outcomes
Use these nursing diagnoses as a guide when developing your plan of care.

Knowledge deficit related to lack of exposure to procedure
Based on this nursing diagnosis, you'll establish the following patient outcomes. The patient will:
• communicate need to increase knowledge.
• state or demonstrate understanding of what is taught.
• state intention to seek help from health professionals when needed.

Health-seeking behaviors related to potential for cervical cancer
Based on this nursing diagnosis, you'll establish the following patient outcomes. The patient will:
• have regularly scheduled tests.
• communicate understanding of need for regular tests.
• attend follow-up sessions with health care professional when test results are abnormal.

Equipment
♦ bivalve vaginal speculum ♦ gloves ♦ Pap stick (wooden spatula) ♦ long cotton-tipped applicator ♦ three glass microscope slides ♦ fixative (a commercial spray or 95% ethyl alcohol solution) ♦ adjustable lamp ♦ drape ♦ laboratory request forms.

Equipment preparation
• Select a speculum of the appropriate size and gather the equipment in the examining room.
• Label the glass slides with the patient's name and "E," "C," and "V" to differentiate endocervical, cervical, and vaginal specimens.

Patient preparation
• Explain the procedure to the patient and wash your hands.

• Instruct the patient to void *to relax the perineal muscles and facilitate bimanual examination of the uterus.*

• Provide privacy and instruct the patient to undress below the waist, but to wear her shoes, if desired, to cushion her feet against the stirrups. Then instruct her to sit on the examining table and to drape her genital region.

Implementation

• Place the patient in the lithotomy position, with her feet in the stirrups and her buttocks extended slightly beyond the edge of the table. Adjust the drape.

• Adjust the lamp *to fully illuminate the genital area.* Then fold back the corner of the drape *to expose the perineum.*

• If you're performing the procedure, first put on gloves. Then take the speculum in your dominant hand, and moisten it with warm water *to ease insertion.* Avoid using water-soluble lubricants, *which can interfere with accurate laboratory testing.*

• Warn the patient that you're about to touch her *to avoid startling her.* Then gently separate the labia with the thumb and forefinger of your nondominant hand.

• Instruct the patient to take several deep breaths, and insert the speculum into the vagina. Once it's in place, slowly open the blades *to expose the cervix.* Then lock the blades in place.

• Insert a cotton-tipped applicator through the speculum $\frac{1}{5}''$ into the cervical os. Rotate it 360 degrees *to obtain an endocervical specimen.* Then remove the cotton-tipped applicator, and gently roll it in a circle across the slide marked "E." Avoid rubbing the applicator on the slide *to prevent cell destruction.* Immediately place the slide in a fixative solution, or spray it with a fixative *to prevent drying of the cells, which interferes with nuclear staining and cytologic interpretation.*

• Insert the small curved end of the Pap stick through the speculum, and place it directly over the cervical os. Rotate the stick gently but firmly *to scrape cells loose.* Remove the stick, spread the specimen across the slide marked "C," and fix it immediately, as before.

• Insert the opposite end of the Pap stick or a cotton-tipped applicator through the speculum, and scrape the posterior fornix or vaginal pool. Remove the stick or applicator, spread the specimen across the slide marked "V," and fix it immediately.

• Unlock the speculum *to ease removal and avoid accidentally pinching the vaginal wall.* Then withdraw the speculum.

• Remove the glove from your nondominant hand to perform the bimanual examination, which usually follows the Pap test. Then remove and discard your other glove.

• Gently remove the patient's feet from the stirrups and assist her to a sitting position. Provide privacy for her to dress.

• Fill out the appropriate laboratory request forms, including the date of the patient's last menses.

Complications

• Failure to unlock the speculum blades before removal can pinch vaginal tissue.

• Although slight cramping normally accompanies this examination, rough handling of the speculum can cause severe cramping.

• Scraping an inflamed cervix with the Pap stick can cause slight bleeding.

Nursing considerations

• *Because many preventable factors can interfere with the Pap test's accuracy,* provide appropriate patient teaching beforehand. For example, caution the patient not to use a vaginal douche in the 48-hour period before specimen collection *because doing so would wash away cellular deposits and prevent adequate sampling.*

• Instillation of vaginal medications in the same period makes cytologic interpretation difficult.

• Collecting a specimen during menstruation prevents adequate sampling *because menstrual flow washes away cells;* ideally, collection should take place 5 to 6 days before menses or 1 week after it.

• Application of topical antibiotics promotes rapid, heavy shedding of cells and requires postponement of the Pap test for at least 1 month.

• If the patient has had a complete hysterectomy, collect test specimens from the vaginal pool and cuff.

Documentation

• On the patient's chart, record the date and time of specimen collection, any complications, and the nursing action taken.

Paracentesis (abdominal)

Abdominal paracentesis is a bedside procedure in which fluid from the peritoneal space is aspirated through a needle, trocar, or cannula inserted in the abdominal wall. It's used in the diagnosis and treatment of massive ascites that's resistant to other therapy. The procedure helps a health care team determine the cause of ascites and, at the same time, relieves the pressure created by ascites. It may be used as a prelude to other procedures, including radiography, peritoneal dialysis, and surgery. It's also used to detect intra-abdominal bleeding after traumatic injury and to obtain a peritoneal fluid specimen for laboratory analysis.

Nursing responsibilities during abdominal paracentesis include preparing the patient, monitoring the patient's condition and providing emotional support during the procedure, assisting the doctor, and obtaining specimens for laboratory analysis.

≫ Key nursing diagnoses and patient outcomes

Use these nursing diagnoses as a guide when developing your plan of care for a patient having an abdominal paracentesis.

Risk for infection related to the procedure

Based on this nursing diagnosis, you'll establish the following patient outcomes. The patient will:

• have vital signs, temperature, and laboratory values within normal limits.

• have no pathogens in cultures.

• show no signs or symptoms of infection at the paracentesis site.

Risk for fluid volume deficit related to paracentesis

Based on this nursing diagnosis, you'll establish the following patient outcomes. The patient will:

Positioning the patient for abdominal paracentesis

Help the patient sit up in bed, or allow the patient to sit on the side of the bed with additional support for his back and arms.

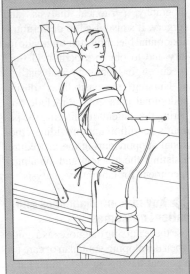

When the patient takes this position, gravity helps fluid to accumulate in the lower abdominal cavity. The internal abdominal structures provide counterresistance and additional pressure to facilitate fluid flow.

• have normal skin color and temperature.
• exhibit no signs of dehydration.
• maintain urine output of at least (specify) ml/hour.
• have electrolyte values within normal ranges.
• have intake equal output.

Equipment

♦ tape measure ♦ sterile gloves ♦ clean gloves ♦ gown ♦ linen-saver pads ♦ goggles ♦ four Vacutainer laboratory tubes ♦ two large glass Vacutainer bottles (1,000 ml or larger) ♦ dry, sterile pressure dressing ♦ laboratory request forms ♦ povidone-iodine solution ♦ local anesthetic (multidose vial of 1% or 2% lidocaine with epinephrine) ♦ sterile $4'' \times 4''$ gauze pads ♦ sterile paracentesis tray (containing needle, trocar, cannula, three-way stopcock) ♦ sterile drapes ♦ marking pen ♦ 5-ml syringe with 22G or 25G needle ♦ optional: povidone-iodine ointment, 50-ml syringe, alcohol sponge, suture materials, salt-poor albumin.

Patient preparation

• Explain the procedure to the patient *to ease his anxiety and promote cooperation.*
• Reassure the patient that the procedure is painless but that he may feel a stinging sensation from the local anesthetic injection and pressure from the needle or trocar and cannula insertion and when the doctor aspirates abdominal fluid.
• Obtain the patient's signed consent form.
• Instruct the patient to void before the procedure. Or insert an indwelling catheter, if ordered, *to minimize the risk of accidental bladder injury from the needle or trocar and cannula insertion.*
• Record baseline values, including the patient's vital signs, weight, and abdominal girth at the umbilical level. Indicate the abdominal area measured with a felt-tipped marking pen.

• Help the patient sit up in bed or in a chair that fully supports his arms and legs *so that fluid accumulates in the lower abdomen.* Or help him sit on the side of the bed and use pillows to support his back. Make the patient as comfortable as possible. (See *Positioning the patient for abdominal paracentesis.*)

• Place a linen-saver pad under the patient *to absorb drainage.*

• Remind the patient to stay as still as possible during the procedure *to prevent injury from the needle or trocar and cannula.*

• Expose the patient's abdomen from diaphragm to pubis.

Implementation

• Wash your hands. Open the paracentesis tray using aseptic technique *to ensure a sterile field.*

• Put on gloves *to assist the doctor with preparing the patient's abdomen with povidone-iodine solution, draping the operative site with sterile drapes, and administering the local anesthetic.*

• If the paracentesis tray doesn't contain a sterile ampule of anesthetic, wipe the top of a multidose vial of anesthetic solution with an alcohol sponge. Invert the vial at a 45-degree angle *so that the doctor can use a syringe to withdraw the anesthetic without touching the nonsterile vial.*

• Using the scalpel, the doctor may make a small incision before inserting the needle or trocar and cannula (usually 1″ to 2″ [2.5 to 5 cm] below the umbilicus). Listen for a popping sound, which indicates that the needle or trocar has pierced the peritoneum.

• Assist the doctor with specimen collection in the appropriate containers.

Wear clean gloves, gown, and goggles *to protect you from possible body fluid contamination.*

• If the doctor orders substantial drainage, connect the three-way stopcock and tubing to the cannula. Run the other end of the tubing to a large sterile Vacutainer collection bottle. Or aspirate the fluid with a three-way stopcock and 50-ml syringe.

• Gently turn the patient from side to side *to enhance drainage,* if necessary.

• As the fluid drains, monitor the patient's vital signs every 15 minutes. Watch closely for vertigo, faintness, diaphoresis, pallor, heightened anxiety, tachycardia, dyspnea, and hypotension — especially if more than 1,500 ml of peritoneal fluid is aspirated at one time. *Substantial drainage may induce a fluid shift and hypovolemic shock.*

• Immediately report signs of shock to the doctor, who may order you to administer salt-poor albumin I.V. *to replace aspirated fluid and to prevent hypovolemia and a decline in renal function.*

• When the procedure ends, wear sterile gloves to apply the dry, sterile pressure dressing and povidone-iodine ointment to the incision.

• Help the patient assume a comfortable position.

• Monitor the patient's vital signs and check the dressing for drainage every 15 minutes for 1 hour, every 30 minutes for 2 hours, every hour for 4 hours, and then every 4 hours for 24 hours. Be sure to note drainage color, amount, and character.

• Label the Vacutainer specimen tubes and send them to the laboratory with the appropriate laboratory request forms. If

BETTER CHARTING

Documenting paracentesis

When caring for a patient during and after paracentesis, be sure to keep a running record of the patient's vital signs and nursing activities related to drainage and to dressing changes. The record should indicate the frequency of drainage checks and the drainage characteristics. Also document daily patient weight and abdominal girth measurements.

If peritoneal fluid leakage occurs, notify the doctor and document that you did so. Be sure to include the time and date.

1/10/97	1100	After procedure explained to pt. and consent obtained. Dr. Mayberry performed paracentesis in RLQ as per protocol. 1500 ml cloudy, pale-yellow fluid drained and sent to lab as ordered. Site sutured with one 3-0 silk suture. Sterile 4" x 4" gauze pad applied. No leakage noted at site. Abd. girth 44" pre-procedure and 42¾" post-procedure. Pt. tolerated procedure w/o difficulty. VSS before and after procedure as per flow sheet. Emotional support given to pt. —— Carol Barton, RN

the patient is receiving antibiotics, note this on the request form for consideration during fluid analysis.

• Make sure that you remove and dispose of all equipment properly.

Complications

• This procedure must be performed cautiously in pregnant patients and in patients with bleeding tendencies or unstable vital signs.

• Removing large amounts of fluid can cause hypotension, oliguria, and hyponatremia. If a large amount of fluid (more than 2 liters) is removed, ascitic fluid tends to form again, drawing fluid from extracellular tissue throughout the body.

• Other possible complications include perforation of abdominal organs by the needle or the trocar and cannula, wound infection, and peritonitis.

Nursing considerations

• Throughout this procedure, help the patient remain still *to prevent accidental perforation of abdominal organs.*

• If the patient shows any signs of hypovolemic shock, reduce the vertical distance between the needle or the trocar and cannula and the drainage collection container *to slow the drainage rate.* If necessary, stop the drainage. *To prevent fluid shifts and hypovolemia,* limit aspirated fluid to between 1,500 and 2,000 ml.

• If peritoneal fluid doesn't flow easily, try repositioning the patient *to facilitate drainage.* Also verify suction in the Vacutainer collection bottle when you connect it to the drainage tubing, and be sure to use macrodrip tubing without a backflow device.

• After the procedure, observe for peritoneal fluid leakage. If this develops, notify the doctor.

Documentation

• Record daily patient weight and abdominal girth records. Compare these values with the baseline figures *to detect recurrent ascites.*

• Record the date and time of the procedure, the puncture site location, and whether the wound was sutured.

• Document the amount, color, viscosity, and odor of aspirated fluid in your notes and in the fluid intake and output record.

• Note the patient's tolerance of the procedure, vital signs, and any signs and symptoms of complications during the procedure.

• Note the number of specimens sent to the laboratory. (See *Documenting paracentesis.*)

Passive range-of-motion exercises

Passive range-of-motion (ROM) exercises are used to move the patient's joints through as full a range of motion as possible to improve or maintain joint mobility and help prevent contractures. These exercises — which are performed by a nurse, a physical therapist, or a caregiver of the patient's choosing — are indicated for the patient with temporary or permanent loss of mobility, sensation, or consciousness. Performed properly, passive ROM exercises require recognition of the patient's limits of motion and support of all joints during movement. (See *Glossary of joint movements,* page 644.)

Passive ROM exercises are contraindicated in patients with septic joints, acute thrombophlebitis, severe arthritic joint inflammation, or recent trauma with possible hidden fractures or internal injuries.

≫ Key nursing diagnoses and patient outcomes

Use these nursing diagnoses as a guide when developing your plan of care for a patient undergoing passive ROM exercises.

Risk for disuse syndrome related to prolonged inactivity

Based on this nursing diagnosis, you'll establish the following patient outcomes. The patient will:

• display no evidence of altered mental, sensory, or motor ability.

• maintain muscle strength and tone and joint range of motion.

• maintain normal neurologic, cardiovascular, respiratory, musculoskeletal, GI, and integumentary functioning during period of inactivity.

Impaired physical mobility related to neuromuscular impairment

Based on this nursing diagnosis, you'll establish the following patient outcomes. The patient will:

• show no evidence of complications, such as contractures, venous stasis, thrombus formation, or skin breakdown.

• have mobility regimen carried out by self or caregiver.

Equipment

No special equipment is necessary to perform passive ROM exercises.

Equipment preparation

• Before you begin, raise the bed to a comfortable working height.

Glossary of joint movements

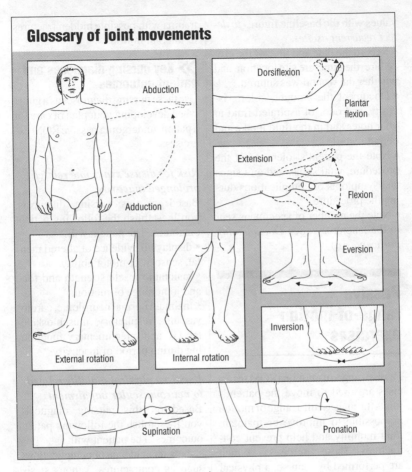

Abduction

Adduction

Dorsiflexion

Plantar flexion

Extension

Flexion

Eversion

Inversion

External rotation

Internal rotation

Supination

Pronation

Patient preparation

• Determine the joints that need ROM exercises, and consult the doctor or physical therapist about limitations or precautions for specific exercises.

Implementation

The exercises below are used to treat all joints, but they don't have to be performed in the order given or all at once. You can schedule them over the course of a day, whenever the patient is in the most convenient position. Perform all exercises slowly, gently, and to the end

of the normal range of motion or to the point of pain, but no further.

Neck

• Support the patient's head with your hands and extend the neck, flex the chin to the chest, and tilt the head laterally toward each shoulder.

• Rotate the head from right to left.

Shoulder

• Support the patient's arm in an extended, neutral position; then extend the forearm and flex it back. Abduct

the arm outward from the side of the body, and adduct it back to the side.
• Rotate the shoulder so that the arm crosses the midline, and bend the elbow so that the hand touches the opposite shoulder, then touches the mattress of the bed for complete internal rotation.
• Return the shoulder to a neutral position and, with elbow bent, push the arm backward so that the back of the hand touches the mattress for complete external rotation.

Elbow
• Place the patient's arm at his side with his palm facing up.
• Flex and extend the arm at the elbow.

Forearm
• Stabilize the patient's elbow, and then twist the hand to bring the palm up (supination).
• Twist it back again to bring the palm down (pronation).

Wrist
• Stabilize the forearm and flex and extend the wrist.
• Rock the hand sideways for lateral flexion and rotate the hand in a circular motion.

Fingers and thumb
• Extend the patient's fingers, and then flex the hand into a fist; repeat extension and flexion of each joint of each finger and thumb separately.
• Spread two adjoining fingers apart (abduction) and then bring them together (adduction).
• Oppose each fingertip to the thumb, and rotate the thumb and each finger in a circle.

Hip and knee
• Fully extend the patient's leg, and then bend the hip and knee toward the chest, allowing full joint flexion.
• Move the straight leg sideways, out and away from the other leg (abduction), and then back, over, and across it (adduction).
• Rotate the straight leg internally toward the midline, and then externally away from the midline.

Ankle
• Bend the patient's foot so that the toes push upward (dorsiflexion), and then bend the foot so that the toes push downward (plantar flexion).
• Rotate the ankle in a circular motion.
• Invert the ankle so that the sole of the foot faces the midline, and evert the ankle so that the sole faces away from the midline.

Toes
• Flex the patient's toes toward the sole of the foot, and then extend them back toward the top of the foot.
• Spread two adjoining toes apart (abduction) and bring them together (adduction).

Complications
• Potential complications include thromboemboli and overextension leading to joint injury or dislocation.

Nursing considerations
• *Because joints begin to stiffen within 24 hours of disuse,* start passive ROM exercises as soon as possible, and perform them at least once a shift, particularly while bathing or turning the patient.
• Use proper body mechanics, and repeat each exercise at least three times.

Learning about isometric exercises

Patients can strengthen and increase muscle tone by contracting muscles against resistance (from other muscles or from a stationary object, such as a bed or a wall) without joint movement. These exercises require only a comfortable position — standing, sitting, or lying down — and proper body alignment. For each exercise, instruct the patient to hold each contraction for 2 to 5 seconds and to repeat it three to four times daily, below peak contraction level for the first week and at peak level thereafter.

Neck rotators
The patient places the heel of his hand above one ear and pushes his head toward the hand as forcefully as possible, without moving the head, neck, or arm. He repeats the exercise on the other side.

Neck flexors
The patient places both palms on his forehead. Without moving his neck, he pushes the head forward while resisting with the palms.

Neck extensors
The patient clasps his fingers behind his head, then pushes the head against the clasped hands without moving his neck.

Shoulder elevators
Holding the right arm straight down at the side, the patient grasps his right wrist with his left hand. He then tries to shrug his right shoulder, but prevents it from moving by holding his arm in place. He repeats this exercise, alternating arms.

Shoulder, chest, and scapular musculature
The patient places his right fist in his left palm and raises both arms to shoulder height. He pushes the fist into the palm as forcefully as possible without moving either arm.

Then, with his arms in the same position, he clasps the fingers and tries to pull the hands apart. He repeats the pattern, beginning with the left fist in the right palm.

Elbow flexors and extensors
With his right elbow bent 90 degrees and his right palm facing upward, the patient places his left fist against his right palm. He tries to bend the right elbow further while resisting with the left fist. He repeats the pattern, bending the left elbow.

Abdomen
The patient assumes a sitting position and bends slightly forward, with his hands in front of the middle of his thighs. He tries to bend forward further, resisting by pressing the palms against the thighs.

Alternatively, in the supine position, he clasps his hands behind his head. Then he raises his shoulders about 1″ (2.5 cm), holding this position for a few seconds.

Back extensors
In a sitting position, the patient bends forward and places his hands under his buttocks. He tries to stand up, resisting with both hands.

Learning about isometric exercises (continued)

Hip abductors
While standing, the patient squeezes his inner thighs together as tightly as possible. Placing a pillow between the knees supplies resistance and increases the effectiveness of this exercise.

Hip extensors
The patient squeezes his buttocks together as tightly as possible.

Knee extensors
The patient straightens his knee fully. Then he vigorously tightens the muscle above the knee so that it moves the kneecap upward. He repeats this exercise, alternating legs.

Ankle flexors and extensors
The patient pulls his toes upward, holding briefly. Then he pushes them down as far as possible, again holding briefly.

Home care
• Patients who experience prolonged bed rest or limited activity without profound weakness can also be taught to perform ROM exercises on their own (called active ROM) or may benefit from isometric exercises. (See *Learning about isometric exercises*.)
• If the disabled patient requires long-term rehabilitation after discharge, consult with a physical therapist and teach a family member or caregiver to perform passive ROM exercises.

Documentation
• Record the joints exercised, the presence of edema or pressure areas, any pain resulting from the exercises, any limitation of ROM, and the patient's tolerance of the exercises.

Perineal care

Perineal care, including the external genitalia and the anal area, should be performed during the daily bath and, if necessary, at bedtime and after urination and bowel movements. The procedure promotes cleanliness and prevents infection. It also removes irritating and odorous secretions, such as smegma, a cheeselike substance that collects under the foreskin of the penis and on the inner surface of the labia. For the patient with perineal skin breakdown, frequent bathing followed by application of an ointment or cream aids healing.

Universal precautions must be followed when providing perineal care, with due consideration given to the patient's privacy.

≫ Key nursing diagnoses and patient outcomes
Use this nursing diagnosis as a guide when developing your plan of care for a patient requiring perineal care.

Bathing or hygiene self-care deficit related to (specify)
Based on this nursing diagnosis, you'll establish the following patient outcomes. The patient will:
• meet self-care needs.
• carry out self-care program daily.

• communicate feelings and concerns.

Equipment

♦ gloves ♦ washcloths ♦ clean basin ♦ mild soap ♦ bath towel ♦ bath blanket ♦ toilet tissue ♦ linen-saver pad ♦ trash bag ♦ optional: bedpan, peri bottle, antiseptic soap, petroleum jelly, zinc oxide cream, vitamin A and D ointment.

Following genital or rectal surgery: ♦ sterile supplies, including sterile gloves, gauze, and cotton balls ♦ ABD pad.

Equipment preparation

• Obtain ointment or cream, as needed.
• Fill the basin two-thirds full with warm water.
• Fill the peri bottle with warm water, if needed.
• Assemble equipment at the patient's bedside.

Patient preparation

• Provide privacy and explain the procedure.
• Adjust the bed to a comfortable working height *to prevent back strain,* and lower the head of the bed, if allowed.
• Help the patient to a supine position.
• Place a linen-saver pad under the patient's buttocks.

Implementation

• Wash your hands thoroughly and put on gloves.

Perineal care for women

• *To minimize the patient's exposure and embarrassment,* place the bath blanket over her with corners head to foot and side to side. Wrap each leg with a side corner, tucking it under the hip. Then fold back the corner between the legs to expose the perineum.
• Ask the patient to bend her knees slightly and to spread her legs.
• Separate the patient's labia with one hand and wash with the other, using gentle downward strokes from the front to the back of the perineum *to prevent intestinal organisms from contaminating the urethra or vagina.* Avoid the area around the anus, and use a clean section of washcloth for each stroke by folding each used section inward. *This prevents the spread of contaminated secretions or discharge.*
• Using a clean washcloth, rinse the area thoroughly from front to back. Pat the area dry with a bath towel.
• Apply ordered ointments or creams.
• Turn the patient on her side in Sims' position, if possible, *to expose the anal area.*
• Clean, rinse, and dry the anal area, starting at the posterior vaginal opening and wiping from front to back.

Perineal care for men

• Drape the patient's legs *to minimize exposure and embarrassment and expose the genital area.*
• Hold the shaft of the penis with one hand and wash with the other, beginning at the tip and working in a circular motion from the center to the periphery *to avoid introducing microorganisms into the urethra.* Use a clean section of washcloth for each stroke *to prevent the spread of contaminated secretions or discharge.*
• Rinse thoroughly, using the same circular motion.

• For the uncircumcised patient, gently retract the foreskin and clean beneath it. Rinse well but don't dry *because moisture provides lubrication and prevents friction when replacing the foreskin.*

• Wash the rest of the penis, using downward strokes toward the scrotum. Rinse well and pat dry with a bath towel.

• Clean the top and sides of the scrotum; rinse thoroughly and pat dry. Handle the scrotum gently *to avoid causing discomfort.*

• Turn the patient on his side. Clean the bottom of the scrotum and the anal area. Rinse well and pat dry.

After providing perineal care

• Return the patient to a comfortable position.

• Remove the bath blanket and linensaver pad, and then replace the bed linens.

• Clean and return the basin and dispose of soiled articles including gloves.

Nursing considerations

• Give perineal care to a patient of the opposite sex in a matter-of-fact way *to minimize embarrassment.*

• If the patient is incontinent, first remove excess feces with toilet tissue. Then position him on a bedpan, and add a small amount of antiseptic soap to a peri bottle *to eliminate odor.* Irrigate the perineal area *to remove any remaining fecal matter.*

• After cleaning the perineum, apply ointment or cream (petroleum jelly, zinc oxide cream, or vitamin A and D ointment) *to prevent skin breakdown.*

• To reduce the number of linen changes, tuck an ABD pad between the patient's buttocks *to absorb oozing feces.*

Documentation

• Record perineal care and any special treatment in your notes.

• Document the need for continued treatment, if necessary, in your care plan.

• Describe perineal skin condition and any odor or discharge.

Peripheral I.V. line insertion

A peripheral line, which allows I.V. access to the patient, is used to administer fluids, medication, blood, and blood components. Insertion of a peripheral line involves selecting a venipuncture device and insertion site, applying a tourniquet, preparing the site, and completing the venipuncture. Selection of a venipuncture device and site depends on the type of solution to be used; the frequency and duration of infusion; the patient's age, size, and condition; the patency and location of accessible veins; and, when possible, the patient's preference.

Typically, a vein in the nondominant arm or hand is selected. The most favorable venipuncture sites are the cephalic and basilic veins in the lower arm and the veins in the dorsum of the hand; least favorable are the leg and foot veins because of the increased risk of thrombophlebitis. Antecubital veins can be used if no other venous access is available, to accommodate a large-bore needle, or to administer drugs requiring large volume dilution.

≫ **Key nursing diagnoses and patient outcomes**

Use these nursing diagnoses as a guide when developing your plan of care for a patient having a peripheral I.V. line inserted.

Risk for infection related to procedure

Based on this nursing diagnosis, you'll establish the following patient outcomes. The patient will:
• have vital signs, temperature, and laboratory values within normal limits.
• have no pathogens appear in cultures.
• show no signs or symptoms of infection at the I.V. insertion site.

Risk for fluid volume deficit related to need for peripheral I.V.

Based on this nursing diagnosis, you'll establish the following patient outcomes. The patient will:
• maintain normal skin color and temperature.
• exhibit no signs of dehydration.
• maintain urine output of at least (specify) ml/hour.
• have electrolyte values within normal range.
• have intake equal output.

Equipment

♦ alcohol sponges ♦ povidone-iodine sponges ♦ antimicrobial ointment, according to hospital policy ♦ gloves ♦ tourniquet (rubber tubing or a blood pressure cuff) ♦ two I.V. needles or I.V. catheter devices ♦ sterile 2″ × 2″ gauze pads or a transparent semipermeable dressing ♦ 1″ hypoallergenic tape ♦ I.V. solution with attached and primed administration set ♦ I.V. pole ♦ sharps container ♦ optional: armboard, roller gauze, tube gauze, warm packs, antimicrobial solution (such as 70% isopropyl alcohol, tincture of iodine, povidone-iodine, or chlorhexidine), local anesthetic (such as 1% lidocaine without epinephrine), U-100 insulin syringe with a 27G needle.

Commercial venipuncture kits are available with or without an I.V. needle or I.V. catheter device. (See *Comparing venipuncture devices.*)

Equipment preparation

• In many hospitals, venipuncture equipment is kept on a tray or cart, allowing choice of the correct needle or catheter and easy replacement of contaminated items.
• Select the smallest gauge needle or catheter device available for the infusion unless subsequent therapy will require a larger one. *Smaller gauges cause less trauma to veins, allow greater blood flow around their tips, and reduce the clotting risk.*
• To use a winged infusion set, connect the adapter to the administration set, and unclamp the line until fluid flows from the open end of the needle cover. Then close the clamp and place the needle on a sterile surface, such as the inside of its packaging.
• To use a catheter device, open the package to allow easy access.
• Place the I.V. pole in the proper slot in the patient's bed frame. If you're using a portable I.V. pole, position it close to the patient.
• Hang the I.V. solution with attached primed administration set on the I.V. pole.

Comparing venipuncture devices

Most I.V. infusions are delivered through one of three basic types of venipuncture devices: an over-the-needle catheter, a through-the-needle catheter, or a winged infusion set. To improve I.V. therapy and guard against accidental needle sticks, you can use an innovative device, such as the Baxter Interlink I.V. system.

Over-the-needle catheter
Purpose: long-term therapy for active or agitated patient.
Advantages: makes accidental puncture of the vein less likely than with a needle; is more comfortable for the patient once it's in place; contains radiopaque thread for easy location; some units come with a syringe that permits easy check of blood return; some units include wings.
Disadvantage: is more difficult to insert than other devices.

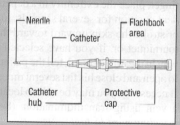

Through-the-needle catheter
Purpose: long-term therapy for active or agitated patient.
Advantages: makes accidental puncture of the vein less likely than with a needle; is more comfortable for the patient once it's in place; is available in many lengths; most plastic catheters contain radiopaque thread for easy location; one variant, the peripherally inserted central catheter, is inserted in the antecubital vein by a specially prepared nurse.

Disadvantages: leaking at the site may occur, especially in an elderly patient; if a needle guard isn't used, the catheter may be severed.

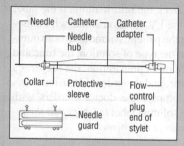

Winged infusion set
Purpose: short-term therapy for any cooperative adult patient; therapy of any duration for an infant or child or for an elderly patient with fragile or sclerotic veins.
Advantages: is easiest intravascular device to insert; is ideal for I.V. push drugs.
Disadvantage: may easily cause infiltration if a rigid-needle winged infusion device is used.

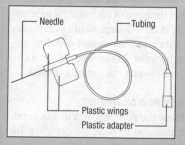

Patient preparation

• Verify the patient's identity by comparing the information on the solution container with the patient's wristband.
• Explain the procedure to the patient *to ensure cooperation and reduce anxiety, which can cause a vasomotor response resulting in venous constriction.*

Implementation

• Wash your hands thoroughly.
• Check the information on the label of the I.V. solution container, including the patient's name and room number, the type of solution, the time and date of its preparation, the preparer's name, and the ordered infusion rate.
• Compare the doctor's orders with the solution label *to verify that the infusion is the correct one.*

Selecting the site

• A vein in the patient's nondominant arm is the preferred site.
• For fluid replacement, choose a small vein unless a large vein will be needed for subsequent therapy; *this leaves the large veins available for emergency infusion.*
• If long-term therapy is anticipated, start with a vein at the most distal site *so you can move proximally as needed for subsequent I.V. insertion sites.*
• For infusion of an irritating medication, choose a large vein (with plenty of subcutaneous tissue) distal to any nearby joint. Make sure the vein can accommodate the cannula if used.

Applying a tourniquet

• Place the patient's arm in a dependent position to increase capillary fill of the lower arms and hands.

• If the patient's skin is cold, warm it by rubbing and stroking the arm, or cover the entire arm with warm packs for 5 to 10 minutes.
• Apply the tourniquet about 6″ (15.2 cm) above the intended puncture site *to dilate the vein.*
• Check for a distal pulse. If it is not present, release the tourniquet and reapply it with less tension *to prevent arterial occlusion.*
• Lightly palpate the vein with your index and middle fingers, while stretching it *to prevent rolling.* If the vein feels hard or ropelike, select another.
• If the vein is easily palpable but not sufficiently dilated, one or more of the following techniques may help raise the vein. Flick the skin over the vein with one or two sharp snaps of your finger, place the extremity in a dependent position for several seconds, rub or stroke the skin upward toward the tourniquet or, if you have selected a vein in the arm or hand, tell the patient to open and close his fist several times. If necessary, you may be able to locate a vein using transillumination. (See *Locating hard-to-find veins.*)
• Leave the tourniquet in place for no longer than 2 minutes. If you can't find a suitable vein and prepare the site in that time, release the tourniquet for a few minutes. Then reapply it and continue the procedure.

Preparing the site

• Put on gloves.
• Clip the hair around the insertion site, if necessary, and clean the site with one of the following antimicrobials: povidone-iodine solution, 70% alcohol solution, tincture of iodine, or chlorhexidine. Do not apply alcohol

Locating hard-to-find veins

You can locate hard-to-find peripheral veins more easily by using a transillumination device such as the Landry Vein Light. This device uses bright light from a pair of adjustable fiber-optic arms to reveal the blood vessels. Secure the light to the patient's limb with tape. Dim the room lights. With the device on its brightest setting, scan the limb below the tourniquet for a vein. The vein appears as a dark line between the fiber-optic arms.

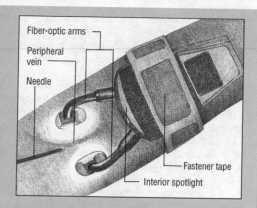

after cleaning with povidone-iodine *because alcohol negates iodine's effect.* Work in a circular motion outward from the site to a diameter of 2″ to 4″ (5 to 10 cm) *to remove flora that would otherwise be introduced into the vascular system with the venipuncture.*

• Allow the antimicrobial solution to dry.

• If ordered, administer a local anesthetic. Make sure the patient is not sensitive to lidocaine. (See *Administering a local anesthetic*, page 654.)

• Grasp the needle or catheter. If you're using a *winged infusion set,* hold the short edges of the wings (with the needle's bevel facing upward) between the thumb and forefinger of your dominant hand. Then squeeze the wings together. If you're using an *over-the-needle catheter,* grasp the plastic hub with your dominant hand,

remove the cover, and examine the catheter tip. If the edge isn't smooth, discard and replace the device. If you're using a *through-the-needle catheter,* grasp the needle hub with one hand, and unsnap the needle cover. Then rotate the catheter device until the bevel faces upward.

• Using the thumb of your opposite hand, stretch the skin taut below the puncture site *to stabilize the vein.*

• Lightly press the vein with your thumb about 1½″ (3.8 cm) from the intended insertion site. The vein should feel round, firm, fully engorged, and resilient.

• Tell the patient that you're about to insert the device.

• For the direct approach, hold the needle bevel up and enter the skin over the vein at a 30- to 45-degree angle. For the indirect approach, enter the skin slightly adjacent to the vein. Di-

Administering a local anesthetic

Although the procedure isn't recommended by the Intravenous Nurses Society, many doctors order a local anesthetic when starting I.V. therapy to numb the infusion site. A local anesthetic may be injected subcutaneously, or a topical anesthetic, such as EMLA cream, may be used.

Injecting a local anesthetic
• Using a U-100 insulin syringe with a 27G needle, draw up 0.1 ml of 1% lidocaine without epinephrine.
• Clean the venipuncture site. Put on gloves. Insert the needle next to the vein, introducing about one-third of it into the skin subcutaneously at a 30-degree angle, as shown here.

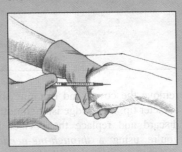

• This lateral approach carries less risk of accidental vein puncture. If the vein is deep, however, inject the lidocaine over the top of it, taking care to avoid injecting the anesthetic into the vein.

• Hold your thumb on the plunger of the syringe during insertion to avoid unnecessary movement once the needle is under the skin.
• Without aspirating, quickly inject the lidocaine until a small wheal appears. You may not have to administer the entire amount in the syringe.
• Quickly withdraw the syringe, and massage the wheal with an alcohol sponge. This will make the wheal disappear so the vein won't be hidden. However, you'll see a small pinprick of blood. The skin will be numb for about 30 minutes. When numbness occurs, insert the venipuncture device into the skin.

Applying a topical anesthetic
• Apply 2.5 g of EMLA cream in a thick layer over a 2″ × 2″ area at the I.V. site. Don't rub the cream into the skin.
• Cover the area with a transparent semipermeable dressing. Seal the edges only.

---

rect the device into the side of the vein wall *to avoid perforating the vein's opposite wall.*
• Advance the device steadily until you meet resistance. Don't penetrate the vein. Lower the needle to a 15- to 20-degree angle, and slowly pierce the vein. You may not always feel a "pop" or a sensation of release when the device enters the vein.

• When you observe blood flashback behind the hub, tilt the needle slightly upward and advance it farther into the vein *to prevent puncture of the posterior vein wall.* (You may not see blood return with a small vein.)
• If you're using a *winged infusion set,* advance the needle fully, if possible, and hold it in place. Release the tourniquet, open the administration set

clamp slightly, and check for free flow or infiltration.

• If you're using an over-the-needle catheter, advance the device to at least half of its length *to ensure that the catheter itself, not just the introducer needle, has entered the vein.* Then remove the tourniquet.

• Grasp the catheter hub *to hold it in place* in the vein, and withdraw the needle. As you withdraw it, press lightly on the catheter tip *to prevent bleeding.*

• Advance the catheter up to the hub or until you meet resistance.

• To advance the catheter while infusing I.V. solution, release the tourniquet and remove the inner needle. Using aseptic technique, attach the I.V. tubing and begin the infusion. While stabilizing the vein with one hand, use the other to advance the catheter into the vein. When the catheter is advanced, decrease the I.V. flow rate. *This method reduces the risk of puncturing the vein's opposite wall because the catheter is advanced without the steel needle and because the rapid flow dilates the vein.*

• To advance the catheter before starting the infusion, first release the tourniquet. While stabilizing the vein with one hand, use the other to advance the catheter up to the hub. Next, remove the inner needle and, using aseptic technique, quickly attach the I.V. tubing. *This method often results in less blood being spilled.*

• If you're using a *through-the-needle catheter*, remove the tourniquet, hold the needle in place with one hand and, with your opposite hand, grasp the catheter through the protective sleeve. Then slowly thread the catheter through the needle until the hub is within the needle collar. Never pull back on the catheter without pulling back on the needle *to avoid severing and releasing the catheter into the circulation, causing an embolus.* If you feel resistance from a valve, withdraw the catheter and needle slightly and reinsert them, rotating the catheter as you pass the valve. Then withdraw the metal needle, and cover it with the protector. Remove the stylet and protective sleeve, and attach the administration set to the catheter hub. Open the administration set clamp slightly, and check for free flow or infiltration.

Dressing the site

• After the venipuncture device has been inserted, clean the skin completely. If necessary, dispose of the inner needle in a needle receptacle. Then regulate the flow rate.

• You may use a transparent semipermeable dressing to secure the device. (See *How to apply a transparent semipermeable dressing*, page 656.)

• If a transparent dressing is not used, apply antiseptic ointment at the insertion site according to hospital policy; cover with a sterile gauze pad or small adhesive bandage.

• Loop the I.V. tubing on the patient's limb, and secure the tubing with tape. *The loop allows some slack to prevent dislodgment of the catheter from tension on the line.* (See *Taping a venipuncture site*, pages 657 and 658.)

• Label the last piece of tape with the type and gauge of needle or catheter, the date and time of insertion, and your initials. Adjust the flow rate, as ordered.

• If the puncture site is near a movable joint, secure an armboard with roller gauze or tape *to prevent movement*

How to apply a transparent semipermeable dressing

To secure the I.V. insertion site, you can apply a transparent semipermeable dressing as follows:
• Make sure the insertion site is clean and dry.
• Remove the dressing from the package and, using aseptic technique, remove the protective seal. Avoid touching the sterile surface.
• Place the dressing directly over the insertion site and the hub, as shown. Don't cover the tubing. Also, don't stretch the dressing; doing so may cause itching.

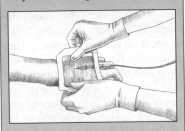

• Tuck the dressing around and under the catheter hub to make the site impervious to microorganisms.
• To remove the dressing, grasp one corner, and then lift and stretch it. If removal is difficult, try loosening the edges with alcohol or water.

that can dislodge the needle or catheter and increase the risk of thrombophlebitis and infection.

Removing a peripheral I.V. line

A peripheral I.V. line is removed after completion of therapy, for needle or catheter changes, and for suspected infection or infiltration. This procedure usually requires an alcohol sponge, a sterile gauze pad, and an adhesive bandage.
• First, clamp the I.V. tubing to stop the flow of solution. Then, gently remove all tape from the skin.
• Using aseptic technique, open the gauze pad and adhesive bandage, and place them within reach. Put on gloves. Hold the sterile gauze pad over the puncture site, and use your other hand to withdraw the needle or catheter slowly and smoothly, keeping it parallel to the skin.
• Inspect the catheter tip; if it's not smooth, assess the patient immediately, and notify the doctor.
• Using the gauze pad, apply firm pressure over the puncture site for 1 to 2 minutes after the device has been removed or until bleeding has stopped.
• Clean the site and apply the adhesive bandage. Or if blood oozes from the site, apply a pressure bandage.
• If drainage appears at the puncture site, send the tip of the device and a sample of the drainage to the laboratory to be cultured according to hospital policy. (A draining site may or may not be infected.) Then clean the area and apply antiseptic ointment and a sterile dressing.
• Instruct the patient to restrict activity for about 10 minutes and to leave the dressing in place for at least 8 hours. If he feels lingering tenderness at the site, apply warm packs.

Complications

• Peripheral line complications can result from the needle or catheter (infection, phlebitis, and embolism) or from the solution (circulatory overload, infiltration, sepsis, and allergic

Taping a venipuncture site

Use one of the four basic methods described below when using tape to secure a venipuncture device.

Chevron method
• Cover the venipuncture site with an adhesive strip or a $2'' \times 2''$ sterile gauze pad. Cut a long strip of $\frac{1}{2}''$ (1.3-cm) tape and place it, sticky side up, under the needle and parallel to the short strip of tape (below).

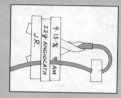

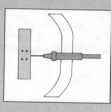

• Cross the ends of the tape over the needle as shown.

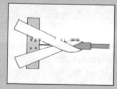

• Apply a piece of 1" (2.5-cm) tape across the two wings of the chevron
• Loop the tubing and secure it with more tape. Write the date and time of insertion, the type and gauge of the needle, and your initials (top, center column).

U method
• Cover the venipuncture site with an adhesive strip or a $2'' \times 2''$ sterile gauze pad. Place a 2" (5-cm) strip of $\frac{1}{2}''$ tape, sticky side up, under the tubing (below).

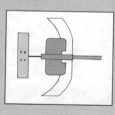

• Fold each side of the tape over the wings, and affix the ends parallel to the tubing (below).

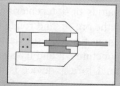

• Finish taping as you would with the chevron method.

• Sign the insertion as you would with the chevron method (below).

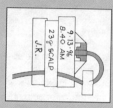

Two tape method
• Cover the venipuncture site with an adhesive strip or a $2'' \times 2''$ gauze pad. Then place a 2" strip of $\frac{1}{2}''$ tape, sticky side up, under the needle (below).

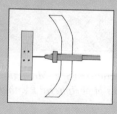

• Fold the tape ends over and affix them to the patient's skin in a U shape (below).

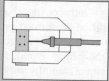

(continued)

Taping a venipuncture site *(continued)*

• Place a second strip of ½ " tape, sticky side down, over the needle hub. On the tape, write the date and time of insertion, the type and gauge of the needle or catheter, and your initials (below).

  With this method, you can remove the upper strip of tape to check the insertion site while the lower strip anchors the needle.

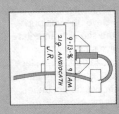

Three tape method
• Cover the venipuncture site with an adhesive strip or a 2″ x 2″ gauze pad (below). Then cut three strips of 1″ tape.

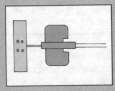

• Place one strip of tape over each wing, keeping the tape parallel to the needle (below).

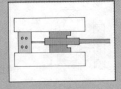

• Place the other strip perpendicular to the first two. Put it either directly on top of the wings or just below the wings, directly on top of the tubing.
• On the last piece of tape, write the date and time of insertion, the type and gauge of the needle or catheter, and your initials (below).

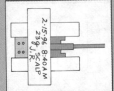

reaction). (See *Managing common risks of peripheral I.V. therapy.*)

Nursing considerations
• I.V. insertion is contraindicated in a sclerotic vein, in an edematous or impaired arm or hand, and in the presence of burns or an arteriovenous fistula. Subsequent venipunctures should be performed proximal to a previously used or injured vein.
• If the patient is elderly, apply the tourniquet carefully *to avoid pinching the skin.* If necessary, apply it over the patient's gown. Make sure skin preparation materials are at room temper-

ature *to avoid vasoconstriction resulting from lower temperatures.* If the patient is allergic to iodine-containing compounds, clean with alcohol.
• If you fail to see blood flashback after entering the vein, pull back slightly and rotate the device. If you still fail to see flashback, remove the cannula and try again. If you suspect that the device is in the vein, try these measures to facilitate blood flashback: position the I.V. container below needle level, or insert the needle and syringe into the injection port closest to the puncture site. Then close the clamp on
(Text continues on page 664.)

PROBLEM SOLVER

Managing common risks of peripheral I.V. therapy

COMPLICATION	SIGNS AND SYMPTOMS	POSSIBLE CAUSES	NURSING INTERVENTIONS
Phlebitis	• Tenderness at tip of and proximal to venipuncture device • Redness at tip of catheter and along vein • Puffy area over vein • Vein hard on palpation • Elevated temperature	• Poor blood flow around venipuncture device • Friction from catheter movement in vein • Venipuncture device left in vein too long • Clotting at catheter tip (thrombophlebitis) • Drug or solution with high or low pH or high osmolarity	• Remove venipuncture device. • Apply warm soaks. • Notify doctor if patient has fever. • Document patient's condition and your interventions. ***Prevention*** • Restart infusion using larger vein for irritating solution, or restart with smaller-gauge device *to ensure adequate blood flow.* • Use filter *to reduce risk of phlebitis.* • Tape device securely *to prevent motion.*
Extravasation	• Swelling at and above I.V. site (may extend along entire limb) • Discomfort, burning, or pain at site (but may be painless) • Tight feeling at site • Decreased skin temperature around site • Blanching at site	• Venipuncture device dislodged from vein, or perforated vein	• Stop the infusion. Infiltrate the site with an antidote, if appropriate. • Apply ice (early) or warm soaks (later) *to aid absorption.* Elevate limb. • Check for pulse and capillary refill periodically *to assess circulation.* • Restart infusion above infiltration site or in another limb. • Document patient's condition and your interventions. *(continued)*

Managing common risks of peripheral I.V. therapy *(continued)*

COMPLICATION	SIGNS AND SYMPTOMS	POSSIBLE CAUSES	NURSING INTERVENTIONS
Extra-vasation *(continued)*	• Continuing fluid infusion even when vein is occluded (although rate may decrease) • Absent backflow of blood		*Prevention* • Check I.V. site frequently. • Don't obscure area above site with tape. • Teach patient to observe I.V. site and report pain or swelling.
Catheter dislodgment	• Loose tape • Catheter partly backed out of vein • Solution infiltrating	• Loosened tape, or tubing snagged in bed linens, resulting in partial retraction of catheter; pulled out by confused patient	• If no infiltration occurs, retape without pushing catheter back into vein. If pulled out, apply pressure to I.V. site with sterile dressing. *Prevention* • Tape venipuncture securely on insertion.
Occlusion	• No increase in flow rate when I.V. container is raised • Blood backflow in line • Discomfort at insertion site	• I.V. flow interrupted • Heparin lock not flushed • Blood backflow in line when patient walks • Line clamped too long	• Use mild flush injection. Don't force it. If unsuccessful, reinsert I.V. line. *Prevention* • Maintain I.V. flow rate. • Flush promptly after intermittent piggyback administration. • Have patient walk with his arm bent at the elbow *to reduce risk of blood backflow.*
Vein irritation or pain at I.V. site	• Pain during infusion • Possible blanching if vasospasm occurs	• Solution with high or low pH or high osmolarity, such as 40 mEq/liter of potassium chloride,	• Decrease the flow rate. • Try using an electronic flow device *to achieve a steady flow.*

Managing common risks of peripheral I.V. therapy *(continued)*

COMPLICATION	SIGNS AND SYMPTOMS	POSSIBLE CAUSES	NURSING INTERVENTIONS
Vein irritation or pain at I.V. site *(continued)*	• Red skin over vein during infusion • Rapidly developing signs of phlebitis	phenytoin, and some antibiotics (vancomycin, erythromycin, and nafcillin)	**Prevention** • Dilute solutions before administration. For example, give antibiotics in 250-ml solution rather than 100 ml. If drug has low pH, ask pharmacist if drug can be buffered with sodium bicarbonate. (Refer to hospital policy.) • If long-term therapy of irritating drug is planned, ask doctor to use central I.V. line.
Severed catheter	• Leakage from catheter shaft	• Catheter inadvertently cut by scissors • Reinsertion of needle into catheter	• If broken part is visible, attempt to retrieve it. If unsuccessful, notify the doctor. • If portion of catheter enters bloodstream, place tourniquet above I.V. site *to prevent progression of broken part.* • Notify doctor and radiology department. • Document patient's condition and your interventions. **Prevention** • Don't use scissors around I.V. site. • Never reinsert needle into catheter. • Remove unsuccessfully inserted catheter and needle together. *(continued)*

Managing common risks of peripheral I.V. therapy *(continued)*

COMPLICATION	SIGNS AND SYMPTOMS	POSSIBLE CAUSES	NURSING INTERVENTIONS
Hematoma	• Tenderness at venipuncture site • Bruised area around site • Inability to advance or flush I.V. line	• Vein punctured through opposite wall at time of insertion • Leakage of blood from needle displacement • Inadequate pressure applied when catheter discontinued	• Remove venipuncture device. • Apply pressure and warm soaks to affected area. • Recheck for bleeding. • Document patient's condition and your interventions. ***Prevention*** • Choose a vein that can accommodate size of venipuncture device. • Release tourniquet as soon as successful insertion achieved.
Venous spasm	• Pain along vein • Flow rate sluggish when clamp completely open • Blanched skin over vein	• Severe vein irritation from irritating drugs or fluids • Administration of cold fluids or blood • Very rapid flow rate (with fluids at room temperature)	• Apply warm soaks over vein and surrounding area. • Decrease flow rate. ***Prevention*** • Use a bloodwarmer for blood or packed red blood cells.
Vasovagal reaction	• Sudden collapse of vein during venipuncture • Sudden pallor, sweating, faintness, dizziness, and nausea • Decreased blood pressure	• Vasospasm from anxiety or pain	• Lower head of bed. • Have patient take deep breaths. • Check vital signs. ***Prevention*** • Prepare patient for therapy *to relieve his anxiety.* • Use local anesthetic *to prevent pain.*

Managing common risks of peripheral I.V. therapy *(continued)*

COMPLICATION	SIGNS AND SYMPTOMS	POSSIBLE CAUSES	NURSING INTERVENTIONS
Thrombosis	• Painful, reddened and swollen vein • Sluggish or stopped I.V. flow	• Injury to endothelial cells of vein wall, allowing platelets to adhere and thrombi to form	• Remove venipuncture device; restart infusion in opposite limb if possible. • Apply warm soaks. • Watch for I.V. therapy-related infection; thrombi provide an excellent environment for bacterial growth. ***Prevention*** • Use proper venipuncture techniques *to reduce injury to vein.*
Thrombophlebitis	• Severe discomfort • Reddened, swollen, and hardened vein	• Thrombosis and inflammation	• Same as for thrombosis. ***Prevention*** • Check site frequently. Remove venipuncture device at first sign of redness and tenderness.
Nerve, tendon, or ligament damage	• Extreme pain (similar to electrical shock when nerve is punctured) • Numbness and muscle contraction • Delayed effects, including paralysis, numbness, and deformity	• Improper venipuncture technique, resulting in injury to surrounding nerves, tendons, or ligaments • Tight taping or improper splinting with armboard	• Stop procedure. ***Prevention*** • Don't repeatedly penetrate tissues with venipuncture device. • Don't apply excessive pressure when taping; don't encircle limb with tape. • Pad armboards and tape securing armboards if possible.

the I.V. tubing and attempt to aspirate. (Keep in mind that, if the device is tightly in place or the patient is extremely dehydrated or hypovolemic, you may not see blood flashback.)
• Change a gauze or transparent dressing when you change the administration set (every 48 hours or according to hospital policy).
• Rotate the I.V. site, usually every 48 to 72 hours or according to hospital policy.
• When a vein cannot be entered percutaneously, venesection may need to be performed.

Home care
• Most patients receiving I.V. therapy at home will have a central venous line. But if the patient is going home with a peripheral line, teach care of the I.V. site and identify possible complications.
• Make sure the patient understands and is willing to observe any necessary movement restrictions.
• Teach the patient how to examine the site, and instruct him to notify the doctor if redness, swelling, or discomfort develops; if the dressing becomes moist; or if blood is in the tubing.
• Tell the patient to report any problems with the I.V. line — for instance, if the solution stops infusing or if an alarm goes off on an infusion pump or controller.
• Explain that the I.V. site will be changed at established intervals by a home care nurse.
• If the patient is using an intermittent infusion device, such as a heparin lock, teach him how and when to flush it.

• Tell the patient to keep a daily record of whether the I.V. site is free from pain, swelling, and redness.

Documentation
• Record the date and time of venipuncture, the type and gauge of needle or catheter, the location of the insertion site, and the reason the site was changed.
• Document the number of attempts at venipuncture (if you made more than one), the type and flow rate of the I.V. solution, the name and amount of medication in the solution (if any), any adverse reactions and actions taken to correct them, patient teaching and evidence of patient understanding, and your initials.

Peripheral I.V. maintenance

Routine maintenance of I.V. sites and systems includes regular assessment and rotation of the site and periodic changes of the dressing, tubing, and solution. These measures help prevent complications, such as thrombophlebitis and infection.

Perform maintenance according to hospital policy. Typically, I.V. dressings are changed every 48 hours or whenever the dressing becomes wet, soiled, or nonocclusive. I.V. tubing is changed every 48 to 72 hours or according to hospital policy, and I.V. solution is changed every 24 hours or as needed. The site should be assessed every 2 hours if a transparent semipermeable dressing is used, otherwise with every dressing change and should be rotated every 48 to 72 hours.

Sometimes limited venous access prevents frequent site changes; if so, be sure to assess the site frequently.

>> Key nursing diagnoses and patient outcomes

Use these nursing diagnoses as a guide when developing your plan of care for a patient who has a peripheral I.V. line.

Risk for infection related to presence of I.V. line

Based on this nursing diagnosis, you'll establish the following patient outcomes. The patient will:
• have vital signs, temperature, and laboratory values within normal limits.
• have no pathogens appear in cultures.
• show no signs or symptoms of infection at the I.V. insertion site.

Risk for fluid volume deficit related to need for peripheral I.V.

Based on this nursing diagnosis, you'll establish the following patient outcomes. The patient will:
• have normal skin color and temperature.
• exhibit no signs of dehydration.
• maintain urine output of at least (specify) ml/hour.
• have electrolyte values within normal range.
• have intake equal output.

Equipment

For dressing changes: ◆ sterile gloves ◆ povidone-iodine or alcohol sponges ◆ povidone-iodine or other antimicrobial ointment, according to hospital policy ◆ adhesive bandage ◆ sterile $2'' \times 2''$ gauze pad or transparent semipermeable dressing ◆ $1''$ adhesive tape.

Commercial kits containing the equipment for dressing changes are available.

For solution changes: ◆ solution container ◆ alcohol sponge.

For tubing changes: ◆ I.V. administration set ◆ sterile $2'' \times 2''$ gauze pad ◆ adhesive tape for labeling ◆ sterile gloves ◆ optional: hemostats.

For I.V. site change: See "Peripheral I.V. Line Insertion," page 649.

Equipment preparation

• If your hospital keeps I.V. equipment and dressings in a tray or cart, have it nearby because you may have to select a new venipuncture site, depending on the current site's condition.
• If you're changing both the solution and the tubing, attach and prime the I.V. administration set before entering the patient's room.

Patient preparation

• Explain the procedure *to allay the patient's fears and ensure cooperation.*

Implementation

• Wash your hands thoroughly, and wear sterile gloves whenever working near the venipuncture site.

To change the dressing

• Remove the old dressing, open all supply packages, and put on sterile gloves.
• Hold the needle or catheter in place with your nondominant hand to prevent accidental movement or dislodgment, which could puncture the vein and cause infiltration.

• Assess the venipuncture site for signs of infection (redness and pain at the puncture site), infiltration (coolness, blanching, and edema at the site), and thrombophlebitis (redness, firmness, pain along the path of the vein, and edema). If any such signs are present, apply pressure to the area with a sterile $2'' \times 2''$ gauze pad and remove the catheter or needle. Maintain pressure on the area until the bleeding stops, and apply an adhesive bandage. Then, using fresh equipment and solution, start the I.V. in another appropriate site, preferably on the opposite extremity.

• If the venipuncture site is intact, hold the needle or catheter and carefully clean around the puncture site with a povidone-iodine or alcohol sponge. Work in a circular motion outward from the site *to avoid introducing bacteria into the clean area.* Allow the area to dry completely.

• Apply povidone-iodine or other antimicrobial ointment if hospital policy dictates, and cover with an adhesive bandage or sterile $2'' \times 2''$ gauze pad. Retape the site, or apply a transparent semipermeable dressing.

• When using a transparent semipermeable dressing, omit the povidone-iodine ointment and place it over the insertion site to halfway up the catheter or needle hub.

To change the solution
• Wash your hands.
• Inspect the new solution container for cracks, leaks, and other damage. Check the solution for discoloration, turbidity, and particulates. Note the date and time the solution was mixed and its expiration date.

• Clamp the tubing when inverting it *to prevent air from entering the tubing.* Keep the drip chamber half full.
• If you're replacing a bag, remove the seal or tab from the new bag and remove the old bag from the pole. Remove the spike, insert it into the new bag, and adjust the flow rate.
• If you're replacing a bottle, remove the cap and seal from the new bottle and wipe the rubber port with an alcohol sponge. Clamp the line, remove the spike from the old bottle, and insert the spike into the new bottle. Then hang the new bottle and adjust the flow rate.

To change tubing
• Reduce the I.V. flow rate, remove the old spike from the container, and hang it on the I.V. pole. Place the cover of the new spike loosely over the old one.
• Keeping the old spike in an upright position above the patient's heart level, insert the new spike into the I.V. container.
• Prime the system. Hang the new I.V. container and primed set on the pole, and grasp the new adapter in one hand. Then stop the flow rate in the old tubing.
• Put on sterile gloves.
• Place a sterile gauze pad under the needle or catheter hub *to create a sterile field.* Press one of your fingers over the catheter *to prevent bleeding.*
• Gently disconnect the old tubing, being careful not to dislodge or move the I.V. device. (If you have trouble disconnecting the old tubing, use a hemostat to hold the hub securely while twisting the tubing to remove it. Or use one hemostat on the venipuncture device and another on the hard plastic end of the tubing. Then pull the hemo-

BETTER CHARTING

Using a flow sheet to document I.V. therapy

This sample shows the typical features of an I.V. therapy flow sheet.

I.V. therapy Flow Sheet

Diagnosis: ® *mastectomy*
Venipuncture limitations: ① *arm only*
Permanent access: *None*

Date and time	1/14/97 1400	1/15 0800					
Patient visit	2	1					
Site status	1	1					
Procedure	R	C					
Gauge I.V. device	20	∨					
Catheter type	J	J					
Location	LPF	LPF					
Date of insertion	1/14	1/14					
Routine site rotation	—	—					
Phlebitis	O	O					
Infiltration	O	O					
Catheter status	4	—					
No. of failed attempts	O	—					
Lock status	—	—					
Flush	—	—					
Tubing: Macrodrip	∨	∨					
Minidrip							
Valleylah							
Filter							
Extension	∨	∨					
Dressing change	∨	—					
Blood sample drawn	—	—					
Subcutaneous	—	—					
Patient response	1	1					
Patient teaching	1	1					
Nurse's initials	CG	TB					

Initials	Signature	Initials	Signature
CG	*Carol Griff, RN*		
TB	*Theresa Butler, RN*		

(continued)

Using a flow sheet to document I.V. therapy *(continued)*

Date	Time	Patient care notes
11/14/97	1400	IV restarted LPF c̄ 20G jelco, D₅ 1/2 NSS c̄ 40 Meq KCL @ 125 ml/hr.———— Carol Graff, RN
11/15/97	0800	IV D₅ 1/2 NSS c̄ 40 meq KCL infusing @ 125 ml/hr.———— Theresa Butler, RN

KEY

Patient visit
1   Routine rounds
2   Unit request
3   Patient not available for rounds

Site status
1   Within normal limits
2   Dressing intact

Procedure
S   Start
R   Restart
C   Check
D   Discontinue

Catheter type
J   Jelco
H   Huber
I   Intima
TC   Twin catheter
BR   Broviac
GR   Groshong catheter
PICC   Peripherelly inserted central catheter
TL   triple luman cartheter
HI   Hickman catheter
SC   subclavian catheter
SG   Swan-Ganz catheter
TE   Tenckhoff catheter

Location
RH   Right hand
RW   Right wrist
RA   Right arm
RPF   Right posterior forearm
RC   Right anticubital
RU   Right upper arm
LH   Left hand

LW   Left wrist
LA   Left arm
LPF   Left posterior forearm
LC   Left anticubital
LU   Left upper arm
RF   Right foot
LF   Left foot
RJ   Right jugular
LJ   Left jugular
AB   Abdomen
CD   Cutdown
IP   Introducer port
SQP   Subq port

Phlebitis
0   No pain to slight pain at site; no erythemia; no edema; no streak; no palpable cord
1+   Pain at site; erythema or edema; no streak; no palpable cord
2+   Pain at site; erythema or edema streak formation; nonpalpable cord
3+   Pain at site; erythema or edema; streak formation; palpable cord

Infiltration
0+   Slight edema; no infiltration
1+   Slight puffiness at site
2+   Swelling above or below site
3+   Skin cool and pale; large area of swelling above or below site

Catheter status
1   Leaking
2   Occluded
3   Patient removed catheter
4   Other (see patient care notes)

Lock status
1   Leaking
2   Occluded
3   Patient removed catheter
4   Other (see patient care notes)

Flush
1   Heparin
2   Saline

Patient response
1   Patient tolerated
2   Patient agitated or combative
3   Unresponsive
4   Other (see patient care notes)

Patient teaching
1   Patient or family member indicates understanding of procedure
2   Instructed to call nurse for signs of redness, swelling, leaking, pain, or problem
3   Patient unable to comprehend; further documentation in patient care notes

stats in opposite directions. Don't clamp the hemostats shut; *this may crack the tubing adapter or the venipuncture device.)*

• Remove the protective cap from the new tubing, and connect the new adapter to the needle or catheter. Hold the hub securely *to prevent dislodging the needle or catheter tip.*

• Observe for blood backflow into the new tubing to verify that the needle or catheter is still in place. (You may not

be able to do this with small-gauge catheters.)

• Adjust the clamp *to maintain the appropriate flow rate.*

• Retape the needle or catheter hub and I.V. tubing, and recheck the I.V. flow rate.

• Label the new tubing and container with the date and time. Label the solution container with a time strip.

Complications
• Peripheral line complications can result from the needle or catheter (infection, phlebitis, and embolism) or from the solution (circulatory overload, infiltration, sepsis, and allergic reaction).

Nursing considerations
• Check the prescribed I.V. flow rate before each solution change *to prevent errors.*
• If you crack the adapter or hub (or if you accidentally dislodge the needle or catheter from the vein), remove the needle or catheter. Apply pressure and an adhesive bandage *to stop any bleeding.* Perform a venipuncture at another site and restart the I.V.
• Keep in mind that flow rates may change 20% to 40% during an infusion. If you're not using an infusion pump, check the flow rate every hour.

Documentation
• Record the time, date, and rate and type of solution (and any additives) on the I.V. flow sheet and in your notes. (See *Using a flow sheet to document I.V. therapy*, pages 667 and 668.)
• Record dressing or tubing changes and appearance of the site in your notes.

Peripherally inserted central catheter placement and removal

For a patient who needs central venous (CV) therapy for 5 days to several months or who requires repeated venous access, a peripherally inserted central catheter (PICC) line may be the best option. It's used when a patient has suffered trauma or burns resulting in chest injury or when respiratory compromise results from chronic obstructive pulmonary disease, a mediastinal mass, cystic fibrosis, or pneumothorax. A PICC line is used to avoid complications that may occur with a CV line and is more biocompatible.

A PICC is made of soft and flexible silicone or polyurethane. It may be 16G to 23G in diameter and from 16" to 24" (40.5 to 61 cm) in length. A PICC is available in single- and double-lumen versions, with or without guide wires. A guide wire stiffens the catheter, easing its advancement through the vein, but it can damage the vessel if used improperly.

PICC lines are used increasingly for patients receiving home care. The device is easier to insert than other CV devices and provides safe, reliable access for drugs and blood sampling. A single catheter may be used for the entire course of therapy (up to 140 days), with greater convenience and at reduced cost.

Infusions commonly given by PICC include total parenteral nutrition, chemotherapy, antibiotics, narcotics, analgesics, and blood products. PICC therapy works best when introduced early in treatment; it shouldn't be considered a last resort for patients with sclerotic or repeatedly punctured veins.

The patient receiving PICC therapy must have a peripheral vein large enough to accept a 14G or 16G introducer needle and a 3.8G to 4.8G catheter. The doctor or nurse inserts a PICC via the basilic, median antecubital, basilic, cubital, or cephalic vein. It's then threaded to the superior vena cava or subclavian vein or to a noncentral site, such as the axillary vein.

PICCs cost from $11 to $60. Insertion may cost from $50 to $300, compared with approximately $500 for insertion of short-term CV catheters and $1,200 for insertion of long-term CV catheters and implantable CV devices.

If your state's nurse practice act permits, you may insert a PICC if you show sufficient knowledge of vascular access devices. To prove your competence in PICC insertion, it's recommended that you complete an 8-hour workshop and demonstrate three successful catheter insertions. You may have to re-demonstrate competence every year.

>> Key nursing diagnoses and patient outcomes

Use these nursing diagnoses as a guide when developing your plan of care for a patient having a PICC inserted.

Risk for infection related to procedure

Based on this nursing diagnosis, you'll establish the following patient outcomes. The patient will have:
• vital signs, temperature, and laboratory values within normal limits.
• no pathogens that appear in cultures.
• no signs or symptoms of infection at the PICC insertion site.

Risk for fluid volume deficit related to need for PICC line

Based on this nursing diagnosis, you'll establish the following patient outcomes. The patient will:

• have normal skin color and temperature.
• exhibit no signs of dehydration.
• maintain urine output of at least (specify) ml/hour.
• have electrolyte values within normal range.
• have intake equal output.

Equipment

♦ catheter insertion kit ♦ three alcohol swabs ♦ three povidone-iodine swabs ♦ povidone-iodine ointment ♦ 3-ml vial of heparin (100 units/ml) ♦ latex injection port with short extension tubing ♦ sterile and nonsterile measuring tape ♦ vial of normal saline solution ♦ sterile gauze pads ♦ tape ♦ linen-saver pad ♦ sterile drapes ♦ tourniquet ♦ sterile transparent semipermeable dressing ♦ two pairs of sterile gloves ♦ gown ♦ mask ♦ goggles.

Equipment preparation

• Gather the necessary supplies.
• If you're administering PICC therapy in the patient's home, bring everything with you.

Patient preparation

• Describe the procedure to your patient, and answer all questions.

Implementation

PICC placement and removal is explained below.

To insert a PICC

• Select the insertion site, and place the tourniquet on the patient's arm. Assess the antecubital fossa.
• Remove the tourniquet.
• Determine catheter tip placement or the spot at which the catheter tip will

rest after insertion. For subclavian vein placement, use the nonsterile measuring tape to measure the distance from the insertion site to the shoulder and from the shoulder to the sternal notch.

• For placement in the superior vena cava, measure the distance from the insertion site to the shoulder and from the shoulder to the sternal notch. Then add 3″ (7.5 cm).

• Have the patient lie in a supine position with his arm at a 90-degree angle to his body. Place a linen-saver pad under his arm.

• Open the PICC tray and drop the rest of the sterile items onto the sterile field. Put on the sterile gown, mask, goggles, and gloves.

• Using the sterile measuring tape, cut the distal end of the catheter to the premeasured length. Cut the tip straight across *to prevent the catheter from lying flush against the intima of the vein and possibly obstructing infusion flow.*

• Using sterile technique, withdraw 5 ml of the normal saline solution and flush the extension tubing and the latex cap.

• Remove the needle from the syringe. Attach the syringe to the hub of the catheter and flush.

• Prepare the insertion site by rubbing three alcohol swabs over it. Use a circular motion, working outward from the site about 6″ (15 cm). Repeat, using three povidone-iodine swabs. Pat the area dry with a sterile 4″ × 4″ gauze pad. Be sure not to touch the intended insertion site.

• Take your gloves off. Then apply the tourniquet about 4″ (10 cm) above the antecubital fossa.

• Put on a new pair of sterile gloves. Then place a sterile drape under the patient's arm and another on top of his arm. Drop a sterile 4″ × 4″ gauze pad over the tourniquet.

• Stabilize the patient's vein. Insert the catheter introducer at a 10-degree angle, directly into the vein.

• After successful vein entry, you should see a blood return in the flashback chamber. Without changing the needle's position, gently advance the plastic introducer sheath until you're sure the tip is well within the vein.

• Carefully withdraw the needle while holding the introducer still. *To minimize blood loss,* try applying finger pressure on the vein just beyond the distal end of the introducer sheath.

• Using sterile forceps, insert the catheter into the introducer sheath, and advance it into the vein. Remove the tourniquet, using the 4″ × 4″ gauze pad.

• When you have advanced the catheter to the shoulder, ask the patient to turn his head toward the affected arm and place his chin on his chest. This will occlude the jugular vein and ease the catheter's advancement into the subclavian vein.

• Advance the catheter until about 4″ (10 cm) remain. Then pull the introducer sheath out of the vein and away from the introducer site.

• Grasp the blue tabs of the introducer sheath, and flex them toward its distal end to split the sheath.

• Pull the blue tabs apart and away from the catheter until the sheath is completely split. Discard the sheath.

• Continue to advance the catheter until about 2″ (5 cm) remain externally. Flush with normal saline solution.

• With the patient's arm below heart level, remove the syringe. Connect the capped extension set to the hub of the catheter.

• Apply a sterile $2'' \times 2''$ gauze pad directly over the site and a sterile transparent semipermeable dressing over that. Leave this dressing in place for 24 hours.

• After the initial 24 hours, apply a new sterile transparent semipermeable dressing. The gauze pad is no longer necessary. You can place Steri-Strips over the catheter wings. Flush with heparin.

To administer drugs

• As with any CV line, be sure to check for blood return and flush with normal saline solution before administering a drug through a PICC line.

• Clamp the $7''$ (17.5 cm) extension tubing, and connect the empty syringe to the tubing. Release the clamp and aspirate slowly *to verify blood return.* Flush with 3 ml of normal saline solution; then administer the drug.

• After giving the drug, flush again with 3 ml of normal saline solution. (And remember to flush with the same solution between infusions of incompatible drugs or fluids.)

To change the dressing

• Change the dressing every 4 days for an inpatient and every 5 to 7 days for a home care patient. If possible, choose a transparent semipermeable dressing, which has a high moisture-vapor transmission rate. Use aseptic technique.

• Wash your hands and assemble the necessary supplies. Position the patient with his arm extended away from

his body at a 45- to 90-degree angle. Put on a sterile mask.

• Open a package of sterile gloves and use the inside of the package as a sterile field. Then open the transparent semipermeable dressing and drop it onto the field. Remove the old dressing by holding your left thumb on the catheter and stretching the dressing parallel to the skin. Repeat this last step with your right thumb holding the catheter. Free the remaining section of the dressing from the catheter by peeling toward the insertion site from the distal end to the proximal end *to prevent catheter dislodgment.*

• Put on the sterile gloves. Clean the area thoroughly with three alcohol swabs, starting at the insertion site and working outward from the site. Repeat this step three times with povidone-iodine swabs and pat dry.

• Apply the dressing carefully. Secure the tubing to the edge of the dressing over the tape with $\frac{1}{4}''$ of adhesive tape.

To remove a PICC

• You'll remove a PICC when therapy is complete, if the catheter becomes damaged or broken and can't be repaired or, possibly, if the line becomes occluded. Measure the catheter after you remove it *to ensure that the line has been removed intact and thus help prevent formation of emboli in the catheter.*

• Assemble the necessary equipment at the patient's bedside.

• Explain the procedure to the patient.

• Wash your hands.

• Place a linen-saver pad under the patient's arm.

• Remove the tape holding the extension tubing. Open two sterile gauze pads on a clean, flat surface. Put on clean gloves. Stabilize the catheter at the hub with one hand. Without dislodging the catheter, use your other hand to gently remove the dressing by pulling it toward the insertion site.

• Next, gently tug on the PICC. It should come out easily. If you feel resistance, apply tension to the line by taping it down. Then try removing it again in a few minutes.

• After you remove the catheter, apply manual pressure to the site with a sterile gauze pad for 1 minute.

• Cover the site with the povidone-iodine ointment, and tape a new folded gauze pad in place. Dispose of used items properly, and wash your hands.

• Measure and inspect the catheter. If any part has broken off during removal, notify the doctor immediately, and monitor the patient for signs of distress.

Complications

PICC therapy causes fewer and less severe complications than conventionally placed CV lines.

• Phlebitis, perhaps the most common complication, can occur during the first 48 to 72 hours after PICC insertion. It's more common in left-sided insertions and when a large-gauge catheter is used.

• Air embolism, always a potential risk of venipuncture, poses less danger in PICC therapy than with traditional CV lines because the line is inserted below heart level.

• Some patients complain of pain at the catheter insertion site, usually from chemical properties of the infused drug or fluid.

• Catheter tip migration may occur with vigorous flushing. Patients re-

ceiving chemotherapy are most vulnerable to this complication because of frequent nausea and vomiting and subsequent changes in intrathoracic pressure.

• Catheter occlusion is a relatively common complication.

Nursing considerations

• A doctor or nurse probably will place the PICC in the superior vena cava if the patient is to receive therapy in the hospital.

• For a hospital patient receiving intermittent PICC therapy, flush the catheter with 6 ml of normal saline solution and 6 ml of heparin (10 units/ml) after each use. For catheters that aren't being used, a weekly flush of 2 ml (1,000 units/ml) of heparin will maintain patency.

• You can use a anticlotting agent, such as urokinase, to clear a clotted PICC line, but be sure to read the manufacturer's recommendations first.

• Remember to add an extension set to all PICC lines *so you can start and stop an infusion away from the insertion site.* An extension set also make a PICC line easier to use for the patient who self-administers infusions.

• If a patient will be receiving blood or blood products through the PICC line, use at least an 18G catheter.

• Assess the catheter insertion site through the transparent semipermeable dressing every 24 hours. Look at the catheter and check for any bleeding, redness, drainage, and swelling. Ask the patient if he's having any pain associated with therapy. Although bleeding is common for the first 24 hours after insertion, excessive bleeding after that must be evaluated.

Documentation
• Document the entire procedure, including the size and type of catheter, the insertion site, and any problems with catheter placement.

Peritoneal dialysis

Peritoneal dialysis is indicated for patients with chronic renal failure who have cardiovascular instability, vascular access problems that prevent hemodialysis, fluid overload, or electrolyte imbalances. In this procedure, dialysate — the solution instilled into the peritoneal cavity by a catheter — draws waste products, excess fluid, and electrolytes from the blood across the semipermeable peritoneal membrane. (See *Principles of peritoneal dialysis.*)

After a prescribed period, the dialysate is drained from the peritoneal cavity, removing impurities with it. The dialysis procedure is then repeated, using a new dialysate each time, until waste removal is complete and fluid, electrolyte, and acid-base balance has been restored.

The catheter is inserted in the operating room or at the patient's bedside with a nurse assisting. With special preparation, the nurse may perform dialysis, either manually or using an automatic or semiautomatic cycle machine.

≫ Key nursing diagnoses and patient outcomes
Use these nursing diagnoses as a guide when developing your plan of care for a patient who's receiving peritoneal dialysis.

Risk for infection related to invasive procedure
Based on this nursing diagnosis, you'll establish the following patient outcomes. The patient will:
• maintain temperature within normal limits.
• state infection risk factors.
• identify signs and symptoms of infection.

Impaired skin integrity related to presence of peritoneal catheter
Based on this nursing diagnosis, you'll establish the following patient outcomes. The patient will:
• communicate understanding of preventive skin care measures.
• demonstrate preventive skin care. measures.

Equipment
For catheter placement and dialysis:
♦ prescribed dialysate (in 1- or 2-liter bottles or bags, as ordered) ♦ heating pad, warmer, or water bath ♦ at least three face masks ♦ medication, such as heparin, if ordered ♦ dialysis administration set with drainage bag ♦ two pairs of sterile gloves ♦ I.V. pole ♦ fenestrated sterile drape ♦ vial of 1% or 2% lidocaine ♦ povidone-iodine sponges ♦ 3-ml syringe with 25G 1″ needle ♦ scalpel (with #11 blade) ♦ ordered type of multi-eyed, nylon, peritoneal catheter (see *Comparing peritoneal dialysis catheters,* pages 676 and 677) ♦ peritoneal stylet ♦ sutures or hypoallergenic tape ♦ povidone-iodine solution (to prepare abdomen) ♦ precut drain dressings ♦ protective cap for catheter ♦ small, sterile plastic clamp ♦ 4″ × 4″ gauze pads ♦ optional: 10-ml syringe with 22G 1½″ needle, protein

Principles of peritoneal dialysis

Peritoneal dialysis works by a combination of diffusion and osmosis.

Diffusion

In this process, particles move through a semipermeable membrane from an area of high-solute concentration to an area of low-solute concentration.

In peritoneal dialysis, the water-based dialysate being infused contains glucose, sodium chloride, calcium, magnesium, acetate or lactate, and no waste products. Therefore, the waste products and excess electrolytes in the blood cross through the semipermeable peritoneal membrane into the dialysate. Removing the waste-filled dialysate and replacing it with fresh solution keeps the waste concentration low and encourages further diffusion.

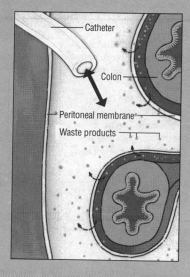

Osmosis

In this process, fluids move through a semipermeable membrane from an area of low-solute concentration to an area of high-solute concentration. In peritoneal dialysis, dextrose is added to the dialysate to give it a higher solute concentration than the blood, creating a high osmotic gradient. Water migrates from the blood through the membrane at the beginning of each infusion, when the osmotic gradient is highest.

---

or potassium supplement, specimen container, label, laboratory request form.

For dressing changes: ♦ one pair of sterile gloves ♦ ten sterile cotton-tipped applicators or sterile $2'' \times 2''$ gauze pads ♦ povidone-iodine ointment ♦ two precut drain dressings ♦ adhesive tape ♦ povidone-iodine solution or normal saline solution ♦ two sterile $4'' \times 4''$ gauze pads.

All equipment must be sterile. Commercially packaged dialysis kits or trays are available.

Equipment preparation

• Bring all equipment to the patient's bedside.

• Make sure the dialysate is at body temperature. This decreases patient discomfort during the procedure and reduces vasoconstriction of the peritoneal capillaries. Dilated capillaries enhance blood flow to the peritoneal membrane surface, increasing waste clearance into the peritoneal cavity. To warm the solution, place the container in a warmer or wrap it in a heating pad set at 98.6° F (37° C) for 30 to 60 min-

Comparing peritoneal dialysis catheters

The first step in any type of peritoneal dialysis is insertion of a catheter to allow instillation of dialyzing solution. The surgeon may insert one of three different catheters described below.

Tenckhoff catheter

To implant a Tenckhoff catheter, the surgeon inserts the first 6¾" (17 cm) of the catheter into the patient's abdomen. The next 2¾" (7-cm) segment, which may have a Dacron cuff at one or both ends, is embedded subcutaneously. Within a few days after insertion, the patient's tissues grow around the cuffs, forming a tight barrier against bacterial infiltration. The remaining 3⅞" (10 cm) of the catheter extends outside of the abdomen and is equipped with a metal adapter at the tip that connects to dialyzer tubing.

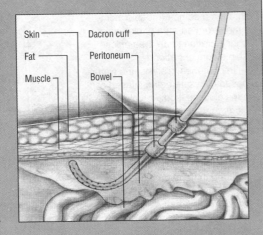

Flanged-collar catheter

To insert this kind of catheter, the surgeon positions its flanged collar just below the dermis so that the device extends through the abdominal wall. He keeps the distal end of the cuff from extending into the peritoneum, where it could cause adhesions.

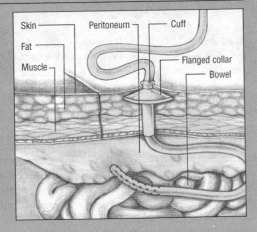

Comparing peritoneal dialysis catheters *(continued)*

Column-disk peritoneal catheter
To insert a column-disk peritoneal catheter (CDPC), the surgeon rolls up the flexible disk section of the implant, inserts it into the peritoneal cavity, and retracts it against the abdominal wall. The implant's first cuff rests just outside the peritoneal membrane, while its second cuff rests just beneath the skin. Because the CDPC doesn't float freely in the peritoneal cavity, it prevents flowing dialyzing solution from being directed at the sensitive organs — which increases patient comfort during dialysis.

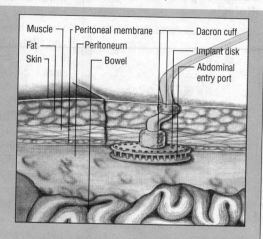

Muscle — Peritoneal membrane — Dacron cuff
Fat — Peritoneum — Implant disk
Skin — Bowel — Abdominal entry port

---

utes. You can also place the container in a water bath at the same temperature for 30 to 60 minutes.

Implementation
• Explain the procedure to the patient. Assess and record vital signs, weight, and abdominal girth *to establish baseline levels.*
• Review recent laboratory values (blood urea nitrogen; serum creatinine, sodium, and potassium; and complete blood count).
• Identify the patient's hepatitis B virus and human immunodeficiency virus status, if known.

For catheter placement and dialysis
• Have the patient try to urinate. *This reduces the risk of bladder perforation during insertion of the peritoneal catheter and also reduces patient discomfort. If he can't urinate, and if you suspect that his bladder isn't empty, obtain an order for straight catheterization to empty his bladder.*
• Place the patient in the supine position, and have him put on one of the sterile face masks.
• Wash your hands.
• Inspect the warmed dialysate, which should appear clear and colorless.
• Put on a sterile face mask. Prepare to add any prescribed medication to the dialysate, using strict aseptic technique *to avoid contaminating the solution.* Medications should be added immediately before the solution will be hung and used. Disinfect multiple-dose vials by soaking them in povidone-iodine solution for 5 minutes. Commonly, heparin is added to

Setup for peritoneal dialysis

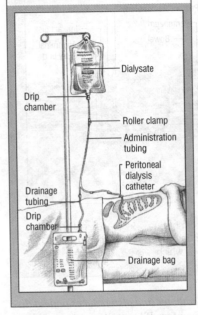

povidone-iodine solution and drapes it with a sterile drape.

• Wipe the stopper of the lidocaine vial with povidone-iodine sponges and allow it to dry. Invert the vial and hand it to the doctor so he can withdraw the lidocaine, using the 3-ml syringe with the 25G 1″ needle.

• The doctor anesthetizes a small area of the patient's abdomen below the umbilicus. He then makes a small incision with the scalpel, inserts the catheter into the peritoneal cavity — using the stylet as a guide — and sutures or tapes the catheter in place.

• Connect the catheter to the administration set, using strict aseptic technique, *to prevent contamination of the catheter and the solution, which could cause peritonitis.*

• Open the drain dressing and the 4″ × 4″ gauze pad packages. Put on the other pair of sterile gloves. Apply the precut drain dressings around the catheter. Cover them with the gauze pads and tape them securely.

• Unclamp the lines to the patient. Rapidly instill 500 ml of dialysate into the peritoneal cavity *to test the catheter's patency.*

• Clamp the lines to the patient. Immediately unclamp the lines to the drainage bag *to allow fluid to drain into the bag.* Outflow should be brisk.

• Having established the catheter's patency, clamp the lines to the drainage bag, and unclamp the lines to the patient *to infuse the prescribed volume of solution over a period of 5 to 10 minutes.* As soon as the dialysate container empties, clamp the lines to the patient immediately *to prevent air from entering the tubing.*

• Allow the solution to dwell in the peritoneal cavity for the prescribed

the dialysate *to prevent accumulation of fibrin in the catheter.*

• Prepare the dialysis administration set. (See *Setup for peritoneal dialysis.*)

• Close the clamps on all lines. Place the drainage bag below the patient *to facilitate gravity drainage,* and connect the drainage line to it. Connect the dialysate infusion lines to the bottles or bags of dialysate. Hang the bottles or bags on the I.V. pole at the patient's bedside. *To prime the tubing,* open the infusion lines and allow the solution to flow until all lines are primed. Then close all clamps.

• At this point, the doctor puts on a mask and a pair of sterile gloves. He cleans the patient's abdomen with

time (10 minutes to 4 hours). *This lets excess fluid, electrolytes, and accumulated wastes move from the blood through the peritoneal membrane and into the dialysate.*

• Warm the solution for the next infusion.

• At the end of the prescribed dwell time, unclamp the line to the drainage bag, and allow the solution to drain from the peritoneal cavity into the drainage bag.

• Repeat the infusion-dwell-drain cycle immediately after outflow until the prescribed number of fluid exchanges has been completed.

• If the doctor or hospital policy requires a dialysate specimen, you'll usually collect one after every 10 infusion-dwell-drain cycles (*always* during the drain phase), after every 24-hour period, or as ordered. To do this, attach the 10-ml syringe to the 22G 1½" needle and insert it into the injection port on the drainage line, using strict aseptic technique, and aspirate the drainage sample. Transfer the sample to the specimen container, label it appropriately, and send it to the laboratory with a request form.

• After completing the prescribed number of exchanges, clamp the catheter, and put on sterile gloves. Disconnect the administration set from the peritoneal catheter. Place the sterile protective cap over the catheter's distal end. (Or the doctor may remove the catheter and place a Deane's prosthesis in its place to maintain the patency of the tract and to simplify reinsertion of the catheter for the next dialysis treatment.)

• Dispose of all used equipment appropriately.

For dressing changes

• Explain the procedure to the patient and wash your hands.

• If necessary, carefully remove the old dressings *to avoid putting tension on the catheter and accidentally dislodging it and to avoid introducing bacteria into the tract through movement of the catheter.*

• Put on the sterile gloves.

• Saturate the sterile applicators or the 2" × 2" gauze pads with povidone-iodine, and clean the skin around the catheter, moving in concentric circles from the catheter site outward. Remove any crusted material carefully.

• Inspect the catheter site for drainage and the tissue around the site for redness and swelling.

• Apply povidone-iodine ointment to the catheter site with a sterile gauze pad.

• Place two precut drain dressings around the catheter site. Tape the 4"× 4" gauze pads over them to secure the dressing.

Complications

• Peritonitis, the most common complication, usually follows contamination of the dialysate, but it may develop if solution leaks from the catheter exit site and flows back into the catheter tract.

• Protein depletion may result from the diffusion of protein in the blood into the dialysate solution through the peritoneal membrane. As much as ½ oz (15 g) of protein may be lost daily, more in patients with peritonitis.

• Respiratory distress may result when dialysate in the peritoneal cavity increases pressure on the diaphragm, which decreases lung expansion.

• Constipation is a major cause of inflow-outflow problems; therefore, *to ensure regular bowel movements,* give a laxative or stool softener, as needed.

• Excessive fluid loss from the use of 4.25% solution may cause hypovolemia, hypotension, and shock. Excessive fluid retention may lead to blood volume expansion, hypertension, peripheral edema, and even pulmonary edema and congestive heart failure.

• Other possible complications include electrolyte imbalance and hyperglycemia, which can be identified by frequent blood tests.

Nursing considerations

• During and after dialysis, monitor the patient and his response to treatment.

• Peritoneal dialysis is usually contraindicated in patients who have had extensive abdominal or bowel surgery or extensive abdominal trauma.

• Monitor the patient's vital signs every 10 to 15 minutes for the first 1 to 2 hours of exchanges, then every 2 to 4 hours, or more frequently if necessary. Notify the doctor of any abrupt changes in the patient's condition.

• *To reduce the risk of peritonitis,* use strict aseptic technique during catheter insertion, dialysis, and dressing changes. Masks should be worn by all personnel in the room whenever the dialysis system is opened or entered. Change the dressing at least every 24 hours or whenever it becomes wet or soiled. *Frequent dressing changes will also help prevent skin excoriation from any leakage.*

• *To prevent respiratory distress,* position the patient for maximal lung expansion. Promote lung expansion through turning and deep-breathing exercises.

Nursing alert: If the patient suffers severe respiratory distress during the dwell phase of dialysis, drain the peritoneal cavity and notify the doctor. Monitor any patient on peritoneal dialysis who's being weaned from a ventilator.

• *To prevent protein depletion,* the doctor may order a high-protein diet or a protein supplement. He will also monitor serum albumin levels.

• Dialysate is available in three concentrations — 4.25% dextrose, 2.5% dextrose, and 1.5% dextrose. The 4.25% solution usually removes the largest amount of fluid from the blood because its glucose concentration is highest. If your patient receives this concentrated solution, monitor him carefully *to prevent excessive fluid loss.* Also, some of the glucose in the 4.25% solution may enter the patient's bloodstream, causing hyperglycemia severe enough to require an insulin injection or an insulin addition to the dialysate.

• Patients with low serum potassium levels may require the addition of potassium to the dialysate solution *to prevent further losses.*

• Monitor fluid volume balance, blood pressure, and pulse *to help prevent fluid imbalance.* Assess fluid balance at the end of each infusion-dwell-drain cycle. Fluid balance is positive if less than the amount infused was recovered; it's negative if more than the amount infused was recovered. Notify the doctor if the patient retains 500 ml or more of fluid for three consecutive cycles or if he loses at least 1 liter of fluid for three consecutive cycles.

• Weigh the patient daily *to help you determine how much fluid is being removed during dialysis treatment.* Note the time and any variations in the weighing technique next to his weight on his chart.

• If inflow and outflow are slow or absent, check the tubing for kinks. You can also try raising the I.V. pole or repositioning the patient *to increase the inflow rate.* Repositioning the patient or applying manual pressure to the lateral aspects of the patient's abdomen may also help increase drainage. If these maneuvers fail, notify the doctor. *Improper positioning of the catheter or an accumulation of fibrin may obstruct the catheter.*

• Always examine outflow fluid (effluent) for color and clarity. Normally, it's clear or pale yellow, but pink-tinged effluent may appear during the first three or four cycles. If the effluent remains pink-tinged, or if it's grossly bloody, suspect bleeding into the peritoneal cavity and notify the doctor. Also notify the doctor if the outflow contains feces, which suggests bowel perforation, or if it's cloudy, which suggests peritonitis. Obtain a sample for culture and Gram stain. Send the fluid in a labeled specimen container to the laboratory with a laboratory request form.

• Patient discomfort at the start of the procedure is normal. If the patient experiences pain during the procedure, determine when it occurs, its quality and duration, and whether it radiates to other body parts. Then notify the doctor. Pain during infusion usually results from a dialysate that's too cool or acidic. Pain may also result from rapid inflow; slowing the inflow rate may reduce the pain. Severe, diffuse pain with rebound tenderness and cloudy effluent may indicate peritoneal infection. Pain that radiates to the shoulder often results from air accumulation under the diaphragm. Severe, persistent perineal or rectal pain can result from improper catheter placement.

• The patient undergoing peritoneal dialysis will require a great deal of assistance in his daily care. *To minimize his discomfort,* perform daily care during a drain phase in the cycle, when the patient's abdomen is less distended.

Documentation

• Record the amount of dialysate infused and drained, any medications added to the solution, and the color and character of effluent.

• Record the patient's daily weight and fluid balance.

• Use a peritoneal dialysis flowchart to compute total fluid balance after each exchange.

• Note the patient's vital signs and tolerance of the treatment and other pertinent observations.

Peritoneal dialysis, continuous ambulatory

In continuous ambulatory peritoneal dialysis (CAPD), a permanent peritoneal catheter (such as a Tenckhoff catheter) is implanted under local anesthetic to constantly circulate dialysate in the peritoneal cavity. The catheter is sutured in place, and its distal portion tunneled subcutaneously to the skin surface. There it serves as a port for the dialysate, which flows in

Three major steps of continuous ambulatory peritoneal dialysis

A bag of dialysate is attached to the tube entering the patient's abdominal area so the fluid flows into the peritoneal cavity.

While the dialysate remains in the peritoneal cavity, the patient can roll up the bag, place it under his shirt, and go about his normal activities.

Unrolling the bag and suspending it below the pelvis allows the dialysate to drain from the peritoneal cavity back into the bag.

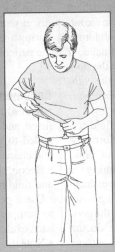
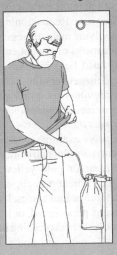

and out of the peritoneal cavity by gravity. (See *Three major steps of continuous ambulatory peritoneal dialysis*.)

CAPD, used most commonly for patients with end-stage renal disease, can be a welcome alternative to hemodialysis because it gives the patient more independence and requires less travel for treatments. It also provides more stable fluid and electrolyte levels than conventional hemodialysis.

Patients or family members can usually learn to perform CAPD after only 2 weeks of training. And because the patient can resume normal daily activities between solution changes, CAPD helps promote independence and a return to a near-normal lifestyle. It also costs less than hemodialysis. (See *Continuous-cycle peritoneal dialysis*.)

Conditions that may prohibit CAPD include recent abdominal surgery, abdominal adhesions, an infected abdominal wall, diaphragmatic tears, ileus, and respiratory insufficiency.

≫ Key nursing diagnoses and patient outcomes

Use these nursing diagnoses as a guide when developing your plan of care for a patient having CAPD.

Risk for infection related to invasive procedure

Based on this nursing diagnosis, you'll establish the following patient outcomes. The patient will:
• have vital signs, temperature, and laboratory values within normal limits.
• have no pathogens appear in cultures.
• show no signs or symptoms of infection at the I.V. insertion site.

Risk for fluid volume deficit related to CAPD

Based on this nursing diagnosis, you'll establish the following patient outcomes. The patient will:
• have normal skin color and temperature.
• exhibit no signs of dehydration.
• maintain urine output of at least (specify) ml/hour.
• have electrolyte values remain within normal range.
• have intake equal output.

Equipment

To infuse dialysate: ◆ prescribed amount of dialysate (usually in 2-liter bags) ◆ basin of hot water or commercial warmer ◆ three face masks ◆ 42″ (106.7-cm) connective tubing with drain clamp ◆ six to eight packages of sterile 4″ × 4″ gauze pads ◆ medication, if ordered ◆ povidone-iodine sponges ◆ hypoallergenic tape ◆ povidone-iodine solution ◆ plastic snap-top container ◆ sterile basin

Continuous-cycle peritoneal dialysis

Continuous ambulatory peritoneal dialysis is easier for the patient who uses an automated continuous cycler system. Once set up, the system runs the dialysis treatment automatically until all dialysate is infused. The system remains closed throughout the treatment, which cuts the risk of contamination. Continuous-cycle peritoneal dialysis (CCPD) can be performed while the patient is awake or asleep. The system's alarms warn about general system, dialysate, and patient problems.

The cycler can be set to an intermittent or continuous dialysate schedule at home or in the hospital. The patient typically initiates CCPD at bedtime and undergoes three to seven exchanges, depending on his prescription. Upon awakening, the patient infuses the prescribed dialysis volume, disconnects himself from the unit, and carries the dialysate in his peritoneal cavity during the day.

The continuous cycler follows the same aseptic care and maintenance procedures as the manual method.

◆ container of alcohol ◆ sterile gloves ◆ belt or fabric pouch ◆ two sterile waterproof paper drapes (one fenestrated) ◆ optional: syringes, labeled specimen container, sterile cotton-tipped applicators.

To discontinue dialysis temporarily: ◆ three sterile waterproof paper barriers (two fenestrated) ◆ 4″ × 4″ gauze pads (for cleaning and dressing the catheter) ◆ two face masks ◆ sterile basin ◆ hypoallergenic tape ◆ povidone-iodine solution ◆ sterile gloves ◆ sterile rubber catheter cap ◆ alcohol sponges.

All equipment for infusing the dialysate and discontinuing the procedure must be sterile. Commercially prepared sterile CAPD kits are available.

Equipment preparation
• Check the concentration of the dialysate against the doctor's order. Also check the expiration date and appearance of the solution, which should be clear, not cloudy.
• Warm the solution to body temperature with a heating pad or a commercial warmer if one is available. Don't warm the solution in a microwave oven *because the temperature is unpredictable.*
• *To minimize the risk of contaminating the bag's port,* leave the dialysate container's wrapper in place. *This also keeps the bag dry, which makes examining it for leakage easier after you remove the wrapper.*
• Wash your hands and put on a surgical mask. Remove the dialysate container from the warming setup, and remove its protective wrapper. Squeeze the bag firmly to check for leaks.
• If ordered, use a syringe to add any prescribed medication to the dialysate, using sterile technique to avoid contamination. (The ideal approach is to add medication under a laminar flow hood.) Disinfect multiple-dose vials in a 5-minute povidone-iodine soak. Insert the connective tubing into the dialysate container. Open the drain clamp to prime the tube. Then close the clamp.

• Place a povidone-iodine sponge on the dialysate container's port.
• Cover the port with a dry gauze pad, and secure the pad with tape.
• Remove and discard the surgical mask.
• Tear the tape *so it will be ready to secure the new dressing.*

Commercial devices with povidone-iodine sponges are available for covering the dialysate container and tubing connection.

Patient preparation
• Weigh the patient *to determine a baseline.* Thereafter, weigh the patient at the same time every day *to monitor fluid balance.*

Implementation
The procedure for administering CAPD is described step-by-step below.

To infuse dialysate
• Assemble all equipment at the patient's bedside, and explain the procedure to him. Prepare the sterile field by placing a waterproof, sterile paper drape on a dry surface near the patient. Take care to maintain the drape's sterility.
• Fill the snap-top container with povidone-iodine solution, and place it on the sterile field. Place the basin on the sterile field. Then place four pairs of sterile gauze pads in the sterile basin, and saturate them with the povidone-iodine solution. Drop the remaining gauze pads on the sterile field. Loosen the cap on the alcohol container, and place it next to the sterile field.
• Put on a clean surgical mask and provide one for the patient.

• Carefully remove the dressing covering the peritoneal catheter and discard it. Be careful not to touch the catheter or skin. Check skin integrity at the catheter site, and look for signs of infection, such as purulent drainage. If drainage is present, obtain a specimen with a sterile applicator, put it in a labeled specimen container, and notify the doctor.

• Put on the sterile gloves and palpate the insertion site and subcutaneous tunnel route for tenderness or pain. If these symptoms occur, notify the doctor.

Nursing alert: If the patient has drainage, tenderness, or pain, don't proceed with the infusion without specific orders.

• Wrap one gauze pad saturated with povidone-iodine solution around the distal end of the catheter, and leave it in place for 5 minutes. Clean the catheter and insertion site with the rest of the gauze pads, moving in concentric circles away from the insertion site. Use straight strokes to clean the catheter, beginning at the insertion site and moving outward. Use a clean area of the pad for each stroke. Loosen the catheter cap one notch and clean the exposed area. Place each used pad at the base of the catheter *to help support it.* After using the third pair of pads, place the fenestrated paper drape around the base of the catheter. Continue cleaning the catheter for another minute with one of the remaining pads soaked with povidone-iodine.

• Next, remove the povidone-iodine sponge on the catheter cap, remove the cap, and use the remaining povidone-iodine sponge to clean the end of the catheter hub. Attach the connective tubing from the dialysate container to the catheter. Be sure to secure the luer-lock connector tightly.

• Open the drain clamp on the dialysate container *to allow solution to enter the peritoneal cavity by gravity* over 5 to 10 minutes. Leave a small amount of fluid in the bag *to make folding it easier.* Close the drain clamp.

• Fold the bag and secure it with a belt, or tuck it into the patient's clothing or a small fabric pouch.

• After the prescribed dwell time (usually 4 to 6 hours), unfold the bag, open the clamp, and allow peritoneal fluid to drain back into the bag by gravity.

• When drainage is complete, attach a new bag of dialysate and repeat the infusion.

• Discard used supplies appropriately.

To discontinue dialysis temporarily

• Wash your hands, put on a surgical mask, and provide one for the patient.

• Explain the procedure to the patient.

• Using sterile gloves, remove and discard the dressing over the peritoneal catheter.

• Set up a sterile field next to the patient by covering a clean, dry surface with a waterproof drape. Be sure to maintain the drape's sterility. Place all equipment on the sterile field, and place the $4'' \times 4''$ gauze pads in the basin. Saturate them with the povidone-iodine solution. Open the $4'' \times 4''$ gauze pads to be used as the dressing, and drop them onto the sterile field. Tear pieces of tape as needed.

• Tape the dialysate tubing to the side rail of the bed *to keep the catheter and tubing off the patient's abdomen.*

• Change to another pair of sterile gloves. Then place one of the fenes-

BETTER CHARTING

Documenting peritoneal dialysis

During and after dialysis, monitor and document the patient's response to treatment. Document any abrupt changes in the patient's condition, notify the doctor, and document doing so. Also record each time that you notify the doctor of an abnormality.

Document the amount of dialysate infused and drained and any medications added. Be sure to complete a peritoneal dialysis flowchart every 24 hours.

Note the condition of the patient's skin at the dialysis catheter site, the patient's reports of unusual discomfort or pain, and your interventions.

1/15/97	0700	Pt. receiving exchanges q 2 hr of 1,500 cc 4.25 dialysate with 500 units heparin and 2 mEq KCL. Dialysate infused over 15 min. Dwell time 75 min. Drain time 30 min. Drainage clear, pale-yellow fluid. (See flow sheet for fluid balance.) VSS. Pt. tolerates procedure. No cramping or discomfort. Skin warm, dry at RLQ catheter site and no redness. Dry split 4" x 4" dressing applied β site cleaned per protocol. ———— Pamela Worth, RN

trated drapes around the base of the catheter.

• Use a pair of povidone-iodine sponges to clean about 6" (15.2 cm) of the dialysis tubing. Clean for 1 minute, moving in one direction only, away from the catheter. Then clean the catheter, moving from the insertion site to the junction of the catheter and dialysis tubing. Place used sponges at the base of the catheter *to prop it up.* Using two more pairs of sponges, clean the junction for a total of 3 minutes.

• Place the second fenestrated paper drape over the first at the base of the catheter. Then, with the fourth pair of sponges, clean the junction of the catheter and 6" of the dialysate tubing for another minute.

• Disconnect the dialysate tubing from the catheter. Pick up the catheter cap and fasten it to the catheter, making sure it fits securely over both notches of the hard plastic catheter tip.

• Clean the insertion site and a 2" (5-cm) radius around it with povidone-iodine sponges, working from the insertion site outward. Let the skin air-dry before applying the dressing.

• Discard used supplies appropriately.

Complications

• Peritonitis is the most frequent complication of CAPD. Although treatable, it can permanently scar the peritoneal membrane, decreasing its permeability and reducing the efficiency of dialysis. Untreated peritonitis can cause septicemia and death.

• Excessive fluid loss may result from a concentrated (4.25%) dialysate solution, improper or inaccurate monitoring of inflow and outflow, or inadequate oral fluid intake.

• Excessive fluid retention may result from improper or inaccurate monitoring of inflow and outflow, or excessive salt or oral fluid intake.

Nursing considerations
• If inflow and outflow are slow or absent, check the tubing for kinks. You can also try raising the solution or repositioning the patient *to increase the inflow rate.* Repositioning the patient or applying manual pressure to the lateral aspects of the patient's abdomen may also help increase drainage.

Home care
• Teach the patient and family how to use sterile technique throughout the procedure, especially for cleaning and dressing changes, *to prevent complications such as peritonitis.*
• Teach them the signs and symptoms of peritonitis — cloudy fluid, fever, abdominal pain, and tenderness — and stress the importance of notifying the doctor immediately if such symptoms arise.
• Tell them to call the doctor if redness and drainage occur; *these are also signs of infection.*
• Instruct the patient to record his weight and blood pressure daily and to check regularly for swelling of the extremities.
• Teach him to keep an accurate record of intake and output.

Documentation
• Record the type and amount of fluid instilled and returned for each exchange, the time and duration of the exchange, and any medications added to the dialysate.
• Note the color and clarity of the returned exchange fluid, and check it for mucus, pus, and blood.
• Note any discrepancy in the balance of fluid intake and output, as well as any signs or symptoms of fluid imbalance, such as weight changes, decreased breath sounds, ascites, peripheral edema, and changes in skin turgor. Record the patient's weight, blood pressure, and pulse rate after his last fluid exchange for the day. (See *Documenting peritoneal dialysis.*)

Peritoneal lavage

Used as a diagnostic procedure in a patient with blunt abdominal trauma, peritoneal lavage helps detect bleeding in the peritoneal cavity. The test may proceed through several steps. Initially, the doctor inserts a catheter through the abdominal wall into the peritoneal cavity and aspirates the peritoneal fluid with a syringe. If he can't see blood in the aspirated fluid, he then infuses a balanced saline solution and siphons the fluid from the cavity. He inspects the siphoned fluid for blood and also sends fluid samples to the laboratory for microscopic examination.

The medical team maintains strict aseptic technique throughout this procedure to avoid introducing microorganisms into the peritoneum and causing peritonitis. (See *Tapping the peritoneal cavity,* page 688.)

Peritoneal lavage is contraindicated in a patient who has had several abdominal operations (adhesions), who has an abdominal wall hematoma, who is unstable and needs immediate surgery, or who can't be catheterized before the procedure. The procedure requires great caution and a different technique if the patient is pregnant.

Tapping the peritoneal cavity

After administering a local anesthetic to numb the area near the patient's navel, the surgeon will make a small incision (about ¾″ [2 cm]) through the skin and subcutaneous tissues of the abdominal wall. He will retract the tissue, ligate severed blood vessels, and use $4'' \times 4''$ gauze pads to absorb and keep incisional blood from entering the wound and producing a false-positive test result. Next, he will direct the trocar through the incision into the pelvic midline until the instrument enters the peritoneum. Then, he will advance the peritoneal catheter (via the trocar) 6″ to 8″ (15.2 to 20.3 cm) into the pelvis.

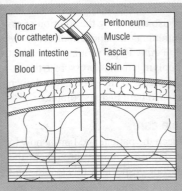

Using a syringe attached to the catheter, he will aspirate fluid from the peritoneal cavity and look for blood or other abnormal findings.

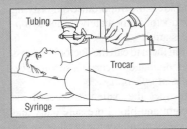

›› Key nursing diagnoses and patient outcomes

Use these nursing diagnoses as a guide when developing your plan of care for a patient who needs peritoneal lavage.

Risk for injury related to invasive procedure

Based on this nursing diagnosis, you'll establish the following patient outcomes. The patient will:
• maintain effective breathing patterns.
• maintain adequate cardiac output.
• show no signs of bleeding from incision site.

Risk for infection related to invasive procedure

Based on this nursing diagnosis, you'll establish the following patient outcomes. The patient will:
• maintain a normal body temperature.
• remain free from signs and symptoms of infection.

Anxiety related to invasive procedure and results of procedure

Based on this nursing diagnosis, you'll establish the following patient outcomes. The patient will:

• communicate any feelings of anxiety.
• verbalize understanding of need for procedure.

Equipment

♦ indwelling catheter, catheter insertion kit, and drainage bag ♦ nasogastric (NG) tube ♦ gastric suction machine ♦ shaving kit ♦ I.V. pole ♦ macrodrip I.V. tubing ♦ I.V. solutions (1 liter of warmed, balanced saline solution, usually lactated Ringer's solution or normal saline solution) ♦ peritoneal dialysis tray ♦ sterile gloves ♦ gown ♦ goggles ♦ antiseptic solution (such as povidone-iodine) ♦ 3-ml syringe with 25G 1″ needle ♦ bottle of 1% lidocaine with epinephrine ♦ 8″ (20.3 cm) #14 intracatheter extension tubing and a small sterile hemostat (to clamp tubing) ♦ 30-ml syringe ♦ one 20G 1½″ needle ♦ sterile towels ♦ three containers for specimen collection, including one sterile tube for a culture and sensitivity specimen ♦ labels ♦ antiseptic ointment ♦ 4″ × 4″ gauze pads ♦ alcohol sponges ♦ 1″ hypoallergenic tape ♦ 00 and 000 sutures.

If you're using a commercially prepared peritoneal dialysis kit (containing a #15 peritoneal dialysis catheter, trocar, and extension tubing with roller clamp), make sure the macrodrip I.V. tubing doesn't have a reverse flow (or backcheck) valve that prevents infused fluid from draining out of the peritoneal cavity.

Patient preparation

• Provide privacy and wash your hands. Reinforce the doctor's explanation of the procedure.

• Put on the gown and goggles.
• Before the procedure, advise the patient to expect a sensation of abdominal fullness.
• Tell the patient he may experience a chill if the lavage solution isn't warmed or doesn't reach his body temperature.

Implementation

• Catheterize the patient with the indwelling urinary catheter, and connect this catheter to the drainage bag.
• Insert the NG tube. Attach this tube to the gastric suction machine (set for low intermittent suction) to drain the patient's stomach contents. *Decompressing the stomach prevents vomiting and subsequent aspiration and minimizes the possibility of bowel perforation during trocar or catheter insertion.*
• Using the shaving kit, clip or shave the hair, as ordered, from the area between the patient's umbilicus and symphysis pubis.
• Set up the I.V. pole. Attach the macrodrip tubing to the lavage solution container, and clear air from the tubing *to avoid introducing air into the peritoneal cavity during lavage.*
• Using aseptic technique, open the peritoneal dialysis tray.
• The doctor will wipe the patient's abdomen from the costal margin to the pubic area and from flank to flank with the antiseptic solution. He will drape the area with sterile towels from the dialysis tray *to create a sterile field.*
• Using aseptic technique, hand the doctor the 3-ml syringe and the 25G 1″ needle. If the peritoneal dialysis tray doesn't contain a sterile ampule of anesthetic, wipe the top of a multi-

Interpreting peritoneal lavage results

With abnormal test findings in peritoneal lavage, your patient may need laparotomy and further treatment. The most common abnormal findings include the following:
• unclotted blood, bile, or intestinal contents in aspirated peritoneal fluid (20 ml in an adult or 10 ml in a child)
• bloody or pinkish red fluid returned from lavage — dark enough to obscure reading newsprint through it (if you can read newsprint through the fluid, test results are considered negative, although the doctor may order more tests)
• green, cloudy, turbid, or milky peritoneal fluid return (normal peritoneal fluid appears clear to pale yellow)
• red blood cell count exceeding 100,000/mm³
• white blood cell count exceeding 500/mm³
• bacteria in fluid (identified by culture and sensitivity testing or Gram stain).

If the patient's condition is stable, borderline positive results may suggest the need for additional tests, such as echography and arteriography.

If test results are questionable or inconclusive, the doctor may leave the catheter in place to repeat the procedure.

dose vial of 1% lidocaine with epinephrine with an alcohol sponge, and invert the vial at a 45-degree angle. *This allows the doctor to insert the needle and withdraw the anesthetic without touching the nonsterile vial.*

• The doctor injects the anesthetic directly below the umbilicus (or at an adjacent site if the patient has a surgical scar). Once the area is numb, he makes an incision, inserts the catheter or trocar, withdraws fluid, and checks the findings. With positive findings, the procedure ends, and you'll prepare the patient for laparotomy and further measures. Even if retrieved fluid looks normal, lavage will continue. (See *Interpreting peritoneal lavage results.*)
• Wearing gloves, connect the catheter extension tubing to the I.V. tubing, if ordered, and instill 500 to 1,000 ml (10 ml/kg body weight) of the warmed I.V. solution into the peritoneal cavity over 5 to 10 minutes. Then clamp the tubing with the hemostat.
• Unless contraindicated by the patient's injuries (such as a spinal cord injury, fractured ribs, or unstable pelvic fracture), gently tilt the patient from side to side *to distribute the fluid throughout the peritoneal cavity.* (If the patient's condition contraindicates tilting, the doctor may gently palpate the sides of the abdomen *to distribute the fluid.*)
• After 5 to 10 minutes, place the I.V. container below the level of the patient's body, and open the clamp on the I.V. tubing. *Lowering the container helps excess fluid to drain.* Gently drain as much of the fluid as possible from the peritoneal cavity to the container. Be careful not to disconnect the tubing from the catheter. The peritoneal cavity may take 20 to 30 minutes to drain completely.
• Although you don't need to vent a plastic bag container, be sure to vent glass I.V. containers with a needle *to promote flow.*

• To obtain a fluid specimen, put on gloves and use a 30-ml syringe and 20G 1½″ needle to withdraw between 25 and 30 ml of fluid from a port in the I.V. tubing. Clean the top of each specimen container with an alcohol sponge. Deposit fluid specimens in the containers, and send the specimens to the laboratory for culture and sensitivity analysis, Gram stain, red and white blood cell counts, amylase and bile level determinations, and spun-down sediment evaluation.

Note: If you didn't obtain the culture and sensitivity specimen first, change the needle before drawing this fluid sample *to avoid contaminating the specimen.*

• Label the specimens, and send them to the laboratory immediately. With positive test results, the doctor will usually perform a laparotomy. If test results are normal, the doctor will close the incision.

• Wearing sterile gloves, apply antiseptic ointment to the site, and dress the incision with a 4″ × 4″ gauze pad secured with 1″ of hypoallergenic tape.

• Discard disposable equipment. Return reusable equipment to the appropriate department for cleaning and sterilization

Complications

• Bleeding from lacerated blood vessels may occur at the incision site or intra-abdominally.

• A visceral perforation causes peritonitis and necessitates laparotomy for repair.

• If the patient has respiratory distress, infusion of a balanced saline solution may cause additional stress and trigger respiratory arrest.

• The bladder may be lacerated or punctured if it isn't emptied completely before peritoneal lavage. Infection may develop at the incision site without strict aseptic technique

Nursing considerations

• After the lavage, monitor the patient's vital signs frequently. Report symptoms of shock, such as tachycardia, decreased blood pressure, diaphoresis, dyspnea or shortness of breath, and vertigo immediately. Assess the incision site frequently for bleeding.

• If the doctor orders abdominal X-rays, they will probably precede peritoneal lavage. *X-ray films made after lavage may be unreliable because of air introduced into the peritoneal cavity.*

Documentation

• Record the type and size of the peritoneal dialysis catheter used, the type and amount of solution instilled and withdrawn from the peritoneal cavity, and the amount and color of fluid returned.

• Document whether the fluid flowed freely into and out of the abdomen.

• Note which specimens were obtained and sent to the laboratory.

• Note any complications encountered and the nursing actions taken to handle them.

Persantine thallium imaging

This imaging test is an alternative method of assessing coronary vessel function for patients who can't tolerate exercise or stress electrocardiography. Persantine (dipyridamole) infusion simulates the effects of exercise by increasing blood flow to the collateral circulation and away from the coronary arteries, thereby inducing ischemia. Then thallium is infused so that the cardiac vessels' response can be evaluated. The heart is scanned immediately after the thallium infusion and again 2 to 4 hours later. Diseased vessels can't deliver thallium to the heart, and thallium lingers in diseased areas of the myocardium.

Normally, Persantine thallium imaging reveals characteristic distribution of the isotope throughout the left ventricle and no visible defects.

The presence of ST-segment depression, angina, and arrhythmias strongly suggests coronary artery disease. Persistent ST-segment depression generally indicates myocardial infarction. In contrast, transient ST-segment depression indicates ischemia from coronary artery disease.

Cold spots are usually due to coronary artery disease, but may result from sarcoidosis, myocardial fibrosis, cardiac contusion, attenuation due to soft tissue (for example, breast and diaphragm) apical cleft, and coronary spasm. Absence of cold spots in the presence of coronary artery disease may indicate insignificant obstruction, single-vessel disease, and collateral circulation.

≫ Key nursing diagnoses and patient outcomes

Use these nursing diagnoses as a guide when developing your plan of care.

Altered cardiopulmonary tissue perfusion related to decreased cellular exchange

Based on this nursing diagnosis, you'll establish the following patient outcomes. The patient will:

• attain hemodynamic stability as evidenced by pulse not less than ___ beats/minute and not greater than ___ beats/minute, blood pressure not less than ___ mm Hg and not greater than ___ mm Hg, respiratory rate ± 5 breaths/minute of baseline rate.

• not exhibit arrhythmias after infusion of Persantine.

Decreased cardiac output related to decreased stroke volume

Based on this nursing diagnosis, you'll establish the following patient outcomes. The patient will:

• have warm and dry skin.
• have a diminished heart workload.
• maintain adequate cardiac output.

Equipment

♦ electrocardiography machine ♦ oral or I.V. Persantine ♦ computed tomography scanner.

Patient preparation

• Tell the patient that a painless, 5- to 10-minute baseline electrocardiogram (ECG) will precede the test.

• Explain what food and fluids restrictions are to be followed before the test. Tell the patient to avoid caffeine and other stimulants, *which may cause arrhythmias.*

• Instruct the patient to continue to take all regular medications, with the possible exception of beta blockers, as prescribed.

• Explain that an I.V. line is used to infuse the medications for study. Tell him who will start the I.V. and when. Explain that the needle insertion and pressure of the tourniquet may cause some discomfort.

• Inform the patient that he may experience mild nausea, headache, dizziness, or flushing after Persantine administration. Reassure him that these temporary adverse reactions rarely need treatment.

• Make sure that the patient or a responsible family member has signed a consent form.

Implementation

• The patient reclines or sits while a resting ECG is performed. Then Persantine is given either orally or I.V. over 4 minutes. Blood pressure, pulse, and cardiac rhythm are monitored continuously.

• After the Persantine is administered, the patient is asked to get up and walk. After Persantine takes effect, thallium is injected.

• The patient is placed in a supine position for about 40 minutes while the scan is performed. Then the scan is reviewed. If necessary, a second scan is performed.

• If the patient must return for further scanning, tell him to rest and to restrict food and fluids in the interim.

Complications

• The patient may experience arrhythmias, angina, ST-segment depression, or bronchospasm.

• More common adverse reactions are nausea, headache, flushing, dizziness, and epigastric pain.

Nursing considerations

• Make sure resuscitation equipment is available.

Documentation

• Begin documenting diagnostic testing with any preliminary assessments you make of a patient's condition. If the patient's age, illness, or disability requires special preparation for the test, enter this information on the chart as well.

• Always prepare the patient for the test, and document any teaching you've done about the test itself and any follow-up care associated with it.

• Also record the administration or withholding of drugs and preparations, special diets, and food or fluid restrictions.

Pneumatic antishock garment

The pneumatic antishock garment (PASG, also known as medical antishock trousers or MAST suit) is made of inflatable bladders lying between double layers of fabric. When inflated, the garment places external pressure on the lower extremities and abdomen, creating an autotransfusion effect by squeezing blood superiorly and increasing blood volume to the heart, lungs, and brain by up to 30%.

The PASG, used to treat shock when systolic blood pressure falls below 80 mm Hg — or below 100 mm Hg when accompanied by signs of shock — can control abdominal and lower extremity hemorrhage by creating internal pressure and external tamponade effects. It can also help stabilize and splint pelvic and femoral fractures.

Use of the PASG is contraindicated in patients with cardiogenic shock, congestive heart failure, pulmonary edema, tension pneumothorax, or increased intracranial pressure. It should be used cautiously during pregnancy.

The PASG must be deflated slowly, with continuous blood pressure monitoring, to prevent potentially irreversible shock from hypovolemia. It shouldn't be removed until the patient's blood volume is restored, his condition has stabilized, or he's being prepared for surgery. If necessary, the PASG can be deflated by stages in the operating room.

≫ Key nursing diagnoses and patient outcomes

Use this nursing diagnosis as a guide when developing your plan of care for a patient using a PASG.

Decreased cardiac output related to decreased stroke volume

Based on this nursing diagnosis, you'll establish the following patient outcomes. The patient will:
• attain hemodynamic stability as evidenced pulse not less than ___ beats/minute and not greater than ___ beats/minute, blood pressure not less than ___ mm Hg and not greater than ___ mm Hg.
• have warm and dry skin.
• have a diminished heart workload.
• maintain adequate cardiac output.

Equipment

♦ PASG with a foot pump is the only necessary equipment. (PASGs come in pediatric size for patients 3½' to 5' [1 to 1.5-m] tall and adult size for patients taller than 5') ♦ optional: resuscitation equipment.

Equipment preparation

• Spread open the PASG on a smooth surface or blanket to avoid puncturing it.
• Make sure all the stopcock valves are open.
• Attach the foot pump.

Patient preparation

• Assess the patient's physical condition to ensure that there are no contraindications to the use of the suit.
• Explain the procedure to the patient to allay fears and promote cooperation.

Implementation

Follow the steps below when using a PASG.

To apply a PASG

• Take vital signs *to establish baseline measurements.*
• Assess the patient's injuries to determine whether he can be turned from side to side. If he can't be turned, slide the PASG under him. If he can be turned, place the PASG next to him and logroll him onto it. You can also set up the PASG on a stretcher, and place the patient on it in a supine position. (See *Applying a pneumatic antishock garment.*)
• Examine the patient for sharp objects, such as pieces of glass, *that could injure him or puncture the suit.*
• Double-check the stopcocks *to make sure they're all open so that the PASG will inflate uniformly.*

Applying a pneumatic antishock garment

After taking the patient's baseline vital signs and explaining the treatment, prepare to apply the antishock garment. On a smooth surface, open the garment with Velcro fasteners down, as shown.

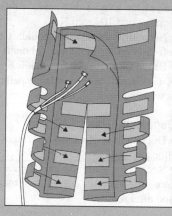

Open all stopcock valves; then attach the foot pump tubing to the valve on the pressure control unit. Can the patient be turned from side to side? If not, slide the garment under him. If he can be turned, place the garment next to him and, with assistance, move him onto it.

Before closing the garment, remove any sharp objects, such as pieces of glass, stones, keys, or a buckle, that could injure the patient

or tear the trousers. As appropriate, pad pressure points and apply lanolin to protect the patient's skin from irritation.

Place the upper edge of the garment just below the patient's lowest rib. Wrap the right leg compartment around the patient's right leg. Secure the compartment by fastening the Velcro straps from the ankle to the thigh.

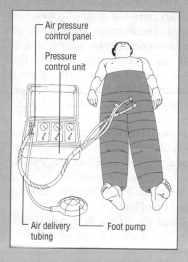

Repeat this procedure for the left leg; then wrap the abdomen. Ensure that all valves are properly positioned.

• Inflate the legs of the PASG first, then the abdominal segment, to about 20 to 30 mm Hg initially.
• Monitor the patient's blood pressure and pulse rate. Continue to inflate the garment slowly while monitoring vital signs. Stop inflating when the patient's systolic blood pressure reaches the desired level, usually 100 mm Hg.

• Close all stopcocks *to prevent accidental air loss.*
• Monitor the patient's blood pressure, pulse rate, and respirations every 5 minutes. Check his pedal pulses and temperature periodically. Notify the doctor if circulation to the patient's feet appears impaired.

To remove a PASG

• Before deflation, make sure that I.V. lines are patent, a doctor is in attendance, and emergency resuscitation equipment is available. Removing a PASG may cause the patient's blood pressure to drop rapidly.

• Open the abdominal stopcock and start releasing small amounts of air. Closely monitor the patient's systolic blood pressure as you do this. If it drops 5 mm Hg, close the stopcock.

Note. Deflating the garment too quickly can allow circulating blood to rush to the abdomen or extremities, causing potentially irreversible shock.

• If you need to stop deflating the PASG because of a drop in blood pressure, increase the flow rate of I.V. solutions to help stabilize blood pressure.

• If blood pressure is stable, continue to deflate the PASG slowly. After deflating the abdominal section, deflate the legs simultaneously.

• When the PASG loosens enough, gently pull it off.

• Clean the PASG, as required, but don't autoclave it or use solvents.

Complications

• Vomiting can result from compression of the abdomen.

• Anaerobic metabolism, which can result from the PASG's pressure being higher than the patient's systolic pressure, can lead to metabolic acidosis.

• Skin breakdown may follow prolonged use. When used with severe leg fractures for long periods, tissue sloughing and necrosis caused by increased compartmental pressures can necessitate amputation.

Nursing considerations

• Generally, you should see a therapeutic response to treatment when the PASG is inflated to 25 mm Hg. A so-called morbidity effect, caused by a change in local circulation, occurs at about 50 mm Hg. Most types of PASGs have Velcro straps, pop-off valves, or gauges that prevent inflation beyond 104 mm Hg.

• Normally, the PASG shouldn't be left inflated for more than 2 hours.

• Because a PASG is radiolucent, X-rays can be taken while the patient is wearing it.

Documentation

• Document application and removal times.

• Record the patient's vital signs before application, during treatment, and after removal.

Positron emission tomography scan

Like computed tomography (CT) scanning and magnetic resonance imaging (MRI), positron emission tomography (PET) provides images of the brain through sophisticated computer reconstruction algorithms. However, PET images detail brain function as well as structure and thus differ significantly from the images provided by these other advanced techniques. PET is also used to detect coronary artery disease, to evaluate myocardial metabolism and contractility, and to distinguish viable from infarcted cardiac tissue, especially during early stages of myocardial infarction.

PET uses radioisotopes of biologically important elements — oxygen, nitrogen, carbon, and fluorine — that emit particles called *positrons*. During positron emissions, gamma rays are detected by the PET scanner and reconstructed to form an image. Positron-emitters can be chemically "tagged" to biologically active molecules, such as carbon monoxide, neurotransmitters, hormones, and metabolites (particularly glucose), allowing study of their uptake and distribution in brain and cardiac tissue. For example, blood tagged with $_{11}$C-carbon monoxide allows study of hemodynamic patterns in brain tissue, whereas tagged neurotransmitters, hormones, and drugs allow mapping of receptor distribution. Isotope-tagged glucose (which penetrates the blood-brain barrier rapidly) allows dynamic study of brain function because PET can pinpoint the sites of glucose metabolism in the brain under various conditions. This may prove useful in the diagnosis of psychiatric disorders, transient ischemic attacks, amyotrophic lateral sclerosis, Parkinson's disease, Wilson's disease, multiple sclerosis, seizure disorders, cerebrovascular disease, and Alzheimer's disease. This is possible because all of these disorders may alter the location and patterns of cerebral glucose metabolism.

PET is used mainly for diagnosing central nervous system disorders, and can also provide information about myocardial perfusion and infarction size. The test distinguishes viable tissue from tissue injured by infarction and may also be used to help assess mitochondrial impairment associated with ischemia or evaluate coronary artery obstruction.

A normal PET scan reveals no areas of ischemic tissue. If the patient receives two injections, the flow and distribution of the two tracers should match, indicating normal tissue.

If the scan reveals reduced blood flow but increased glucose use, ischemia is present. Decreased blood flow and glucose use indicate necrotic, scarred tissue.

PET is a costly test because the radioisotopes used have very short half-lives and must be produced at an on-site cyclotron and attached quickly to the desired tracer molecules. So far, this prohibitive cost has limited PET's use. However, PET has already provided significant information about the brain and may someday have widespread clinical applications.

≫ Key nursing diagnoses and patient outcomes

Use these nursing diagnoses as a guide when developing your plan of care.

Knowledge deficit related to lack of exposure to procedure

Based on this nursing diagnosis, you'll establish the following patient outcomes. The patient will:
• communicate a need to increase knowledge about the procedure.
• state or demonstrate understanding of what has been taught.
• state intention to make needed changes in lifestyle, including seeking help from health professionals when needed.

Anxiety related to situational crisis
Based on this nursing diagnosis, you'll establish the following patient outcomes. The patient will:
• identify factors that elicit anxious behaviors.
• practice progressive relaxation techniques during procedure.
• cope with current medical situation (specify) without demonstrating signs of severe anxiety (specify for individual).

Equipment
♦ PET scanner ♦ a cyclotron ♦ the appropriate radioisotope.

Patient preparation
• Explain that the patient will be given a radioactive substance, either by injection, inhalation, or I.V., and that a highly specialized camera will detect the radioactive decay of this substance and send this data to a computer, which converts it to a visual image.
• Describe the test, including who will administer it, where it will take place, and its duration (typically 60 to 90 minutes). Take time to describe the equipment.
• Tell the patient that the test is painless, unless an I.V. infusion is planned, in which case there may be some discomfort from the needle puncture and tourniquet. If the radioisotope is to be inhaled, explain this painless procedure.
• If a fast is ordered, describe food and fluid restrictions.
• Caution the patient to remain still during the procedure *because lack of patient cooperation can hinder accurate imaging.*

Implementation
• While lying in the supine position with arms above head, the patient undergoes an attenuation scan for about 30 minutes. The appropriate positron emitter is then injected and undergoes PET scanning.
• If comparative studies are needed, the patient may receive an additional injection of a different positron emitter.
• Encourage the patient to drink plenty of fluids *to help flush the radioisotope from the bladder.*

Complications
• An allergic reaction to the radioisotope may occur as well as postural hypotension.
• The radioisotope may be harmful to a fetus, so women of childbearing age should be screened carefully before undergoing this procedure.

Nursing considerations
• After the test, instruct the patient to move slowly immediately after the procedure *to avoid postural hypotension.*

Documentation
• Begin documenting diagnostic testing with any preliminary assessments you make of a patient's condition.
• If the patient's age, illness, or disability requires special preparation for the test, enter this information on the chart as well.
• Always prepare the patient for the test, and document any teaching you've done about the test itself and any follow-up care associated with it.
• Include the administration or withholding of drugs and preparations, special diets, and food or fluid restrictions.

Postoperative care

This phase of care begins when the patient arrives in the postanesthesia care unit (PACU) and continues in the short procedure unit, medical-surgical unit, or critical care area. The goal of postoperative care is to minimize postoperative complications by early detection and prompt treatment. The patient recovering from anesthesia may experience pain, inadequate oxygenation, or adverse physiologic effects caused by sudden movement.

Recovery from general anesthesia takes longer than induction because the anesthetic is retained in fat and muscle. Fat has a meager blood supply; thus, it releases the anesthetic slowly, providing enough anesthesia to maintain adequate blood and brain levels during surgery. Recovery time varies with the patient's amount of body fat, overall condition, premedication regimen, and the type, dosage, and duration of anesthesia.

≫ Key nursing diagnoses and patient outcomes

Use these nursing diagnoses as a guide when developing your plan of care for a postoperative patient.

Impaired skin integrity related to surgery

Based on this nursing diagnosis, you'll establish the following patient outcomes. The patient will:
• exhibit no evidence of skin breakdown.
• show normal skin turgor.
• regain skin integrity; surgical wound heals.

• communicate understanding of skin protection measures.
• demonstrate skill in care of wound or incision.

Risk for infection related to procedure

Based on this nursing diagnosis, you'll establish the following patient outcomes. The patient will:
• have vital signs, temperature, and laboratory values within normal limits.
• have no pathogens in cultures.
• show no signs or symptoms of infection at the surgical site.

Equipment

♦ thermometer ♦ watch with second hand ♦ stethoscope ♦ sphygmomanometer ♦ postoperative flowchart or other documentation tool.

Equipment preparation

• Assemble equipment at the patient's bedside.

Implementation

• Obtain the patient's record from the PACU nurse. This should include a summary of operative procedures and pertinent findings; type of anesthesia; vital signs (preoperative, intraoperative and postoperative); medical history; medication history, including preoperative, intraoperative, and postoperative medications; fluid therapy, including estimated blood loss, type and number of drains, catheters, and characteristics of drainage; and notes on the condition of the surgical wound. If the patient had vascular surgery, for example, knowing the location and duration of blood vessel clamping is important for preventing postoperative complications.

• Transfer the patient from the PACU stretcher to the bed and position him properly. Get a coworker to help, if necessary. When moving the patient, keep transfer movements smooth *to minimize pain and postoperative complications and avoid back strain by team members.*

• If the patient has had orthopedic surgery, always get a coworker to help transfer him. Ask the coworker to move only the affected extremity.

• If the patient is in skeletal traction, you may have to follow special orders for moving him. If you must move him, have a coworker move the weights as you and another coworker move the patient.

• Make the patient comfortable and raise the bed's side rails *to ensure the patient's safety.*

• Assess the patient's level of consciousness, skin color, and mucous membranes.

• Monitor the patient's respiratory status by assessing his airway. Note breathing rate and depth, and auscultate breath sounds. Administer oxygen and initiate oximetry *to monitor oxygen saturation if ordered.*

• Monitor the patient's pulse rate. It should be strong and easily palpable. The postoperative heart rate should be within 20% of the preoperative heart rate.

• Compare postoperative blood pressure to preoperative blood pressure. It should be within 20% of the preoperative level unless the patient suffered a hypotensive episode during surgery.

• Assess the patient's temperature *because anesthesia lowers body temperature.* Body temperature should be at least 95° F (35° C). If it's lower, apply blankets *to warm the patient.*

• Assess the patient's infusion sites for redness, pain, swelling, or drainage.

• Assess surgical wound dressings. Dressings should be clean and dry. If they're soiled, assess the characteristics of the drainage and outline the soiled area. Note the date and time of assessment on the dressing. Assess the soiled area frequently; if it enlarges, reinforce the dressing and alert the doctor.

• Note the presence and condition of any drains and tubes. Note the color, type, odor, and amount of drainage. Make sure all drains are properly connected and free of kinks and obstructions.

• If the patient has had vascular or orthopedic surgery, assess the appropriate extremity, or all extremities, depending on the surgical procedure. Assess color, temperature, sensation, movement, and presence and quality of pulses, and notify the doctor of any abnormalities.

• As the patient recovers from anesthesia, monitor respiratory and cardiovascular status closely. Be alert for signs of airway obstruction and hypoventilation caused by laryngospasm, or for sedation, which can lead to hypoxemia. *Cardiovascular complications — such as arrhythmias and hypotension — may result from the anesthetic agent or the operative procedure.*

• Encourage coughing and deep-breathing exercises, but *not* if the patient has just had nasal, ophthalmic, or neurologic surgery *(to avoid increasing intracranial pressure).*

• Administer postoperative medications, such as antibiotics, analgesics, antiemetics, or reversal agents, as ordered and appropriate.

• Remove all fluids from the bedside until the patient is alert enough to eat and drink. Before giving liquids, assess the patient's gag reflex *to prevent aspiration.* To do this, lightly touch the back of the patient's throat with a cotton-tipped applicator. The patient will gag if the reflex has returned. Do this test quickly *to prevent a vagal reaction.*

Complications

Postoperative complications may include:

• arrhythmias
• hypotension
• hypovolemia
• septicemia
• septic shock
• atelectasis
• pneumonia
• thrombophlebitis
• pulmonary embolism
• urine retention
• wound infection
• wound dehiscence
• evisceration
• abdominal distention
• paralytic ileus
• constipation
• altered body image
• postoperative psychosis.

Nursing considerations

• *Fear, pain, anxiety, hypothermia, confusion, and immobility can upset the patient and jeopardize his safety and postoperative status.* Offer emotional support to the patient and his family. Keep in mind that the patient who has lost a body part or who has been diagnosed with an incurable disease will need ongoing emotional support. Refer him and his family to appropriate clerical or psychological counseling.

• As the patient recovers from general anesthesia, reflexes appear in reverse order to that in which they disappeared. *Hearing recovers first,* so avoid holding inappropriate conversations near the patient.

• The patient under general anesthesia can't protect his own airway because of muscle relaxation. As he recovers, his cough and gag reflexes reappear. If he can lift his head without assistance, he's usually able to breathe on his own and protect his airway.

• If the patient received spinal anesthesia, he will need to remain supine with the bed adjusted to between 0 degrees and 20 degrees for at least 6 hours to reduce the risk of spinal head ache from leakage of cerebrospinal fluid. The patient will also be unable to move his legs so be sure to explain this to him, and reassure him that sensation and mobility will return.

• If the patient has had epidural anesthesia for postoperative pain control, monitor his respiratory status closely. Respiratory arrest may result from paralysis of the diaphragm by the anesthetic. The patient may also experience nausea, vomiting, or itching.

• If a patient-controlled anesthesia (PCA) unit is to be used, make sure the patient understands how to use it. Caution him to activate it only when he has pain, not when he feels sleepy or is pain-free. Review your hospital criteria for PCA.

BETTER CHARTING

Documenting postoperative status

When your patient recovers from the effects of anesthesia, he can be transferred from the operating room-postanesthesia care unit (OR-PACU) to his assigned unit. As the nurse on this service, you're responsible for the four-part documentation that travels with the patient. Here are some tips for making sure all parts of the record are complete.

Part 1: History
Make sure this section of the report includes the patient's pertinent medical and surgical history.

Include drug allergies, medication history, chronic illnesses, significant surgical history and hospitalizations, and smoking history.

Part 2: Operation
Check that the following information is recorded in this section of the report, describing the surgery itself:
• the procedure performed
• the type and dosage of anesthetics administered
• the length of time the patient was anesthetized
• the patient's vital signs throughout surgery
• the volume of fluid lost and replaced
• drugs administered
• surgical complications
• tourniquet time
• any drains, tubes, implants, or dressings used in surgery and removed or still in place.

Part 3: Postanesthesia period
Be certain that this part of the record includes information about:
• pain medications and pain control devices that the patient received and how he responded to them.

• interventions that should continue on the unit. For example, if the patient underwent leg surgery and had a tourniquet on for a long time, he will need more frequent circulatory, motor, and neurologic checks. Or, if the anesthesiologist inserted an epidural catheter, the record should note any doctor's orders regarding medication administration or special care procedures.
• a flow sheet showing the patient's postanesthesia recovery scores on arrival and discharge in these areas: activity level, respiration, circulation, level of consciousness (LOC), and color.
• an account of unusual events or complications that occured on the PACU — for instance, nausea or vomiting, shivering, hypothermia, arrythmias, central anticholinergic syndrome, sore throat, back or neck pain, corneal abrasion, tooth loss during intubation, swollen lips or tongue, pharyngeal or laryngeal abrasion, and postspinal headache.

Part 4: Current status
Expect this section to describe the patient's status at the time of transfer. Information should include the patient's vital signs, LOC, and sensorium.

Documentation
• Document vital signs on the appropriate flowchart.
• Record the condition of dressings, and drains, and characteristics of drainage.
• Document all interventions taken to alleviate pain and anxiety and the patient's responses to them.
• Document any complications that may have occurred and interventions taken. (See *Documenting postoperative status*.)

Postpartum fundal assessment

After delivery, the uterus gradually shrinks and descends into its prepregnancy position in the pelvis — a process known as involution. The nurse evaluates normal involutional progress by palpating and massaging the uterus to identify uterine size, firmness, and descent. (See *Hand placement for fundal palpation and massage*, page 704.)

Involution normally begins immediately after delivery, when the firmly contracted uterus lies midway between the umbilicus and the symphysis pubis. Soon the uterus rises to the umbilicus and, after the first postpartum day, begins returning to the pelvis. The average descent rate is 1 fingerbreadth or centimeter daily — slightly slower if the patient had a cesarean section. By the 10th postpartum day the now nonpalpable uterus lies deep in the pelvis, either at or below the symphysis pubis.

When the uterus fails to contract or remain firm during involution, uterine bleeding, or hemorrhage can result. That's because placental separation after delivery exposes large uterine blood vessels, which uterine contractions close off (like a tourniquet). Fundal massage, synthetic oxytocic therapy, or natural oxytocic substances released during breastfeeding help to maintain or stimulate contraction.

Typical nursing procedures that coincide with fundal palpation and massage include caring for the perineum and evaluating healing.

≫ Key nursing diagnoses and patient outcomes
Use these nursing diagnoses as a guide when developing your plan of care.

Pain related to incision (if a cesarean section was performed)
Based on this nursing diagnosis, you'll establish the following patient outcomes. The patient will:
• give verbal and nonverbal cues of decreasing pain within 24 hours.
• require less pain medication (specify).

Altered urinary elimination related to decreased bladder tone
Based on this nursing diagnosis, you'll establish the following patient outcomes. The patient will:
• void spontaneously within 3 hours.
• have her uterine fundus palpated centrally and below the umbilicus.

Equipment
♦ gloves ♦ analgesics ♦ perineal pad ♦ optional: urinary catheter.

Patient preparation
• Explain the procedure.

Hand placement for fundal palpation and massage

A full-term pregnancy stretches the ligaments supporting the uterus, placing the uterus at risk for inversion during palpation and massage. To guard against this, use your hands to support and fix the uterus in a safe position. Here's how.

Place one hand against the patient's abdomen at the symphysis pubis level. This steadies the fundus and prevents downward displacement.

Place the other hand at the top of the fundus, cupping it.

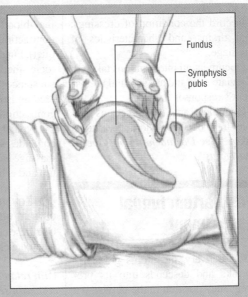

Fundus

Symphysis pubis

• Provide privacy.
• Schedule fundal assessments (unless the doctor orders otherwise) every 15 minutes for the first hour after delivery, every 30 minutes for the next 2 to 3 hours, every hour for the next 4 hours, every 4 hours for the rest of the first postpartum day, and every 8 hours until the patient's discharge.
• Give prescribed analgesics before fundal checks, if indicated. Teach her relaxation techniques (deep breathing) *to help her cope with discomfort.*

Implementation
• Encourage the patient's efforts to urinate *because bladder distention impairs uterine contraction by pushing the uterus up and aside.* You may need to catheterize the patient if she can't urinate or if the uterus becomes displaced with increased bleeding.
• Lower the head of the bed until the patient lies supine. If she reports discomfort in this position — especially if she's had a cesarean section — keep the head of the bed slightly elevated.
• Expose the abdomen for palpation and the perineum for observation. You'll watch for bleeding, clots, and tissue expulsion as you massage the fundus.
• Gently compress the uterus between both hands *to evaluate uterine firmness.* Note the level of the fundus above or below the umbilicus in fingerbreadths or centimeters.
• If the uterus seems soft and boggy, gently massage the fundus with a circular motion until it becomes firm. Simply cupping the uterus between

your hands may also stimulate contraction.

Alternatively, massage the fundus with the side of the hand above the fundus. Without digging into the abdomen, gently compress and release, always supporting the lower uterine segment with the other hand. Observe for lochia flow during massage.

• Massage long enough to produce firmness. The sensitive and tender fundus needs only gentle pressure. *This should produce desired results without causing excessive discomfort.*

• Notify the doctor or nurse-midwife immediately should the uterus fail to contract and should heavy bleeding occur. If the fundus becomes firm after massage, keep one hand on the lower uterus and press gently toward the pubis *to help expel any clots.*

• Clean the perineum and apply a clean perineal pad. Help the patient into a comfortable position.

Complications

• Because the uterus and its supporting ligaments are usually tender after delivery, pain is the most common complication of fundal palpation and massage. Excessive massage can stimulate premature uterine contractions, causing undue muscle fatigue and leading to uterine atony or inversion.

Nursing considerations

• Because incision pain makes fundal palpation uncomfortable for the patient who has had a cesarean section, provide pain medication beforehand, as ordered. If the lochia flow diminishes after 4 hours, the doctor may permit fewer fundal checks than usual,

especially if the patient is receiving oxytocin.

• Beware if no lochia appears. *This may signal a clot blocking the cervical os. Subsequent heavy bleeding may result if a position change dislodges the clot.* Take vital signs *to assess for signs of hypovolemic shock.*

Documentation

• Record vital signs, fundal height in fingerbreadths or centimeters, and also record position (midline or off-center) and tone (firm or soft and boggy).

• Document massage and note passage of any clots. Record excessive bleeding and your notification of the doctor or nurse-midwife.

Preoperative care

Preoperative care begins when the patient's surgery is planned and ends when anesthesia is administered. This phase of care includes a preoperative interview and assessment to collect baseline subjective and objective data from the patient and members of the patient's family; diagnostic tests such as urinalysis, electrocardiogram (ECG), and chest radiography; preoperative teaching; securing informed consent from the patient; and physical preparation.

≫ Key nursing diagnoses and patient outcomes

Use these nursing diagnoses as a guide when developing your plan of care for a preoperative patient.

Knowledge deficit related to lack of exposure to procedure
Based on this nursing diagnosis, you'll establish the following patient outcomes. The patient will:
• communicate a need to increase knowledge.
• state or demonstrate understanding of what has been taught.
• state intention to make needed changes in lifestyle, including seeking help from health professionals when needed.

Anxiety related to situational crisis
Based on this nursing diagnosis, you'll establish the following patient outcomes. The patient will:
• identify factors that elicit anxious behaviors.
• practice progressive relaxation techniques during procedure.
• cope with current medical situation (specify) without demonstrating signs of severe anxiety (specify for individual).

Equipment
◆ gloves ◆ thermometer ◆ sphygmomanometer ◆ stethoscope ◆ watch with second hand ◆ weight scale ◆ tape measure.

Equipment preparation
• Assemble all needed equipment at the patient's bedside or in the admission area.

Patient preparation
• If the patient is having same day surgery, make sure he knows ahead of time not to eat or drink anything for 8 hours prior to surgery.
• Confirm with him what time he's scheduled to arrive at the hospital, and

tell him to leave all jewelry and valuables at home.
• Make sure the patient has arranged for someone to accompany him home after surgery.

Implementation
• Obtain a health history and assess the patient's knowledge, perceptions, and expectations about surgery.
• Ask about previous medical and surgical interventions.
• Determine the patient's psychosocial needs; ask about occupational well-being, financial matters, support systems, mental status, and cultural beliefs.
• Use your facility's preoperative surgical assessment data base, if available, to gather this information.
• Obtain a drug history. Ask about current prescription and over-the-counter medications and about known allergies to foods and drugs.
• Measure the patient's height, weight, and vital signs.
• Identify risk factors that might interfere with a positive expected outcome. Be sure to consider age, general health, medications, mobility, nutritional status, fluid and electrolyte disturbances, and lifestyle. Also consider the duration and location of the primary disorder, and the nature and extent of the surgical procedure.
• Explain preoperative procedures to the patient. Include typical events that the patient can expect. *Preoperative teaching can help reduce postoperative anxiety and pain, increase patient compliance, hasten recovery, and decrease length of hospital stay.*
• Discuss equipment that may be used postoperatively, such as nasogastric tubes and I.V. equipment. Explain the

typical incision, dressings, and staples or sutures that will be used.

• Talk the patient through the sequence of events from operating room to recovery room (postanesthesia care unit or PACU) and back to patient's room. Some patients may be transferred from the PACU to an intensive care unit or surgical care unit. Your patient may also benefit from a tour of the areas he will see during the perioperative events.

• Tell the patient about exercises that he may be expected to perform after surgery (to minimize respiratory and circulatory complications), such as deep-breathing, coughing (while splinting the incision if necessary), extremity exercises, and movement and ambulation. If the patient is to undergo ophthalmic or neurologic surgery, he won't be asked to cough *because coughing increases intracranial pressure.*

• On the day of surgery, important interventions include giving morning care, administering ordered preoperative medications, completing the preoperative checklist and chart, and providing support to the patient and family members.

• Verify that the patient has signed an informed consent form. (See *Obtaining informed consent.*)

• Other immediate preoperative interventions may include preparing the GI tract (restricting food and fluids for about 8 hours before surgery) *to reduce vomiting and the risk of aspiration,* cleaning the lower GI tract of fecal material by enemas before abdominal or GI surgery, and giving antibiotics for 2 or 3 days preoperatively *to prevent contamination of the peritoneal cavity by GI bacteria.*

Obtaining informed consent

Informed consent means that the patient is entitled to a full explanation of the procedure, its risks and complications, and the risk if the procedure isn't performed at this time. Although obtaining informed consent is the doctor's responsibility, the nurse is responsible for verifying that this step has been taken.

You may be asked to witness the patient's signature. However, if you didn't hear the doctor's explanation to the patient, you must sign that you are witnessing the patient's signature only.

Consent forms must be signed before the patient receives his preoperative medication because forms signed after sedatives are given are legally invalid. Adults and emancipated minors can sign their own consent forms. Children's consent forms, or those of adults with impaired mental status, must be signed by a parent or guardian.

• Just before the patient is moved to the surgical area, make sure he's wearing a hospital gown, has his identification band in place, and has his vital signs recorded. Check to see that hairpins, nail polish, and jewelry have been removed. Note whether dentures, contact lenses, or prosthetic devices have been removed or left in place.

Nursing considerations
• Give preoperative medications on time *to enhance the effect of ordered anesthesia.* The patient should take

nothing by mouth preoperatively. Do not give oral medications unless ordered. Be sure to raise the bed's side rails immediately after giving preoperative medications.

• If the patient's family members or others are present, direct them to the appropriate waiting area and offer support as needed.

Documentation
• Complete the preoperative checklist used by your hospital.
• Record all nursing care measures and preoperative medications, results of diagnostic tests, and the time the patient is transferred to the surgical area.
• The chart and the surgical checklist must accompany the patient to surgery.

Pressure dressings

For effective control of capillary or small-vein bleeding, temporary application of pressure directly over a wound may be achieved with a bulk dressing held by a glove-protected hand, bound into place with a pressure bandage, or held under pressure by an inflated air splint. A pressure dressing requires frequent checks for wound drainage to determine its effectiveness in controlling bleeding. Patients who need a pressure dressing may have such diagnoses as fluid volume deficit, impaired skin integrity, impaired tissue integrity, or altered tissue perfusion.

≫ Key nursing diagnoses and patient outcomes
Use these nursing diagnoses as a guide when developing your plan of care for a patient with pressure dressings.

Risk for fluid volume deficit related to excessive loss
Based on this nursing diagnosis, you'll establish the following patient outcomes. The patient will:
• have vital signs remain stable.
• have electrolyte values remain within normal range.

Altered tissue perfusion (specify) related to decreased cellular exchange
Based on this nursing diagnosis, you'll establish the following patient outcomes. The patient will:
• attain hemodynamic stability as evidenced by pulse not less than ___ beats/minute or more than ___ beats/minute; blood pressure not less than ___ mm Hg or more than ___ mm Hg.
• not exhibit arrhythmias.

Equipment
♦ two or more sterile gauze pads ♦ roller gauze ♦ adhesive tape ♦ clean disposable gloves ♦ metric ruler.

Obtain the pressure dressing as quickly as possible *to avoid excessive blood loss.* Use clean cloth for the dressing if sterile gauze pads are unavailable.

Implementation
• Quickly explain the procedure to the patient *to help decrease his anxiety,* and put on gloves.
• Elevate the injured body part *to help reduce bleeding.*

• Place enough gauze pads over the wound to cover it. Don't clean the wound; *you can do this when the bleeding stops.*

• For an extremity or trunk wound, hold the dressing firmly over the wound, and wrap the roller gauze tightly across it and around the body part *to provide pressure on the wound.* Secure the bandage with adhesive tape.

• To apply a dressing to the neck, the shoulder, or another location that can't be tightly wrapped, don't use roller gauze. Instead, apply tape directly over the dressings *to provide the necessary pressure at the wound site.*

• Check pulse, temperature, and skin condition distal to the wound site *because excessive pressure can obstruct normal circulation.*

• Check the dressing frequently *to monitor wound drainage.* Use the metric standard of measurement to determine the amount of drainage, and document these serial measurements for later reference. Do not circle a potentially wet dressing with ink *because this provides no permanent documentation in the medical record and also runs the risk of contaminating the dressing.*

• If the dressing becomes saturated, do not remove it *because this will interfere with the pressure.* Instead, apply an additional dressing over the saturated one and continue to monitor and record drainage.

• Obtain additional medical care as soon as possible.

Complications

• Excessively tight application of a pressure dressing can impair circulation.

Nursing considerations

• Cover the wound with your gloved hand if sterile gauze pads and clean cloth are unavailable.

• Avoid using an elastic bandage to bind the dressing *because it can't be wrapped tightly enough to create pressure on the wound site.*

Documentation

• Once the bleeding is controlled, record the date and time of dressing application, the presence or absence of distal pulses, the integrity of distal skin, the amount of wound drainage, and any complications.

Pressure ulcer care

As the name implies, pressure ulcers result when pressure — applied with great force for a short period or with less force over a longer period — impairs circulation, depriving tissues of oxygen and other life-sustaining nutrients. This process damages skin and underlying structures. Untreated, these ischemic lesions can lead to serious infection.

Most pressure ulcers develop over bony prominences, where friction and shearing force combine with pressure to break down skin and underlying tissues. Common sites include the sacrum, coccyx, ischial tuberosities, and greater trochanters. Other common sites include the skin over the vertebrae, scapulae, elbows, knees, and heels in bedridden and relatively immobile patients. (See *Pressure ulcers: Who's at risk?*, page 710.)

Successful pressure ulcer treatment involves relieving pressure, restoring circulation, and, if possible,

Pressure ulcers: Who's at risk?

Assess every patient for signs of developing pressure ulcers. To determine your patient's risk, you may use a formal risk assessment scale, such as the Braden, Norton, or Gosnell scale. At greatest risk for pressure ulcers are elderly patients and those with the following conditions:
- poor circulation
- diabetes mellitus
- malnutrition
- immunosuppression
- dehydration
- incontinence
- significant obesity or thinness
- paralysis
- diminished pain awareness
- history of corticosteroid therapy
- previous pressure ulcers
- chronic illness that requires bed rest
- mental impairment, possibly related to coma, altered level of consciousness, sedation, confusion, or use of restraints.

resolving or managing related disorders. Typically, the effectiveness and duration of treatment depend on the characteristics of the pressure ulcer. (See *Staging pressure ulcers*.)

Ideally, prevention is the key to avoiding extensive therapy. Preventive measures include ensuring adequate nourishment and mobility to relieve pressure and promote circulation.

When a pressure ulcer develops despite preventive efforts, treatment includes methods to decrease pressure. These include frequent repositioning to shorten pressure duration and use of special equipment to reduce pressure intensity. Treatment may involve special pressure-reducing devices, such as beds, mattresses, mattress overlays, and chair cushions. Other therapeutic measures include decreasing risk factors and use of topical treatments, wound cleansing, debridement, and dressing application to support moist wound healing. (See *Guide to topical agents for pressure ulcers*, pages 712 and 713, and *Choosing an ulcer dressing*, page 714.)

Nurses usually perform or coordinate treatments according to hospital policy. The procedures detailed below address cleaning and dressing the pressure ulcer.

⟩⟩ Key nursing diagnoses and patient outcomes

Use these nursing diagnoses as a guide when developing your plan of care for a patient with a pressure ulcer.

Impaired skin integrity related to pressure ulcer

Based on this nursing diagnosis, you'll establish the following patient outcomes. The patient will:
- exhibit no evidence of further skin breakdown.
- show normal skin turgor.
- regain skin integrity (the pressure ulcer will heal).
- communicate understanding of skin protection measures.
- demonstrate skill in care of wound or incision.

Risk for infection related to pressure ulcer

Based on this nursing diagnosis, you'll establish the following patient outcomes. The patient will:

Staging pressure ulcers

To select the most effective treatment for a pressure ulcer, you first need to assess its characteristics. The pressure ulcer stages described below, used by the National Pressure Ulcer Advisory Panel and the Agency for Health Care Policy and Research, reflect the anatomic depth of exposed tissue. Keep in mind that if the wound contains necrotic tissue, you won't be able to determine the stage until you can see the wound base.

Stage 1

The heralding lesion of a pressure ulcer is a reddened area of intact skin that does not blanch.

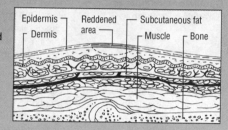

Stage 2

This stage is marked by partial-thickness skin loss involving the epidermis, dermis, or both. The ulcer is superficial and appears as an abrasion, a blister, or a shallow crater.

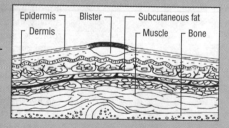

Stage 3

The ulcer constitutes a full-thickness wound penetrating the subcutaneous tissue, which may extend to — but not through — underlying fascia. It looks like a deep crater and may or may not undermine adjacent tissue.

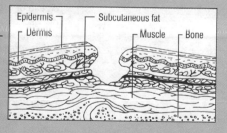

Stage 4

The ulcer extends through the skin, accompanied by extensive destruction, tissue necrosis, or damage to muscle, bone, or supporting structures

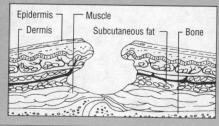

Guide to topical agents for pressure ulcers

TOPICAL AGENTS	NURSING CONSIDERATIONS
Antibiotics bacitracin, Neosporin Ointment, Polysporin Ointment	• Use only for early ulcers because these agents may not penetrate sufficiently to kill deeper bacterial colonies.
Circulatory stimulants (Granulex, Proderm)	• Use these agents to promote blood flow. Both contain balsam of Peru and castor oil, but Granulex also contains trypsin, an enzyme that facilitates debridement.
Enzymes collagenase (Santyl), fibrinolysin and desoxyribonuclease (Elase), sutilains (Travase)	• Apply collagenase in thin layers after cleaning the wound with normal saline solution. • Promote effectiveness by avoiding concurrent use of collagenase with agents that decrease enzymatic activity, including detergents, hexachlorophene, iodine, antiseptics with heavy-metal ions, or such acid solutions as Burow's solution. • Use collagenase cautiously near the patient's eyes. If contact occurs, flush the eyes repeatedly with normal saline solution or sterile water. • Use fibrinolysin and desoxyribonuclease only after surgical removal of dry eschar. • If using sutilains and topical antibacterials, apply sutilains ointment first. • Avoid applying sutilains to ulcers in major body cavities, to areas with exposed nerve tissue, or to fungating neoplastic lesions. Do not use sutilains in women of childbearing age or in patients with limited cardiopulmonary reserve. • Store sutilains at a cool temperature: $35.6°$ to $50°$ F ($2°$ to $10°$ C). • Use sutilains cautiously near the patient's eyes. If contact occurs, flush the eyes repeatedly with normal saline solution or sterile water.

Guide to topical agents for pressure ulcers *(continued)*

TOPICAL AGENTS	NURSING CONSIDERATIONS
Exudate absorbers dextranomer beads (Debrisan)	• Use dextranomer beads on secreting ulcers. Discontinue use when secretions stop. • Clean, but don't dry, the ulcer before applying dextranomer beads. Don't use in tunneling ulcers. • Remove gray-yellow beads (which indicate saturation) by irrigating with sterile water or normal saline solution. • Use cautiously near the eyes. If contact occurs, flush the eyes repeatedly with normal saline solution or sterile water.
Isotonic solutions normal saline solution	• This agent moisturizes tissue without injuring cells.

• have vital signs, temperature, and laboratory values that remain within the patient's normal limits.

• have no pathogens in cultures.

• show no signs or symptoms of worsening infection at the pressure ulcer site.

Equipment

♦ hypoallergenic tape or elastic netting ♦ overbed table ♦ piston syringe for irrigation ♦ two pairs of gloves ♦ normal saline solution, as ordered ♦ sterile 4″ × 4″ gauze pads ♦ selected topical dressing ♦ linensaver pads ♦ impervious plastic trash bag ♦ disposable wound-measuring device.

Equipment preparation

• Assemble equipment at the patient's bedside.

• Cut tape into strips for securing dressings.

• Loosen lids on cleaning solutions and medications for easy removal.

• Loosen existing dressing edges and tapes before putting on gloves.

• Attach an impervious plastic trash bag to the overbed table *to hold used dressings and refuse.*

Patient preparation

• Provide privacy and explain the procedure to the patient *to allay fears and promote cooperation.*

• Position the patient to increase his comfort but be sure that the position allows you easy access to the pressure ulcer site.

Implementation

• Before any dressing change, wash your hands and review the principles of universal precautions.

Choosing an ulcer dressing

The patient's individual needs and the ulcer characteristics determine which type of dressing to use on a pressure ulcer.

Gauze dressings
Made of absorptive cotton or synthetic fabric, these dressings are permeable to water, water vapor, and oxygen and may be impregnated with petroleum jelly or another agent. When uncertain about which dressing to use, you may apply a gauze dressing moistened in saline solution until a wound specialist recommends definitive treatment.

Hydrocolloid dressings
These adhesive, moldable wafers are made of a carbohydrate-based material and usually have waterproof backings. They are impermeable to oxygen, water, and water vapor, and most have some absorptive properties.

Transparent film dressings
Clear, adherent, and nonabsorptive, these polymer-based dressings are permeable to oxygen and water vapor but not to water. Their transparency allows visual inspection. Because they can't absorb drainage, transparent film dressings are used on partial-thickness wounds with minimal exudate.

Alginate dressings
Made from seaweed, these nonwoven, absorptive dressings are available as soft, white sterile pads or ropes. They absorb excessive exudate and may be used on infected wounds. As the dressing absorbs exudate, it turns into a gel that keeps the wound bed moist and promotes healing. When exudate is no longer excessive, switch to another type of dressing.

Foam dressings
These spongelike polymer dressings may be impregnated or coated with other materials. Somewhat absorptive, they may or may not be adherent. Foam dressings promote moist wound healing and are useful when a nonadherent surface is desired.

Hydrogel dressings
Water-based and nonadherent, these polymer-based dressings have some absorptive properties. They are available as a gel in a tube or in flexible sheets, and may have a cooling effect that eases pain.

To clean the pressure ulcer
• Cover the bed linens with a linen-saver pad *to prevent soiling.*
• Open the normal saline solution container and the piston syringe. Carefully pour normal saline solution into an irrigation container *to avoid splashing.* (This container may be clean or sterile, depending on hospital policy.) Put the piston syringe into the opening provided in the irrigation container.
• Open packages of supplies.
• Put on gloves to remove the old dressing and expose the pressure ulcer. Discard the soiled dressing in the impervious plastic trash bag *to avoid*

contaminating the sterile field and spreading infection.

• Inspect the wound. Note color, amount, and odor of any drainage and necrotic debris. Measure the wound perimeter with the disposable wound-measuring device (a square, transparent card with concentric circles arranged in bull's-eye fashion and bordered with a straight-edge ruler).

• Using the piston syringe, apply full force to irrigate the pressure ulcer *to remove necrotic debris and help decrease bacteria in the wound.*

• Remove and discard your soiled gloves and put on a fresh pair.

• Insert a gloved finger into the wound *to assess wound tunneling or undermining.* Tunneling usually signals wound extension along fascial planes. Gauge tunnel depth by determining how far you can insert your finger.

• Next, reassess the condition of the skin and the ulcer. Note the character of the clean wound bed and the surrounding skin.

• If you observe adherent necrotic material, notify a wound care specialist or a doctor *to ensure appropriate debridement.* (See *Understanding pressure ulcer debridement,* page 716.)

• Prepare to apply the appropriate topical dressing. Directions for typical moist saline gauze, hydrocolloid, transparent, alginate, foam, and hydrogel dressings follow. For other dressings or topical agents, follow your hospital's protocol or the supplier's instructions.

To apply a moist saline gauze dressing

• Irrigate the pressure ulcer with normal saline solution. Blot the surrounding skin dry.

• Moisten the gauze dressing with saline solution.

• Gently place the dressing over the surface of the ulcer. *To separate surfaces within the wound,* gently place a dressing between opposing wound surfaces. Don't pack the gauze tightly, however, *to avoid damaging tissues.*

• Change the dressing often enough *to keep the wound moist.*

To apply a hydrocolloid dressing

• Irrigate the pressure ulcer with normal saline solution. Blot the surrounding skin dry.

• Choose a clean, dry, presized dressing, or cut one to overlap the pressure ulcer by about 1″ (2.5 cm). Remove the dressing from its package, pull the release paper from the adherent side of the dressing, and apply the dressing to the wound. *To minimize irritation,* carefully smooth out wrinkles as you apply the dressing.

• If the dressing's edges need to be secured with tape, apply a skin sealant to the intact skin around the ulcer. After the area dries, tape the dressing to the skin; avoid using tension or pressure.

• Remove your gloves and discard them in the impervious trash bag. Dispose of refuse according to hospital policy, and wash your hands.

• Change a hydrocolloid dressing every 2 to 7 days, as needed — for example, if the patient complains of pain, the dressing no longer adheres, or leakage occurs.

To apply a transparent dressing

• Irrigate the pressure ulcer with normal saline solution. Blot the surrounding skin dry.

Understanding pressure ulcer debridement

Because moist, necrotic tissue promotes the growth of pathologic organisms, removing such tissue aids pressure ulcer healing. A pressure ulcer can be debrided using various methods. The patient's condition and the goals of care determine which method to use. Sharp debridement is indicated for patients with an urgent need for debridement, such as those with sepsis or cellulitis. Otherwise, another method, such as mechanical, enzymatic, or autolytic debridement, may be used. Sometimes, several methods are used in combination.

Sharp debridement
The most rapid method, sharp debridement removes thick, adherent eschar and devitalized tissue through use of a scalpel, scissors, or another sharp instrument. Small amounts of necrotic tissue can be debrided at the bedside; extensive amounts must be debrided in the operating room.

Mechanical debridement
Typically, this method involves the use of wet-to-dry dressings. Gauze moistened with normal saline solution is applied to the wound and then removed after it dries and adheres to the wound bed. The goal is to debride the wound as the dressing is removed. Mechanical debridement has certain disadvantages; for example, it is often painful and it

may take a long time to completely debride the ulcer.

Enzymatic debridement
This method removes necrotic tissue by breaking down tissue elements. Topical enzymatic debriding agents are placed on the necrotic tissue. If eschar is present, it must be crosshatched to allow the enzyme to penetrate the tissue.

Autolytic debridement
This technique involves the use of moisture-retentive dressings to cover the wound bed. Necrotic tissue is then removed through self-digestion of enzymes in the wound fluid. Although autolytic debridement takes longer than other debridement methods, it's appropriate for patients who can't tolerate any other method.

• Clean and dry the wound as described above.
• Select a dressing to overlap the ulcer by 2″ (5 cm).
• Gently lay the dressing over the ulcer. *To prevent shearing force,* do not stretch the dressing. Press firmly on the edges of the dressing *to promote adherence.* Although these dressings are self-adhesive, you may have to

tape the edges to prevent them from curling.
• If necessary, aspirate accumulated fluid with a 21G needle and syringe. After aspirating the pocket of fluid, clean the aspiration site with an alcohol sponge, and cover it with another strip of transparent dressing.
• Change the dressing every 3 to 7 days, depending on the amount of drainage.

To apply an alginate dressing
• Irrigate the pressure ulcer with normal saline solution. Blot the surrounding skin dry.
• Apply the alginate to the ulcer surface. Cover the area with a second dressing, such as gauze pads, as ordered. Secure the dressing with tape or elastic netting.
• If the wound is draining heavily, change the dressing once or twice daily for the first 3 to 5 days. As drainage decreases, change the dressing every 2 to 4 days, or as ordered. When the drainage stops or the wound bed looks dry, stop using alginate dressing.

To apply a foam dressing
• Irrigate the pressure ulcer with normal saline solution. Blot the surrounding skin dry.
• Gently lay the foam dressing over the ulcer.
• Use tape, elastic netting, or gauze *to hold the dressing in place.*
• Change the dressing when the foam no longer absorbs exudate.

To apply a hydrogel dressing
• Irrigate the pressure ulcer with normal saline solution. Blot the surrounding skin dry.
• Apply gel to the wound bed.
• Cover with a secondary dressing.
• Change the dressing daily, or as needed, *to keep the wound bed moist.*

To prevent pressure ulcers
• Turn and reposition the patient every 1 to 2 hours unless contraindicated. For patients who can't turn themselves or who are turned on a schedule, use pressure-reducing devices, such as air, gel, or a 4″ foam mattress overlay. Low- or high-air-loss therapy may be indicated to reduce excessive pressure and promote evaporation of excess moisture. As appropriate, implement active or passive range-of-motion exercises *to relieve pressure and promote circulation.* To save time, combine these exercises with bathing if applicable.
• When turning the patient, lift him rather than slide him, *to avoid friction and shear.* Use a turning sheet and get help from coworkers if necessary.
• Use pillows to position the patient and increase his comfort. Be sure to eliminate sheet wrinkles that could increase pressure and cause discomfort.
• Post a turning schedule at the patient's bedside. Adapt position changes to the patient's situation. Emphasize the importance of regular position changes to the patient and members of his family, and encourage their participation in treating and preventing pressure ulcers by having each of them perform a position change correctly after you've demonstrated how.
• Avoid placing the patient directly on the trochanter. Instead, position him on his side, at an angle of about 30 degrees.
• Except for brief periods, avoid raising the head of the bed more than 30 degrees, *to prevent shearing pressure.*
• Direct the patient who is confined to a chair or wheelchair to shift his weight every 30 minutes *to promote blood flow to compressed tissues.* Show a paraplegic patient how to shift his weight by doing push-ups in the wheelchair. If the patient needs help, sit next to him and help him shift his weight to one buttock for 60 seconds; then repeat the procedure on the other side. Provide pressure-relieving cush-

ions, as appropriate. However, avoid seating the patient on a rubber or plastic doughnut, *which can increase localized pressure at vulnerable points.*

• Adjust or pad appliances, casts, and splints, as needed, *to ensure proper fit and avoid increased pressure and impaired circulation.*

• Tell the patient to avoid heat lamps and harsh soaps *because they dry the skin.* Lotion applied after bathing will help keep the patient's skin moist.

• Tell the patient to avoid vigorous massage because it can damage capillaries.

• If the patient's condition permits, recommend a diet that includes adequate calories, protein, and vitamins. Dietary therapy may involve nutritional consultation, food supplements, enteral feeding, or total parenteral nutrition.

• If diarrhea develops or if the patient is incontinent, clean and dry soiled skin. Then apply a protective moisture barrier *to prevent skin maceration.*

Complications

• Infection may cause foul-smelling drainage, persistent pain, severe erythema, induration, and elevated skin and body temperatures. Advancing infection or cellulitis can lead to septicemia. Severe erythema may signal worsening cellulitis, which indicates that the offending organisms have invaded the tissue and are no longer localized.

Nursing considerations

• Avoid using elbow and heel protectors that fasten with a single narrow strap. *The strap could impair neurovascular function in the involved hand or foot.*

• Avoid using artificial sheepskin. *It doesn't reduce pressure and may create a false sense of security.*

Documentation

• Record the date and time of initial and subsequent treatments.

• Note the specific treatment given.

• Detail preventive strategies.

• Document the pressure ulcer's location and size (length, width, and depth); color and appearance of the wound bed; amount, odor, color, and consistency of drainage; and condition of the surrounding skin.

• Update the care plan as required.

• Note any change in the condition or size of the pressure ulcer and any elevation of skin temperature on the clinical record.

• Document when the doctor was notified of any pertinent abnormal observations.

• Record the patient's temperature daily on the graphic sheet to allow easy assessment of body temperature patterns.

Pulmonary artery and pulmonary artery wedge pressure monitoring

Continuous pulmonary artery pressure (PAP) and intermittent pulmonary artery wedge pressure (PAWP) measurements provide important information about left ventricular function and preload. You can use this information not only for monitoring but also for aiding diagnosis, refining your assessment, guiding interventions, and projecting patient outcome.

Nearly all acutely ill patients are candidates for PAP monitoring, especially those who are hemodynamically unstable, need fluid management or continuous cardiopulmonary assessment, or who are receiving multiple or frequently administered cardioactive drugs. PAP monitoring also is crucial for patients with shock, trauma, pulmonary or cardiac disease, or multiorgan disease.

The PAWP reading accurately reflects left atrial pressure and left ventricular end-diastolic pressure, although the catheter itself never enters the left side of the heart. Obtaining this information is possible because the heart momentarily relaxes during diastole as it fills with blood from the pulmonary veins; at this instant, the pulmonary vasculature, left atrium, and left ventricle act as a single chamber, and all have identical pressures. Thus, changes in PAP and PAWP reflect changes in left ventricular filling pressure, permitting detection of left ventricular impairment.

After the insertion of a pulmonary artery catheter and initial pressure readings are recorded, record subsequent PAP values and monitor waveforms. These values will be used to calculate other important hemodynamic indices.

Normal pressures are as follows:
• Right atrial: 1 to 6 mm Hg
• Systolic right ventricular (RV): 20 to 30 mm Hg
• End-diastolic RV: less than 5 mm Hg
• Systolic PAP: 20 to 30 mm Hg
• Diastolic PAP: about 10 mm Hg
• Mean PAP: less than 20 mm Hg
• PAWP: 6 to 12 mm Hg

• Left atrial: about 10 mm Hg.

An abnormally high right atrial pressure can indicate pulmonary disease, failure of the right side of the heart, fluid overload, cardiac tamponade, tricuspid stenosis and insufficiency, or pulmonary hypertension.

Elevated right ventricular pressure can result from pulmonary hypertension, pulmonary valvular stenosis, right ventricular failure, pericardial effusion, constrictive pericarditis, chronic congestive heart failure, or ventricular septal defects.

An abnormally high PAP is characteristic in increased pulmonary blood flow, as occurs in a left-to-right shunt secondary to atrial or ventricular septal defect; increased pulmonary artery resistance, as occurs in pulmonary hypertension or mitral stenosis; chronic obstructive pulmonary disease; pulmonary edema or embolus; and left ventricular failure from any cause. Pulmonary artery systolic pressure is the same as right ventricular systolic pressure. Pulmonary artery diastolic pressure is the same as left atrial pressure, except in patients with severe pulmonary disease causing pulmonary hypertension.

Elevated PAWP can result from left ventricular failure, mitral stenosis and insufficiency, cardiac tamponade, or cardiac insufficiency; low PAWP can result from hypovolemia.

≫ Key nursing diagnoses and patient outcomes

Use these nursing diagnoses as a guide when developing your plan of care for a patient undergoing pulmonary artery and pulmonary artery wedge pressure monitoring.

Altered cardiopulmonary tissue perfusion related to decreased cellular exchange

Based on this nursing diagnosis, you'll establish the following patient outcomes. The patient will:
• have warm and dry skin.
• maintain adequate cardiac output.
• not exhibit arrhythmias.

Decreased cardiac output related to decreased stroke volume

Based on this nursing diagnosis, you'll establish the following patient outcomes. The patient will:
• attain hemodynamic stability as evidenced by pulse not less than __ beats/minute and not greater than __ beats/minute, blood pressure not less than __ mm Hg and not greater than __ mm Hg.
• exhibit PAP and PAWP measurements within normal limits.
• have a diminished heart workload.
• maintain adequate cardiac output.

Equipment

♦ pressure cuff ♦ balloon-tipped, flow-directed PA catheter ♦ bag of heparin flush solution (usually 500 ml normal saline with 500 or 1,000 units heparin) ♦ alcohol sponges ♦ medication-added label ♦ preassembled disposable pressure tubing with flush device and disposable transducer ♦ monitor and monitor cable ♦ I.V. pole with transducer mount ♦ emergency resuscitation equipment ♦ electrocardiogram (ECG) monitor ♦ ECG electrodes ♦ armboard (for antecubital insertion) ♦ lead aprons (if fluoroscope is used during insertion) ♦ sutures ♦ sterile 4″ × 4″ gauze pads or other dry occlusive dressing material ♦ prepackaged introducer kit ♦ op-

tional: dextrose 5% in water, shaving materials (if femoral insertion site is used).

If a prepackaged introducer kit is unavailable, obtain the following:
♦ an introducer one size larger than the catheter ♦ sterile tray containing instruments for procedure ♦ masks ♦ sterile gowns ♦ sterile gloves ♦ povidone-iodine ointment ♦ sutures ♦ two 10-ml syringes ♦ local anesthetic (1% to 2% lidocaine) ♦ one 5-ml syringe ♦ 25G ½″ needle ♦ 1″ and 3″ tape.

Equipment preparation

• To obtain reliable pressure readings and clear waveforms, the pressure monitoring system and bedside monitor must be properly calibrated and zeroed.
• Make sure the monitor has the correct pressure modules; then calibrate it according to the manufacturer's instructions.

Implementation

• If possible, obtain PAP at end expiration (when the patient completely exhales). *At this time, intrathoracic pressure approaches atmospheric pressure and has the least effect on PAP.* If you obtain a reading during other phases of the respiratory cycle, respiratory interference may occur. For instance, during inspiration, when intrathoracic pressure drops, PAP may be falsely low because the negative pressure is transmitted to the catheter. During expiration, when intrathoracic pressure rises, PAP may be falsely high.
• For patients with a rapid respiratory rate and subsequent variations, you may have trouble identifying end ex-

piration. The monitor displays an average of the digital readings obtained over time as well as the readings from a full respiratory cycle. If possible, obtain a printout. Use the averaged values obtained through the full respiratory cycle. *To analyze trends accurately,* be sure to record values at consistent times during the respiratory cycle.

To take a PAWP reading

PAWP is recorded by inflating the balloon and letting it float in a distal artery. Some hospitals allow only doctors or specially trained nurses to take a PAWP reading because of the risk of pulmonary artery rupture, a rare but life-threatening complication. If hospital policy permits you to perform this procedure, do so with extreme caution and make sure you're thoroughly familiar with intracardiac waveform interpretation. Refer to the following procedure.

• To begin, verify that the transducer is properly leveled and zeroed. Detach the syringe from the balloon inflation hub. Draw 1.5 cc of air into the syringe, and then reattach the syringe to the hub. Watching the monitor, inject the air through the hub slowly and smoothly. When you see a wedge tracing on the monitor, immediately stop inflating the balloon. Never inflate the balloon beyond the volume needed to obtain a wedge tracing.

• Take the pressure reading at end expiration. Note the amount of air needed to change the pulmonary artery tracing to a wedge tracing (normally, 1.25 to 1.5 cc). If the wedge tracing appeared with injection of less than 1.25 cc, suspect that the catheter has migrated into a more distal branch and

requires repositioning. If the balloon is in a more distal branch, the tracings might move up the oscilloscope, indicating that the catheter tip is recording balloon pressure rather than PAWP. This can lead to pulmonary artery rupture.

Complications

• Complications of pulmonary artery catheter insertion include pulmonary artery perforation, pulmonary infarction, catheter knotting, local or systemic infection, cardiac arrhythmias, and heparin-induced thrombocytopenia.

Nursing considerations

• Advise the patient to use caution when moving about in bed *to avoid dislodging the catheter.*

• Be sure to tell the patient and members of his family not to be alarmed if they see the pressure waveform on the monitor move around. Explain that the cause usually is artifact.

• Never leave the balloon inflated *because this may cause pulmonary infarction.* To determine if the balloon is inflated, check the monitor for a wedge tracing, which indicates inflation. (A pulmonary artery tracing confirms balloon deflation.)

• Never inflate the balloon with more than the recommended air volume (specified on the catheter shaft) *because this may cause loss of elasticity or balloon rupture.* With appropriate inflation volume, the balloon floats easily through the heart chambers and rests in the main branch of the pulmonary artery, producing accurate waveforms. If the patient has a suspected left-to-right shunt, use carbon dioxide to inflate the balloon, as ordered, *because it diffuses more quickly than air.* Never inflate the balloon with fluids *because it may not be possible to retrieve it from inside the balloon, thus preventing deflation.*

• Be aware that the catheter may slip back into the right ventricle. *Because the tip may irritate the ventricle,* be sure to detect this problem promptly by checking the monitor for a right ventricular waveform.

• *To minimize valvular trauma,* make sure the balloon is deflated whenever the catheter is withdrawn from the pulmonary artery to the right ventricle or from the right ventricle to the right atrium.

• The Centers for Disease Control and Prevention (CDC) recommends changing the dressing whenever it's moist or every 24 to 48 hours, redressing the site according to hospital policy, changing the catheter every 72 hours, changing the pressure tubing every 48 hours, and changing the flush solution every 24 hours. However, these recommendations were issued in 1982. Since then, some hospitals have maintained closed-pressure monitoring systems for longer than the recommended times with no increase in infection rates. Nonetheless, before departing from CDC recommendations, determine your hospital's policy.

Documentation

• Document PAP waveforms at the beginning of each shift, and monitor them frequently throughout each shift and with changes in treatment.

• Check and document PAWP and cardiac output regularly (usually every 6 hours).

Pulmonary artery catheterization

The original catheter for pulmonary artery catheterization, which had two lumens, was invented by two doctors, Swan and Ganz. The device still bears their names (Swan-Ganz catheter) but is commonly referred to as a pulmonary artery (PA) catheter. Current versions have as many as six lumens, allowing more hemodynamic information to be gathered. Besides distal and proximal lumens used to measure pressures, a PA catheter has a balloon inflation lumen that inflates the balloon for pulmonary artery wedge pressure (PAWP) measurement and a thermistor connector lumen that allows cardiac output measurement. Some catheters also have a pacemaker wire lumen that provides a port for pacemaker electrodes and measures continuous mixed venous oxygen saturation. (See *PA catheter: From basic to complex.*)

PA catheterization is usually performed at bedside in an intensive care unit. The catheter is inserted through the cephalic vein in the antecubital fossa or the subclavian (sometimes femoral) vein. In addition to measuring atrial and pulmonary arterial pressures, this procedure is used to evaluate pulmonary vascular resistance and tissue oxygenation, as indicated by mixed venous oxygen content. It should be performed cautiously in patients with left bundle-branch block or implanted pacemakers.

PA catheter: From basic to complex

Depending on the intended uses, a pulmonary artery (PA) catheter may be simple or complex. The basic PA catheter has a distal and proximal lumen, a thermistor, and a balloon inflation gate valve. The *distal lumen,* which exits in the pulmonary artery, monitors PA pressure. Its hub usually is marked "PA distal" or is color-coded yellow. The *proximal lumen* exits in the right atrium or vena cava, depending on the size of the patient's heart. It monitors right atrial pressure and can be used as the injected solution lumen for cardiac output determination and infusing solutions. The proximal lumen hub usually is marked "Proximal" or is color-coded blue.

The *thermistor,* located about 1½" (4 cm) from the distal tip, measures temperature (aiding core temperature evaluation) and allows cardiac output measurement. The thermistor connector attaches to a cardiac output connector cable, then to a cardiac output monitor. Typically, it's red.

The *balloon inflation gate valve* is used for inflating the balloon tip with air. A stopcock connection, typically color-coded red, may be used.

Additional lumens

Some PA catheters have additional lumens used to obtain other hemodynamic data or permit certain interventions. For instance, a *proximal infusion port,* which exits in the right atrium or vena cava, allows additional fluid administration. A *right ventricular lumen,* exiting in the right ventricle, allows fluid administration, right ventricular pressure measurement, or use of a temporary ventricular pacing lead.

Some catheters have additional right atrial and right ventricular lumens for atrioventricular pacing. A *right ventricular ejection fraction fast-response thermistor,* with PA and right ventricular sensing electrodes, allows volumetric and ejection fraction measurements. Fiberoptic filaments, such as those used in pulse oximetry, exit into the pulmonary artery and permit measurement of continuous mixed venous oxygen saturation.

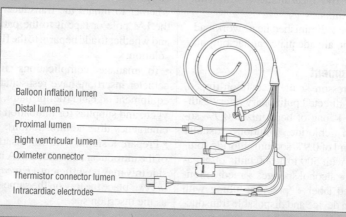

Balloon inflation lumen
Distal lumen
Proximal lumen
Right ventricular lumen
Oximeter connector
Thermistor connector lumen
Intracardiac electrodes

≫ Key nursing diagnoses and patient outcomes

Use these nursing diagnoses as a guide when developing your plan of care for a patient undergoing pulmonary artery catheterization.

Altered cardiopulmonary tissue perfusion related to decreased cellular exchange

Based on this nursing diagnosis, you'll establish the following patient outcomes. The patient will:
• have warm and dry skin.
• maintain adequate cardiac output.
• not exhibit arrhythmias.

Decreased cardiac output related to decreased stroke volume

Based on this nursing diagnosis, you'll establish the following patient outcomes. The patient will:
• attain hemodynamic stability as evidenced by pulse not less than __ beats/minute and not greater than __ beats/minute, blood pressure not less than __ mm Hg and not greater than __ mm Hg.
• exhibit pulmonary artery pressure and PAWP measurements within normal limits.
• have a diminished heart workload.
• maintain adequate cardiac output.

Equipment

♦ pressure cuff ♦ balloon-tipped, flow-directed pulmonary artery catheter ♦ bag of heparinized 0.9% sodium chloride solution (usually 500 ml of 0.9% sodium chloride solution with 500 to 1,000 units of heparin) ♦ alcohol sponges ♦ medication-added label ♦ pressure tubing with flush device and disposable transducer ♦ I.V. pole with transducer mount ♦ emergency resuscitation equipment ♦ armboard (for antecubital insertion) ♦ lead aprons (if fluoroscope is used during insertion) ♦ sutures ♦ 4″ × 4″ gauze pads or other dry occlusive dressing material ♦ prepackaged introducer kit ♦ dextrose 5% in water ♦ shaving materials (optional).

If a prepackaged introducer kit is not available, obtain the following: ♦ introducer (one size larger than the catheter) ♦ sterile tray containing instruments for procedure ♦ masks ♦ sterile gowns and gloves ♦ povidone-iodine ointment ♦ sutures ♦ two 10-ml syringes ♦ local anesthetic (1% to 2% lidocaine) ♦ one 5-ml syringe ♦ 25G ½″ needle and 3″ tape.

Equipment preparation

• Turn the monitor on before gathering the equipment to give it sufficient time to warm up. Be sure to check the operations manual for the monitor you're using; some older monitors may need 20 minutes to warm up.
• Prepare the pressure monitoring system according to hospital policy. Hospital guidelines also may specify whether to mount the transducer on the I.V. pole or tape it to the patient and whether to add heparin to the flush solution.
• To manage complications from catheter insertion, have resuscitation equipment on hand (defibrillator, oxygen, and supplies for intubation and emergency drug administration).
• Prepare a sterile field for insertion of the introducer and catheter. (A bedside tray may be sufficient.) *For easier access,* place the tray on the same side as the insertion site.

• Maintain aseptic technique and use universal precautions throughout catheter preparation and insertion.

• Wash your hands. Clean the insertion site with povidone-iodine ointment and drape it appropriately.

• Put on a mask. Help the doctor put on a sterile mask, gown, and gloves.

• Open the outer packaging of the catheter, revealing the inner sterile wrapping. Using aseptic technique, the doctor opens the inner wrapping and picks up the catheter. Take the catheter lumen hubs as the doctor hands them to you.

• *To remove air from the catheter and verify its patency,* flush the catheter. In the more common flushing method, you connect the syringes aseptically to the appropriate pressure lines, and then flush them before insertion. *This method makes pressure waveforms easier to identify on the monitor during insertion.*

• Alternatively, you may flush the lumens after catheter insertion with sterile I.V. solution from sterile syringes attached to the lumens. Leave the filled syringes on during insertion.

• If the system has multiple pressure lines (such as a distal line to monitor PA pressure and a proximal line to monitor right atrial pressure), make sure the distal PA lumen hub is attached to the pressure line that will be observed on the monitor. *Inadvertently attaching the distal PA line to the proximal lumen hub would prevent the proper waveform from appearing during insertion.*

• Observe the diastolic values carefully during insertion. Make sure the scale is appropriate for lower pressures. A scale of 0 to 25 or 0 to 50 mm Hg (more common) is preferred.

(With a higher scale, such as 0 to 100 or 0 to 250 mm Hg, waveforms appear too small and the location of the catheter tip is difficult to identify.)

• *To verify the integrity of the balloon,* the doctor inflates it with air (usually 1.5 cc) before handing you the lumens to attach to the pressure monitoring system. The doctor then observes the balloon for symmetrical shape. He also may submerge it in a small, sterile basin filled with sterile water and observe it for bubbles, which indicate a leak.

• *To obtain reliable pressure values and clear waveforms,* the pressure monitoring system and bedside monitor must be properly calibrated and zeroed. Make sure the monitor has the correct pressure modules; then calibrate it according to the manufacturer's instructions.

Patient preparation

• Explain to the patient that this test is used to evaluate heart function and provides information necessary to determine appropriate therapy or to manage fluid status.

• Tell the patient that there are no food or fluid restrictions.

• Describe the test, including who will perform it and where.

• Tell the patient that he'll be conscious during catheterization and may feel transient local discomfort from the administration of the local anesthetic.

• Explain that catheter insertion takes about 30 minutes but that the catheter will remain in place, causing little or no discomfort, for 48 to 72 hours. Tell him that he will need to stay in bed *to avoid dislodging the catheter.*

• Instruct the patient to report any discomfort immediately.

• Make sure the patient or a responsible family member has signed a consent form.

• Assist the patient to a supine position. For antecubital insertion, his arm is abducted with palm upward on an overbed table for support; for subclavian insertion, the patient is placed in the supine position with his head and shoulders slightly lower than his trunk to make the vein more accessible. If the patient can't tolerate the supine position, assist him to semi-Fowler's position. During the test, monitor all pressures with the patient in the same position.

Implementation

• Assist the doctor as the introducer is inserted to gain access to the vessel. The doctor may perform a cutdown or (more commonly) insert the catheter percutaneously, as with a modified Seldinger technique.

• After the introducer is placed, and the catheter lumens are flushed, the doctor inserts the catheter through the introducer. In the internal jugular or subclavian approach, the catheter is inserted into the end of the introducer sheath with the balloon deflated, directing the curl of the catheter toward the patient's midline.

• As insertion begins, observe the bedside monitor for waveform variations. (See *Normal PA waveforms*.)

• When the catheter exits the introducer sheath and reaches the junction of the superior vena cava and right atrium (at the 15- to 20-cm mark on the catheter shaft), the monitor shows oscillations that correspond to the patient's respirations. The balloon is then inflated with the recommended volume of air. *This allows normal blood flow and aids catheter insertion.*

• Using a gentle, smooth motion, the doctor advances the catheter through the heart chambers, moving rapidly to the PA to avoid prolonged manipulation, which can reduce catheter stiffness.

• When the mark on the catheter shaft reaches 15 to 20 cm, the catheter enters the right atrium. The waveform shows two small, upright waves; pressure is low (from 2 to 4 mm Hg). Read pressure values in the mean mode *because systolic and diastolic values are similar.*

• The doctor advances the catheter into the right ventricle, working quickly to minimize irritation. The waveform now shows sharp systolic upstrokes and lower diastolic dips. Depending on the size of the patient's heart, the catheter should reach the 30- to 35-cm mark. (The smaller the heart, the less catheter length will be needed to reach the right ventricle.) Record both systolic and diastolic pressures. Systolic pressure normally ranges from 15 to 25 mm Hg; diastolic pressure, from 0 to 8 mm Hg.

• As the catheter floats into the pulmonary artery, note that the upstroke from right ventricular systole is smoother, and systolic pressure is nearly the same as right ventricular systolic pressure. Record systolic, diastolic, and mean pressures (typically ranging from 8 to 15 mm Hg). A dicrotic notch on the diastolic portion of the waveform indicates pulmonic valve closure.

Normal PA waveforms

During pulmonary artery (PA) catheter insertion, the monitor shows various waveforms as the catheter advances through the heart chambers.

Right atrium

When the catheter tip enters the right atrium, the first heart chamber on its route, a waveform like the one shown below appears on the monitor. Note the two small upright waves. The *a* waves represent left atrial contraction; the *v* waves, increased pressure or volume in the left atrium during left ventricular systole.

like the one shown below. Note that the upstroke is smoother than on the right ventricular waveform. The dicrotic notch indicates pulmonic valve closure.

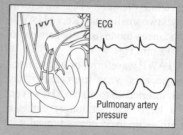

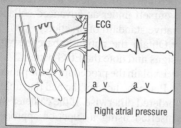

Right ventricle

As the catheter tip reaches the right ventricle, you'll see a waveform with sharp systolic upstrokes and lower diastolic dips.

PAWP

Floating into a distal branch of the pulmonary artery, the balloon wedges where the vessel becomes too narrow for it to pass. The monitor now shows a pulmonary artery wedge pressure (PAWP) waveform, with two small uprises from left atrial systole and diastole. The balloon is then deflated and the catheter is left in the pulmonary artery.

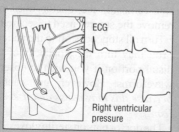

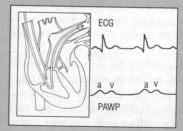

Pulmonary artery

The catheter then floats into the pulmonary artery, causing a waveform

To wedge the catheter

• To obtain a wedge tracing, the doctor lets the inflated balloon float downstream with venous blood flow to a smaller, more distal branch of the PA. Here, the catheter lodges, or wedges, causing occlusion of right ventricular and PA diastolic pressures. The tracing resembles the right atrial tracing because the catheter tip is recording left atrial pressure. The waveform shows two small peaks. Record PAWP in the mean mode (usually between 6 and 12 mm Hg).

• A PAWP waveform, or wedge tracing, appears when the catheter has been inserted 45 to 50 cm. (However, in a large heart, a longer catheter length — up to 55 cm — typically is required. A catheter should never be inserted more than 60 cm.) Usually, 30 to 45 seconds elapse from the time the doctor inserts the introducer until the wedge tracing appears.

• The doctor deflates the balloon, and the catheter drifts out of the wedge position and into the PA, its normal resting place.

• If the appropriate waveforms don't appear at the expected times during catheter insertion, the catheter may be coiled in the right atrium and ventricle. To correct this problem, deflate the balloon. To do this, unlock the gate valve or turn the stopcock to the ON position, and then detach the syringe from the balloon inflation port. Back pressure in the pulmonary artery causes the balloon to deflate on its own. (Active air withdrawal may compromise balloon integrity.) *To verify balloon deflation,* observe the monitor for return of the PA tracing.

• Typically, the doctor orders a portable chest X-ray to confirm catheter position.

• Apply a sterile occlusive dressing to the insertion site.

• Set alarms on the electrocardiogram (ECG) and pressure monitors.

• Monitor vital signs.

• Take routine aseptic precautions to prevent infection.

To remove the catheter

• To assist the doctor, inspect the chest X-ray for signs of catheter kinking or knotting. (In some states, you may be permitted to remove a PA catheter yourself under an advanced collaborative standard of practice.)

• Obtain the patient's baseline vital signs and note the ECG pattern.

• Explain the procedure to the patient.

• Place the head of the bed flat, unless ordered otherwise. If the catheter was inserted using a superior approach, turn the patient's head to the side opposite the insertion site. Gently remove the dressing.

• The doctor removes any sutures securing the catheter. However, the introducer is to be left in place after catheter removal, the doctor does not remove the sutures used to secure it.

• Turn all stopcocks off to the patient. (You may turn the stopcocks of the distal port on if you wish to observe waveforms. However, use caution *because this may cause an air embolism.*)

• The doctor puts on sterile gloves. After verifying that the balloon is deflated, the catheter is withdrawn slowly and smoothly. If any resistance is felt as the catheter is withdrawn, the doctor stops immediately.

- Watch the ECG monitor for arrhythmias.
- If the introducer was removed, apply pressure to the site, and check it frequently *for signs of bleeding.* Dress the site again, as necessary. If the introducer is left in place, observe the diaphragm for any blood backflow, *which verifies the integrity of the hemostasis valve.*
- Return all equipment to the appropriate location. You may turn off the bedside pressure modules but leave the ECG module on.
- Reassure the patient and family members that he will be observed closely. Make sure the patient understands that the catheter was removed because his condition has improved and he no longer needs it.

Complications
- Complications may include pulmonary emboli, PA perforation, heart murmurs, thrombi, and arrhythmias.

Nursing considerations
- Maintain 300 mm Hg of pressure in the pressure bag to permit fluid flow of 3 to 6 ml/hour. Instruct the patient to extend the appropriate arm (or leg, if the catheter is inserted in the femoral vein).
- If a damped waveform occurs, the catheter may need to be withdrawn slightly. Pulmonary infarct may occur if the catheter is allowed to remain in a wedged position.
- Make sure stopcocks are properly positioned and connections are secure. *Loose connections may allow air into the system or cause blood backup, leakage of deoxygenated blood, or inaccurate pressure readings.*

- Be sure the lumen hubs are properly identified to serve the appropriate catheter ports. Don't add or remove fluids from the distal pulmonary artery port; *this may cause pulmonary extravasation or damage the artery.*
- If the catheter was not sutured to the skin, tape it securely to prevent dislodgment.

Documentation
- Document the date and time of catheter insertion, the doctor who performed the procedure, the catheter insertion site, pressure waveforms and values for the various heart chambers, balloon inflation volume required to obtain a wedge tracing, any arrhythmias occurring during or after the procedure, type of flush solution used and its heparin concentration (if any), type of dressing applied, and the patient's tolerance of the procedure. Remember to initial and date the dressing.
- After catheter removal, document the patient's tolerance for the removal procedure, and note any problems encountered during removal.

Pulse amplitude monitoring

Determining the presence and strength of peripheral pulses, an essential part of cardiovascular assessment, helps you to evaluate the adequacy of peripheral perfusion. A pulse amplitude monitor simplifies this procedure. A sensor taped to the patient's skin over a pulse point sends signals to a monitor, which measures the amplitude of the pulse and displays it as a waveform on a screen. The system continuously monitors the patient's peripheral pulse so you can perform other patient care duties.

The pulse amplitude monitor can be used after peripheral vascular reconstruction on the upper or lower extremities or after percutaneous transluminal peripheral or coronary angioplasty (either with the sheaths in place or after they've been removed).

Because the sensor monitors only relatively flat pulse points, it can't be used for the posterior tibial pulse point. Also, movement distorts the waveform, so the patient must stay as still as possible during monitoring. The patient shouldn't have lesions on the skin where the pulse will be monitored because the sensor must be placed directly on this site. The sensor and tape could irritate the lesion, or the lesion could impair transmission of the pulse amplitude. If the patient has a strong peripheral pulse, you'll see an adequate waveform.

》 Key nursing diagnoses and patient outcomes
Use these nursing diagnoses as a guide when developing your plan of care.

Altered peripheral tissue perfusion related to (specify)
Based on this nursing diagnosis, you'll establish the following patient outcomes. The patient will:
• express a feeling of comfort or absence of pain at rest.
• have peripheral pulses that are present and strong.
• have skin color and temperature that remain unchanged.
• have no evidence of pressure ulcers.
• maintain tissue perfusion and cellular oxygenation.

Decreased cardiac output related to decreased stroke volume
Based on this nursing diagnosis, you'll establish the following patient outcomes. The patient will:
• attain hemodynamic stability, as evidenced by pulse not less than __ beats/minute and not greater than __ beats/minute, blood pressure not less than __ mm Hg and not greater than __ mm Hg.
• have warm and dry skin.
• have a diminished heart workload.
• maintain adequate cardiac output.

Equipment
♦ pulse amplitude display monitor with sensor.

Equipment preparation
• Plug the monitor into a grounded outlet. Although the monitor has battery power for up to 24 hours, it should be plugged in when the battery isn't needed.
• Turn on the monitor and allow it to warm up, which may take up to 10 seconds. Plug the sensor cable into the monitor; then tap the sensor gently. If tapping causes interference on the display screen, assume the sensor-monitor connection is functioning properly.

Patient preparation
• Explain to the patient how the pulse amplitude monitor works.
• Locate the pulse you want to monitor. Mention that you'll tape the sensor to a selected site, usually the foot.

Implementation
• Place the sensor over the strongest point of the pulse you're going to monitor. While observing the display

screen, move the sensor until you see a strong upright waveform.
• Without moving the sensor from this site, peel off the adhesive strips and affix the sensor securely to the patient's foot. *The sensor must maintain proper skin contact, so be sure to tape it firmly.*
• Adjust the height of the pulse wave signal to half the height of the display screen. *This will give the waveform room to fluctuate as the pulse amplitude increases and decreases.*
• Set the low and high waveform amplitude alarms *so you'll be alerted to any waveform changes.*

To discontinue monitor use
• Peel the sensor tapes from the patient's skin.
• Turn the machine off but keep it plugged in.
• Discard the sensor and, if necessary, wipe the monitor with a mild soap solution.

Nursing considerations
• Be aware that although the waveform displayed by a pulse amplitude monitor may resemble an ECG or blood pressure waveform, it's not the same.
• Don't apply much pressure on the pulse sensor film or press on it with a sharp object *because such stress may warp or destroy the sensor.*
• Never place the sensor over an open wound or ulcerated skin.
• If waveform amplitude decreases, assess the patient's leg for capillary refill time, temperature, color, and sensation. *The amplitude change may stem from a malfunction in the monitor itself (such as a low battery) or from a thrombus, a hematoma, or a*

significant change in the patient's hemodynamic status.
• If the display screen is blank when you turn on the machine, make sure that the monitor is plugged in. If it's plugged in but the screen remains blank, *the screen may need repair.*
• If the screen is functioning but no waveform appears on it, first check the sensor-monitor connection. Then check the sensor by gently tapping it to see if interference appears on the screen. If the sensor is working properly, relocate the peripheral pulse on the patient's foot, and reapply the sensor. If your interventions don't work, the screen may need servicing.

Documentation
• Print out a strip of the patient's waveform, and place the strip in the patient's medical record during every shift and whenever you note a change in the waveform or the patient's condition.
• Along the left side of the strip is a reference scale that's used to measure pulse amplitude height. Include this scale in your documentation.

Pulse and ear oximetry

Oximetry is a relatively simple procedure that's used to noninvasively monitor arterial oxygen saturation. It may be performed intermittently or continuously.

Pulse oximeters usually denote arterial oxygen saturation values with the symbol SpO_2 to differentiate electronically measured from invasively measured arterial oxygen saturation (SaO_2). Two diodes send red and infrared light through a pulsating arterial vascular bed, like the one in the fingertip. A photodetector slipped over the finger measures the transmitted light as it passes through the vascular bed, detects the relative amount of color absorbed by arterial blood, and calculates the exact SaO_2 without interference from surrounding venous blood, skin, connective tissue, or bone.

Ear oximetry works by monitoring the transmission of light waves through the vascular bed of a patient's earlobe. However, results may be inaccurate if the patient's earlobe is poorly perfused, as from a low cardiac output. (See *How oximetry works*.)

≫ Key nursing diagnoses and patient outcomes

Use these nursing diagnoses as a guide when developing your plan of care.

Impaired gas exchange related to altered oxygen supply

Based on this nursing diagnosis, you'll establish the following patient outcomes. The patient will:
• maintain respiratory rate within ± 5 breaths/minute of baseline.
• express feeling of comfort in maintaining air exchange.
• have normal breath sounds.
• have arterial blood gas levels return to baseline, as evidenced by (specify) pH; (specify) partial pressure of arterial oxygen; and (specify) partial pressure of arterial carbon dioxide.

Ineffective breathing pattern related to (specify)

Based on this nursing diagnosis, you'll establish the following patient outcomes. The patient will:

• have pulse and ear oximetry levels that remain between 95% and 100% for adults, and 93.8% to 100% by 1 hour after birth in healthy, full-term neonates.
• report feeling comfortable when breathing.
• achieve maximum lung expansion with adequate ventilation.

Equipment

♦ oximeter ♦ finger or ear probe ♦ alcohol sponges ♦ nail polish remover, if necessary.

Equipment preparation

• Review the manufacturer's instructions for assembling the oximeter.

Patient preparation

• Explain the procedure to the patient.

Implementation

To perform pulse oximetry

• Select a finger for the test. Although the index finger is commonly used, a smaller finger may be selected if the patient's fingers are too large for the equipment.
• Make sure the patient isn't wearing false fingernails, and remove any nail polish from the test finger.
• Place the transducer (photodetector) probe over the patient's finger so that light beams and sensors oppose each other. If the patient has long fingernails, position the probe perpendicular to the finger, if possible, or clip the fingernail.
• Always position the patient's hand at heart level *to eliminate venous pulsations and to promote accurate readings*.
• When testing a neonate or small infant, wrap the probe around the foot

How oximetry works

The pulse oximeter allows noninvasive monitoring of a patient's arterial oxygen saturation (SaO_2) levels by measuring the absorption (amplitude) of light waves as they pass through areas of the body that are highly perfused by arterial blood. Oximetry also monitors pulse rate and amplitude.

Light-emitting diodes in a transducer (photodetector) attached to the patient's body (shown here on the index finger) send red and infrared light beams through tissue. The photodetector records the relative amount of each color absorbed by arterial blood and transmits the data to a monitor, which displays the information with each heartbeat. If the SaO_2 level or pulse rate varies from preset limits, the monitor triggers visual and audible alarms.

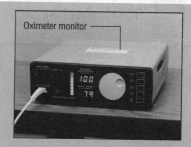

Oximeter monitor

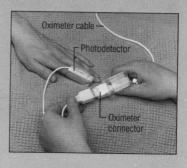

Oximeter cable
Photodetector
Oximeter connector

so that light beams and detectors oppose each other.

• For a large infant, use a probe that fits on the great toe and secure it to the foot.

• Turn on the power switch. If the device is working properly, a beep sounds, a display lights momentarily, and the pulse searchlight flashes. The SpO_2 and pulse rate displays show stationary zeros. After four to six heartbeats, the SpO_2 and pulse rate displays supply information with each beat, and the pulse amplitude indicator begins tracking the pulse.

To perform ear oximetry

• Using an alcohol sponge, massage the patient's earlobe for 10 to 20 seconds. Mild erythema indicates adequate vascularization.

• Following the manufacturer's instructions, attach the ear probe to the patient's earlobe or pinna. Use the ear probe stabilizer for prolonged or exercise testing. Be sure to establish good contact on the ear; *an unstable probe may set off the low-perfusion alarm.* After the probe has been attached for a few seconds, a saturation reading and pulse waveform appear on the oximeter's screen.

• Leave the ear probe in place for 3 or more minutes until readings stabilize at the highest point, or take three sep-

PROBLEM SOLVER

 Troubleshooting pulse oximeter problems

To maintain a continuous display of SaO$_2$ levels, you'll need to keep the monitoring site clean and dry. Make sure the skin doesn't become irritated from adhesives used to keep disposable probes in place. You may need to change the site if this happens. Disposable probes that irritate the skin also can be replaced by nondisposable models that don't need tape.

Another common problem with pulse oximeters is the failure of the devices to obtain a signal. Your first reaction if this happens should be to check the patient's vital signs. If they're sufficient to produce a signal, then check for the following problems:

• *Poor connection.* See if the sensors are properly aligned. Make sure that wires are intact and securely fastened and that the pulse oximeter is plugged into a power source.

• *Inadequate or intermittent blood flow to the site.* Check the patient's pulse rate and capillary refill time, and take corrective action if blood flow to the site is decreased. This may mean loosening restraints, removing tight-fitting clothes, taking off a blood pressure cuff, or checking arterial and I.V. lines. If none of these interventions works, you may need to find an alternate site. Finding a site with proper circulation may also prove challenging when a patient is receiving vasoconstrictive drugs.

• *Equipment malfunctions.* Remove the pulse oximeter from the patient, put the alarm limits at 85% and 100%, and try the instrument on yourself or another healthy person. This will tell you if the equipment is working correctly.

arate readings and average them. Make sure you revascularize the patient's earlobe each time.

• After the procedure, remove the probe, turn off and unplug the unit, and clean the probe by gently rubbing it with an alcohol sponge.

Nursing considerations

• If oximetry is performed properly, readings are typically accurate. However, certain factors may interfere with accuracy. For example, an elevated bilirubin level may falsely lower SpO$_2$ readings, while elevated carboxyhemoglobin or methemoglobin levels (such as occur in heavy smokers or urban dwellers) can cause a falsely elevated SpO$_2$ reading.

• Certain intravascular substances — such as lipid emulsions and dyes — can also prevent accurate readings.

• Other factors that may interfere with accurate results include excessive light (such as from phototherapy, surgical lamps, direct sunlight, and excessive ambient lighting), excessive patient movement, dense ear pigment, hypothermia, hypotension, and vasoconstriction.

• If light is a problem, cover the probes; if patient movement is a problem, move the probe or select a different probe; if ear pigment is a problem, reposition the probe, revascularize the site, or use a finger probe. (See *Troubleshooting pulse oximeter problems*.)

• Normal SpO_2 levels for ear and pulse oximetry are 95% to 100% for adults, and 93.8% to 100% by 1 hour after birth for healthy, full-term neonates. Lower levels may indicate hypoxemia that warrants intervention. For such patients, follow hospital policy or the doctor's orders, which may include increasing oxygen therapy.

• If SaO_2 levels decrease suddenly, you may need to resuscitate the patient immediately.

• Notify the doctor of any significant change in the patient's condition.

Documentation

• Document the date, time, and type of procedure; oximetric measurement; and any action taken.

• Record reading on appropriate flowcharts if indicated.

Pulse measurement

Blood pumped by the heart into an already-full aorta during ventricular contraction creates a fluid wave that travels from the heart to the peripheral arteries. This recurring wave — called a pulse — can be palpated at locations on the body where an artery crosses over bone or firm tissue. (See *Pulse points*, page 736.)

In adults and children over age 3, the radial artery in the wrist is the most common palpation site because it's easily accessible and the artery can be compressed readily against the radius. In infants and children under age 3, a stethoscope is used to listen to the heart itself rather than palpating a pulse. Because auscultation is done at the heart's apex, this is called the apical pulse.

An apical-radial pulse is taken by simultaneously counting apical and radial beats — the first by auscultation at the apex of the heart, the second by palpation at the radial artery. Some heartbeats detected at the apex aren't strong enough to be detected at peripheral sites. When this occurs, the apical pulse rate is higher than the radial; the difference between the two rates is the pulse deficit.

Pulse measurement involves determining the rate (number of beats per minute), rhythm (pattern or regularity of the beats), and volume (amount of blood pumped with each beat). If the pulse is faint or weak, use a Doppler ultrasound blood flow detector if available. (See *Detecting blood flow with Doppler ultrasound*, page 737.)

≫ Key nursing diagnoses and patient outcomes

Use these nursing diagnoses as a guide when developing your plan of care.

Altered peripheral tissue perfusion related to (specify)

Based on this nursing diagnosis, you'll establish the following patient outcomes. The patient will:

• express a feeling of comfort or absence of pain at rest.

• have peripheral pulses that are present and strong.

Pulse points

Shown below are anatomic locations where an artery crosses bone or firm tissue and can be palpated for a pulse.

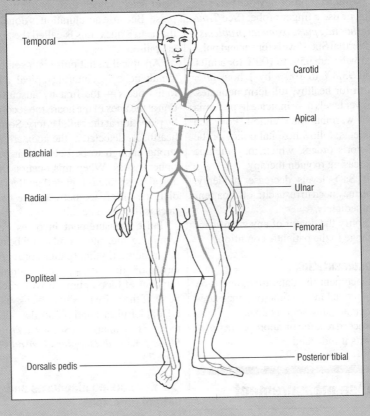

• have skin color and temperature that remain unchanged.
• have no evidence of pressure ulcers.
• maintain tissue perfusion and cellular oxygenation.

Decreased cardiac output related to decreased stroke volume

Based on this nursing diagnosis, you'll establish the following patient outcomes. The patient will:

• attain hemodynamic stability, as evidenced by pulse not less than __ beats/minute and not greater than __ beats/minute, blood pressure not less than __ mm Hg and not greater than __ mm Hg.
• have warm and dry skin
• have a diminished heart workload
• maintain adequate cardiac output.

Detecting blood flow with Doppler ultrasound

More sensitive than palpation for determining pulse rate, the Doppler ultrasound blood flow detector is especially useful when a pulse is faint or weak. Unlike palpation, which detects arterial wall expansion and retraction, this instrument detects the motion of red blood cells.

To use the Doppler device

• Apply a small amount of coupling gel or transmission gel (not water-soluble lubricant) to the ultrasound probe.

• Position the probe on the skin directly over the selected artery. In the top illustration, the probe is over the posterior tibial artery.

• When using a Doppler model like the one pictured top right, turn the instrument on and, moving counterclockwise, set the volume control to the lowest setting. If your model doesn't have a speaker, plug in the earphones and slowly raise the volume. The Doppler ultrasound stethoscope shown at lower right is basically a stethoscope fitted with an audio unit, volume control, and transducer, which amplifies the movement of red blood cells.

• To obtain the best signals with either device, tilt the probe 45 degrees from the artery, making sure to put gel between the skin and the probe. Slowly move the probe in a circular motion to locate the center of the artery and the Doppler signal — a hissing noise at the heartbeat. Avoid moving the probe rapidly because this distorts the signal.

• Count the signals for 60 seconds to determine the pulse rate.

• After you've measured the pulse rate, clean the probe with a soft cloth soaked in antiseptic solution or soapy water. Don't immerse the probe or bump it against a hard surface.

Doppler probe with amplifier

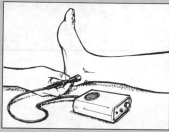

Doppler ultrasound stethoscope

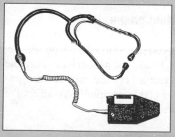

Equipment

♦ watch with second hand ♦ stethoscope (for auscultating apical pulse) ♦ Doppler ultrasound blood flow detector, if necessary.

Equipment preparation

• If you're not using your own stethoscope, disinfect the earpieces with an alcohol sponge before and after use to prevent cross-contamination.

Identifying pulse patterns

TYPE	RATE
Normal	60 to 80 beats/minute; in neonates, 120 to 140 beats/minute
Tachycardia	Above 100 beats/minute
Bradycardia	Below 60 beats/minute
Irregular	Uneven time intervals between beats (for example, periods of regular rhythm interrupted by pauses or premature beats)

Patient preparation
• Wash your hands, and tell the patient that you intend to take his pulse.
• Make sure the patient is comfortable and relaxed because an awkward, uncomfortable position may affect the heart rate.

Implementation
Follow the steps below to measure a patient's pulse.

Taking a radial pulse
• Place the patient in a sitting or supine position, with his arm at his side or across his chest.
• Gently press your index, middle, and ring fingers on the radial artery,

inside the patient's wrist. You should feel a pulse with only moderate pressure; *excessive pressure may obstruct blood flow distal to the pulse site.* Don't use your thumb to take the patient's pulse *because the strong pulse in your thumb may be confused with the patient's.*
• After you've located the pulse, count the beats for 60 seconds, or, if it's more convenient, count for 30 seconds and multiply by 2. *Counting for a full minute provides a more accurate picture of irregularities.* While counting the rate, assess pulse rhythm and volume by noting the pattern and strength of the beats. If you detect an irregularity, repeat the count *because pulse irreg-*

RHYTHM (PER 3 SECONDS)	CAUSES AND INCIDENCE
● ● ● ●	• Varies with such factors as age, physical activity, and sex (men usually have lower pulse rates than women)
●●●●●●●	• Accompanies stimulation of the sympathetic nervous system by emotional stress — anger, fear, anxiety — or certain drugs, such as caffeine • May result from exercise and from certain health conditions, such as congestive heart failure, anemia, and fever (which increases oxygen requirements and therefore pulse rate)
● ● ●	• Accompanies stimulation of the parasympathetic nervous system by drugs — especially digitalis — and such conditions as cerebral hemorrhage and heart block • May also be present in fit athletes
●●●● ●●●	• May indicate cardiac irritability, hypoxia, digitalis overdose, potassium imbalance, or sometimes more serious arrhythmias if frequent premature beats • Occasional premature beats normal

ularities are important signs. Note if the irregularity occurs in a pattern or randomly. If doubt remains, take an apical pulse. (See *Identifying pulse patterns.*)

Taking an apical pulse
• Help the patient to a supine position and drape him if necessary.
• Warm the diaphragm or bell of the stethoscope in your hand before applying it to the patient's chest. *Keep in mind that the bell transmits low-pitched sounds more effectively than the diaphragm.*
• Place the diaphragm or bell of the stethoscope over the apex of the heart, which normally is located at the fifth

intercostal space left of the midclavicular line. Then insert the earpieces into your ears. Count the beats for 60 seconds (or count for 30 seconds and multiply by 2) and note their rhythm and volume. Also evaluate the intensity (loudness) of heart sounds.
• Remove the stethoscope and make sure the patient is comfortable.

Taking an apical-radial pulse
• Two nurses work together to obtain the apical-radial pulse; one palpates the radial pulse while the other auscultates the apical pulse with a stethoscope. Both must use the same watch when counting beats.

• Help the patient to a supine position and drape him if necessary.
• Locate the apical and radial pulses.
• Determine a time to begin counting. Then each nurse counts beats for 60 seconds.

Nursing considerations
• When the peripheral pulse is irregular, take an apical pulse *to measure the heartbeat more directly.*
• If the pulse is faint or weak, use a Doppler ultrasound blood flow detector, if available.
• If a second nurse is not available to help take an apical-radial pulse, hold the stethoscope in place with the hand that holds the watch while palpating the radial pulse with the other hand. *You can then feel any discrepancies between the apical and radial pulses.*

Documentation
• Record pulse rate, rhythm, and volume and the time of measurement. "Full" or "bounding" describes a pulse of increased volume; "weak" or "thready," decreased volume.
• When recording apical pulse, include intensity of heart sounds.
• When recording apical-radial pulse, chart the rate according to the pulse site, for example, A/R pulse of 80/76.

R

Radiation implant therapy

In this treatment, also called brachytherapy, the doctor uses implants of radioactive isotopes (encapsulated in seeds, needles, or sutures) to deliver ionizing radiation within a body cavity or interstitially to a tumor site. The implants may be permanent or temporary. They deliver a continuous radiation dose over several hours or days to a specific site while minimizing exposure to adjacent tissues. Isotopes such as cesium 137, gold 198, iodine 125, iridium 192, palladium 103, and phosphorus 32 (^{32}P) are used to treat cancers. (See *Radioisotopes and their uses,* pages 742 and 743.)

Common implant sites include the brain, breast, cervix, endometrium, lung, neck, oral cavity, prostate gland, and vagina. For treatment, the patient is usually placed in a private room (with its own bathroom) located as far away from high-traffic areas as is practical. If monitoring shows an increased radiation hazard, adjacent rooms and hallways may also need to be restricted. Consult your hospital's radiation safety policy for specific guidelines.

Brachytherapy is commonly combined with external radiation therapy (teletherapy) for increased effectiveness.

≫ Key nursing diagnoses and patient outcomes

Use these nursing diagnoses as a guide when developing your plan of care for a patient undergoing radiation implant therapy.

Body image disturbance related to presence of implants

Based on this nursing diagnosis, you'll establish the following patient outcomes. The patient will:
• acknowledge change in body image.
• participate in decision making about his radiation implant therapy.
• express positive feelings about self.

Decisional conflict related to perceived threat to value system

Based on this nursing diagnosis, you'll establish the following patient outcomes. The patient will:
• state feelings about current situation.
• identify desirable and undesirable consequences of available options.
• accept assistance from family, friends, clergy, and other supportive persons.

Equipment

♦ film badge or pocket dosimeter ♦ RADIATION PRECAUTION sign for door ♦ RADIATION PRECAUTION warning labels ♦ masking tape ♦ lead-lined container ♦ long-handled forceps ♦ male T-binder and two sanitary napkins with safety pin(if Burnett applicator is being used) ♦ optional: lead shield and lead strip.

Equipment preparation

• Place the lead-lined container and long-handled forceps in a corner of the patient's room.
• Mark a *safe line* on the floor with masking tape 6′ (2 m) from the pa-

Radioisotopes and their uses

Unstable elements, radioisotopes emit three kinds of energy particles as they "decay" to a stable state. These particles are ranked by their penetrating power. *Alpha particles* possess the lowest energy level and are easily stopped by a sheet of paper. More powerful *beta particles* can be stopped by the skin's surface. *Gamma rays*, the most powerful, can only be stopped by dense shielding, such as lead. Some isotopes commonly used in cancer treatments are listed below.

ISOTOPE AND INDICATIONS	DESCRIPTION	NURSING CONSIDERATIONS
Cesium 137 (^{137}Cs) Gynecologic cancers	• 30-year half-life • Emits gamma particles • Encased in steel capsules which are placed temporarily in the patient in the operating room	• Elevate the head of the bed no more than 45 degrees. • Encourage fluids and implement a low-residue diet. • Encourage quiet activities; enforce strict bed rest, as ordered.
Gold 198 (^{198}Au) Localized male genitourinary tumors	• 3-day half-life • Emits gamma particles • Permanently implanted as tiny seeds directly into the tumor or tumor bed	• If a seed is dislodged and found, call the radiation oncology department for disposal.
Iodine 125 (^{125}I) Localized or unresectable tumors; slow-growing tumors; recurrent disease	• 60-day half-life • Emits gamma particles • Permanently implanted as tiny seeds or sutures directly into the tumor or tumor bed	• Because seeds may become dislodged, no linens, body fluids, instruments, or utensils may leave the patient's room until they're monitored. • If a seed is dislodged and found, call the radiation department; use long-handled forceps to put it in a lead-lined container in the room. • Monitor body fluids to detect displaced seeds. Give the patient a 24-hour urine container that can be closed.

Radioisotopes and their uses *(continued)*

ISOTOPE AND INDICATIONS	DESCRIPTION	NURSING CONSIDERATIONS
Iridium 192 (^{192}Ir) Localized or unresectable tumors	• 74-day half-life • Emits gamma particles • Temporarily implanted as seeds strung inside special catheters that are implanted around the tumor	• If a catheter is dislodged, call the radiation department; use long-handled forceps to put the implant in a lead-lined container in the room.
Palladium 103 (^{103}Pd) Superficial, localized or unresectable intrathoracic or intra-abdominal tumors	• 17-day half-life • Emits gamma particles • Permanently implanted as seeds in the tumor or tumor bed	• See Iodine 125.
Phosphorus 32 (^{32}P) Polycythemia, leukemia, bone metastasis, and malignant ascites	• 14-day half-life • Emits beta particles • Used as an I.V. solution rather than an implant because of its low energy level	• No shielding is required other than a lucite syringe shield. • Patients receiving ^{32}P are placed in a private room with a separate bathroom.

tient's bed to warn visitors to keep clear of the patient to minimize their radiation exposure.

• If desired, place a portable lead shield in the back of the room to use when providing care.

• Place an emergency tracheotomy tray in the room if an implant is to be inserted in the oral cavity or neck.

Patient preparation

• Explain the treatment and its goals to the patient.

• Review radiation safety procedures, visitation policies, potential adverse effects, and interventions for those ef-

fects. Also review long-term concerns and home care issues.

Implementation

• Place the RADIATION PRECAUTION sign on the door.

• Check to see that informed consent has been obtained.

• Ensure that all laboratory tests are performed before beginning treatment. If laboratory work is required during treatment, the badged technician obtains the specimen, labels the collection tube with a radioactive precaution label, and alerts the laboratory personnel before bringing it. If urine tests are needed for ^{32}P therapy, ask the radiation oncology department or laboratory technician how to transport these specimens safely.

• Affix a RADIATION PRECAUTION warning label to the patient's identification wristband.

• Affix warning labels to the patient's chart and Kardex *to ensure staff awareness of the patient's radioactive status.*

• Wear a film badge or dosimeter at waist level during the entire shift. Turn in the radiation badge monthly or according to your hospital's protocol. *Pocket dosimeters measure immediate exposures.* In many centers, these measurements aren't part of the permanent exposure record but are used to ensure that nurses receive the lowest possible exposure.

• Each nurse must have a personal, nontransferable film badge or ring badge. *Badges document each person's cumulative lifetime radiation exposure.* Only primary caregivers are badged and allowed into the patient's room.

• To minimize exposure to radiation, use the three principles of *time, distance,* and *shielding*: give care in the shortest time possible; work as far away from the radiation source as possible (give care from the side opposite the implant or from a position allowing the greatest working distance possible); and use a portable shield, if needed and desired.

• Give essential nursing care only; omit bed baths. If ordered, provide perineal care, making sure that wipes, sanitary pads, and similar items are bagged correctly and monitored. (Refer to your hospital's radiation policy.)

• Dressing changes over an implanted area must be supervised by the radiation technician or another designated caregiver.

• Before discharge, a patient's temporary implant must be removed and properly stored by the radiation oncology department. *A patient with a permanent implant may not be released until his radioactivity level is less than 5 millirems (mrem) per hour at one meter's distance.*

Complications

Depending on the implant site and total radiation dosage, complications of implant therapy may include:

• dislodgment of the radiation source or applicator
• tissue fibrosis
• xerostomia
• radiation pneumonitis
• muscle atrophy
• sterility
• vaginal dryness or stenosis
• fistulas
• hypothyroidism
• altered bowel habits
• infection
• airway obstruction
• diarrhea
• cystitis
• myelosuppression
• neurotoxicity
• secondary cancers.

Nursing considerations

• Nurses and visitors who are pregnant or trying to conceive or father a child must not attend patients receiving radiation implant therapy *because the gonads and developing embryo and fetus are highly susceptible to the damaging effects of ionizing radiation.*

• If the patient must be moved out of his room, notify the appropriate department of the patient's status *to give receiving personnel time to make appropriate preparations to receive the patient.* When moving the patient, ensure that the route is clear of equipment and other persons, and that the elevator, if there is one, is keyed and ready to receive the patient. Move the patient in a bed or wheelchair, accompanied by two badged caregivers. If the patient is delayed along the way, stand as far away from the bed as possible until you can proceed.

• The patient's room must be monitored daily by the radiation oncology department, and disposables must be monitored and removed according to hospital guidelines.

• If a code is called on a patient with an implant, follow your hospital's code procedures as well as these steps: Notify the code team of the patient's radioactive status *to exclude any team member who is pregnant or trying to conceive or father a child.* Also notify the radiation oncology department. Cover the implant site with a strip of lead shielding if possible. Don't allow anything to leave the patient's room until it is monitored for radiation. The primary care nurse must remain in the room (as far away from the patient as possible) *to act as a resource person for the patient and to provide film badges or dosimeters to code team members.*

• If an implant becomes dislodged, notify the radiation oncology department staff and follow their instructions. Typically, the dislodged implant is collected with long-handled forceps and placed in a lead-shielded canister.

• Refer the patient for sexual or psychological counseling if needed.

• If a patient with an implant dies on the unit, notify the radiation oncology department *so they can remove a temporary implant and store it properly.* If the implant was permanent, radiation oncology staff members will determine which precautions to follow before postmortem care can be provided and before the body can be moved to the morgue.

Home care

• Tell the patient who has had a cervical implant to expect slight to moderate vaginal bleeding after being discharged from the hospital. This flow normally changes color from pink to brown to white.

• Instruct her to notify the doctor if bleeding increases, persists for more than 48 hours, or has a foul odor.

• Explain to the patient that she may resume most normal activities but that she should avoid sexual intercourse and the use of tampons until after her follow-up visit to the doctor (about 6 weeks after discharge).

• Instruct her to take showers rather than baths for 2 weeks, to avoid douching unless allowed by the doctor, and to avoid activities that cause abdominal strain for 6 weeks.

• Encourage the patient and family members to keep in contact with the radiation oncology department and to notify them if concerns or physical changes occur.

Documentation

Record the following information:

• radiation precautions taken during treatment

• adverse effects of therapy

• teaching given to the patient and family and their responses to it
• patient's tolerance of isolation procedures and the family's compliance with procedures
• referrals to local cancer services.

Radiation therapy, external

Approximately 60% of all cancer patients are treated with some form of external radiation therapy. Also called radiotherapy, this treatment delivers radiation — X-rays or gamma rays — directly to the cancer site. Its effects are local, since only the area being treated experiences direct effects.

Radiation doses are based on the type, stage, and location of the tumor as well as on the patient's size, condition, and treatment goals. Doses are given in increments, usually three to five times a week until the total dose is reached.

The goals of radiation therapy include *cure*, in which the cancer is completely destroyed and not expected to recur; *control*, in which the cancer does not progress or regress, but is expected to progress at some later time; or *palliation*, in which radiation is given to relieve symptoms (such as bone pain, seizures, bleeding, headache) caused by the cancer.

External beam radiation therapy is delivered by machines that aim a concentrated beam of high-energy particles (photons and gamma rays) at the target site. Two types of machines are commonly used: units containing cobalt or cesium as radioactive sources for gamma rays, and linear accelera-

tors that use electricity to produce X-rays. Linear accelerators produce high energy with great penetrating ability. Some (known as orthovoltage machines) produce less powerful electron beams that may be used for superficial tumors.

Radiation therapy may be augmented by chemotherapy, brachytherapy (radiation implant therapy), or surgery, as needed.

≫ Key nursing diagnoses and patient outcomes

Use these nursing diagnoses as a guide when developing your plan of care for a patient undergoing external radiation therapy.

Body image disturbance related to presence of implants
Based on this nursing diagnosis, you'll establish the following patient outcomes. The patient will:
• acknowledge change in body image.
• participate in decision making about his radiation therapy.
• express positive feelings about self.

Decisional conflict related to perceived threat to value system
Based on this nursing diagnosis, you'll establish the following patient outcomes. The patient will:
• state feelings about current situation.
• identify desirable and undesirable consequences of available options.
• accept assistance from family, friends, clergy, and other supportive persons.

Equipment
♦ radiation therapy machine ♦ film badge or pocket dosimeter.

Patient preparation

- Explain the treatment to the patient and his family.
- Review the treatment goals, and discuss the range of potential adverse effects and interventions to minimize them.
- Discuss possible long-term complications and treatment issues.
- Educate the patient and his family about local cancer services.
- Check to see that the radiation oncology department has obtained informed consent.
- Review the patient's clinical record for recent laboratory and imaging results, and alert the radiation oncology staff to any abnormalities or pertinent results (such as myelosuppression, paraneoplastic syndromes, oncologic emergencies, and tumor progression).

Implementation

- Transport the patient to the radiology department.
- The patient first undergoes simulation (treatment planning), in which the target area is mapped out on the body using a machine similar to the radiotherapy machine. Then the target area is tattooed or marked in ink to ensure accurate treatments.
- The doctor and radiation oncologist determine the duration and frequency of treatments, depending on the patient's body size, size of portal, extent and location of cancer, and treatment goals.
- The patient is positioned on the treatment table beneath the machine. Treatments last from a few seconds to a few minutes. Reassure the patient that he won't feel anything and that he will not be radioactive. After treat-

ment is complete, the patient may return home or to his room.

Complications

- Adverse effects arise gradually and diminish gradually after treatments. They may be acute, subacute (accumulating as treatment progresses), chronic (following treatment), and long-term (arising months to years after treatment). Adverse effects are localized to the area of treatment, and their severity depends on the total radiation dosage, underlying organ sensitivity, and the patient's overall condition.
- Common acute and subacute adverse effects can include altered skin integrity (wet or dry desquamation), altered GI and genitourinary function, altered fertility and sexual function, altered bone marrow production, fatigue, and alopecia.
- Long-term complications or adverse effects may include radiation pneumonitis, neuropathy, skin and muscle atrophy, telangiectasia, fistulas, altered endocrine function, and secondary malignant disease.
- Other complications of treatment include headache, xerostomia, dysphagia, stomatitis, vomiting, heartburn, diarrhea, cystitis, and fatigue.

Nursing considerations

- Explain to the patient that the full benefit of radiation treatments may not occur until several weeks or months after treatments begin. Instruct him to report any long-term adverse effects.
- Emphasize the importance of keeping follow-up appointments with the doctor.

• Refer the patient to a support group, such as a local chapter of the American Cancer Society.

Home care
• Instruct the patient and his family on proper skin care and management of the adverse effects of treatment.

Documentation
Record the following information:
• radiation precautions taken during treatment
• interventions used and evaluation of them
• grading of adverse effects
• teaching given to the patient and family and their responses to it
• patient's tolerance of isolation procedures and the family's compliance with procedures
• discharge plans and teaching
• referrals to local cancer services.

Radioactive iodine therapy

Because the thyroid gland concentrates iodine, radioactive iodine 131 (^{131}I) can be used to treat thyroid cancer. This isotope emits beta and gamma radiation, and its half-life (the time required for it to decay to 50% of its original activity) is 8 days. Usually administered orally, ^{131}I is used to treat postoperative residual cancer, recurrent disease, inoperable primary thyroid tumors, invasion of the thyroid capsule, or thyroid ablation as well as cancers that have metastasized to cervical or mediastinal lymph nodes or other distant sites.

Because ^{131}I is absorbed systemically, all body secretions, especially urine, must be considered radioactive. For ^{131}I treatments, the patient usually is placed in a private room (with its own bathroom) located as far away from high-traffic areas as is practical. If monitoring shows increased radiation hazard, adjacent rooms and hallways may also need to be restricted. Consult your hospital's radiation safety policy for specific guidelines.

In lower doses, radioactive ^{131}I also may be used to treat hyperthyroidism. Most patients receive this treatment on an outpatient basis and are sent home with appropriate home care instructions.

⟫ Key nursing diagnoses and patient outcomes
Use these nursing diagnoses as a guide when developing your plan of care for a patient undergoing external radioactive iodine therapy.

Body image disturbance related to need for therapy
Based on this nursing diagnosis, you'll establish the following patient outcomes. The patient will:
• acknowledge change in body image.
• participate in decision making about his iodine therapy.
• express positive feelings about self.

Decisional conflict related to perceived threat to value system
Based on this nursing diagnosis, you'll establish the following patient outcomes. The patient will:
• state feelings about current situation.
• identify desirable and undesirable consequences of available options.

• accept assistance from family, friends, clergy, and other supportive persons.

Equipment

♦ film badges, pocket dosimeters, or ring badges ♦ RADIATION PRECAUTION sign for door ♦ RADIATION PRECAUTION warning labels ♦ waterproof gowns ♦ clear and red plastic bags for contaminated articles ♦ plastic wrap ♦ absorbent plastic-lined pads ♦ masking tape ♦ radioresistant gloves ♦ trash cans ♦ optional: portable lead shield.

Equipment preparation

• Assemble all necessary equipment in the patient's room. Keep an emergency tracheotomy tray just outside the room or in a handy place at the nurses' station.

• Place the RADIATION PRECAUTION sign on the door. Affix warning labels to the patient's chart and Kardex *to ensure staff awareness of the patient's radioactive status.*

• Place an absorbent plastic back pad on the bathroom floor and under the sink; if the patient's room is carpeted, cover it with such a pad as well.

• Place an additional pad over the bedside table.

• Secure plastic wrap over the telephone, TV controls, bed controls, mattress, call button, and toilet. *These measures prevent radioactive contamination of working surfaces.*

• Keep large trash cans in the room lined with plastic bags (two clear bags inserted inside an outer red bag). Monitor all objects before they leave the room.

• Notify the dietitian to supply foods and beverages only in disposable containers and with disposable utensils.

Patient preparation

• Explain the procedure and review treatment goals with the patient and his family.

• Before treatment begins, review radiation safety procedures, visitation policies, potential adverse effects, interventions, and home care procedures.

• Verify that the doctor has obtained informed consent.

• Check for allergies to iodine-containing substances, such as contrast media or shellfish.

• Review the medication history for thyroid-containing or thyroid-altering drugs and for lithium carbonate, which may increase ^{131}I uptake.

• Review the patient's health history for vomiting, diarrhea, productive cough, and sinus drainage, *which could increase the risk of radioactive secretions.*

• If necessary, remove the patient's dentures *to avoid contaminating them and to reduce radioactive secretions.*

• Tell him they'll be replaced 48 hours after treatment.

• Affix a RADIATION PRECAUTION label to the patient's identification wristband.

Implementation

• Encourage the patient to use the toilet rather than a bedpan or urinal, and to flush it three times after each use *to reduce radiation levels.*

• Instruct the patient to remain in his room except for tests or other special reasons.

• Allow him to ambulate.

• Unless contraindicated, instruct the patient to increase his fluid intake to 3 liters (or quarts) daily.

• Encourage the patient to chew or suck on hard candy to keep salivary glands stimulated and to prevent them from becoming inflamed, which may occur in the first 24 hours.

• Ensure that all laboratory tests are performed before beginning treatment. If laboratory work is required, the badged laboratory technician obtains the specimen, labels the collection tube with a RADIOACTIVE PRECAUTION label, and alerts the laboratory personnel before transporting it. If urine tests are needed, ask the radiation oncology department or laboratory technician how to transport these specimens safely.

• Wear a film badge or dosimeter at waist level during the entire shift. Turn in the radiation badge monthly or according to your hospital's protocol, and be sure to record your exposures accurately. *Pocket dosimeters measure immediate exposures.* These measurements may not be part of the permanent exposure record but *help to ensure that nurses receive the lowest possible exposure.*

• Each nurse must have a personal, nontransferable film badge or ring badge. *Badges document each person's cumulative lifetime radiation exposure.* Only primary caregivers are badged and allowed into the patient's room.

• Wear gloves to touch the patient or objects in the room.

• Allow visitors to spend no more than 30 minutes every 24 hours with the patient. Stress that no visitors will be allowed who are under age 18 or who are pregnant or trying to conceive or father a child.

• Restrict direct contact to no more than 30 minutes or 20 millirems (mrem) per day. If the patient is receiving 200 millicuries (mCi) of ^{131}I, remain with him only 2 to 4 minutes and stand no closer than 1' (30 cm) away. If standing 3' (1 m) away, the time limit is 20 minutes; if standing 5' (1.5 m) away, the limit is 30 minutes.

• Give essential nursing care only; omit bed baths. If ordered, provide perineal care, making sure that wipes, sanitary pads, and similar items are bagged correctly and monitored.

• If the patient vomits or urinates on the floor, notify the nuclear medicine department and use nondisposable radioresistant gloves when cleaning the spill. After cleanup, wash your gloved hands, remove the gloves and leave them in the room; then rewash your hands.

• If the patient must be moved from his room, notify the appropriate department of the patient's status so that receiving personnel can make appropriate arrangements to receive him. When moving the patient, ensure that the route is clear of equipment and other persons and that the elevator, if there is one, is keyed and ready to receive the patient. Move the patient in a bed or wheelchair, accompanied by two badged caregivers. If the patient is delayed along the way, stand as far away from him as possible until you can continue.

• The patient's room must be cleaned by the radiation oncology department, not by housekeeping. The room must be monitored daily, and disposables must be monitored and removed according to hospital guidelines.

• At discharge, schedule the patient for a follow-up examination. Also arrange for a whole-body scan approximately 7 to 10 days after ^{131}I treatment.

• Inform the patient and his family of community support services for cancer patients.

Complications

• Myelosuppression is common in patients who have extensive disease or who undergo repeated ^{131}I treatments.

• Radiation pulmonary fibrosis may develop if extensive lung metastasis was present when ^{131}I was administered.

• Other complications may include nausea, vomiting, headache, radiation thyroiditis, fever, sialadenitis, or pain and swelling at metastatic sites.

Nursing considerations

• Nurses and visitors who are pregnant or trying to conceive or father a child must not attend or visit patients receiving ^{131}I therapy *because the gonads and developing embryo and fetus are highly susceptible to the damaging effects of ionizing radiation.*

• If a code is called on a patient undergoing ^{131}I therapy, follow your hospital's code procedures as well as these steps. Notify the code team of the patient's radioactive status *to exclude any team member who is pregnant or trying to conceive or father a child.* Also notify the radiation oncology department. Don't allow anything out of the patient's room until it's monitored. The primary care nurse must remain in the room (as far as possible from the patient) *to act as a resource person for the patient and to*

What to do after ^{131}I treatment

After your patient has undergone treatment with ^{131}I, teach him the necessary precautions to take:

• Instruct the patient to report any long-term adverse reactions. In particular, review signs and symptoms of hypothyroidism and hyperthyroidism. Also ask him to report any signs and symptoms of thyroid cancer, such as enlarged lymph nodes, dyspnea, bone pain, nausea, vomiting, and abdominal discomfort.

• Although the patient's radiation level at discharge will be safe, suggest that he take extra precautions during the first week, such as using separate eating utensils, sleeping in a separate bedroom, and avoiding bodily contact.

• Sexual intercourse may be resumed 1 week after ^{131}I treatment. However, urge a female patient to avoid pregnancy for 6 months after treatment, and tell a male patient to avoid impregnating his partner for 3 months after treatment.

---

provide film badges or dosimeters to code team members.

• If the patient dies on the unit, notify the radiology safety officer who will determine which precautions to follow before postmortem care can be provided and the body moved to the morgue.

Home care

• See *What to do after ^{131}I treatment.*

Documentation

Record the following information:

• radiation precautions taken during treatment
• teaching given to the patient and family and their responses to it
• patient's tolerance of isolation procedures and the family's compliance with procedures
• referrals to local cancer counseling services.

Radiographic testing

Radiographic testing includes cardiac, chest, kidney-ureter-bladder, mammography, paranasal sinus, and skull examinations.

Cardiac radiography

Cardiac radiography — among the most frequently used tests for evaluating cardiac disease and its effects on the pulmonary vasculature — provides images of the thorax, mediastinum, heart, and lungs. In a routine evaluation, posteroanterior and left lateral views are taken. Cardiac radiography may be performed on a bedridden patient using portable equipment, but such equipment can provide only anteroposterior views. It is used to help detect cardiac disease and abnormalities that change the size, shape, or appearance of the heart and lungs and to ensure correct positioning of pulmonary artery and cardiac catheters and of pacemaker wires.

Chest radiography

In chest radiography, X-rays or electromagnetic waves penetrate the chest and cause an image to form on specially sensitized film. Normal pulmonary tissue is radiolucent, whereas abnormalities — such as infiltrates, foreign bodies, fluids, and tumors — appear as densities on the film. A chest X-ray is most useful when compared with prior films to detect changes.

Kidney-ureter-bladder radiography

Kidney-ureter-bladder (KUB) radiography is used to survey the abdomen to determine the position of the kidneys, ureters, and bladder and to detect gross abnormalities. It's usually the first step in diagnostic testing of the urinary system.

This test does not require intact renal function and may aid differential diagnosis of urologic and GI diseases, which often produce similar signs and symptoms. However, KUB radiography has limitations and nearly always must be followed by more elaborate tests, such as excretory urography or renal computed tomography. KUB radiography should not follow recent instillation of barium.

Mammography

This radiographic technique is used to help to detect breast cysts or tumors, especially those not palpable on physical examination. Biopsy of suspicious areas may be required to confirm malignant disease. Mammography can detect 90% to 95% of malignant breast disease.

Paranasal sinus radiography

The paranasal sinuses, air-filled cavities lined with mucous membrane, lie within the maxillary, ethmoid, sphenoid, and frontal bones. Sinus abnormalities, resulting from inflammation, trauma, cysts, mucoceles, granulomatosis, and other conditions, may include distorted bony sinus walls, altered mucous membranes, and fluid or masses within the cavities. In paranasal sinus radiography, X-rays or electromagnetic waves penetrate the paranasal sinuses and react on specially sensitized film, forming a film image that differentiates sinus structures.

Skull radiography

Although of limited value in assessing patients with head injuries, skull X-rays are extremely valuable for studying abnormalities of the base of the skull and the cranial vault, congenital and perinatal anomalies, and systemic diseases that produce bone defects of the skull.

Skull radiography is used to evaluate the three groups of bones that comprise the skull: the calvaria (vault), the mandible (jaw bone), and the facial bones. The calvaria and the facial bones are closely connected by immovable joints with irregular serrated edges called sutures. The bones of the skull form an anatomic structure so complex that a complete skull examination requires several radiologic views of each area.

≫ Key nursing diagnoses and patient outcomes

Use this nursing diagnosis as a guide when developing your plan of care.

Knowledge deficit related to procedure

Based on this nursing diagnosis, you'll establish the following patient outcomes. The patient will:
• communicate a need to increase knowledge.
• state or demonstrate understanding of what has been taught.

• seek help from health professionals when needed.

Equipment
♦ X-ray machine.

Patient preparation
• Describe the test, including who will perform it, where it will take place, and its expected duration.
• Provide a gown without snaps, and instruct the patient to remove jewelry that may be in the X-ray field.

Cardiac radiography
• Explain to the patient that this test is used to determine the size and shape of the heart. Provide reassurance that little radiation is used and that the test is harmless.

Chest radiography
• Explain that this test is used to assess respiratory status.
• Tell the patient he need not restrict food or fluid before the test.
• Explain that he'll be asked to take a deep breath and to hold it momentarily while the film is being taken *to provide a clearer view of pulmonary structures.*

KUB radiography
• Explain to the patient that this test is used to detect urinary system abnormalities.
• Inform the patient that he needn't restrict food or fluids. Tell him that the test takes only a few minutes.

Mammography
• Inform her that although the test takes only about 15 minutes to perform, she may be asked to wait while

the films are checked to make sure that they're readable.

• Just before the test, give the patient a gown to wear that opens in the front, and ask her to remove all jewelry and clothing above the waist.

Paranasal sinus radiography

• Explain that this test is used to evaluate abnormalities of the paranasal sinuses.

• The expected duration of the test is usually 10 to 15 minutes.

• Tell the patient that his head may be immobilized in a foam vise during the test *to help maintain the correct position* but that the vise doesn't hurt.

• Tell the patient that he'll be asked to sit upright and avoid moving while the X-rays are being taken *to prevent blurring of the image and to allow visualization of air-fluid levels, if present.* Emphasize the importance of cooperation.

Skull radiography

• Explain to the patient that his head will be immobilized and that several X-rays of his skull will be taken from various angles.

• Tell him that this test is used to determine the presence of fractures, tumors, or other anomalies.

• Tell the patient that the test takes about 15 minutes and does not cause discomfort.

• Explain that he need not restrict food or fluid before the test.

Implementation

The steps below show you how various radiographs are taken.

Cardiac and chest radiography

• Move cardiac monitoring cables, I.V. tubing from subclavian lines, pulmonary artery catheter lines, and safety pins as far from the X-ray field as possible.

For a posteroanterior view

• The patient stands erect about 6′ (1.8 m) from the X-ray machine with his back to the machine and his chin resting on top of the film cassette holder.

• The holder is adjusted to slightly hyperextend the patient's neck. The patient places his hands on his hips, with his shoulders touching the holder, and centers his chest against it.

• The patient is asked to take a deep breath and hold it during the X-ray film exposure.

For a left lateral view

• The patient is positioned with his arms extended over his head and his left torso flush against the cassette and centered.

• The patient is asked to take a deep breath and hold it during the X-ray film exposure.

For an anteroposterior view of a bedridden patient

• The head of the bed is elevated as much as possible.

• The patient is assisted to an upright position to reduce visceral pressure on the diaphragm and other thoracic structures.

• The film cassette is centered under the patient's back. Although the distance between the patient and the X-ray machine may vary, the path between the two should be clear.

• The patient is instructed to take a deep breath and hold it during the X-ray film exposure.

KUB radiography
- The patient is placed in a supine position in correct body alignment on an X-ray table. His arms are extended overhead, and the iliac crests are checked for symmetrical positioning.
- If the patient can't extend his arms or stand, he may lie on his left side with his right arm up.
- A single X-ray is taken.

Mammography
- The patient stands and is asked to rest one of her breasts on a table above an X-ray cassette.
- The compression plate is placed on the breast, and the patient is told to hold her breath. A radiograph is taken of the craniocaudal view.
- The machine is rotated, the breast is compressed again, and a radiograph of the lateral view is taken.
- The procedure is repeated on the other breast.
- After the films are developed, they are checked to make sure they're readable.

Paranasal sinus radiography
- Have the patient sit upright (his head may be placed in a foam vise) between the X-ray tube and a film cassette.
- During the test, the X-ray tube is positioned at specific angles, and the patient's head is placed in various standard positions, while his paranasal sinuses are filmed from different angles. If necessary, assist with positioning the patient.

Skull radiography
- Have the patient recline on the X-ray table or sit in a chair.
- Tell him to remain still during the procedure.

- Use foam pads, sandbags, or a headband to immobilize the patient's head and increase comfort.
- Five views of the skull are routinely taken: left and right lateral, anteroposterior Townes, posteroanterior Caldwell, and axial (or base).
- Films are developed and checked for quality before the patient leaves the area.

Nursing considerations
- Radiography is usually contraindicated during the first trimester of pregnancy. If it's performed during pregnancy, a lead shield or apron should cover the abdomen and pelvic area during the X-ray exposure.

Cardiac and chest radiography
- When testing an ambulatory patient, make sure the radiographic order stipulates a posteroanterior view and not an anteroposterior view. Include on the order any pertinent findings from previous cardiac radiographs as well as the indication for this test.
- When testing a bedridden patient, make sure anyone else in the room is protected from X-rays by a lead shield, a room divider, or sufficient distance.
- If the patient is intubated, check that no tubes have been dislodged during positioning.

KUB radiography
- Male patients should have gonadal shielding *to prevent irradiation of the testes.* Female patients' ovaries can't be shielded because they're too close to the kidneys, ureters, and bladder.

Mammography

• Tell the patient to remove powder, deodorant, or salves from the breasts or underarms before the test. *These substances may cause false-positive results.*

• Have the patient remove jewelry and clothing within the X-ray field. *These objects can cause false-positive results or unsatisfactory films.*

Paranasal sinus radiography

• When surrounding facial structures that are superimposed on the paranasal sinuses interfere with visualization of relevant areas, computed tomography scanning may be performed to obtain further information.

Documentation

• Record preliminary assessments you made of the patient's condition.
• Note whether the patient's age, illness, or disability requires special preparation for the test.
• Document teaching you've done about the test and follow-up care.

Rectal suppository and ointment administration

A rectal suppository is a small, solid, medicated mass, usually cone-shaped, with a cocoa butter or glycerin base. It may be inserted to stimulate peristalsis and defecation or to relieve pain, vomiting, and local irritation. Rectal suppositories commonly contain drugs that reduce fever or induce relaxation; the drugs interact poorly with digestive enzymes, or have a taste too offensive for oral use. Rectal suppositories melt at body temperature and are absorbed slowly.

Because insertion of a rectal suppository may stimulate the vagus nerve, this drug route is contraindicated in patients with potential cardiac arrhythmias. It may have to be avoided in patients with recent rectal or prostate surgery because of the risk of local trauma or discomfort during insertion.

An ointment is a semisolid medication used to produce local effects. It may be applied externally to the anus or internally to the rectum. Rectal ointments commonly contain drugs that reduce inflammation or relieve pain and itching.

≫ Key nursing diagnoses and patient outcomes

Use these nursing diagnoses as a guide when developing your plan of care for a patient receiving a rectal suppository or ointment.

Constipation related to (specify)

Based on this nursing diagnosis, you'll establish the following patient outcomes. The patient will:
• have elimination return to normal.
• state understanding of causes of constipation.
• move bowels every (specify) days without suppository.

Impaired tissue integrity related to (specify)

Based on this nursing diagnosis, you'll establish the following patient outcomes. The patient will:
• express feelings of rectal comfort.
• show symptoms of rectal tissue healing without evidence of infection.

Equipment

♦ rectal suppository or tube of ointment and ointment applicator ♦ patient's medication record and chart ♦ $4'' \times 4''$ gauze pads ♦ water-soluble lubricant ♦ gloves ♦ optional: bedpan.

Equipment preparation

• Store rectal suppositories in the refrigerator until needed to prevent softening and possible decreased effectiveness of the medication. A softened suppository is also difficult to handle and insert.

• To harden it again, hold the suppository (in its wrapper) under cold running water.

Patient preparation

• Verify the order on the patient's medication record by checking it against the doctor's order.

• Wash your hands with warm soap and water.

• Confirm the patient's identity by asking his name and checking the name, room number, and bed number on his wristband.

• Explain the procedure and the purpose of the medication to the patient.

• Provide privacy.

Implementation

Here's how to administer a rectal suppository or ointment.

Inserting a rectal suppository

• Place the patient on his left side in Sims' position. Drape him with the bedcovers *to expose only the buttocks.*

• Put on gloves. Remove the suppository from its wrapper, and lubricate it with water-soluble lubricant.

• Lift the patient's upper buttock with your nondominant hand *to expose the anus.*

• Instruct the patient to take several deep breaths through his mouth *to help relax the anal sphincters and reduce anxiety or discomfort during insertion.*

• Using the index finger of your dominant hand, insert the suppository — tapered end first — about $3''$ (7.6 cm), until you feel it pass the internal anal sphincter. Try to direct the tapered end toward the side of the rectum so it contacts the membranes. (See *How to administer a rectal suppository or a rectal ointment,* page 758.)

• Ensure the patient's comfort. Encourage him to lie quietly and, if applicable, to retain the suppository for the appropriate length of time. A suppository administered to relieve constipation should be retained as long as possible (at least 20 minutes) to be effective. Press on the anus with a gauze pad if necessary until the urge to defecate passes.

• Discard the used equipment.

Applying an ointment

• To apply externally, wear gloves or use a gauze pad to spread medication over the anal area.

• To apply internally, attach the applicator to the tube of ointment and coat the applicator with water-soluble lubricant.

• Expect to use approximately $1''$ (2.5 cm) of ointment. To gauge how much pressure to use during application, try squeezing a small amount from the tube before you attach the applicator.

• Lift the patient's upper buttock with your nondominant hand *to expose the anus.*

How to administer a rectal suppository or a rectal ointment

When inserting a suppository, direct its tapered end toward the side of the rectum so it contacts the membranes, enhancing absorption of the medication.

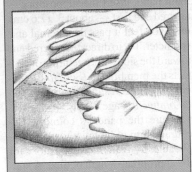

When applying an ointment, be sure to lubricate the applicator to minimize pain on insertion. Direct the applicator tip toward the patient's umbilicus.

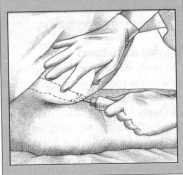

• Instruct the patient to take several deep breaths through his mouth *to relax the anal sphincters and reduce anxiety or discomfort during insertion.*

• Gently insert the applicator, directing it toward the umbilicus.
• Slowly squeeze the tube to eject the medication.
• Remove the applicator and place a folded $4'' \times 4''$ gauze pad between the patient's buttocks *to absorb excess ointment.*
• Disassemble the tube and applicator. Recap the tube, and clean the applicator thoroughly with soap and warm water.

Complications
• Complications can result from an allergic reaction to the medications in the suppositories or ointments.
• Diarrhea may occur.

Nursing considerations
• Because the intake of food and fluid stimulates peristalsis, a suppository for relieving constipation should be inserted about 30 minutes before mealtime *to help soften the feces in the rectum and facilitate defecation.* A medicated retention suppository should be inserted between meals.
• Instruct the patient to avoid expelling the suppository. However, if he has difficulty retaining it, place him on a bedpan.
• Make sure the patient's call button is handy, and watch for his signal *because he may be unable to suppress the urge to defecate.* For example, a patient with proctitis has a highly sensitive rectum and may not be able to retain a suppository for long.
• Be sure to inform the patient that the suppository may discolor his next bowel movement. Anusol suppositories, for example, can give feces a silver-gray pasty appearance.

Documentation
• Record the administration time, the dose, and the patient's response.

Reflex evaluation, deep tendon and superficial

Assessment of deep tendon and superficial reflexes provides information about the integrity of the sensory receptor organ and is used to evaluate how well afferent nerves relay sensory messages to the spinal cord. It's also used to evaluate how well the spinal cord or brain stem segment mediates the reflex, how well the lower motor neurons transmit messages to the muscles, and how well the muscles respond to the motor message.

Reflex evaluation is usually reserved for a complete neurologic assessment and indirectly provides information about the presence or absence of inhibiting brain messages. These messages travel along the corticospinal tract to modify reflex strength.

Deep tendon reflexes, or muscle-stretch reflexes, occur when a sudden stimulus causes the muscle to stretch. *Superficial reflexes,* or cutaneous reflexes, are elicited by light, rapid, tactile stimulation, such as stroking or scratching the skin.

Pathologic superficial reflexes, or primitive reflexes, usually occur in early infancy and disappear with maturity. In adults, they usually indicate an underlying central nervous system (CNS) disease.

Abnormal reflex findings include the following:

• increased (hyperactive) reflexes, which may indicate upper motor neuron disorders. Examples include spasticity associated with spinal cord injuries or other upper motor neuron disorders, such as multiple sclerosis.
• decreased or absent reflexes, which signal a disorder of the lower motor neurons or the anterior horn of the spinal cord, where the peripheral nerve originates. Examples of lower motor neuron disorders characterized by hyporeflexia (or areflexia) include Guillain-Barré syndrome and amyotrophic lateral sclerosis.
• diminished reflex associated with a particular cord level, which may reflect a compressed spinal nerve root. For example, a herniated intervertebral disk at L3 or L4 may decrease the knee-jerk reflex.
• Babinski's reflex, which in adults is associated with disorders of the pyramidal tract (such as cerebrovascular accident). The patient responds to the stimulus by dorsiflexion of the great toe.
• absent cremasteric reflex, which may occur in upper or lower motor neuron disease
• absent abdominal reflex, which may reflect aging and diseases of the upper and lower motor neurons.

≫ Key nursing diagnoses and patient outcomes
Use this nursing diagnosis as a guide when developing your plan of care.

Risk for injury related to neural disorder
Based on this nursing diagnosis, you'll establish the following patient outcomes. The patient will:

• identify factors that increase potential for injury.
• assist in identifying and applying safety measures to prevent injury.
• perform activities of daily living optimally within sensorimotor limitations.

Equipment

♦ reflex hammer ♦ applicator stick, tongue blade, or a key.

Implementation

• Position the patient comfortably and encourage him to relax and become limp. Place the patient's extremities in a neutral position, with the muscle you're testing in a slightly stretched position.
• Hold the reflex hammer loosely, yet securely, between your thumb and fingers so that it can swing freely in a controlled direction.
• To elicit the reflex, tap the tendon lightly but firmly with the reflex hammer. Then grade the briskness of the response on a scale of 0 (no response) to 4+ (hyperactive).

Deep tendon reflexes

• These reflexes include the biceps, triceps, brachioradialis, patellar, and Achilles reflexes. Test deep tendon reflexes from head to toe, and compare reflexes on opposite body sides for symmetry of movement and muscle strength.

Before you test a deep tendon reflex, make sure the limb is relaxed and the joint is in the mid-position; for instance, the knee or elbow should be flexed at a 45-degree angle. Then distract the patient by asking him to focus on an object across the room. *If he focuses on his performance, the cerebral cortex may dampen his response.* You can also distract the patient by using Jendrassik's maneuver: Instruct him to clench his teeth or to squeeze his thigh.

Biceps reflex
• Position the patient's arm so the elbow is flexed at a 45-degree angle and the arm is relaxed.
• Place your thumb or index finger over the biceps tendon and your remaining fingers loosely over the triceps muscle.
• Strike your thumb or index finger with the pointed tip of the reflex hammer, and watch and feel for contraction of the biceps muscle and flexion of the forearm.

Triceps reflex
• Have the patient abduct his arm and place his forearm across his chest.
• Strike the triceps tendon about 2″ (5 cm) above the olecranon process on the extensor surface of the upper arm.
• Watch for contraction of the triceps muscle and extension of the forearm.
• If you don't elicit the triceps reflex, try this alternative technique: Ask the patient to abduct his arm at the shoulder. If you're right-handed, support his upper arm with your left arm. Ask him to let his arm hang loosely over yours. With the hammer in your right hand, strike the triceps tendon briskly, using either the blunt or the pointed end. Again, watch for contraction of the triceps and extension of the forearm at the elbow.

Brachioradialis reflex
• Instruct the patient to rest the ulnar surface of his hand on his knee and to partially flex his elbow.
• With the tip of the hammer, strike the radius about 2″ proximal to the radial styloid.

• Watch for supination of the hand and flexion of the forearm at the elbow.

Patellar reflex

• Have the patient sit on the side of the bed with his legs dangling freely.

• If he can't sit up, flex his knee at a 45-degree angle, and place your nondominant hand behind it for support.

• Strike the patellar tendon just below the patella, and look for contraction of the quadriceps muscle in the anterior thigh and for extension of the leg.

Achilles reflex

• Slightly flex the foot and support the plantar surface.

• Using the pointed end of the reflex hammer, strike the Achilles tendon.

• Watch for plantar flexion of the foot at the ankle.

• If the patient is bedridden, position him with his hip externally rotated and his foot resting on his other knee. Slightly flex the foot at the ankle and strike the tendon briskly.

Superficial reflexes

These reflexes include the plantar, cremasteric, and abdominal reflexes. To elicit these reflexes, you'll stimulate the patient's skin or mucous membranes.

Plantar reflex

• Using an applicator stick, a tongue blade, or a key, slowly stroke the lateral side of the patient's sole from the heel to the great toe.

• The normal response is plantar flexion of the toes. In an elderly patient, this normal response may be diminished because of arthritic deformities of the toe or foot.

Cremasteric reflex

• When testing a male patient, use an applicator stick to lightly stimulate the inner thigh.

• Watch for contraction of the cremaster muscle in the scrotum and prompt elevation of the testicle on the side of the stimulus.

Abdominal reflex

• Place the patient in the supine position with his arms at his sides and his knees slightly flexed.

• Using the tip of the reflex hammer, a key, or an applicator stick, briskly stroke both sides of the abdomen above and below the umbilicus, moving from the periphery toward the midline.

• After each stroke, watch for abdominal muscle contraction and movement of the umbilicus toward the stimulus.

• When evaluating an obese patient, retract the umbilicus to the side opposite the stimulus and note whether it pulls toward the stimulus.

Pathologic superficial reflexes

Although normal in infants, primitive reflexes are considered abnormal in adults. They include the grasp, snout, sucking, and glabellar reflexes.

Grasp reflex

• Apply gentle pressure to the patient's palm with your fingers.

• If he grasps your fingers between his thumb and index finger, suspect cortical (pre-motor cortex) damage.

Snout reflex

• Tap lightly on the patient's upper lip.

• Lip pursing, known as the snout reflex, indicates frontal lobe damage.

Sucking reflex

• Observe the patient while you are feeding him or suctioning his mouth.

• If he begins sucking, you've elicited the sucking reflex — an indication of cortical damage typically seen in the patient with advanced dementia.

Grading deep tendon reflexes

This figure indicates normal deep tendon reflex activity. When testing the patient's deep tendon reflexes, use the following grading scale.

0 absent
1+ present but diminished
2+ normal
3+ increased but not necessarily pathologic
4+ hyperactive; clonic
Record the patient's reflex scores by drawing a stick figure and entering the scores at the proper location.

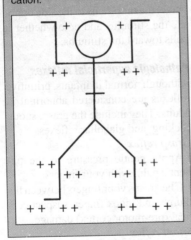

Glabellar reflex
• Repeatedly tap the bridge of the patient's nose. A persistent blinking response indicates diffuse cortical dysfunction.

Nursing considerations
• Make sure the patient is relaxed and comfortable during assessment *be-*

cause tension or anxiety could diminish the reflex.
• Ask the patient who seems to have depressed reflexes to perform isometric muscle contractions, as follows:

To improve leg reflexes, have the patient clench both hands together and tense the arm muscles during the reflex assessment.

To improve arm reflexes, have him clench his teeth or squeeze one thigh with the hand not being evaluated.

Both of these maneuvers force the patient to concentrate on something other than the reflexes being tested, which may eliminate unintentional cognitive inhibition. If reflexes still remain depressed, evaluate further.

Documentation
• Use a grading scale to rate each reflex. Then document the rating for each reflex at the appropriate site on a stick figure. (See *Grading deep tendon reflexes.*)
• Be sure to document which technique you used to distract the patient.
• To document your findings, use a plus sign (+) to indicate that a reflex is present and a minus sign (-) to indicate that it's absent.

Respiratory assessment

Respiration is the exchange of oxygen and carbon dioxide between the atmosphere and body cells. It's controlled by the respiratory center in the lateral medulla oblongata. External respiration, or breathing, is accomplished by the diaphragm and chest muscles and delivers oxygen to the lower respiratory tract and alveoli.

Four measures of respiration — rate, rhythm, depth, and sound — reflect the body's metabolic state, diaphragm and chest-muscle condition, and airway patency. Respiratory rate is recorded as the number of cycles (with inspiration and expiration comprising one cycle) per minute; rhythm, as the regularity of these cycles; depth, as the volume of air inhaled and exhaled with each respiration; and sound, as the audible digression from normal, effortless breathing.

≫ Key nursing diagnoses and patient outcomes

Use these nursing diagnoses as a guide when developing your plan of care.

Impaired gas exchange related to altered oxygen supply.

Based on this nursing diagnosis, you'll establish the following patient outcomes. The patient will:
• maintain respiratory rate within ± 5 breaths/minute of baseline.
• express feeling of comfort in maintaining air exchange.
• have normal breath sounds.
• have arterial blood gas levels return to baseline: (specify) pH; (specify) partial pressure of arterial oxygen; (specify) partial pressure of arterial carbon dioxide.

Ineffective breathing pattern related to (specify)

Based on this nursing diagnosis, you'll establish the following patient outcomes. The patient will:
• report feeling comfortable when breathing.
• achieve maximum lung expansion with adequate ventilation.

Equipment

♦ watch with second hand ♦ optional: stethoscope.

Patient preparation

• The best time to assess your patient's respirations is immediately after taking the pulse rate. Keep your fingertips over the radial artery, and don't tell the patient you're counting respirations. If you tell him, he'll become conscious of his respirations and the rate may change.

Implementation

• Count respirations by observing the rise and fall of the patient's chest as he breathes. Or position the patient's opposite arm across his chest and count respirations by feeling its rise and fall. Consider one rise and one fall as one respiration.
• Count respirations for 30 seconds and multiply by 2 or count for 60 seconds if respirations are irregular to account for variations in respiratory rate and pattern.
• As you count respirations, be alert for and record such breath sounds as stertor, stridor, wheezing, and an expiratory grunt. *Stertor* is a snoring sound resulting from secretions in the trachea and large bronchi. Listen for it in patients with neurologic disorders and in those who are comatose. *Stridor* is an inspiratory crowing sound that occurs with upper airway obstruction in laryngitis, croup, or the presence of a foreign body. When listening for stridor in infants and children with croup, also observe for sternal, substernal, or intercostal retractions. *Wheezing* is caused by partial obstruction in the smaller bronchi and bronchioles. This high-pitched, musical

Identifying respiratory patterns

TYPE	CHARACTERISTICS
Apnea	Periodic absence of breathing
Apneustic	Prolonged, gasping inspiration, followed by extremely short, inefficient expiration
Bradypnea	Slow, regular respirations of equal depth
Cheyne-Stokes	Fast, deep respirations of 30 to 170 seconds punctuated by periods of apnea lasting 20 to 60 seconds
Eupnea	Normal rate and rhythm
Kussmaul's	Fast (over 20 breaths/minute), deep (resembling sighs), labored respirations without pause
Tachypnea	Rapid respirations. Rate rises with body temperature — about four breaths/minute for every degree Fahrenheit above normal

sound is common in patients with emphysema or asthma. In infants, an *expiratory grunt* indicates imminent respiratory distress. In older patients, it may result from partial airway obstruction or neuromuscular reflex.

• Use a stethoscope to detect other breath sounds, such as crackles and rhonchi, or the lack of sound in the lungs.

• Observe chest movements for depth of respiration. If the patient inhales a small volume of air, record this as shallow; if he inhales a large volume, record this as deep.

• Watch chest movements and listen to breathing *to determine the rhythm and sound of respiration.* (See *Identifying respiratory patterns.*)

Nursing considerations

• Respiratory rates below 8 and above 40 breaths/minute usually are considered abnormal; report the sudden onset of such rates promptly.

• Observe for signs of dyspnea, such as an anxious facial expression, flaring nostrils, a heaving chest wall, and cyanosis. *To detect cyanosis,* look for characteristic bluish discoloration in the nail beds or the lips, under the tongue, in the buccal mucosa, or in the conjunctiva.

• In assessing the patient's respiratory status, consider his personal and fam-

PATTERN	POSSIBLE CAUSES
	• Mechanical airway obstruction • Conditions affecting the brain's respiratory center in the lateral medulla oblongata
	• Lesions of the respiratory center
	• Normal pattern during sleep • Conditions affecting the respiratory center: tumors, metabolic disorders, respiratory decompensation; use of opiates and alcohol
	• Increased intracranial pressure, severe congestive heart failure, renal failure, meningitis, drug overdose, cerebral anoxia
	• Normal respiration
	• Renal failure or metabolic acidosis, particularly diabetic ketoacidosis
	• Pneumonia, compensatory respiratory alkalosis, respiratory insufficiency, lesions of the respiratory center, and salicylate poisoning

ily history. Ask if he smokes and, if so, for how many years and how many packs a day.

• A child's respiratory rate may double in response to exercise, illness, or emotion. Normally, the rate for newborns is 30 to 80 breaths/minute; for toddlers, 20 to 40; and for children of school age and older, 15 to 25. Children usually reach the adult rate (12 to 20) at about age 15.

Documentation

• Record the rate, depth, rhythm, and sound of the patient's respirations.

Restraints

Various soft restraints limit movement to prevent a confused, disoriented, or combative patient from injuring himself or others. Vest and belt restraints, used to prevent falls from a bed or a chair, permit full movement of arms and legs. Limb restraints, used to prevent the patient from removing supportive equipment — such as I.V. lines, indwelling catheters, and nasogastric tubes — allow only slight limb motion. Like limb restraints, mitts prevent removal of supportive equipment, keep the patient from scratching rashes or sores, and prevent the combative patient from injuring himself or others. Body restraints, used to control the combative or hysterical patient, immobilize all or most of the body.

When soft restraints aren't sufficient and sedation is dangerous or ineffective, leather restraints can be used. Depending on the patient's behavior, leather restraints may be applied to all limbs (four-point restraints) or to one arm and one leg (two-point restraints). The duration of such restraint is governed by state law and by hospital policy.

Because a patient rarely submits readily to leather restraints, safe and speedy application requires teamwork by several staff members, the availability of all equipment, proper patient positioning, and a brief, clear explanation of the procedure to the patient.

Restraints must be used cautiously in seizure-prone patients because they increase the risk of fracture and trauma. And because restraints can cause skin irritation and restrict blood flow, they shouldn't be applied directly over wounds or I.V. catheters. Vest restraints should be used with caution in patients who have congestive heart failure or respiratory disorders. Such restraints can tighten with movement, further limiting circulation and respiratory function.

➤➤ Key nursing diagnoses and patient outcomes

Use these nursing diagnoses as a guide when developing your plan of care for a patient requiring restraints.

Risk for injury related to neural disorders

Based on this nursing diagnosis, you'll establish the following patient outcomes. The patient will:
• identify factors that increase potential for injury.
• assist in identifying and applying safety measures to prevent injury.
• perform activities of daily living optimally, within sensorimotor limitations.

Impaired memory related to (specify)

Based on this nursing diagnosis, you'll establish the following patient outcomes. The patient will:
• remain free of injury.
• have family members or other caregivers contact appropriate resources as needed.

Equipment

For soft restraints: ♦ restraint (vest, limb, mitt, belt, or body, as needed) ♦ gauze pads if needed.

For leather restraints: ♦ two wrist and two ankle leather restraints ♦ four straps ♦ key ♦ large gauze pads to cushion each extremity.

Equipment preparation

• Before entering the patient's room, make sure the restraints are the correct size, using the patient's build and weight as a guide. (For children, who typically are too small for standard restraints, see *Types of child restraints*.)
• If the restraints are too loose and you can't obtain smaller ones, build them up with gauze pads or washcloths and tape them down securely.

Types of child restraints

You may need to restrain an infant or a child to prevent injury or to facilitate examination, diagnostic tests, or treatment. If so, follow these steps.

• Provide a simple explanation, reassurance, and constant observation to minimize the child's fear.
• Explain the restraint to the parents and enlist their help. Reassure them that it will not hurt the child.

• Make sure restraint ties or safety pins are secured outside the child's reach to prevent injury.
• When using a mummy restraint, secure the infant's arms in proper alignment with the body to avoid dislocation and other injuries.

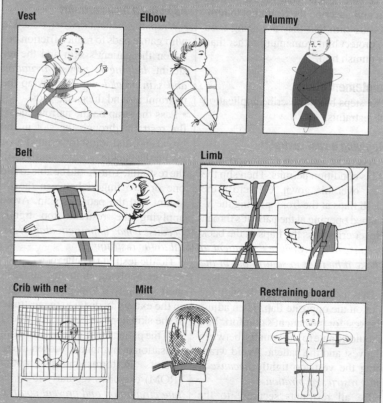

Vest

Elbow

Mummy

Belt

Limb

Crib with net

Mitt

Restraining board

• If you use leather restraints, be sure the straps are unlocked and the key fits the locks.

Patient preparation
• Obtain a doctor's order for the restraint if required. However, never leave a confused or combative patient

unattended or unrestrained while attempting to secure the order.

• If necessary, obtain adequate assistance to restrain the patient before entering his room. Enlist the aid of several coworkers and organize their effort, giving each person a specific task; for example, one person explains the procedure to the patient and applies the restraints while the others immobilize the patient's arms and legs.

• Tell the patient what you're about to do and describe the restraints to him. Assure him that they are being used to protect him from injury rather than to punish him.

Implementation

The steps below describe application of restraints.

Applying a vest restraint

• Assist the patient to a sitting position if his condition permits. Then slip the vest over his gown. Crisscross the cloth flaps at the front, placing the V-shaped opening at the patient's throat. Never crisscross the flaps in the back *because this may cause the patient to choke if he tries to squirm out of the vest.*

• Pass the tab on one flap through the slot on the opposite flap. Then adjust the vest for the patient's comfort. You should be able to slip your fist between the vest and the patient. Avoid wrapping the vest too tightly *because it may restrict respiration.*

• Tie all restraints securely to the frame of the bed, chair, or wheelchair and out of the patient's reach. Use a bow or a knot that can be released quickly and easily in an emergency. Never tie a regular knot to secure the straps. Leave 1″ to 2″ (2.5 to 5 cm) of

slack in the straps to allow room for movement. (See *Knots for securing soft restraints.*)

• After applying the vest, check the patient's respiratory rate and breath sounds regularly. Be alert for signs of respiratory distress. Also, make sure the vest hasn't tightened with the patient's movement. Loosen the vest frequently, if possible, *so the patient can stretch, turn, and breathe deeply.*

Applying a limb restraint

• Wrap the patient's wrist or ankle with gauze pads to reduce friction between the patient's skin and the restraint, *helping to prevent irritation and skin breakdown.* Then wrap the restraint around the gauze pads.

• Pass the strap on the narrow end of the restraint through the slot in the broad end, and adjust for a snug fit. Or fasten the buckle or Velcro cuffs to fit the restraint. You should be able to slip one or two fingers between the restraint and the patient's skin. Avoid applying the restraint too tightly *because it may impair circulation distal to the restraint.*

• Tie the restraint as above.

• After applying limb restraints, be alert for signs of impaired circulation in the extremity distal to the restraint. If the skin appears blue or feels cold, or if the patient complains of a tingling sensation or numbness, loosen the restraint. Perform range-of-motion (ROM) exercises regularly *to stimulate circulation and prevent contractures and loss of mobility.*

Applying a mitt restraint

• Wash and dry the patient's hands.

• Roll up a washcloth or gauze pad, and place it in the patient's palm. Have him form a loose fist, if possible; then pull the mitt over it and secure the closure.

• *To restrict the patient's arm movement,* attach the strap to the mitt and tie it securely, using a bow or a knot that can be released quickly and easily in an emergency.

• When using mitts made of transparent mesh, check hand movement and skin color frequently *to assess circulation.* Remove the mitts regularly *to stimulate circulation,* and perform passive ROM exercises *to prevent contractures.*

Applying a belt restraint

• Center the flannel pad of the belt on the bed. Then wrap the short strap of the belt around the bed frame and fasten it under the bed.

• Position the patient on the pad. Then have him roll slightly to one side while you guide the long strap around his waist and through the slot in the pad.

• Wrap the long strap around the bed frame and fasten it under the bed.

• After applying the belt, slip your hand between the patient and the belt *to ensure a secure but comfortable fit.* A loose belt can be raised to chest level; a tight one can cause abdominal discomfort.

Applying a body (Posey net) restraint

• Place the restraint flat on the bed, with arm and wrist cuffs facing down and the V at the head of the bed.

• Place the patient in the prone position on top of the restraint.

• Lift the V over the patient's head. Thread the chest belt through one of the loops in the V to ensure a snug fit.

Knots for securing soft restraints

When securing soft restraints, use knots that can be released quickly and easily. Remember, never secure restraints to the bed's side rails.

To secure the restraint to the bed frame, use one of these hitches.

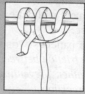

Magnus hitch   **Clove hitch**

Loop

To secure the limb restraint to the patient, use the reverse clove hitch.

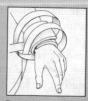

Reverse clove hitch

• Secure the straps around the patient's chest, thighs, and legs. Then turn the patient on his back.

• Secure the straps to the bed frame to anchor the restraint. Then secure the straps around the patient's arms and wrists.

Applying leather restraints

• Position the patient supine on the bed, with each arm and leg securely held down *to minimize combative behavior and to prevent injury to the patient and others.* Immobilize the patient's arms and legs at the joints — knee, ankle, shoulder, and wrist — to minimize his movement without exerting excessive force.

• Apply pads to the patient's wrists and ankles *to reduce friction between his skin and the leather, preventing skin irritation and breakdown.*

• Wrap the restraint around the gauze pads. Then insert the metal loop through the hole that gives the best fit. Apply the restraints securely but not too tightly. You should be able to slip one or two fingers between the restraint and the patient's skin. *A tight restraint can compromise circulation; a loose one can slip off or move up the patient's arm or leg, causing skin irritation and breakdown.*

• Thread the strap through the metal loop on the restraint, close the metal loop, and secure the strap to the bed frame, out of the patient's reach.

• Lock the restraint by pushing in the button on the side of the metal loop, and tug it gently to be sure it's secure. Once it's secure, a coworker can release the arm or leg. Flex the patient's arm or leg slightly before locking the strap *to allow room for movement and to prevent frozen joints and dislocations.*

• Place the key in an accessible location at the nurse's station.

• After applying leather restraints, observe the patient regularly *to give emotional support and to reassess the need for continued use of the restraint.* Check his pulse rate and vital signs at least every 2 hours. Remove or loosen the restraints one at a time, every 2 hours, and perform passive ROM exercises if possible. Watch for signs of impaired peripheral circulation, such as cool, cyanotic skin. To unlock the restraint, insert the key into the metal loop, opposite the locking button. This releases the lock, and the metal loop can be opened.

Complications

• Excessively tight limb restraints can reduce peripheral circulation; tight vest restraints can impair respiration. Apply restraints carefully and check them regularly.

• Skin breakdown can also occur under limb restraints. To prevent this, pad the patient's wrists and ankles, loosen or remove the restraints frequently, and provide regular skin care.

• Long periods of immobility can predispose the patient to pneumonia, urine retention, constipation, and sensory deprivation. Reposition the patient and attend to his elimination requirements as needed.

• Some patients resist restraints by biting, kicking, scratching, or head butting, possibly injuring themselves or others.

Nursing considerations

• Because the authority to use restraints varies among hospitals, learn your hospital's policy. You may be able to apply restraints without a doctor's order in an emergency. Also, be sure to know your state's regulations governing such restraints. For example, some states prohibit the use of four-point restraints.

• When the patient is at high risk for aspiration, restrain him on his side. Never secure all four restraints to one side of the bed *because the patient may fall out of bed.*

• When loosening restraints, have a coworker on hand to assist in restraining the patient if necessary.

• After assessing the patient's behavior and condition, you may decide to use a two-point restraint, which should restrain one arm and the opposite leg — for example, the right arm and the left leg. Never restrain the arm and leg on the same side *because the patient could fall out of bed.*

• Don't apply a limb restraint above an I.V. site *because the constriction may occlude the infusion or cause infiltration into surrounding tissue.*

• Never secure restraints to the side rails *because someone might inadvertently lower the rail before noticing the attached restraint.* This may jerk the patient's limb or body, causing discomfort and trauma.

• Don't restrain a patient in the prone position. *This position limits his field of vision, intensifies feelings of helplessness and vulnerability, and impairs respiration, especially if the patient has been sedated.*

• *Because the restrained patient has limited mobility,* his nutrition, elimination, and positioning become your responsibility. *To prevent pressure ulcers,* reposition the patient regularly, and massage and pad bony prominences and other vulnerable areas.

• When using washable restraints, place them in the laundry as your hospital directs. Many hospitals separate restraints from other linens to avoid losing them.

Documentation

• Record the behavior that necessitated restraints, when the restraints were applied and removed, and the type of restraints used.

• If you expect a continued need for restraints, document their use in the Kardex.

• Record vital signs, skin condition, respiratory status, peripheral circulation, and mental status.

S

Self-catheterization instruction

A patient with impaired or absent bladder function may catheterize himself for routine bladder drainage. Called intermittent self-catheterization, this procedure requires thorough and careful teaching by the nurse. The patient is usually taught to use clean technique for self-catheterization at home, but must use sterile technique in the hospital because of the increased risk of infection.

>> Key nursing diagnoses and patient outcomes

Use these nursing diagnoses as a guide when developing your plan of care for a patient needing intermittent self-catheterization.

Urinary retention related to sensory or neuromuscular impairment

Based on this nursing diagnosis, you'll establish the following patient outcomes. The patient will:
• maintain fluid balance; have equal intake and output.
• express a feeling of increased comfort.
• demonstrate skill in performing self-catheterization.
• identify resources to assist with care following discharge.

Risk for infection related to self-catheterization

Based on this nursing diagnosis, you'll establish the following patient outcomes. The patient will:
• have vital signs, temperature, and laboratory values that remain within normal limits.
• have no pathogens appear in cultures.
• show no signs or symptoms of urinary tract infection.

Equipment

♦ rubber catheter ♦ washcloth ♦ soap and water ♦ small packet of water-soluble lubricant ♦ plastic storage bag ♦ optional: drainage container, paper towels, deodorant (such as Diaparene), rubber or plastic sheets, gooseneck lamp, catheterization record.

Equipment preparation

• Instruct the patient to keep a supply of catheters at home and to use each catheter only once before cleaning it.
• Advise the patient to wash the used catheter in warm, soapy water, rinse it inside and out; then dry it with a clean towel, and store it in a plastic bag until the next time it's needed.
• Catheters become brittle with repeated use, so tell the patient to check them often and to order a new supply well in advance.

Patient preparation

• Tell the patient to begin by trying to urinate into the toilet or, if a toilet's not available or he needs to measure urine quantity, into a drainage container.

• The patient should then wash his hands thoroughly with soap and water and dry them.

Implementation
• Demonstrate how the patient is to perform the catheterization, explaining each step clearly and carefully.
• Position a gooseneck lamp nearby if room lighting is inadequate to make the urinary meatus clearly visible.
• Arrange the patient's clothing so it's out of the way.

Teaching a woman
• Demonstrate and explain to the female patient how to separate the vaginal folds as widely as possible with the fingers of her nondominant hand to fully expose the urinary meatus. Ask if she's right- or left-handed and then tell her which is her nondominant hand.
• While holding her labia open with the nondominant hand, she uses the dominant hand to wash the perineal area thoroughly with a soapy washcloth, using downward strokes. Tell her to rinse the area with the washcloth, using downward strokes as well.
• Show her how to squeeze some lubricant onto the first 3″ (7.6 cm) of the catheter and then how to insert the catheter.
• When the urine stops draining, tell her to remove the catheter slowly, get dressed, and wash the catheter with warm, soapy water. Then she should rinse it inside and out and dry it with a paper towel.

Teaching a man
• Tell a male patient to wash and rinse the end of his penis thoroughly with soap and water, pulling back the foreskin if appropriate. He should keep the foreskin pulled back during the procedure.
• Show him how to squeeze lubricant onto a paper towel and have him roll the first 7″ to 10″ (17.8 to 25 cm) of the catheter in the lubricant. Tell him that copious lubricant will make the procedure more comfortable for him. Then show him how to insert the catheter.
• When the urine stops draining, tell him to remove the catheter slowly and, if necessary, pull the foreskin forward again. Have him get dressed and wash and dry the catheter as described above.

Complications
• Overdistention of the bladder can lead to urinary tract infection and urine leakage.
• Improper hand washing or equipment cleaning can cause urinary tract infection.
• Incorrect catheter insertion can injure the urethral or bladder mucosa.

Nursing considerations
• Impress on the patient that the timing of catheterization is critical to preventing overdistention of the bladder, which can lead to infection. Intermittent self-catheterization usually occurs every 4 to 6 hours around the clock (or more often at first).
• Female patients should be able to identify the body parts involved in self-catheterization: labia majora, labia minora, vagina, and urinary meatus.
• Keep in mind the difference between boiling and sterilization. Boiling kills bacteria, viruses and fungi, but does

Teaching self-catheterization

Teach a woman to hold the catheter in her dominant hand as if it were a pencil or a dart, about ½" (1.3 cm) from its tip. Keeping the vaginal folds separated, she should slowly insert the lubricated catheter about 3" (7.6 cm) into the urethra. Tell her to press down with her abdominal muscles to empty the bladder, allowing all urine to drain through the catheter and into the toilet or drainage container.

Teach a man to hold his penis in his nondominant hand, at a right angle to his body. He should hold the catheter in his dominant hand as if it were a pencil or a dart and slowly insert it 7" to 10" (17.8 to 25 cm) into the urethra until urine begins flowing. Then he should gently advance the catheter about 1" (2.5 cm) farther, allowing all urine to drain into the toilet or drainage container.

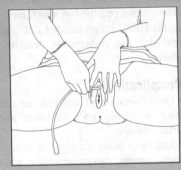
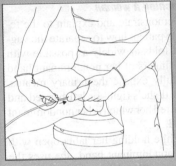

not kill spores, whereas sterilization does. However, *because catheter cleaning will be done in the patient's home, boiling provides sufficient safeguard against spreading infections.*
• Advise the patient to store cleaned catheters only after they are completely dry *to prevent growth of gram-negative organisms.*
• Stress the importance of regulating fluid intake, as ordered, *to prevent incontinence while maintaining adequate hydration.* However, explain that incontinent episodes may occur occasionally. For managing incontinence, the doctor or a home health care nurse can help develop a plan, such as more frequent catheteriza-

tions. After an incontinent episode, tell the patient to wash with soap and water, pat the area dry with a towel, and expose the skin to the air for as long as possible. Urine odor can be reduced by putting methylbenzethonium chloride (Diaparene) or cornstarch on the skin. Bedding and furniture can be protected by covering them with rubber or plastic sheets and then covering the rubber or plastic with fabric.
• Stress the importance of taking medications as ordered *to increase urine retention and help prevent incontinence.* The patient should avoid calcium-rich and phosphorus-rich foods,

as ordered, to reduce the chance of renal calculus formation.

Home care
• See *Teaching self-catheterization.*

Documentation
• Record the date and times of catheterization, character of the urine (odor, color, clarity, presence of particles or blood), the amount of urine (increase, decrease, no change), and any problems encountered during the procedure.
• Note whether the patient has difficulty performing a return demonstration.

Sequential compression therapy

Sequential compression therapy helps prevent deep vein thrombosis in surgical patients. The technique involves massaging the legs in a wavelike, milking motion that promotes blood flow and deters thrombosis. It's a safe, effective, and noninvasive type of therapy.

Typically, sequential compression therapy complements other preventive measures, such as antiembolism stockings and anticoagulant medications. Although patients at low risk for deep vein thrombosis may require only antiembolism stockings, those at moderate to high risk may require both antiembolism stockings and sequential compression therapy. These preventive measures will be administered for as long as the patient remains at risk.

Both antiembolism stockings and sequential compression sleeves are commonly used preoperatively because blood clots tend to form during surgery. About 20% of blood clots form in the femoral vein. Sequential compression therapy counteracts blood stasis and coagulation changes, which are two of the three major factors that promote deep vein thrombosis. It reduces stasis by increasing peak blood flow velocity and helping to empty the femoral vein's valve cusps of pooled or static blood. Also, the compressions cause an anticlotting effect by increasing fibrinolytic activity, which stimulates the release of a plasminogen activator.

≫ Key nursing diagnoses and patient outcomes
Use these nursing diagnoses as a guide when developing your plan of care for a patient using sequential compression therapy.

Impaired physical mobility related to (specify)
Based on this nursing diagnosis, you'll establish the following patient outcomes. The patient will:
• maintain muscle strength and joint range of motion.
• show no evidence of complications, such as contractures, venous stasis, thrombus formation, or skin breakdown.
• have mobility regimen carried out by a family member or another caregiver.

Risk for peripheral neurovascular dysfunction

Based on this nursing diagnosis, you'll establish the following patient outcomes. The patient will:
• maintain circulation in extremities.
• demonstrate correct body positioning techniques.
• have no symptoms of neurovascular compromise.

Equipment

♦ measuring tape and sizing chart for the brand of sleeves you're using ♦ pair of compression sleeves in correct size ♦ connecting tubing ♦ compression controller.

Patient preparation

• Explain the procedure to the patient to increase her cooperation.

Implementation

Follow these steps.

To determine proper sleeve size

Before applying the compression sleeve, determine the proper size of sleeve that you need.
• Begin by washing your hands.
• Measure the circumference of the upper thigh while the patient rests in bed. Do this by placing the measuring tape under the thigh at the gluteal furrow.
• Hold the tape snugly, but not tightly, around the patient's leg. Note the exact circumference.
• Find the patient's thigh measurement on the sizing chart, and locate the corresponding size of the compression sleeve.
• Remove the compression sleeves from the package and unfold them.

• Lay the unfolded sleeves on a flat surface with the cotton lining facing up.
• Notice the markings on the lining denoting the ankle and the area behind the knee at the popliteal pulse point. Use these markings to position the sleeve at the appropriate landmarks.

To apply the sleeves

• Place the patient's leg on the sleeve lining. Position the back of the knee over the popliteal opening.
• Make sure that the back of the ankle is over the ankle marking.
• Starting at the side opposite the clear plastic tubing, wrap the sleeve snugly around the patient's leg.
• Fasten the sleeve securely with the Velcro fasteners. For the best fit, first secure the ankle and calf sections, then the thigh.
• The sleeve should fit snugly but not tightly. Check the fit by inserting two fingers between the sleeve and the patient's leg at the knee opening. Loosen or tighten the sleeve by readjusting the Velcro fastener.
• Using the same procedure, apply the second sleeve.

To operate the system

• Connect each sleeve to the tubing leading to the controller. Both sleeves must connect to the compression controller for the system to operate. Line up the blue arrows on the sleeve connector with the arrows on the tubing connectors; push the ends together firmly. Listen for a click signaling a firm connection. Make sure that the tubing has no kinks.
• Plug the compression controller into the proper wall outlet. Turn the power on.

• The controller automatically sets the compression sleeve pressure at 45 mm Hg, which is the midpoint of the normal range (35 to 55 mm Hg).
• Observe the patient *to see how well he tolerates the therapy and the controller as the system completes its first cycle.* Typically, each cycle lasts 71 seconds — 11 seconds of compression and 60 seconds of decompression.
• The cycle monitor displays the sequence status continuously. During compression, the words *ankle, calf,* and *thigh* light up as the respective chambers inflate. Besides regulating sequential compressions, the controller supplies pressure in increments, starting at 45 mm Hg in the ankle, dropping to 40 mm Hg in the calf, and leveling off at 30 mm Hg in the thigh.
• During decompression — or the vent cycle — you'll see the word *vent* displayed on the monitor.
• Check the AUDIBLE ALARM key. The green light should be lit, indicating that the alarm is working.
• The compression sleeves should function continuously (24 hours a day) until the patient is fully ambulatory. Check the sleeves at least once each shift *to ensure proper fit and inflation.*

To remove the sleeves

• You may remove the sleeves when the patient is walking, bathing, or leaving the room for tests or other procedures. Reapply them immediately after any of these activities.
• To disconnect the sleeves from the blue tubing, depress the latches on each side of the connectors and pull the connectors apart.
• Store the blue tubing and compression controller according to hospital protocol. This equipment is not disposable.

Complications

Don't use this therapy in patients with any of the following conditions:
• acute deep vein thrombosis (or deep vein thrombosis diagnosed within the last 6 months)
• severe arteriosclerosis or any other ischemic vascular disease
• massive edema of the legs resulting from pulmonary edema or congestive heart failure
• any local condition that the compression sleeves would aggravate, such as dermatitis, vein ligation, gangrene, or recent skin grafting. (A patient with a pronounced leg deformity also would be unlikely to benefit from the compression sleeves.)

Nursing considerations

• Although pressure adjustments are seldom necessary, they can be made if directed by the doctor. Push either the up or down arrow keys labeled PRESSURE ADJUST on the front of the controller.
• If directed to adjust the settings, remember to stay within the clinically effective pressure range of 35 to 55 mm Hg.
• The compression controller also has a mechanism to help cool the patient. To activate it, push the SLEEVE COOLING key, and a small green light will appear to the right of this key.
• Avoid activating the sleeve-cooling feature in the operating room, where it may cause undesirable air movement.
• If you are applying only one sleeve — for example, if the patient has a cast — leave the unused sleeve folded in

the plastic bag. Cut a small hole in the bag's sealed bottom edge, and pull the sleeve connector (the part that holds the connecting tubing) through the hole. Then join both sleeves to the compression controller.

• If a malfunction triggers the instrument's alarm, you'll hear beeping and see a fault code in the display window that originally presented the pressure, for example, *Fault Sh*. The system shuts off whenever the alarm is activated.

• To respond to the alarm, remove the operator's card from the slot on the top of the compression controller. Match the fault code in the display window with the matching code listed on the operator's card.

• Follow the instructions printed on the card next to the matching code. For example, if *Sh* appears, check the tubing for kinks. If *Sl* appears, check for loose connections.

Documentation

• Document the procedure, the patient's response to and understanding of the procedure, and the status of the alarm and cooling settings.

Sinus palpation

Four pairs of paranasal sinuses open into the internal nose. The largest pair, the maxillary sinuses, lie within the maxilla. The smaller ethmoid sinuses are located between the orbits and the upper nasal cavity. The frontal sinuses lie within the frontal bone, whereas the sphenoid sinuses lie within the sphenoid bone. The small openings between the sinuses and the nasal cavity can easily become obstructed because they are lined with mucous membrane that can become inflamed and swollen.

You'll be able to examine the frontal and maxillary sinuses, but not the ethmoid and sphenoid sinuses.

≫ Key nursing diagnoses and patient outcomes

Use these nursing diagnoses as a guide when developing your plan of care.

Risk for infection related to inflamed sinuses

Based on this nursing diagnosis, you'll establish the following patient outcomes. The patient will:

• have vital signs, temperature, and laboratory values that remain within normal limits.

• have no pathogens appear in cultures.

• show no signs or symptoms of infection when the sinuses are palpated.

Pain related to inflamed sinuses

Based on this nursing diagnosis, you'll establish the following patient outcomes. The patient will:

• identify pain characteristics.

• state and carry out appropriate interventions for pain relief.

• express a feeling of comfort and relief from pain.

Equipment

No special equipment is necessary for sinus palpation.

Patient preparation

• Explain the procedure *to ensure cooperation and reduce the patient's anxiety.*

• Position the patient sitting upright and facing you.

Implementation
- Wash your hands.
- Inspect for swelling around the eyes.
- To palpate the frontal sinuses, place your thumbs above the patient's eyes, just under the bony ridges of the upper orbits. Place your fingertips on the forehead and apply gentle pressure (top photo, below).
- Palpate over the frontal sinuses for tenderness. Avoid pressing on the eyeball.
- Palpate the maxillary sinuses by gently pressing your thumbs (or index and middle fingers) on each side of the nose just below the zygomatic bone (bottom photo, below). Note any tenderness.

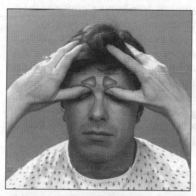

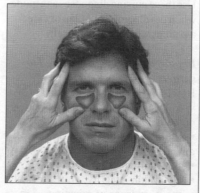

- Lightly percuss over the frontal and maxillary sinus areas (as shown below). Note any tenderness.

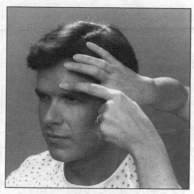

Nursing considerations
- Local sinus tenderness accompanied by fever and nasal drainage suggests acute sinusitis. This form of sinusitis usually involves the frontal or maxillary sinuses.

Documentation
- Document the presence of redness, edema, or tenderness.
- Note the date and time of the examination.

Skin graft care

A skin graft consists of healthy skin taken either from the patient (autograft) or a donor (allograft) and applied to a part of the patient's body. There the graft resurfaces an area damaged by burns, traumatic injury, or surgery. Care procedures for an autograft or allograft are essentially the same. However, an autograft requires care for two sites: the graft site and the donor site.

Understanding graft types

A burn patient may receive one or more of the graft types described below.

Split-thickness
The type used most commonly for covering open burns, a split-thickness graft includes the epidermis and part of the dermis. It may be applied as a sheet (usually on the face or neck to preserve the cosmetic result) or as a mesh. A mesh graft has tiny slits cut in that allow the graft to expand up to nine times its original size. Mesh grafts prevent fluids from collecting under the graft and typically are used over extensive full-thickness burns.

Full-thickness
This graft type includes the epidermis and the entire dermis. Consequently, the graft contains hair follicles, sweat glands, and sebaceous glands, which typically aren't included in split-thickness grafts. Full-thickness grafts usually are used for small burns that cause deep wounds.

Pedicle-flap
This full-thickness graft includes not only skin and subcutaneous tissue, but also subcutaneous blood vessels to ensure a continued blood supply to the graft. Pedicle-flap grafts may be used during reconstructive surgery to cover previous defects.

The graft may be one of several types: split-thickness, full-thickness, or pedicle-flap. (See *Understanding graft types*.)

Successful grafting depends on various factors, including clean wound granulation with adequate vascularization; complete contact of the graft with the wound bed; aseptic technique to prevent infection; adequate graft immobilization; and skilled care.

The size and depth of the patient's burns determine whether they will require grafting.

Grafting is usually done at the completion of wound debridement. The goal is to cover all wounds with an autograft or allograft within 2 weeks. With enzymatic debridement, grafting may be performed 5 to 7 days after debridement is complete; with surgical debridement, grafting can occur the same day as the surgery.

Depending on hospital policy, a doctor or a specially trained nurse may change graft dressings. The dressings usually stay in place for 3 to 5 days after surgery to avoid disturbing the graft site. Meanwhile, the donor graft site needs diligent care. (See *How to care for a donor graft site*.)

≫ Key nursing diagnoses and patient outcomes
Use these nursing diagnoses as a guide when developing your plan of care for a patient who has a skin graft.

Impaired skin integrity related to surgery
Based on this nursing diagnosis, you'll establish the following patient outcomes. The patient will:
• exhibit no evidence of skin breakdown.
• show normal skin turgor.
• regain skin integrity; graft site heals without evidence of rejection.

How to care for a donor graft site

Autografts are usually taken from another area of the patient's body with a dermatome. This instrument cuts uniform, split-thickness skin portions — typically, about 0.013 to 0.05 cm thick. Essentially, autografting makes the donor site a partial-thickness wound, which may bleed, drain, and cause pain.

This site needs scrupulous care to prevent infection, which could convert the site to a full-thickness wound. Depending on the graft's thickness, tissue may be obtained from the donor site again in as few as 10 days.

Usually, Xeroflo gauze is applied postoperatively. The outer gauze dressing can be taken off on the first postoperative day; the Xeroflo will protect the new epithelial proliferation.

Care for the donor site as you care for the autograft, using dressing changes at the initial stages to prevent infection and promote healing. Follow the guidelines below.

Dressing the wound
• Wash your hands and put on sterile gloves.
• Remove the outer gauze dressings within 24 hours. Inspect the Xeroflo for signs of infection; then leave it open to the air to speed drying and healing.
• Leave small amounts of fluid accumulation alone. Using aseptic technique, aspirate larger amounts through the dressing with a small-gauge needle and syringe.
• Apply a lanolin-based cream daily to completely healed donor sites to keep skin tissue pliable and to remove crusts.

• communicate understanding of skin protection measures.
• demonstrate skill in care of graft site.

Risk for infection related to presence of graft
Based on this nursing diagnosis, you'll establish the following patient outcomes. The patient will:
• have vital signs, temperature, and laboratory values that remain within normal limits.
• have no pathogens that appear in cultures.
• show no signs or symptoms of infection at the graft site.

Equipment
♦ ordered analgesic ♦ clean and sterile gloves ♦ sterile gown ♦ cap ♦ mask ♦ sterile forceps ♦ sterile scissors ♦ sterile scalpel ♦ sterile 4″ × 4″ gauze pads ♦ Xeroflo gauze ♦ elastic gauze dressing ♦ warm normal saline solution ♦ moisturizing cream ♦ topical medication (such as micronized silver sulfadiazine cream) ♦ optional: sterile cotton-tipped applicators.

Equipment preparation
• Assemble the equipment on the dressing cart.

Patient preparation
• Explain the procedure to the patient and provide privacy.

Evacuating fluid from a sheet graft

When small pockets of fluid (called blebs) accumulate beneath a sheet graft, you'll need to evacuate the fluid using a sterile scalpel and cotton-tipped applicators. First, carefully perforate the center of the bleb with the scalpel.

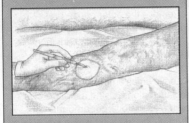

Gently express the fluid with cotton-tipped applicators.

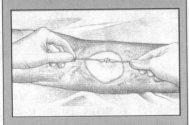

Never express fluid by rolling the bleb to the edge of the graft. This would disturb healing in other areas.

• Administer an analgesic, as ordered, 20 to 30 minutes before beginning the procedure. Alternatively, give an I.V. analgesic immediately before the procedure.

Implementation
• Wash your hands.
• Put on the sterile gown and clean mask, cap, and gloves.

• Gently lift off all outer dressings.
• Soak the middle dressings with warm saline solution. Remove these carefully and slowly *to avoid disturbing the graft site.*
• Leave the Xeroflo intact *to avoid dislodging the graft.*
• Remove and discard the clean gloves, wash your hands, and put on the sterile gloves.
• Assess the condition of the graft. If you see purulent drainage, notify the doctor.
• Remove the Xeroflo with sterile forceps, and clean the area gently. If necessary, soak the Xeroflo with warm saline solution *to facilitate removal.*
• Inspect an allograft for signs of rejection, such as infection and delayed healing. Inspect a sheet graft frequently for blebs. If ordered, evacuate them carefully with a sterile scalpel. (See *Evacuating fluid from a sheet graft.*)
• Place fresh Xeroflo over the site *to promote wound healing and prevent infection.* Cover this with burn gauze and a roller bandage.
• Clean any completely healed areas, and apply a moisturizing cream to them *to keep the skin pliable and to retard scarring.*

Complications
• Graft failure may result from traumatic injury, hematoma or seroma formation, infection, an inadequate graft bed, rejection, or compromised nutritional status.

Nursing considerations
• *To avoid dislodging the graft,* hydrotherapy is usually discontinued, as ordered, for 3 to 4 days after grafting.
• Avoid using a blood pressure cuff over the graft.

• Don't tug or pull dressings during dressing changes.
• Keep the patient from lying on the graft.
• If the graft dislodges, apply sterile skin compresses *to keep the area moist until the surgeon reapplies the graft.*
• If the graft affects an arm or a leg, elevate the affected extremity *to reduce postoperative edema.*
• Check for bleeding and signs of neurovascular impairment: increasing pain, numbness or tingling, coolness, and pallor.

Home care
• Teach the patient how to apply moisturizing cream.
• Emphasize the importance of using a sunscreen with a sun protection factor of 20 or higher on all grafted areas to avoid sunburn and discoloration.
• Tell the patient to call the doctor if there are any signs of infection or rejection.

Documentation
• Record the time and date of all dressing changes.
• Document all medications used, and note the patient's response to the medications.
• Describe the condition of the graft, and note any signs of infection or rejection.
• Record any additional treatment.
• Note the patient's reaction to the graft.

Skin, hair, and nail inspection

The largest and heaviest body system, the skin and its appendages (the hair,

nails, and certain glands) perform many vital functions: they protect the inner organs, bones, muscles, and blood vessels; they help to regulate body temperature and provide sensory information; they prevent body fluids from escaping while allowing body wastes to escape through more than 2 million pores.

Assessment of the skin, hair, and nails begins with a complete health history. Remember that skin disorders may involve or stem from disorders in other body systems.

Examining the patient's nails is a vital part of your assessment because they can be a critical indicator of a systemic illness. Plus, their overall condition tells you much about the patient's grooming habits and level of self-care.

≫ Key nursing diagnoses and patient outcomes
Use these nursing diagnoses as a guide when developing your plan of care for a patient who has a skin disorder.

Impaired skin integrity related to (specify)
Based on this nursing diagnosis, you'll establish the following patient outcomes. The patient will:
• exhibit no evidence of skin breakdown.
• show normal skin turgor.
• regain skin integrity; wound heals without evidence of infection.
• communicate understanding of skin protection measures.
• demonstrate skill in skin care.

Risk for infection related to altered skin integrity

Based on this nursing diagnosis, you'll establish the following patient outcomes. The patient will:
• have vital signs, temperature, and laboratory values that remain within normal limits.
• have no pathogens appear in cultures.
• show no signs or symptoms of skin infections.

Equipment
♦ centimeter ruler ♦ disposable gloves.

Patient preparation
• Make sure the lighting is adequate for the assessment.
• Because the patient will be partially undressed, make sure the room temperature is comfortably warm.

Implementation
• Wash your hands.
• Put on a pair of gloves to protect yourself during palpation.

Skin
• To examine the patient's skin, use inspection and palpation, sometimes simultaneously.
• Begin by systematically inspecting the skin's overall appearance. Observe general coloring and pigmentation, keeping in mind racial differences as well as normal variations from one part of the body to another.
• Examine all the exposed areas of the skin, including the face, ears, back of the neck, the axillae, and the backs of the hands and arms.
• Always ask the patient if he has noticed any changes in skin color anywhere on his body.

• Inspect and palpate the texture of the skin, noting thickness and mobility.
• *To determine if the skin over a joint is supple or taut,* have the patient bend the joint as you palpate.
• Assessing the turgor, or elasticity, of the patient's skin helps you to evaluate hydration. To assess turgor, gently squeeze the skin on the forearm. If it quickly returns to its original shape, the patient has normal turgor. If it resumes its original shape slowly or maintains a tented shape, the skin has poor turgor.
• Observe the skin for excessive dryness or moisture.
• *To assess skin temperature,* touch the surface, using the backs of your fingers.
• If you detect a lesion, identify the type and provide an accurate description. Classify it as primary or secondary. A primary lesion is the initial lesion that develops. When changes take place in a primary lesion, it's considered a secondary lesion. (See *Identifying primary and secondary skin lesions.*)
• Note whether the primary lesion is solid or fluid-filled. Macules, papules, nodules, wheals, and hives are examples of solid lesions. Vesicles, bullae, pustules, and cysts are fluid-filled lesions. (See *Macule or papule? page 787.*)
• Inspect the patient's skin daily and document findings, particularly noting any change in status, *to prevent or minimize skin breakdown.*

Hair
• Examine the hair over the patient's entire body, not just on the head.
• Assess the distribution, quantity, texture, and color.

Identifying primary and secondary skin lesions

Use these descriptions and drawings to help identify your patient's lesion. When examining a lesion, remember to keep your centimeter (cm) ruler with you so that measurements will be accurate.

Primary lesions
Macule

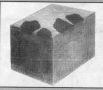

A flat, circumscribed area of altered skin color; generally less than 1 cm. Examples: freckles, flat nevus

Patch

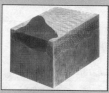

A macule larger than 1 cm. Example: herald patch (pityriasis rosea)

Papule

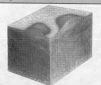

Raised, circumscribed, solid area; generally less than 1 cm. Examples: elevated nevus, wart

Pustule

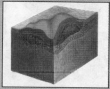

Raised lesion containing purulent fluid; varying in size. Examples: impetigo, furuncle

Nodule

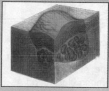

Raised or solid area; generally greater than 1 cm. Examples: acne pustulosa, epithelioma

Tumor

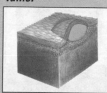

Solid lesion extending into dermal and subcutaneous layers; can be raised, level with skin, or beneath skin; larger than 1 cm. Example: tumor stage of mycosis fungoides

Plaque

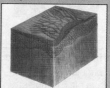

Circumscribed, superficial, solid elevation; larger than 1 cm. Examples: localized mycosis fungoides, neurodermatitis

Vesicle

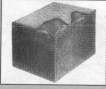

Circumscribed, elevated lesion; contains serous fluid; less than 1 cm. Examples: early chicken pox, contact dermatitis

Bulla

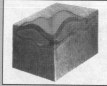

Vesicle larger than 2 cm. Examples: pemphigus, second-degree burn

(continued)

Identifying primary and secondary skin lesions *(continued)*

Secondary lesions
Scale

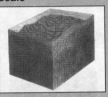

Thickened, desiccated epithelial cells that flake off. Examples: dandruff, psoriasis

Crust

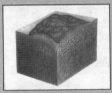

Dried serum, blood, or purulent exudate. Examples: impetigo, infectious dermatitis

Fissure

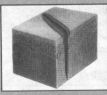

Deep linear break in the skin, extending into the dermis. Examples: congenital syphilis, athlete's foot

Erosion

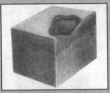

Circumscribed, moist, depressed lesion. Example: abrasion

Keloid

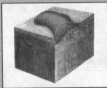

Thick, firm, reddened scar formed by hyperplasia of fibrous tissue; more common among blacks and Asians. Example: surgical incision

Ulcer

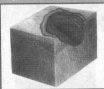

Localized tissue destruction that can extend into mucous membrane or through epidermis, dermis, and underlying tissue. Example: tertiary syphilis

Scar

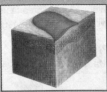

Area of replacement connective tissue, resulting from damage or disease. Example: healed surgical incision

Excoriation

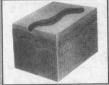

Abrasion or scratch mark. Example: eczema

Lichenification

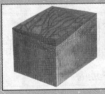

Thickened, rough skin with obvious lines. Example: chronic atopic dermatitis

• Examine the pattern of the patient's hair growth and loss. If you note patchy hair loss, look for regrowth.
• Check the scalp for erythema, scaling, and encrustations.

Nails

• Note the nail color. Light-skinned patients generally have pinkish nails, and dark-skinned patients typically have brown nails with longitudinal lines.
• Inspect the shape and texture of the patient's nails, noting brittleness, cracking, peeling, striations, ridges, or depressions.
• *To detect finger clubbing,* inspect and palpate. With clubbed fingers, the nail is thickened, hard, shiny, and curved at the end.
• Press the nail base to determine firmness, and press the nail to determine the strength of its attachment to the nailbed.
• *To assess capillary refill,* press the tip of the nail plate and check for blanching. The color should return in less than 1 second after you release the pressure. A delay could indicate cardiovascular disease.

Nursing considerations

• *To detect color variations in dark-skinned and black patients,* examine the sclerae, conjunctivae, buccal mucosa, tongue, lips, nail beds, palms, and soles. A yellowish brown color in dark-skinned patients or an ashen gray color in black patients indicates pallor.
• Changes may indicate local irritation or trauma, or can be a result of problems in other body systems. For example, rough, dry skin is common in hypothyroidism; soft, smooth skin is common in hyperthyroidism.

Macule or papule?

To determine whether a lesion is a macule or a papule, try this test. Reduce direct light, and shine a penlight or flashlight at a right angle to the lesion. If the light casts a shadow, the lesion is a papule. Macules are flat and won't produce a shadow.

• *To accurately assess skin turgor in an elderly patient,* try squeezing the skin of the sternum or forehead instead of the forearm. In an elderly patient, the skin of the forearm tends to be flaccid, so using this site doesn't permit accurate evaluation of the patient's hydration.
• Use proper hand washing and universal precautions when providing direct care *to minimize the patient's risk of infection.*
• Help the patient turn every 2 hours. Provide skin care, particularly over bony prominences, *to help prevent venous stasis and skin breakdown.*
• Ensure adequate nutritional intake. Offer high-protein supplements, unless contraindicated, *to aid healing, help stabilize weight, and improve muscle tone and mass.*

Home care

• If there is an alteration in skin integrity, discuss precipitating factors, if known.
• Explain dietary restrictions if the patient has an allergy to food.
• Instruct the patient and family members in skin care regimen. Supervise the patient's skin care regimen and provide feedback.
• Educate the patient regarding good hand-washing technique, factors that

increase risk of infection, and infection signs and symptoms.
• Encourage adherence to other aspects of health care management to control or minimize effects on skin.

Documentation
• Note the location of any bruising, discoloration, or erythema.
• Document skin color (noting pallor, a dusky appearance, jaundice, and cyanosis), texture, turgor, moisture, and temperature. Note generalized and localized warmth or coolness.
• When you palpate local edema, be sure to document any associated discolorations or lesions. Note the lesion's location, distribution pattern (local or generalized), and configuration (separate or fused together) as well as any associated symptoms. Document a primary lesion as solid or fluid-filled.
• Use the *ABCD* mnemonic device to describe a lesion:
  A: *A*symmetry. Is the lesion symmetrical or asymmetrical?
  B: *B*order. Note whether the border is well defined.
  C: *C*olor.
  D: *D*iameter. Measure the diameter using a centimeter ruler. Don't estimate.
• If you note drainage from a lesion, document the type and amount and if it is malodorous.
• Note the distribution, quality, texture, and color of the hair and scalp.
• Document the shape, texture, and color of the patient's nails.
• Note capillary refill.
• Document the presence of finger clubbing.

Skull tongs

Applying skeletal traction with skull tongs immobilizes the cervical spine after a fracture or dislocation, invasion by tumor or infection, or surgery. Three types of skull tongs are commonly used: Crutchfield, Gardner-Wells, and Vinke. Crutchfield tongs are applied by incising the skin with a scalpel, drilling a hole in the exposed skull, and inserting the pins on the tongs into the hole. Gardner-Wells tongs and Vinke tongs are applied less invasively. Gardner-Wells tongs have spring-loaded pins that are advanced gently into the scalp; then the tongs are tightened to secure the apparatus. (See *Types of skull tongs*, page 790.)

After any tongs are applied, traction is created by extending a rope from the center of the tongs over a pulley and attaching weights to it. With the help of X-ray monitoring, the weights are then adjusted to establish reduction, if necessary, and to maintain alignment. Nursing care of the patient with skull tongs requires meticulous pin site care (three times a day to prevent infection) and frequent observation of the traction apparatus to make sure it's working properly.

❯❯ Key nursing diagnoses and patient outcomes
Use these nursing diagnoses as a guide when developing your plan of care for a patient with skull tongs.

Risk for infection related to presence of invasive appliance

Based on this nursing diagnosis, you'll establish the following patient outcomes. The patient will:
• have vital signs, temperature, and laboratory values remain within normal limits.
• have no pathogens appear in cultures.
• show no signs or symptoms of infection at insertion sites.

Impaired physical mobility related to skeletal traction

Based on this nursing diagnosis, you'll establish the following patient outcomes. The patient will:
• maintain muscle strength and joint range of motion.
• show no evidence of complications, such as contractures, venous stasis, thrombus formation, or skin break down.

Equipment

♦ three medicine cups ♦ one bottle each of ordered cleaning solution, normal saline solution, and povidone-iodine solution ♦ sterile, cotton-tipped applicators ♦ sandbags or cervical collar (hard or soft) ♦ fine mesh gauze strips ♦ $4'' \times 4''$ gauze pads ♦ sterile gloves ♦ sterile basin ♦ sterile scissors ♦ hair clippers ♦ optional: turning frame, antibacterial ointment.

Equipment preparation

• Bring the equipment to the patient's room.
• Place the medicine cups on the bedside table.
• Fill one cup with a small amount of cleaning solution, one with normal saline solution, and one with povidone-iodine solution. Then set out the cotton-tipped applicators.
• Keep the sandbags or cervical collar handy for emergency immobilization of the head and neck if the pins in the tongs should slip.

Patient preparation

• Explain the procedure to the patient.
• Inform the patient that pin sites usually feel tender for several days after the tongs are applied, and that he'll feel some muscular discomfort in the injured area.
• Before providing care, observe each pin site carefully for signs of infection, such as loose pins, swelling or redness, or purulent drainage. Use hair clippers to trim the patient's hair around the pin sites, when necessary.

Implementation

• Wash your hands.
• Put on gloves.
• Gently wipe each pin site with a cotton-tipped applicator dipped in cleaning solution *to loosen and remove crusty drainage*. Repeat with a fresh applicator, as needed, for thorough cleaning. Use a separate applicator for each site. Next, wipe each site with normal saline solution *to remove excess cleaning solution*. Finally, wipe with povidone-iodine *to provide asepsis at the site and prevent infection*.
• After providing care, discard all pin-site cleaning materials.
• If the pin sites are infected, apply a povidone-iodine wrap, as ordered. First, obtain strips of fine mesh gauze, or cut a $4'' \times 4''$ gauze pad into strips (using sterile scissors and wearing sterile gloves). Soak the strips in a sterile basin of povidone-iodine solu-

Types of skull tongs

Skull (or cervical) tongs consist of a stainless steel body with a pin at the end of each arm. Each pin is about $1/8''$ (0.3 cm) in diameter with a sharp tip.

On **Crutchfield tongs,** the pins are placed about $5''$ (12.7 cm) apart in line with the long axis of the cervical spine.

On **Gardner-Wells tongs,** the pins are farther apart. They are inserted slightly above the patient's ears.

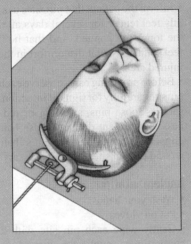

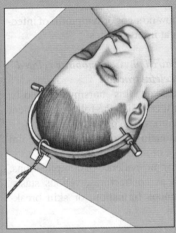

tion or normal saline solution, and squeeze out the excess solution. Wrap one strip securely around each pin site. Leave the strip in place to dry until you provide care again. *Removing the dried strip aids in debridement and helps clear the infection.*

• Check the traction apparatus — rope, weights, and pulleys — at the start of each shift, every 4 hours, and as necessary (for example, after position changes). Make sure the rope hangs freely and that the weights never rest on the floor or become caught under the bed.

Complications

• Infection, excessive traction force, or osteoporosis can cause the skull pins to slip or pull out. Because this interrupts traction, the patient must receive immediate attention to prevent further injury.

Nursing considerations

• At times, the doctor may prefer an antibacterial ointment for pin site care instead of povidone-iodine solution. *To remove old ointment,* wrap a cotton-tipped applicator with a $4'' \times 4''$ gauze pad, moisten it with cleaning solution, and gently clean each site. Keep a box of sterile gauze pads handy at the patient's bedside.

On *Vinke tongs,* the pins are placed at the parietal bones, near the widest transverse diameter of the skull, about 1″ (2.5 cm) above the helix.

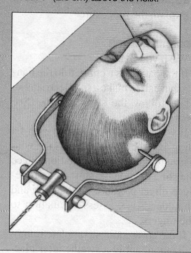

• Watch for signs and symptoms of loose pins, such as persistent pain or tenderness at pin sites, redness, and drainage. The patient may also report feeling or hearing the pins move.
• If you suspect a pin has loosened or slipped, don't turn the patient until the doctor examines the skull tongs and fixes them as needed.
• If the pins fall out, immobilize the patient's head and neck with sandbags or apply a cervical collar. Then carefully remove the traction weights. Apply manual traction to the patient's head by placing your hands on each side of the mandible and pulling very gently, while maintaining proper alignment. Once you stabilize the

alignment, have someone send for the doctor immediately. Remain calm and reassure the patient. Once traction is reestablished, take the patient's neurologic vital signs.

Nursing alert: Never add or subtract weights to the traction apparatus without an order from the doctor. *This can cause neurologic impairment.*
• Take neurologic vital signs at the beginning of each shift, every 4 hours, and as necessary (for example, after turning or transporting the patient). Carefully assess the function of cranial nerves, which may be impaired by pin placement. Note any asymmetry, deviation, or atrophy. Review the patient's chart *to determine baseline neurologic vital signs on admission to the hospital and immediately after the tongs were applied.*
• Monitor respirations closely and keep suction equipment handy. Remember, *injury to the cervical spine may affect respiration.* So be alert for signs of respiratory distress, such as unequal chest expansion and an irregular or altered respiratory rate or pattern.
• Patients with skull tongs may be placed on a turning frame *to facilitate turning without disrupting vertebral alignment.* Establish a turning schedule for the patient — usually a supine position for 2 hours and then a prone position for 1 hour — *to help prevent complications of immobility.*

Documentation
• Record the date, time, and type of pin site care and the patient's response to the procedure in your notes.
• Describe any signs of infection.
• Note if any weights were added or subtracted.

• Record the patient's neurologic vital signs, respiratory status, and the turning schedule on the Kardex.

Sling application

A sling — made from a triangular piece of muslin, canvas, or cotton — supports and immobilizes an injured arm, wrist, or hand, and thereby facilitates healing. It may be applied to restrict movement of a fracture or dislocation or to support a muscle sprain. A sling can also support the weight of a splint or help secure dressings.

≫ Key nursing diagnoses and patient outcomes

Use these nursing diagnoses as a guide when developing your plan of care for a patient with a triangular sling.

Impaired physical mobility related to triangular sling

Based on this nursing diagnosis, you'll establish the following patient outcomes. The patient will:
• maintain muscle strength and joint range of motion.
• show no evidence of complications, such as contractures, venous stasis, thrombus formation, or skin breakdown.

Dressing or grooming self-care deficit related to need for triangular sling

Based on this nursing diagnosis, you'll establish the following patient outcomes. The patient will:
• have self-care needs met daily.
• have minimal or no complications.

• identify resources to help cope with problems after discharge.

Equipment
♦ triangular bandage or commercial sling ♦ gauze (for padding) ♦ safety pins (tape for children under age 7).

Patient preparation
• Explain the procedure.

Implementation
• Wash your hands.
• If the patient is a child, fold the bandage in half to make a smaller triangle. Then follow the steps shown. (See *Making a sling*, page 229.)
• If you anticipate prolonged use of a sling, pad the area under the knot with gauze to prevent skin irritation. Place the sling outside the shirt collar to reduce direct pressure on the neck and shoulder. Also, assess circulation to the fingers.
• If the arm requires complete immobilization, apply a swathe after placing the arm in a sling. (See *Applying a swathe*.)

Nursing considerations
• At regular intervals, check to make sure the sling stays in proper position.

Home care
• Before the patient leaves the hospital, provide an extra triangular bandage.
• Teach the patient and a family member or friend how to change the sling. If appropriate, tell the patient to change the sling regularly because a soiled sling can cause irritation and infection.

• Teach the patient how to check periodically for axillary skin breakdown.

Documentation
• Record the date, time, and location of sling application.
• Describe the patient's tolerance of the procedure.
• Document circulation to the fingers, noting color and temperature.

Soaks

A soak involves immersion of a body part in warm water or a medicated solution. This treatment is used to soften exudates, facilitate debridement, enhance suppuration, clean wounds or burns, rehydrate wounds, apply medication to infected areas, and increase local blood supply and circulation.

Most soaks are applied with clean tap water and clean technique. Sterile solution and sterile equipment are required for treating wounds, burns, or other breaks in the skin.

⟫ Key nursing diagnoses and patient outcomes
Use these nursing diagnoses as a guide when developing your plan of care for a patient requiring soaks.

Impaired skin integrity related to (specify)
Based on this nursing diagnosis, you'll establish the following patient outcomes. The patient will:
• show no evidence of skin breakdown.
• have normal skin turgor.
• regain skin integrity; have his wound site heal.

Applying a swathe

To further immobilize an arm after applying a sling, wrap a folded triangular bandage or wide elastic bandage around the patient's upper torso and the upper arm on the injured side. Don't cover the patient's uninjured arm. Make the swathe just tight enough to secure the injured arm to the body. Tie or pin the ends of the bandage just in front of the axilla on the uninjured side.

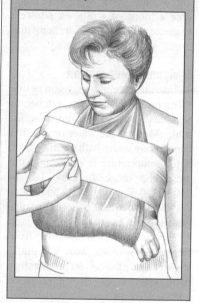

• communicate understanding of skin protection measures.
• demonstrate skill in care of wound site.

Risk for infection related to altered skin integrity
Based on this nursing diagnosis, you'll establish the following patient outcomes. The patient will:

• have vital signs, temperature, and laboratory values that remain within normal limits.

• have no pathogens appear in cultures.

• show no signs or symptoms of infection at the wound site.

Equipment

♦ basin, or arm or foot tub ♦ bath (utility) thermometer ♦ hot tap water or prescribed solution ♦ pitcher ♦ cup ♦ linen-saver pad ♦ overbed table ♦ footstool ♦ pillows ♦ towels ♦ gauze pads and other dressing materials ♦ gloves, if necessary.

Equipment preparation

• Clean and disinfect the basin or tub.

• Run hot tap water into a pitcher, or heat the prescribed solution, as applicable. Measure the water or solution temperature with a bath thermometer. If the temperature is not within the prescribed range (usually 105° to 110° F [40.6° to 43.3° C]), add hot or cold water or reheat or cool the solution, as needed.

• When preparing the soak away from the patient's room, heat the liquid slightly above the correct temperature to allow for cooling during transport.

• If the solution for a medicated soak isn't premixed, prepare the dilution and heat it.

• If the soak basin or tub is to be placed in bed, make sure the bed is flat beneath it to prevent spills.

Patient preparation

• Provide privacy.

• Check the doctor's order and assess the patient's condition.

• Explain the procedure to the patient and, if necessary, check his history for previous allergic reactions to the medicated solution.

• For an arm soak, have the patient sit erect. For a leg or foot soak, ask the patient to lie down and bend the appropriate knee. For a foot soak in the sitting position, let him sit on the edge of the bed or transfer him to a chair.

Implementation

• Wash your hands thoroughly.

• Place a linen-saver pad under the treatment site and, if necessary, cover the pad with a towel *to absorb spillage.*

• Expose the treatment site.

• Put on gloves before removing any dressing; dispose of the soiled dressing properly. If the dressing is encrusted and stuck to the wound, leave it in place and proceed with the soak. Remove the dressing several minutes later, after it begins to loosen.

• Position the soak basin under the treatment site on the bed, overbed table, footstool, or floor, as appropriate. Pour the heated liquid into the soak basin or tub. Then lower the arm or leg into the basin gradually *to allow adjustment to the temperature change.* Make sure the soak solution covers the treatment site.

• Support other body parts with pillows or towels as needed *to prevent discomfort and muscle strain.* Make the patient comfortable and ensure proper body alignment.

• Check the temperature of the soak solution with the bath thermometer every 5 minutes. If the temperature drops below the prescribed range, remove some of the cooled solution with a cup. Then lift the patient's arm or leg from the basin *to avoid burns,* and add hot water or solution to the basin. Mix the liquid thoroughly and then check the temperature; if it's within the prescribed range, lower the patient's affected part back into the basin.

• Observe the patient for signs of tissue intolerance: extreme redness at the treatment site, excessive drainage, bleeding, or maceration. If such signs develop or the patient complains of pain, discontinue the treatment and notify the doctor.

• After 15 to 20 minutes, or as ordered, lift the patient's arm or leg from the basin and remove the basin.

• Dry the arm or leg thoroughly with a towel. If the patient has a wound, dry the skin around it without touching the wound.

• While the skin is hydrated from the soak, use gauze pads *to remove loose scales or crusts.*

• Observe the treatment area for general appearance, degree of swelling, debridement, suppuration, and healing. Re-dress the wound, if appropriate.

• Remove the towel and linen-saver pad and make the patient comfortable in bed.

• Discard the soak solution, dispose of soiled materials properly, and clean and disinfect the basin.

• If the treatment is to be repeated, store the equipment in the patient's room, out of his reach; otherwise, return it to the central supply department.

Nursing considerations

• To treat large areas, particularly burns, a soak may be administered in a whirlpool or Hubbard tank.

Documentation

• Record the date, time, and duration of the soak.

• Record location of the treatment site.

• Document the type of solution and its temperature.

• Note skin and wound appearance before, during, and after treatment.

• Document the patient's tolerance of the treatment.

Spirometry, bedside

This procedure is used to measure forced vital capacity (FVC) and forced expiratory volume (FEV), allowing calculation of other pulmonary function indices, such as timed forced expiratory flow rate. Depending on the type of spirometer used, bedside spirometry can also allow direct measurement of vital capacity and tidal volume.

Bedside spirometry aids in diagnosing pulmonary dysfunction before it appears on an X-ray or physical examination, evaluating its severity, and determining the patient's response to therapy. By allowing assessment of the relationship of flow rate to vital capacity, it helps the caregiver distinguish between obstructive and restrictive pulmonary disease. It's also useful for evaluating preoperative anesthesia risk. Because the required breathing patterns can aggravate conditions such as bronchospasm, use of the bedside spirometer requires a review of the patient's history and close observation during testing.

≫ Key nursing diagnoses and patient outcomes

Use these nursing diagnoses as a guide when developing your plan of care.

Impaired gas exchange related to altered oxygen supply

Based on this nursing diagnosis, you'll establish the following patient outcomes. The patient will:
• maintain respiratory rate within ± 5 breaths/minute of baseline.
• express feeling of comfort in maintaining air exchange.
• have normal breath sounds.
• have arterial blood gas levels return to baseline, as evidenced by (specify) pH; (specify) partial pressure of arterial oxygen; (specify) partial pressure of arterial carbon dioxide.

Ineffective breathing pattern related to (specify)

Based on this nursing diagnosis, you'll establish the following patient outcomes. The patient will:
• report feeling comfortable when breathing.
• achieve maximum lung expansion with adequate ventilation.

Equipment

♦ spirometer ♦ disposable mouthpiece ♦ breathing tube, if required ♦ spirographic chart, if required ♦ chart and pen, if required ♦ noseclips ♦ optional: vital capacity predicted-values table.

Equipment preparation

• Review the manufacturer's instructions for assembly and use of the spirometer. If necessary, firmly insert the breathing tube to ensure a tight connection. If the tube comes pre-connected, check the seals for tightness and the tubing for leaks.
• Check the operation of the recording mechanism, and insert a chart and pen if necessary.
• Insert the disposable mouthpiece and make sure it's tightly sealed.

Patient preparation

• Explain the procedure.
• Emphasize that cooperation is essential to ensure accurate results.
• Instruct the patient to remove or loosen any constricting clothing, such as a brassiere, to prevent alteration of test results from restricted thoracic expansion and abdominal mobility.
• Instruct the patient to void to prevent abdominal discomfort.
• Don't perform pulmonary function tests immediately after a large meal because the patient will experience abdominal discomfort.
• If the patient wears dentures that fit poorly, remove them to prevent incomplete closure of his mouth, which could allow air to leak around the mouthpiece. If the dentures fit well, leave them in place to promote a tight seal.

Implementation

• Plug in the spirometer and set the baseline time.
• If desired, allow the patient to practice the required breathing with the breathing tube unhooked. After practice, replace the tube and check the seal.
• Tell the patient not to breathe through his nose. If the patient has difficulty complying, apply nose clips.
• To measure vital capacity, instruct the patient to inhale as deeply as possible, and then insert the mouthpiece

so that his lips are sealed tightly around it to prevent air leakage and ensure an accurate digital readout or spirogram recording.

• Tell the patient to exhale completely. Then remove the mouthpiece to prevent recording his next inspiration.

• Allow the patient to rest and repeat the procedure twice.

• To measure FEV and FVC, repeat this procedure with the chart or timer on, but instruct the patient to exhale as quickly and completely as possible. Tell him when to start, and turn on the recorder or timer at the same time.

• Allow the patient to rest and repeat the procedure twice.

• After completing the procedure, discard the mouthpiece, remove the spirographic chart, and follow the manufacturer's instructions for cleaning and sterilizing.

Complications

Forced exhalation can cause dizziness or light-headedness, precipitate or worsen bronchospasm, rapidly increase exhaustion (possibly to where the patient will require mechanical support), and increase air trapping in the emphysemic patient.

Nursing considerations

• Encourage the patient during the test; this may help him to exhale more forcefully, which can be significant. If the patient coughs during expiration, wait until coughing subsides before repeating the measurement.

• Read the vital capacity directly from the readout or spirogram chart. The FVC is the highest volume recorded on the curve. Of the three trials, accept the highest recorded exhalation as the vital capacity result.

• To determine the percentage of predicted vital capacity, first determine the patient's predicted value from the vital capacity predicted-values table, then calculate the percentage by using the following formula:

$$\frac{\text{observed vital capacity}}{\text{predicted vital capacity}} \times 100 =$$

$$\% \text{ predicted vital capacity}$$

• To determine the FEV for a specified time, mark the point on the spirogram where it crosses the desired time, and draw a straight line from this point to the side of the chart, which indicates volume in liters. This measurement is usually calculated for 1, 2, and 3 seconds and reported as a percentage of vital capacity. A healthy patient will have exhaled 75%, 85%, and 95% respectively of his FVC. Calculate this percentage by using the following formula:

$$\frac{\text{observed forced expiratory volume}}{\text{observed vital capacity}}$$

$$\times 100 = \% \text{ vital capacity}$$

Documentation

• Record the procedure date and time.

• Document observed and calculated values, including FEV at 1, 2, and 3 seconds.

• Document complications and nursing actions taken.

• Note the patient's tolerance of the procedure.

Spirometry, incentive

This procedure involves using a breathing device to help the patient achieve maximal ventilation. The de-

TECHNOLOGY UPDATE

Measuring pulmonary function with spirometry

Compact spirometers such as the Spirolite 323 can measure and analyze more than 22 different pulmonary function parameters by testing forced vital capacity, slow vital capacity, and maximal voluntary ventilation. The spirometer compares actual measures values to predicted values and can suggest diagnosis and print results with an optional printer. Other functions include report customization, automatic calibration, patient name and identification input, and memory for 16 patients. It can also communicate with a personal computer via an optional software package.

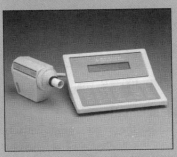

Photo courtesy of Medical Systems Corp., Greenvale, N.Y.

vice measures respiratory flow or respiratory volume and induces the patient to take a deep breath and hold it for several seconds. This deep breath increases lung volume, boosts alveolar inflation, and promotes venous return. This exercise also establishes alveolar hyperinflation for a longer time than is possible with a normal deep breath, thus preventing and reversing the alveolar collapse that causes atelectasis and pneumonitis.

Devices used for incentive spirometry provide a visual incentive to breathe deeply. Some are activated when the patient inhales a certain volume of air; the device then estimates the amount of air inhaled. Others contain plastic floats, which rise according to the amount of air the patient pulls through the device when he inhales.

Patients at low risk for developing atelectasis may use a flow incentive spirometer. Patients at high risk may need a volume incentive spirometer, which measures lung inflation more precisely. (See *Spirometers that analyze pulmonary function*, page 798.)

Incentive spirometry benefits the patient on prolonged bed rest, especially the postoperative patient who may regain his normal respiratory pattern slowly because of such predisposing factors as abdominal or thoracic surgery, advanced age, inactivity, obesity, smoking, and decreased ability to cough effectively and expel lung secretions.

≫ Key nursing diagnoses and patient outcomes

Use these nursing diagnoses as a guide when developing your plan of care for a patient who is being treated with incentive spirometry.

Ineffective breathing pattern related to decreased energy

Based on this nursing diagnosis, you'll establish the following patient outcomes. The patient will:
• achieve maximum lung expansion with adequate ventilation.

• report feeling comfortable with breathing.

Impaired gas exchange related to altered oxygen supply
Based on this nursing diagnosis, you'll establish the following patient outcomes. The patient will:
• cough effectively.
• expectorate sputum.

Equipment
♦ flow or volume incentive spirometer, as indicated, with sterile disposable tube and mouthpiece ♦ stethoscope ♦ watch ♦ nose clip (optional) ♦ tape.

Equipment preparation
• Assemble the ordered equipment at the patient's bedside.
• Read the manufacturer's instructions for spirometer setup and operation.
• Remove the sterile flow tube and mouthpiece from the package and attach them to the device. (The tube and mouthpiece are sterile on first use and clean on subsequent uses.)
• Set the flow rate or volume goal as determined by the doctor or respiratory therapist and based on the patient's preoperative performance.
• Turn on the machine if necessary.

Patient preparation
• Explain the procedure, making sure the patient understands the importance of performing this exercise regularly *to maintain alveolar inflation.*
• Assist the patient to a comfortable sitting or semi-Fowler's position *to promote optimal lung expansion.* If you're using a flow incentive spirometer and the patient is unable to as-

sume or maintain this position, he can perform the procedure in any position as long as the device remains upright. *Tilting a flow incentive spirometer decreases the required patient effort and reduces the exercise's effectiveness.*

Implementation
• Wash your hands.
• Assess the patient's condition.
• Auscultate the patient's lungs *to provide a baseline for comparison with posttreatment auscultation.*
• Instruct the patient to insert the mouthpiece and close his lips tightly around it *because a weak seal may alter flow or volume readings.* (*Note:* Some patients may need to use a nose clip to prevent air leakage.)
• Instruct the patient to exhale normally and then inhale as slowly and

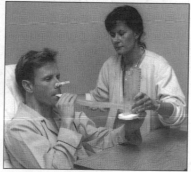

as deeply as possible. If the patient has difficulty with this step, tell him to suck as he would through a straw, but to do so more slowly. Ask the patient to retain the entire volume of air he inhaled for 3 seconds or, if you're using a device with a light indicator, until the light turns off. This deep breath creates sustained transpulmonary pressure near the end of inspiration and is sometimes called a sustained maximal inspiration.

• Tell the patient to remove the mouthpiece and exhale normally. Allow him to relax and take several normal breaths before attempting another breath with the spirometer. Repeat this sequence 5 to 10 times during every waking hour. Note tidal volumes.

• Evaluate the patient's ability to cough effectively, and encourage him to cough after each effort *because deep lung inflation may loosen secretions and facilitate their removal.* Observe any expectorated secretions.

• Auscultate the patient's lungs, and compare findings with the first auscultation.

• Instruct the patient to remove the mouthpiece.

• Wash the device in warm water, and shake it dry. Avoid immersing the spirometer itself *because this enhances bacterial growth and impairs the internal filter's effectiveness in preventing inhalation of extraneous material.*

• Place the mouthpiece in a plastic storage bag between exercises, and label it and the spirometer, if applicable, with the patient's name *to avoid inadvertent use by another patient.*

Nursing considerations

• If the patient is scheduled for surgery, make a preoperative assessment of his respiratory pattern and capability to ensure the development of appropriate postoperative goals. Then teach the patient to use the spirometer before surgery *so that he can concentrate on your instructions and practice the exercise.* A preoperative evaluation will also help in establishing a postoperative therapeutic goal.

• Avoid exercising at mealtime *to prevent nausea.* If the patient has difficulty breathing only through his mouth, provide a noseclip *to fully measure each breath.* Provide paper and pencil so the patient can note exercise times. Exercise frequency varies with condition and ability.

• Immediately after surgery, monitor the exercise frequently *to ensure compliance and assess achievement.*

Documentation

• Record any preoperative teaching and preoperative flow or volume levels; date and time of the procedure; type of spirometer; flow or volume levels achieved; number of breaths taken; patient's condition before and after the procedure; his tolerance of the procedure; and results of both auscultations.

• If you've used a flow incentive spirometer, compute *volume* by multiplying the setting by the duration the patient kept the ball (or balls) suspended, as follows. If the patient suspended the ball for 3 seconds at a setting of 500 cc during each of 10 breaths, multiply 500 cc by 3 seconds and then record this total (1,500 cc) and the number of breaths: 1,500 cc × 10 breaths. If you've used a volume incentive spirometer, take the volume reading directly from the spirometer. For example, record 1,000 cc × 5 breaths.

Splint application

By immobilizing the site of an injury, a splint alleviates pain and allows the injury to heal in proper alignment. It also minimizes possible complications, such as excessive bleeding into tissues, restricted blood flow caused by bone pressing against vessels, and possible paralysis from a spinal cord injury. In cases of multiple serious injuries, a splint or spine board allows caretakers to move the patient without risking further damage to bones, muscles, nerves, blood vessels, and skin.

A splint can be applied to immobilize a simple or compound fracture, a dislocation, or a subluxation. (See *Types of splints*, page 802.)

During an emergency, any injury even suspected of being a fracture, dislocation, or subluxation should be splinted. No contraindications exist for rigid splints; traction splints are contraindicated for upper extremity injuries and open fractures.

≫ Key nursing diagnoses and patient outcomes
Use these nursing diagnoses as a guide when developing your plan of care for a patient who is being treated with a splint.

Impaired physical mobility related to neuromuscular impairment
Based on this nursing diagnosis, you'll establish the following patient outcomes. The patient will:
• maintain muscle strength and joint range of motion.
• show no evidence of complications, such as contractures, venous stasis, thrombus formation or skin breakdown.

Pain related to physical agents
Based on this nursing diagnosis, you'll establish the following patient outcomes. The patient will:
• express a feeling of comfort and relief from pain.

• state and carry out appropriate interventions for pain relief.

Equipment
♦ rigid splint, Velcro support splint, spine board, or traction splint ♦ bindings ♦ padding ♦ sandbags or rolled towels or clothing ♦ optional: roller gauze, cloth strips, sterile or clean compress, ice bag.

Several commercial splints are available. In an emergency, any long, sturdy object, such as a tree limb, mop handle, or broom — even a magazine or newspaper — can be used to make a rigid splint for an extremity; a door can be used as a spine board.

Velcro straps, 2″ roller gauze, or 2″ cloth strips can be used as bindings. When improvising, avoid using twine or rope, if possible, *because they can restrict circulation.*

An inflatable semirigid splint, called an air splint, sometimes can be used to secure an injured extremity. (See *Using an air splint*, page 803.)

Patient preparation
• Explain what you'll be doing while examining the patient, *to allay his fears.*

Implementation
• Obtain a complete history of the injury, if possible, and begin a thorough head-to-toe assessment, inspecting for obvious deformities, swelling, or bleeding.
• Ask the patient if he can move the injured area (typically an extremity). Compare it bilaterally with the uninjured extremity, where applicable. Gently palpate the injured area; inspect for swelling, obvious deformities, bleeding, discoloration, and evidence of fracture or dislocation.

Types of splints

Three kinds of splints are commonly used to help provide support for injured or weakened limbs, or to help correct deformities.

A rigid splint can be used to immobilize a fracture or dislocation in an extremity, as shown. Ideally, two people should apply a rigid splint to an extremity.

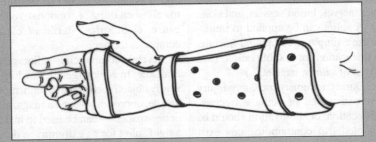

A *traction splint* immobilizes a fracture and exerts a longitudinal pull that reduces muscle spasms, pain, and arterial and neural damage. Used primarily for femoral fractures, a traction splint may also be applied for a fractured hip or tibia. Two trained people should apply a traction splint.

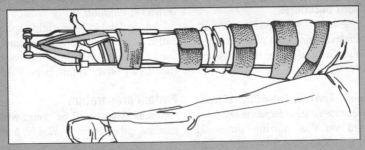

A *spine board,* applied for a suspected spinal fracture, is a rigid splint that supports the injured person's entire body. Three people should apply a spine board.

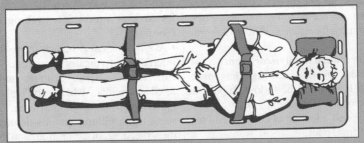

• Remove or cut away clothing from the injury site, if necessary.

• Check neurovascular integrity distal to the site.

• If an obvious bone misalignment causes the patient acute distress or severe neurovascular problems, align the extremity in its normal anatomic position, if possible. Stop doing this, however, if the action causes further neurovascular deterioration. Don't attempt to straighten a dislocation *because movement may damage displaced vessels and nerves.* Also, don't attempt reduction of a contaminated bone end *because this may cause additional laceration of soft tissues, vessels, and nerves, and also may cause gross contamination of deep tissues.*

• Choose a splint that will immobilize the joints above and below the fracture; pad the splint, as necessary, *to prevent excessive pressure over bony prominences.*

To apply a rigid splint

• Support the injured extremity, and apply firm, gentle traction.

• Have an assistant place the splint under, beside, or on top of the extremity, as ordered.

• Tell the assistant to apply the bindings *to secure the splint.* Make sure the bindings don't obstruct circulation.

To apply a spine board

• Pad the spine board (or door) carefully, especially the areas that will support the lumbar region and knees, to prevent uneven pressure and discomfort.

• If the patient is lying on his back, place one hand on each side of his head and apply gentle traction to the head and neck, keeping the head aligned

Using an air splint

In an emergency, an air splint can be applied to immobilize a fracture or control bleeding, especially from a forearm or lower leg. This compact, comfortable splint is made of double-walled plastic and provides gentle, diffuse pressure over an injured area. The appropriate splint is wrapped around the affected extremity, secured with Velcro or other strips, then inflated. The fit should be snug enough to immobilize the extremity without impairing circulation.

An air splint may actually control bleeding better than a local pressure bandage. The device's clear plastic construction simplifies inspection of the affected site for bleeding, pallor, or cyanosis. An air splint also allows the patient to be moved without further damage to the injured limb.

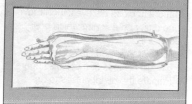

with the body. Have one assistant logroll the patient onto his side while another slides the spine board under the patient. Then instruct the assistants to roll the patient onto the board while you maintain traction and alignment.

• If the patient is in a prone position, logroll him onto the board so he ends up in a supine position.

• *To maintain body alignment,* use strips of cloth to secure the patient on the spine board; *to keep head and neck aligned,* place sandbags or rolled towels or clothing on both sides of his head.

Assessing neurovascular status

When assessing an injured extremity, always include the following steps, and compare your findings bilaterally.
• Inspect the color of fingers or toes.
• To detect edema, note the size of the digits.
• Simultaneously touch the digits of the affected and unaffected extremities, and compare temperature.
• Check capillary refill by pressing on the distal tip of one digit until it's white. Then release the pressure and note how soon the normal color returns. It should return quickly in the affected and unaffected extremities.
• Check sensation by touching the fingers or toes and asking the patient how the touch feels. Note reports of any numbness or tingling.
• To check proprioception, tell the patient to close his eyes; then move one digit and ask him which position it's in.
• To test movement, tell the patient to wiggle his toes or move his fingers.
• Palpate the distal pulses to assess vascular patency.

Warmth, free movement, rapid capillary refill, and normal color, sensation, and proprioception indicate sound neurovascular status. Record your findings for the affected and unaffected extremities, using standard terminology to avoid ambiguity.

To apply a traction splint
• Place the splint beside the injured leg. (Never use a traction splint on an arm *because the major axillary plexus of nerves and blood vessels can't tolerate countertraction.*) Adjust the splint to the correct length, and then open and adjust the Velcro straps.
• Have an assistant keep the leg motionless while you pad the ankle and foot and fasten the ankle hitch around them. (You may leave the shoe on.)
• Tell the assistant to lift and support the leg at the injury site, as you apply firm, gentle traction.
• While you maintain traction, instruct the assistant to slide the splint under the leg, pad the groin *to avoid excessive pressure on external genitalia,* and gently apply the ischial strap.
• Have the assistant connect the loops of the ankle hitch to the end of the splint.
• Adjust the splint to apply enough traction *to secure the leg comfortably in the corrected position.*
• After applying traction, fasten the Velcro support splints *to secure the leg closely to the splint.*

   Note: Don't use a traction splint for a severely angulated femur or knee fracture.

Complications
• Multiple transfers and repeated manipulation of a fracture may result in fat embolism, indicated by shortness of breath, agitation, and irrational behavior. This complication usually occurs within 24 to 72 hours of injury or manipulation.

Nursing considerations
• At the scene of an accident, always examine the patient completely for other injuries.
• Avoid unnecessary movement or manipulation *that may cause additional pain or injury.*
• Always consider the possibility of cervical injury in an unconscious pa-

tient. If possible, apply the splint before repositioning the patient.

If the patient requires a rigid splint but one isn't available, use another body part as a splint. To splint a leg in this manner, pad its inner aspect and secure it to the other leg with roller gauze or cloth strips.

• After applying any type of splint, monitor vital signs frequently *because bleeding in fractured bones and surrounding tissues may cause shock.* Also monitor the neurovascular status of the fractured limb by assessing skin color and checking for numbness in the fingers or toes. *Numbness or paralysis distal to the injury indicates pressure on nerves.* (See *Assessing neurovascular status.*)

• Transport the patient as soon as possible to a medical facility. Apply ice to the injury. Regardless of the apparent extent of the patient's injury, don't allow him to eat or drink anything until the doctor evaluates him.

• Indications for removal of a splint include evidence of improper application or vascular impairment. Apply gentle traction, and remove the splint carefully under a doctor's direct supervision.

Documentation

• Record the circumstances and cause of the injury.

• Document the patient's complaints, noting whether symptoms are localized.

• Record neurovascular status before and after applying the splint.

• Note the type of wound and the amount and type of drainage, if any.

• Document the time of splint application.

• Note whether the bone end slips into surrounding tissue or transportation causes change in degree of dislocation.

Sputum collection

Secreted by mucous membranes lining the bronchioles, bronchi, and trachea, sputum helps protect the respiratory tract from infection. When expelled from the respiratory tract, sputum carries with it saliva, nasal and sinus secretions, dead cells, and normal oral bacteria. Sputum specimens may be cultured for identification of respiratory pathogens.

Expectoration, which may require ultrasonic nebulization, hydration, or chest percussion and postural drainage, is the usual method of sputum-specimen collection. Less common methods include tracheal suctioning and, rarely, bronchoscopy. Tracheal suctioning is contraindicated within 1 hour of eating and in patients with esophageal varices, nausea, facial or basilar skull fractures, laryngospasm, or bronchospasm. It should be performed cautiously in patients with cardiac disease because it may precipitate cardiac arrhythmias.

❯❯ Key nursing diagnoses and patient outcomes

Use these nursing diagnoses as a guide when developing your plan of care.

Ineffective breathing pattern related to decreased energy

Based on this nursing diagnosis, you'll establish the following patient outcomes. The patient will:

• achieve maximum lung expansion with adequate ventilation.

• report feeling comfortable with breathing.

Attaching a specimen trap to a suction catheter

Wearing gloves, push the suction tubing onto the male adapter of the in-line trap.

Next, insert the suction catheter into the rubber tubing of the trap.

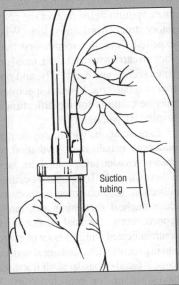

Suction tubing

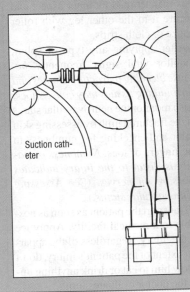

Suction catheter

Impaired gas exchange related to altered oxygen supply

Based on this nursing diagnosis, you'll establish the following patient outcomes. The patient will:
• cough effectively.
• expectorate sputum.

Equipment

For expectoration: ◆ sterile specimen container with tight-fitting cap ◆ label ◆ laboratory request form ◆ aerosol (10% sodium chloride, propylene glycol, acetylcysteine, or sterile or distilled water) to induce coughing, as ordered ◆ facial tissues ◆ emesis basin ◆ gloves, if necessary.

For tracheal suctioning: ◆ #12 to #14 French sterile suction catheter

◆ water-soluble lubricant ◆ laboratory request form ◆ sterile gloves ◆ sterile in-line specimen trap (Lukens trap) ◆ 3-ml syringe, if necessary ◆ normal saline solution ◆ portable suction machine, if wall unit is unavailable ◆ oxygen therapy equipment. ◆ optional: nasal airway, to obtain a nasotracheal specimen with suctioning, if needed. (Commercial suction kits are available containing all equipment except the suction machine and an in-line specimen container.)

Patient preparation

• Tell the patient you will collect a specimen of sputum (not saliva), and explain the procedure *to ease his anxiety and promote cooperation.*

After suctioning, disconnect the in-line trap from the suction tubing and catheter. To seal the container, connect the rubber tubing to the male adapter of the trap.

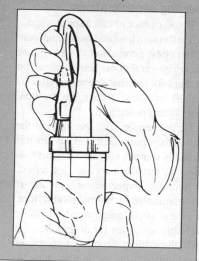

Implementation

• Collect the specimen early in the morning, before breakfast, if possible, *to obtain an overnight accumulation of secretions.*

Collecting sputum by expectoration

• Put on gloves.

• Instruct the patient to sit on a chair or at the edge of the bed. If he can't sit up, place him in high Fowler's position.

• Ask the patient to rinse his mouth with water *to reduce specimen contamination by oral bacteria and food particles.* (Avoid mouthwash and toothpaste *because they may affect the mobility of organisms in the sputum sample.*) Tell him to cough deeply and expectorate directly into the specimen container. Ask him to produce at least 15 ml of sputum, if possible.

• Cap the container and, if necessary, clean its exterior *to prevent cross-contamination.* Label the container with the patient's name and room number, the doctor's name, date and time of collection, and initial diagnosis. Also include on the laboratory request form whether the patient was febrile or was taking antibiotics, and whether sputum was induced *(because such specimens commonly appear watery and may resemble saliva).*

• Send the specimen to the laboratory immediately.

Collecting sputum by tracheal suctioning

• If the patient can't produce an adequate specimen by coughing, prepare to suction him to obtain the specimen.

• Explain the suctioning procedure to him and tell him that he may cough, gag, or feel short of breath during the procedure.

• Check the suction machine to be sure it's functioning properly. Then, place the patient in a high or semi-Fowler's position.

• Administer oxygen to the patient before beginning the procedure.

• Wash your hands thoroughly.

• Put on sterile gloves.

• Consider one hand sterile and the other hand clean, *to prevent cross-contamination.*

• Connect the suction tubing to the male adapter of the in-line trap.

• Attach the sterile suction catheter to the rubber tubing of the trap. (See *Attaching a specimen trap to a suction catheter.*)

• Position a mask over your face *because the patient may cough violently during suctioning.*
• Tell the patient to tilt his head back slightly. Then lubricate the catheter with normal saline solution, and gently pass it through the patient's nostril without suction.
• When the catheter reaches the larynx, the patient will cough. As he does, quickly advance the catheter into the trachea. Tell the patient to take several deep breaths through his mouth *to help ease insertion.*
• To obtain the specimen, apply suction for 5 to 10 seconds but never longer than 15 seconds *because prolonged suctioning can cause hypoxia.* If the procedure must be repeated, let the patient rest for four to six breaths. When collection is completed, discontinue the suction, gently remove the catheter, and administer oxygen.
• Detach the catheter from the in-line trap, gather it up in your dominant hand, and pull the glove cuff inside out and down around the used catheter to enclose it for disposal.
• Remove and discard the other glove and your mask.
• Detach the trap from the tubing connected to the suction machine.
• Seal the trap tightly by connecting the rubber tubing to the male adapter of the trap.
• Label the trap's container as an expectorated specimen, and send it to the laboratory immediately with a completed laboratory request form.
• Offer the patient a glass of water or mouthwash.

Complications
• Patients with cardiac disease may develop arrhythmias during the pro-

cedure as a result of coughing, especially when the specimen is obtained by suctioning.
• Other complications may include tracheal trauma or bleeding, vomiting, aspiration, and hypoxemia.

Nursing considerations
• If you cannot obtain a sputum specimen through tracheal suctioning, perform chest percussion *to loosen and mobilize secretions,* and position the patient for optimal drainage. After 20 to 30 minutes, repeat the tracheal suctioning procedure.
• Before sending the specimen to the laboratory, examine it to make sure it is actually sputum, not saliva, *because saliva will produce inaccurate test results.*
• Because expectorated sputum is contaminated by normal mouth flora, tracheal suctioning provides a more reliable specimen for diagnosis.
• If the patient becomes hypoxic or cyanotic during suctioning, remove the catheter immediately and administer oxygen.
• If the patient has asthma or chronic bronchitis, watch for aggravated bronchospasms with use of more than a 10% concentration of sodium chloride or acetylcysteine in an aerosol. If he has suspected tuberculosis, don't use more than 20% propylene glycol with water when inducing a sputum specimen *because a higher concentration inhibits growth of the pathogen and causes erroneous test results.* If propylene glycol isn't available, use 10% to 20% acetylcysteine with water or sodium chloride.

Documentation
• In your notes, record the method used to obtain the specimen, the time

and date of collection, how the patient tolerated the procedure, the color and consistency of the specimen, and its proper disposition.

Stool collection

Stool is collected to determine the presence of blood, ova and parasites, bile, fat, pathogens, or such substances as ingested drugs. Gross examination of stool characteristics, such as color, consistency, and odor, can reveal such conditions as GI bleeding and steatorrhea. Stool specimens are collected randomly or for specific periods, such as 72 hours. Because stool specimens can't be obtained on demand, their proper collection necessitates careful instructions to the patient to ensure an uncontaminated specimen.

≫ Key nursing diagnoses and patient outcomes

Use these nursing diagnoses as a guide when developing your plan of care.

Diarrhea related to irritation of bowel

Based on this nursing diagnosis, you'll establish the following patient outcomes. The patient will:
• have elimination pattern return to normal.
• regain and maintain fluid and electrolyte balance.

Pain related to physical, biological, or chemical agents

Based on this nursing diagnosis, you'll establish the following patient outcomes. The patient will:

• express a feeling of comfort and relief from pain.
• state and carry out appropriate interventions for pain relief.

Equipment

♦ specimen container with lid ♦ two tongue blades ♦ paper towel or paper bag ♦ bedpan or portable commode ♦ two patient care reminders (for timed specimens) ♦ laboratory request form ♦ gloves.

Patient preparation

• Explain the procedure to the patient and to family members, if possible, *to ensure their cooperation and prevent inadvertent disposal of timed stool specimens.*

Implementation

Follow the steps below for stool collection.

Collecting a random specimen

• Tell the patient to notify you when he has the urge to defecate. Have him defecate into a clean, dry bedpan or commode. Instruct him not to contaminate the specimen with urine or toilet tissue *because urine inhibits fecal bacterial growth and toilet tissue contains bismuth, which interferes with test results.*
• Don gloves.
• Using a tongue blade, transfer the most representative stool specimen from the bedpan to the container, and cap the container. If the patient passes blood, mucus, or pus with the stool, be sure to include this with the specimen.
• Wrap the tongue blade in a paper towel and discard it.

• Remove your gloves, and wash your hands thoroughly *to prevent cross-contamination.*

• Label the specimen container with the patient's name and room number and the date and time of collection.

• Send the specimen to the laboratory with a laboratory request form immediately *because a fresh specimen provides the most accurate results.*

• Refrigerate the specimen if it can't be transported to the laboratory immediately.

Note: Some pathogens are killed by refrigeration. (Do not refrigerate stool collected to confirm the presence of ova and parasites; such a specimen must be examined immediately or discarded.)

Collecting a timed specimen

• Place a patient care reminder stating SAVE ALL STOOL over the patient's bed, in his bathroom, and in the utility room.

• After donning gloves, collect the first defecation, and include this in the total specimen.

• Obtain the timed specimen as you would a random specimen, but remember to transfer all stool to the specimen container.

• If stool must be obtained with an enema, use only tap water or normal saline solution.

• As ordered, send each specimen to the laboratory immediately with a laboratory request form or, if permitted, refrigerate the specimens collected during the test period and send them when collection is complete.

• Remove and discard gloves.

• Make sure the patient is comfortable after the procedure and that he has the opportunity to clean his hands and perianal area thoroughly. Perineal care may be necessary for some patients.

Nursing considerations

• Never place a stool specimen in a refrigerator that contains food or medication *to prevent contamination.*

• Notify the doctor if the stool appears unusual.

Home care

• If the patient is to collect a specimen at home, instruct him to collect it in a clean container with a tight-fitting lid, wrap the container in a brown paper bag, and keep it in the refrigerator (separate from any food items) until it can be transported.

Documentation

• Record the time of specimen collection and transport to the laboratory.

• Note stool color, odor, consistency, and any unusual characteristics; also note if the patient had difficulty passing the stool.

Stump and prosthesis care

Patient care immediately after limb amputation includes monitoring drainage from the stump, positioning the affected limb, assisting with exercises prescribed by a physical therapist, and wrapping and conditioning the stump. Postoperative care of the stump will vary slightly, depending on the amputation site (arm or leg) and the type of dressing applied to the stump (elastic bandage or plaster cast).

After the stump heals, it requires only routine daily care, such as proper hygiene and continued muscle-strengthening exercises. The prosthesis also requires daily care once the patient begins to use it. Typically, a plastic prosthesis, the most common type, must be cleaned and lubricated and checked for proper fit. As the patient recovers from the physical and psychological trauma of amputation, he will need to learn correct procedures for routine daily care of the stump and the prosthesis.

≫ Key nursing diagnoses and patient outcomes

Use these nursing diagnoses as a guide when developing your plan of care for a patient who requires stump and prosthesis care.

Impaired physical mobility related to neuromuscular impairment

Based on this nursing diagnosis, you'll establish the following patient outcomes. The patient will:
• maintain muscle strength and joint range of motion.
• show no evidence of complications, such as contractures, venous stasis, thrombus formation, or skin breakdown.

Pain related to physical agents

Based on this nursing diagnosis, you'll establish the following patient outcomes. The patient will:
• express a feeling of comfort and relief from pain.
• state and carry out appropriate interventions for pain relief.

Equipment

For postoperative stump care: ◆ pressure dressing ◆ tourniquet ◆ ABD pad ◆ suction equipment, if ordered ◆ overhead trapeze ◆ 1″ adhesive tape, bandage clips, or safety pins ◆ sandbags or trochanter roll (for a leg) ◆ elastic stump shrinker or 4″ elastic bandage ◆ optional: tourniquet (as last resort to control bleeding).

For stump and prosthesis care: ◆ mild soap or alcohol pads ◆ stump socks or athletic tube socks ◆ two washcloths ◆ two towels ◆ appropriate lubricating oil.

Implementation

• Perform routine postoperative care, frequently assessing respiratory status and level of consciousness, monitoring vital signs and I.V. infusions, checking tube patency, and providing for the patient's comfort and safety.

Monitoring stump drainage

• *Because gravity causes fluid to accumulate at the stump,* frequently check the amount of blood and drainage on the dressing. Notify the doctor if accumulations of drainage or blood increase rapidly. If excessive bleeding occurs, notify the doctor immediately and apply a pressure dressing or compress the appropriate pressure points. If this doesn't control bleeding, use a tourniquet only as a last resort. Keep a tourniquet available, if needed.
• Tape the ABD pad over the moist part of the dressing, as necessary. *This provides a dry area to help prevent bacterial infection.*
• Monitor suction drainage equipment, and note the amount and type of drainage.

Wrapping a stump

Proper stump care helps protect the limb, reduces swelling, and prepares the limb for a prosthesis. As you perform the procedure, teach it to the patient. Start by obtaining two 4″ elastic bandages. Center the end of the first 4″ bandage at the top of the patient's thigh. Unroll the bandage downward over the stump and to the back of the leg, as shown here.

Make three figure-eight turns to adequately cover the ends of the stump. As you wrap, be sure to include the roll of flesh in the groin area. Use enough pressure to ensure that the stump narrows toward the end so that it fits comfortably into the prosthesis.

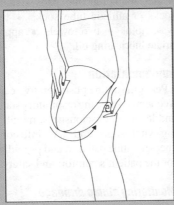
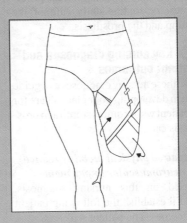

Positioning the extremity

• *To prevent contractures,* position an arm with the elbow extended and the shoulder abducted.

• *To correctly position a leg,* elevate the foot of the bed slightly and place sandbags or a trochanter roll against the hip *to prevent external rotation.*

• Don't place a pillow under the thigh to flex the hip *because this can cause hip flexion contracture.* For the same reason, tell the patient to avoid prolonged sitting.

• After a below-the-knee amputation, maintain knee extension *to prevent hamstring muscle contractures.*

• After any leg amputation, place the patient on a firm surface in the prone position for at least 4 hours a day, with his legs close together and without pillows under his stomach, hips, knees, or stump, unless this position is contraindicated. *This position helps prevent hip flexion, contractures, and abduction; it also stretches the flexor muscles.*

Assisting with prescribed exercises

• After arm amputation, encourage the patient to exercise the remaining arm *to prevent muscle contractures.* Help the patient perform isometric

Use the second 4″ bandage to anchor the first bandage around the waist. For a below-the-knee amputation, use the knee to anchor the bandage in place. Secure the bandage with clips, safety pins, or adhesive tape. Check the stump bandage regularly, and rewrap it if it bunches at the end.

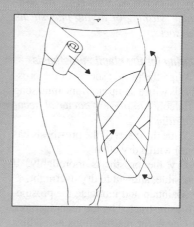

and range-of-motion (ROM) exercises for both shoulders, as prescribed by the physical therapist, *because use of the prosthesis requires both shoulders.*

• After leg amputation, stand behind the patient and, if necessary, support him with your hands at his waist during balancing exercises.

• Instruct the patient to exercise the affected and unaffected limbs *to maintain muscle tone and increase muscle strength.* The patient with a leg amputation may perform push-ups, as ordered (in the sitting position, arms at his sides), or pull-ups on the overhead trapeze *to strengthen his arms, shoul-*

ders, and back in preparation for using crutches.

Wrapping and conditioning the stump

• If the patient doesn't have a rigid cast, apply an elastic stump shrinker *to prevent edema and shape the limb in preparation for the prosthesis.* Wrap the stump so that it narrows toward the distal end. *This helps to ensure comfort when the patient wears the prosthesis.*

• Instead of using an elastic stump shrinker, you can wrap the stump in a 4″ elastic bandage. To do this, stretch the bandage to about two-thirds its maximum length as you wrap it diagonally around the stump, with the greatest pressure distally. (Depending on the size of the leg, you may need to use two 4″ bandages.) Secure the bandage with clips, safety pins, or adhesive tape. Make sure the bandage covers all portions of the stump smoothly *because wrinkles or exposed areas encourage skin breakdown.* (See *Wrapping a stump.*)

• If the patient experiences throbbing after the stump is wrapped, remove the bandage immediately and reapply it less tightly. *Throbbing indicates impaired circulation.* (See *Stump sock reduces pain, edema,* page 814.)

• Check the bandage regularly. Rewrap it when it begins to bunch up at the end (usually about every 12 hours for a moderately active patient) or every 24 hours.

• After removing the bandage to rewrap it, massage the stump gently, always pushing toward the suture line rather than away from it. *This stimulates circulation and prevents scar tissue from adhering to the bone.*

TECHNOLOGY UPDATE

Stump sock reduces pain, edema

A new stretchable sock can be used to prepare stumps for prosthesis fittings. The sock can be molded to fit any shape, and spreads pressure evenly over the limb end for total prosthesis-to-limb contact. The sock exerts 11.5 mm Hg of controlled surface counter pressure, thereby limiting postoperative edema and providing greater patient comfort than traditional elastic strapping.

• When healing begins, instruct the patient to push the stump against a pillow. Then have him gradually progress to pushing against harder surfaces, such as a padded chair, then a hard chair. *These conditioning exercises will help the patient adjust to experiencing pressure and sensation in the stump.*

Caring for the healed stump

• Bathe the stump, but never shave it *because a rash or irritation may result.* If possible, bathe the stump at the end of the day *because the warm water may cause swelling, making reapplication of the prosthesis difficult.*

• Rub the stump with alcohol daily *to toughen the skin, reducing the risk of skin breakdown.* (Avoid using powders or lotions *because they can soften or irritate the skin.) Because alcohol may cause severe irritation in some patients,* instruct the patient to watch for and report this sign.

• Inspect the stump for redness, swelling, irritation, and calluses. Report any of these to the doctor. Tell the patient to avoid putting weight on the stump. (The skin should be firm but not taut over the bony end of the limb.)

• Continue muscle-strengthening exercises *so the patient can build the strength he'll need to control the prosthesis.*

• Change the patient's stump socks, as necessary, *to avoid exposing the skin to excessive perspiration, which can be irritating.* Wash the socks in warm water and gentle nondetergent soap; lay them flat on a towel to dry. *Machine washing or drying may shrink the socks.*

Caring for the plastic prosthesis

• Wipe the plastic socket of the prosthesis with a damp cloth and mild soap or alcohol *to prevent bacterial accumulation.*

• Wipe the insert (if the prosthesis has one) with a dry cloth.

• Dry the prosthesis thoroughly; if possible, allow it to dry overnight.

• Maintain and lubricate the prosthesis as instructed by the manufacturer.

• Check for malfunctions and adjust or repair the prosthesis, as necessary, *to prevent further damage.*

• Check the condition of the shoe on a foot prosthesis frequently, and change it as necessary.

Applying the prosthesis

• Apply a stump sock. Keep the seams away from bony prominences.

• If the prosthesis has an insert, remove it from the socket, place it over the stump, and insert the stump into the prosthesis.

• If it has no insert, merely slide the prosthesis over the stump. Secure the prosthesis onto the stump according to the manufacturer's directions.

Complications

The most common postoperative complications include:
- hemorrhage
- stump infection
- contractures
- swollen or flabby stump.

Complications that may develop at any time after an amputation include:
- skin breakdown or irritation from lack of ventilation or friction from an irritant in the prosthesis
- a sebaceous cyst or boil from tight socks
- psychological problems, such as denial, depression, or withdrawal
- phantom limb pain caused by stimulation of nerves that once carried sensations from the distal part of the extremity.

Nursing considerations

- If a patient arrives at the hospital with a traumatic amputation, the amputated part may be saved for possible reimplantation. (See *Caring for an amputated body part*, page 816.)
- Teach the patient how to care for his stump and prosthesis properly. Make sure he knows the signs and symptoms that indicate problems in the stump. Explain that a 10-lb (4.5-kg) change in body weight will alter his stump size and require a new prosthesis socket *to ensure a correct fit.*
- Exercise of the remaining muscles in an amputated limb must begin the day after surgery. A physical therapist will direct these exercises. For example, arm exercises progress from isometrics to assisted ROM to active ROM. Leg exercises include rising from a chair, balancing on one leg, and ROM exercises of the knees and hips.

- For a below-the-knee amputation, you may substitute an athletic tube sock for a stump sock by cutting off the elastic band. If the patient has a rigid plaster of Paris dressing, perform normal cast care. Check the cast frequently *to make sure it doesn't slip off.* If it does, apply an elastic bandage immediately and notify the doctor *because edema will develop rapidly.*

Home care

- Emphasize to the patient that proper care of his stump can speed healing.
- Tell the patient to inspect his stump carefully every day, using a mirror.
- Instruct him to call the doctor if the incision appears to be opening, looks red or swollen, feels warm, is painful to touch, or is seeping drainage.
- Instruct him to continue proper daily stump care.
- Tell the patient to massage the stump toward the suture line *to mobilize the scar and prevent its adherence to bone.* Advise him to avoid exposing the skin around the stump to excessive perspiration, *which can be irritating.* Tell him to change his elastic bandages or stump socks during the day to avoid this.
- Tell the patient that he may experience twitching, spasms, or phantom limb pain as his stump muscles adjust to amputation. Advise him that he can decrease these symptoms with heat, massage, or gentle pressure. If his stump is sensitive to touch, tell him to rub it with a dry washcloth for 4 minutes three times a day.
- Stress the importance of performing prescribed exercises *to help minimize complications, maintain muscle strength and tone, prevent contractures, and promote independence.*

Caring for an amputated body part

After traumatic amputation, a surgeon may be able to reimplant the severed body part through microsurgery. The chance of successful reimplantation is much greater if the amputated part has received proper care.

• If a patient arrives at the hospital with a severed body part, first make sure that bleeding at the amputation site has been controlled. Then follow these guidelines for preserving the body part.

• Put on sterile gloves. Place several sterile gauze pads and an appropriate amount of sterile roller gauze in a sterile basin, and pour sterile normal saline or sterile lactated Ringer's solution over them. *Never* use any other solution, and don't try to scrub or debride the part.

• Holding the body part in one gloved hand, carefully pat it dry with sterile gauze. Place saline-soaked gauze pads over the stump; then wrap the whole body part with saline-soaked roller gauze. Wrap the gauze with a sterile towel, if available. Then put this package in a watertight container or bag and seal it.

• Fill another plastic bag with ice and place the part, still in its watertight container, inside. Seal the outer bag. (Always protect the part from direct contact with the ice — and never

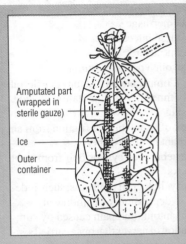

Amputated part (wrapped in sterile gauze)

Ice

Outer container

use dry ice — to prevent irreversible tissue damage, which would make the part unsuitable for reimplantation.) Keep this bag ice-cold until the doctor's ready to do the reimplantation surgery.

• Label the bag with the patient's name, identification number, identification of the amputated part, hospital identification number, and date and time when cooling began.

Note: The body part must be wrapped and cooled quickly. Irreversible tissue damage occurs after only 6 hours at ambient temperature. However, hypothermic management seldom preserves tissues for more than 24 hours.

Also stress the importance of positioning *to prevent contractures and edema.*

Documentation

• Record the date, time, and specific procedures of all postoperative care, including amount and type of drainage, condition of the dressing, need for dressing reinforcement, and appearance of the suture line and surrounding tissue.

• Note any signs of skin irritation or infection, any complications and the

nursing action taken, the patient's tolerance for exercises, and his psychological reaction to the amputation.
• During routine daily care, document the date, time, type of care given, and condition of the skin and suture line, noting any signs of irritation, such as redness or tenderness. Also note the patient's progress in caring for the stump or prosthesis.

Subcutaneous drug administration

When injected into the fatty tissues beneath the skin, a drug moves into the bloodstream more rapidly than if given by mouth. Subcutaneous injection allows slower, more sustained drug administration than intramuscular injection. It also causes minimal tissue trauma and carries little risk of the needle through which the drug is being administered striking large blood vessels and nerves.

Absorbed mainly through the capillaries, drugs recommended for subcutaneous injection include nonirritating aqueous solutions and suspensions contained in 0.5 to 2.0 ml of fluid. Heparin and insulin, for example, are usually administered subcutaneously.

Drugs and solutions for subcutaneous injection are injected through a relatively short needle, using meticulous sterile technique. The most common subcutaneous injection sites are the outer aspect of the upper arm, anterior thigh, loose tissue of the lower abdomen, buttocks, and upper back. Injection is contraindicated in sites that are inflamed, edematous, scarred, or covered by a mole, birthmark, or other lesion. It may also be contraindicated in patients with impaired coagulation mechanisms.

≫ Key nursing diagnoses and patient outcomes

Use these nursing diagnoses as a guide when developing your plan of care for a patient who is receiving subcutaneous injections.

Knowledge deficit related to lack of exposure
Based on this nursing diagnosis, you'll establish the following patient outcomes. The patient will:
• state or demonstrate understanding of what has been taught.
• demonstrate ability to perform new health-related behaviors as they are taught.

Risk for injury related to improper technique
Based on this nursing diagnosis, you'll establish the following patient outcomes. The patient will:
• identify factors that increase risk for injury.
• assist in identifying safety measures to prevent injury.

Equipment
♦ prescribed medication ♦ patient's medication record and chart ♦ needle of appropriate gauge and length ♦ gloves ♦ 1- to 3-ml syringe ♦ alcohol pads ♦ optional: antiseptic cleaning agent, filter needle, insulin syringe, insulin pump.

Equipment preparation
• Verify the order on the patient's medication record by checking it against the doctor's order.

• Inspect the medication *to make sure it's not abnormally discolored or cloudy and that it doesn't contain precipitates.*
• Select a needle of the proper gauge and length. An average adult patient requires a 25G ⅝″ needle; an infant, a child, or an elderly or thin patient, a 25G to 27G ½″ needle.
• Remember to check the label on the medication against the medication record. Read the label again as you draw up the medication for injection.

For single-dose ampules

• Wrap the ampule's neck in an alcohol pad and snap off the top, directing the force away from your body. If desired, attach a filter needle to the needle and withdraw the medication. Tap the syringe *to clear air from it.* Cover the needle with the needle sheath.
• Before discarding the ampule, check the label against the patient's medication record.
• Discard the filter needle and the ampule. Attach the appropriate needle to the syringe.

For single-dose or multidose vials

• Reconstitute powdered drugs according to the label's instructions. Make sure that all crystals have dissolved in the solution. Warming the vial by holding it and rolling it between your palms may help to dissolve the drug more quickly.
• Clean the vial's rubber stopper with an alcohol pad. Pull the syringe plunger back until the volume of air in the syringe equals the volume of drug to be withdrawn from the vial.
• Insert the needle into the vial. Inject the air, invert the vial, and keep the needle's bevel tip below the level of the solution as you withdraw the prescribed amount of medication. Cover the needle with the needle sheath. Tap the syringe *to clear any air from it.*
• Check the drug label against the patient's medication record before returning the multidose vial to the shelf or drawer or before discarding the single-dose vial.

Patient preparation

• Explain the procedure to the patient and provide privacy.
• Confirm the patient's identity by asking his name and checking the name, room number, and bed number on his wristband.

Implementation

• Wash your hands.
• Select an appropriate injection site. (See *Locating subcutaneous injection sites.*)

Rotate sites according to a schedule for patients who require repeated injections. Use different areas of the body unless contraindicated by the specific drug. (Heparin, for example, should be injected only in certain sites.)
• Put on gloves.
• Position and drape the patient if necessary.
• Clean the injection site with an alcohol pad, beginning at the center of the site and moving outward in a circular motion. Allow the skin to dry before injecting the drug *to avoid a stinging sensation from introducing alcohol into subcutaneous tissues.*
• Loosen the protective needle sheath.
• With your nondominant hand, grasp the skin around the injection site firmly to elevate the subcutaneous tissue, forming a 1″ (2.5-cm) fat fold.

• Holding the syringe in your dominant hand, insert the loosened needle sheath between the fourth and fifth fingers of your other hand while still pinching the skin around the injection site. Pull back the syringe with your dominant hand *to uncover the needle by grasping the syringe like a pencil.* Don't touch the needle.

• Position the needle with its bevel up.

• Tell the patient he'll feel a prick as the needle is inserted.

• Insert the needle quickly in one motion. (See *Technique for subcutaneous injections,* page 820.)

Release the patient's skin *to avoid injecting the drug into compressed tissue and irritating nerve fibers.*

• Pull back the plunger slightly *to check for blood return.* If none appears, begin injecting the drug slowly. If blood appears upon aspiration, withdraw the needle, prepare another syringe, and repeat the procedure.

• Don't aspirate for blood return when giving insulin or heparin. *It's not necessary with insulin and may cause a hematoma with heparin.*

• After injection, remove the needle gently but quickly at the same angle used for insertion.

• Cover the site with an alcohol pad, and massage the site gently (unless you have injected a drug that contraindicates massage, such as heparin or insulin) *to distribute the drug and facilitate absorption.*

• Remove the alcohol pad, and check the injection site for bleeding or bruising.

• Dispose of injection equipment according to hospital policy. *To avoid needle-stick injuries,* don't resheath the needle.

Locating subcutaneous injection sites

Subcutaneous injection sites (shown by dotted areas) include the fat pads on the abdomen, upper hips, upper back, and lateral upper arms and thighs. For subcutaneous injections administered repeatedly such as insulin, rotate sites. Choose one injection site in one area, move to a corresponding injection site in the next area, and so on. When returning to an area, choose a new site in that area. Preferred injection sites for insulin are the arms, abdomen, thighs, and buttocks. Preferred injection sites for heparin injections are in the lower abdominal fat pad just below the umbilicus.

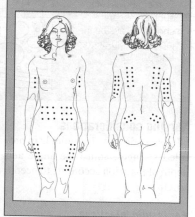

Complications

• Concentrated or irritating solutions may cause formation of sterile abscesses.

• Repeated injections in the same site can cause lipodystrophy.

• A natural immune response, this complication can be minimized by rotating injection sites.

Technique for subcutaneous injections

Before giving the injection, elevate the subcutaneous tissue at the site by grasping it firmly.

Insert the needle at a 45- or 90-degree angle to the skin surface, depending upon needle length and the amount of subcutaneous tissue at the site. Some medications, such as heparin, should always be injected at a 90-degree angle.

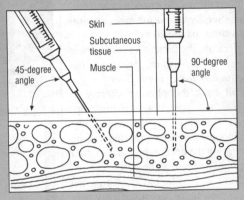

Nursing considerations

• If the medication is available in pre-filled syringes, adjust the angle and depth of insertion according to needle length.

For insulin injections

• To establish more consistent blood insulin levels, rotate insulin injection sites within anatomic regions. Absorption varies from one region to another. Preferred insulin injection sites are the arms, abdomen, thighs, and buttocks.

• Make sure the type of insulin, unit dosage, and syringe are correct.

• When combining insulins in a syringe, make sure they are compatible.

Regular insulin can be mixed with all other types. Prompt insulin zinc suspension (semilente insulin) cannot be mixed with NPH insulin. Follow hospital policy regarding which insulin to draw up first.

• Before drawing up insulin suspension, gently roll and invert the bottle to ensure even drug particle distribution. Don't shake the bottle *because this can cause foam or bubbles to develop in the syringe.*

• Some patients may benefit from an insulin infusion pump. (See *Types of insulin infusion pumps* .)

Types of insulin infusion pumps

A continuous subcutaneous insulin infusion pump provides long-term insulin therapy for patients with insulin-dependent diabetes mellitus. Complications include infection at the injection site, catheter clogging, and insulin loss from loose reservoir-catheter connections. Insulin pumps work on either a closed-loop or an open-loop system.

Open-loop system
The open-loop pump is used most commonly. It infuses insulin but can't respond to blood glucose changes. It is portable, self-contained, programmable, and the size of a credit card.

The pump delivers insulin in small (basal) doses every few minutes and large bolus doses that the patient sets manually. The system consists of a reservoir containing the insulin syringe, a small pump, an infusion rate selector that allows insulin release adjustments, a battery, and a plastic catheter with an attached needle leading from the syringe to the subcutaneous injection site. The needle is typically held in place with waterproof tape. The patient can wear the pump on his belt or in his pocket.

The infusion rate selector releases half the total daily insulin requirement. The patient releases the remainder in bolus amounts before meals and snacks. The patient must change the syringe daily; he must change the needle, catheter, and injection site every other day.

Closed-loop system
The self-contained closed-loop system detects and responds to changing blood glucose levels. The typical closed-loop system includes a glucose sensor, a programmable computer, a power supply, a pump, and an insulin reservoir. The computer triggers continuous insulin delivery in appropriate amounts from the reservoir.

Nonneedle catheter system
In this system, a tiny plastic catheter is inserted into the skin over a needle. The needle is then withdrawn, leaving the catheter in place. This pump can be placed in the abdomen, thigh, or flank and should be changed every 2 or 3 days.

For heparin injections
• The preferred site for heparin injection is the lower abdominal fat pad, 2″ (5 cm) beneath the umbilicus, between the right and the left iliac crests. *Injecting heparin into this area, which isn't involved in muscular activity, reduces the risk of local capillary bleeding.* Always rotate the sites from one side to the other.

• Don't administer any injections within 2″ of a scar, a bruise, or the umbilicus.
• Don't aspirate to check for blood return *because this may cause bleeding into the tissues at the site.*
• Don't rub or massage the site after the injection. *Rubbing can cause localized minute hemorrhages or bruises.*

• If the patient bruises easily, apply ice to the site for the first 5 minutes after the injection *to minimize local hemorrhage,* then apply pressure.

Documentation
• Record the time and date of the injection, the medication administered and the dose, the injection site and route, and the patient's reaction to the medication.

Sublingual drug administration

Certain drugs are given subligually to prevent their destruction or transformation in the stomach or small intestine. These drugs act quickly because the oral mucosa's thin epithelium and abundant vasculature allow direct absorption into the bloodstream. Sublingual drugs include ergotamine tartrate, erythrityl tetranitrate, isoproterenol hydrochloride, isosorbide dinitrate, and nitroglycerin.

≫ Key nursing diagnoses and patient outcomes
Use these nursing diagnosis as a guide when developing your plan of care for a patient receiving sublingual medications.

Knowledge deficit related to lack of exposure
Based on this nursing diagnosis, you'll establish the following patient outcomes. The patient will:
• state or demonstrate understanding of what has been taught.
• demonstrate ability to perform new health-related behaviors as they are

Placing drugs in the oral mucosa

Sublingual administration routes allow some drugs such as nitroglycerin to enter the bloodstream rapidly without being degraded in the GI tract. To give a drug sublingually, place it under the patient's tongue, as shown below, and ask him to leave it there until it's dissolved.

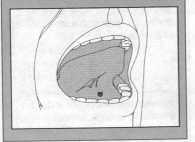

taught and list specific skills and realistic target dates for each.

Risk for injury related to improper technique
Based on this nursing diagnosis, you'll establish the following patient outcomes. The patient will:
• identify factors that increase the risk of injury.
• assist in identifying and applying safety measures to prevent injury.

Equipment
♦ patient's medication record and chart ♦ prescribed medication ♦ medication cup.

Equipment preparation
• Have the drug ready to administer.
• Verify the order on the patient's medication record by checking it

BETTER CHARTING

Guidelines for documenting medication administration

When using the medication administration record (MAR), follow these guidelines:
• Know and follow your hospital's policies and procedures for recording drug orders and charting drug administration.
• Make sure that all drug orders include the patient's full name, the date, the drug's name, dose, administration route or method, and frequency. When appropriate include the specific number of doses given or the stop date. When administering a drug dose immediately, or stat, make sure to record the time. Also be certain to include drug allergy information.
• Write legibly.
• Use only standard abbreviations approved by the hospital. When doubtful about an abbreviation, write out the word or phrase.

• After administering the first dose, sign your full name, licensure status, and your initials in the appropriate space on the MAR.
• Record drugs immediately after administration so that another nurse doesn't give the drug again.
• If you document medication administration by computer, chart your information for each drug right after you give it. This is particularly important if you don't use printouts as a backup. By keying in information immediately, you ensure that all health care team members have access to the latest drug administration data for the patient.
• Document the reason the drug was not given (for example, if the patient is having a test, which requires him not to take the drug).

against the doctor's order on the patient's chart.
• Check the label on the medication before administering it *to make sure you'll be giving the prescribed medication.*
• Confirm the patient's identity by asking his name and checking the name and room and bed number on his wristband.

Patient preparation
• Explain the procedure to the patient if he's never taken a drug sublingually.

Implementation
• Wash your hands with warm water and soap.

Sublingual administration
• Place the tablet under the patient's tongue. (See *Placing drugs in the oral mucosa.*)
• Instruct the patient to keep the medication in place until it dissolves completely *to ensure absorption.*
• Caution him against chewing the tablet or touching it with his tongue *to prevent accidental swallowing.*
• Tell him not to smoke before the drug has dissolved *because nicotine's*

vasoconstrictive effects slow absorption.

Complications
• Sublingual medications, such as erythrityl tetranitrate, may cause a tingling sensation under the tongue. If the patient finds this annoying, try placing the drug in the buccal pouch instead.

Nursing considerations
• Tell the angina patient to wet the nitroglycerin tablet with saliva and keep it under the tongue until fully absorbed.

Documentation
• Your employer probably includes a medication administration record (MAR) in your documentation system. Commonly included in a card file (medication Kardex) or on a separate medication administration sheet, the MAR serves as the central record of medication orders and their execution and is part of the patient's permanent record.
• Record the medication administered, the dose, the date and time, and the patient's reaction, if any. (See *Guidelines for documenting medication administration*, page 823.)

Swab specimen collection

Correct collection and handling of swab specimens helps the laboratory staff identify pathogens accurately, with a minimum of contamination from normal bacterial flora. Collection normally involves sampling inflamed tissues and exudates from the throat, nasopharynx, wounds, eye, ear, or rectum with sterile swabs of cotton or other absorbent material. Such swabs are immediately placed in a sterile tube containing a transport medium and, in the case of sampling for anaerobes, an inert gas. These specimens are usually collected to identify pathogens and sometimes to identify asymptomatic carriers of certain easily transmitted disease organisms.

≫ Key nursing diagnoses and patient outcomes
Use these nursing diagnoses as a guide when developing your plan of care.

Anxiety related to situational crisis
Based on this nursing diagnosis, you'll establish the following patient outcomes. The patient will:
• state at least two ways to eliminate or minimize anxious behaviors.
• report being able to cope with current situation without experiencing severe anxiety.

Knowledge deficit related to lack of exposure
Based on this nursing diagnosis, you'll establish the following patient outcomes. The patient will:
• communicate a need to know.
• state or demonstrate understanding of procedure.

Equipment
For a throat specimen: ♦ sterile swab ♦ tongue blade ♦ sterile culture tube with transport medium (or commercial collection kit) ♦ penlight ♦ gloves ♦ label ♦ laboratory request form.

For a nasopharyngeal specimen:
♦ sterile, flexible cotton-tipped wire swab ♦ gloves ♦ tongue blade ♦ sterile culture tube with transport medium ♦ penlight ♦ label ♦ laboratory request form ♦ optional: small open-ended Pyrex tube or nasal speculum.

For a wound specimen: ♦ sterile gloves ♦ alcohol pads or povidone-iodine sponges ♦ sterile swabs ♦ sterile 10-ml syringe ♦ sterile 21G needle ♦ sterile forceps ♦ sterile culture tube with transport medium (or commercial collection kit for aerobic culture) ♦ labels ♦ special anaerobic culture tube containing carbon dioxide or nitrogen ♦ fresh dressings for the wound ♦ laboratory request form ♦ optional: rubber stopper for needle.

For an ear specimen: ♦ gloves ♦ sterile swabs ♦ sterile culture tube with transport medium ♦ normal saline solution ♦ two $2'' \times 2''$ gauze pads ♦ label ♦ 10-ml syringe and 22G 1" needle (for tympanocentesis) ♦ label ♦ laboratory request form.

For an eye specimen: ♦ sterile gloves ♦ sterile swabs ♦ sterile wire culture loop (for corneal scraping) ♦ sterile culture tube with transport medium ♦ sterile normal saline solution ♦ two $2'' \times 2''$ gauze pads ♦ label ♦ laboratory request form.

For a rectal specimen: ♦ gloves ♦ sterile swab ♦ soap and water ♦ washcloth ♦ normal saline solution ♦ sterile culture tube with transport medium ♦ label ♦ laboratory request form.

Patient preparation
• Explain the procedure to the patient *to ease his anxiety and ensure cooperation.*

Implementation
Follow the steps below to obtain various types of specimens with a swab.

Collecting a throat specimen
• Tell the patient that he may gag during the swabbing but that the procedure will probably take less than a minute.
• Instruct the patient to sit erect at the edge of the bed or on a chair, facing you. Then wash your hands and don gloves.
• Ask the patient to tilt his head back. Depress his tongue with the tongue blade, and illuminate his throat with the penlight *to check for inflamed areas.*
• If the patient starts to gag, withdraw the tongue blade and tell him to breathe deeply. Once he's relaxed, reinsert the tongue blade, but not as deeply as before.
• Using the cotton-tipped wire swab, wipe the tonsillar areas from side to side, including any inflamed or purulent sites. Make sure you don't touch the tongue, cheeks, or teeth with the swab *to avoid contaminating it with oral bacteria.*
• Withdraw the swab and immediately place it in the culture tube. If you're using a commercial kit, crush the ampule of culture medium at the bottom of the tube, and then push the swab into the medium *to keep the swab moist.*
• Discard gloves and wash your hands.
• Label the specimen with the patient's name and room number, the doctor's name, and the date, time, and site of collection.
• On the laboratory request form, indicate whether any organism is strongly

Obtaining a nasopharyngeal specimen

After you've passed the swab into the nasopharynx, *gently* but quickly rotate the swab to collect the specimen. Then remove the swab, taking care not to injure the nasal mucous membrane.

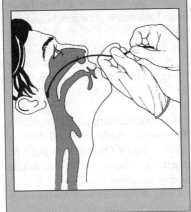

suspected, especially *Corynebacterium diphtheriae* (requires two swabs and special growth medium), *Bordetella pertussis* (requires a nasopharyngeal culture and special growth medium), and *Neisseria meningitidis* (requires enriched selective media).

• Send the specimen to the laboratory immediately *to prevent growth or deterioration of microbes.*

Collecting a nasopharyngeal specimen

• Tell the patient that he may gag or feel the urge to sneeze during the swabbing but that the procedure takes less than 1 minute.

• Have the patient sit erect at the edge of the bed or on a chair, facing you.

Then wash your hands and don gloves.

• Ask the patient to blow his nose *to clear his nasal passages.* Then check his nares for patency with a penlight.

• Tell the patient to occlude one nostril first and then the other as he exhales. Listen for the more patent nostril *because you'll insert the swab through it.*

• Ask the patient to cough *to bring organisms to the nasopharynx for a better specimen.*

• Bend the sterile wire swab in a curve and then open the package without contaminating the swab.

• Ask the patient to tilt his head back, and gently pass the swab through the more patent nostril about 3″ to 4″ (8 to 10 cm) into the nasopharynx, keeping the swab near the septum and the floor of the nose. (See *Obtaining a nasopharyngeal specimen.*) Rotate the swab quickly and remove it.

• Alternatively, depress the patient's tongue with a tongue blade, and pass the bent wire swab up behind the uvula. Rotate the swab and withdraw it.

• Remove the cap from the culture tube, insert the swab, and break off the contaminated end. Close the tube tightly, label it for throat culture, fill out laboratory request form, and send the specimen and form to the laboratory immediately. If you're collecting the specimen to isolate a possible virus, check with the laboratory for the recommended collection technique.

• Discard gloves and wash your hands.

Collecting a wound specimen

• Wash your hands, prepare a sterile field, and put on sterile gloves. With sterile forceps, remove the dressing to expose the wound. Dispose of the soiled dressings properly.

• Clean the area around the wound with an alcohol pad or a povidone-iodine sponge to reduce the risk of contaminating the specimen with skin bacteria. Then allow the area to dry.

• For an aerobic culture, use a sterile cotton-tipped swab to collect as much exudate as possible, or insert the swab deeply into the wound and gently rotate it. Remove the swab from the wound and immediately place it in the aerobic culture tube. Send the tube to the laboratory immediately with a completed laboratory request form. Never collect exudate from the skin and then insert the same swab into the wound; *this could contaminate the wound with skin bacteria.*

• For an anaerobic culture, insert the sterile cotton-tipped swab deeply into the wound, rotate it gently, remove it, and immediately place it in the anaerobic culture tube. (See *Anaerobic specimen collection*, page 828.)

Or insert a sterile 10-ml syringe, without a needle, into the wound, and aspirate 1 to 5 ml of exudate into the syringe. Then attach the 21G needle to the syringe, and immediately inject the aspirate into the anaerobic culture tube. If an anaerobic culture tube is unavailable, obtain a rubber stopper, attach the needle to the syringe, and gently push all the air out of the syringe by pressing on the plunger. Stick the needle tip into the rubber stopper, and send the syringe of aspirate to the laboratory immediately with a completed laboratory request form.

• Apply a new dressing to the wound.

Collecting an ear specimen
• Wash your hands and put on gloves.

• Gently clean excess debris from the patient's ear with normal saline solution and gauze pads.

• Insert the swab into the ear canal, and rotate it gently along the walls of the canal *to avoid damaging the eardrum.*

• Withdraw the swab, being careful not to touch other surfaces *to prevent contaminating the specimen.*

• Place the swab in the culture tube with transport medium.

• Remove the gloves and dispose of them properly. Wash your hands.

• Label the specimen for culture, complete a laboratory request form, and send the specimen to the laboratory immediately.

Collecting a middle ear specimen
• Put on gloves and clean the outer ear with normal saline solution and gauze pads. After the doctor punctures the eardrum with a needle and aspirates fluid into the syringe, label the container, complete a laboratory request form, and send the specimen to the laboratory immediately.

Collecting an eye specimen
• Wash your hands and put on sterile gloves.

• Gently clean excess debris from the outside of the eye with normal saline solution and gauze pads, wiping from the inner to the outer canthus.

• Retract the lower eyelid *to expose the conjunctival sac.* Gently rub the sterile swab over the conjunctiva, being careful not to touch other surfaces *to avoid contaminating the specimen.* Hold the swab parallel to the eye, rather than pointed directly at it, *to prevent corneal irritation or trauma due to sudden movement.* (If a corneal scrap-

Anaerobic specimen collection

Because most anaerobes die when exposed to oxygen, they must be transported in tubes filled with carbon dioxide or nitrogen. The anaerobic specimen collector shown here includes a rubber-stoppered tube filled with carbon dioxide, a small inner tube, and a swab attached to a plastic plunger.

Before specimen collection, the small inner tube containing the swab is held in place with the rubber stopper (as shown below left). After collecting the specimen, quickly replace the swab in the inner tube and depress the plunger to separate the inner tube from the stopper (as shown below right), forcing it into the larger tube and exposing the specimen to a carbon dioxide-rich environment.

Before   **After**

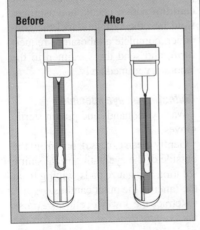

ing is required, this procedure is performed by a doctor using a wire culture loop.)
• Immediately place the swab or wire loop in the culture tube with transport medium.

• Remove the gloves and dispose of them properly.
• Wash your hands.
• Label the specimen for culture, complete a laboratory request form, and send the specimen to the laboratory immediately.

Collecting a rectal specimen
• Wash your hands and put on gloves.
• Clean the area around the patient's anus using a washcloth and soap and water.
• Insert the swab, moistened with normal saline solution or sterile broth medium, through the anus and advance it about $\frac{3}{8}''$ (1 cm) for infants or $1\frac{1}{2}''$ (4 cm) for adults. While withdrawing the swab, gently rotate it against the walls of the lower rectum to sample a large area of the rectal mucosa.
• Place the swab in a culture tube with transport medium. Then label the tube for rectal culture, complete a laboratory request form, and send the specimen to the laboratory immediately.
• Remove your gloves and dispose of them properly.
• Wash your hands.

Nursing considerations
• Note recent antibiotic therapy on the laboratory request form.

For a wound specimen
• Although you would normally clean the area around a wound to prevent contamination by normal skin flora, you should not clean a perineal wound with alcohol *because this could cause irritation to sensitive tissues.* Also, make sure none of the antiseptic enters the wound.

For an eye specimen

• Don't use an antiseptic before culturing *to avoid irritating the eye and inhibiting growth of organisms in culture.* If the patient is a child or an uncooperative adult, ask a coworker to restrain the patient's head *to prevent eye trauma resulting from sudden movement.*

Documentation

• Record the time, date, and site of specimen collection and any recent or current antibiotic therapy.

• Make sure that you note whether the specimen has an unusual appearance or odor.

T

Temperature measurement

Body temperature represents the balance between heat produced by metabolism, muscular activity, and other factors and heat lost through the skin, lungs, and body wastes. A stable temperature pattern promotes proper function of cells, tissues, and organs; a change in this pattern usually signals the onset of illness.

Temperature can be measured with a mercury, a digital electronic, or a chemical-dot thermometer. Normal oral temperature in adults typically ranges from 97° to 99.5° F (36.1° to 37.5° C); rectal temperature, the most accurate reading, is usually 1° F higher; axillary temperature, the least accurate, is usually 1° to 2° F (0.6° to 1.1° C) lower.

Temperature normally fluctuates with rest and activity. Lowest readings typically occur between 4 and 5 a.m., highest readings between 4 and 8 p.m. Sex, age, emotional condition, and environment also influence temperature.

Keep the following principles in mind: Women normally have higher temperatures than men, especially during ovulation. Normal temperature is highest in neonates and lowest in elderly persons. Heightened emotions raise temperature; depressed emotions lower it. A hot external environment raises temperature; a cold environment lowers it.

≫ Key nursing diagnoses and patient outcomes

Use these nursing diagnoses as a guide when developing your plan of care.

Anxiety related to situational crisis

Based on this nursing diagnosis, you'll establish the following patient outcomes. The patient will:
• state at least two ways to eliminate or minimize anxious behaviors.
• report being able to cope with current situation without experiencing severe anxiety.

Knowledge deficit related to lack of exposure

Based on this nursing diagnosis, you'll establish the following patient outcomes. The patient will:
• communicate a need to know.
• state or demonstrate understanding of procedure.

Equipment

♦ mercury or electronic thermometer for oral or rectal use, chemical-dot thermometer, or tympanic thermometer ♦ water-soluble lubricant or petroleum jelly (for rectal temperature) ♦ facial tissue ♦ disposable thermometer sheath or probe cover (except for chemical-dot thermometer) ♦ alcohol pad.

Equipment preparation

• A thermometer may be included as part of the admission pack. If it is, keep it at the patient's bedside and, on discharge, allow him to take it home. Otherwise, obtain a thermometer from the nurses' station or central supply department, and bring it to the patient's bedside. If you use an electronic thermometer, make sure it has been recharged. (See *Types of thermometers.*)

Patient preparation
• Explain the procedure.

Implementation
• Wash your hands.

Using a mercury thermometer
• Hold the thermometer between your thumb and index finger at the end opposite the bulb.
• If the thermometer has been soaking in a disinfectant, rinse it in cold water. *Rinsing removes chemicals that may irritate oral or rectal mucous membranes or axillary skin.* Avoid using hot water *because it expands the mercury, which could break the thermometer.* Using a twisting motion, wipe the thermometer from the bulb upward.
• Then quickly snap your wrist several times while holding the thermometer to shake it down. *Shaking causes the mercury to descend into the bulb.* The mercury will then expand in response to the patient's body temperature and be forced upward.
• To use a disposable sheath over the mercury thermometer, disinfect the thermometer with an alcohol pad. Insert it into the disposable sheath opening; then twist to tear the seal at the dotted line. Pull it apart.

Using an electronic thermometer
• Insert the probe into a disposable probe cover. If taking a rectal temperature, lubricate the probe cover *to reduce friction and ease insertion.* Leave the probe in place until the max-

imum temperature appears on the digital display.

Using a chemical-dot thermometer
• Remove the thermometer from its protective dispenser case by grasping the handle end with your thumb and forefinger, moving the handle up and down to break the seal, and pulling the handle straight out. Be sure to keep the thermometer sealed until use *because opening it activates the dye dots.*

Using a tympanic thermometer
• Stabilize the head; then gently pull the ear straight back for children up to age 1 or up and back for children age 1 or older to adults.
• Insert the thermometer as far as possible until the ear canal is sealed off. Then press the activation button and hold it for 1 second. The temperature will appear on the display. For infants under age 3 months, take three readings and use the highest.

Taking an oral temperature
• Position the tip of the thermometer under the patient's tongue, as far back as possible, on either side of the frenulum linguae. *Placing the tip in this area promotes contact with abundant superficial blood vessels and contributes to an accurate reading.*
• Instruct the patient to close his lips but to avoid biting down with his teeth. *Biting can break a mercury thermometer, cutting the mouth or lips or causing ingestion of broken glass or mercury.*
• Leave a mercury thermometer in place for at least 2 minutes or a chemical-dot thermometer for 45 seconds *to register temperature,* or wait until

Types of thermometers

You can take an oral, rectal, or axillary temperature with such instruments as a mercury glass thermometer, a chemical-dot device, or various electronic digital thermometers. You may even have access to a tympanic thermometer.

You'll use the oral route most for adults who are awake, alert, oriented, and cooperative. For infants, young children, and confused or unconscious patients, you may need to take the temperature rectally.

Chemical-dot thermometer

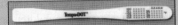

Individual electronic digital thermometer

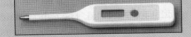

Tympanic thermometer

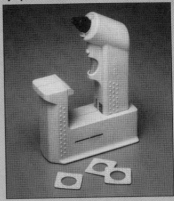

Institutional electronic digital thermometer

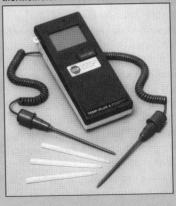

the maximum temperature is displayed on the electronic thermometer.
• For a mercury thermometer, remove and discard the disposable sheath; then read the temperature at eye level, noting it before shaking down the thermometer. For an electronic thermometer, note the temperature, then remove and discard the probe cover. For the chemical-dot thermometer, read the temperature as the last dye dot that has changed color, or fired; then discard the thermometer and its dispenser case.

Taking a rectal temperature
• Position the patient on his side with his top leg flexed, and drape him to provide privacy. Then fold back the bed linens to expose the anus.

TECHNOLOGY UPDATE

New skin sensor measures temperature continuously

A new device, the Premier Series adult skin sensor, allows continuous measurement of a patient's skin temperature. The adult skin sensor, compatible with most monitors, features hypoallergenic adhesive and a positive locking hub for secure cable connections.

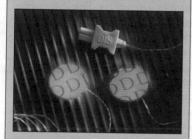

Photo courtesy of DeRoyal Industries, Powell, Tenn.

• Squeeze the lubricant onto a facial tissue *to prevent contamination of the lubricant supply.*

• Lubricate about ½" (1.3 cm) of the thermometer tip for an infant or about 1½" (4 cm) for an adult. *Lubrication reduces friction and thus eases insertion.* This step may be unnecessary when using disposable rectal sheaths *because they're prelubricated.*

• Lift the patient's upper buttock, and insert the thermometer about ½" for an infant or 1½" for an adult. Gently direct the thermometer along the rectal wall toward the umbilicus. *This will avoid perforating the anus or rectum or breaking the thermometer. It*

also will help ensure an accurate reading because the thermometer will register hemorrhoidal artery temperature instead of fecal temperature.

• Hold the mercury thermometer in place for 2 to 3 minutes or the electronic thermometer until the maximum temperature is displayed. *Holding it prevents damage to rectal tissues caused by displacement or loss of the thermometer into the rectum.*

• Carefully remove the thermometer, wiping it as necessary. Then wipe the patient's anal area *to remove any lubricant or feces.*

Taking an axillary temperature

• Position the patient with the axilla exposed.

• Gently pat the axilla dry with a facial tissue *because moisture conducts heat.* Avoid harsh rubbing, *which generates heat.*

• Ask the patient to place his hand over his chest and to grasp his opposite shoulder, lifting his elbow.

• Position the thermometer in the axilla, with the tip pointing toward the patient's head.

• Tell the patient to continue grasping his shoulder and to lower his elbow and hold it against his chest. *This promotes skin contact with the thermometer.*

• Leave a mercury thermometer in place for 10 minutes; leave an electronic thermometer in place until it displays the maximum temperature. Axillary temperature takes longer to register than oral or rectal temperature *because the thermometer isn't enclosed in a body cavity.*

• Grasp the end of the thermometer and remove it from the axilla.

Nursing considerations
• Oral measurement is contraindicated in patients who are unconscious, disoriented, or seizure-prone; in young children and infants; and in patients with oral or nasal impairment that necessitates mouth breathing.
• Rectal measurement is contraindicated in patients with diarrhea, recent rectal or prostatic surgery or injury *because it may injure inflamed tissue,* or recent myocardial infarction *because anal manipulation may stimulate the vagus nerve, causing bradycardia or another rhythm disturbance.*
• Drinking hot or cold liquids, chewing gum, or smoking may alter oral temperature readings. Wait 15 minutes after these activities before taking a temperature. *Bathing may alter axillary temperature.*
• Use the same thermometer for repeated temperature taking *to avoid spurious variations caused by equipment differences.* Store chemical-dot thermometers in a cool area *because exposure to heat activates the dye dots.*
• Don't avoid taking an oral temperature when the patient is receiving nasal oxygen *because oxygen administration raises oral temperature by only about 0.3° F (0.17° C).* (See *New skin sensor measures temperature continuously.*)

Documentation
• Record the time, route, and temperature on the patient's chart.

Thallium imaging

Also called cold spot myocardial imaging or thallium scintigraphy, this test evaluates myocardial blood flow after I.V. injection of the radioisotope thallium-201 (thallous chloride Tl 201, or $^{201}TlCl$). Because thallium, the physiologic analogue of potassium, concentrates in healthy myocardial tissue but not in necrotic or ischemic tissue, areas of the heart with normal blood supply and intact cells take it up rapidly. Areas with poor blood flow and ischemic cells fail to take up the isotope and appear as cold spots on a scan.

This test is performed in a resting state or after stress. Possible complications of stress testing include arrhythmias, angina pectoris, and myocardial infarction (MI).

The purpose of resting imaging is to assess myocardial scarring and perfusion and to demonstrate the location and extent of acute or chronic MI, including transmural and postoperative infarction. The purposes of stress imaging are to diagnose coronary artery disease (CAD), to evaluate the patency of grafts after coronary artery bypass surgery, and to evaluate the effectiveness of antianginal therapy or balloon angioplasty.

≫ Key nursing diagnoses and patient outcomes
Use these nursing diagnoses as a guide when developing your plan of care.

Anxiety related to situational crisis
Based on this nursing diagnosis, you'll establish the following patient outcomes. The patient will:
• state at least two ways to eliminate or minimize anxious behaviors.
• report being able to cope with current situation without experiencing severe anxiety.

Knowledge deficit related to lack of exposure to procedure
Based on this nursing diagnosis, you'll establish the following patient outcomes. The patient will:
• communicate a need to know.
• state or demonstrate understanding of procedure.

Equipment

For the resting test: ♦ thallium scanner ♦ prepared thallium for I.V. injection ♦ normal saline solution.

For the stress test: ♦ thallium scanner ♦ prepared thallium for I.V. injection ♦ normal saline solution ♦ ECG machine ♦ cardiac electrodes ♦ treadmill.

Patient preparation

• Explain to the patient that these tests help determine if any areas of the heart muscle aren't receiving an adequate supply of blood.
• For stress imaging, instruct him to restrict alcohol, tobacco, and unprescribed medications for 24 hours before the test and to have nothing by mouth for 3 hours before the test (advise him to eat a light meal beforehand).
• Describe the test, including who will perform it, where it will take place, and how long it's expected to take (45 to 90 minutes). Explain that additional scans may be required.
• Tell him that he will receive a radioactive tracer I.V. and that multiple images of his heart will be scanned.
• Warn him that he may experience discomfort from skin abrasion during preparation for electrode placement. Assure him the test involves minimal radiation exposure.

• Make sure the patient or a responsible family member has signed a consent form.
• For stress imaging, instruct the patient to wear walking shoes during the treadmill exercise and to report fatigue, pain, or shortness of breath immediately.

Implementation

Follow the steps outlined below for a patient undergoing thallium imaging.

Resting imaging

• Within the first few hours of symptoms of MI, the patient receives an injection of thallium I.V. and scanning begins after 3 to 5 minutes.
• If further scanning is required, have the patient rest and restrict food and fluids.

Stress imaging

• The patient, wired with electrodes, walks on a treadmill at a regulated pace that's gradually increased, while the electrocardiogram (ECG), blood pressure, and heart rate are monitored.
• When the patient reaches peak stress, the examiner injects 1.5 to 3 mC of thallium into the antecubital vein and then flushes it with 10 to 15 ml of normal saline solution.
• The patient exercises an additional 45 to 60 seconds to permit circulation and uptake of the isotope, and then lies on his back under the scintillation camera.
• If the patient is asymptomatic, the precordial leads are removed. Scanning begins after 3 to 5 minutes with the patient in anterior, 45-degree and 60-degree left anterior oblique, and left lateral positions.

• Additional scans may be taken after the patient rests 3 to 6 hours.

Complications
• Stop stress imaging at once if the patient develops chest pain, dyspnea, fatigue, syncope, hypotension, ischemic ECG changes, significant arrhythmias, or critical signs (pale, clammy skin, confusion, or staggering).

Nursing considerations
• Contraindications include impaired neuromuscular function, pregnancy, locomotor disturbances, acute MI and myocarditis, aortic stenosis, acute infection, unstable metabolic conditions (like diabetes), digitalis toxicity, and recent pulmonary infarction.
• Tell the patient to avoid heavy meals, cigarette smoking, and strenuous activity before the test. If your patient is scheduled for an exercise thallium scan, advise him to wear comfortable clothes or pajamas and snug-fitting shoes or slippers.
• Imaging should show normal distribution of the isotope throughout the left ventricle and no defects (cold spots).
• Persistent defects indicate MI; transient defects (which disappear after a 3- to 6-hour rest) indicate ischemia from CAD. After coronary artery bypass surgery, improved regional perfusion suggests patency of the graft. Increased perfusion after ingestion of antianginal drugs can show that they relieve ischemia. Improved perfusion after balloon angioplasty suggests increased coronary flow.

Documentation
• Record allergies on patient's chart and allergy band clearly, and alert ra-diologist and involved doctors of the patient's allergies.
• Record any preparation and instruction given to the patient and his responses.
• Record any premedication given to the patient and its effects.
• Document toleration of procedure and any reactions to the thallium.
• Document type of needle used to start I.V., site location, appearance, and solution used and rate of flow.

Thermoregulation

A large body surface-to-mass ratio, reduced metabolism per unit area, limited amounts of insulating subcutaneous fat, vasomotor instability, and limited metabolic capacity make all neonates susceptible to hypothermia. To stay warm when he is cold-stressed, the neonate metabolizes brown fat. Unique to neonates, brown fat has energy-producing mitochondria in its cells, which enhances its capacity for heat production.

Brown fat metabolism effectively warms the body — but only within a narrow temperature range. Without careful external thermoregulation, the neonate may become chilled. Acidosis, hypoxia, hypoglycemia, pulmonary vasoconstriction, and even death may result.

Thermoregulation provides a neutral thermal environment that helps the neonate maintain a normal core temperature with minimal oxygen consumption and caloric expenditure. Although it varies with each neonate, average core temperature is 97.7° F (36.5° C).

Understanding thermoregulators

Thermoregulators preserve neonatal body warmth in various ways. A radiant warmer maintains the neonate's temperature by *radiation*. An incubator maintains the neonate's temperature by *conduction* and *convection*.

Temperature settings
Radiant warmers and incubators have two operating modes: *nonservo* and *servo*. Whereas the nurse manually sets temperature controls on nonservo equipment, a probe on the neonate's skin controls temperature settings on servo models.

Other features
Most thermoregulators come with alarms. Incubators have the additional advantage of providing a stable, enclosed environment that protects the neonate from evaporative heat loss.

Two kinds of thermoregulators are common in the hospital nursery: radiant warmers and incubators. The radiant warmer controls environmental temperature while the nurse gives initial care in the delivery room. Then when the neonate arrives in the nursery, another radiant warmer may be used until his temperature stabilizes and he can occupy a bassinet. If the temperature doesn't stabilize or if the neonate has a condition that affects thermoregulation, a temperature-controlled incubator will house him. (See *Understanding thermoregulators*.)

≫ Key nursing diagnoses and patient outcomes
Use these nursing diagnoses as a guide when developing your plan of care for a neonate who is undergoing thermoregulation.

Ineffective thermoregulation related to trauma or illness
Based on this nursing diagnosis, you'll establish the following patient outcomes. The patient will:
• maintain body temperature at normothermic levels.
• demonstrate no signs of shivering.
• express feelings of comfort.

Altered peripheral tissue perfusion related to decreased arterial blood flow
Based on this nursing diagnosis, you'll establish the following patient outcomes. The patient will:
• have no arrhythmias.
• have skin color and temperature within normal limits.

Equipment
♦ radiant warmer or incubator (if necessary) ♦ blankets ♦ washcloths or towels ♦ skin probe ♦ adhesive pad ♦ water-soluble lubricant ♦ thermometer ♦ clothing (including a cap) ♦ optional: stockinette gauze.

Equipment preparation
• Turn on the radiant warmer in the delivery room, and set the desired temperature. Warm the blankets, washcloths, or towels under a heat source.

Implementation
• Continue nursing measures to conserve neonatal body warmth until the patient's discharge.

In the delivery room

• Place the neonate under the radiant warmer, and dry him with the warm washcloths or towels *to prevent heat loss by evaporation.*

• Pay special attention to drying his scalp and hair. Then if you take him off the warmer, make sure you cover his head (which makes up about 25% of neonatal body surface) with a ready-made cap *to prevent heat loss.*

• Perform required procedures quickly *to reduce the neonate's exposure to cool delivery room air.*

• Wrap him in the warmed blankets. If his condition permits, give him to his parents *to promote bonding.*

• Transport the neonate to the nursery in the warmed blankets. Use a transport incubator when the nursery is far from the delivery room.

In the nursery

• Remove the blankets and cap, and place the neonate under the radiant warmer.

• Use the adhesive pad to attach the temperature control probe to his skin in the upper-right abdominal quadrant. *This lets the servo control maintain neonatal skin temperature between 96.8° and 97.7° F (36° and 36.5° C).* If the neonate will lie in a prone position, put the skin probe on his back *to ensure accurate temperature control and avoid false-high readings from the neonate lying on the probe.* Don't cover the device with anything *because this could interfere with the servo control.* Be sure to raise the warmer's side panels *to prevent accidents.*

• Lubricate the thermometer and take the neonate's rectal temperature on admission *to identify core tempera-*

ture. Take axillary temperatures thereafter *to avoid injuring delicate rectal mucosa.* Usually, axillary temperature readings are lower than the core temperature (see "Neonatal vital sign measurement," page 567). Take axillary temperatures every 15 to 30 minutes until the temperature stabilizes, then every 4 hours *to ensure stability.*

• Sponge-bathe the neonate under the warmer only after his temperature stabilizes and his glucose level is normal, and leave him under the warmer until his temperature remains stable.

• Take appropriate action if the temperature doesn't stabilize. For example, place the neonate under a plastic heat shield or in a warmed incubator — depending on hospital policy. Look for objects such as a phototherapy unit that may be blocking the heat source. Also check for signs of infection, which can cause hypothermia.

• Apply a skin probe to the neonate in an incubator as you would for a neonate in a radiant warmer. Move the incubator away from cold walls or objects.

• Perform all required procedures quickly *to maintain a neutral thermal environment and to minimize heat loss.* Close portholes in the hood immediately after completing any procedure, *also to reduce heat loss.* If procedures must be performed outside the incubator, do them under a radiant warmer.

• To leave the hospital or to move to a bassinet, a neonate must be weaned from the incubator. Slowly reduce the incubator's temperature to that of the nursery. Check periodically for hypothermia. *To ensure temperature stability,* never discharge the neonate to home directly from an incubator.

• When the normal neonate's temperature stabilizes, dress him, put him in a bassinet, and cover him with a blanket.

Complications

• Hypothermia from ineffective natural or external thermoregulation can inhibit weight gain because the neonate must use caloric energy to maintain his temperature.

• Hyperthermia can cause increased oxygen consumption and apnea. Both conditions can result from equipment failures or insufficient monitoring.

Nursing considerations

• Always warm oxygen before administering it to a neonate *to avoid initiating heat loss from his head and face.*

• *To prevent conductive heat loss,* preheat the radiant warmer bed and linen; warm stethoscopes and other instruments before use; and pad the scale with paper or a preweighed, warmed sheet before weighing the neonate.

• *To avoid convective heat loss,* place the neonate's bed out of direct line with an open window, a fan, or an air-conditioning vent.

• *To control evaporative heat loss,* dry the neonate immediately after delivery. When bathing the neonate, expose only one body part at a time, wash each part thoroughly, then dry it immediately.

• Review the reasons for regulating body temperature with the neonate's family. Instruct them to keep him wrapped in a blanket and out of drafts when he's not in the bassinet — both in the hospital and at home. In a warm place, guard against overheating the neonate.

Documentation

• Name the heat source, and record its temperature and the neonate's temperature, whenever taken.

• Document any complications that result from using thermoregulatory equipment.

Thoracentesis

This procedure involves aspiration of fluid or air from the pleural space. It relieves pulmonary compression and respiratory distress by removing accumulated air or fluid that results from injury or such conditions as tuberculosis or cancer. It also provides a specimen of pleural fluid or tissue for analysis, and allows instillation of chemotherapeutic agents or other medications into the pleural space.

Thoracentesis is contraindicated in patients with bleeding disorders.

≫ Key nursing diagnoses and patient outcomes

Use these nursing diagnoses as a guide when developing your plan of care for a patient who is undergoing thoracentesis.

Ineffective breathing pattern related to decreased energy

Based on this nursing diagnosis, you'll establish the following patient outcomes. The patient will:

• achieve maximum lung expansion with adequate ventilation.

• report feeling comfortable with breathing.

Impaired gas exchange related to altered oxygen supply
Based on this nursing diagnosis, you'll establish the following patient outcomes. The patient will:
• cough effectively.
• expectorate sputum.

Equipment

Most hospitals use a prepackaged thoracentesis tray that typically includes the following: ♦ sterile gloves ♦ sterile drapes ♦ 70% isopropyl alcohol or povidone-iodine solution ♦ 1% or 2% lidocaine ♦ 5-ml syringe with 21G and 25G needles for anesthetic injection ♦ 17G thoracentesis needle for aspiration ♦ 50-ml syringe ♦ three-way stopcock and tubing ♦ sterile specimen containers ♦ sterile hemostat ♦ sterile 4″ × 4″ gauze pads.

You'll also need the following: ♦ adhesive tape ♦ sphygmomanometer ♦ gloves ♦ stethoscope ♦ laboratory request slips ♦ drainage bottles ♦ optional: Teflon catheter, shaving supplies, biopsy needle, prescribed sedative with 3-ml syringe and 21G needle, drainage bottles (if the doctor expects a large amount of drainage).

Equipment preparation

• Assemble all equipment at the patient's bedside or in the treatment area.
• Check the expiration date on each sterile package and inspect for tears.
• Prepare the necessary laboratory request form.
• Be sure to list current antibiotic therapy on the laboratory forms *because this will be considered in analyzing the specimens.*
• Make sure the patient has signed an appropriate consent form.

• Note any drug allergies, especially to the local anesthetic.
• Have the patient's chest X-rays available.

Patient preparation

• Explain the procedure to the patient.
• Inform him that he may feel some discomfort and a sensation of pressure during the needle insertion.
• Provide privacy and emotional support.

Implementation

• Wash your hands.
• Administer the prescribed sedative.
• Obtain baseline vital signs and assess respiratory function.
• Position the patient. Make sure he's firmly supported and comfortable. Although the choice of position varies, you'll usually seat the patient on the edge of the bed with his legs supported and his head and folded arms resting on a pillow on the overbed table, or have him straddle a chair backward and rest his head and folded arms on the back of the chair. If the patient is not able to sit, turn him on the unaffected side with the arm of the affected side raised above his head. Elevate the head of the bed 30 to 45 degrees if such elevation isn't contraindicated. *Proper positioning stretches the chest or back and allows easier access to the intercostal spaces.*
• Remind the patient not to cough, breathe deeply, or move suddenly during the procedure *to avoid puncture of the visceral pleura or lung.* If the patient coughs, the doctor will briefly halt the procedure and withdraw the needle slightly *to prevent puncture.*
• Expose the patient's entire chest or back as appropriate.

BETTER CHARTING

Documenting thoracentesis

Document the date, time, name of the doctor performing the procedure, the amount and quality of fluid aspirated, and the patient's response to the procedure.

If later symptoms of pneumothorax, subcutaneous emphysema, or infection occur, notify the doctor immediately and document your observations and interventions on the chart.

Also note whether you sent a fluid specimen to the laboratory for analysis.

• Shave the aspiration site as ordered.
• Wash your hands again before touching the sterile equipment. Then using sterile technique, open the thoracentesis tray, and assist the doctor as necessary in disinfecting the site.
• If an ampule of local anesthetic is not included in the sterile tray and a multidose vial of local anesthetic is to be used, assist the doctor by wiping the rubber stopper with an alcohol pad and holding the inverted vial while the doctor withdraws the anesthetic solution.
• After draping the patient and injecting the local anesthetic, the doctor attaches a three-way stopcock with tubing to the aspirating needle and turns the stopcock to prevent air from entering the pleural space through the needle.
• Attach the other end of the tubing to the drainage bottle.
• The doctor then inserts the needle into the pleural space and attaches a 50-ml syringe to the needle's stop-

cock. A hemostat may be used *to hold the needle in place and prevent pleural tear or lung puncture.* As an alternative, the doctor may introduce a Teflon catheter into the needle, remove the needle, and attach a stopcock and syringe or drainage tubing to the catheter *to reduce the risk of pleural puncture by the needle.*
• Provide emotional support throughout the procedure, and keep the patient informed of each step. Assess him for signs of anxiety and provide reassurance as necessary.
• Check vital signs regularly during the procedure. Continually observe the patient for such signs of distress as pallor, vertigo, faintness, weak and rapid pulse, decreased blood pressure, dyspnea, tachypnea, diaphoresis, chest pain, blood-tinged mucus, and excessive coughing. Alert the doctor if such signs develop *because they may indicate complications, such as hypovolemic shock or tension pneumothorax.*
• Put on gloves and assist the doctor as necessary in collecting the specimen, draining the fluid, and dressing the site.
• After the doctor withdraws the needle or catheter, apply pressure to the puncture site, using a sterile $4'' \times 4''$ gauze pad. Then apply a new sterile gauze pad, and secure it with tape.
• Place the patient in a comfortable position, take his vital signs, and assess his respiratory status.
• Label the specimens properly, and send them to the laboratory.
• Discard disposable equipment. Clean nondisposable items, and return them for sterilization.
• Check the patient's vital signs and the dressing for drainage every 15 minutes for 1 hour. Then continue to

assess the patient's vital signs and respiratory status as indicated by his condition.

Complications
• Pneumothorax (possibly leading to mediastinal shift and requiring chest tube insertion) can occur if the needle punctures the lung and allows air to enter the pleural cavity.
• Pyogenic infection can result from contamination during the procedure.
• Other potential difficulties include pain, cough, anxiety, dry taps, and subcutaneous hematoma.

Nursing considerations
• To prevent postthoracentesis pulmonary edema and hypovolemic shock, fluid is removed slowly, and no more than 1,000 ml of fluid is removed during the first 30 minutes. *Removing the fluid increases the negative intrapleural pressure, which can lead to edema if the lung doesn't reexpand to fill the space.*
• Pleuritic or shoulder pain may indicate pleural irritation by the needle point.
• A chest X-ray is usually ordered after the procedure *to detect pneumothorax and evaluate the results of the procedure.*

Documentation
• Record the date and time of thoracentesis; location of the puncture site; volume and description (color, viscosity, odor) of the fluid withdrawn; specimens sent to the laboratory; vital signs and respiratory assessment before, during, and after the procedure; any postprocedural tests such as chest X-ray; any complications and the nursing action taken; and the patient's

reaction to the procedure. (See *Documenting thoracentesis,* page 841.)

Thorax inspection

To detect either subtle or obvious respiratory changes, you need to perform a systematic assessment. The depth of the assessment will depend on factors such as the patient's primary health problem and his risk of developing complications.

›› Key nursing diagnosis and patient outcomes
Use these nursing diagnoses as a guide when developing your plan of care.

Ineffective breathing pattern related to decreased energy
Based on this nursing diagnosis, you'll establish the following patient outcomes. The patient will:
• achieve maximum lung expansion with adequate ventilation.
• report feeling comfortable with breathing.

Impaired gas exchange related to altered oxygen supply
Based on this nursing diagnosis, you'll establish the following patient outcomes. The patient will:
• cough effectively.
• expectorate sputum.

Equipment
♦ stethoscope ♦ marking pen ♦ tape measure or ruler.

Use an area that's well lighted, preferably with natural light.

Patient preparation

• Position the patient so you'll have access to his posterior and anterior chest. If his condition permits, have him sit on the edge of the bed or examination table or on a chair, leaning slightly forward with his arms folded across his chest.

If this isn't possible, place him in semi-Fowler's position for the anterior chest examination. Then ask him to lean forward slightly and use the side rails or mattress for support while you quickly examine his posterior chest. If he can't lean forward, place him in a lateral position or ask another staff member to help him sit up.

Implementation

• First inspect the patient's chest. Quickly observe the patient's overall appearance for signs and symptoms of acute respiratory difficulty. Restlessness, anxiety, or a decreased level of consciousness may indicate hypoxemia (low blood O_2 levels) or hypercapnia (high blood CO_2 levels).

• Continue your inspection by observing the patient's respiratory rate and pattern. Then examine his head, neck, and shoulders, and his chest, skin, and fingers.

• Next, observe the patient at rest as he breathes naturally and effortlessly. *To avoid altering his natural breathing pattern,* don't make it obvious that you're counting his respirations. Count an adult's respirations for at least 1 minute. For an infant or a patient with periodic or irregular breathing, monitor the respirations for more than 1 minute to ensure accuracy. Note the duration of any periods of apnea. (The normal respiratory rate is 12 to

20 breaths/minute in adults and as much as 44 breaths/minute in infants.)

• Assess the quality of respirations by observing the type and depth of breathing. Remember that men, children, and infants are usually diaphragmatic (abdominal) breathers, as are athletes and singers. Most women are intercostal (chest) breathers.

• Examine the patient's mouth, noting the color of the mucous membranes. They should be pale pink to pink. Bluish or gray oral mucosa may indicate central cyanosis due to prolonged hypoxia. Central cyanosis may appear in other highly vascular areas as well: the lips, conjunctivae, earlobes, and tip of the nose.

• Observe the neck and shoulders *to determine whether the patient is using his accessory muscles — the sternocleidomastoid, scalene, and trapezius muscles — to breathe.* Typically, the diaphragm and external intercostal muscles should easily maintain the breathing process. Hypertrophy of any of the accessory muscles may indicate frequent use, although it may be normal in a well-conditioned athlete. *Use of accessory muscles as well as pursed-lip breathing, mouth breathing, and nasal flaring may indicate respiratory difficulty.*

• Examine the chest for wounds, bruises, scars, rib deformities, and masses. Then observe the shape of the thorax. In an adult, the transverse diameter (side to side) should be greater than the anteroposterior diameter (front to back).

• Note the angle between the ribs and the sternum at the point immediately above the xiphoid process. This angle, called the costal angle, should be less than 90 degrees in an adult. If the patient's chest wall is chronically expanded because of intercostal muscle hypertrophy, the costal angle will be wider.

• Inspect first the anterior chest and then the posterior chest for symmetrical movement. Carefully observe the patient's quiet, deep breathing for equal expansion of the chest wall. Be alert for paradoxical movement — the abnormal collapse of part of the chest wall during inspiration, and the abnormal expansion of the same area during expiration. *Such movement indicates a loss of normal chest wall function.*

• Inspect the patient's entire thorax for shape, size, symmetry, obvious pulsations, and retractions. Look for an apical impulse, or point of maximal impulse (PMI), normally located in the fifth intercostal space at about the midclavicular line. You can see the PMI as a pulsation produced by the thrust of the contracting left ventricle against the chest wall. The apical impulse reflects cardiac size, especially left ventricular size and location, and is evident in about half the normal adult population. Because it occurs almost simultaneously with the carotid pulse, palpating this pulse can help you identify it.

Nursing considerations

• Watch for use of the sternocleidomastoid, scalene, or trapezius muscles to breathe or for supraclavicular retractions. *If they're present, the patient's inhalation may be impeded. Similarly, watch for prolonged exhalation.*

• Make sure the room temperature is comfortable for the patient.

Documentation

• Document your findings and inform the doctor about them.

Thorax and lung field palpation

If possible, perform palpation immediately after your inspection. Using the palmar surface of your hands, including the base of your fingers, palpate the anterior and posterior chest. Assess skin temperature and turgor, identify thoracic structures, and evaluate tactile fremitus and respiratory excursion. Note any tenderness, swelling, or abnormalities such as masses.

⟫ Key nursing diagnoses and patient outcomes

Use these nursing diagnoses as a guide when developing your plan of care.

Ineffective breathing pattern related to decreased energy
Based on this nursing diagnosis, you'll establish the following patient outcomes. The patient will:

• achieve maximum lung expansion with adequate ventilation.

• report feeling comfortable with breathing.

Impaired gas exchange related to altered oxygen supply
Based on this nursing diagnosis, you'll establish the following patient outcomes. The patient will:

• cough effectively.

• expectorate sputum.

Equipment

No special equipment is needed to palpate the thorax and lung fields.

Patient preparation

• Assist the patient to a sitting position, unless contraindicated, with his chest and back exposed. Explain the procedure to the patient before beginning the assessment.

Implementation

• Begin by palpating the skin for temperature, moisture, turgor, tender areas, and masses. Cold, clammy skin results from increased sympathetic stimulation, which may be caused by hypoxia or circulatory failure. Warm, dry, or moist skin may indicate infection. Decreased turgor indicates dehydration, whereas edema suggests inadequate circulation that could involve the respiratory system.

• Palpate bony structures, including the thoracic spine, scapulae, and sternum, noting any tenderness, swelling, or deformities. A normal spine feels straight from the cervical area through the beginning of the thoracic area. Normal scapulae are symmetrical, with well-developed surrounding musculature. A normal chest wall feels stable at the junctions of the ribs, spine, and sternum. Note any deviations that may interfere with ventilation.

Gentle palpation shouldn't elicit pain. If it does, note the location, any radiation, and the severity. Note any other unusual findings, including skin irregularities and crepitus — a crackling feeling under the patient's skin that may indicate subcutaneous emphysema. Also, note any masses.

• To palpate for tactile fremitus (vibrations in the thorax), place your open palms against the upper portion of the anterior chest, making sure your fingers don't touch the chest. Avoid placing your palms over bony promi-nences or organs such as the heart by starting above the clavicles anteriorly. Ask the patient to repeat "ninety-nine" or another resonant phrase while you systematically move your palms over the chest from the central airways to each lung's periphery and back. You should feel vibrations of equal intensity on both sides of the chest. Assess the posterior thorax in a similar manner.

Fremitus typically occurs in the upper chest close to the bronchi and feels strongest at the second intercostal space on either side of the sternum. Little or no fremitus should occur in the lower chest. The intensity of the vibrations varies according to the thickness and structure of the patient's chest wall as well as the patient's voice intensity and pitch.

Increased fremitus indicates consolidation, possibly from pneumonia. Decreased fremitus, which commonly occurs with chronic obstructive pulmonary disease, indicates increased physiologic dead space (pulmonary space that doesn't participate in gas exchange).

• Assess respiratory excursion in three areas on the patient's anterior chest. To assess the first area, place your hands on the upper chest with your thumbs at the second intercostal spaces. Your thumbs should barely touch at the midline, and your palms and fingers should be flat on the chest wall. Don't apply pressure; *this could alter the patient's inspiratory effort.* As the patient inhales deeply, observe your thumbs. They should separate simultaneously and equally to a distance several centimeters from the sternum. Repeat the procedure with your thumbs at the fifth intercostal

spaces and again with your thumbs at the tenth intercostal spaces.
• Assess respiratory excursion in two areas on the posterior chest. Stand behind the patient and place your thumbs at the infrascapular areas on either side of the spine at the level of the tenth rib. Grasp the lateral rib cage and rest your palms gently over the lateroposterior surface. As the patient inhales, the posterior chest should move upward and outward, and your thumbs should move apart. When the patient exhales, your thumbs should return to the midline and touch. Repeat the procedure, placing your thumbs lateral to the vertebral column in the interscapular area, with your fingers extending into the axillary area.

Unequal excursion may be caused by conditions that cause pain on deep inspiration or by underlying structural problems, such as fractures or masses.

Nursing considerations
• Provide for patient privacy. Ensure that patient is comfortable by adjusting room temperature appropriately.

Documentation
• Document your findings in the nursing assessment flow sheet, and inform the doctor of your findings.

Thorax and lung field percussion

Indirect percussion, the most frequently used percussion technique, allows you to assess structures $1\frac{3}{4}''$ to $3''$ (4 to 8 cm) deep. You'll use indirect percussion to identify the boundaries of the lungs and determine if they contain gas, liquid, or solid matter. You'll also use indirect percussion to determine diaphragmatic excursion, the distance that the diaphragm travels between inhalation and exhalation. To interpret your findings, you must be able to recognize five percussion sounds:
• resonance — a low-pitched, moderate to loud sound with a hollow quality
• tympany — a high-pitched loud sound with a drumlike quality
• dullness — a high-pitched, soft to moderate sound with a thudlike quality
• hyperresonance — a low-pitched, loud sound with a booming quality
• flatness — a high-pitched, soft sound with an extremely dull quality.

Be sure to work systematically, percussing the anterior, lateral, and posterior chest over the intercostal spaces.

⟫ Key nursing diagnoses and patient outcomes
Use these nursing diagnoses as a guide when developing your plan of care.

Ineffective breathing pattern related to decreased energy
Based on this nursing diagnosis, you'll establish the following patient outcomes. The patient will:
• achieve maximum lung expansion with adequate ventilation.
• report feeling comfortable with breathing.

Impaired gas exchange related to altered oxygen supply
Based on this nursing diagnosis, you'll establish the following patient outcomes. The patient will:
• cough effectively.
• expectorate sputum.

Equipment

No equipment is needed to percuss the thorax and lung fields.

Patient preparation

• Ask the patient to sit upright, unless contraindicated, with his chest and back exposed.
• Explain the procedure to the patient before assessing him.

Implementation

• Place your nondominant hand on the patient's anterior thorax. Use the tip of the middle finger of your dominant hand to tap on the middle finger of your other hand just below the distal joint. Percuss the patient's anterior thorax at the left clavicle, then at the right.
• Begin by percussing the lung apices (in the supraclavicular areas), comparing the right and left sides. Then percuss downward in $1\frac{1}{4}''$ to $2''$ (3- to 5-cm) intervals. You should hear resonance, which indicates normal lung tissue, until you reach the third or fourth intercostal space to the left of the sternum, where you'll hear a dull sound produced by the heart. This sound should continue as you percuss down toward the fifth intercostal space and laterally toward the midclavicular line. At the sixth intercostal space at the left midclavicular line, you'll hear resonance again. As you percuss downward, you'll hear tympany over the stomach.

On the right side, you should hear resonance, indicating normal lung tissue. Near the fifth to seventh intercostal spaces, you'll hear dullness, marking the superior border of the liver.
• To percuss the lateral chest, instruct the patient to raise his arms over his head. Percuss laterally, comparing the right and left sides as you proceed. These areas should also be resonant.
• Percuss the posterior chest, following the percussion sequence. Start percussing across the top of each shoulder, and move downward toward the patient's diaphragm at $1\frac{1}{4}''$ to $2''$ intervals. The area from the shoulders to the level of the 10th thoracic vertebra should be resonant.

Nursing considerations

• Provide for patient privacy and adjust room temperature to comfort.
• Be alert for these abnormal sounds: *hyperresonance* (low-pitched, loud, longer than normal, and booming) over emphysematous areas and pneumothorax; *tympany* (high-pitched, loud, musical, and drumlike) over a stomach or abdomen distended with air; *dullness* (high-pitched, soft, and thudlike) over solid areas such as a pleural effusion; and *flatness* (high-pitched, soft, extremely dull, and brief) over areas of atelectasis and extensive pleural effusion.

Documentation

• Document findings in nursing assessment and notify physician of findings.

Thyroid gland palpation

The thyroid gland lies directly below the larynx, partially in front of the trachea. Two lobes, one on either side of the trachea, join with a narrow tissue bridge called the isthmus to give the thyroid its butterfly shape. The lobes function as one unit to produce the

Palpating the thyroid

To palpate the thyroid from the front, stand in front of the patient and place your index and middle fingers below the cricoid cartilage on both sides of the trachea. Palpate for the thyroid isthmus as he swallows. Then ask the patient to flex his neck to the side being examined as you gently palpate each lobe. In most cases, you'll feel only the isthmus connecting the two lobes. However, if the patient has a thin neck, you may feel the whole gland. If he has a short stocky neck, you may have trouble palpating even an enlarged thyroid.

To locate the right lobe, use your right hand to displace the thyroid cartilage slightly to your left. Hook your left index and middle fingers around the sternocleidomastoid muscle to palpate for thyroid enlargement. Then examine the left lobe, using your left hand to displace the thyroid cartilage and your right hand to palpate the lobe.

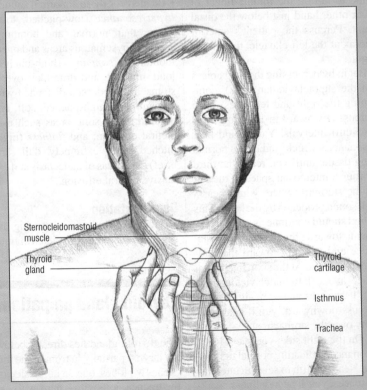

hormones triiodothyronine (T_3), thyroxine (T_4), and thyrocalcitonin. T_3 and T_4 are referred to collectively as thyroid hormone.

≫ Key nursing diagnoses and patient outcomes

Use these nursing diagnoses as a guide when developing your plan of care.

Body image disturbance related to medical condition
Based on this nursing diagnosis, you'll establish the following patient outcomes. The patient will:
• express positive feelings about self.
• demonstrate ability to practice two new coping behaviors.

Ineffective individual coping related to personal vulnerability
Based on this nursing diagnosis, you'll establish the following patient outcomes. The patient will:
• become actively involved in planning own care.
• identify effective and ineffective coping techniques.

Equipment
♦ stethoscope.

Patient preparation
• Assist the patient to a sitting position, unless contraindicated, and expose his neck area.
• Explain the procedure to the patient before the assessment.

Implementation
• Palpate the trachea, which is normally positioned midline in the neck. Place your thumbs along each side of the trachea near the lower portion of the neck. Determine whether the dis-

tance between the trachea's outer edge and the sternocleidomastoid muscle is equal on both sides.
• Now feel the thyroid *to detect deviation or displacement from the midline.*
• Inspect the trachea while the patient swallows. It should move symmetrically during swallowing. Then position yourself behind the patient. Place two fingers from each hand on the sides of the trachea, and ask the patient to swallow. Expect to feel the thyroid move freely. (See *Palpating the thyroid.*)
• Displace the thyroid to the right and ask the patient to swallow again. Palpate the right lobe, noting enlargement, nodules, tenderness, or a gritty sensation.
• Displace the thyroid to the left and palpate the left lobe as the patient swallows.
• If you detect an enlarged thyroid, auscultate the area with the bell of your stethoscope. Listen for a bruit or a soft, rushing sound indicating a hypermetabolic state.

Nursing considerations
• In most cases, you will feel only the isthmus connecting the two lobes. However, if the patient has a thin neck, you may feel the whole gland. If he has a short, stocky neck, you may have trouble palpating even an enlarged thyroid.

Documentation
• Document your nursing assessment findings, and inform the doctor of the results.

Topical drug administration

Topical drugs are applied directly to the skin surface. They include lotions, pastes, ointments, creams, powders, shampoos, and aerosol sprays. The medication is absorbed through the epidermal layer into the dermis. The extent of absorption depends on the vascularity of the region. Except for nitroglycerin and certain supplemental hormone replacements, topical medications are commonly used for local, rather than systemic, effects. Ointments have a fatty base, which is an ideal vehicle for such drugs as antimicrobials and antiseptics. Typically, topical medications should be applied two or three times a day to achieve their therapeutic effect.

≫ Key nursing diagnoses and patient outcome

Use these nursing diagnoses as a guide when developing your plan of care for a patient receiving topical medications.

Knowledge deficit related to lack of exposure

Based on this nursing diagnosis, you'll establish the following patient outcomes. The patient will:
• state or demonstrate understanding of what has been taught.
• demonstrate ability to perform new health-related behaviors as they are taught.

Risk for injury related to improper technique

Based on this nursing diagnosis, you'll establish the following patient outcomes. The patient will:
• identify factors that increase risk for injury.
• assist in identifying and applying safety measures to prevent injury.

Equipment

♦ patient's medication record and chart ♦ prescribed medication ♦ sterile tongue blades ♦ gloves ♦ sterile 4″ × 4″ gauze pads ♦ transparent semipermeable dressing ♦ adhesive tape ♦ solvent (such as cottonseed oil).

Equipment preparation

• Verify the order on the patient's medication record by checking it against the doctor's order on the chart.
• Make sure the label on the medication agrees with the medication order. Read the label again before you open the container and as you remove the medication from the container.
• Confirm the patient's identity by asking his name and checking the name, room number, and bed number on his wristband.

Patient preparation

• Provide privacy.
• Explain the procedure thoroughly to the patient *because, after discharge, he may have to apply the medication by himself.*

Implementation

• Wash your hands *to prevent cross-contamination,* and glove your dominant hand.

• Help the patient assume a comfortable position that provides access to the area to be treated.

• Expose the area to be treated. Make sure the skin or mucous membrane is intact (unless the medication has been ordered to treat a skin lesion such as an ulcer). *Application of medication to broken or abraded skin may cause unwanted systemic absorption and result in further irritation.*

• If necessary, clean the skin of debris, including crusts, epidermal scales, and old medication. You may have to change the glove if it becomes soiled.

Applying a paste, a cream, or an ointment

• Open the container. Place the lid or cap upside down *to prevent contamination of the inside surface.*

• Remove a tongue blade from its sterile wrapper, and cover one end with medication from the tube or jar. Then, transfer the medication from the tongue blade to your gloved hand.

• Apply the medication to the affected area with long, smooth strokes that follow the direction of hair growth. *This technique avoids forcing medication into hair follicles, which can cause irritation and lead to folliculitis.* Avoid excessive pressure when applying the medication *because it could abrade the skin.*

• *To prevent contamination of the medication,* use a new tongue blade each time you remove medication from the container.

Removing an ointment

• To remove ointment, wash your hands; then rub solvent on them and apply it liberally to the treated area in the direction of hair growth. Alterna-

tively, saturate a sterile gauze pad with the solvent and use this pad to gently remove the ointment. Remove excess oil by gently wiping the area with the sterile gauze pad. Don't rub too hard to remove the medication *because you could irritate the skin.*

Applying other topical medications

• To apply *shampoos,* follow package directions. (See *Using medicated shampoos,* page 852.)

• To apply *aerosol sprays,* shake the container, if indicated, *to mix the medication.* Hold the container 6″ to 12″ (15 to 30.5 cm) from the skin or follow the manufacturer's recommendation. Spray the medication evenly over the treatment area *to apply a thin film.*

• To apply *powders,* dry the skin surface, making sure to spread skin folds where moisture collects. Then apply a thin layer of powder over the treatment area.

• *To protect applied medications and prevent them from soiling the patient's clothes,* tape an appropriate amount of sterile gauze pad or a transparent semipermeable dressing over the treated area. If you're applying topical medication to the patient's hands or feet, cover the site with white cotton gloves for the hands or terry cloth scuffs for the feet.

• Assess the patient's skin for signs of irritation, allergic reaction, or breakdown.

Complications

• Skin irritation, a rash, or an allergic reaction may occur.

Nursing considerations

• Never apply medication without first removing previous applications

Using medicated shampoos

Medicated shampoos include keratolytic and cytostatic agents, coal tar preparations, and lindane (gamma benzene hexachloride) solutions. They can be used to treat such conditions as dandruff, psoriasis, and head lice. However, they're contraindicated in patients with broken or abraded skin.

Because application instructions may vary among brands, check the label on the shampoo before starting the procedure *to ensure use of the correct amount.* Keep the shampoo away from the patient's eyes. If any shampoo should accidentally get in his eyes, irrigate promptly with water. Selenium sulfide, used in cytostatic agents, is extremely toxic if ingested.

To apply a medicated shampoo, follow these steps:
• Prepare the patient for shampoo treatment.
• Shake the bottle of shampoo well *to mix the solution evenly.*
• Wet the patient's hair thoroughly, and wring out excess water.
• Apply the proper amount of shampoo as directed on the label.
• Work the shampoo into a lather, adding water as necessary. Part the hair and work the shampoo into the scalp, taking care not to use your fingernails.
• Leave the shampoo on the scalp and hair for as long as instructed (usually 5 to 10 minutes). Then rinse the hair thoroughly.
• Towel-dry the patient's hair.
• After the hair is dry, comb or brush it. Use a fine-tooth comb to remove nits if necessary.

to prevent skin irritation from an accumulation of medication.
• Be sure to wear gloves *to prevent absorption by your own skin.* If the patient has an infectious skin condition, use sterile gloves, and dispose of old dressings according to your hospital's policy.
• Don't apply ointments to mucous membranes as liberally as you would to skin *because mucous membranes are usually moist and absorb ointment more quickly than skin does.* Also, don't apply too much ointment to any skin area. *It may cause irritation and discomfort, stain clothing and bedding, and make removal difficult.*
• Never apply ointment to the eyelids or ear canal unless ordered. *The ointment may congeal and occlude the tear duct or ear canal.*
• Inspect the treated area frequently for adverse effects such as signs of an allergic reaction.

Documentation
• Record the medication applied; the time, date, and site of application; and the condition of the patient's skin at the time of application. Note subsequent effects of the medication, if any.

Total parenteral nutrition administration

When a patient can't meet nutritional needs by oral or enteral feedings, I.V. nutritional support, or parenteral nutrition, may be required. The patient's diagnosis, history, and prognosis determine the need for parenteral nutrition. Generally, this treatment is pre-

scribed for any patient who can't absorb nutrients through the GI tract for more than 10 days. More specific indications include:
• debilitating illness lasting longer than 2 weeks.
• loss of 10% or more of pre-illness weight.
• serum albumin level below 3.5 g/dl.
• excessive nitrogen loss from wound infection, fistulas, or abscesses.
• renal or hepatic failure.
• a nonfunctioning GI tract for 5 to 7 days in a severely catabolic patient.

Common illnesses that make parenteral nutrition needed include inflammatory bowel disease, radiation enteritis, severe diarrhea, intractable vomiting, and moderate to severe pancreatitis. A massive small-bowel resection, a bone marrow transplant, high-dose chemotherapy or radiation therapy, or major surgery can also hinder a patient's ability to absorb nutrients and necessitate parenteral nutrition.

Infants with congenital or acquired disorders may need parenteral nutrition to promote their growth and development. Specific disorders that could require parenteral nutrition include tracheoesophageal fistula, gastroschisis, duodenal atresia, cystic fibrosis, meconium ileus, diaphragmatic hernia, volvulus, malrotation of the gut, and annular pancreas.

However, parenteral nutrition has limited value for well-nourished patients whose GI tracts will resume normal function within 10 days. It also shouldn't be given if the patient has a normally functioning GI tract. It may be inappropriate for a patient with a poor prognosis or if the risks of parenteral nutrition outweigh the benefits.

Parenteral nutrition may be given through a peripheral or central venous (CV) line. Depending on the solution, it may be used to boost the patient's caloric intake, to supply full caloric needs, or to surpass the patient's caloric requirements.

The type of parenteral solution that's prescribed depends on the patient's condition and metabolic needs and on whether it's to be given through a peripheral or CV line. The solution usually contains protein, carbohydrates, electrolytes, vitamins, and trace minerals. A lipid emulsion provides the necessary fat. (See *Types of parenteral nutrition*, pages 854 to 857.)

Total parenteral nutrition (TPN) refers to any nutrient solution, including lipids, given through a central line. Peripheral parenteral nutrition (PPN), which is given through a peripheral line, supplies full caloric needs while avoiding the risks that accompany a CV line. However, to keep from sclerosing the vein through which it's administered, the dextrose in PPN solution must be limited to 10%. Therefore, the success of PPN depends on the patient's tolerance for the large volume of fluid necessary to supply his nutritional needs.

Often, you'll need to increase the glucose content beyond the level a peripheral vein can handle. For example, most TPN solutions are six times more concentrated than blood. As a result, they must be delivered into a vein with a high rate of blood flow to dilute the solution.

The most common delivery route for TPN is through a CV catheter into the superior vena cava. The catheter

(Text continues on page 856.)

Types of parenteral nutrition

TYPE	SOLUTION COMPONENTS/LITER
Standard I.V. therapy	• Dextrose, water, electrolytes in varying amounts—for example: — Dextrose 5% in water (D_5W) = 170 cal/L, — $D_{10}W$ = 340 cal/L, — Normal saline = 0 calories • Vitamins as ordered
Total parenteral nutrition (TPN) via central venous (CV) line	• $D_{15}W$ to $D_{25}W$ (1 L dextrose 25% = 850 nonprotein cal) • Crystalline amino acids 2.5% to 8.5% • Electrolytes, vitamins, trace elements, and insulin, as ordered • Lipid emulsion 10% to 20% (usually infused as a separate solution)
Total nutrient admixture	• One day's nutrients are contained in a single, 3-L bag (also called 3:1 solution) • Combines lipid emulsion with other parenteral solution components
Peripheral parenteral nutrition (PPN)	• D_5W to $D_{10}W$ • Crystalline amino acids 2.5% to 5% • Electrolytes, minerals, vitamins, and trace elements, as ordered

Types of parenteral nutrition *(continued)*

USES	SPECIAL CONSIDERATIONS
• Less than 1 week as nutrition source • Maintains hydration (main function) • Facilitates and maintains normal metabolic function	• Nutritionally incomplete; does not provide sufficient calories to maintain adequate nutritional status
• 2 weeks or more • For patients with large caloric and nutrient needs • Provides calories, restores nitrogen balance, and replaces essential vitamins, electrolytes, minerals, and trace elements • Promotes tissue synthesis, wound healing, and normal metabolic function • Allows bowel rest and healing; reduces activity in the gallbladder, pancreas, and small intestine • Improves tolerance of surgery	**Basic solution** • Nutritionally complete • Requires minor surgical procedure for CV line insertion (can be done at bedside by the doctor) • Highly hypertonic solution • May cause metabolic complications (glucose intolerance, electrolyte imbalance, essential fatty acid deficiency) **I.V. lipid emulsion** • May not be used effectively in severely stressed patients (especially burn patients) • May interfere with immune mechanisms; in patients suffering respiratory compromise, reduces carbon dioxide buildup • Given via CV line; irritates peripheral vein in long-term use
• 2 weeks or more • For relatively stable patients because solution components can be adjusted just once daily • For other uses, see TPN (above)	• See TPN (above) • Reduces need to handle bag, cutting risk of contamination • Decreases nursing time and reduces need for infusion sets and electronic devices, lowering hospital costs, increasing patient mobility, and allowing easier adjustment to home care • Precludes use of certain infusion pumps because they can't accurately deliver large volumes of solution; precludes use of standard I.V. tubing filters because a 0.22-micron filter blocks lipid and albumin molecules • Has limited use because not all types and amounts of components are compatible
• 2 weeks or less • Provides up to 2,000 cal/day	**Basic solution** • Nutritionally complete for a short time • Can't be used in nutritionally depleted patients *(continued)*

Types of parenteral nutrition *(continued)*

TYPE	SOLUTION COMPONENTS/LITER
Peripheral parenteral nutrition (PPN) *(continued)*	• Lipid emulsion 10% or 20% (1 L of dextrose 10% and amino acids 3.5% infused at the same time as 1 L of lipid emulsion = 1,440 nonprotein cal) • Heparin or hydrocortisone as ordered
Protein-sparing therapy	• Crystalline amino acids in same amounts as TPN • Electrolytes, vitamins, minerals, and trace elements, as ordered

may also be placed through the infraclavicular approach or, less commonly, through the supraclavicular, internal jugular, or antecubital fossa approach.

≫ Key nursing diagnoses and patient outcomes

Use these nursing diagnoses as a guide when developing your plan of care for a patient who is receiving total parenteral nutrition.

Altered nutrition: less than body requirements related to inability to digest or absorb nutrients
Based on this nursing diagnosis, you'll establish the following patient outcomes. The patient will:
• tolerate oral, tube or I.V. feedings without adverse effects.
• show no evidence of further weight loss.

USES	SPECIAL CONSIDERATIONS
• Maintains adequate nutritional status in patients who can tolerate relatively high fluid volume, in those who usually resume bowel function and oral feedings after a few days, and in those who are susceptible to infections associated with the CV catheter	• Can't be used in volume-restricted patients because PPN exceeds CV-line volume • Doesn't cause weight gain • Avoids insertion and care of CV line, but requires adequate venous access; site must be changed every 72 hours • Delivers less hypertonic solutions than CV-line TPN • May cause phlebitis and increases risk of metabolic complications • Less chance of metabolic complications than with CV-line TPN **I.V. lipid emulsion** • As effective as dextrose for caloric source • Diminishes phlebitis if infused at the same time as basic nutrient solution • Irritates vein in long-term use • Reduces carbon dioxide buildup when pulmonary compromise is present
• 2 weeks or less • May preserve body protein in a stable patient • Augments oral or tube feedings	• Nutritionally complete • Requires little mixing • May be started or stopped any time during the hospital stay • Other I.V. fluids, medications, and blood by-products may be administered through the same I.V. line • Not as likely to cause phlebitis as PPN • Adds a major expense; has limited benefits

Risk for fluid volume deficit related to active loss

Based on this nursing diagnosis, you'll establish the following patient outcomes. The patient will:
• have fluid volume remain adequate.
• have electrolyte levels stay within normal range.

Equipment

♦ bag or bottle of prescribed parenteral nutrition solution ♦ sterile I.V. tubing with attached extension tubing

♦ 0.22-micron filter (or 1.2-micron filter if solution contains lipids or albumin) ♦ reflux valve ♦ time tape ♦ alcohol pads ♦ electronic infusion pump ♦ test kit for urine glucose and ketone levels (or glucose enzymatic test strip if patient is receiving cephalosporins, methyldopa, aspirin, or large doses of ascorbic acid) ♦ scale ♦ intake and output record.

Equipment preparation

• Remove the bag or bottle of solution from the refrigerator at least 1 hour before use to avoid the pain, hypothermia, venous spasm, and venous constriction that can result from delivery of a chilled solution.

• Check the solution against the doctor's order for correct patient name, expiration date, and formula components.

• Look for cracks in the container and for cloudiness, turbidity, or particles in the solution. If you detect any of these, return the solution to the pharmacy.

• If you'll be administering a total nutrient admixture solution, look for a brown layer on the solution, *which can indicate that the lipid emulsion has "cracked," or separated from the solution.* If you see a brown layer, return the solution to the pharmacy.

• In sequence, connect the pump tubing, the micron filter with attached extension tubing (if the tubing doesn't contain an in-line filter), and the reflux valve. Be sure to insert the filter so that it will be as close to the catheter site as possible. If the tubing doesn't have luer-lock connections, tape all connections *to prevent accidental separation, which could lead to air embolism, exsanguination, and sepsis.*

• Next, squeeze the I.V. drip chamber and, holding the drip chamber upright, insert the tubing spike into the I.V. bag or bottle. Then release the drip chamber.

• Squeezing the drip chamber before spiking an I.V. bottle prevents accidental dripping of the parenteral nutrition solution. An I.V. bag, however, shouldn't drip.

• Next, prime the tubing. Invert the filter at the distal end of the tubing, and open the roller clamp. Let the solution fill the tubing and the filter. Gently tap it *to dislodge air bubbles trapped in the Y-ports.*

• If indicated, attach a time tape to the parenteral nutrition container *for accurate measurement of fluid intake.*

• Record the date and time you hung the fluid, and initial the parenteral nutrition solution container.

• Next, attach the setup to the infusion pump and prepare it according to the manufacturer's instructions.

• With the patient in the supine position, flush the catheter with heparin or normal saline solution, according to hospital policy.

• Put on gloves and clean the catheter injection cap with an alcohol pad.

• If specified by hospital policy, put on a mask.

Patient preparation

• Explain the procedure.

• Check the name on the solution container against the name on the patient's wristband.

Implementation

• Throughout the procedure, use strict aseptic technique.

• If you'll be attaching the container of parenteral nutrition solution to a CV line, clamp the CV line before disconnecting it *to prevent air from entering the catheter.* If a clamp isn't available, ask the patient to perform Valsalva's maneuver just as you change the tubing, if possible. Or, if the patient is being mechanically ventilated, change the I.V. tubing immediately after the machine delivers a breath at peak inspiration. *Both of*

these measures increase intrathoracic pressure and prevent air embolism.
• Using aseptic technique, insert the tubing with the needle into the injection cap. Once you've connected the tubing, remove the clamp if applicable.
• Set the infusion pump at the ordered flow rate, and start the infusion. Check to make sure the catheter junction is secure.
• Tag the tubing, indicating the date and time of change.

To start the infusion
• *Because parenteral nutrition solution often contains large amounts of glucose,* you may need to start the infusion slowly to allow the patient's pancreatic beta cells time to increase their output of insulin. Depending on the patient's tolerance, parenteral nutrition is usually initiated at a rate of 40 to 50 ml/hour and then advanced by 25 ml/hour every 6 hours until the desired infusion rate is achieved. However, when the glucose concentration is low, as occurs in most PPN formulas, you can initiate the rate necessary to infuse the complete 24-hour volume. In this instance, you can also discontinue the solution without tapering.
• You may allow a parenteral nutrition solution container to hang for 24 to 72 hours or according to hospital policy. However, if the patient has a 3-in-1 solution (a solution that contains lipids in addition to carbohydrates and protein), you'll need to hang a new solution container every 24 hours.

To change solutions
• Prepare the new solution and I.V. tubing as described earlier. Put on sterile gloves. Remove the protective caps from the solution containers, and wipe the tops of the containers with alcohol pads.
• Turn off the infusion pump and close the flow clamps. Using strict aseptic technique, remove the spike from the solution container that's hanging, and insert it into the new container.
• Hang the new container and tubing alongside the old. Turn on the infusion pump, set the flow rate, and open the flow clamp completely.
• If you'll be attaching the solution to a peripheral line, examine the skin above the insertion site for signs of phlebitis, such as redness and warmth, and assess for pain. If such signs exist, remove the existing I.V. line and start a line in a different vein. Also insert a new line if the present I.V. catheter has been in place for 72 hours or more *to reduce the risk of phlebitis and infiltration.*
• Next, turn off the infusion pump and close the flow clamp on the old tubing. Disconnect the tubing from the needle or catheter hub, and connect the new tubing. Open the flow clamp on the new container to a keep-vein-open rate *to prevent clot formation in the needle or catheter while you insert the tubing into the infusion pump.*
• Remove the old tubing from the infusion pump, and insert the new tubing according to the manufacturer's instructions. Then turn on the infusion pump, set it to the desired flow rate, and open the flow clamp completely. Remove the old equipment and dispose of it properly.

Complications
• Catheter-related sepsis is the most serious complication of parenteral nutrition.

• Although rare, a malpositioned subclavian or jugular vein catheter may lead to thrombosis or sepsis.

• An air embolism, a potentially fatal complication, can occur during I.V. tubing changes if the tubing is inadvertently disconnected. An embolism may also result from undetected hairline cracks in the tubing.

• Extravasation of parenteral nutrition solution can cause necrosis, with sequential sloughing of the epidermis and dermis.

Nursing considerations

• Always infuse a parenteral nutrition solution at a constant rate without interruption *to avoid fluctuations in blood glucose levels.* If the infusion slows, consult the doctor before changing the infusion rate.

• Monitor the patient's vital signs every 4 hours, or more often if necessary. Be alert for an increased temperature, *which may be an early sign of catheter-related sepsis.*

• Check the patient's urine for glucose and ketones every 4 to 6 hours. Some patients may require supplementary insulin throughout parenteral nutrition feeding, which the pharmacist may add directly to the solution.

• Because most patients receiving PPN are in a protein-wasted state, the therapy causes marked changes in electrolyte and fluid states and in levels of glucose, amino acids, minerals, and vitamins. Therefore, record daily fluid intake and output accurately. Specify the volume and type of each fluid, and calculate the daily caloric intake.

• Monitor the results of routine laboratory tests, and report any abnormal findings to the doctor *to allow for appropriate changes in the parenteral nutrition solution.* Typical laboratory tests include measurement of serum electrolytes, calcium, blood urea nitrogen, creatinine, and blood glucose levels at least three times weekly; serum magnesium and phosphorus levels twice weekly; liver function studies, complete blood count and differential, and serum albumin and transferrin levels weekly; and urine nitrogen balance and creatinine-height index studies weekly. A serum zinc level is obtained at the start of parenteral nutrition therapy. Other studies the doctor may order include serum prealbumin, total lymphocyte count, aminogram, skin testing, fatty acid-phospholipid fraction, and expired gas analysis.

• Physically assess the patient daily. If ordered, measure arm circumference and skinfold thickness over the triceps. Weigh the patient at the same time each morning after he voids; he should be weighed in similar clothing and on the same scale. Suspect fluid imbalance if the patient gains more than 1 lb (0.5 kg) daily.

• Change the dressing over the catheter according to hospital policy or whenever the dressing becomes wet, soiled, or nonocclusive. Always use strict aseptic technique. When performing dressing changes, watch for signs of phlebitis or catheter retraction from the vein. Measure the catheter length from the insertion site to the hub for verification.

• Change the tubing and filters every 24 to 72 hours or according to hospital policy.

• Closely monitor the catheter site for any sign of swelling, which may indicate infiltration. *Extravasation of parenteral nutrition solution can lead to tissue necrosis.*

• Use caution when using the parenteral nutrition line for other functions. If you're using a single-lumen CV catheter, don't use the line to infuse blood or blood products, to give a bolus injection, to administer simultaneous I.V. solutions, to measure CV pressure, or to draw blood for laboratory tests. Never add medication to a parenteral nutrition solution container. Also, don't use a three-way stopcock, if possible, *because add-on devices increase the risk of infection.* (See *What to avoid during TPN.*)

• Don't administer parenteral nutrition solution through a pulmonary artery catheter *because of the high risk of phlebitis.* After the infusion, flush the catheter with heparin or normal saline solution, according to hospital policy.

• Provide regular mouth care.

• Provide emotional support.

• Keep in mind that patients commonly associate eating with positive feelings and become disturbed when they can't eat.

Home care

• Patients who require prolonged or indefinite parenteral nutrition may be able to receive the therapy at home.

• Home parenteral nutrition reduces the need for long hospitalizations and allows the patient to resume many of his normal activities.

• Meet with a home care patient before discharge to make sure he knows how to perform the administration procedure and how to handle complications.

• Teach the patient the potential adverse effects and complications of parenteral nutrition.

What to avoid during TPN

The following are contraindicated when using a central venous line for TPN:

• infusion of blood or blood products
• bolus injection of drugs
• simultaneous administration of I.V. solutions
• measurement of central venous pressure
• aspiration of blood for routine laboratory tests
• addition of medication to a TPN solution container
• use of three-way stopcocks.

• Encourage him to inspect his mouth regularly for signs of parotitis, glossitis, or oral lesions.

• Tell him that he may have fewer bowel movements while receiving parenteral nutrition therapy.

• Encourage him to remain physically active to help his body use the nutrients more fully.

Documentation

• Document the times of the dressing, filter, and solution changes; the condition of the catheter insertion site; your observations of the patient's condition; and any complications and resulting treatments.

Total parenteral nutrition monitoring

Total parenteral nutrition (TPN) requires careful monitoring to assess the patient's response to the nutrient solution and to detect early signs of complications. Because the typical patient is in a protein-wasting state, TPN therapy causes marked changes in fluid and electrolyte status and in glucose, amino acid, mineral, and vitamin levels. If the patient displays an adverse reaction or signs of complications, the TPN regimen can be changed as needed.

Assessment of the patient's nutritional status includes a physical examination, anthropometric measurements, biochemical determinations, and tests of cell-mediated immunity. Assessment of the patient's condition to detect complications requires recognition of the signs and symptoms of possible complications, understanding of laboratory test results, and careful record keeping.

Because TPN solution is high in glucose, infusion must start slowly to allow the patient's pancreatic beta cells to adapt by increasing insulin output. Within the first 3 to 5 days of TPN, the typical adult patient can tolerate 3 L of solution daily without adverse reactions. Lipid emulsions also require monitoring.

≫ Key nursing diagnoses and patient outcomes

Use these nursing diagnoses as a guide when developing your plan of care.

Altered nutrition: less than body requirements related to inability to digest or absorb nutrients

Based on this nursing diagnosis, you'll establish the following patient outcomes. The patient will:
• tolerate oral, tube or I.V. feedings without adverse effects.
• show no further evidence of weight loss.

Risk for fluid volume deficit related to active loss

Based on this nursing diagnosis, you'll establish the following patient outcomes. The patient will:
• have fluid volume remain adequate.
• have electrolyte levels stay within normal range.

Equipment

♦ blood glucose meter ♦ stethoscope ♦ sphygmomanometer ♦ watch with second hand ♦ scale ♦ input and output chart ♦ time tape ♦ additional equipment for nutritional assessment as ordered.

Equipment preparation

• For preparation of infusion pump and TPN solution, see "Total parenteral nutrition administration."
• Attach a time tape to the TPN container to allow approximate measurement of fluid intake.
• Make sure each bag or bottle has a label listing the expiration date, glucose concentration, and total volume of solution. (If the bag or bottle is damaged and you don't have an immediate replacement, hang a bag of dextrose 10% in water until the new container is ready.)

Patient preparation

• Explain the procedure *to diminish patient anxiety and encourage cooperation.*
• Tell the patient to inform you if he feels any unusual sensations during infusion.

Implementation

• Record vital signs every 4 hours, or more often if necessary, *because in-*

creased temperature is one of ... *liest signs of catheter-related seps...*

• Perform I.V. site care and dressing changes at least three times a week (once a week for transparent semipermeable dressings) or whenever the dressing becomes wet, soiled, or nonocclusive. Use strict aseptic technique.

• Physically assess the patient daily. If ordered, measure arm circumference and skinfold thickness over the triceps.

• Weigh the patient at the same time each morning (after voiding), in similar clothing, and on the same scale. Compare this data with his fluid intake and output record. *Weight gain, particularly early in treatment, may indicate fluid overload, rather than an increase in fat and protein stores.* A patient shouldn't gain more than 3 lb (1.5 kg) a week; a gain of 1 lb (0.5 kg) a week is a reasonable goal for most patients. Suspect fluid imbalance if the patient gains more than 1 lb daily. Assess for peripheral and pulmonary edema.

• Monitor the patient for signs and symptoms of glucose metabolism disturbance, fluid and electrolyte imbalances, and nutritional aberrations. Remember that some patients may require supplemental insulin for the duration of TPN; the pharmacy usually adds insulin directly to the TPN solution.

• Monitor electrolyte and protein levels frequently — daily at first for electrolytes and twice a week for serum albumin. Later, as the patient's condition stabilizes, you won't need to monitor these values quite as closely. (Be aware that in a severely dehydrated patient, albumin levels may actual-

... initially as treatment ... an... lytes ... attention to magnesium lution, the ... els. If these electro- to maintain nor... ded to the TPN so- sess the patient for ... need adjusting toms of magnesium and ... levels. As- balances. ... symp- ... im-

• Monitor serum glucose levels every 6 hours initially, then once a day, and stay alert for signs and symptoms of hyperglycemia, such as thirst and polyuria. Periodically confirm blood glucose meter readings with laboratory tests.

• Check renal function by monitoring blood urea nitrogen and creatinine levels — *increases can indicate excess amino acid intake.* Also assess nitrogen balance with 24-hour urine collection.

• Assess liver function by periodically monitoring liver enzyme, bilirubin, triglyceride, and cholesterol levels. *Abnormal values may indicate an intolerance or an excess of lipid emulsions or problems with metabolizing the protein or glucose in the TPN formula.*

• Change the I.V. administration set according to hospital policy. Use aseptic technique and coordinate the change with a solution change. Keep in mind that the tubing, injection caps, stopcocks, catheter, and even the patient's skin are potential sources of microbial contamination. The catheter hub, where most manipulations take place, is especially vulnerable. (The TPN formula itself, which is prepared aseptically in the pharmacy, is rarely the source of infection.)

BETTER CHARTING

Docu... ...PN

If a patient ...PN), document the teral nut...ing total paren-...ation of the central line, type ...ition of the insertion site, the ... and the ...olume and rate of the solu-tion ...used. Monitor any patient re-...iving TPN for adverse reactions and document your observations and interventions. When you discon-tinue a central or peripheral I.V. line for TPN, record the date and time and the type of dressing applied. Also describe the appearance of the administration site.

• Many hospitals require changing I.V. administration sets every 24 hours, which is what most infection-control practitioners recommend for TPN infusions. However, some now wait 48 to 72 hours. *Because the risk of contamination is so high with TPN,* each hospital should continuously evaluate protocols based on quality-control findings.

• Monitor for signs of inflammation, infection, or sepsis, the most common complications of TPN. Microbial con-tamination of the venous access de-vice is the usual cause. Watch for red-ness and drainage at the venous access site, and monitor the patient for fever and other signs and symptoms of sep-sis.

• While weaning the patient from TPN, document his dietary intake and work with the nutritionist to deter-mine the total calorie and protein in-take. Also teach other health care staff

caring for the patient the importance of recording food intake. Using per-centages of food consumed ("ate 50% of a baked potato") instead of subjec-tive descriptions ("had a good appe-tite") gives a more accurate account of patient intake.

• Provide emotional support. Keep in mind that patients often associate eat-ing with positive feelings and become disturbed when eating is prohibited.

• Provide frequent mouth care.

• Keep the patient active *to enable him to use nutrients more fully.*

• When discontinuing TPN, decrease the infusion rate slowly, depending on the patient's current glucose intake, *to minimize the risk of hyperinsulinemia and resulting hypoglycemia.* Weaning usually takes place over 24 to 48 hours but can be completed in 4 to 6 hours if the patient receives sufficient oral or I.V. carbohydrates.

Complications

• Catheter-related, metabolic, and mechanical complications can occur during TPN administration.

Nursing considerations

• Always maintain strict aseptic tech-nique when handling the equipment used to administer therapy. *Because the TPN solution serves as a medium for bacterial growth and the central venous (CV) line provides systemic access,* the patient risks infection and sepsis.

• When using a filter, position it as close to the access site as possible. Check the filter's porosity and pounds-per-square-inch (psi) capaci-ty to make sure it exceeds the number of psi exerted by the infusion pump.

tion to a TPN solution container. Also, don't use a three-way stopcock, if possible *because add-on devices increase the risk of infection.*

• When a patient is severely malnourished, starting TPN may spark "refeeding syndrome," which includes a rapid drop in potassium, magnesium, and phosphorus levels. *To avoid compromising cardiac function,* initiate feeding slowly and monitor the patient's blood values especially closely until they stabilize.

Documentation
• Record serial monitoring indices on the appropriate flowchart to determine the patient's progress and response.
• Note any abnormal, adverse, or altered responses. (See *Documenting TPN.*)

Tracheal suction

This procedure involves the removal of secretions from the trachea or bronchi by means of a catheter inserted through the mouth, nose, tracheal stoma, tracheostomy tube, or endotracheal tube (ET). Besides removing secretions, tracheal suctioning also stimulates the cough reflex. This procedure helps maintain a patent airway

[...] ote optimal exchange of oxygen [...] carbon dioxide and to prevent [...] that results from pooling [...] formed as frequently [...] ndition warrants, strict aseptic [...]

Use these nursing diagnoses as a guide when developing your plan of care for a patient requiring tracheal suctioning.

Ineffective breathing pattern related to decreased energy
Based on this nursing diagnosis, you'll establish the following patient outcomes. The patient will:
• achieve maximum lung expansion with adequate ventilation.
• report feeling comfortable with breathing.

Impaired gas exchange related to altered oxygen supply
Based on this nursing diagnosis, you'll establish the following patient outcomes. The patient will:
• cough effectively.
• expectorate sputum.

Equipment
♦ oxygen source (wall or portable unit, and handheld resuscitation bag with a mask, 15-mm adapter, or a positive end-expiratory pressure [PEEP] valve, if indicated) ♦ wall or portable suction apparatus ♦ collection container ♦ connecting tube ♦ suction catheter kit, or a sterile suction catheter ♦ one sterile glove, one clean glove ♦ a disposable sterile solution container ♦ 1-L bottle of sterile water or

normal saline so'
• soluble lubric;
• syringe f'
tracheosto
bag • o..ion catheter of appro-

Equi
• C..Le. The diameter should be no larger than half the inside diameter of the tracheostomy or ET tube *to minimize hypoxia during suctioning.* (A #12 or #14 French catheter may be used for an 8-mm or larger tube.) Place the suction apparatus on the patient's overbed table or bedside stand.

• Position the table or stand on your preferred side of the bed *to facilitate suctioning.*

• Attach the collection container to the suction unit and the connecting tube to the collection container.

• Label and date the normal saline solution or sterile water.

• Open the waterproof trash bag.

Patient preparation

• Explain the procedure, even if the patient is unresponsive.

• Tell the patient that suctioning usually causes transient coughing or gagging, but that coughing helps remove secretions.

• If the patient has been suctioned previously, summarize the reasons for suctioning.

• Continue to reassure the patient throughout the procedure *to minimize anxiety, promote relaxation, and decrease oxygen demand.*

Implementation

• Before suctioning, determine whether your hospital requires a doctor's order and obtain one if necessary.

appear-
*...aseline for com-
... suctioning.*

..eview the patient's arterial blood gas values and oxygen saturation levels if they're available.

• Evaluate the patient's ability to cough and deep breathe *because this will help move secretions up the tracheobronchial tree.*

• If you'll be performing nasotracheal suctioning, check the patient's history for a deviated septum, nasal polyps, nasal obstruction, nasal trauma, epistaxis, or mucosal swelling.

• Wash your hands.

• Unless contraindicated, place the patient in the semi-Fowler or high Fowler position *to promote lung expansion and productive coughing.*

• Remove the top from the normal saline solution or water bottle.

• Open the package containing the sterile solution container.

• Using strictly aseptic technique, open the suction catheter kit and put on the gloves. If using individual supplies, open the suction catheter and the gloves, placing the nonsterile glove on your nondominant hand and then the sterile glove on your dominant hand.

• Using your nondominant (nonsterile) hand, pour the normal saline solution or sterile water into the solution container.

• Place a small amount of water-soluble lubricant on the sterile area. *Lubricant may be used to facilitate passage of the catheter during nasotracheal suctioning.*

• Place a sterile towel over the patient's chest, if desired, *to provide an additional sterile area.*

the resusc...
flow meter at 15 L/m...
the patient from the ventila...
liver three to six breaths with the re...
suscitation bag.

• If the patient is being maintained on PEEP, evaluate the need to use a resuscitation bag with a PEEP valve.

• To preoxygenate using the ventilator, first adjust the fraction of inspired oxygen (FIO_2) and tidal volume according to hospital policy and patient need. Then, either use the sigh mode or manually deliver three to six breaths. If you have an assistant for the procedure, the assistant can manage the patient's oxygen needs while you perform the suctioning.

Nasotracheal insertion in a nonintubated patient

• Disconnect the oxygen from the patient, if applicable.

• Using your nondominant hand, raise the tip of the patient's nose *to straighten the passageway and facilitate insertion of the catheter.*

• Insert the catheter into the patient's nostril while gently rolling it between your fingers *to help it advance through the turbinates.*

• As the patient inhales, quickly advance the catheter as far as possible. Do not apply suction during insertion *to avoid oxygen loss and tissue trauma.*

• If the patient coughs as the catheter passes through the larynx, briefly hold

---

the ... and, set
the ... ing to hospital ... pressure may
be set b... and 120 mm Hg.
Higher pre...res don't enhance secretion removal and may cause traumatic injury. Occlude the suction port *to assess suction pressure.*

• Dip the catheter tip in the saline solution *to lubricate the outside of the catheter and reduce tissue trauma during insertion.*

• With the catheter tip in the sterile solution, occlude the control valve with the thumb of your nondominant hand. Suction a small amount of solution through the catheter, *to lubricate the inside of the catheter to facilitate passage of secretions through it.*

• For nasal insertion of the catheter, lubricate the tip of the catheter with the sterile, water-soluble lubricant *to reduce tissue trauma during insertion.*

• If the patient is not intubated, or is intubated but is not receiving supplemental oxygen or aerosol, instruct him to take three to six deep breaths *to help minimize or prevent hypoxia during suctioning.*

• If the patient is not intubated but is receiving oxygen, evaluate his need for preoxygenation. If indicated, instruct the patient to take three to six deep breaths while using his supplemental oxygen. (If needed, the patient may continue to receive supplemental oxygen during suctioning by leaving his nasal cannula in one nostril or by

...eal
...d 870.
...terile hand, discon-
...patient from the ventilator.
Using your sterile hand, gently insert the suction catheter into the artificial airway, as shown at upper right. Advance the catheter, without applying suction, until you meet resistance. If the patient coughs, pause briefly and then resume advancement.

Suctioning the patient

• After inserting the catheter, apply suction intermittently by removing and replacing the thumb of your nondominant hand over the control valve. Simultaneously use your dominant hand to withdraw the catheter as you roll it between your thumb and forefinger. *This rotating motion prevents the catheter from pulling tissue into the tube as it exits, thus avoiding tissue trauma.* Never suction more than 5 to 10 seconds at a time *to prevent hypoxia.*

• If the patient is intubated, use your nondominant hand to stabilize the tip of the ET tube as you withdraw the catheter *to prevent mucous membrane irritation or accidental extubation.*

• If applicable, resume oxygen delivery by reconnecting the source of oxygen or ventilation, and hyperoxygenating the patient's lungs before continuing *to prevent or relieve hypoxia.*

• Observe the patient and allow him to rest for a few minutes before the next suctioning. The timing of each

...each rest
...tolerance for the
...the absence of compli-
...*To enhance secretion removal,* encourage the patient to cough between suctioning attempts.

• Observe the secretions. If they're thick, clear the catheter periodically by dipping the tip in the saline solution and applying suction. Normally, sputum is watery and tends to be sticky. Tenacious or thick sputum usually indicates dehydration. Watch for color variations. White or translucent color is normal; yellow indicates pus; green indicates retained secretions or *Pseudomonas* infection; brown usually indicates old blood; red indicates fresh blood; and a "red currant jelly" appearance indicates *Klebsiella* infection. When sputum contains blood, note whether it is streaked or well mixed. Also indicate how often blood appears.

If the patient's heart rate and rhythm are being monitored, observe for arrhythmias. Should they occur, stop suctioning and ventilate the patient.

After suctioning

• After the procedure, hyperoxygenate the patient being maintained on a ventilator with the handheld resuscitation bag or by using the ventilator's sigh mode, as described earlier.

• Readjust the FIO_2 and, for ventilated patients, the tidal volume, to the ordered settings.

• After suctioning the lower airway, assess the patient's need for upper airway suctioning. If the cuff of the ET or tracheostomy tube is inflated, suction the upper airway before deflating the cuff with a syringe. Always change

cheal suctioning

sisting ... in a clear plastic sleeve ... system permits the patient to remain connected to the ventilator during suctioning.

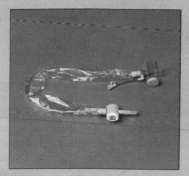

As a result, the patient can maintain the tidal volume, oxygen concentration, and positive end-expiratory pressure delivered by the ventilator while being suctioned. In turn, this reduces the occurrence of suction-induced hypoxemia.

Another advantage of this system is a reduced risk of infection, even when the same catheter is used many times. Because the catheter remains in a protective sleeve, gloves aren't required. The caregiver doesn't need to touch the catheter, and the ventilator circuit remains closed.

To perform the procedure, gather a closed suction control valve, a T-piece to connect the artificial airway to the ventilator breathing circuit, and a catheter sleeve that encloses the catheter and has connections at each end for the

ing valve and the T-piece. Then ... steps:

• Depress the thumb suction control valve and keep it depressed while setting the suction pressure to the desired level.

• Connect the T-piece to the ventilator breathing circuit, making sure that the irrigation port is closed (below); then connect the T-piece to the patient's endotracheal or tracheostomy tube.

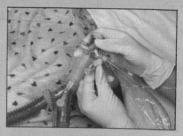

• With one hand keeping the T-piece parallel to the patient's chin, use the thumb and index finger of the other hand to advance the catheter through the tube and into the patient's tracheobronchial tree, as shown.

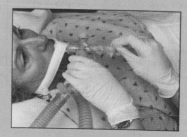

TRACHEAL SUCTION

How to perform clos...

It may be ne...
tract the cat...valve, apply inter-
vance th...
• Wh...ction and withdraw the
catheter until it reaches its fully extended length in the sleeve. Repeat
the procedure as necessary.
• After you have finished suctioning, flush the catheter by maintain-

...ile slowly introducing
...al saline solution or sterile water into the irrigation port.
• Place the thumb control valve in
the off position.
• Dispose of and replace the suction equipment and supplies according to hospital policy.
• Change the closed suction system every 24 hours to minimize the
risk of infection.

the catheter and sterile glove before
resuctioning the lower airway *to avoid
introducing microorganisms into the
lower airway.*
• Discard the gloves and the catheter
in the waterproof trash bag. Clear the
connecting tubing by aspirating the
remaining saline solution or water.
Discard and replace suction equipment and supplies according to hospital policy. Wash your hands.
• Auscultate lungs bilaterally and take
vital signs, if indicated, *to assess the
procedure's effectiveness.*

Complications
• Because oxygen is removed along
with secretions, the patient may experience hypoxemia and dyspnea.
• Anxiety may alter respiratory patterns.
• Cardiac arrhythmias can result from
hypoxia and stimulation of the vagus
nerve in the tracheobronchial tree.
Tracheal or bronchial trauma can result from traumatic or prolonged
suctioning.
• Patients with a compromised cardiovascular or pulmonary state are at

risk for hypoxemia, arrhythmias, hypertension, or hypotension.
• Patients with a history of nasopharyngeal bleeding, who are taking anticoagulants, who have had a tracheostomy recently, or who have a blood
dyscrasia incur an increased risk of
bleeding as a result of suctioning. Use
caution when suctioning patients who
have increased intracranial pressure
because it may increase pressure further.
• If the patient experiences laryngospasm or bronchospasm (rare complications) during suctioning, disconnect
the suction catheter from the connecting tubing and allow the catheter to
act as an airway. Discuss with the patient's doctor the use of bronchodilators or lidocaine to reduce the risk
of this complication.

Nursing considerations
• Raising the patient's nose into the
sniffing position helps align the larynx
and pharynx and may facilitate passing the catheter during nasotracheal
suctioning. If the patient's condition
permits, have an assistant extend the
patient's head and neck above his

...patient's lower jaw
insertion, ...d up and forward.
• During suctioning, the... ask him to ...not be
ically is advanced as far as... ...
mainstem bronchi. However, because
of tracheobronchial anatomy, the
catheter tends to enter the right
mainstem bronchi instead of the left.
Using an angled catheter (such as a
Coude or Bronchitrac L) may help
you guide the catheter into the left
mainstem bronchus. Rotating the patient's head to the right seems to have
a limited effect.

• Studies show that instillation of normal saline solution into the trachea before suctioning may stimulate the patient's cough but does not liquefy the
patient's secretions. Keeping the patient adequately hydrated and using
bronchial hygiene techniques seems
to have a greater effect on mobilizing
secretions.

• In addition to the closed tracheal
method, oxygen insufflation offers a
new approach to suctioning. Oxygen
insufflation suctioning uses a double
lumen catheter that allows oxygen insufflation during the suctioning procedure.

• Do not allow the collection container on the suction machine to become
more than ¾ full *to keep from damaging the machine.*

Home care

• Teach patient how to perform tracheal suctioning using clean technique (thorough hand washing and
use of clean gloves).

Documentation

• Record the date and time of...
cedure, the technique used, an...
reason for suctioning.

• Note the amount, color, consistency,
...d odor (if any) of the secretions.

• Record any complications and
...n taken.

patient's subjective data regarding the
procedure ...sponse to the

Tracheostomy care

Whether a tracheotomy is performed
in an emergency situation or as a permanent measure or as temporary therapy, tracheostomy care has identical
goals: to ensure airway patency by
keeping the tube free from mucus
buildup, to maintain mucous membrane and skin integrity, to prevent infection, and to provide psychological
support.

The patient may have one of three
types of tracheostomy tube — uncuffed, cuffed, or fenestrated. Tube selection depends on the patient's condition and the doctor's preference.

The *uncuffed* tube, which may be
plastic or metal, allows air to flow
freely around the tracheostomy tube
and through the larynx, reducing the
risk of tracheal damage. It's a safer
choice for children, but increases the
risk of aspiration in adults. The *cuffed*
tube, made of plastic, is disposable.
The cuff and the tube won't separate
accidentally inside the trachea
because the cuff is bonded to the tube.
Also, a cuffed tube doesn't require periodic deflating to lower pressure
because cuff pressure is low and eve...

y distributed against the tracheal wall. Although cuffed tubes may cost more than other tubes, cuffed tubes reduce the risk of tracheal damage. The plastic *fenestrated* tube permits speech through the upper airway when the external opening is capped and the cuff is deflated. The inner cannula for easy removal of the fenestrated tube for cleaning. However, the fenestrated tube may become occluded.

Whichever tube is used, tracheostomy care should be performed using aseptic technique until the stoma has healed. For recently performed tracheostomies, use sterile gloves for all manipulations at the tracheostomy site. Once the stoma has healed, clean gloves may be substituted for sterile ones.

≫ Key nursing diagnoses and patient outcomes

Use these nursing diagnoses as a guide when developing your plan of care for a patient who requires tracheostomy care.

Ineffective breathing pattern related to decreased energy

Based on this nursing diagnosis, you'll establish the following patient outcomes. The patient will:
• achieve maximum lung expansion with adequate ventilation.
• report feeling comfortable with breathing.

Impaired gas exchange related to altered oxygen supply

Based on this nursing diagnosis, you'll establish the following patient outcomes. The patient will:
• cough effectively.
• expectorate sputum.

Equipment

For cannula ... bag ◆ two pipe cleaners ◆ normal saline solution ◆ hydrogen peroxide ◆ sterile cotton-tipped applicators ◆ sterile 4″ × 4″ gauze pads ◆ sterile gloves ◆ prepackaged sterile tracheostomy dressing (or 4″ × 4″ gauze pad) ◆ equipment and supplies for suctioning and mouth care ◆ water-soluble lubricant or topical antibiotic cream ◆ materials as needed for cuff procedures and for changing tracheostomy ties (see below).

For aseptic inner-cannula care: ◆ all of the preceding equipment plus a prepackaged commercial tracheostomy-care set, or sterile forceps ◆ sterile nylon brush ◆ sterile 6″ (15-cm) pipe cleaners ◆ clean gloves ◆ a third sterile solution container ◆ disposable temporary inner cannula (for a patient on a ventilator).

For changing tracheostomy ties: ◆ 30″ (76-cm) length of tracheostomy twill tape ◆ bandage scissors ◆ sterile gloves ◆ hemostat.

For emergency tracheostomy tube replacement: ◆ sterile tracheal dilator or sterile hemostat ◆ sterile obturator that fits the tracheostomy tube in use ◆ extra sterile tracheostomy tube and obturator in appropriate size ◆ suction equipment and supplies.

Keep these supplies in full view in the patient's room at all times for easy access in case of emergency. Consider taping an emergency sterile tracheostomy tube in a sterile wrapper to the head of the patient's bed for easy access in an emergency.

For cuff procedures: ◆ 5- or 10-ml syringe ◆ padded hemostat ◆ stethoscope.

Equip

- Wash you
equipment and s.
tient's room.
- Check the expiration date on
sterile package and inspect the package for tears.
- Open the waterproof trash bag and
place it next to you, *so you can avoid
reaching across the sterile field or the
patient's stoma when discarding
soiled items.*
- Establish a sterile field near the patient's bed (usually on the overbed table), and place equipment and supplies on it.
- Pour normal saline solution, hydrogen peroxide, or a mixture of equal
parts of both solutions into one of the
sterile solution containers; then pour
normal saline solution into the second
sterile container for rinsing.
- For inner cannula care, you may use
a third sterile solution container to
hold the gauze pads and cotton-tipped
applicators saturated with cleaning
solution.
- If you'll be replacing the disposable
inner cannula, open the package containing the new inner cannula while
maintaining sterile technique.
- Obtain or prepare new tracheostomy
ties if indicated.

Patient preparation
- Explain the procedure to the patient,
even if he is unresponsive.
- Provide privacy.

Implementation
- Place the patient in semi-Fowler's
position (unless it's contraindicated)
*to decrease abdominal pressure on the
diaphragm, thereby promoting lung
expansion.*

- Remove any humidification or ventilation device.
Assess the patient's condition *to de-*
ing his need for care.
ite sterile technique, suction the
that may of the tracheostomy tube
ay of any secretions
- Reconnect the genation.
ifier or ventilator, if the humid-

To clean a stoma and outer cannula
- Put on sterile gloves if you're not already wearing them.
- With your dominant hand, saturate
a sterile gauze pad with the cleaning
solution. Squeeze out the excess liquid *to prevent accidental aspiration.*
Then wipe the patient's neck under the
tracheostomy tube flanges and twill
tapes.
- Saturate a second pad, and wipe until the skin surrounding the tracheostomy is cleaned. Use additional pads
or cotton-tipped applicators to clean
the stoma site and the tube's flanges.
Wipe only once with each pad and
then discard it *to prevent contamina-*
tion of a clean area with a soiled pad.
- Rinse debris and peroxide (if used)
with one or more sterile $4'' \times 4''$ gauze
pads dampened in normal saline solution. Dry the area thoroughly with additional sterile gauze pads; then apply
a new sterile tracheostomy dressing.
- Remove and discard your gloves.

To clean a nondisposable inner cannula
- Put on sterile gloves.
- Using your nondominant hand, remove and discard the patient's tracheostomy dressing. Then, with the same
hand, disconnect the ventilator or humidification device and unlock the

tracheostomy tube's inner cannula by rotating it counterclockwise. Place the inner cannula in the container of hydrogen peroxide.
• Working quickly, use your dominant hand to scrub the cannula with a sterile nylon brush. If the cannula doesn't slide easily into the container, use a sterile pipe cleaner.
• Immerse the cannula in the container of normal saline solution, and agitate it for about 10 seconds *to rinse it thoroughly.*
• Inspect the cannula for cleanliness. Repeat the cleaning process if necessary. When the cannula is clean, tap it gently against the inside edge of the sterile container *to remove excess liquid and prevent aspiration.* Don't dry the outer surface *because a thin film of moisture acts as a lubricant during insertion.*
• Reinsert the inner cannula into the patient's tracheostomy tube. Lock it in place and then gently pull on it *to be sure it's positioned securely.* Reconnect the mechanical ventilator. Apply a new sterile tracheostomy dressing.
• If the patient can't tolerate being disconnected from the ventilator for the time it takes to clean the inner cannula, replace the existing inner cannula with a clean one, and reattach the mechanical ventilator. Then clean the cannula just removed from the patient, and store it in a sterile container until the next time tracheostomy care is performed.

To care for a disposable inner cannula
• Put on clean gloves.
• Using your dominant hand, remove the patient's inner cannula. After evaluating the secretions, discard it following the manufacturer's instructions, lock it securely.

To change tracheostomy ties
• Obtain assistance from another nurse or a respiratory therapist *because of the risk of accidental tube expulsion during this procedure.* Patient movement or coughing can dislodge the tube.
• Wash your hands thoroughly and put on sterile gloves, if you're not already wearing them.
• If you're not using commercially packaged tracheostomy ties, prepare new ties from a 30″ (76-cm) length of twill tape by folding one end back 1″ (2.5 cm) on itself. Then, with the bandage scissors, cut a ½″ (1.3-cm) slit down the center of the tape from the folded edge.
• Prepare the other end of the tape in the same way.
• Hold both ends together and, using scissors, cut the resulting circle of tape so that one piece is approximately 10″ (25 cm) long, and the other is about 20″ (51 cm) long.
• Assist the patient into semi-Fowler's position if possible.
• After your assistant puts on gloves, instruct her to hold the tracheostomy tube in place *to prevent its expulsion during replacement of the ties.* However, if you must perform the procedure without assistance, fasten the clean ties in place before removing the old ties *to prevent tube expulsion.*
• With the assistant's gloved fingers holding the tracheostomy tube in

place, cut the soiled tracheostomy ties with the bandage scissors or untie them and discard the ties. Be careful not to cut the tube of the pilot balloon.
• Thread the slit end of one new tie a short distance through the eye of one tracheostomy tube flange from the underside; use the hemostat, if necessary, to pull the tie through. Then thread the other end of the tie completely through the slit end, and pull it taut so it loops firmly through the tube's flange. *This avoids knots that can cause discomfort, tissue irritation, pressure, and necrosis at the patient's throat.*
• Fasten the second tie to the opposite flange in the same manner.
• Instruct the patient to flex his neck while you bring the ties around to the side and tie them together with a square knot. *Flexion produces the same neck circumference as coughing and helps prevent an overly tight tie.* Instruct your assistant to place one finger under the tapes as you tie them *to ensure that they're tight enough to avoid slippage but loose enough to prevent choking or jugular vein constriction.* Placing the closure on the side *allows easy access and prevents pressure necrosis at the back of the neck when the patient is recumbent.*
• After securing the ties, cut off the excess tape with the scissors, and instruct your assistant to release the tracheostomy tube.
• Make sure the patient is comfortable and can reach the call button easily.
• For the patient with traumatic injury, radical neck dissection, or cardiac failure, check tracheostomy-tie tension frequently *because neck diameter can increase from swelling and cause constriction;* also check fre-

quently for the neonatal or restless patient *because ties can loosen,* possibly predisposing to tube misplacement.

To conclude tracheostomy care
• Replace any humidification device.
• Give oral care, as needed, *because the oral cavity can become dry and malodorous or develop sores from encrusted secretions.*
• Observe soiled dressings and suctioned secretions for amount, color, consistency, and odor.
• Properly clean or dispose of all equipment, supplies, solutions, and trash, according to hospital policy.
• Take off and discard your gloves.
• Make sure that the patient is comfortable and that he can easily reach the call button.
• Make sure all necessary supplies are readily available at the bedside.
• Repeat the procedure at least once every 8 hours or as needed. Change the dressing as often as necessary, whether or not you also perform the entire cleaning procedure, *because a dressing wet with exudate or secretions predisposes the patient to skin excoriation, breakdown, and infection.*

To deflate and inflate a tracheostomy cuff
• Read the cuff manufacturer's instructions *because cuff types and procedures vary widely.*
• Assess the patient's condition, explain the procedure to him, and reassure him. Thoroughly wash your hands.
• Help the patient into semi-Fowler's position, if possible, or place him in a supine position, *so that secretions above the cuff site will be pushed up*

into the mouth if the patient is receiving positive-pressure ventilation.
• Suction the oropharyngeal cavity *to prevent any pooled secretions from descending into the trachea after cuff deflation.*
• Release the padded hemostat clamping the cuff inflation tubing if a hemostat is present.
• Insert a 5- or 10-cc syringe into the cuff pilot balloon, and slowly withdraw all air from the cuff. Leave the syringe attached to the tubing *for later reinflation of the cuff. Slow deflation allows positive lung pressure to push secretions upward from the bronchi. Cuff deflation may also stimulate the patient's cough reflex, producing additional secretions.*
• Remove any ventilation device. Suction the lower airway through any existing tube *to remove all secretions.* Then return the patient to the ventilation device.
• Maintain cuff deflation for the prescribed period of time. Observe the patient for adequate ventilation, and suction as necessary. If the patient has difficulty breathing, reinflate the cuff immediately by depressing the syringe plunger very slowly. Inject the least amount of air necessary to achieve an adequate tracheal seal.
• When inflating the cuff, you may use the minimal-leak technique or the minimal occlusive volume technique *to help gauge the proper inflation point.*
• If you're inflating the cuff using cuff-pressure measurement, be careful not to exceed 25 mm Hg. If the pressure exceeds 25 mm Hg, notify the doctor *because you may need to change to a larger size tube, use higher inflation pressures, or permit a larger air leak.*

A cuff pressure of about 18 mm Hg is usually recommended.
• After you've inflated the cuff, if the tubing doesn't have a one-way valve at the end, clamp the inflation line with a padded hemostat (to protect the tubing), and remove the syringe.
• Check for a minimal-leak cuff seal. With minimal cuff inflation, you shouldn't feel air coming from the patient's mouth, nose, or tracheostomy site, and a conscious patient shouldn't be able to speak.
• Be alert for air leaks from the cuff itself. Suspect a leak if injection of air fails to inflate the cuff or increase cuff pressure, if you're unable to inject the amount of air you withdrew, if the patient can speak, if ventilation fails to maintain adequate respiratory movement with pressures or volumes previously considered adequate, or if air escapes during the ventilator's inspiratory cycle.
• Note the amount of air used to inflate the cuff *to detect tracheal malacia if more air is consistently needed.*
• Make sure the patient is comfortable and can easily reach the call button and communication aids.
• Properly clean or dispose of all equipment, supplies, and trash, according to hospital policy.
• Replenish any used supplies and make sure all necessary emergency supplies are at the bedside.

Complications
The following complications can occur within the first 48 hours after tracheostomy tube insertion:
• hemorrhage at the operative site, causing drowning
• bleeding or edema within the tracheal tissue, causing airway obstruction

• aspiration of secretions
• introduction of air into the pleural cavity, causing pneumothorax
• hypoxia or acidosis, triggering cardiac arrest
• introduction of air into surrounding tissues, causing subcutaneous emphysema.

Watch also for the following problems.

• Secretions collecting under dressings and twill tape can encourage skin excoriation and infection.
• Hardened mucus or a slipped cuff can occlude the cannula opening and obstruct the airway.
• Tube displacement can stimulate the cough reflex if the tip rests on the carina or cause blood vessel erosion and hemorrhage.
• Just the presence of the tube or cuff pressure can produce tracheal erosion and necrosis.

Nursing considerations

• Keep appropriate equipment at the patient's bedside for immediate use in an emergency.
• Consult the doctor about first-aid measures you can use for your tracheostomy patient should an emergency occur. Follow hospital policy, for instance, on what to do if a tracheostomy tube is expelled or if the outer cannula becomes blocked. If the patient's breathing is obstructed — for example, when the tube is blocked with mucus that can't be removed by suctioning or by withdrawing the inner cannula — call the appropriate code and provide manual resuscitation with a handheld resuscitation bag, or reconnect the patient to the ventilator. Don't remove the tracheostomy tube entirely *because this may*

TECHNOLOGY UPDATE

Preventing aspiration with a Passy-Muir Valve

The Passy-Muir Valve (PMV) is a one-way speaking valve that enhances communication and reduces the risk of aspiration in tracheostomy patients. The one-way valve opens only when the patient inhales. It acts the way vocal cords do, allowing the patient to speak when a tracheostomy tube is in place. Also, recent studies have shown that the PMV reduces aspiration during swallowing of liquids and semisolid and pureed foods.

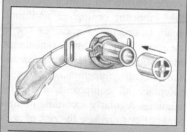

Photo courtesy of Passy-Muir, Inc., Irvine, Calif.

allow the airway to close completely. Use extreme caution when attempting to reinsert an expelled tracheostomy tube *because of the risk of tracheal trauma, perforation, compression, and asphyxiation.* Reassure the patient until the doctor arrives (usually a minute or less in this type of code or emergency).

• In some cases, patients who cannot readily be decannulated for oral feeding due to the risk of aspiration can be fed with the aid of a one way valve (See *Preventing aspiration with a Passy-Muir Valve.*)

• Refrain from changing tracheostomy ties unnecessarily during the immediate postoperative period before the stoma track is well formed (usually 4 days) *to avoid accidental dislodgment and expulsion of the tube.* Unless secretions or drainage is a problem, ties can be changed once a day.

• Refrain from changing a single-cannula tracheostomy tube or the outer cannula of a double-cannula tube. Because of the risk of tracheal complications, the doctor usually changes the cannula, with the frequency of change depending on the patient's condition.

• If the patient's neck or stoma is excoriated or infected, apply a water-soluble lubricant or topical antibiotic cream as ordered. Remember not to use a powder or an oil-based substance on or around a stoma *because aspiration can cause infection and abscess.*

• Replace all equipment, including solutions, regularly according to hospital policy *to reduce the risk of nosocomial infections.*

Home care

• If the patient is being discharged with a tracheostomy, start self-care teaching as soon as he's receptive.

• Teach the patient how to change and clean the tube.

• If he's being discharged with suction equipment (a few patients are), make sure he and his family feel knowledgeable and comfortable about using this equipment.

Documentation

• Record the date and time of the procedure.

• Record the type of procedure.

• Note the amount, consistency, color, and odor of secretions.

• Document stoma and skin condition.

• Document the patient's respiratory status.

• Make note of any change of tracheostomy tube by the doctor, duration of any cuff deflation and degree of any cuff inflation.

• Record cuff pressure readings and specific body position.

• Note any complications and the nursing action taken, any patient or family teaching and their comprehension and progress, and the patient's tolerance of the treatment.

Transabdominal tube feeding and care

To access the stomach, duodenum, or jejunum, the doctor may place a tube through the patient's abdominal wall. This may be done surgically or percutaneously.

Gastrostomy or jejunostomy tubes are usually placed during intra-abdominal surgery. The tube may be used for feeding during the immediate postoperative period or it may provide long-term enteral access, depending on what type of surgery the patient had. Typically, the doctor will suture the tube in place to prevent gastric contents from leaking.

In contrast, a percutaneous endoscopic gastrostomy (PEG) or jejunostomy (PEJ) tube can be inserted endoscopically without the need for laparotomy or general anesthesia. Typically, the insertion is done in the endoscopy suite or at the patient's bedside. A PEG or PEJ tube may be used for nutrition, drainage, and decompression. Contraindications to endoscopic placement include obstruction (such as an esophageal stricture or duodenal blockage), previous gastric surgery, morbid obesity, and ascites. These conditions necessitate surgical placement.

With either type of tube placement, feedings may begin after about 24 hours (or when peristalsis resumes).

Eventually, the tube may need replacement, and the doctor may recommend a similar tube, such as an indwelling urinary or a mushroom catheter, or a gastrostomy button — a skin-level feeding tube.

Nursing care includes providing skin care at the tube site, maintaining the feeding tube, administering feeding, monitoring the patient's response to feeding, adjusting the feeding schedule, and preparing the patient for self-care after discharge.

≫ Key nursing diagnoses and patient outcomes

Use these nursing diagnoses as a guide when developing your plan of care for a patient who is being treated with transabdominal tube feeding.

Altered nutrition: less than body requirements related to inability to absorb nutrients

Based on this nursing diagnosis, you'll establish the following patient outcomes. The patient will:
• tolerate oral, tube or I.V. feedings without adverse effects.
• show no further evidence of weight loss.

Risk for fluid volume deficit related to active loss

Based on this nursing diagnosis, you'll establish the following patient outcomes. The patient will:
• have fluid volume remain adequate.
• have electrolyte levels stay within normal range.

Equipment

For feeding: ♦ feeding formula ♦ large-bulb or catheter-tip syringe ♦ 120 ml of water ♦ 4″ × 4″ gauze pads ♦ soap ♦ skin protectant ♦ antibacterial ointment ♦ hypoallergenic tape ♦ gravity-drip administration bags ♦ mouthwash, toothpaste, or mild salt solution ♦ gloves ♦ optional: enteral infusion pump.

For decompression: ♦ suction apparatus with tubing and straight drainage collection set.

Equipment preparation

• Check the expiration date on commercially prepared feeding formulas. If the formula has been prepared by the dietitian or pharmacist, check the preparation time and date. Discard any opened formula or solution that's more than 1 day old.
• Commercially prepared administration sets and enteral pumps allow continuous formula administration. Place the desired amount of formula into the gavage container, and purge air from the tubing.
• To avoid formula contamination, hang only a 4- to 6-hour supply of formula at a time.

Patient preparation

• Provide privacy.
• Explain the procedure to the patient. Tell him, for example, that feedings

usually start at a slow rate and increase as tolerated.

• Tell him that after he tolerates continuous feedings, he may progress to intermittent feedings to prepare him for home management as ordered.

Implementation

• Wash your hands.

• Assess for bowel sounds before feeding, and monitor for abdominal distention.

• Ask the patient to sit, or assist him into semi-Fowler's position, for the entire feeding. *This helps to prevent esophageal reflux and pulmonary aspiration of the formula.* For an intermittent feeding, have the patient maintain this position throughout the feeding and for 30 minutes to 1 hour afterward.

• Put on gloves. Before starting the feeding, measure residual gastric contents. Attach the syringe to the feeding tube and aspirate. If the contents measure more than twice the amount infused, hold the feeding and recheck in 1 hour. Then, if residual contents remain too high, notify the doctor. Chances are the formula isn't being absorbed properly.

• With PEJ or jejunostomy tube feedings, keep in mind that residual contents will be minimal.

• Allow 1 oz (30 ml) of water to flow into the feeding tube *to establish patency.*

• Be sure to administer formula at room temperature. *Cold formula may cause cramping.*

Intermittent feedings

• Allow gravity to help the formula flow over 30 to 45 minutes. *Faster infusions may cause bloating, cramps, or diarrhea.*

• Begin intermittent feeding with a low volume (7 oz [200 ml]) daily. According to the patient's tolerance, increase the volume per feeding, as needed, *to reach the desired calorie intake.*

• When the feeding finishes, flush the feeding tube with 1 to 2 oz (30 to 60 ml) of water. *This maintains patency and provides hydration.*

• Cap the tube *to prevent leakage.*

• Rinse the feeding administration set thoroughly with hot water *to avoid contaminating subsequent feedings.* Allow the feeding set to dry between feedings.

Continuous feedings

• Measure residual gastric contents every 4 hours.

• To administer the feeding with a pump, set up the equipment according to the manufacturer's guidelines, and fill the feeding bag. To administer the feeding by gravity, fill the container with formula and purge air from the tubing.

• Monitor the gravity drip rate or pump infusion rate frequently *to ensure accurate delivery of formula.*

• Flush the feeding tube with 1 to 2 oz (30 to 60 ml) of water every 4 hours *to maintain patency and to provide hydration.*

• Monitor intake and output *to anticipate and detect fluid or electrolyte imbalances.*

Decompression

• To decompress the stomach, connect the PEG port to the suction device with tubing or straight gravity drainage tubing. Jejunostomy feeding may be given simultaneously via the PEJ port of the dual-lumen tube.

Tube exit site care

• Provide daily skin care.

• Gently remove the dressing by hand. Never cut away the dressing over the catheter because *you may inadvertently cut the tube or the sutures holding the tube in place.*

• At least daily and as needed, clean the skin around the tube's exit site using a $4'' \times 4''$ gauze pad soaked in the prescribed cleaning solution. When healed, wash the skin around the exit site daily with soap. Rinse the area with water, and pat dry. Apply skin protectant, if necessary, and antibacterial ointment to the catheter at the exit site *to prevent or treat skin maceration.*

• Anchor a gastrostomy or jejunostomy tube to the skin with hypoallergenic tape *to prevent peristaltic migration of the tube.* This also prevents tension on the suture anchoring the tube in place.

• Coil the tube, if necessary, and tape it to the abdomen *to prevent pulling and contamination of the tube.* PEG and PEJ tubes have toggle-bolt-like internal and external bumpers that make tape anchors unnecessary (See *Caring for the PEG or PEJ site*, page 882.)

Complications

• Common complications related to transabdominal tubes include GI or other systemic problems, mechanical malfunction, and metabolic disturbances.

• Cramping, nausea, vomiting, bloating, and diarrhea may be related to medication; rapid infusion rate; formula contamination, osmolarity, or temperature (too cold or too warm); fat malabsorption; or intestinal atrophy from malnutrition.

• Constipation may result from inadequate hydration, or insufficient exercise.

• Systemic problems may be caused by pulmonary aspiration, infection at the tube exit site, or contaminated formula. Proper positioning during feeding, verification of tube placement, meticulous skin care, and aseptic formula preparation are ways to prevent these complications.

• Typical mechanical problems include tube dislodgment, obstruction, or impairment. For example, a PEG or PEJ tube may migrate if the external bumper loosens. Occlusion may result from incompletely crushed and liquefied medication particles or inadequate tube flushing. Further, the tube may rupture or crack from age, drying, or frequent manipulation.

• Monitor the patient for vitamin and mineral deficiencies, glucose tolerance, and fluid and electrolyte imbalances, which may follow bouts of diarrhea or constipation.

Nursing considerations

• If the patient vomits, stop the feeding immediately and assess his condition. Also stop the feeding if he complains of nausea, feeling too full, or regurgitation. Flush the feeding tube and attempt to restart the feeding again in 1 hour (measure residual gastric contents first). You may have to decrease the volume or rate of feedings. If dumping syndrome develops, which includes nausea, vomiting, cramps, pallor, and diarrhea, the feedings may have been given too quickly.

• Provide oral hygiene frequently. Brush all surfaces of the teeth, gums, and tongue at least twice daily using mouthwash, toothpaste, or mild salt solution.

Caring for the PEG or PEJ site

The exit site of a percutaneous endoscopic gastrostomy (PEG) or percutaneous endoscopic jejunostomy (PEJ) tube requires routine observation and care. Follow these care guidelines:
• Change the dressing daily while the tube is in place.
• After removing the dressing, carefully slide the tube's outer bumper away from the skin about ½" (1 cm), as shown below.

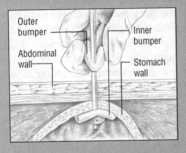

Outer bumper
Inner bumper
Abdominal wall
Stomach wall

• Examine the skin around the tube. Look for redness and other signs of infection or erosion.
• Gently depress the skin surrounding the tube and inspect for drainage, as shown above right. Expect minimal wound drainage after implantation. This should subside in about 1 week.

• Inspect the tube for wear and tear. (A tube that wears out will need replacement.)

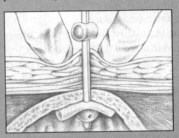

• Clean the site with the prescribed cleaning solution. Then apply povidone-iodine ointment over the exit site, according to your hospital's guidelines.
• Rotate the outer bumper 90 degrees *(to prevent repeating the same tension on the same skin area)*, and slide the outer bumper back over the exit site.
• If leakage appears at the PEG site, or if the patient risks dislodging the tube, apply a sterile gauze dressing over the site. Do not put sterile gauze underneath the outer bumper. Loosening the anchor in this way allows the feeding tube free play, which could lead to wound abscess.
• Write the date and time of the dressing change on the tape.

• You can administer most tablets and pills through the tube by crushing them and diluting as necessary. (The exception is enteric-coated or sustained-released drugs, which lose their effectiveness when crushed.) Medications should be in liquid form for administration.

• Control diarrhea resulting from dumping syndrome by using continuous pump or gravity-drip infusions, diluting the feeding formula, or adding antidiarrheal medications.

Home care
• Instruct the patient and family members or other caregivers in all aspects

of enteral feedings, including tube maintenance and site care.
• Specify signs and symptoms to report to the doctor, define emergency situations, and review actions to take.
• When the tube needs replacement, advise the patient that the doctor may insert a replacement gastrostomy button or a latex, indwelling, or mushroom catheter after removing the initial feeding tube. The procedure may be done in the doctor's office or the hospital endoscopy suite.
• As the patient's tolerance to tube feeding improves, he may wish to try syringe feedings, rather than intermittent feedings. If appropriate, teach him how to feed himself by this method.

Documentation
• On the intake and output record, note the date, time, and amount of each feeding and the water volume instilled. Maintain total volumes for nutrients and water separately to allow calculation of nutrient intake.
• In your notes, document the type of formula, the infusion method and rate, the patient's tolerance of the procedure and formula, and the amount of residual gastric contents.
• Record complications and abdominal assessment findings. Note patient-teaching topics covered and the patient's progress in self-care.

Transcutaneous electrical nerve stimulation

Transcutaneous electrical nerve stimulation (TENS) is based on the gate the-

ory of pain, which proposes that painful impulses pass through a "gate" in the brain. TENS is done with a portable, battery-powered device that transmits painless electrical current to peripheral nerves or directly to a painful area over relatively large nerve fibers. This treatment alters the patient's perception of pain by blocking painful stimuli traveling over smaller nerve fibers. Used for patients after surgery and those with chronic pain, a TENS device reduces the need for analgesic drugs and may allow the patient to resume normal activities. (See *Positioning TENS electrodes,* page 884.)

Typically, a course of TENS treatments lasts 3 to 5 days. Some conditions such as phantom limb pain may require continuous stimulation; other conditions such as a painful arthritic joint require shorter periods (3 to 4 hours).
• The TENS device is contraindicated for patients with cardiac pacemakers because it can interfere with pacemaker function. The procedure is also contraindicated for pregnant patients because its effect on the fetus is unknown. It's also contraindicated in patients who are senile. TENS should be used cautiously in all patients with cardiac disorders. TENS electrodes should not be placed on the head or neck of patients with vascular disorders or seizure disorders.

≫ Key nursing diagnoses and patient outcomes
Use these nursing diagnoses as a guide when developing your plan of care for a patient who is receiving TENS.

Positioning TENS electrodes

In transcutaneous electrical nerve stimulation (TENS), electrodes placed around peripheral nerves (or an incisional site) transmit mild electrical pulses to the brain. The current is thought to block pain impulses. The patient can influence the level and frequency of his pain relief by adjusting the controls on the device.

Typically, electrode placement varies, even though patients may have similar complaints. Electrodes can be placed:
• to cover the painful area or surround it, as with muscle tenderness or spasm or painful joints.

• to "capture" the painful area between electrodes, as with incisional pain.

In peripheral nerve injury, electrodes should be placed proximal to the injury (between the brain and the injury site) to avoid increasing pain. Placing electrodes in a hypersensitive area also increases pain. In an area lacking sensation, electrodes should be placed on adjacent dermatomes.

The illustrations show combinations of electrode placement (black squares) and areas of nerve stimulation (shaded) for low back and leg pain.

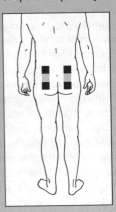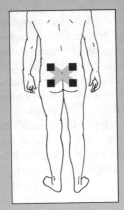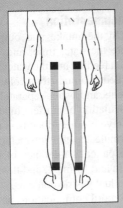

Impaired physical mobility related to neuromuscular impairment
Based on this nursing diagnosis, you'll establish the following patient outcomes. The patient will:
• maintain muscle strength and joint range of motion.
• show no evidence of complications, such as skin breakdown.

Pain related to physical agents
Based on this nursing diagnosis, you'll establish the following patient outcomes. The patient will:
• express a feeling of comfort and relief from pain.
• state and carry out appropriate interventions for pain relief.

Equipment

♦ TENS device ♦ alcohol pads ♦ electrodes ♦ electrode gel ♦ warm water and soap ♦ leadwires ♦ charged battery pack ♦ battery recharger ♦ adhesive patch or hypoallergenic tape.

Commercial TENS kits are available. They include the stimulator, leadwires, electrodes, spare battery pack, battery recharger, and sometimes the adhesive patch.

Equipment preparation

• Before beginning the procedure, always test the battery pack to make sure it's fully charged.

Patient preparation

• Provide privacy.
• If the patient has never seen a TENS unit before, show him the device and explain the procedure.

Implementation

• Wash your hands.

Before TENS treatment

• With an alcohol pad, thoroughly clean the skin where the electrode will be applied. Then dry the skin.
• Apply electrode gel to the bottom of each electrode.
• Place the ordered number of electrodes on the proper skin area, leaving at least 2″ (5 cm) between them. Then secure them with the adhesive patch or hypoallergenic tape. Tape all sides evenly *so that the electrodes are firmly attached to the skin.*
• Plug the pin connectors into the electrode sockets. *To protect the cords,* hold the connectors — not the cords themselves — during insertion.

• Turn the channel controls to the "off" position or to the position recommended in the operator's manual.
• Plug the leadwires into the jacks in the control box.
• Turn the amplitude and rate dials slowly, as the manual directs. (The patient should feel a tingling sensation.) Then adjust the controls on this device to the prescribed settings or to settings that are most comfortable. Most patients select stimulation frequencies of 60 to 100 Hertz.
• Attach the TENS control box to part of the patient's clothing, such as a belt, pocket, or bra.
• *To make sure the device is working effectively,* monitor the patient for signs of excessive stimulation such as muscular twitches or signs of inadequate stimulation, signaled by the patient's inability to feel any mild tingling sensation.

After TENS treatment

• Turn off the controls and unplug the electrode leadwires from the control box.
• If another treatment will be given soon, leave the electrodes in place; if not, remove them.
• Clean the electrodes with soap and water, and clean the patient's skin with alcohol pads. (Don't soak the electrodes in alcohol *because it will damage the rubber.*)
• Remove the battery pack from the unit, and replace it with a charged battery pack.
• Recharge the used battery pack *so that it's always ready for use.*

Nursing considerations

• If you must move the electrodes during the procedure, turn off the controls

first. Follow the doctor's orders regarding electrode placement and control settings. *Incorrect placement of the electrodes will result in inappropriate pain control. Setting the controls too high can cause pain; setting them too low will fail to relieve pain.* Never place the electrodes near the patient's eyes or over the nerves that innervate the carotid sinus or laryngeal or pharyngeal muscles *to avoid interference with critical nerve function.*
• If TENS is used continuously for postoperative pain, remove the electrodes at least daily *to check for skin irritation, and provide skin care.*
• If appropriate, let the patient study the operator's manual. Teach him how to place the electrodes properly and how to take care of the TENS unit.

Documentation
• On the medical record of the patient and the nursing plan of care, record electrode sites and control settings.
• Document the patient's tolerance to the treatment.
• Evaluate pain control.

Transdermal drug administration

Through an adhesive disk or patch or a measured dose of ointment applied to the skin, transdermal drugs deliver constant, controlled medication directly into the bloodstream for prolonged systemic effect. Medications available in transdermal form include: nitroglycerin, used to control angina; scopolamine, used to treat motion sickness; estradiol for postmenopausal hormone replacement; clonidine,

used to treat hypertension; nicotine, for smoking cessation; and fentanyl, a narcotic analgesic used to control chronic pain. Nitroglycerin ointment dilates coronary vessels for up to 4 hours; a nitroglycerin disk can produce the same effect for as long as 24 hours. The scopolamine disk can relieve motion sickness for as long as 72 hours, transdermal estradiol lasts for up to 1 week, clonidine and the nicotine patch last for 24 hours, and fentanyl lasts for up to 72 hours.

Contraindications for transdermal application include skin allergies or skin reactions to the drug. Transdermal drugs should not be applied to broken or irritated skin because they increase irritation, or to scarred or calloused skin because they may impair absorption.

≫ Key nursing diagnoses and patient outcomes
Use these nursing diagnoses as a guide when developing your plan of care for a patient who is receiving transdermal medication.

Knowledge deficit related to lack of exposure
Based on this nursing diagnosis, you'll establish the following patient outcomes. The patient will:
• state or demonstrate understanding of what has been taught.
• demonstrate ability to perform new health-related behaviors as they are taught.

Risk for injury related to improper technique
Based on this nursing diagnosis, you'll establish these patient outcomes. The patient will:

• identify factors that increase risk for injury.
• assist in identifying and applying safety measures to prevent injury.

Equipment

♦ patient's medication record and chart ♦ prescribed medication (disk or ointment) ♦ application strip or measuring paper (for nitroglycerin ointment) ♦ adhesive tape ♦ plastic wrap (optional for nitroglycerin ointment) or semipermeable dressing ♦ optional: gloves.

Equipment preparation

• Verify the order on the patient's medication record by checking it against the doctor's order.
• Check the label on the medication *to make sure you'll be administering the correct drug in the correct dose.*

Patient preparation

• Wash your hands and, if necessary, don gloves.
• Confirm the patient's identity by asking his name and checking the name, room number, and bed number on his wristband.
• Explain the procedure to the patient and provide privacy.
• As needed, remove any previously applied medication.

Implementation

Follow the steps below to administer drugs transdermally.

Applying transdermal ointment

• Place the prescribed amount of ointment on the application strip or measuring paper, taking care not to get any on your skin. (See *Applying nitroglycerin ointment*, page 888.)

• Apply the strip to any dry, hairless area of the body. Don't rub the ointment into the skin.
• Tape the application strip and ointment to the skin.
• If desired, cover the application strip with the plastic wrap, and tape the wrap in place.

Applying a transdermal disk

• Open the package, and remove the disk.
• Without touching the adhesive surface, remove the clear plastic backing.
• Apply the disk to any dry, hairless area — behind the ear, for example, as with scopolamine. (See *Applying a transdermal medication disk*, page 889.)

After applying transdermal medications

• Store the medication as ordered.
• Instruct the patient to keep the area around the disk or ointment as dry as possible.
• If you didn't wear gloves, wash your hands immediately after applying the disk or ointment *to avoid absorbing the drug yourself.*

Complications

• Skin irritation, such as pruritus or a rash, may occur.
• The patient may also suffer adverse effects of the drug administered. For example, transdermal nitroglycerin medications may cause headaches and, in elderly patients, postural hypotension.
• Scopolamine has various adverse effects; dry mouth and drowsiness are the most common.
• Transdermal estradiol carries an increased risk of endometrial cancer,

Applying nitroglycerin ointment

Unlike most topical medications, nitroglycerin ointment is used for its transdermal *systemic* effect. It's used to dilate the veins and arteries, thus improving cardiac perfusion in a patient with cardiac ischemia or angina pectoris.

To apply nitroglycerin ointment, start by taking the patient's baseline blood pressure *so that you can compare it with later readings.* Gather your equipment. Nitroglycerin ointment, which is prescribed by the inch, comes with a rectangular piece of ruled paper, to be used in applying the medication. Squeeze the prescribed amount of ointment onto the ruled paper, as shown below. Put on gloves, if desired, to avoid contact *with the medication.*

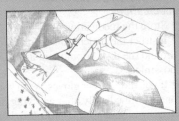

After measuring the correct amount of ointment, tape the paper — drug side down — directly to the skin, as

shown below. (Some hospitals require you to use the paper to apply the medication to the patient's skin, usually on the chest or arm. Spread a thin layer of the ointment over a 3″ [7.6 cm] area.) For increased absorption, the doctor may request that you cover the site with plastic wrap or a transparent semipermeable dressing.

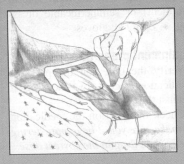

After 5 minutes, record the patient's blood pressure. If it has dropped significantly and he has a headache (from vasodilation of blood vessels in his head), notify the doctor immediately. He may reduce the dose. If the patient's blood pressure has dropped, but he has no symptoms, instruct him to lie still until it returns to normal.

thromboembolic disease, and birth defects.
• Clonidine may cause severe rebound hypertension, especially if withdrawn suddenly.

Nursing considerations
• Reapply daily transdermal medications at the same time every day *to ensure a continuous effect,* but alternate the application sites *to avoid skin ir-*

ritation. Before reapplying nitroglycerin ointment, remove the plastic wrap, application strip, and any remaining ointment from the patient's skin at the previous site.
• When applying a scopolamine disk, instruct the patient not to drive or operate machinery until his response to the drug has been determined.
• Warn a patient using clonidine disks to check with his doctor before using

Applying a transdermal medication disk

If the patient will be receiving medication by transdermal disk, instruct him in its proper use, as described below:

• Explain to the patient that the disk consists of several layers. The layer closest to his skin contains a small amount of the drug and allows prompt introduction of the drug into the bloodstream (as indicated by the dots). The next layer controls release of the drug from the main portion of the patch. The third layer contains the main dose of the drug, and the outermost layer provides an aluminized polyester barrier.

• Teach the patient to apply the disk to appropriate skin areas, such as on the upper arm or chest or behind the ear. Warn him to avoid touching the gel or surrounding tape. Tell him to use a different site for each application to avoid skin irritation. If necessary, he can shave the site. Tell him to avoid any area

that may cause uneven absorption, such as skin folds, scars, and calluses or any irritated or damaged skin areas. Also, tell him not to apply the disk below the elbow or knee.

• Instruct the patient to wash his hands after application to remove any medication that may have rubbed off.

• Warn the patient not to get the disk wet. Tell him to discard the disk if it leaks or falls off, and then to clean the site and apply a new disk at a different site.

• Instruct the patient to apply the disk at the same time at the prescribed interval to ensure continuous drug delivery. Bedtime application is ideal because body movement is reduced during the night. Finally, tell him to apply a new disk about 30 minutes before removing the old one.

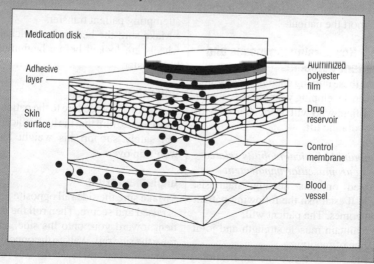

any over-the-counter cough preparations *because these may counteract the effects of the drug.*

Documentation
• Record the type of medication, the date, time, and site of application, and the dose. Also note any adverse effects and the patient's response.

Transferring a patient with a hydraulic lift

Using a hydraulic lift to raise the immobile patient from the supine to the sitting position allows safe, comfortable transfer between bed and chair. It's indicated for the obese or immobile patient for whom manual transfer poses the potential for nurse or patient injury. Although most hydraulic lift models can be operated by one person, it's better to have two staff members present during transfer to stabilize and support the patient.

≫ Key nursing diagnoses and patient outcomes
Use these nursing diagnoses as a guide when developing your plan of care for a patient who will be transferred with a hydraulic lift.

Impaired physical mobility related to neuromuscular impairment
Based on this nursing diagnosis, you'll establish the following patient outcomes. The patient will:
• maintain muscle strength and joint range of motion.
• show no evidence of complications, such as contractures, venous stasis, thrombus formation, or skin breakdown.
• have mobility regimen carried out by significant other.

Risk for injury related to sensory deficits
Based on this nursing diagnosis, you'll establish the following patient outcomes. The patient will:
• identify factors that increase potential for injury.
• identify and apply safety measures to prevent injury.
• optimize activities of daily living within sensorimotor limitations.

Equipment
♦ hydraulic lift with sling, chains or straps, and hooks ♦ chair or wheelchair.

Equipment preparation
• Because hydraulic lift models may vary in weight capacity, check the manufacturer's specifications before attempting patient transfer.
• Make sure the bed and wheelchair wheels are locked before beginning the transfer.

Patient preparation
• Explain the procedure to the patient, and reassure him that the hydraulic lift can safely support his weight and won't tip over.

Implementation
• Make sure the side rail opposite you is raised and secure. Then roll the patient toward you, onto his side, and raise the side rail. Walk to the opposite side of the bed and lower the side rail.
• Place the sling under the patient's buttocks with its lower edge below the

Using a hydraulic lift

After placing the patient in a supine position in the center of the sling, position the hydraulic lift above him, as shown here. Then attach the chains to the hooks on the sling.

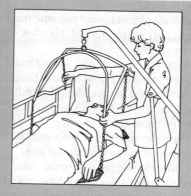

Turn the lift handle clockwise to raise the patient to the sitting position. If he's positioned properly, continue to raise him until he's suspended just above the bed.

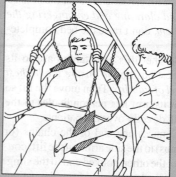

After positioning the patient above the wheelchair, turn the lift handle counterclockwise to lower him onto the seat. When the chains become slack, stop turning and unhook the sling from the lift.

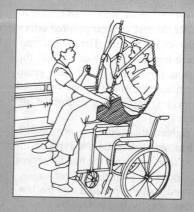

greater trochanter. Then fanfold the far side of the sling against the back and buttocks.

• Roll the patient toward you onto the sling, and raise the side rail. Then lower the opposite side rail.

• Slide your hands under the patient and pull the sling from beneath him, smoothing out all wrinkles. Then roll the patient onto his back and center him on the sling.

• Place the appropriate chair next to the head of the bed, facing the foot.

• Lower the side rail next to the chair, and raise the bed only until the base of the lift can extend under the bed. *To avoid alarming and endangering the patient,* don't raise the bed completely.

• Set the lift's adjustable base to its widest position *to ensure the highest level of stability.* Then move the lift so that its arm lies perpendicular to the bed, directly over the patient.

• Connect one end of the chains (or straps) to the side arms on the lift; connect the other, hooked end to the sling. Face the hooks away from the patient *to prevent them from slipping and to avoid the risk of their pointed edges injuring the patient.* The patient may place his arms inside or outside the chains (or straps) or he may grasp them once the slack is gone (to avoid injury). (See *Using a hydraulic lift,* page 891.)

• Tighten the turnscrew on the lift. Then, depending on the type of lift you're using, pump the handle or turn it clockwise until the patient has assumed a sitting position and his buttocks clear the bed surface by $1''$ or $2''$ (2.5 or 5 cm). Momentarily suspend the patient above the bed *until he feels secure in the lift and sees that it can bear his weight.*

• Steady the patient as you move the lift or, preferably, have another coworker guide the patient's body while you move the lift. Depending on the type of lift you're using, the arm should now rest in front or to one side of the chair.

• Release the turnscrew. Then depress the handle or turn it counterclockwise *to lower the patient into the chair.* While lowering him, push gently on his knees *to maintain the correct sitting posture.* After lowering the patient into the chair, fasten the seat belt *to ensure his safety.*

• Remove the hooks or straps from the sling, but leave the sling in place under the patient so you'll be able to transfer him back to the bed from the chair. Then move the lift away from the patient.

• To return the patient to bed, reverse the procedure.

Nursing considerations

• If the patient has an altered center of gravity (caused by a halo vest or lower-extremity cast, for example), obtain help from a coworker before transferring him with a hydraulic lift.

• If the patient will require use of a hydraulic lift for transfers after discharge, teach his family how to use this device correctly, and allow them to practice with supervision.

Documentation

• If necessary, record the time of transfer in your notes.

• Complete other required forms as necessary.

Transfusion reaction management

A transfusion reaction typically stems from a major antigen-antibody reaction and can result from a single or massive transfusion of blood or blood products. Although many reactions occur during transfusion or within 96 hours afterward, infectious diseases transmitted during a transfusion may go undetected until days, weeks, or months later, when signs and symptoms appear.

Nursing alert. A transfusion reaction requires immediate recognition and prompt nursing action to prevent further complications and possible death — particularly if the patient is unconscious or so heavily sedated that he can't report the common symptoms. (See *Managing transfusion reactions,* page 894 to 897.)

≫ Key nursing diagnoses and patient outcomes

Use these nursing diagnoses as a guide when developing your plan of care for a patient who is having a transfusion reaction.

Fluid volume deficit related to active loss

Based on this nursing diagnosis, you'll establish the following patient outcomes. The patient will:
• have vital signs remain stable.
• have fluid and blood volume return to normal.

Altered (specify type) tissue perfusion related to decreased cellular exchange

Based on this nursing diagnosis, you'll establish the following patient outcomes. The patient will:
• attain hemodynamic stability: pulse not __ and not __ (specify). Blood pressure not __ and not __ (specify).
• not exhibit arrhythmias.

Equipment

♦ normal saline solution ♦ I.V. administration set ♦ sterile urine specimen container ♦ needle, syringe, and tubes for blood samples ♦ transfusion reaction report form ♦ optional: oxygen, epinephrine, hypothermia blanket, leukocyte removal filter.

Equipment preparation
• Gather needed equipment.

Patient preparation
• Assess the patient's airway, breathing, and circulation.
• Make the patient comfortable and provide reassurance as necessary.
• Explain the procedure.

Implementation
• As soon as you suspect an adverse reaction, stop the transfusion and start the saline infusion at a keep-vein-open rate *to maintain venous access.* Don't discard the blood bag or administration set.
• Notify the doctor.
• Monitor vital signs every 15 minutes or as indicated by the severity and type of reaction.
• Compare the labels on all blood containers to corresponding patient identification forms *to verify that the*
(Text continues on page 897.)

PROBLEM SOLVER

Managing transfusion reactions

Any patient receiving a transfusion of processed blood products risks certain complications — hemosiderosis and hypothermia, for example. The chart below describes how to recognize and manage *endogenous reactions,* those caused by an antigen-antibody reaction in the recipient, and *exogenous reactions,* those caused by external factors in administered blood.

REACTION AND CAUSES	SIGNS AND SYMPTOMS	NURSING INTERVENTIONS
Endogenous		
Allergic • Allergen in donor blood • Donor blood hypersensitive to certain drugs	• Anaphylaxis (chills, facial swelling, laryngeal edema, pruritus, urticaria, wheezing), fever, nausea and vomiting	• Administer antihistamines as prescribed. • Monitor patient for anaphylactic reaction, and administer epinephrine and corticosteroids if indicated. • As prescribed, premedicate patient with diphenhydramine before subsequent transfusion.
Bacterial contamination • Organisms that can survive the cold, such as *Pseudomonas* or *Staphylococcus*	• Chills, fever, vomiting, abdominal cramping, diarrhea, shock, signs of renal failure	• Provide broad-spectrum antibiotics, corticosteroids, or epinephrine, as prescribed. • Maintain strict blood-storage control. • Change blood administration set and filter every 4 hours or after every two units. • Infuse each unit of blood over 2 to 4 hours; stop the infusion if the time span exceeds 4 hours. • Maintain sterile technique when administering blood products.

Managing transfusion reactions (continued)

REACTION AND CAUSES	SIGNS AND SYMPTOMS	NURSING INTERVENTIONS
Febrile • Bacterial lipo-polysaccharides • Antileukocyte recipient antibodies directed against donor white blood cells	• Fever up to 104° F (40° C), chills, headache, facial flushing, palpitations, cough, chest tightness, increased pulse rate, flank pain	• Relieve symptoms with an antipyretic, an antihistamine, or meperidine, as ordered. • If the patient requires further transfusions, use frozen red blood cells (RBCs), add a special leukocyte removal filter to the blood line, or premedicate him with acetaminophen, as ordered, before starting another transfusion.
Hemolytic • ABO or Rh incompatibility • Intradonor incompatibility • Improper cross-matching • Improperly stored blood	• Chest pain, dyspnea, facial flushing, fever, chills, hypotension, flank pain, hemoglobinuria, oliguria, bloody oozing at the infusion site or surgical incision site, burning along vein receiving blood, shock, renal failure	• Monitor blood pressure. • Manage shock with I.V. fluids, oxygen, epinephrine, a diuretic, and a vasopressor, as ordered. • Obtain posttransfusion-reaction blood samples and urine specimens for analysis. • Observe for signs of hemorrhage resulting from disseminated intravascular coagulation.
Plasma protein incompatibility • Immunoglobulin-A incompatibility	• Abdominal pain, diarrhea, dyspnea, chills, fever, flushing, hypotension	• Administer oxygen, fluids, epinephrine, or a corticosteroid, as ordered.
Bleeding tendencies • Low platelet count in stored blood, causing thrombocytopenia	• Abnormal bleeding from a cut, a break in the skin surface, or the gums; abnormal bruising and petechiae	• Administer platelets, fresh frozen plasma, or cryoprecipitate, as ordered. • Monitor platelet count.
Circulatory overload • May result from infusing whole blood too rapidly	• Increased plasma volume, back pain, chest tightness, chills, fever, dyspnea, flushed feeling headache hypertension, increased central venous pressure and jugular vein pressure	• Monitor blood pressure. • Use packed RBCs instead of whole blood. • Administer diuretics, as ordered.

(continued)

Managing transfusion reactions (continued)

REACTION AND CAUSES	SIGNS AND SYMPTOMS	NURSING INTERVENTIONS
Elevated blood ammonia level • Increased ammonia level in stored donor blood	• Confusion, forgetfulness, lethargy	• Monitor ammonia level in blood. • Decrease the amount of protein in the patient's diet. • If indicated, give neomycin.
Hemosiderosis • Increased level of hemosiderin (iron-containing pigment) from RBC destruction, especially after many transfusions	• Iron plasma level exceeding 200 mg/dl	• Perform a phlebotomy to remove excess iron.
Hypocalcemia • Citrate toxicity occurs when citrate-treated blood is infused rapidly. Citrate binds with calcium, causing a calcium deficiency, or normal citrate metabolism becomes impeded by hepatic disease.	• Arrhythmias, hypotension, muscle cramps, nausea and vomiting, seizures, tingling in fingers	• Slow or stop the transfusion, depending on the patient's reaction. Expect a more severe reaction in hypothermic patients or patients with elevated potassium levels. • Slowly administer calcium gluconate I.V. if ordered.
Hypothermia • Rapid infusion of large amounts of cold blood, which decreases body temperature	• Chills; shaking; hypotension; arrhythmias, especially bradycardia; cardiac arrest, if core temperature falls below 86° F (30° C)	• Stop the transfusion. • Warm the patient with blankets. • Place the patient in a warm environment if necessary. • Obtain an electrocardiogram (ECG). • Warm blood if the transfusion is resumed.

Managing transfusion reactions *(continued)*

REACTION AND CAUSES	SIGNS AND SYMPTOMS	NURSING INTERVENTIONS
Increased oxygen affinity for hemo-globin • Decreased level of 2,3-diphospho-glycerate in stored blood, causing an increase in the oxygen's hemoglobin affinity. Oxygen then stays in the bloodstream and isn't released into tissues.	• Depressed respiratory rate, especially in patients with chronic lung disease	• Monitor arterial blood gas levels, and provide respiratory support, as needed.
Potassium intoxi-cation • An abnormally high level of potassium in stored plasma caused by hemolysis of RBCs	• Diarrhea, intestinal colic, flaccidity, muscle twitching, oliguria, renal failure, bradycardia progressing to cardiac arrest, ECG changes with tall, peaked T waves	• Obtain an ECG. • Administer sodium polystyrene sulfonate (Kayexalate) orally or by enema. • Administer glucose 50% and insulin, bicarbonate, or calcium, as ordered, to force vitamin K into cells.

transfusion was the correct blood or blood product.
• Notify the blood bank of a possible transfusion reaction and collect blood samples, as ordered. Immediately send these samples, all transfusion containers (even if empty), and the administration set to the blood bank. *The blood bank will test these materials to further evaluate the reaction.*
• Collect the first posttransfusion urine specimen, mark the collection slip "Possible transfusion reaction," and send it to the laboratory immediately. *The laboratory tests this urine specimen for the presence of hemo-*

globin, which indicates a hemolytic reaction.
• Closely monitor intake and output. Note evidence of oliguria or anuria *because hemoglobin deposition in the renal tubules can cause renal damage.*
• If ordered, administer oxygen, epinephrine, or other drugs. If ordered, apply a hypothermia blanket *to reduce fever.*

Nursing considerations
• Treat all transfusion reactions as serious until proven otherwise. If the doctor anticipates a transfusion reaction such as one that may occur in a leukemia patient, he may order pro-

BETTER CHARTING

Documenting transfusion reactions

If the patient develops a transfusion reaction, stop the transfusion immediately, and notify the doctor. Be sure to document the time and date of the reaction, the type and amount of infused blood or blood products, the time you started the transfusion, and the time you stopped it. Also record the clinical signs of the reaction in order of occurrence, the patient's vital signs, any urine specimen and blood samples sent to the laboratory for analysis, any treatment given, and the patient's response to the treatment. If required by the health care facility, complete a transfusion reaction form.

phylactic treatment with antihistamines or antipyretics to precede blood administration.

• To avoid a possible febrile reaction, the doctor may order the blood washed *to remove as many leukocytes as possible,* or a leukocyte removal filter may be used during the transfusion.

Documentation
• Record the time and date of the transfusion reaction.
• Document the type and amount of infused blood or blood products.
• Note clinical signs of the transfusion reaction in order of occurrence.
• Record the patient's vital signs.
• Document any specimens sent to the laboratory for analysis.
• Note any treatment given and the patient's response to it.

• If required by hospital policy, complete the transfusion reaction form. (See *Documenting transfusion reactions.*)

T-tube care

The T tube (or biliary drainage tube) may be placed in the common bile duct after cholecystectomy or choledochostomy, to facilitate biliary drainage during healing. The surgeon inserts the short end (crossbar) of the T tube in the common bile duct and draws the long end through the incision. The tube then connects to a closed gravity-drainage system. (See *Understanding T-tube placement.*)

The tube remains in place for 1 to 2 weeks postoperatively.

⟩⟩ Key nursing diagnoses and patient outcomes
Use these nursing diagnoses as a guide when developing your plan of care for a patient with a T tube.

Risk for infection related to presence of T tube
Based on this nursing diagnosis, you'll establish the following patient outcomes. The patient will:
• have temperature stay within normal limits.
• have white blood cell count and differential stay within normal range.

Risk for fluid volume deficit related to excessive loss through indwelling tube
Based on this nursing diagnosis, you'll establish the following patient outcomes. The patient will:

Understanding T-tube placement

The T tube is placed in the common bile duct, anchored to the abdominal wall, and connected to a closed drainage system.

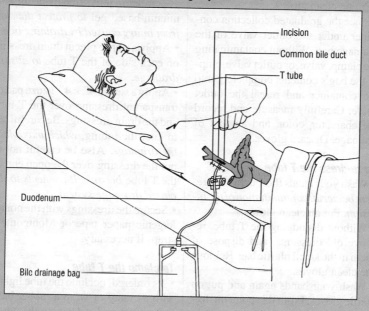

- have vital signs remain stable.
- have electrolyte values remain within normal range.

Equipment

◆ graduated collection container ◆ small plastic bag ◆ sterile gloves and clean gloves ◆ clamp ◆ sterile 4″ × 4″ gauze pads ◆ transparent dressings ◆ rubber band ◆ normal saline solution ◆ sterile cleaning solution ◆ two sterile basins ◆ povidone-iodine sponges ◆ sterile precut drain dressings ◆ hypoallergenic paper tape ◆ skin protectant, such as petroleum jelly, zinc oxide, or aluminum-based gel ◆ optional: Montgomery straps.

Equipment preparation
- Assemble equipment at bedside.
- Open all sterile equipment.
- Place one sterile 4″ × 4″ gauze pad in each sterile basin.
- Using sterile technique, pour 50 ml of cleaning solution into one basin and 50 ml of normal saline into the other basin.
- Tape a small plastic bag on the table to use for refuse.

Patient preparation
- Provide privacy.
- Explain the procedure to the patient.

Implementation
• Wash your hands thoroughly.

To empty drainage
• Put on clean gloves.
• Place the graduated collection container under the outlet valve of the drainage bag. Without contaminating the clamp, valve, or outlet valve, empty the bag's contents completely into the container and reseal the outlet valve. Carefully measure and record the character, color, and amount of drainage. Discard gloves.

To re-dress the T tube
• Wash your hands thoroughly *to prevent bacterial contamination of the incision.* Put on clean gloves.
• Without dislodging the T tube, remove old dressings, and dispose of them in the small plastic bag. Remove the clean gloves.
• Wash your hands again and put on sterile gloves. From this point on, follow strict aseptic technique *to prevent bacterial contamination of the incision.*
• Inspect the incision and tube site for signs of infection, including redness, edema, warmth, tenderness, induration, or skin excoriation. Assess for wound dehiscence or evisceration.
• Use sterile cleaning solution as prescribed to clean and remove dried matter or drainage from around the tube. Always start at the tube site and gently wipe outward in a continuous motion *to prevent recontamination of the incision.*
• Use normal saline solution to rinse off the prescribed cleaning solution. Dry the area with a sterile 4″ × 4″ gauze pad and discard all used materials.

• Using a circular motion, wipe the incision site with a povidone-iodine sponge. Allow the area to dry.
• Lightly apply a skin protectant, such as petroleum jelly, zinc oxide, or aluminum-based gel *to protect the skin from injury caused by draining bile.*
• Apply a sterile precut drain dressing on each side of the T tube *to absorb drainage.*
• Apply a sterile 4″ × 4″ gauze pad or transparent dressing over the T tube and the drain dressings. Be careful not to kink the tubing, *which may block the drainage.* Also be careful not to put the dressing over the open end of the T tube *because it connects to the closed drainage system.*
• Secure the dressings with the nonallergenic paper tape or Montgomery straps if necessary.

To clamp the T tube
• As ordered, occlude the tube lightly with a clamp or wrap a rubber band around the end. *Clamping the tube 1 hour before and after meals diverts bile back to the duodenum to aid digestion.*
• *To ensure patient comfort and safety,* check bile drainage amounts regularly. Be alert for such signs of obstructed bile flow as chills, fever, tachycardia, nausea, right-upper-quadrant fullness and pain, jaundice, dark foamy urine, and clay-colored stools. Report them immediately. (See *Managing T-tube obstruction.*)

Complications
The most common complications are:
• obstructed bile flow
• skin excoriation or breakdown
• tube dislodgment
• drainage reflux
• infection.

Nursing considerations
• Normal daily bile drainage ranges from 500 to 1,000 ml of viscous, green-brown liquid. The T tube usually drains 300 to 500 ml of blood-tinged bile in the first 24 hours after surgery. Report drainage that exceeds 500 ml in the first 24 hours after surgery. This amount typically declines to 200 ml or less after 4 days. Monitor fluid, electrolyte, and acid-base status carefully.
• To prevent excessive bile loss (over 500 ml in first 24 hours) or backflow contamination, secure the T-tube drainage system at abdominal level. Bile will flow into the bag only when biliary pressure increases. As ordered, return excessive bile drainage (between 1,000 and 1,500 ml daily) to the patient mixed with chilled fruit juice or, if possible, through a nasogastric tube.
• Provide meticulous skin care and frequent dressing changes. Observe for bile leakage, which may indicate obstruction. Assess tube patency and site condition hourly for the first 8 hours and then every 4 hours until the doctor removes the tube. Protect the skin edges and avoid excessive taping *to prevent shearing the skin.*
• Monitor all urine and stools for color changes. Assess for icteric skin and sclera, *which may signal jaundice.*

Documentation
• Record the date and time of each dressing change.
• Note the appearance of the wound and surrounding skin.
• Write down the color, character, and volume of bile collected.

PROBLEM SOLVER

Managing T-tube obstruction

If your patient's T tube becomes obstructed after cholecystectomy, notify the doctor and take the following steps while you wait for him to arrive.
• Unclamp the T tube (if it was clamped before and after a meal) and connect the tube to a closed gravity-drainage system.
• Inspect the tube carefully for kinks or obstructions.
• Prepare the patient for possible T-tube irrigation or direct X-ray of the common bile duct (cholangiography). Briefly describe these measures to reduce the patient's apprehension and promote cooperation.

• Record the color of skin and mucous membranes around the T tube.
• Keep a precise record of temperature trends and the amount and frequency of urination and bowel movements.

Tube feeding

This procedure involves delivery of a liquid feeding formula directly to the stomach (known as gastric gavage), duodenum, or jejunum. Gastric gavage is typically indicated for a patient who can't eat normally because of dysphagia or oral or esophageal obstruction or injury. Gastric feedings also may be given to an unconscious or intubated patient or to a patient recovering from GI tract surgery who can't ingest food orally.

Duodenal or jejunal feedings decrease the risk of aspiration because the formula bypasses the pylorus. Jejunal feedings result in reduced pancreatic stimulation; thus, the patient may require an elemental diet.

Usually, patients receive gastric feedings on an intermittent schedule. For duodenal or jejunal feedings, however, most patients seem to better tolerate a continuous slow drip.

Liquid nutrient solutions come in various formulas for administration through a nasogastric tube, small-bore feeding tube, gastrostomy or jejunostomy tube, percutaneous endoscopic gastrostomy or jejunostomy tube, or gastrostomy feeding button. (See *Managing tube feeding problems.*)

Tube feeding is contraindicated in patients who have no bowel sounds or suspected intestinal obstruction.

≫ Key nursing diagnoses and patient outcomes

Use these nursing diagnoses as a guide when developing your plan of care for a patient receiving tube feedings.

Altered nutrition: less than body requirements related to inability to digest or absorb nutrients

Based on this nursing diagnosis, you'll establish the following patient outcomes. The patient will:
• tolerate oral, tube or I.V. feedings without adverse effects.
• show no further evidence of weight loss.

Risk for fluid volume deficit related to active loss

Based on this nursing diagnosis, you'll establish the following patient outcomes. The patient will:
• have fluid volume remain adequate.
• have electrolyte levels stay within normal range.

Equipment

For gastric feedings: ♦ feeding formula ♦ graduated container ♦ 120 ml of water ♦ gavage bag with tubing and flow regulator clamp ♦ towel or linen-saver pad ♦ 60-ml syringe ♦ stethoscope ♦ optional: infusion controller and tubing set (for continuous administration), adapter to connect gavage tubing to feeding tube.

For duodenal or jejunal feedings: ♦ feeding formula ♦ enteral administration set containing a gavage container, drip chamber, roller clamp or flow regulator, and tube connector ♦ I.V. pole ♦ 60-ml syringe with adapter tip ♦ water ♦ optional: pump administration set (for an enteral infusion pump), Y-connector.

For nasal and oral care: ♦ cotton-tipped applicators ♦ water-soluble lubricant ♦ lemon-glycerin swabs ♦ petroleum jelly.

Equipment preparation

• A bulb syringe or large catheter-tip syringe may be substituted for a gavage bag after the patient demonstrates tolerance for a gravity drip infusion. The doctor may order an infusion pump *to ensure accurate delivery of the prescribed formula.*
• Be sure to refrigerate formulas prepared in the dietary department or pharmacy. Refrigerate commercial formulas only after opening them.

PROBLEM SOLVER

Managing tube feeding problems

COMPLICATION	INTERVENTIONS
Aspiration of gastric secretions	• Discontinue feeding immediately. • Perform tracheal suction of aspirated contents if possible. • Notify the doctor. Prophylactic antibiotics and chest physiotherapy may be ordered. • Check tube placement before feeding to prevent complication.
Tube obstruction	• Flush the tube with warm water. If necessary, replace the tube. • Flush the tube with 50 ml of water after each feeding to remove excess sticky formula, which could occlude the tube.
Nasal or pharyngeal irritation or necrosis	• Provide frequent oral hygiene using mouthwash or lemon-glycerin swabs. Use petroleum jelly on cracked lips. • Change the tube's position. If necessary, replace the tube.
Vomiting, bloating, diarrhea, or cramps	• Reduce the flow rate. • Administer metoclopramide to increase GI motility. • Warm the formula. • For 30 minutes after feeding, position the patient on his right side with his head elevated to facilitate gastric emptying. • Notify the doctor. He may want to reduce the amount of formula being given during each feeding.
Constipation	• Provide additional fluids if the patient can tolerate them. • Administer a bulk-forming laxative. • Increase fruit, vegetable, or sugar content of the feeding.
Electrolyte imbalance	• Monitor serum electrolyte levels. • Notify the doctor. He may want to adjust the formula content to correct the deficiency.
Hyperglycemia	• Monitor blood glucose levels. • Notify the doctor of elevated levels. • Administer insulin if ordered. • The doctor may adjust the sugar content of the formula.

• Check the date on all formula containers. Discard expired commercial formula. Use powdered formula within 24 hours of mixing. Always shake the container well *to mix the solution thoroughly.*

• Allow the formula to warm to room temperature before administration. Never warm it over direct heat or in a microwave *because heat may curdle the formula or change its chemical composition. Also, hot formula may injure the patient.*

• Pour 60 ml of water into the graduated container. After closing the flow clamp on the administration set, pour the appropriate amount of formula into the gavage bag. Hang no more than a 4- to 6-hour supply at one time *to prevent bacterial growth.*

• Open the flow clamp on the administration set *to remove air from the lines. This keeps air from entering the patient's stomach and causing distention and discomfort.*

Patient preparation

• Provide privacy.

• Inform the patient that he will receive nourishment through the tube.

• Explain the procedure.

• If possible, give him a schedule of subsequent feedings.

• If the patient has a nasal or oral tube, cover his chest with a towel or linen-saver pad *to protect him and the bed linens from spills.*

Implementation

• Wash your hands.

• Assess the patient's abdomen for bowel sounds and distention.

To deliver a gastric feeding

• Elevate the bed to a semi-Fowler or high Fowler position *to prevent aspiration by gastroesophageal reflux and to promote digestion.*

• Check placement of the feeding tube *to be sure it hasn't slipped out since the last feeding.* Never give a tube feeding until you're sure the tube is properly positioned in the patient's stomach. *Administering a feeding through a misplaced tube can cause formula to enter the patient's lungs.*

• *To check tube patency and position,* remove the cap or plug from the feeding tube, and use the syringe to inject 5 to 10 cc of air through the tube. At the same time, auscultate the patient's stomach with the stethoscope. Listen for a whooshing sound to confirm tube positioning in the stomach. Also aspirate stomach contents to confirm tube patency and placement.

• *To assess gastric emptying,* aspirate and measure residual gastric contents. Reinstill any aspirate obtained.

• Connect the gavage bag tubing to the feeding tube. Depending on the type of tube used, you may need to use an adapter to connect the two.

• If you're using a bulb or catheter-tip syringe, remove the bulb or plunger and attach the syringe to the pinched-off feeding tube *to prevent excess air from entering the patient's stomach, causing distention.* If you're using an infusion controller, thread the tube from the formula container through the controller according to the manufacturer's directions. Purge the tubing of air and attach it to the feeding tube.

• Open the regulator clamp on the gavage bag tubing, and adjust the flow rate appropriately. When using a bulb syringe, fill the syringe with formula and release the feeding tube *to allow formula to flow through it.* The height at which you hold the syringe will determine flow rate. When the syringe is three-quarters empty, pour more formula into it.

• *To prevent air from entering the tube and the patient's stomach,* never allow the syringe to empty completely. If you're using an infusion controller, set the flow rate according to the manufacturer's directions. *To prevent sudden stomach distention, which can cause nausea, vomiting, cramps, or diarrhea,* always administer a tube feeding slowly — typically 7 to 12 oz (200 to 350 ml) over 15 to 30 minutes, depending on the patient's tolerance and the doctor's order.

• After administering the appropriate amount of formula, flush the tubing by adding about 2 oz (60 ml) of water to the gavage bag or bulb syringe, or manually flush it using a barrel syringe. *This maintains the tube's patency by removing excess formula, which could occlude the tube.*

• If you're administering a continuous feeding, flush the feeding tube every 4 hours *to help prevent tube occlusion.* Monitor gastric emptying every 4 hours.

• To discontinue gastric feeding (depending on the equipment you're using), close the regulator clamp on the gavage bag tubing, disconnect the syringe from the feeding tube, or turn off the infusion controller.

• Cover the end of the feeding tube with its plug or cap *to prevent leakage and contamination of the tube.*

• Leave the patient in a semi-Fowler or high Fowler position for at least 30 minutes.

• Rinse all reusable equipment with warm water. Dry it and store it in a convenient place for the next feeding. Change equipment every 24 hours or according to the hospital's policy.

To deliver a duodenal or jejunal feeding

• Elevate the head of the bed and place the patient in low Fowler's position.

• Open the enteral administration set and hang the gavage container on the I.V. pole.

• If you're using a nasoduodenal tube, measure its length *to check tube placement.* Remember that you may not get any residual when you aspirate the tube.

• Open the flow clamp and regulate the flow to the desired rate. To regulate the rate using a volumetric infusion pump, follow the manufacturer's directions for setting up the equipment. Most patients receive small amounts initially, with volumes increasing gradually once tolerance is established.

• Flush the tube every 4 hours with water *to maintain patency and provide hydration.* A needle catheter jejunostomy tube may require flushing every 2 hours *to prevent formula buildup inside the tube.* A Y-connector may be useful for frequent flushing. Attach the continuous feeding to the main port and use the side port for flushes.

Complications

• Erosion of esophageal, tracheal, nasal, and oropharyngeal mucosa can result if tubes are left in place for a long time. If possible, use smaller-lumen tubes *to prevent such irritation. Check hospital policy regarding the frequen-*

cy of changing feeding tubes to prevent complications.
• Using the gastric route, frequent or large-volume feedings can cause bloating and retention.
• Dehydration, diarrhea, and vomiting can cause metabolic disturbances. Glycosuria, cramping, and abdominal distention usually indicate intolerance.
• Clogging of the feeding tube is common when the duodenal or jejunal route is used.
• The patient may experience metabolic, fluid, and electrolyte abnormalities including hyperglycemia, glycosuria, hyperosmolar dehydration, coma, edema, hypernatremia, and essential fatty acid deficiency.
• The patient also may experience dumping syndrome, in which a large amount of hyperosmotic solution in the duodenum causes excessive diffusion of fluid through the semipermeable membrane and results in diarrhea. In a patient with low serum albumin levels, these symptoms may result from low oncotic pressure in the duodenal mucosa.

Nursing considerations
• If the feeding solution doesn't initially flow through a bulb syringe, attach the bulb and squeeze it gently to start the flow. Then remove the bulb. Never use the bulb to force the formula through the tube.
• If the patient becomes nauseated or vomits, stop the feeding immediately. The patient may vomit if the stomach becomes distended from overfeeding or delayed gastric emptying.
• *To reduce oropharyngeal discomfort from the tube,* allow the patient to brush his teeth or care for his dentures

regularly, and encourage frequent gargling. If the patient is unconscious, administer oral care with lemon-glycerin swabs every 4 hours. Use petroleum jelly on dry, cracked lips. (Remember: Dry mucous membranes may indicate dehydration, which requires increased fluid intake.) Clean the patient's nostrils with cotton-tipped applicators, apply lubricant along the mucosa, and assess the skin for signs of breakdown.
• During continuous feedings, assess the patient frequently for abdominal distention. Flush the tubing by adding about 50 ml of water to the gavage bag or bulb syringe. *This maintains the tube's patency by removing excess formula, which could occlude the tube.*
• If the patient develops diarrhea, administer small, frequent, less concentrated feedings, or administer bolus feedings over a longer time. Also, make sure that the formula isn't cold and that proper storage and sanitation practices have been followed. The loose stools associated with tube feedings make extra perineal and skin care necessary. Giving paregoric, tincture of opium, or diphenoxylate hydrochloride may improve the condition. Changing to a formula with more fiber may eliminate liquid stools.
• If the patient becomes constipated, the doctor may increase the fruit, vegetable, or sugar content of the formula. Assess the patient's hydration status *because dehydration may produce constipation.* Increase fluid intake as necessary. If the condition persists, administer an appropriate drug or enema as ordered.
• Drugs can be administered through the feeding tube. Except for enteric-

coated drugs or sustained-release medications, crush tablets or open and dissolve capsule contents in water before administering them. Be sure to flush the tubing afterward *to ensure full instillation of medication.* Keep in mind that some drugs may change the osmolarity of the feeding formula and cause diarrhea.

• Small-bore feeding tubes may kink, making instillation impossible. If you suspect this problem, try changing the patient's position, or withdraw the tube a few inches and restart. Never use a guide wire to reposition the tube.

• Constantly monitor the flow rate of a blended or high-residue formula *to determine if the formula is clogging the tubing as it settles. To prevent such clogging,* squeeze the bag frequently to agitate the solution.

• Glycosuria, hyperglycemia, and diuresis can indicate an excessive carbohydrate level, leading to hyperosmotic dehydration, which may be fatal. Collect urine specimens every 4 to 6 hours, and blood specimens as ordered. Monitor urine and blood glucose levels *to assess glucose tolerance.* (A patient with a serum glucose level of less than 200 mg/100 ml and without glycosuria is considered stable.) Also monitor serum electrolytes, blood urea nitrogen, serum glucose, serum osmolality, and other pertinent findings *to determine the patient's response to therapy and assess his hydration status.*

• Check the flow rate hourly to ensure correct infusion. (With an improvised administration set, use a time tape to record the rate *because it's difficult to get precise readings from an irrigation container or enema bag.*)

• For duodenal or jejunal feeding, most patients tolerate a continuous drip better than bolus feedings. *Bolus feedings can cause such complications as hyperglycemia, glycosuria, and diarrhea.*

• Until the patient acquires a tolerance for the formula, you may need to dilute it to half or three-quarters strength to start, and increase it gradually. Patients under stress or who are receiving steroids may experience a pseudodiabetic state. Assess them frequently to determine the need for insulin.

Home care

• Patient education for home tube feeding includes instructions on an infusion control device to maintain accuracy, use of the syringe or bag and tubing, care of the tube and insertion site, and formula mixing. Formula may be mixed in an electric blender according to package directions. Formula not used within 24 hours must be discarded. If the formula must hang for more than 8 hours, advise the patient to use a gavage or pump administration set with an ice pouch to decrease the incidence of bacterial growth. Tell him to use a new bag every day.

• Family members should be instructed in signs and symptoms to report to the doctor or home care nurse, as well as measures to take in an emergency.

Documentation

• On the intake and output sheet, record the date, volume of formula, and volume of water.

• In your notes, include abdominal assessment (including tube exit site, if appropriate); amount of residuals;

verification of tube placement; amount, type, and time of feeding; and tube patency.

• Discuss the patient's tolerance of the feeding, including nausea, vomiting, cramping, diarrhea, and distention.

• Note the result of blood and urine tests, hydration state, and any drugs given through the tube. Include the date and time of administration set changes, oral and nasal hygiene, and results of specimen collections.

U

Ultrasonography

These noninvasive diagnostic procedures show the size, shape, and motion of internal structures. They are useful for evaluating many different conditions. All forms of ultrasonography use sound waves and the echoes they produce to "see" structures in the body. Results are interpreted by studying tracings made on a strip chart or videotape.

Echocardiography. In this procedure, a transducer directs ultrahigh-frequency sound waves toward cardiac structures, which reflect these waves. The echoes are converted to images displayed on an oscilloscope screen and recorded on a strip chart or videotape. Results are correlated with clinical history, physical examination, and findings from other tests.

Transesophageal echocardiography (TEE). This procedure combines ultrasound with endoscopy to obtain a better view of cardiac structures. In TEE, a small transducer is attached to the end of a gastroscope and inserted into the esophagus, which allows images to be taken from the posterior aspect of the heart. This causes less interference from chest wall structures and produces high-quality images of the thoracic aorta, except for the superior ascending aorta, which is shadowed by the trachea.

Thyroid ultrasonography. This procedure can differentiate between a cyst and a tumor larger than ⅜" (1 cm). This procedure is also used to evaluate thyroid nodules during pregnancy because it doesn't require use of radioactive iodine.

Doppler ultrasonography. This procedure is used to evaluate blood flow in the major veins and arteries of the arms and legs, and to evaluate blood flow in the extracranial cerebrovascular system. Although it can accurately detect arteriovenous disease that impairs blood flow by at least 50%, it may not reveal mild arteriosclerotic plaques, small thrombi, or major calf-vein thrombosis.

Measurement of systolic pressure during this procedure is used to detect the presence, location, and extent of peripheral arterial occlusive disease. Changes in sound wave frequency during respiration are observed to detect venous occlusive disease. Compression maneuvers can also help detect occlusion of the veins and occlusion or stenosis of carotid arteries. Pulse volume recorder testing may be performed with Doppler ultrasonography to record changes in blood volume or flow in an extremity or organ.

Ultrasonography of the abdominal aorta. This procedure uses a transducer to direct high-frequency sound waves into the abdomen over a wide area from the xiphoid process to the umbilical region. The echoing sound waves indicate organs, the vertebral column, and the size and course of the abdominal aorta and other major vessels.

Ultrasonography of the gallbladder and biliary system. This procedure confirms diagnosis of cholelithiasis (oral cholecystography may be performed if ultrasound is inconclusive) and acute cholecystitis. Ultrasonography also distinguishes between obstructive and nonobstructive jaundice.

Ultrasonography of the liver. This procedure shows intrahepatic structures and liver size, shape, and position. It is indicated in patients with:
• jaundice of unknown etiology.
• unexplained hepatomegaly and abnormal biochemical test results.
• suspected metastatic tumors and elevated serum alkaline phosphatase levels.
• recent abdominal trauma.

When used with liver-spleen scanning, ultrasonography can define cold spots (focal defects that fail to pick up the radionuclide), such as tumors, abscesses, or cysts, and can provide better views of the periportal and perihepatic spaces than liver-spleen scanning.

Ultrasonography of the spleen. This technique indicates size, shape, and position of the spleen and surrounding viscera. The test is indicated in patients with:
• an upper left quadrant mass of unknown origin.
• known splenomegaly.
• local tenderness.
• recent abdominal trauma.

Ultrasonography of the pancreas. This ultrasound technique indicates size, shape, and position of the pancreas and surrounding viscera.

Renal ultrasonography. This procedure can be used to detect abnormalities or to clarify abnormalities detected by other tests. It is especially useful in cases where excretory urography is ruled out. Unlike excretory urography, this test is not dependent on renal function and so may be useful in patients with renal failure.

Transcranial Doppler studies provide information about the presence, quality, and changing nature of circulation to an area of the brain by measuring velocity of blood flow through cerebral arteries. Narrowed blood vessels produce high velocities, indicating possible stenosis or vasospasm. High velocities may also indicate an arteriovenous malformation.

Pelvic ultrasonography is used to obtain images of the interior pelvic area. Purposes of pelvic ultrasonography include:
• evaluation of symptoms suggesting pelvic disease and confirmation of tentative diagnosis
• detection of foreign bodies and distinction between cystic and solid masses (tumors)
• measurement of organ size
• evaluation of fetal viability, position, gestational age, and growth rate
• detection of multiple fetuses
• confirmation of fetal and maternal abnormalities
• guidance of amniocentesis by determining placental location and fetal position.

Techniques of sound imaging include A-mode (amplitude modulation, recorded as spikes), B-mode (brightness modulation), gray scale (a representation of organ texture in shades of gray), and real-time imaging (instantaneous images of the tissues in motion, similar to fluoroscopic examination). Selected views may be photographed for later examination and to provide a permanent record.

⟫ Key nursing diagnoses and patient outcomes

Use these nursing diagnoses as a guide when developing your plan of care.

Anxiety related to situational crisis
Based on this nursing diagnosis, you'll establish the following patient outcomes. The patient will:
• state at least two ways to eliminate or minimize anxious behaviors.
• report being able to cope with current situation without experiencing severe anxiety.

Knowledge deficit related to lack of exposure to ultrasonography
Based on this nursing diagnosis, you'll establish the following patient outcomes. The patient will:
• communicate a need to know.
• state or demonstrate understanding of procedure.

Equipment

For TEE: ♦ cardiac monitor ♦ sedative ♦ topical anesthetic ♦ bite block ♦ gastroscope ♦ ultrasonography equipment ♦ suction equipment ♦ resuscitation equipment.

For thyroid ultrasonography: ♦ sonographic equipment ♦ camera and film or videotape. ♦ water-soluble contact solution.

For Doppler ultrasonography: ♦ handheld transducer ♦ water-soluble conductive jelly ♦ sphygmomanometer.

For abdominal aorta ultrasonography: ♦ acoustic coupling gel or mineral oil ♦ sonographic equipment ♦ camera and film or videotape.

For gallbladder and biliary system, liver, spleen, and pancreas ultrasonography: ♦ sonographic equipment ♦ camera and film ♦ water-soluble contact solution.

For renal ultrasonography: ♦ transducer and jelly ♦ cathode ray tube and amplifier ♦ oscilloscope ♦ camera ♦ dynamic or real-time imaging equipment.

For transcranial Doppler ultrasonography: ♦ transcranial Doppler unit ♦ Doppler probe ♦ water-soluble conductive jelly.

For pelvic ultrasonography: ♦ Mineral oil or water-soluble conductive jelly ♦ ultrasound machine and transducer ♦ camera and film ♦ oscilloscope.

Equipment preparation

• Gather equipment at the patient's bedside.
• Attach transducer cable to the monitor if necessary.
• Apply conductive jelly or solution to the probe surface.

Patient preparation

For general ultrasonography (including thyroid, Doppler, and renal procedures)
• Explain what the purpose of the test is and who will perform it and where.
• Tell the patient the test may take 15 to 30 minutes and that it is safe and painless.
• Explain that the room may be darkened slightly to aid visualization on the oscilloscope screen or other monitoring device and that other procedures may be performed simultaneously.
• Describe the procedure and instruct the patient to remain still during the test because movement may distort results.

• Ask the patient about any allergies and note them on the chart.

• Make sure the patient or a responsible family member signs a consent form if required.

• Instruct the patient to remove all clothing above or below the waist, depending on the test site, and place the patient in supine position on the examining table or bed, with the arms at the sides.

For TEE

• Explain the purpose of the test and who will perform it. Instruct the patient to fast for 6 hours beforehand.

• Review the patient's medical history for possible contraindications to the test, such as esophageal obstruction or varices, GI bleeding, previous mediastinal radiation therapy, or severe cervical arthritis.

• Before the test, have the patient remove any dentures or oral prostheses, and note any loose teeth.

• Explain to the patient that a topical anesthetic will be sprayed in his throat before the procedure and that he may gag when the tube is inserted.

• Tell him that an I.V. line will be inserted to administer sedation before the procedure and that he may feel some discomfort from the needle puncture and the pressure of the tourniquet. Reassure him that he'll be made as comfortable as possible during the procedure and that his blood pressure and heart rate will be monitored continuously.

For ultrasonography of the abdominal aorta

• Instruct the patient to fast for 12 hours before the test *to minimize bowel gas and motility.*

• Describe the procedure and reassure the patient with a known aneurysm that the sound waves will not cause rupture.

• Give simethicone *to reduce bowel gas.*

For ultrasonography of the gallbladder and biliary system

• Instruct the patient to eat a fat-free meal in the evening and then to fast for 8 to 12 hours before the procedure if possible; *this promotes accumulation of bile in the gallbladder and enhances ultrasonic visualization.*

For ultrasonography of the liver, spleen, and pancreas

• Instruct the patient to fast for 8 to 12 hours before the test *to reduce bowel gas, which hinders transmission of ultrasound.*

For transcranial Doppler ultrasonography

• Be sure to remove turban head dressings or thick dressings over the test site.

For pelvic ultrasonography

• *Because this test requires a full bladder as a landmark to define pelvic organs,* instruct the patient to drink liquids and not to void before the test.

• Tell her who will perform the procedure and where, and that it can vary in length from a few minutes to several hours.

• Explain that a water enema may be necessary *to produce a better outline of the large intestine.*

• Reassure the patient that the test will not harm the fetus, and provide emotional support throughout.

Implementation

Follow the steps below to administer different types of ultrasound tests.

Echocardiography

• The patient is placed in supine position.

• Conductive jelly is applied to the test area and the transducer is placed directly over it.

• The transducer is systematically angled to direct ultrasonic waves at specific parts.

• Significant oscilloscopic findings are recorded on a strip chart recorder.

• For a left lateral view, the patient may be positioned on his left side.

• To record heart function under various conditions, the patient is asked to inhale and exhale slowly, to hold his breath, or to inhale amyl nitrite.

• Conductive jelly is removed from the patient's skin.

Thyroid ultrasonography

• The patient is placed in a supine position, with a pillow under the shoulder blades to hyperextend the neck.

• The patient's neck is coated with water-soluble gel, and scanning proceeds.

• The image on the oscilloscope screen is photographed for subsequent examination.

TEE

• Connect the patient to a cardiac monitor so that his blood pressure and pulse oximetry can be assessed during the procedure.

• Help him lie down on his left side, and administer the prescribed sedative.

• The back of the patient's throat is sprayed with a topical anesthetic.

• A bite block is placed in his mouth, and he's instructed to close his lips around it.

• A gastroscope is introduced and advanced 12″ to 14″ (31 to 36 cm) to the level of the right atrium. To visualize the left ventricle, the scope is advanced 16″ to 18″ (41 to 46 cm).

• Ultrasound images are recorded and then reviewed after the procedure.

Doppler ultrasonography

• During lower extremity tests, a blood pressure cuff is wrapped around the calf, pressure readings are obtained, and waveforms recorded from the dorsalis pedis and posterior tibial arteries. Then the cuff is wrapped around the thigh, and waveforms are recorded at the popliteal artery.

• In upper extremity tests, examination is performed on one arm, with the patient first in a supine position and then sitting; it's then repeated on the other arm. A blood pressure cuff is wrapped around the forearm, pressure readings are taken, and waveforms are recorded over both the radial and ulnar arteries. Then, the cuff is wrapped around the upper arm, pressure readings are taken, and waveforms are recorded with the transducer over the brachial artery. Blood pressure readings and waveform recordings are repeated with the arm in extreme hyperextension and hyperabduction to check for possible compression factors that may interfere with arterial blood flow.

• During lower extremity tests, the patient is asked to perform Valsalva's maneuver, and venous blood flow is recorded.

Ultrasonography of the abdominal aorta

• The patient is placed in a supine position, and acoustic coupling gel or mineral oil is applied to his abdomen.
• Longitudinal scans are made at 0.5- to 1-cm intervals left and right of the midline until the entire abdominal aorta is outlined; transverse scans are made at $\frac{3}{8}''$ to $\frac{3}{4}''$ (1- to 2-cm) intervals from the xiphoid to the bifurcation at the common iliac arteries.
• The patient may be placed in right and left lateral positions.
• Appropriate views are photographed or videotaped.
• Remove the acoustic coupling gel.
• Instruct the patient to resume his usual diet and medications.
• Aneurysms may expand and dissect rapidly, so check the patient's vital signs frequently.

Note: Remember that sudden onset of constant abdominal or back pain accompanies rapid expansion of the aneurysm; sudden, excruciating pain with weakness, sweating, tachycardia, and hypotension signals rupture.

Ultrasonography of the gallbladder and biliary system

• Transverse and longitudinal oblique scans of the gallbladder are taken.
• During each scan, the patient is asked to exhale deeply and hold his breath. (If the gallbladder is positioned deeply under the right costal margin, a scan may be taken through the intercostal spaces, while the patient inhales deeply and holds his breath.)
• The patient is then placed in a left lateral decubitus position and is scanned beneath the right costal margin. (This position and scanning angle

may displace and allow detection of stones lodged in the cystic duct region.)
• Scanning with the patient erect helps demonstrate mobility or fixedness of suspicious echogenic areas. Oscilloscopic views may be photographed for later study.

Ultrasonography of the liver

• Transverse scans between the costal margins demonstrate the left lobe of the liver and part of the right lobe; sector scans through the intercostal spaces are used to view the remainder of the right lobe.
• Scans are taken longitudinally from the right border of the liver to the left.
• For better demonstration of the right lateral dome, oblique cephalad-angled scans may be taken beneath the right costal margin.
• Scans are then taken parallel to the hepatic portal, at a 45-degree angle toward the superior right lateral dome, to examine the peripheral anatomy, portal venous system, common bile duct, and biliary tree. Clear images are photographed for later study.
• During each scan, the patient is asked to hold his breath briefly in deep inspiration *to displace the liver caudally from the costal margin and the ribs to aid visualization.*

Ultrasonography of the spleen

• Generally, the patient is first placed in supine position, with his chest uncovered.
• A water-soluble lubricant is applied to the face of the transducer, and transverse scans of the spleen are taken at $\frac{3}{8}''$ to $\frac{3}{4}''$ (1- to 2-cm) intervals.
• The patient is then placed in right lateral decubitus position, and trans-

verse scans are taken through the intercostal spaces using a sectoring motion.

• A pillow may be placed under the patient's right side to help separate the intercostal spaces, making it easier to position the transducer face between them.

• Longitudinal scans are taken from the axilla toward the iliac crest.

• To prevent rib artifacts and obtain the best view of the splenic parenchyma, oblique scans are taken by passing the transducer face along the intercostal spaces.

• During each scan, the patient may be asked to hold his breath briefly at various stages of inspiration.

• Good views are photographed for later study.

Ultrasonography of the pancreas

• A water-soluble lubricant or mineral oil is applied to the abdomen and, with the patient at full inspiration, transverse scans are taken at 1-cm intervals, starting from the xiphoid and moving caudally; longitudinal scans are taken to view the head, body, and tail of the pancreas in sequence; scanning the right anterior oblique view allows imaging of the head and body of the pancreas; oblique sagittal scans are used to view the portal vein; and scanning from the sagittal view images the vena cava.

• Good oscilloscopic views are photographed for later study.

Renal ultrasonography

• The patient is placed in prone position, the area to be scanned is exposed, and ultrasound jelly is applied to the area.

• The longitudinal axis of the kidneys is located by using measurements from excretory urography or by performing transverse scans through the upper and lower renal poles.

• These points are marked on the skin and connected with straight lines. Sectional images $\frac{3}{8}''$ to $\frac{3}{4}''$ (1 to 2 cm) apart can then be obtained.

• During the test, the patient may be asked to breathe deeply to assess the kidneys' movement during respiration.

Transcranial Doppler ultrasonography

• A small amount of gel is applied to the transcranial window (an area where bone is thin enough to allow the Doppler signal to enter and be detected); the most common approaches are temporal, transorbital, and through the foramen magnum.

• The technician directs the signal toward the artery being studied and records the velocities detected; waveforms may be printed for later analysis.

• The Doppler signal can be transmitted to varying depths.

Pelvic ultrasonography

• With the patient in supine position, the pelvic area is coated with mineral oil or water-soluble jelly to increase sound wave conduction.

• The transducer is guided over the area, images are observed on the oscilloscope screen, and a good image is photographed.

• The patient is allowed to empty her bladder immediately after the test.

Nursing considerations

For general ultrasonography (including thyroid, Doppler, and renal procedures)
• Remove gel or paste from the patient's skin after the procedure.

For TEE
• Keep resuscitation equipment available.
• Have suction equipment nearby *to avoid aspiration if vomiting occurs.*
• Vasovagal responses may occur with gagging, so observe the cardiac monitor closely.
• Use pulse oximetry *to detect hypoxia.*
• If bleeding occurs, stop the procedure immediately.
• Laryngospasm, arrhythmias, and bleeding increase the risk of complications. If any of these occurs, postpone the test.
• Do not place the Doppler probe over an open or draining lesion.
• Monitor the patient's vital signs and oxygen levels for any changes.
• Keep the patient in a supine position until the sedative wears off.
• Encourage the patient to cough after the procedure, either while lying on his side or sitting upright.
• Do not give food or water until the patient's gag response returns.
• If the procedure is done on an outpatient basis, make sure someone is available to drive the patient home.
• Treat sore throat symptomatically.

Documentation
• Document the specific procedure and note the patient's tolerance to it on the nursing documentation flow sheet.

Upper GI and small-bowel series

This diagnostic procedure is the fluoroscopic examination of the esophagus, stomach, and small intestine after the patient ingests barium sulfate, a contrast agent. As the barium passes through the digestive tract, fluoroscopy outlines peristalsis and the mucosal contours of the respective organs, and spot films record significant findings. This test is indicated in patients who have upper GI symptoms (difficulty in swallowing, regurgitation, burning or gnawing epigastric pain), signs of small-bowel disease (diarrhea, weight loss), and signs of GI bleeding (hematemesis, melena). Although this test can detect various mucosal abnormalities, subsequent biopsy is often necessary to rule out malignancy or distinguish specific inflammatory diseases. Oral cholecystography, barium enema, and routine radiography should always precede this test because retained barium clouds anatomic detail on X-ray films.

❯❯ Key nursing diagnoses and patient outcomes
Use these nursing diagnoses as a guide when developing your plan of care.

Pain related to physical or chemical agents
Based on this nursing diagnosis, you'll establish the following patient outcomes. The patient will:
• express a feeling of comfort and relief from pain.

• state and carry out appropriate interventions for pain relief.

Diarrhea related to irritation of bowel

Based on this nursing diagnosis, you'll establish the following patient outcomes. The patient will:
• have elimination pattern return to normal.
• regain and maintain fluid and electrolyte balance.

Equipment

♦ contrast agent ♦ enema administration equipment ♦ cathartic, such as castor oil.

Patient preparation

• Explain to the patient that this procedure uses ingested barium and X-ray films to examine the esophagus, stomach, and small intestine.
• Tell him to consume a low-residue diet for 2 or 3 days before the test and then to fast and avoid smoking after midnight the night before the test.
• Describe the test, including who will perform it, where it will take place, and how long it's expected to take (up to 6 hours).
• Encourage the patient to bring reading material.
• Inform the patient that he'll be placed on an X-ray table that rotates into vertical, semivertical, and horizontal positions.
• Explain that he'll be adequately secured and that he will be assisted to supine, prone, and side-lying positions.
• Describe the barium mixture's milk shake consistency and chalky taste. Although it's flavored, he may find its taste unpleasant. Tell him he must drink 16 to 20 oz (475 to 590 ml) for a complete examination.
• Inform him that his abdomen may be compressed to ensure proper coating of the stomach or intestinal walls with barium, or to separate overlapping bowel loops.
• As prescribed, withhold most oral medications after midnight and anticholinergics and narcotics for 24 hours *because these drugs affect small intestinal motility.* Antacids are also sometimes withheld for several hours if gastric reflux is suspected.
• Just before the procedure, instruct the patient to put on a hospital gown without snap closures and to remove jewelry, dentures, hair clips, or other objects that might obscure anatomic detail on the X-ray films.

Implementation

• After the patient is secured in a supine position on the radiographic table, the table is tilted until the patient is erect. The heart, lungs, and abdomen are examined fluoroscopically.
• The patient is instructed to take several swallows of the barium suspension, and its passage through the esophagus is observed. (Occasionally, the patient is given a thick barium suspension, especially when esophageal pathology is strongly suspected.)
• During fluoroscopic examination, spot films of the esophagus are taken from lateral angles and from right and left posteroanterior angles.
• When barium enters the stomach, the patient's abdomen is palpated or compressed *to ensure adequate coating of the gastric mucosa with barium.*
• To perform a double-contrast examination, the patient is instructed to sip the barium through a perforated straw.

As he does so, a small amount of air is also introduced into the stomach, which permits detailed examination of the gastric rugae, and spot films of significant findings are then taken. The patient is then instructed to ingest the remaining barium suspension and the filling of the stomach and emptying into the duodenum are observed fluoroscopically.

• Two series of spot films of the stomach and duodenum are taken from posteroanterior, anteroposterior, lateral, and oblique angles, with the patient erect and then in a supine position.

• The passage of barium into the remainder of the small intestine is then observed fluoroscopically and spot films are taken at 30- to 60-minute intervals until the barium reaches the ileocecal valve region. If abnormalities in the small intestine are detected, the area is palpated and compressed to help clarify the defect, and a spot film is taken. The examination ends when the barium enters the cecum.

• Make sure that additional X-rays haven't been ordered before allowing the patient to have food, fluids, and oral medications (if applicable).

Complications

• The upper GI and small-bowel series is contraindicated in patients with digestive tract obstruction or perforation. Barium may intensify the obstruction or seep into the abdominal cavity. If a perforation is suspected, gastrografin may be used instead of barium.

Nursing considerations

• Administer a cathartic or enema to the patient. Tell him his stool will be lightly colored for 24 to 72 hours. Record and describe any stool passed by the patient in the hospital. *Retention of barium in the intestine may cause obstruction or fecal impaction. Also, it may affect scheduling of other GI studies.*

Documentation

• Document patient tolerance of procedure, type of cathartic given, and results.

Urinary catheter care

Routine catheter care is intended to prevent infection and other complications by keeping the catheter insertion site clean. It is is typically performed daily after the patient's morning bath and immediately after perineal care. (Bedtime catheter care may have to be performed before perineal care.)

Because some studies suggest that catheter care increases the risk of infection and other complications instead of lowering it, many hospitals don't recommend daily catheter care. Therefore, individual hospital policy dictates whether or not a patient receives such care. Regardless of the catheter care policy, the equipment and the patient's genitalia require inspection twice daily.

⟫ Key nursing diagnoses and patient outcomes

Use these nursing diagnoses as a guide when developing your plan of care for a patient who is having indwelling urinary catheter care.

Altered urinary elimination related to presence of an indwelling catheter

Based on this nursing diagnosis, you'll establish the following patient outcomes. The patient will:
• maintain fluid balance; intake equals output.
• have complications avoided or minimized.
• describe feelings and concerns regarding indwelling urinary catheter.

Risk for infection related to presence of indwelling urinary catheter

Based on this nursing diagnosis, you'll establish the following patient outcomes. The patient will:
• have no pathogens appear in cultures.
• remain afebrile.
• show no evidence of urinary tract infection, such as urine that is cloudy, malodorous, or with sediment.

Equipment

For catheter care: ◆ povidone-iodine (or other antiseptic cleaning agent) ◆ sterile gloves ◆ basin ◆ eight sterile $4'' \times 4''$ gauze pads ◆ sterile absorbent cotton balls or cotton-tipped applicators ◆ leg bag ◆ collection bag ◆ adhesive tape ◆ waste receptacle ◆ optional: safety pin, rubber band, gooseneck lamp or flashlight, adhesive remover, antibiotic ointment, specimen container.

For perineal cleaning: ◆ washcloth ◆ additional basin ◆ soap and water.

Commercially prepared catheter care kits containing all necessary supplies are available.

Equipment preparation

• Wash your hands, and bring all equipment to the patient's bedside. Open the gauze pads, place several in the first basin, and pour some povidone-iodine or other cleaning agent over them.
• Some hospitals specify that, after wiping the urinary meatus with cleaning solution, you should wipe it off with wet, sterile gauze pads *to prevent possible irritation from the cleaning solution.* If this is your hospital's policy, pour water into the second basin, and moisten three more gauze pads.

Patient preparation

• Explain the procedure and its purpose to the patient.
• Provide privacy, and make sure that the lighting is adequate *so you can see the perineum and catheter tubing clearly.* Place a gooseneck lamp at the bedside if needed.

Implementation

• Inspect the catheter for any problems, and check the urine drainage for mucus, blood clots, sediment, and turbidity. Then pinch the catheter between two fingers *to determine if the lumen contains any material.* If you notice any of these conditions (or if hospital policy requires it), obtain a urine specimen (about 6 oz [17.4 ml]), and notify the doctor.
• Inspect the outside of the catheter where it enters the urinary meatus *for encrusted material and suppurative drainage.* Also inspect the tissue around the meatus for irritation or swelling.
• Remove any adhesive tape securing the catheter to the patient's thigh or abdomen. Inspect the area for signs of

Avoiding injury when cleaning a catheter

When cleaning your patient's indwelling catheter, be sure not to pull on it. Pulling on the catheter can cause injury to the urethra and the bladder wall. It can also expose a section of the catheter that was inside the urethra, so that when you release the catheter, the newly contaminated section will reenter the urethra, introducing potentially infectious organisms.

Before securing the catheter, provide enough slack to prevent tension on the tubing. This will help you to avoid injuring the urethral lumen or bladder wall.

adhesive burns — redness, tenderness, or blisters.

• Put on the sterile gloves. Then use a saturated, sterile gauze pad or cotton-tipped applicator to clean the outside of the catheter and the tissue around the meatus. *To avoid contaminating the urinary tract,* always clean by wiping away from — never toward — the urinary meatus. Use a dry gauze pad to remove encrusted material. (See *Avoiding injury when cleaning a catheter.*)

• Remove your gloves, and tear a piece of adhesive tape from the roll.

• *To prevent skin hypersensitivity or irritation,* retape the catheter to the other thigh or opposite side of the abdomen.

• Most drainage bags have a plastic clamp on the tubing to attach them to the sheet. If this isn't available, wrap a rubber band around the drainage tubing, insert the safety pin through a loop of the rubber band, and pin the tubing to the sheet below the patient's bladder level. Then attach the collection bag, below bladder level, to the bed frame.

• If necessary, clean residue from the previous tape site with adhesive remover. Then dispose of all used supplies in a waste receptacle.

Complications

• Sediment buildup, such as casts or mucus plugs, can occur anywhere in a catheterization system, especially in bedridden and dehydrated patients. *To prevent sediment buildup,* keep the patient well hydrated if he's not on fluid restriction. Change the indwelling catheter as ordered or when malfunction, obstruction, or contamination occurs.

• Acute renal failure may result from a catheter obstructed by sediment. Be alert for sharply reduced urine flow from the catheter. Assess for bladder discomfort or distention.

• Urinary tract infection is caused by endogenous or exogenous bacteria introduced into the urethra. This can occur during catheter insertion or from intraluminal or extraluminal migration of bacteria up the catheter. Signs and symptoms vary but may include cloudy urine, hematuria, fever, malaise, tenderness over the bladder, and flank pain.

Nursing considerations

• Your hospital may require the use of specific cleaning agents for catheter care, so check the policy manual before beginning this procedure. A doctor's order will also be needed to apply antibiotic ointments to the urinary meatus after cleaning.

• Avoid raising the drainage bag above bladder level. *This prevents reflux of urine, which may contain bacteria. To avoid damaging the urethral lumen or bladder wall,* always disconnect the drainage bag and tubing from the bed linen and bed frame before helping the patient out of bed.

• Encourage patients with unrestricted fluid intake to increase intake to at least 3,000 ml per day. *This helps flush the urinary system and reduces sediment formation. To prevent urinary sediment and calculi from obstructing the drainage tube,* some patients are placed on an acid-ash diet to acidify the urine. Cranberry juice, for example, may help to promote urinary acidity.

Home care
• When possible, attach a leg bag *to allow the patient greater mobility.* If the patient will be discharged with an indwelling catheter, teach him how to use a leg bag.

• Instruct patients discharged with indwelling catheters to wash the urinary meatus and perineal area with soap and water twice daily and the anal area after each bowel movement.

Documentation
• Record the care you performed, any necessary modifications in technique, any patient complaints or comments, and the condition of the perineum and urinary meatus.

• Note the character of the urine in the drainage bag, any sediment buildup, and whether a specimen was sent for laboratory analysis.

• Record fluid intake and output. An hourly record is usually necessary for critically ill patients and those with re-

nal insufficiency who are hemodynamically unstable.

Urinary catheter insertion

Also known as a Foley or retention catheter, an indwelling catheter remains in the bladder to provide continuous urine drainage. A balloon inflated at the catheter's distal end prevents it from slipping out of the bladder after insertion. Indwelling catheters are used most often to relieve bladder distention caused by urine retention and to allow continuous urine drainage when the urinary meatus is swollen from childbirth, surgery, or local trauma. Other indications for an indwelling catheter include urinary tract obstruction (by a tumor or enlarged prostate), urine retention or infection from neurogenic bladder paralysis caused by spinal cord injury or disease, and any illness in which the patient's urine output must be monitored closely.

An indwelling catheter is inserted using sterile technique and only when absolutely necessary. Insertion should be performed with extreme care to prevent injury and infection.

» Key nursing diagnoses and patient outcomes
Use these nursing diagnoses as a guide when developing your plan of care for a patient who is having an indwelling urinary catheter inserted.

Altered urinary elimination related to presence of an indwelling catheter

Based on this nursing diagnosis, you'll establish the following patient outcomes. The patient will:
• maintain fluid balance; intake equals output.
• have complications avoided or minimized.
• describe feelings and concerns regarding indwelling urinary catheter.

Risk for infection related to presence of indwelling urinary catheter

Based on this nursing diagnosis, you'll establish the following patient outcomes. The patient will:
• have no pathogens in cultures.
• remain afebrile.
• show no evidence of urinary tract infection, such as urine that is cloudy, malodorous, or with sediment.

Equipment

♦ sterile indwelling catheter (latex or silicone #10 to #22 French [average adult sizes are #16 to #18 French]) ♦ syringe filled with 5 to 8 ml of normal saline solution ♦ washcloth ♦ towel ♦ soap and water ♦ two linen-saver pads ♦ sterile gloves ♦ sterile drape ♦ sterile fenestrated drape ♦ sterile cotton-tipped applicators (or cotton balls and plastic forceps) ♦ povidone-iodine or other antiseptic cleaning agent ♦ urine receptacle ♦ sterile water-soluble lubricant ♦ sterile drainage collection bag ♦ intake and output sheet ♦ adhesive tape ♦ optional: urine-specimen container and laboratory request form, leg band with Velcro closure, gooseneck lamp.

Prepackaged sterile disposable kits are available and usually contain all the necessary equipment. The syringes in these kits are prefilled with normal saline solution.

Equipment preparation

• Check the order on the patient's chart *to determine if a catheter size or type has been specified.* Then wash your hands, select the appropriate equipment, and assemble it at the patient's bedside.

Patient preparation

• Explain the procedure.
• Check the patient's chart and ask when the patient last voided.
• Percuss and palpate the bladder *to establish baseline data.*
• Ask the patient if the urge to void is present.

Implementation

• So that you can see the urinary meatus clearly in poor lighting, place a gooseneck lamp next to the patient's bed.
• Place the female patient in the supine position, with her knees flexed and separated and her feet flat on the bed, about 2′ (61 cm) apart. If she finds this position uncomfortable, have her flex one knee and keep the other leg flat on the bed. You may need an assistant to help the patient stay in position or to direct the light. Place the male patient in the supine position with his legs extended and flat on the bed. Ask the patient to hold the position *to give you a clear view of the urinary meatus and to prevent contamination of the sterile field.*
• Use the washcloth to clean the patient's genital area and perineum thor-

oughly with soap and water. Dry the area with the towel. Then, wash your hands.

• Place the linen-saver pads on the bed between the patient's legs and under the hips. *To create the sterile field,* open the prepackaged kit or equipment tray and place it between the female patient's legs or next to the male patient's hip. If the sterile gloves are the first item on the top of the tray, put them on. Place the sterile drape under the patient's hips. Then drape the patient's lower abdomen with the sterile fenestrated drape so that only the genital area remains exposed. Take care not to contaminate your gloves.

• Open the rest of the kit or tray. Put on the sterile gloves if you haven't already done so.

• Tear open the packet of povidone-iodine or other antiseptic cleaning agent, and use it to saturate the sterile cotton balls or applicators. Be careful not to spill the solution on the equipment.

• Open the packet of water-soluble lubricant and apply it to the catheter tip; attach the drainage bag to the other end of the catheter. (If you're using a commercial kit, the drainage bag may be attached.) Make sure all tubing ends remain sterile, and be sure the clamp at the emptying port of the drainage bag is closed *to prevent urine leakage from the bag.* Some drainage systems have an air-lock chamber *to prevent bacteria from traveling to the bladder from urine in the drainage bag.*

• Before inserting the catheter, inflate the balloon with normal saline solution *to inspect it for leaks.* To do this, attach the saline-filled syringe to the luer-lock, then push the plunger and check for seepage as the balloon expands. Aspirate the saline *to deflate the balloon.* Also inspect the catheter for resiliency. *Rough, cracked catheters can injure the urethral mucosa during insertion, which can predispose the patient to infection.*

• For the female patient, separate the labia majora and labia minora as widely as possible with the thumb, middle, and index fingers of your nondominant hand (as shown) *so you have*

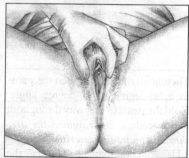

a full view of the urinary meatus. Keep the labia well separated throughout the procedure, *so they don't obscure the urinary meatus or contaminate the area once it's cleaned.*

• With your dominant hand, use a sterile, cotton-tipped applicator (or pick up a sterile cotton ball with the plastic forceps) and wipe one side of the urinary meatus with a single downward motion. Wipe the other side with an-

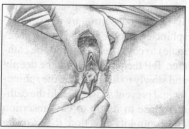

other sterile applicator or cotton ball in the same way. Then wipe directly

over the meatus with still another sterile applicator or cotton ball. Take care not to contaminate your sterile glove.
• For the male patient, hold the penis with your nondominant hand. If he's uncircumcised, retract the foreskin.

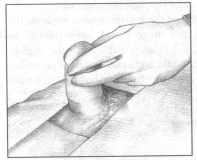

Then gently lift and stretch the penis to a 60-degree to 90-degree angle. Hold the penis in this way throughout the procedure *to straighten the urethra and maintain a sterile field*.
• Use your dominant hand to clean the glans with a sterile cotton-tipped applicator or a sterile cotton ball held in forceps. Clean in a circular motion, starting at the urinary meatus and working outward.
• Repeat the procedure using another sterile applicator or cotton ball. Take care to avoid contaminating your sterile glove.
• Pick up the catheter with your dominant hand and prepare to insert the lubricated tip into the urinary meatus. To facilitate insertion by relaxing the sphincter, ask the patient (male or female) to cough as you insert the catheter. Tell the patient to breathe deeply and slowly to further relax the sphincter and prevent spasms. Hold the catheter close to its tip to ease insertion and control its direction. (See *Easing catheter insertion*.)

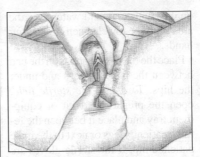

• For the female patient, advance the catheter about 2″ to 3″ (5 to 75 cm) — while continuing to hold the labia apart — until urine begins to flow (as shown at top of next page).

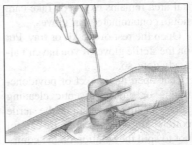

• For the male patient, advance the catheter about 6″ to 8″ (15 to 20 cm) until urine begins to flow. If the foreskin was retracted, be sure to replace it *to prevent compromised circulation and painful swelling*.

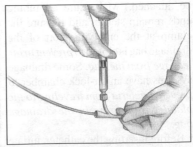

• When urine stops flowing, attach the saline-filled syringe to the luer-lock.

• Push the plunger, and inflate the balloon *to keep the catheter in place in the bladder*.

• Hang the collection bag below bladder level *to prevent urine reflux into the bladder, which can cause infection, and to facilitate gravity drainage of the bladder.* Make sure the tubing doesn't get tangled in the bed's side rails.

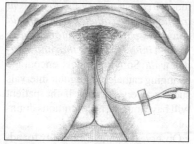

• Tape the catheter to the female patient's thigh *to prevent possible tension on the urogenital trigone.*

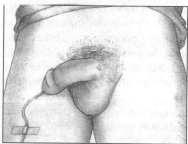

• Tape the catheter to the male patient's thigh or lower abdomen *to prevent pressure on the urethra at the penoscrotal junction, which can lead to formation of urethrocutaneous fistulas.*

• Also tape the catheter, as stated, to prevent traction on the bladder and alteration in the normal direction of urine flow in males.

• As an alternative, secure the catheter to the patient's thigh using a leg band

Easing catheter insertion

Never force a catheter during insertion. Maneuver it gently as the patient bears down or coughs. If you still meet resistance, stop the procedure and notify the doctor. Strictures, sphincter spasms, misplacement in the vagina (in females), or an enlarged prostate (in males) may cause resistance.

with a Velcro closure. *This decreases skin irritation, especially in patients with long-term indwelling catheters.*

• Properly dispose of all used supplies.

Complications

• Urinary tract infection can result from the introduction of bacteria into the bladder.

• Improper insertion can cause traumatic injury to the urethral and bladder mucosa.

• Bladder atony or spasms can result from rapid decompression of a severely distended bladder.

Nursing considerations

• Never inflate a balloon without first establishing urine flow, which assures you that the catheter is in the bladder, not in the urethral channel.

• Several types of catheters are available with balloons of various sizes. Each type has its own method of inflation and closure. For example, in one type of catheter, sterile solution or air is injected through the inflation lumen; then the end of the injection port is folded over itself and fastened with a clamp or rubber band.

Note. Injecting a catheter with air makes identifying leaks difficult and doesn't guarantee deflation of the balloon for removal.

• A similar catheter is inflated by penetrating a seal in the end of the inflation lumen with a needle or the hub of the solution-filled syringe. Another type of balloon catheter self-inflates when a prepositioned clamp is loosened. The balloon size determines the amount of solution needed for inflation, and the exact amount is usually printed on the distal extension of the catheter used for inflating the balloon.

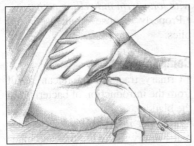

• If necessary, ask the female patient to lie on her side with her knees drawn up to her chest during the catheterization procedure. This position may be especially helpful for elderly or disabled patients, such as those with severe contractures.

• If the doctor orders a urine specimen for laboratory analysis, obtain it from the urine receptacle with a specimen collection container at the time of catheterization, and send it to the laboratory with the appropriate laboratory request form. Connect the drainage bag when urine stops flowing.

• Inspect the catheter and tubing periodically while they're in place *to detect compression or kinking that could obstruct urine flow.* Explain the basic principles of gravity drainage so that the patient realizes the importance of keeping the drainage tubing and collection bag lower than his bladder at all times. If necessary, provide the patient with detailed instructions for performing clean intermittent self-catheterization.

• For monitoring purposes, empty the collection bag at least every 8 hours. Excessive fluid volume may require more frequent emptying *to prevent traction on the catheter, which would cause the patient discomfort, and to prevent injury to the urethra and bladder wall.* Some hospitals encourage changing catheters at regular intervals such as every 30 days if the patient will have long-term continuous drainage.

• Observe the patient carefully for adverse reactions such as hypovolemic shock, caused by removing excessive volumes of residual urine. Check the hospital's policy beforehand to determine the maximum amount of urine that may be drained at one time (some limit the amount to 24 to 34 oz [700 to 1,000 ml]). Whether or not to limit the amount of urine drained is currently controversial. Clamp the catheter at the first sign of an adverse reaction, and notify the doctor.

Home care

• If the patient will be discharged with a long-term indwelling catheter, teach him and his family all aspects of daily catheter maintenance, including care of the skin and urinary meatus, signs and symptoms of urinary tract infection or obstruction, how to irrigate the catheter (if appropriate), and the importance of adequate fluid intake to maintain patency.

• Explain that a home care nurse should visit every 4 to 6 weeks, or more often if needed, to change the catheter.

• If appropriate, the patient or family can learn to perform intermittent self-catheterization. (See *Teaching self-catheterization,* page 774.)

Documentation

• Record the date, time, and size and type of indwelling catheter used.

• Describe the amount, color, and other characteristics of urine emptied from the bladder. Your hospital may require only the intake and output sheet for fluid-balance data. If large volumes of urine have been emptied, describe the patient's tolerance for the procedure.

• Note whether a urine specimen was sent for laboratory analysis.

Urinary catheter irrigation

To avoid introducing microorganisms into the bladder, the nurse irrigates an indwelling catheter only to remove an obstruction, such as a blood clot that develops after bladder, kidney, or prostate surgery.

≫ Key nursing diagnoses and patient outcomes

Use these nursing diagnoses as a guide when developing your plan of care for a patient who is having an indwelling urinary catheter irrigated.

Altered urinary elimination related to possible obstruction

Based on this nursing diagnosis, you'll establish the following patient outcomes. The patient will:

• maintain fluid balance; intake equals output.

• have complications avoided or minimized.

• describe feelings and concerns regarding indwelling urinary catheter.

Risk for infection related to presence of indwelling urinary catheter

Based on this nursing diagnosis, you'll establish the following patient outcomes. The patient will:

• have no pathogens appear in cultures.

• remain afebrile.

• show no evidence of urinary tract infection, such as urine that is cloudy, malodorous, or with sediment.

Equipment

♦ ordered irrigating solution (such as normal saline solution) ♦ sterile graduated receptacle or emesis basin ♦ sterile bulb syringe or 50-ml catheter-tip syringe ♦ two alcohol pads ♦ sterile gloves ♦ linen-saver pad ♦ intake-output sheet ♦ optional: basin of warm water.

Commercially packaged sterile irrigating kits are available and usually include irrigating solution, a graduated receptacle, and a bulb or 50-ml catheter-tip syringe.

If the volume of irrigating solution instilled must be measured, use a graduated syringe instead of a non-calibrated bulb syringe.

Equipment preparation

- Check the expiration date on the irrigating solution.
- To prevent vesical spasms during instillation of solution, warm it to room temperature. If necessary, place the container in a basin of warm water.
- Never heat the solution on a burner or in a microwave oven. Hot irrigating solution can injure the patient's bladder.
- Assemble equipment at bedside.

Patient preparation

- Explain the procedure.
- Provide privacy.

Implementation

- Wash your hands.
- Place the linen-saver pad under the patient's buttocks *to protect the bed linens.*
- Create a sterile field at the patient's bedside by opening the sterile equipment tray or commercial kit. Using aseptic technique, clean the lip of the solution bottle by pouring a small amount of solution into a sink or waste receptacle. Then pour the prescribed amount of solution into the graduated receptacle or emesis basin.
- Place the syringe hub into the solution. Squeeze the bulb or pull back the plunger (depending on the type of syringe), and fill the syringe with the appropriate amount of solution (usually 30 ml).
- Open the alcohol pads; then put on the sterile gloves. Clean the juncture of the catheter and drainage tube with an alcohol pad *to remove as many bacterial contaminants as possible.*
- Disconnect the catheter and drainage tube by twisting them in opposite directions and carefully pulling them

apart without creating tension on the catheter. Do not let go of the catheter; hold it in your nondominant hand. Then place the end of the drainage tube on the sterile field, making sure not to contaminate the tube.

- Twist the bulb syringe or catheter-tip syringe onto the catheter's distal end.
- Squeeze the bulb, or slowly push the plunger of the syringe to instill the irrigating solution through the catheter. If necessary, refill the syringe and repeat this step until you've instilled the prescribed amount of irrigating solution.
- Remove the syringe, and direct the return flow from the catheter into a graduated receptacle or emesis basin. Don't let the catheter end touch the drainage in the receptacle or become contaminated in any other way.
- Wipe the end of the drainage tube and catheter with the remaining alcohol pad.
- Wait a few seconds until the alcohol evaporates; then reattach the drainage tubing to the catheter.
- Properly dispose of all used supplies.

Complications

- Interruptions in a continuous irrigation system can predispose the patient to infection.

Nursing considerations

- Catheter irrigation requires strict aseptic technique to prevent bacteria from entering the bladder. The catheter and drainage tube ends and syringe hub must be kept sterile throughout this procedure.
- If you encounter any resistance during instillation of the irrigating solution, do not try to force the solution

into the bladder. Instead, stop the procedure, and notify the doctor. If an indwelling catheter becomes totally obstructed, obtain an order to remove it, and replace it with a new one *to prevent bladder distention, acute renal failure, urinary stasis, and subsequent infection.*

• Encourage catheterized patients not on restricted fluid intake to increase intake to 3,000 ml per day *to help flush the urinary system and reduce sediment formation. To keep the patient's urine acidic and help prevent calculus formation,* tell the patient to eat foods containing ascorbic acid, including citrus fruits and juices, cranberry juice, and dark green and deep yellow vegetables.

Documentation
• Note the amount, color, and consistency of return urine flow, and document the patient's tolerance for the procedure.
• Note any resistance during instillation of the solution. If the return flow volume is less than the amount of solution instilled, note this on the intake and output balance sheets and in your notes.

Urinary catheter removal

An indwelling catheter should be removed when bladder decompression is no longer necessary, when the patient can resume voiding, or when the catheter is obstructed. Depending on how long the patient was catheterized, the doctor may order bladder retraining before catheter removal.

⟫ Key nursing diagnoses and patient outcomes
Use these nursing diagnoses as a guide when developing your plan of care for a patient who is having an indwelling urinary catheter removed.

Altered urinary elimination related to presence of an indwelling catheter
Based on this nursing diagnosis, you'll establish the following patient outcomes. The patient will:
• maintain fluid balance; intake equals output.
• have complications avoided or minimized.
• describe feelings and concerns regarding indwelling urinary catheter and its removal.

Risk for infection related to presence of indwelling urinary catheter
Based on this nursing diagnosis, you'll establish the following patient outcomes. The patient will:
• have no pathogens in cultures.
• remain afebrile.
• show no evidence of urinary tract infection, such as urine that is cloudy, malodorous, or with sediment.

Equipment
♦ absorbent cotton ♦ gloves ♦ alcohol pad ♦ 10-ml syringe with a luer-lock ♦ bedpan ♦ optional: clamp for bladder retraining.

Equipment preparation
• If the doctor orders bladder retraining, follow these steps: Clamp the catheter for 2 hours; then release it for 5 minutes to empty the bladder. Repeat the procedure. *This gradual fill-*

ing and emptying helps restore the bladder's muscle tone.
• Assemble the equipment at the patient's bedside.

Patient preparation
• Explain the procedure.
• Tell the patient he may feel slight discomfort.
• Tell him that you'll check him periodically during the first 8 to 24 hours after catheter removal to make sure he resumes voiding.
• Provide privacy.

Implementation
• Wash your hands.
• Put on gloves. Attach the syringe to the luer-lock mechanism on the catheter.
• Pull back on the plunger of the syringe. *This deflates the balloon by aspirating the fluid injected at the time of catheter insertion.* The amount of fluid injected is usually indicated on the tip of the catheter's balloon lumen; it should also be noted on the Kardex and the patient's chart.
• Grasp the catheter with the absorbent cotton, and gently pull it from the urethra. Before doing so, offer the patient a bedpan because catheter removal typically creates a desire to void.
• Measure and record the amount of urine in the collection bag before discarding it.

Complications
• Major complications in removing an indwelling catheter are failure of the balloon to deflate and rupture of the balloon. If the balloon ruptures, cystoscopy is usually performed to en-

sure removal of any balloon fragments.

Nursing considerations
• Encourage fluid intake *to stimulate urine production, dilute the urine, and help decrease the patient's discomfort when he begins voiding.*
• Within 24 hours, the patient should be voiding normally (10 to 14 oz [300 to 400 ml] at a time), depending on fluid intake. If he's voiding small amounts (1 to 3 oz [30 to 100 ml] every 30 minutes to 1 hour), he's not emptying his bladder completely. Report this to the doctor. He may order a postvoiding catheterization to remove residual urine.
• After catheter removal, assess the patient for incontinence (or dribbling), urgency, persistent dysuria or bladder spasms, fever, chills, or palpable bladder distention. Report any such findings to the doctor.

Documentation
• For bladder retraining, record the date and time the catheter was clamped, the time it was released, and the volume and appearance of the urine.
• For catheter removal, record the date and time the catheter was removed and the patient's tolerance for the procedure.
• Record when and how much the patient voided after catheter removal and any problems associated with voiding.

Urinary diversion stoma care

Urinary diversions provide an alternative route for urine flow when a disorder such as an invasive bladder tumor impedes normal drainage. A permanent urinary diversion is indicated in any condition that requires a total cystectomy. In conditions requiring temporary urinary drainage or diversion, a suprapubic or urethral catheter is usually inserted to divert the flow of urine temporarily. The catheter remains in place until the incision heals.

Urinary diversions may also be indicated for patients with neurogenic bladder, congenital anomaly, traumatic injury to the lower urinary tract, or severe chronic urinary tract infection.

Three types of permanent urinary diversions can be created: ureterostomy, ileal conduit, and continent urinary diversion. (See *Types of permanent urinary diversion,* page 932.) Most require the patient to wear a urine-collection appliance and to care for the stoma created during surgery.

>> Key nursing diagnoses and patient outcomes

Use these nursing diagnoses as a guide when developing your plan of care for a patient who is receiving stoma care for a urinary diversion.

Ineffective individual coping related to personal vulnerability

Based on this nursing diagnosis, you'll establish the following patient outcomes. The patient will:
• become actively involved in planning own care.

• identify effective and ineffective coping techniques.

Knowledge deficit related to lack of exposure to care of a urinary diversion stoma

Based on this nursing diagnosis, you'll establish the following patient outcomes. The patient will:
• communicate a need to know.
• state or demonstrate understanding of what has been taught.

Equipment

♦ soap and warm water ♦ waste receptacle (such as an impervious or wax-coated bag) ♦ linen-saver pad ♦ hypoallergenic paper tape ♦ urine collection container ♦ povidone-iodine sponges ♦ rubber catheter (usually #14 or #16 French) ♦ ruler ♦ scissors ♦ urine-collection appliance (with or without antireflux valve) ♦ graduated cylinder ♦ cottonless gauze pads (some rolled, some flat) ♦ washcloth ♦ skin barrier in liquid, paste, wafer, or sheet form ♦ appliance belt ♦ stoma covering (nonadherent gauze pad or panty liner) ♦ two pairs of gloves ♦ optional: adhesive solvent, irrigating syringe, tampon, hair dryer, electric razor, regular gauze pads, vinegar, deodorant tablets.

• Commercially packaged stoma care kits are available.

• In place of soap and water, you can use adhesive remover pads, if available, or cotton gauze saturated with adhesive solvent.

• Some appliances come with a semipermeable skin barrier (impermeable to liquid but permeable to vapor and oxygen, which is essential for maintaining skin integrity). Wafer-type

Types of permanent urinary diversion

The types of permanent urinary diversion with stomas include ureterostomy, ileal conduit, and continent urinary diversion.

Ureterostomy
A stoma or stomas are formed when ureters are diverted to the abdominal wall or flank. There are five different types of ureterostomy:
• *Flank loop ureterostomy:* Ureters loop as they are brought to the skin surface, forming a stoma.
• *Double-barrel ureterostomy:* Both ureters are brought to the skin surface to form side-by-side stomas.
• *Transureteroureterostomy:* One ureter is anastomosed to the other, which is then brought to the skin surface to form a stoma.
• *Bilateral ureterostomy:* Both ureters are brought to the skin surface to form stomas.
• *Unilateral ureterostomy:* One ureter is brought to the skin surface to form a stoma.

Ileal conduit
A segment of the ileum is excised, and the two ends of the ileum that result from excision of the segment are sutured closed. Then the ureters are dissected from the bladder and anastomosed to the ileal segment. One end of the ileal segment is closed with sutures; the opposite end is brought through the abdominal wall, thereby forming a stoma.

Continent urinary diversion
A tube is formed from part of the bladder wall. One end of the tube is brought to the skin to form the stoma. At the internal end of this tube, a nipple valve is created from the bladder wall so urine won't drain out unless a catheter is inserted through the stoma into the bladder pouch. The urethral neck is sutured closed.

Another recently developed type of continent urinary diversion (not pictured here) is "hooked" back to the urethra, obviating the need for a stoma.

Flank loop ureterostomy

Double-barrel ureterostomy

Transuretero-ureterostomy

Bilateral ureterostomy

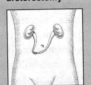

Unilateral ureterostomy

Ileal conduit

Continent urinary diversion

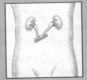
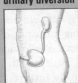

barriers may offer more protection against irritation than adhesive appliances. For example, a carbon-zinc barrier is economical and easy to apply. Its puttylike consistency allows it to be rolled between the palms to form a "washer" that can encircle the base of the stoma. This barrier can withstand enzymes, acids, and other damaging discharge material. All semipermeable barriers are easily removed along with the adhesive, causing less damage to the skin.

Equipment preparation
• Assemble all the equipment on the patient's overbed table.
• Tape the waste receptacle to the table for ready access.
• Measure the diameter of the stoma with a ruler.
• Cut the opening of the appliance with the scissors — it shouldn't be more than $1/16''$ to $1/8''$ larger than the diameter of the stoma.
• Moisten the faceplate of the appliance with a small amount of solvent or water to prepare it for adhesion. Performing these preliminary steps at the bedside allows you *to demonstrate the procedure and show the patient that it's not difficult, which will help him relax.*

Patient preparation
• Provide privacy for the patient, and wash your hands.
• Explain the procedure to the patient as you go, and offer constant reinforcement and reassurance *to counteract negative reactions that may be elicited by stoma care.*

Wicking urine from a stoma

Use a piece of rolled, cottonless gauze or a tampon to wick urine from a stoma. Working by capillary action, wicking absorbs urine while you prepare the patient's skin to hold a urine-collection appliance.

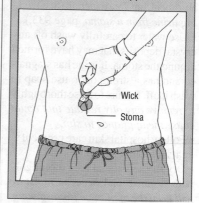

Implementation
• Place the bed in a low Fowler's position so the patient's abdomen is flat. *This position eliminates skin folds that could cause the appliance to slip or irritate the skin and allows the patient to observe or participate.*
• Put on the gloves, and place the linen-saver pad under the patient's side, near the stoma. Open the drain valve of the appliance being replaced *to empty the urine into the graduated cylinder.* Then, *to remove the appliance,* apply soap and water or adhesive solvent as you gently push the skin back from the pouch. If the appliance is disposable, discard it into the waste receptacle. If it's reusable, clean it with soap and lukewarm water and let it air-dry.

Note. To avoid irritating the patient's stoma, avoid touching it with adhesive solvent. If adhesive remains on the skin, gently rub it off with a dry gauze pad. Discard used gauze pads in the waste receptacle.

• *To prevent a constant flow of urine onto the skin while you're changing the appliance,* wick the urine with an absorbent, lint-free material. (See *Wicking urine from a stoma,* page 933.)

• Use water to carefully wash off any crystal deposits that may have formed around the stoma. If urine has stagnated and has a strong odor, use soap to wash it off. Be sure to rinse thoroughly *to remove any oily residue that could cause the appliance to slip.*

• Follow hospital skin care protocol to treat any minor skin problems.

• Dry the peristomal area thoroughly with a gauze pad *because moisture will keep the appliance from sticking.* Use a hair dryer if you wish. Remove any hair from the area with scissors or an electric razor *to prevent hair follicles from becoming irritated when the pouch is removed, which can cause folliculitis.*

• Inspect the stoma *to see if it's healing properly and to detect complications.* Check the color and appearance of the suture line, and examine any moisture or effluent. Inspect the peristomal skin for redness, irritation, and intactness.

• Apply the skin barrier. If you apply a wafer or sheet, cut it to fit over the stoma. Remove any protective backing and set the barrier aside with the adhesive side up. If you apply a liquid barrier (such as Skin-Prep), saturate a gauze pad with it and coat the peristomal skin. Move in concentric circles outward from the stoma until you've covered an area 2″ (5 cm) larger than the wafer. Let the skin dry for several minutes; it should feel tacky. Gently press the wafer around the stoma, sticky side down, smoothing from the stoma outward.

• If you're using a barrier paste, open the tube, squeeze out a small amount, and then discard it. Then squeeze a ribbon of paste directly onto the peristomal skin about ½″ (1.3 cm) from the stoma, making a complete circle. Make several more concentric circles outward. Dip your fingers into lukewarm water, and smooth the paste until the skin is completely covered from the edge of the stoma to 3″ to 4″ (7.6 to 10.2 cm) outward. The paste should be ¼″ to ½″ (0.6 to 1.3 cm) thick. Then discard the gloves, wash your hands, and put on new gloves.

• Remove the material used for wicking urine, and place it in the waste receptacle.

• Now place the appliance over the stoma, leaving only a small amount (⅜″ to ¾″ [1 to 2 cm]) of skin exposed.

• Secure the faceplate of the appliance to the skin with paper tape if recommended. To do this, place a piece of tape lengthwise on each edge of the faceplate so that the tape overlaps onto the skin.

• Apply the appliance belt. Be sure that it's on a level with the stoma. *Applied above or below the stoma, the belt can break the bag's seal, or it can rub or injure the stoma.* The belt should be loose enough for you to insert two fingers between the skin and the belt. *If the belt is too tight, it can irritate the skin or cause internal damage.*

• Dispose of the used materials appropriately.

Complications

• Because intestinal mucosa is delicate, an ill-fitting appliance can cause bleeding. This is especially likely with an ileal conduit, the most common urinary diversion stoma, *because a segment of the intestine forms the conduit.*

• Peristomal skin may become reddened or excoriated from too-frequent changing or improper placement of the appliance, poor skin care, or allergic reaction to the appliance or adhesive. Constant leakage around the appliance can result from improper placement of the appliance or from poor skin turgor.

Nursing considerations

• The patient's attitude toward his urinary diversion stoma plays a big part in determining how well he'll adjust to it. *To encourage a positive attitude,* help him get used to the idea of caring for his stoma and the appliance as though they are natural extensions of himself. When teaching him to perform the procedure, give him written instructions and provide positive reinforcement after he completes each step. Suggest that he perform the procedure in the morning when urine flows most slowly.

• Help the patient choose between disposable and reusable appliances by telling him the advantages and disadvantages of each.

• Emphasize the importance of correct placement and of a well-fitted appliance *to prevent seepage of urine onto the skin.* When positioned correctly, most appliances remain in place for at least 3 days and for as long as 5 days if no leakage occurs. After 5 days, the appliance should be changed. With the improved adhesives and pouches available, belts aren't always necessary.

• Because urine flows constantly, it accumulates quickly, becoming even heavier than stools. *To prevent the weight of the urine from loosening the seal around the stoma and separating the appliance from the skin,* tell the patient to empty the appliance through the drain valve when it is one-third to one-half full.

• Instruct the patient to connect his appliance to a urine-collection container before he goes to sleep. *The continuous flow of urine into the container during the night prevents the urine from accumulating and stagnating in the appliance.*

• Teach the patient sanitary and dietary measures that can protect the peristomal skin and control the odor that commonly results from alkaline urine, infection, or poor hygiene.

• Reusable appliances should be washed with soap and lukewarm water, then air-dried thoroughly *to prevent brittleness.*

• Soaking the appliance in vinegar and water or placing deodorant tablets in it can further dissipate stubborn odors. An acid-ash diet that includes ascorbic acid and cranberry juice may raise urinary acidity, reducing bacterial action and fermentation (the underlying causes of odor). Generous fluid intake also helps to reduce odors by diluting the urine.

• If the patient has a continent urinary diversion, be sure you know how to meet his special needs. (See *Caring for the patient with a continent urinary diversion,* page 936.)

• Tell the patient about ostomy clubs and the American Cancer Society.

Caring for the patient with a continent urinary diversion

In this procedure, an alternative to the traditional ileal conduit, a pouch created from the ascending colon and the terminal ileum serves as a new bladder, which empties through a stoma. To drain urine continuously, several drains are inserted into this reconstructed bladder and left in place for 3 to 6 weeks until the new stoma heals. The patient will be discharged from the hospital with the drains in place. He'll return to have them removed and to learn how to catheterize his stoma.

First hospitalization
• Immediately after surgery, monitor intake and output from each drain. Be alert for decreased output, which may indicate that urine flow is obstructed.
• Watch for common postoperative complications, such as infection or bleeding. Also watch for signs of urinary leakage, which include increased abdominal pain, decreased urine output from the drains, increased abdominal distention, and urine appearing around the drains or midline incision.
• Irrigate the drains, as ordered.
• Clean the area around the drains daily — first with povidone-iodine solution and then with sterile water. Apply a dry, sterile dressing to the area. Use precut 4″ × 4″ drain dressings around the drain to absorb leakage.
• To increase the patient's mobility and comfort, connect the drains to a leg bag.

Second hospitalization or outpatient
• After the patient's drains are removed, teach the patient how to catheterize the stoma. Begin by gathering the following equipment on a clean towel: rubber catheter (usually #14 or #16 French), water-soluble lubricant, washcloth, stoma covering (nonadherent gauze pad or panty liner), nonallergenic adhesive tape, and an irrigating syringe (optional).
• Apply water-soluble lubricant to the catheter tip to facilitate insertion.
• Remove and discard the stoma cover. Using the washcloth, clean the stoma and the area around it, starting at the stoma and working outward in a circular motion.
• Hold the urine collection container under the catheter; then slowly insert the catheter into the stoma. Urine should begin to flow into the container. If it doesn't, gently rotate the catheter or redirect its angle. If the catheter drains slowly, it may be plugged with mucus. Irrigate it with sterile saline solution or sterile water to clear it. When the flow stops, pinch the catheter closed and remove it.
• Dry the skin if necessary. Apply a sterile gauze pad over the stoma to keep it clean, and secure the pad with tape. Alternatively, secure a panty liner to the patient's underwear.

Home care
• Teach the patient how to care for the drains and their insertion sites during the 3 to 6 weeks he'll be at home before their removal, and

(continued)

Caring for the patient with a continent urinary diversion (continued)

teach him how to attach them to a leg bag. Also teach him to recognize the signs of infection and obstruction.

• After the drains are removed, teach the patient how to empty the pouch, and establish a schedule. Initially, he should catheterize the stoma and empty the pouch every 2 to 3 hours. Later, he should catheterize every 4 hours while awake and also irrigate the pouch each morning and evening, if ordered. Instruct him to empty the pouch whenever he feels a sensation of fullness.

• Tell the patient that catheters are reusable, but only after they're cleaned. He should clean the catheter thoroughly with warm, soapy water, rinse it thoroughly, and hang it to dry over a clean towel. He should store cleaned and dried catheters in plastic bags. Tell him he can reuse catheters for up to 1 month before discarding them. However, he should immediately discard any catheter that becomes discolored or cracked.

Members of these organizations routinely visit hospitals to explain ostomy care and the types of appliances available and to help patients learn to function normally with a stoma.

Home care

• The patient or a family member can learn to care for a urinary diversion stoma at home. However, the patient's emotional adjustment to the stoma must be given special consideration before he can be expected to maintain it properly. Arrange for a visiting nurse or an enterostomal therapist to assist the patient at home.

Documentation

• Record the appearance and color of the stoma and whether it's inverted, flush with the skin, or protruding. If it protrudes, note by how much it protrudes above the skin. (The normal range is $\frac{1}{2}''$ to $\frac{3}{4}''$ [1.3 to 2 cm].)

• Record the appearance and condition of the peristomal skin, noting any redness or irritation or complaints by the patient of itching or burning.

Urine collection

A random urine specimen, usually collected as part of the physical examination or at various times during hospitalization, permits laboratory screening for urinary and systemic disorders; it also allows for drug screening. A clean-catch midstream specimen, once used only to confirm urinary tract infection, is replacing random collection because it provides a virtually uncontaminated specimen without the need for bladder catheterization.

An indwelling catheter specimen is obtained by clamping the drainage tube and emptying the accumulated urine into a container or by aspirating a sample with a syringe and requires sterile technique to prevent catheter contamination and urinary tract infection. This method is contraindicated in patients who have recently undergone genitourinary surgery.

>> Key nursing diagnoses and patient outcomes

Use these nursing diagnoses as a guide when developing your plan of care.

Altered urinary elimination related to medical condition

Based on this nursing diagnosis, you'll establish the following patient outcomes. The patient will:
• voice understanding of treatment.
• avoid or minimize complications.

Knowledge deficit related to lack of exposure to procedure

Based on this nursing diagnosis, you'll establish the following patient outcomes. The patient will:
• state or demonstrate what has been taught.
• demonstrate ability to perform new health-related behaviors as they are taught.

Equipment

For a random specimen: ◆ bedpan or urinal with cover if necessary ◆ gloves ◆ graduated container ◆ specimen container with lid ◆ label ◆ laboratory request form.

For a clean-catch midstream specimen: ◆ basin ◆ soap and water ◆ towel ◆ gloves ◆ three sterile 2″ × 2″ gauze pads ◆ povidone-iodine solution ◆ sterile specimen container with lid ◆ label ◆ bedpan or urinal if necessary ◆ laboratory request form.

Commercial clean-catch kits containing antiseptic towelettes, sterile specimen container with lid and label,

and instructions for use in several languages are widely used.

For an indwelling catheter specimen: ◆ 10-ml syringe ◆ 21G or 22G 1 ½″ needle ◆ tube clamp ◆ sterile specimen cup with lid ◆ gloves ◆ alcohol pad ◆ label ◆ laboratory request form.

Patient preparation

• Explain the procedure to him and his family, if necessary, *to promote cooperation and prevent accidental disposal of specimens.*

Implementation

• Tell the patient that you need a urine specimen for laboratory analysis.

Collecting a random specimen

• Provide privacy.
• Instruct the patient on bed rest to void into a clean bedpan or urinal, or ask the ambulatory patient to void into either one in the bathroom.
• Don gloves. Then pour at least 4 oz [120 ml] of urine into the specimen container, and cap the container securely. If the patient's urine output must be measured and recorded, pour the remaining urine into the graduated container. Otherwise, discard the remaining urine. If you inadvertently spill urine on the outside of the container, clean and dry it *to prevent possible cross-contamination.*
• Label the sample container with the patient's name and room number and the date and time of collection. Then attach the request form and send it to the laboratory immediately. *Delaying the sample may alter test results.*
• Clean the graduated container and urinal or bedpan, and return these to their proper storage.

• Discard disposable items.
• Wash your hands thoroughly *to prevent cross-contamination.* Offer the patient a washcloth, soap, and water to wash his hands.

Collecting a clean-catch midstream specimen

• Because the goal of this method is a virtually uncontaminated specimen, explain the procedure to the patient carefully.
• Provide illustrations to emphasize the correct collection technique if possible.
• Tell the male patient to remove all clothing from the waist down and to stand in front of the toilet as for urination.
• Tell the female patient to sit far back on the toilet seat and spread her legs.
• Tell the patient to clean the periurethral area (tip of the penis or labial folds, vulva, and urethral meatus) with soap and water and then wipe the area three times, each time with a fresh 2″× 2″ gauze pad soaked in povidone-iodine solution, or with wipes provided in a commercial kit.
• Instruct the female patient to separate her labial folds with the thumb and forefinger. Tell her to wipe down one side with the first pad and discard it, to wipe the other side with the second pad and discard it and, finally, to wipe down the center over the urinary meatus with the third pad and discard it. Stress the importance of cleaning from front to back *to avoid contaminating the genital area with fecal matter.*
• For the uncircumcised male patient, emphasize the need to retract his foreskin *to effectively clean the meatus*

and to keep the foreskin retracted during voiding.
• Tell the female patient to straddle the bedpan or toilet *to allow labial spreading.* She should continue to keep her labia separated with her fingers while voiding.
• Instruct the patient to begin voiding into the bedpan, urinal, or toilet *because the urine stream washes bacteria from the urethra and urinary meatus.* Then, without stopping the urine stream, the patient should move the collection container into the stream, collecting about 1 to 1.5 oz (30 to 50 ml) at the midstream portion of the voiding. The patient can then finish voiding into the bedpan, urinal, or toilet.
• Don gloves before discarding the first and last portions of the voiding, and measure the remaining urine in a graduated cylinder for intake and output records if necessary. Be sure to include the amount in the specimen container when recording the total amount voided.
• Take the sterile container from the patient, and cap it securely. Avoid touching the inside of the container or the lid.
• If the outside of the container is soiled, clean it and wipe it dry.
• Remove gloves and discard them properly.
• Wash your hands thoroughly *to prevent cross-contamination.* Tell the patient to wash his hands also.
• Label the container with the patient's name and room number, name of test, type of specimen, collection time, and suspected diagnosis, if known. If a urine culture has been ordered, note any current antibiotic therapy on the laboratory request form.

Aspirating a urine specimen

If the patient has an indwelling urinary catheter in place, clamp the tube distal to the aspiration port for about 30 minutes. Wipe the port with an alcohol pad, and insert a needle and a 20- or 30-ml syringe into the port perpendicular to the tube. Aspirate the required amount of urine, and expel it into the specimen container. Remove the clamp on the drainage tube.

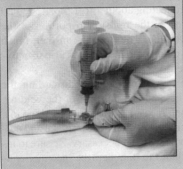

Send the container to the laboratory immediately, or place it on ice *to prevent specimen deterioration and altered test results.*

Collecting an indwelling catheter specimen

• About 30 minutes before collecting the specimen, clamp the drainage tube *to allow urine to accumulate.*
• Put on gloves.
• If the drainage tube has a built-in sampling port, wipe the port with an alcohol pad.
• Uncap the needle on the syringe, and insert the needle into the sampling port at a 90-degree angle to the tubing. Aspirate the specimen into the syringe. (See *Aspirating a urine specimen.*)
• If the drainage tube doesn't have a sampling port and the catheter is made of rubber, obtain the specimen from the catheter. *Other types of catheters will leak after you withdraw the needle.* To withdraw the specimen from a rubber catheter, wipe it with an alcohol pad just above the point where it connects to the drainage tube. Insert the needle into the rubber catheter at a 45-degree angle and withdraw the specimen. Never insert the needle into the shaft of the catheter *because this may puncture the lumen leading to the catheter balloon.*
• Transfer the specimen to a sterile container, label it, and send it to the laboratory immediately or place it on ice. If a urine culture is to be performed, be sure to list any antibiotic therapy on the laboratory request form.
• If the catheter is not made of rubber or has no sampling port, wipe the area where the catheter joins the drainage tube with an alcohol pad. Disconnect the catheter, and allow urine to drain into the sterile specimen container. Avoid touching the inside of the sterile container with the catheter, and don't touch anything with the catheter drainage tube *to avoid contamination.* When you have the specimen, wipe both connection sites with an alcohol pad and join them. Cap the specimen container, label it, and send it to the laboratory immediately or place it on ice.

Nursing considerations

• Make sure you unclamp the drainage tube after collecting the specimen *to prevent urine backflow that may cause bladder distention and infection.*

Home care
• Instruct the patient to collect the sample in a clean container with a tight-fitting lid, and to keep it on ice or in the refrigerator (separate from any food items) for up to 24 hours.

Documentation
• Record the times of specimen collection and transport to the laboratory.
• Specify the test, and the appearance, odor, color, and any unusual characteristics of the specimen.
• If necessary, record the urine volume on the patient's intake and output record.

Urine collection, timed

Because hormones, proteins, and electrolytes are excreted in small variable amounts in urine, specimens for measuring these substances must typically be collected over an extended time to yield quantities of diagnostic value.

A 24-hour specimen is used most commonly because it provides an average excretion rate for substances eliminated during this period. Timed specimens may also be collected for shorter periods, such as 2 or 12 hours, depending on the specific information needed.

A timed urine specimen may also be collected after administering a challenge dose of a chemical — inulin, for example — to detect various renal disorders.

⟫ Key nursing diagnoses and patient outcomes
Use these nursing diagnoses as a guide when developing your plan of care.

Altered urinary elimination related to medical condition
Based on this nursing diagnosis, you'll establish the following patient outcomes. The patient will:
• voice understanding of treatment.
• avoid or minimize complications.

Knowledge deficit related to lack of exposure to procedure
Based on this nursing diagnosis, you'll establish the following patient outcomes. The patient will:
• state or demonstrate what has been taught.
• demonstrate ability to perform new health-related behaviors as they are taught.

Equipment
♦ large collection bottle with a cap or stopper, or a commercial plastic container ♦ preservative if necessary ♦ gloves ♦ bedpan or urinal, if patient does not have an indwelling catheter ♦ graduated container, if patient is on intake and output measurement ♦ gloves ♦ ice-filled container, if a refrigerator isn't available ♦ label ♦ laboratory request form ♦ four patient care reminders.

Check with the laboratory to see what preservatives may be needed in the urine specimen, or if a dark collection bottle is required.

Implementation
• Explain the procedure to the patient and his family members, as necessary, *to enlist their cooperation and prevent*

accidental disposal of urine during the collection period. Emphasize that loss of even *one* urine specimen during the collection period invalidates the test and requires that it begin again.

• Place patient care reminders over the patient's bed, in his bathroom, on the bedpan hopper in the utility room, and on the urinal or indwelling catheter collection bag. Include the patient's name and room number, the date, and the collection interval.

• Instruct the patient to save all urine during the collection period, to notify you after each voiding, and to avoid contaminating the urine with stool or toilet tissue. Explain any dietary or drug restrictions, and be sure he understands and is willing to comply with them.

For 2-hour collection

• If possible, instruct the patient to drink two to four 8-oz glasses (475 to 946 ml) of water about 30 minutes before collection begins. After 30 minutes, tell him to void. Don gloves and discard this specimen *so the patient starts the collection period with an empty bladder.*

• If ordered, administer a challenge dose of medication (such as glucose solution or corticotropin) and record the time.

• If possible, offer the patient a glass of water at least every hour during the collection period *to stimulate urine production.* After each voiding, don gloves and add the specimen to the collection bottle.

• Instruct the patient to void about 15 minutes before the end of the collection period, if possible, and add this specimen to the collection bottle.

• At the end of the collection period, remove and discard gloves, and send the appropriately labeled collection bottle to the laboratory immediately, along with a properly completed laboratory request form.

For 12- and 24-hour collection

• Put on gloves and ask the patient to void. Then discard this urine *so he starts the collection period with an empty bladder.* Record the time.

• After putting on gloves and pouring the first urine specimen into the collection bottle, add the required preservative. Then refrigerate the bottle or keep it on ice until the next voiding as appropriate.

• Collect all urine voided during the prescribed period. Just before the collection period ends, ask the patient to void again if possible. Add this last specimen to the collection bottle, pack it in ice *to inhibit deterioration of the specimen,* and remove and discard gloves. Send the specimen to the laboratory. Include a properly completed laboratory request form.

Nursing considerations

• The patient should be hydrated before and during the test *to ensure adequate urine flow.*

• Before collection of a timed specimen, make sure the laboratory will be open when the collection period ends *to help ensure prompt, accurate results.* Never store a specimen in a refrigerator containing food or medication *to avoid contamination.* If the patient has an indwelling catheter in place, put the collection bag in an ice-filled container at his bedside.

• Instruct the patient to avoid exercise, ingestion of coffee or tea, or any drugs

(unless otherwise directed by the doctor) before the test *to avoid altering test results.*
• If you accidentally discard a specimen during the collection period, restart the collection. Accidentally discarding a specimen during the test period may result in an additional day of hospitalization, possibly causing the patient personal and financial hardship. Therefore, emphasize the need to save all the patient's urine during the collection period to all persons involved in his care as well as to family or other visitors.

Home care
• If the patient must continue collecting urine at home, provide written instructions for the appropriate method.
• Tell the patient he can keep the specimens in a brown bag in his refrigerator at home, separate from other refrigerator contents.

Documentation
• In the Kardex and in your notes, record the date and interval of collection and that the specimen was sent to the laboratory.

Urine glucose and ketone tests

Reagent tablet and strip tests are used to monitor urine glucose and ketone levels and to screen for diabetes. *Urine ketone tests* monitor fat metabolism, help diagnose carbohydrate deprivation and diabetic ketoacidosis, and help distinguish between diabetic and nondiabetic coma. However, urine glucose tests are less accurate than blood glucose tests, and are now used less frequently because of the increasing convenience of blood self-testing.

The *copper reduction test* (Clinitest) measures the concentration of reducing substances in the urine through the reactions of these substances with a tablet composed of sodium hydroxide, cupric sulfate, and other reagents. When this tablet is added to a test tube containing drops of water and urine, the reaction generates heat. Simultaneously, reduction of cupric ions in the presence of glucose causes a color change. Comparison of this test color with a standardized color chart gives the approximate level of urine glucose. Similarly, the *Acetest tablet test* produces a color reaction that allows an estimate of urine ketone levels by comparison to a standardized chart.

Glucose oxidase tests (such as Clinistix, Diastix, Tes-Tape, and Chemstrip UG strips) produce color changes when patches of reagents implanted in handheld plastic strips react with glucose in the patient's urine; *urine ketone strip tests* (such as Chemstrip K and Ketostix) are similar. All test results are read by comparing color changes against a standardized reference chart.

≫ Key nursing diagnoses and patient outcomes
Use these nursing diagnoses as a guide when developing your plan of care.

Knowledge deficit related to lack of exposure to procedure
Based on this nursing diagnosis, you'll establish the following patient outcomes. The patient will:

• verbalize understanding of need for procedure.
• demonstrate correct procedure for obtaining urine specimen.

Anxiety related to lack of exposure to procedure
Based on this nursing diagnosis, you'll establish the following patient outcome. The patient will:
• communicate feelings of anxiety.

Equipment
For reagent tablet tests: ◆ specimen container ◆ 10-ml test tube ◆ medicine dropper ◆ gloves ◆ Clinitest or Acetest tablets ◆ Clinitest or Acetest color chart.

For reagent strip tests: ◆ specimen container ◆ gloves ◆ glucose or ketone test strips ◆ reference color chart.

Wear gloves as barrier protection when performing all urine tests.

Patient preparation
• Explain the test to the patient. If he's a newly diagnosed diabetic patient, teach him to perform the test himself.
• Check his history for medications that may interfere with test results.
• Before each test, instruct the patient not to contaminate the urine specimen with stool or toilet tissue.

Implementation
Follow these steps.

Clinitest tablet test
• Ask the patient to void, and then ask him to drink a glass of water if possible. Don gloves and collect a second-voided urine specimen 30 to 45 minutes later.

• Perform the 5-drop test: With the medicine dropper, transfer 5 drops of urine from the specimen container to the test tube. Rinse the dropper and add 10 drops of water to the test tube. Then add one Clinitest tablet to the tube.
• Hold the test tube near the top during the reaction *because the test solution will come to a boil.* Observe the color change that occurs during the reaction.
• Fifteen seconds after effervescence subsides, shake the tube gently. Observe the solution's color, and compare it with the Clinitest color chart.
• Remove and discard gloves, and record the test results. Ignore any changes that develop after 15 seconds.
• If the color changes rapidly in the 5-drop test, record the result as "over 2%" glycosuria.
• Alternately, perform the 2-drop test: Transfer 2 drops of urine from the specimen container to the test tube, and then add 10 drops of water and a Clinitest tablet. After the reaction, observe the color of the test solution, and compare it with the Clinitest color chart.
• Remove and discard your gloves, and record the test results.
• Rapid color change in the 2-drop test indicates glycosuria up to 5%.

Acetest tablet test
• Don gloves and collect a second-voided specimen, as for the Clinitest tablet test.
• Place the Acetest tablet on a piece of white paper, and add 1 drop of urine to the tablet.
• After 30 seconds, compare the tablet's color (white, lavender, or purple)

with the Acetest color chart. Remove gloves and record the test results.

Glucose oxidase strip test
• Explain the test to the patient. If he's diagnosed with diabetes, teach him to perform it himself. Check his history for medications that may interfere with test results. Don gloves before collecting specimens for each of these tests, and remove them to record test results.
• Instruct the patient to void. Ask him to drink a glass of water, if possible, and collect a second-voided specimen after 30 to 45 minutes.
• If you're using Clinistix, dip the reagent end of the strip into the urine for 2 seconds. Remove excess urine by tapping the strip against the container's rim, wait for exactly 10 seconds, and then compare its color with the color chart on the container. Ignore color changes that occur after 10 seconds. Record the result.
• If you're using a Diastix strip, dip the reagent end of the strip into the urine for 2 seconds. Tap off excess urine, wait for exactly 30 seconds, and then compare its color with the standardized color chart on the container. Ignore color changes that occur after 30 seconds. Record the result.
• If you're using a Tes-Tape strip, pull about $1\frac{1}{2}''$ (3.8 cm) of the reagent strip from the dispenser, and dip one end about $\frac{1}{4}''$ (0.6 cm) into the specimen for 2 seconds. Tap off excess urine, wait exactly 60 seconds, and then compare the darkest part of the tape with the standardized color chart. If the test result exceeds 0.5%, wait an additional 60 seconds and make a final comparison. Record the result.

Ketone strip test
• Explain the procedure to the patient. If he's diagnosed with diabetes, teach him to perform the test. Check his medication history. If he's receiving phenazopyridine or levodopa, use Acetest tablets instead *because reagent strips will give inaccurate results.*
• Don gloves, and collect a second-voided midstream specimen.
• If you're using Ketostix, dip the reagent end of the strip into the specimen and remove it immediately. Wait exactly 15 seconds, and then compare the color of the strip with the standardized color chart on the container. Ignore color changes that occur after 15 seconds. Record the result.
• If you're using Keto-Diastix, dip the reagent end of the strip into the specimen and remove it immediately. Tap off excess urine, and hold the strip horizontally *to prevent mixing of chemicals between the two reagent squares.* Wait exactly 15 seconds, and then compare the color of the ketone part of the strip with the standardized color chart. After 30 seconds, compare the color of the glucose part of the strip with the chart. Record the results.

Nursing considerations
• Test the urine specimen immediately after the patient voids.
• Keep reagent strips in a cool, dry place at a temperature below 86° F (30° C), but don't refrigerate them.
• Keep the containers tightly closed. Don't use discolored or outdated strips.
   Note. Because Clinitest tablets contain caustic soda, keep the container tightly closed and in a dry place. If you must handle these tablets, keep

your fingers dry *to prevent the tablet from leaving a deposit, which could then be accidentally ingested or brought into contact with eyes, skin, mucous membranes, or clothing, causing caustic burns.*

Documentation

• In your notes, record color changes according to the information on the charts on the reagent containers, or use special flowcharts designed to record this information.

• If you're teaching a patient how to perform the test, keep a record of his progress.

V

Vagal maneuvers

When a patient suffers sinus, atrial, or junctional tachyarrhythmias, vagal maneuvers — Valsalva's maneuver and carotid sinus massage — can slow his heart rate. These maneuvers work by stimulating nerve endings, which respond as they would to an increase in blood pressure. They send this message to the brain stem, which in turn stimulates the autonomic nervous system to increase vagal tone and decrease the heart rate.

In *Valsalva's maneuver,* the patient holds his breath and bears down, raising his intrathoracic pressure. When this pressure increase is transmitted to the heart and great vessels, venous return, stroke volume, and systolic blood pressure decrease. Within seconds, the baroreceptors respond to these changes by increasing the heart rate and causing peripheral vasoconstriction.

When the patient exhales at the end of the maneuver, his blood pressure rises to its previous level. This increase, combined with the peripheral vasoconstriction caused by bearing down, stimulates the vagus nerve, decreasing the heart rate.

In *carotid sinus massage,* manual pressure applied to the left or right carotid sinus slows the heart rate. This method is used both to diagnose and treat tachyarrhythmias.

The patient's response to carotid sinus massage depends on the type of arrhythmia. If he has sinus tachycardia, his heart rate will slow gradually during the procedure and speed up again after it. If he has atrial tachycardia, the arrhythmia may stop and the heart rate may remain slow because the procedure increases atrioventricular (AV) block. With atrial fibrillation or flutter, the ventricular rate may not change; AV block may even worsen. With paroxysmal atrial tachycardia, reversion to sinus rhythm occurs only 20% of the time. Nonparoxysmal tachycardia and ventricular tachycardia won't respond.

Vagal maneuvers are contraindicated for patients with severe coronary artery disease, acute myocardial infarction, or hypovolemia. Carotid sinus massage is contraindicated for patients with cardiac glycoside toxicity or cerebrovascular disease and for patients who have had carotid surgery.

Although usually performed by a doctor, vagal maneuvers may also be done by a specially prepared nurse under a doctor's supervision.

▶ Key nursing diagnoses and patient outcomes

Use these nursing diagnoses as a guide when developing your plan of care for a patient who requires vagal maneuvers.

Anxiety related to situational crisis

Based on this nursing diagnosis, you'll establish the following patient outcomes. The patient will:

• state at least two ways to eliminate or minimize anxious behaviors.

• report being able to cope with current situation without experiencing severe anxiety.

Knowledge deficit related to lack of exposure to vagal maneuvers
Based on this nursing diagnosis, you'll establish the following patient outcomes. The patient will:
• communicate a need to know.
• state or demonstrate understanding of procedure.

Equipment

♦ crash cart with emergency medications and airway equipment ♦ electrocardiogram (ECG) monitor and electrodes ♦ I.V. catheter and tubing ♦ tourniquet ♦ dextrose 5% in water ♦ optional: shaving supplies if needed, cardiotonic drugs.

Patient preparation

• Explain the procedure to the patient *to ease his fears and promote cooperation.* Ask him to let you know if he feels light-headed.
• Place the patient in a supine position. Insert an I.V. line if necessary. Then administer dextrose 5% in water at a keep-vein-open rate as ordered. *This line will be used if emergency drugs become necessary.*
• Prepare the patient's skin, shaving it if necessary, and attach ECG electrodes. Adjust the size of the ECG complexes on the monitor *so that you can see the arrhythmia clearly.*

Implementation

• Ask the patient to take a deep breath and bear down, as if he were trying to defecate. If he doesn't feel light-headed or dizzy, and if no new arrhythmias occur, have him hold his breath and bear down for 10 seconds.
• If he does feel dizzy or light-headed, or if you see a new arrhythmia on the monitor — asystole for more than 6 seconds, frequent premature ventricular contractions (PVCs), or ventricular tachycardia or ventricular fibrillation — allow him to exhale and stop bearing down.
• After 10 seconds, ask him to exhale and breathe quietly. If the maneuver is successful, the monitor will show his heart rate slowing before he exhales.

Carotid sinus massage

• Begin by obtaining a rhythm strip, using the lead that shows the strongest P waves.
• Auscultate both carotid sinuses. If you detect bruits, inform the doctor and don't perform carotid sinus massage. If you don't detect bruits, proceed as ordered. (See *Location and technique for carotid sinus massage.*)
• Monitor the ECG throughout the procedure. Stop massaging when the ventricular rate slows sufficiently to permit diagnosis of the rhythm. Or stop as soon as any evidence of a rhythm change appears. Have the crash cart handy to give emergency treatment if a dangerous arrhythmia occurs.
• If the procedure has no effect within 5 seconds, stop massaging the right carotid sinus and begin to massage the left. If this also fails, administer cardiotonic drugs as ordered.

Complications

• Use caution when performing carotid sinus massage on elderly patients, patients receiving cardiac glycosides, and patients with heart block, hypertension, coronary artery disease, diabetes mellitus, or hyperkalemia. The procedure may cause arterial pressure

Location and technique for carotid sinus massage

Before applying manual pressure to the patient's right carotid sinus, locate the carotid artery bifurcation on the right side of the neck. Turn the patient's head slightly to the left and hyperextend the neck. This brings the carotid artery closer to the skin and moves the sternocleidomastoid muscle away from the carotid artery.

Then, using a circular motion, gently massage the right carotid sinus between your fingers and the transverse processes of the spine for 3 to 5 seconds. Don't massage for more than 5 seconds *to avoid risking life-threatening complications.*

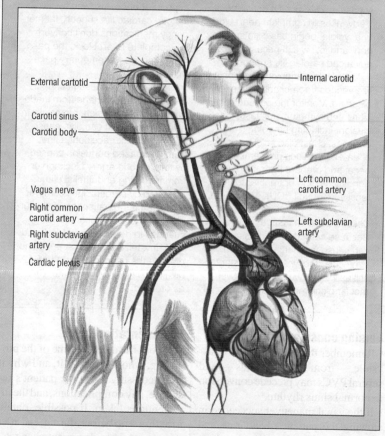

to plummet in these patients, although it usually rises quickly afterward. This is particularly true of elderly patients with heart disease. Vagal maneuvers can occasionally cause bradycardia or complete heart block, so monitor the patient closely. (See *Adverse effects of vagal maneuvers,* page 950.)

Adverse effects of vagal maneuvers

Both Valsalva's maneuver and carotid sinus massage are useful for slowing heart rate. However, they can cause complications, some of which are life-threatening.

Valsalva's maneuver

This maneuver can cause bradycardia, accompanied by a decrease in cardiac output, possibly leading to syncope. The bradycardia will usually pass quickly, but if it doesn't or if it advances to complete heart block or asystole, begin basic life support, and follow it, if necessary, by advanced cardiac life support.

Valsalva's maneuver can mobilize venous thrombi and cause bleeding. Monitor the patient for signs and symptoms of vascular occlusion, including neurologic changes, chest discomfort, and dyspnea. Report such problems at once, and prepare the patient for diagnostic testing or transfer to the intensive care unit (ICU), as ordered.

Carotid sinus massage

Because carotid sinus massage can cause ventricular fibrillation, ventricular tachycardia, and standstill as well as worsening atrioventricular block that leads to junctional or ventricular escape rhythms, you'll need to monitor the patient's electrocardiogram (ECG) closely. If his ECG indicates complete heart block or asystole, start basic life support at once, followed by advanced cardiac life support. If emergency medications don't convert the complete heart block, the patient may need a temporary pacemaker.

Carotid sinus massage can cause cerebral damage from inadequate tissue perfusion, especially in elderly patients. It can also cause a cerebrovascular accident, either from decreased perfusion caused by total carotid artery blockage or from migrating endothelial plaque loosened by carotid sinus compression. Watch the patient carefully during and after the procedure for changes in neurologic status. If you note any, tell the doctor at once and prepare the patient for further diagnostic tests or transfer to the ICU, as ordered.

Nursing considerations

• Remember that a brief period of asystole — from 3 to 6 seconds — and several PVCs may precede conversion to normal sinus rhythm.
• If the vagal maneuver succeeded in slowing the patient's heart rate and converting the arrhythmia, continue monitoring him for several hours.

Documentation

• Record the date and time of the procedure, who performed it, and why it was necessary. Note the patient's response, any complications, and the interventions taken. If possible, obtain a rhythm strip before, during, and after the procedure to document changes.

Vaginal drug administration

Vaginal medications include suppositories, creams, gels, and ointments. These medications can be inserted as topical treatment for infection (particularly *Trichomonas vaginalis* and monilial vaginitis) or inflammation, or as a contraceptive. Suppositories melt on contact with the vaginal mucosa, and their medication diffuses topically — as effectively as creams, gels, and ointments.

Vaginal medications usually come with a disposable applicator that enables placement of medication in the anterior and posterior fornices. Vaginal administration is most effective when the patient can remain lying down afterward to retain the medication.

≫ Key nursing diagnoses and patient outcomes
Use these nursing diagnoses as a guide when developing your plan of care.

Knowledge deficit related to lack of exposure to procedure
Based on this nursing diagnosis, you'll establish the following patient outcomes. The patient will:
• state or demonstrate understanding of what has been taught.
• demonstrate ability to perform new health-related behaviors as they are taught.

Risk for injury related to improper technique
Based on this nursing diagnosis, you'll establish the following patient outcomes. The patient will:
• identify factors that increase risk for injury.
• assist in identifying and applying safety measures to prevent injury.

Equipment
♦ patient's medication record and chart ♦ prescribed medication and applicator if necessary ♦ gloves ♦ water-soluble lubricant ♦ small sanitary pad.

Implementation
• If possible, plan to give vaginal medications at bedtime, when the patient is recumbent.
• Verify the order on the patient's medication record by checking it against the doctor's order.
• Confirm the patient's identity by asking her name and checking the name, room number, and bed number on her wristband.
• Wash your hands, explain the procedure to the patient, and provide her with privacy.
• Ask the patient to void.
• Ask the patient if she would rather insert the medication herself. If so, provide appropriate instructions. If not, proceed with the following steps.
• Help her into the lithotomy position.
• Expose only the perineum.

Inserting a suppository
• Remove the suppository from the wrapper, and lubricate it with water-soluble lubricant.
• Put on gloves and expose the vagina.

How to insert a vaginal suppository

If the suppository is small, place it in the applicator tip. Then, lubricate the applicator, hold it by the cylinder, and insert it into the vagina. To ensure the patient's comfort, direct the applicator down initially (toward the spine), and then up and back (toward the cervix), as shown here. When the suppository reaches the distal end of the vagina, depress the plunger.

Remove the applicator while the plunger is still depressed.

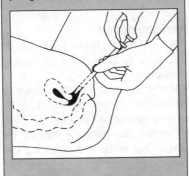

• With an applicator or the forefinger of your free hand, insert the suppository about 2″ (5 cm) into the vagina. (See *How to insert a vaginal suppository.*)

Inserting ointments, creams, or gels

• Insert the plunger into the applicator. Then fit the applicator to the tube of medication.
• Gently squeeze the tube to fill the applicator with the prescribed amount of medication. Lubricate the applicator.
• Put on gloves and expose the vagina.

• Insert the applicator as you would a small suppository and administer the medication by depressing the plunger on the applicator.

After vaginal insertion

• Remove and discard your gloves.
• Wash the applicator with soap and warm water and store it, unless it is disposable. If the applicator can be used again, label it *so it will be used only for the same patient.*
• *To prevent the medication from soiling the patient's clothing and bedding,* provide a sanitary pad.
• Help the patient return to a comfortable position, and advise her to remain in bed as much as possible for the next several hours.
• Wash your hands thoroughly.

Complications

• Vaginal medications may cause local irritation.

Nursing considerations

• Refrigerate vaginal suppositories that melt at room temperature. If possible, teach the patient how to insert vaginal medication. *She may have to administer it herself after discharge.* Give her a patient-teaching sheet if one is available. Instruct the patient not to wear a tampon after inserting vaginal medication *because it would absorb the medication and decrease its effectiveness.*

Documentation

• Record the medication administered, the time, and the date. Note adverse effects and any other pertinent information.

Vaginal examination

During first-stage labor, a doctor or a nurse with special skills performs a vaginal examination to assess cervical dilation, effacement, membrane status, and fetal presentation, position, and engagement.

Important considerations during the examination include respecting the patient's privacy, providing simple explanations for her and her support person, maintaining eye contact when possible, and using aseptic technique. With experience, the typical examiner develops a well-honed routine for collecting necessary information. This enables the examination to proceed precisely and efficiently.

Contraindications to a vaginal examination include excessive vaginal bleeding, which may signal placenta previa.

>> Key nursing diagnoses and patient outcomes

Use these nursing diagnoses as a guide when developing your plan of care.

Anxiety related to situational crisis
Based on this nursing diagnosis, you'll establish the following patient outcomes. The patient will:
• state at least two ways to eliminate or minimize anxious behaviors.
• report being able to cope with current situation without experiencing severe anxiety.

Knowledge deficit related to lack of exposure to a vaginal examination
Based on this nursing diagnosis, you'll establish the following patient outcomes. The patient will:
• communicate a need to know.
• state or demonstrate understanding of procedure.

Equipment

♦ sterile gloves ♦ sterile, water-soluble lubricant or sterile water ♦ mild soap and water or cleaning solution ♦ linen-saver pads ♦ antiseptic solution ♦ sterile gauze.

Patient preparation

• Explain the procedure to the patient, and give her an opportunity to empty her bladder. *A distended bladder may interfere with accurate examination findings.*
• Use Leopold's maneuvers to identify the fetal presenting part and position. Then help the patient into a lithotomy position for the vaginal examination.
• Place a linen-saver pad under the patient's buttocks, and put on sterile gloves.
• Inform the patient when you are about to touch her *to avoid startling her*.

Implementation

• Clean the perineum with mild soap and water or cleaning solution, spreading the labia with your independent hand *to avoid contaminating your examining hand*.
• Lubricate the index and middle fingers of your examining hand with sterile water or sterile water-soluble lubricant *to facilitate insertion*. If the

Step-by-step vaginal examination

Begin the vaginal examination — usually in early labor — by inserting your gloved index and middle fingers palm side down into the vagina. Use your nondominant hand to gently but firmly press on the uterus *to steady the fetal presenting part against the cervix for examination.*

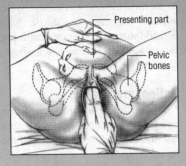

Presenting part

Pelvic bones

Confirm the presenting part and position

Rotate your fingers to palpate and confirm the fetal presenting part (a fetal head feels firm, the buttocks soft) and position (left, right, anterior, posterior, or transverse) identified by using Leopold's maneuvers.

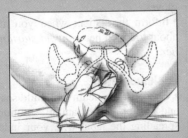

Assess cervical effacement and dilation

Estimate cervical dilation by palpating the internal os. Each fingerbreadth of dilation averages $5/8''$ to

$3/4''$ (1.5 to 2 cm), depending on the width of the examiner's finger.

Next, determine the percentage of effacement by palpating the ridge of tissue around the cervix. Assign a low percentage of effacement to defined and thick cervical tissue. Indistinct, wafer-thin cervical tissue scores 100%.

Assess fetal engagement and station

Estimate the extent of fetal engagement (descent of the fetal presenting part into the pelvis).

Then palpate the presenting part and grade the fetal station (where the presenting part lies in relation to the ischial spines of the maternal pelvis). A zero grade indicates that the presenting part lies level with the ischial spine.

Station grades range from -3 (3 cm above the maternal ischial spines) to +4 (4 cm below the maternal ischial spines, causing the perineum to bulge).

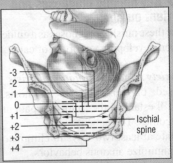

-3
-2
-1
0
+1
+2
+3
+4

Ischial spine

Evaluate membrane status

If appropriate, also check amniotic membrane status. If you feel a bulging, slick surface over the presenting fetal part, you know the membranes remain intact.

membranes are ruptured, use an antiseptic solution.

• Ask the patient to relax by taking several deep breaths and slowly releasing the air. Then insert your lubricated fingers (palmar surface down) into the vagina. Keep your uninserted fingers flexed *to avoid the rectum.* (See *Step-by-step vaginal examination.*)

• Palpate the cervix, keeping in mind that the cervix may assume a posterior position in early labor and be difficult to locate. Once you find the cervix, however, note its consistency. Throughout pregnancy, the cervix gradually softens, reaching a buttery consistency before labor begins.

• After identifying the presenting fetal part and position, evaluating dilation and effacement, assessing fetal engagement and station, and verifying membrane status, gently withdraw your fingers. Let the patient clean her perineum herself with sterile gauze if she can walk to the bathroom. If she's confined to bed, you can clean her perineum and change the linen-saver pad.

• Describe how labor progresses, and define the patient's stage and phase, if appropriate, *to encourage her and help reduce her anxiety.*

Nursing considerations

• In early labor, perform the vaginal examination between contractions, focusing primarily on the extent of cervical dilation and effacement.

• At the end of first-stage labor, perform the examination during a contraction, when the uterine muscle pushes the fetus downward. This examination will focus on assessing fetal descent.

• If the amniotic membrane ruptures during the examination, record the fetal heart rate (FHR). Then note the time and describe the color, odor, and approximate amount of fluid. If FHR becomes unstable, notify the doctor, determine fetal station, and check for umbilical cord prolapse. After the membranes rupture, perform the vaginal examination only when labor changes significantly *to minimize the risk of introducing intrauterine infection.*

Documentation

• After each examination, record the percentage of effacement, dilation, the station of the presenting fetal part, amniotic membrane status, and the patient's tolerance of the procedure.

Vascular access device maintenance

An implanted vascular access device is surgically implanted under local anesthesia by a doctor. The device consists of a silicone catheter attached to a reservoir, which is covered with a self-sealing silicone rubber septum. Such a device is most commonly used when an external central venous (CV) catheter is not desirable for long-term I.V. therapy. The most common type of vascular access device is a vascular access port (VAP). One- and two-piece units with single or double lumens are available. (See *Understanding VAPs,* page 956.)

VAPs come in two basic types: top entry (such as Med-i-Port, Port-A-Cath, and Infuse-A-Port) and side entry (such as S.E.A. Port). The VAP res-

Understanding VAPs

Typically, a vascular access port (VAP) is used to deliver intermittent infusion of medication, chemotherapy, or blood products. Because the device is completely covered by the patient's skin, it reduces the risk of extrinsic contamination. Patients may prefer this type of central line because it doesn't alter the body image and requires less routine catheter care.

The VAP consists of a catheter connected to a small reservoir. A septum designed to withstand multiple punctures seals the reservoir.

VAPs come in two basic designs: top entry and side entry. In a top-entry port, the needle is inserted perpendicular to the reservoir. In a side-entry port, the needle is inserted into the septum nearly parallel to the reservoir. (A needle stop prevents the needle from coming out the other side.)

Top-entry VAP

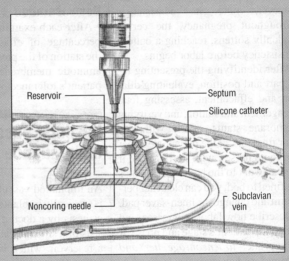

Side-entry VAP

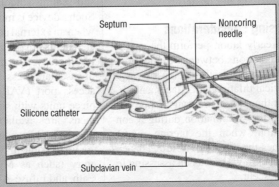

ervoir can be made of titanium (such as Port-A-Cath), stainless steel (such as Q-Port), or molded plastic (such as Infuse-A-Port). The type and lumen size selected depend on the patient's therapeutic needs.

Implanted in a pocket under the skin, a VAP functions much like a long-term CV catheter, except that it has no external parts. The attached indwelling catheter tunnels through the subcutaneous tissue so that the catheter tip lies in a central vein (the subclavian vein, for example). A VAP can also be used for arterial access or can be implanted into the epidural space, peritoneum, or pericardial or pleural cavity.

Typically, VAPs deliver intermittent infusions. Most often used for chemotherapy, a VAP can also deliver I.V. fluids, medications, or blood products. You can also use a VAP to obtain blood samples.

VAPs offer several advantages, including minimal activity restrictions, few self-care measures for the patient to learn and perform, and few dressing changes (except when used to maintain continuous infusions or intermittent infusion devices). Implanted devices are easier to maintain than external devices. For instance, they require heparinization only once after each use (or periodically if not in use). They also pose less risk of infection because they have no exit site to serve as an entry for microorganisms.

Because VAPs create only a slight protrusion under the skin, many patients find them easier to accept than external infusion devices. Because the device is implanted, however, it may be more difficult for the patient to manage, particularly if he'll be admin-

istering medication or fluids daily or frequently. And because accessing the device requires inserting a needle through subcutaneous tissue, patients who fear or dislike needle punctures may be uncomfortable using a VAP and may require a local anesthetic. In addition, implantation and removal of the device requires surgery and hospitalization. The comparatively high cost of VAPs makes them worthwhile only for patients who require infusion therapy for at least 6 months.

Implanted VAPs are contraindicated in patients who have been unable to tolerate other implanted devices and in those who may develop an allergic reaction.

≫ Key nursing diagnoses and patient outcomes

Use these nursing diagnoses as a guide when developing your plan of care for a patient who is being treated with a vascular access device.

Risk for infection related to presence of indwelling tube

Based on this nursing diagnosis, you'll establish the following patient outcomes. The patient will:
• have temperature stay within normal limits.
• have white blood cells and differential stay within range.

High risk for fluid volume deficit related to excessive loss through indwelling tube

Based on this nursing diagnosis, you'll establish the following patient outcomes. The patient will:
• have vital signs remain stable.
• have electrolyte values remain within normal range.

Equipment

To implant a VAP: ◆ noncoring needles of appropriate type and gauge (a noncoring needle has a deflected point, which slices the port's septum instead of scoring it) ◆ VAP ◆ sterile gloves ◆ alcohol pads ◆ extension set tubing if needed ◆ povidone-iodine swabs ◆ local anesthetic (lidocaine without epinephrine) ◆ ice pack ◆ 5-, 10-, and 20-ml syringes ◆ normal saline and heparin flush solutions ◆ I.V. solution ◆ sterile dressings ◆ luer-lock injection cap ◆ clamp ◆ adhesive skin closures ◆ suture removal set.

To administer a bolus injection: ◆ extension set ◆ 10-ml syringe filled with normal saline solution ◆ clamp ◆ syringe containing the prescribed medication ◆ optional: sterile needle filled with heparin flush solution.

To administer a continuous infusion: ◆ prescribed I.V. solution or medication ◆ I.V. administration set ◆ filter if ordered ◆ extension set ◆ clamp ◆ 10-ml syringe filled with normal saline solution ◆ antimicrobial ointment (such as povidone-iodine ointment) ◆ adhesive tape ◆ sterile 2″ × 2″ gauze pad ◆ sterile tape ◆ transparent semipermeable dressing.

Some hospitals use an implantable port access kit.

Equipment preparation

• Confirm the size and type of the device and the insertion site with the doctor.

• Attach the tubing to the solution container, prime the tubing with fluid, fill the syringes with saline or heparin flush solution, and prime the noncoring needle and extension set.

• All priming must be done using strict aseptic technique, and all tubing must be free from air.

• After you've primed the tubing, recheck all connections for tightness.

• Make sure that all open ends are covered with sealed caps.

Implementation

• Wash your hands *to prevent spread of microorganisms.*

Assisting with implantation of a VAP

• Reinforce to the patient the doctor's explanation of the procedure, its benefit to the patient, and what's expected of him during and after implantation.

• Although the doctor is responsible for obtaining consent for the procedure, make sure the written document is signed, witnessed, and on the chart.

• Allay the patient's fears and answer questions about movement restrictions, cosmetic concerns, and management regimens.

• Check the patient's history for hypersensitivity to local anesthetics or iodine.

• The doctor will surgically implant the VAP, most likely using a local anesthetic (similar to insertion of a CV catheter). Occasionally, a patient may receive a general anesthetic for VAP implantation.

• During the implantation procedure, you may be responsible for handing equipment and supplies to the doctor. First, the doctor makes a small incision and introduces the catheter, typically into the superior vena cava through the subclavian, jugular, or cephalic vein. After fluoroscopy verifies correct placement of the catheter tip, the doctor creates a subcutaneous pocket over a bony prominence in the chest wall. Then, he tunnels the catheter to the pocket. Next, he connects the catheter to the reservoir, places the reservoir in the pocket, and flushes it with heparin solution. Finally, he sutures the reservoir to the underlying fascia and closes the incision.

Preparing to access the port

• The VAP can be used immediately after placement, although some edema and tenderness may persist for about 72 hours. This makes the device initially difficult to palpate and slightly uncomfortable for the patient.

• Prepare to access the port, following the specific steps for top-entry or side-entry ports.

• Using aseptic technique, inspect the area around the port for signs of infection or skin breakdown.

• Place an ice pack over the area for several minutes *to alleviate possible discomfort from the needle puncture.* Alternatively, administer a local anesthetic after cleaning the area.

• Wash your hands thoroughly and put on sterile gloves. Remember to keep these gloves on throughout the procedure.

• Clean the area with an alcohol pad, starting at the center of the port and working outward with a firm, circular motion over a 4″ to 5″ (10- to 13-cm) diameter. Repeat this procedure twice.

• If hospital policy calls for a local anesthetic, check the patient's record for possible allergies. As indicated, anesthetize the insertion site by injecting 0.1 ml of lidocaine (without epinephrine).

Accessing a top-entry port

• Palpate the area over the port to locate the port septum.

• Anchor the port with your nondominant hand. Then, using your dominant hand, aim the needle at the center of the device.

• Insert the needle perpendicular to the port septum. Push the needle through the skin and septum until you reach the bottom of the reservoir.

• Check needle placement by aspirating for blood return.

• If you're unable to obtain blood, remove the needle and repeat the procedure. *Inability to obtain blood may indicate that the catheter is lodged against the vessel's wall.* Ask the patient to raise his arms, perform Valsalva's maneuver, or change position to free the catheter. If you still don't get a blood return, notify the doctor; a fibrin sleeve on the distal end of the catheter may be occluding the opening.

• Flush the device with normal saline solution. If you detect swelling or if the patient reports pain at the site, remove the needle and notify the doctor.

Accessing a side-entry port

• To gain access to a side-entry port, you'll follow the same procedure as with a top-entry port; however, you'll insert the needle parallel to the reservoir instead of perpendicular to it.

Administering a bolus injection

• Attach the 10-ml syringe filled with saline solution to the end of the extension set, and remove all the air. Now attach the extension set to the noncoring needle. Check for blood return. Then flush the port with normal saline solution, according to your hospital's

Continuous infusion: Securing the needle

When starting a continuous infusion, you must secure the right-angle noncoring needle to the skin. If the needle hub isn't flush with the skin, place a folded sterile dressing under the hub. Then apply adhesive skin closures across it, as shown.

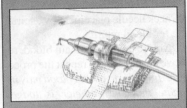

Secure the needle and tubing, using the chevron-taping technique.

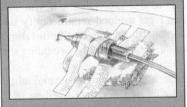

Apply a transparent semipermeable dressing over the entire site.

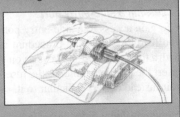

policy. (Some hospitals require flushing the port with a sterile needle of heparin solution first.)
• Clamp the extension set, and remove the saline syringe.

• Connect the medication syringe to the extension set. Open the clamp and inject the drug as ordered.
• Examine the skin surrounding the needle for signs of infiltration, such as swelling or tenderness. If you note these signs, stop the injection and intervene appropriately.
• When the injection is complete, clamp the extension set and remove the medication syringe.
• Open the clamp and flush with 5 ml of normal saline solution after each drug injection to minimize drug incompatibility reactions.
• Flush with heparin solution as hospital policy directs.

Administering a continuous infusion

• Remove all air from the extension set by priming it with an attached syringe of normal saline solution. Now attach the extension set to the noncoring needle.
• Flush the port system with normal saline solution. Clamp the extension set, and remove the syringe.
• Connect the administration set, and secure the connections with sterile tape if necessary.
• Unclamp the extension set, and begin the infusion.
• Apply a small amount of antimicrobial ointment to the insertion site.
• Affix the needle to the skin. (See *Continuous infusion: Securing the needle*.) Then apply a transparent semipermeable dressing.
• Examine the site carefully for infiltration. If the patient complains of stinging, burning, or pain at the site, discontinue the infusion and intervene appropriately.

• When the solution container is empty, obtain a new I.V. solution container as ordered.

• Flush with heparin solution as hospital policy directs.

Complications

• A patient who has a VAP faces risks similar to those associated with CV catheters. These include such complications as infection and infiltration. (See *Understanding the risks of VAP therapy,* page 962.)

Nursing considerations

• After implantation, monitor the site for signs of hematoma and bleeding. Edema and tenderness may persist for about 72 hours. The incision site requires routine postoperative care for 7 to 10 days. You'll also need to assess the implantation site for signs of infection, device rotation, or skin erosion. You don't need to apply a dressing to the wound site except during infusions or to maintain an intermittent infusion device.

• While the patient is hospitalized, a luer-lock injection cap may be attached to the end of the extension set to provide ready access for intermittent infusions. *Besides saving nursing time, a luer-lock cap will reduce the discomfort of accessing the port as well as prolong the life of the port septum by decreasing the number of needle punctures.*

• If your patient is receiving a continuous or prolonged infusion, you'll need to change the dressing and needle every 5 to 7 days. You'll also need to change the tubing and solution, as you would for a long-term CV infusion. If your patient is receiving an intermittent infusion, you'll need to flush the port periodically with heparin solution. When the VAP isn't being used, flush it every 4 weeks. During the course of therapy, you may have to clear a clotted VAP as ordered.

• If clotting threatens to occlude the VAP, the doctor may order a fibrinolytic agent such as urokinase to clear the catheter. The usual dose is 1 ml (5,000 IU/ml of sterile water) of urokinase. Because such agents increase the risk of bleeding, urokinase may be contraindicated in patients who have had surgery within the previous 10 days; who have active internal bleeding such as GI bleeding; or who have experienced central nervous system damage, such as infarction, hemorrhage, traumatic injury, surgery, or primary or metastatic disease, within the past 2 months.

• Besides performing routine care measures, you must be prepared to handle several common problems that may arise during an infusion with a VAP. These common problems include an inability to flush the VAP, withdraw blood from it, or palpate it. (See *Managing common VAP problems,* page 964.)

Home care

• A home care patient needs thorough teaching about procedures and follow-up visits from a home care nurse to ensure safety and successful treatment. If the patient will be accessing the port himself, explain that the most uncomfortable part of the procedure is the actual insertion of the needle into the skin.

• Once the needle has penetrated the skin, the patient will feel mostly pressure. Eventually, the skin over the port will become desensitized from fre-

Understanding the risks of VAP therapy

COMPLICATION	SIGNS AND SYMPTOMS	POSSIBLE CAUSES	NURSING INTERVENTIONS
Site infection or skin breakdown	• Erythema and warmth at the port site • Oozing or purulent drainage at vascular access port (VAP) site or pocket • Fever	• Infected incision or VAP pocket • Poor postoperative healing	• Assess the site daily for redness; note any drainage. • Notify the doctor. • Administer antibiotics as ordered. • Apply warm soaks for 20 minutes four times a day. ***Prevention*** • Teach the patient to inspect for and report any redness, swelling, drainage, or skin breakdown at the port site.
Extravasation	• Burning sensation or swelling in subcutaneous tissue	• Needle dislodged into subcutaneous tissue • Needle incorrectly placed in VAP • Needle position not confirmed; needle pulled out of septum • Use of vesicant drugs	• Stop the infusion. • Notify the doctor; prepare to administer an antidote if ordered. • Follow hospital protocol for removing the needle. ***Prevention*** • Teach the patient how to gain access to the device, verify its placement, and secure the needle before initiating an infusion.
Thrombosis	• Inability to flush port or administer infusion	• Frequent blood sampling • Infusion of packed red blood cells (PRBCs)	• Notify the doctor; obtain an order to administer urokinase. ***Prevention*** • Flush the VAP thoroughly right after obtaining a blood sample.

Understanding the risks of VAP therapy (continued)

COMPLICATION	SIGNS AND SYMPTOMS	POSSIBLE CAUSES	NURSING INTERVENTIONS
Thrombosis (continued)			• Administer PRBCs as a piggyback with normal saline solution and use an infusion pump; flush with saline solution between units.
Fibrin sheath formation	• Blocked port and catheter lumen • Inability to flush port or administer infusion • Possible swelling, tenderness, and erythema in neck, chest, and shoulder	• Adherence of platelets to catheter	• Notify the doctor; add heparin (1,000 to 2,000 U) to continuous infusions as ordered. (Urokinase may also be ordered.) **Prevention** • Use the port only to infuse fluids and medications; don't use it to obtain blood samples. • Administer only compatible substances through the port.

quent needle punctures. Until then, the patient may want to use a topical anesthetic.

• Stress the importance of pushing the needle into the port until the patient feels the needle bevel touch the back of the port. Many patients tend to stop short of the back of the port, leaving the needle bevel in the rubber septum.

• Also stress the importance of monthly flushes when no more infusions are scheduled. If possible, instruct a family member in all aspects of care.

Documentation

• Record your assessment findings and interventions according to hospital policy. Include the following information: type, amount, rate, and duration of the infusion; appearance of the site; development of problems, if any, and steps taken to resolve them.

• Keep a record of all needle and dressing changes for continuous infusions; blood samples obtained, including the type and amount; and patient-teaching topics covered.

PROBLEM SOLVER

 Managing common VAP problems

PROBLEM AND POSSIBLE CAUSE	NURSING INTERVENTIONS
Inability to flush the device or draw blood	
Kinked tubing or closed clamp	• Check tubing or clamp.
Catheter lodged against vessel wall	• Reposition the patient. • Teach the patient to change his position to free the catheter from the vessel wall. • Raise the arm that's on the same side as the catheter. • Roll the patient to his opposite side. • Have the patient cough, sit up, or take a deep breath. • Infuse 10 ml of normal saline solution into the catheter. • Regain access to the catheter or vascular access port (VAP) using a new needle.
Incorrect needle placement or needle not advanced through septum	• Regain access to the device. • Teach the home care patient to push down firmly on the noncoring needle device in the septum and to verify needle placement by aspirating for a blood return.
Clot formation	• Assess patency by trying to flush the VAP while the patient changes position. • Notify the doctor; obtain an order for urokinase instillation. • Teach the patient to recognize clot formation, to notify the doctor if it occurs, and to avoid forcibly flushing the VAP.
Kinked catheter, catheter migration, or port rotation	• Notify the doctor immediately. • Tell the patient to notify the doctor if he has trouble using the VAP.
Inability to palpate the device	
Deeply implanted port	• Note portal chamber scar. • Use deep palpation technique. • Ask another nurse to try locating the VAP. • Use a 1 ½" or 2" (4- or 5-cm) noncoring needle to gain access to the VAP.

• Document the removal of the infusion needle, the status of the site, the use of the heparin flush, and any problems you encountered and resolved.

Venipuncture

Performed to obtain a venous blood sample, venipuncture involves piercing a vein with a needle and collecting blood in a syringe or evacuated tube. Typically, venipuncture is performed via the antecubital fossa. If necessary, however, it can be performed from other locations, such as a vein in the wrist and the dorsum of the hand or foot. Usually, laboratory personnel carry out the procedure in the hospital setting; however, a nurse may perform it occasionally.

≫ Key nursing diagnoses and patient outcomes
Use these nursing diagnoses as a guide when developing your plan of care for a patient who is receiving a venipuncture.

Risk for infection related to presence of an indwelling tube
Based on this nursing diagnosis, you'll establish the following patient outcomes. The patient will:
• have temperature stay within normal limits.
• have white blood cells and differential stay within range.

Risk for fluid volume deficit related to excessive loss through an indwelling tube
Based on this nursing diagnosis, you'll establish the following patient outcomes. The patient will:
• have vital signs remain stable.
• have electrolyte values remain within normal range.

Equipment
♦ tourniquet ♦ gloves ♦ syringe or evacuated tubes and needle holder ♦ 70% ethyl alcohol pads or povidone-iodine sponges ♦ 20G or 21G needle for the forearm or 25G for the wrist, hand, ankle, or for children ♦ color-coded tubes containing appropriate additives (See *Guide to color-top collection tubes*, page 966.) ♦ labels ♦ laboratory request form ♦ 2″ × 2″ gauze pads ♦ adhesive bandage.

If you're using evacuated tubes, open the needle packet, attach the needle to its holder, and select the appropriate tubes.

If you're using a syringe, attach the appropriate needle to it. Be sure to choose a syringe large enough to hold all the blood required for the test.

Label all collection tubes clearly with the patient's name and room number, the doctor's name, and the date and time of collection.

Patient preparation
• Tell the patient that you're about to take a blood sample, and explain the procedure to ease his anxiety and encourage his cooperation. Ask him if he's ever felt faint, sweaty, or nauseated when having blood drawn.

Guide to color-top collection tubes

TUBE COLOR	DRAW VOLUME	ADDITIVE	PURPOSE
Red	2 to 20 ml	None	Serum studies
Lavender	2 to 10 ml	Ethylenediaminetet-raacetic acid	Whole blood studies
Green	2 to 15 ml	Heparin (sodium, lithium, or ammonium)	Plasma studies
Blue	2.7 or 4.5 ml	Sodium citrate and citric acid	Coagulation studies on plasma
Black	2.7 or 4.5 ml	Sodium oxalate	Coagulation studies on plasma
Gray	3 to 10 ml	Glycolytic inhibitor, such as sodium fluoride, powdered oxalate, or glycolytic-microbial inhibitor	Glucose determinations on serum or plasma
Yellow	12 ml	Acid-citrate-dextrose	Whole blood studies

Implementation

• Wash your hands thoroughly, and don *gloves to prevent cross-contamination.*

• If the patient is on bed rest, ask him to lie in a supine position, with his head slightly elevated and his arms at his sides. Ask the ambulatory patient to sit in a chair and support his arm securely on an armrest or table.

• Assess the patient's veins *to determine the best puncture site.* (See *Common venipuncture sites.*)

• Observe the skin for the vein's blue color, or palpate the vein for a firm rebound sensation.

• Tie a tourniquet 2″ (5 cm) proximal to the area chosen. *By impeding venous return to the heart while still allowing arterial flow, a tourniquet produces venous dilation.* If arterial perfusion remains adequate, you'll be able to feel the radial pulse. (If the tourniquet fails to dilate the vein, have the patient open and close his fist repeatedly. Then ask him to close his fist as you insert the needle and to open it again when the needle is in place.)

• Clean the venipuncture site with a povidone-iodine sponge or with an alcohol pad. Don't wipe off the povidone-iodine with alcohol *because alcohol cancels the effect of povidone-iodine.* Wipe in a circular motion, spiraling outward from the site *to avoid introducing potentially infectious skin flora into the vessel during the procedure.* If you use alcohol, apply it with friction for 30 seconds, or until the final pad comes away clean. Allow the skin to dry before performing venipuncture.

Common venipuncture sites

These illustrations show common anatomic locations of veins used for venipuncture. The most commonly used sites are on the forearm, followed by those on the hand.

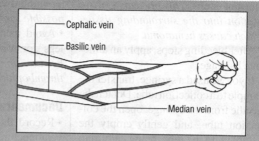

Cephalic vein
Basilic vein
Median vein

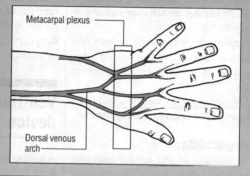

Metacarpal plexus
Dorsal venous arch

• Immobilize the vein by pressing just below the venipuncture site with your thumb and drawing the skin taut.
• Position the needle holder or syringe with the needle bevel up and the shaft parallel to the path of the vein and at a 30-degree angle to the arm. Insert the needle into the vein. If you're using a syringe, venous blood will appear in the hub; withdraw the blood slowly, pulling the plunger of the syringe gently *to create steady suction* until you obtain the required sample. *Pulling the plunger too forcibly may collapse the vein.* If you're using a needle holder and an evacuated tube, grasp the holder securely to stabilize it in the vein, and push down on the collection tube until the needle punc-

tures the rubber stopper. Blood will flow into the tube automatically.
• Remove the tourniquet as soon as blood flows adequately *to prevent stasis and hemoconcentration, which can impair test results.* If the flow is sluggish, leave the tourniquet in place longer, but always remove it before withdrawing the needle.
• Continue to fill the required tubes, removing one and inserting another. Gently rotate each tube as you remove it *to help mix the additive.*
• After you've drawn the sample, place a gauze pad over the puncture site, and slowly and gently remove the needle from the vein. When using an evacuated tube, remove it from the needle holder *to release the vacuum before withdrawing the needle from the vein.*

• Apply gentle pressure to the puncture site for 2 or 3 minutes or until bleeding stops. *This prevents extravasation into the surrounding tissue, which causes hematoma.*
• After bleeding stops, apply an adhesive bandage.
• If you've used a syringe, transfer the sample to a collection tube. Detach the needle from the syringe, open the collection tube, and gently empty the sample into the tube, being careful to avoid foaming, *which may cause hemolysis.*
• Finally, check the venipuncture site *to make sure a hematoma hasn't developed.* If it has, then apply warm soaks.
• Discard syringes, needles, and used gloves in the appropriate containers.

Complications
• Hematoma at the needle insertion site is the most common complication of venipuncture. Infection may result from poor technique.

Nursing considerations
• Never draw a venous sample from an arm or leg already being used for I.V. therapy or blood administration *because this may affect test results.* Don't draw a venous sample from an infection site *because this risks introduction of pathogens into the vascular system.* Likewise, avoid drawing blood from edematous areas, arteriovenous shunts, or sites of previous hematoma or vascular injury.
• If the patient has large, distended, highly visible veins, perform venipuncture without a tourniquet *to minimize the risk of hematoma.*
• If the patient has a clotting disorder or is receiving anticoagulant therapy,

maintain firm pressure on the venipuncture site for at least 5 minutes after withdrawing the needle *to prevent possible formation of a hematoma.*
• Avoid using veins in the patient's legs for venipuncture, if possible, *because this increases the risk of thrombophlebitis.*

Documentation
• Record the date, time, and site of venipuncture; name of the test; the time the sample was sent to the laboratory; and any adverse effects the patient experiences, such as a hematoma or anxiety.

Ventricular assist device

A temporary life-sustaining treatment for a failing heart, the ventricular assist device (VAD) diverts systemic blood flow from a diseased ventricle into a centrifugal pump. It temporarily reduces ventricular work, allowing the myocardium to rest and contractility to improve. Although used most commonly to assist the left ventricle, this device may also assist the right ventricle or both ventricles. (See *VAD: Help for the failing heart.*)

Candidates for VAD include patients with massive myocardial infarction, irreversible cardiomyopathy, acute myocarditis, an inability to be weaned from cardiopulmonary bypass, valvular disease, infective endocarditis, or heart transplant rejection. The device may also be used in those awaiting a heart transplant.

VAD: Help for the failing heart

The ventricular assist device (VAD) functions somewhat like an artificial heart. The major difference is that the VAD assists the heart, whereas the artificial heart replaces it. The VAD is designed to aid one or both ventricles. The pumping chambers themselves aren't usually implanted in the patient.

The permanent VAD is implanted in the patient's chest cavity, although it still provides only temporary support. The device receives power through the skin by a belt of electrical transformer coils (worn externally as a portable battery pack). It can also operate off an implanted, rechargeable battery for up to 1 hour at a time.

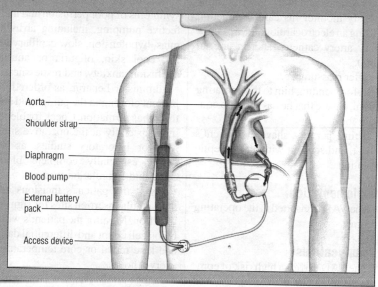

Aorta
Shoulder strap
Diaphragm
Blood pump
External battery pack
Access device

≫ Key nursing diagnoses and patient outcomes

Use these nursing diagnoses as a guide when developing your plan of care for a patient who is being treated with a ventricular assist device.

Decreased cardiac output related to decreased stroke volume
Based on this nursing diagnosis, you'll establish the following patient outcomes. The patient will:
• have no arrhythmias.

• have cardiac output remain adequate.

Altered (specify type) tissue perfusion related to decreased cellular exchange
Based on this nursing diagnosis, you'll establish the following patient outcomes. The patient will:
• attain hemodynamic stability as evidenced by pulse not less than __ and not more than __ and blood pressure not less than __/__ and not more than __/__.

• have heart rate remain within prescribed limits while he carries out activities of daily living.

Equipment
♦ VAD.

Patient preparation
• Before surgery, explain to the patient that food and fluid intake must be restricted and that you will continuously monitor his cardiac function (using an electrocardiogram, a pulmonary artery catheter, and an arterial line).
• Offer reassurance.
• Before sending him to the operating room, ensure that he has signed a consent form.
• If time permits, shave the patient's chest, and scrub it with an antiseptic solution.

Implementation
• The VAD is inserted in the operating room.

Complications
• The VAD carries a high risk of complications, including damaged blood cells, which can increase the likelihood of thrombus formation and subsequent pulmonary embolism or cerebrovascular accident.

Nursing considerations
• When the patient returns from surgery, administer analgesics as ordered.
• Frequently monitor vital signs, intake, and output.
• Keep the patient immobile *to prevent accidental extubation, contamination, or disconnection of the VAD.* Use soft restraints as necessary.

• Monitor pulmonary artery pressures. If you've been prepared to adjust the pump, maintain cardiac output at about 5 to 8 L/minute, central venous pressure at about 8 to 16 mm Hg, pulmonary artery wedge pressure at about 10 to 20 mm Hg, mean arterial pressure at greater than 60 mm Hg, and left arterial pressure between 4 and 12 mm Hg.
• Monitor the patient for signs and symptoms of poor perfusion and ineffective pumping, including arrhythmias, hypotension, slow capillary refill, cool skin, oliguria or anuria, confusion, anxiety, and restlessness.
• Administer heparin, as ordered, to prevent clotting in the pump head and thrombus formation. Check for bleeding, especially at the operative sites. Monitor laboratory studies, as ordered, especially complete blood count and coagulation studies.
• Assess the patient's incisions and the cannula insertion sites for signs of infection. Monitor the patient's white blood cell count and differential daily, and take rectal or core temperatures every 4 hours.
• Change the dressing over the cannula sites daily or according to hospital policy.
• Provide supportive care, including range-of-motion exercises and mouth and skin care.
• If ventricular function fails to improve within 4 days, the patient may need a transplant. If so, provide psychological support for the patient and family as they endure referral. You may also initiate the transplant process by contacting the appropriate agency.

• The psychological effects of the VAD can produce stress in the patient, his family, and his close friends. If appropriate, refer them to other support personnel.

Documentation
• Note the patient's condition following insertion of the VAD.
• Document any pump adjustments as well as any complications and interventions.

W X Y Z

Wound care, closed-wound drainage

Typically inserted during surgery in anticipation of substantial postoperative drainage, a closed-wound drain promotes healing and prevents swelling by suctioning the serosanguineous fluid that accumulates at the wound site. By removing this fluid, the closed-wound drain helps reduce the risk of infection and skin breakdown as well as the number of dressing changes. Hemovac and Jackson-Pratt closed-wound drainage systems are used most commonly.

A closed-wound drain consists of perforated tubing connected to a portable vacuum unit. The distal end of the tubing lies within the wound and usually leaves the body from a site other than the primary suture line to preserve the integrity of the surgical wound. The tubing exit site is treated as an additional surgical wound; the drain is usually sutured to the skin.

If the wound produces heavy drainage, the closed-wound drain may be left in place for longer than 1 week. Drainage must be emptied and measured frequently to maintain maximum suction and prevent strain on the suture line.

≫ Key nursing diagnoses and patient outcomes

Use these nursing diagnoses as a guide when developing your plan of care for a patient with a closed-wound drainage system.

Risk for infection related to surgical incision

Based on this nursing diagnosis, you'll establish the following patient outcomes. The patient will:
• exhibit vital signs, temperature and lab values within the patients normal limits.
• have no signs or symptoms of infection at incision site.

Impaired skin integrity related to presence of drain

Based on this nursing diagnosis, you'll establish the following patient outcomes. The patient will:
• exhibit improved or healing wound.
• avoid or minimize complications.

Equipment

♦ graduated biohazard cylinder ♦ sterile laboratory container, if needed ♦ alcohol pads ♦ gloves ♦ gown ♦ face shield ♦ trash bag ♦ sterile gauze pads ♦ antiseptic cleaning agent ♦ prepackaged povidone-iodine swabs.

Implementation

• Check the doctor's order, and assess the patient's condition.
• Explain the procedure to the patient, provide privacy, and wash your hands.
• Unclip the vacuum unit from the patient's bed or gown.
• Using aseptic technique, release the vacuum by removing the spout plug on the collection chamber. The container expands completely as it draws in air.
• Empty the unit's contents into a graduated biohazard cylinder, and note the amount and appearance of the

Using a closed-wound drainage system

The portable closed-wound drainage system draws drainage from a wound site, such as the chest wall postmastectomy shown at left, by means of a Y-tube. To empty the drainage, remove the plug and empty it into a graduated cylinder. To reestablish suction, compress the drainage unit against a firm surface to expel air and, while holding it down, replace the plug with your other hand, as shown at right.

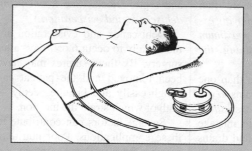 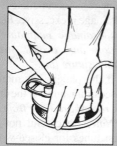

drainage. If diagnostic tests will be performed on the fluid specimen, pour the drainage directly into a sterile laboratory container, note the amount and appearance, and send it to the laboratory.

• Maintaining aseptic technique, use an alcohol pad to clean the unit's spout and plug.

• *To reestablish the vacuum that creates the drain's suction power,* fully compress the vacuum unit. With one hand holding the unit compressed *to maintain the vacuum,* replace the spout plug with your other hand. (See *Using a closed-wound drainage system.*)

• Check the patency of the equipment. Make sure the tubing is free from twists, kinks, and leaks *because the drainage system must be airtight to work properly.* The vacuum unit should remain compressed when you release manual pressure; rapid reinflation indicates an air leak. If this oc-

curs, recompress the unit and make sure the spout plug is secure.

• Secure the vacuum unit to the patient's bedding or, if she is ambulatory, to her gown. Fasten it below wound level *to promote drainage.* Do not apply tension on drainage tubing when fastening the unit *to prevent possible dislodgement.* Remove and discard your gloves and wash your hands thoroughly.

• Observe the sutures that secure the drain to the patient's skin; look for signs of pulling or tearing, and for swelling or infection of surrounding skin. Gently clean the sutures with sterile gauze pads soaked in an antiseptic cleaning agent or with a povidone-iodine swab.

• Properly dispose of drainage, solutions, and trash bag, and clean or dispose of soiled equipment and supplies according to institutional policy.

Complications
• Occlusion of the tubing by fibrin, clots, or other particles can reduce or obstruct drainage.

Nursing considerations
• Empty the system and measure its contents once during each shift if drainage has accumulated, more often if drainage is excessive. *Removing excess drainage maintains maximum suction and avoids straining the drain's suture line.*

If the patient has more than one closed drain, number the drains *so you can record drainage from each site.*

Note. Be careful not to mistake chest tubes for closed-wound drains *because the vacuum of a chest tube should never be released.*

Documentation
• Record the date and time you empty the system, the appearance of the drain site and presence of swelling or signs of infection, any equipment malfunction and consequent nursing action, and the patient's tolerance of the treatment.
• On the intake and output sheet, record drainage color, consistency, type, and amount.
• If the patient has more than one closed-wound drain, number the drains and record the above information separately for each drainage site.

Wound dehiscence and evisceration

Although the typical surgical wound heals without incident, occasionally the edges of a wound may fail to join, or may separate even after they seem to be healing normally. This development, called wound dehiscence, may lead to an even more serious complication: evisceration, where a portion of the viscera (usually a bowel loop) protrudes through the incision. Evisceration, in turn, can lead to peritonitis and septic shock. (See *Recognizing dehiscence and evisceration.*)

Dehiscence and evisceration are most likely to occur 6 or 7 days after surgery. By then, sutures may have been removed and the patient can cough easily and breathe deeply — both of which strain the incision.

Several factors can contribute to these complications. Poor nutrition, whether from inadequate intake or a condition such as diabetes mellitus, may hinder wound healing. Chronic pulmonary or cardiac disease can also slow healing because the injured tissue doesn't get needed nutrients and oxygen. Localized wound infection may limit closure, delay healing, and weaken the incision. And stress on the incision from coughing or vomiting may cause abdominal distention or severe stretching. A midline abdominal incision, for instance, has a high risk of wound dehiscence.

⟫ Key nursing diagnoses and patient outcomes
Use these nursing diagnoses as a guide when developing your plan of care for a patient who has wound dehiscence and evisceration.

Fluid volume deficit related to active loss
Based on this nursing diagnosis, you'll establish the following patient outcomes. The patient will:

- have vital signs remain stable.
- have fluid and blood volume return to normal.

Altered (specify type) tissue perfusion related to decreased cellular exchange

Based on this nursing diagnosis, you'll establish the following patient outcomes. The patient will:
- attain hemodynamic stability. Pulse not less than (specify) and not more than (specify). Blood pressure not more than (specify) and not less than (specify).
- not exhibit arrhythmias.

Equipment

◆ two sterile towels ◆ 1 L of normal sterile saline solution ◆ sterile irrigation set, including a basin, a solution container, and a 50-ml catheter-tip syringe ◆ several large abdominal dressings ◆ sterile, waterproof drape ◆ linen-saver pads ◆ sterile gloves.

If the patient will return to the operating room, make sure you also gather the following equipment: ◆ I.V. administration set and I.V. fluids ◆ equipment for nasogastric intubation ◆ sedative as ordered ◆ suction apparatus.

Equipment preparation

- Using sterile technique, unfold a sterile towel to create a sterile field. Open the package containing the irrigation set, and place the basin, solution container, and 50-ml syringe on the sterile field.
- Open the bottle of normal saline solution, and pour about 14 oz (400 ml) into the solution container. Also pour about 8 oz (200 ml) into the sterile basin.

Recognizing dehiscence and evisceration

In wound dehiscence, the layers of the surgical wound separate. With evisceration, the viscera (in this case, a bowel loop) protrude through the surgical incision.

Wound dehiscence

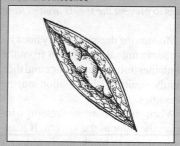

Evisceration of a bowel loop

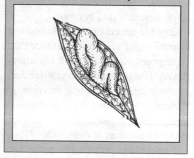

- Open several large abdominal dressings, and place them on the sterile field.
- Put on the sterile gloves, and place one or two of the large abdominal dressings into the basin *to saturate them with saline solution.*

Patient preparation

- Provide reassurance and support *to ease the patient's anxiety.* Tell him to stay in bed. If possible, stay with him

while someone else notifies the doctor and collects the necessary equipment.
• Place a linen-saver pad under the patient *to keep the sheets dry when you moisten the exposed viscera.*

Implementation
• Place the moistened dressings over the exposed viscera. Then place a sterile, waterproof drape over the dressings *to prevent the sheets from getting wet.*
• Moisten the dressings every hour by withdrawing saline solution from the container through the syringe and then gently squirting the solution on the dressings.
• When you moisten the dressings, inspect the color of the viscera. If it appears dusky or black, notify a doctor immediately. *With its blood supply interrupted, a protruding organ may become ischemic and necrotic.*
• Keep the patient on absolute bed rest in low Fowler's position (no more than 20 degrees elevation) with his knees flexed. *This prevents injury and reduces stress on an abdominal incision.*
• Monitor the patient's pulse, respirations, blood pressure, and temperature every 15 minutes *to detect shock.*
• If necessary, prepare the patient to return to the operating room. Gather the equipment and start an I.V. infusion as ordered.
• Insert a nasogastric tube, and connect it to continuous or intermittent low suction as ordered.
• Also administer preoperative medications to the patient as ordered.
• Depending on the circumstances, some of these procedures may not be done at the bedside. For instance, nasogastric intubation may make the patient gag or vomit, causing further eviscerate. For this reason, the doctor may choose to have the tube inserted in the operating room with the patient under anesthesia.
• Continue to reassure the patient while you prepare him for surgery. Be sure he has signed a consent form and the operating room staff has been informed about the procedure.

Complications
• Infection, which can lead to peritonitis and possibly septic shock, is the most severe and most common complication of wound dehiscence and evisceration. Caused by bacterial contamination or by drying of normally moist abdominal contents, infection can impair circulation and lead to necrosis of the affected organ.

Nursing considerations
• As always, the best treatment is prevention. If you're caring for a postoperative patient who's at risk for poor healing, be sure he gets an adequate supply of protein, vitamins, and calories. Monitor his dietary deficiencies, and discuss any problems with a doctor and a dietitian.
• When changing wound dressings, always use sterile technique. Inspect the incision with each dressing change and, if you recognize the early signs of infection, start treatment before dehiscence or evisceration can occur. If local infection develops, clean the wound as necessary to eliminate a buildup of purulent drainage. Always make sure bandages aren't so tight that they limit blood supply to the wound.

Documentation
• Note when the problem occurred, the patient's activity preceding the

problem, his condition, and the time the doctor was notified.
• Describe the appearance of the wound or eviscerated organ; the amount, color, consistency, and odor of any drainage; and any nursing actions taken.
• Record the patient's vital signs, his response to the incident, and the doctor's actions.
• Be sure you change the patient care plan to reflect nursing actions needed to promote proper healing.

Wound irrigation

Irrigation cleans tissues and flushes cell debris and drainage from an open wound. Irrigation with an antiseptic or antibiotic solution helps the wound heal properly from the inside tissue layers outward to the skin surface; it also helps prevent premature surface healing over an abscess pocket or infected tract. Performed properly, wound irrigation requires strict sterile technique. After irrigation, open wounds usually are packed to absorb additional drainage.

≫ Key nursing diagnoses and patient outcomes
Use these nursing diagnoses as a guide when developing your plan of care for a patient who is undergoing wound irrigation.

Risk for infection related to surgical incision
Based on this nursing diagnosis, you'll establish the following patient outcomes. The patient will:

• have vital signs, temperature, and lab values remain within patient's normal limits.
• have incision site free from signs and symptoms of infection.

Anxiety related to situational crisis
Based on this nursing diagnosis, you'll establish the following patient outcomes. The patient will:
• state at least two ways to eliminate or minimize anxious behaviors.
• report being able to cope with current situation without experiencing severe anxiety.

Equipment
♦ waterproof trash bag ♦ linen-saver pad ♦ emesis basin ♦ clean gloves ♦ sterile gloves ♦ goggles ♦ gown if indicated ♦ prescribed irrigant, such as sterile normal saline solution, hydrogen peroxide, or antibiotic solutions ♦ sterile water or normal saline solution ♦ soft rubber or plastic catheter ♦ 50- to 60-ml piston syringe ♦ sterile container ♦ antiseptic cleaning agent ♦ materials as needed for wound care ♦ sterile irrigation and dressing set ♦ povidone-iodine sponges ♦ sterile petroleum jelly.

Equipment preparation
• Assemble all equipment in the patient's room.
• Check the expiration date on each sterile package, and inspect for tears.
• Check the sterilization date and the date that each bottle of irrigating solution was opened; don't use any solution that's been open longer than 24 hours.
• Using aseptic technique, dilute the prescribed irrigant to the correct proportions with sterile water or normal saline solution if necessary. Let the so-

Irrigating a deep wound

When preparing to irrigate a deep wound, attach a soft rubber catheter to a piston-type syringe. Soft rubber minimizes tissue trauma, irritation, and bleeding. Then gently insert the catheter into the recesses of the wound until you feel resistance. Avoid forcing the catheter into the wound to prevent tissue damage or, in an abdominal wound, intestinal perforation.

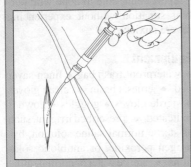

Irrigate the wound with gentle pressure until the solution returns clean. Then position the emesis basin under the wound to collect any remaining drainage.

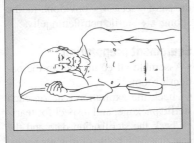

lution stand until it reaches room temperature, or warm it to 90° to 95° F (32.2° to 35° C).
• Open the waterproof trash bag and place it near the patient's bed *to avoid*

reaching across the sterile field or the wound when disposing of soiled articles. Form a cuff by turning down the top of the trash bag *to provide a wide opening and prevent contamination by touching the bag's edge.*

Patient preparation
• Explain the procedure.
• Provide privacy.
• Position the patient correctly.

Implementation
• Check the doctor's order, and assess the patient's condition. Identify the patient's allergies, especially to povidone-iodine or other topical solutions or medications.
• Place the linen-saver pad under the patient *to catch any spills and avoid linen changes.* Place the emesis basin below the wound *so the irrigating solution flows from the wound into the basin.*
• Wash your hands thoroughly. If necessary, put on a gown *to protect your clothing from wound drainage and contamination.* Put on clean gloves.
• Remove the soiled dressing; then discard the dressing and gloves in the trash bag.
• Establish a sterile field with all the equipment and supplies you'll need for irrigation and wound care. Pour the prescribed amount of irrigating solution into a sterile container *so that you don't contaminate your sterile gloves later by picking up unsterile containers.* Put on sterile gloves, gown, and goggles, if indicated.
• Fill the syringe with the irrigating solution; then connect the catheter to the syringe. Gently instill a slow, steady stream of irrigating solution into the wound until the syringe empties. (See *Irrigating a deep wound.*)

Make sure the solution flows from the clean to the dirty area of the wound *to prevent contamination of clean tissue by exudate*. Also make sure the solution reaches all areas of the wound.

• Refill the syringe, reconnect it to the catheter, and repeat the irrigation.

• Continue to irrigate the wound until you've administered the prescribed amount of solution or until the solution returns clear. Note the amount of solution administered. Then remove and discard the catheter and syringe in the waterproof trash bag.

• Keep the patient positioned *to allow further wound drainage into the basin.*

• Clean the area around the wound with povidone-iodine sponges or an antiseptic cleaning agent *to help prevent skin breakdown and infection.*

• Pack the wound, if ordered, and apply a sterile dressing. Remove and discard your gloves and gown

• Make sure the patient is comfortable.

• Properly dispose of drainage, solutions, and trash bag, and clean or dispose of soiled equipment and supplies according to hospital policy. *To prevent contamination of other equipment,* don't return unopened sterile supplies to the sterile supply cabinet.

Complications
• Wound irrigation increases the risk of infection. Excoriation and increased pain may also occur.

Nursing considerations
• Try to coordinate wound irrigation with the doctor's visit *so that he can inspect the wound.* Use only the irrigant specified by the doctor *because others may be erosive or otherwise harmful.* When using an irritating irrigant such as Dakin's solution, spread

sterile petroleum jelly around the wound site *to protect the patient's skin.* Remember to follow your institution's policy concerning wound and skin precautions when appropriate. Irrigate with a bulb syringe only if a piston syringe is unavailable; *the piston syringe reduces the risk of aspirating drainage.* If the wound is small or not particularly deep, you may want to use just the syringe for irrigation.

Home care
• If the wound must be irrigated at home, teach the patient or a family member how to perform irrigation using strict aseptic technique.

• Ask for a return demonstration of the proper technique. Provide written instructions.

• Arrange for home health supplies and nursing visits as appropriate.

• Urge the patient to call his doctor if he detects signs of infection.

Documentation
• Record the date and time of irrigation, amount and type of irrigant, appearance of the wound, any sloughing tissue or exudate, amount of solution returned, any skin care performed around the wound, any dressings applied, and the patient's tolerance of the treatment.

Wound management, surgical

When caring for a surgical wound, you carry out procedures that help prevent infection by stopping pathogens from entering the wound. Besides promoting patient comfort, such procedures also protect the skin surface from maceration and excoriation caused by contact with irritating drainage. They also allow you to measure wound drainage to monitor fluid and electrolyte balance.

The two primary methods used to manage a draining surgical wound are dressing and pouching. Dressing is preferred unless caustic or excessive drainage is compromising your patient's skin integrity. Usually, lightly seeping wounds with drains and wounds with minimal purulent drainage can be managed with packing and gauze dressings. Some wounds such as those that become chronic may require an occlusive dressing.

A wound with copious, excoriating drainage calls for pouching to protect the surrounding skin. If your patient has a surgical wound, you must monitor him, and choose the appropriate dressing.

Dressing a wound calls for sterile technique and sterile supplies to prevent contamination. You may use the color of the wound to help determine which type of dressing to apply. (See *Tailoring wound care to wound color*.)

Be sure to change the dressing often enough to keep the skin dry.

›› Key nursing diagnoses and patient outcomes

Use these nursing diagnoses as a guide when developing your plan of care for a patient who has a surgical wound.

Risk for infection related to surgical incision
Based on this nursing diagnosis, you'll establish the following patient outcomes. The patient will:

• have vital signs, temperature, and lab values remain within patient's normal limits.
• have incision site free from signs and symptoms of infection.

Anxiety related to situational crisis
Based on this nursing diagnosis, you'll establish the following patient outcomes. The patient will:
• state at least two ways to eliminate or minimize anxious behaviors.
• report being able to cope with current situation without experiencing severe anxiety.

Equipment
♦ waterproof trash bag ♦ clean gloves ♦ sterile gloves ♦ gown and face shield or goggles if indicated ♦ sterile $4'' \times 4''$ gauze pads ♦ ABD pads if indicated ♦ sterile cotton-tipped applicators ♦ sterile dressing set ♦ povidone-iodine swabs ♦ topical medication if ordered ♦ adhesive or other tape ♦ soap and water ♦ optional: skin protectant; nonadherent pads; collodion spray, acetone-free adhesive remover, or baby oil; sterile normal saline solution; graduated container; and Montgomery straps, a fishnet tube elasticized dressing support, or a T-binder.

For a wound with a drain: ♦ sterile scissors ♦ sterile $4'' \times 4''$ gauze pads without cotton lining ♦ sump drain ♦ ostomy pouch or another collection bag ♦ precut tracheostomy pads or drain dressings ♦ adhesive tape (paper or silk tape if the patient is hypersensitive) ♦ surgical mask.

For pouching a wound: ♦ collection pouch with drainage port ♦ sterile gloves ♦ skin protectant ♦ sterile gauze pads.

Tailoring wound care to wound color

With any wound, promote healing by keeping it moist, clean, and free from debris. If your patient has an open wound, you can assess how well it's healing by inspecting its color and then use wound color to guide the specific management approach.

Red wounds
Red, the color of healthy granulation tissue, indicates normal healing. When a wound begins to heal, a layer of pale pink granulation tissue covers the wound bed. As this layer thickens, it becomes beefy red. Cover a red wound, keep it moist and clean, and protect it from trauma. Use a transparent dressing (such as Tegaderm or Op-Site), a hydrocolloid dressing (such as DuoDerm), or a gauze dressing moistened with sterile normal saline solution or impregnated with petroleum jelly or an antibiotic.

Yellow wounds
Yellow is the color of exudate produced by microorganisms in an open wound. When a wound heals without complications, the immune system removes microorganisms. But if there are too many microorganisms to remove, exudate accumulates and becomes visible. Exudate usually appears whitish yellow, creamy yellow, yellowish green, or beige. Water content influences the shade: Dry exudate appears darker.

If your patient has a yellow wound, clean it and remove exudate using high-pressure irrigation; then cover it with a moist dressing. Use absorptive products (for example, Debrisan beads and paste) or a moist gauze dressing with or without an antibiotic. You may also use hydrotherapy with whirlpool or high-pressure irrigation.

Black wounds
Black, the least healthy color, signals necrosis. Dead, avascular tissue slows healing and provides a site for microorganisms to proliferate.

You should debride a black wound. After removing dead tissue, apply a dressing to keep the wound moist and guard against external contamination. As ordered, use enzyme products (such as Elase or Travase), surgical debridement, hydrotherapy with whirlpool or high-pressure irrigation, or a moist gauze dressing.

Multicolored wounds
You may note two or even all three colors in a wound. In this case, you'd classify the wound according to the least healthy color present. For example, if your patient's wound is both red and yellow, classify it as a yellow wound.

Equipment preparation
• Assemble all equipment in the patient's room.
• Check the expiration date on each sterile package, and inspect for tears.

• Open the waterproof trash bag, and place it near the patient's bed.
• Position the bag to avoid reaching across the sterile field or the wound when disposing of soiled articles.

• Form a cuff by turning down the top of the trash bag to provide a wide opening and to prevent contamination of instruments or gloves by touching the bag's edge.

Patient preparation
• Explain the procedure to the patient to allay his anxiety *and to enlist his cooperation.*
• Ask the patient about allergies to tapes and dressings.

Implementation
Follow the steps below when managing surgical wounds.

Removing the old dressing
• Check the doctor's order for specific wound care and medication instructions. Be sure to note the location of surgical drains *to avoid dislodging them during the procedure.*
• Assess the patient's condition.
• Identify the patient's allergies, especially to adhesive tape, povidone-iodine or other topical solutions, or medications.
• Provide the patient with privacy, and position him as necessary. *To avoid chilling him,* expose only the wound site.
• Wash your hands thoroughly. Put on a gown and a face shield if necessary. Then put on clean gloves.
• Loosen the soiled dressing by holding the patient's skin and pulling the tape or dressing toward the wound. *This protects the newly formed tissue and prevents stress on the incision.* Moisten the tape with acetone-free adhesive remover or baby oil, if necessary, *to make the tape removal less painful (particularly if the skin is hairy).* Don't apply solvents to the incision *because they could contaminate the wound.*
• Slowly remove the soiled dressing. If the gauze adheres to the wound, loosen the gauze by moistening it with sterile normal saline solution.
• Observe the dressing for the amount, type, color, and odor of drainage.
• Discard the dressing and gloves in the waterproof trash bag.

Caring for the wound
• Wash your hands. Establish a sterile field with all the equipment and supplies you'll need for suture-line care and the dressing change, including a sterile dressing set and povidone-iodine swabs. If the doctor has ordered ointment, squeeze the needed amount onto the sterile field. If you're using an antiseptic from an unsterile bottle, pour the antiseptic cleaning agent into a sterile container *so you don't contaminate your gloves.* Then put on sterile gloves. (See *How to put on sterile gloves.*)
• Saturate the sterile gauze pads with the prescribed cleaning agent. Avoid using cotton balls *because they may shed fibers in the wound, causing irritation, infection, or adhesion.*
• If ordered, obtain a wound culture; then proceed to clean the wound.
• Pick up the moistened gauze pad or swab, and squeeze out the excess solution.
• Working from the top of the incision, wipe once to the bottom and then discard the gauze pad. With a second moistened pad, wipe from top to bottom in a vertical path next to the incision.
• Continue to work outward from the incision in lines running parallel to it. Always wipe from the clean area to-

How to put on sterile gloves

Using your nondominant hand, pick up the opposite glove by grasping the exposed inside of the cuff.

Slip the gloved fingers of your dominant hand under the cuff of the loose glove to pick it up.

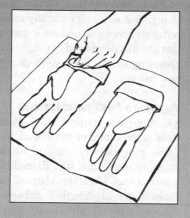

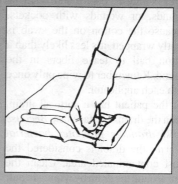

Put the glove onto your dominant hand. Be sure to keep your thumb folded inward to avoid touching the sterile part of the glove. Allow the glove to come uncuffed as you finish inserting your hand, but don't touch the outside of the glove.

Slide your nondominant hand into the glove, holding your dominant thumb as far away as possible to avoid brushing against your arm. Allow the glove to come uncuffed as you finish putting it on, but don't touch the skin side of the cuff with your other gloved hand.

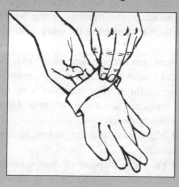

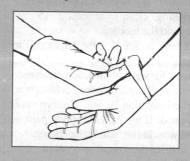

ward the less clean area (usually from top to bottom). Use each gauze pad or swab for only one stroke *to avoid tracking wound exudate and normal* *body flora from surrounding skin to the clean areas.* Remember that the suture line is cleaner than the adjacent skin and the top of the suture line is usually cleaner than the bottom *because more drainage collects at the bottom of the wound.*

• Use sterile cotton-tipped applicators for efficient cleaning of tight-fitting wire sutures, deep and narrow wounds, or wounds with pockets. Because the cotton on the swab is tightly wrapped, it's less likely than a cotton ball to leave fibers in the wound. Remember to wipe only once with each applicator.

• If the patient has a surgical drain, clean the drain's surface last. *Because moist drainage promotes bacterial growth,* the drain is considered the most contaminated area. Clean the skin around the drain by wiping in half or full circles from the drain site outward.

• Clean all areas of the wound to wash away debris, pus, blood, and necrotic material. Try not to disturb sutures or irritate the incision. Clean to at least 1″ (2.5 cm) beyond the end of the new dressing. If you aren't applying a new dressing, clean to at least 2″ (5 cm) beyond the incision.

• Check to see that the edges of the incision are lined up properly, and check for signs of infection (heat, redness, swelling, and odor), dehiscence, or evisceration. If you observe such signs or if the patient reports pain at the wound site, notify the doctor.

• Irrigate the wound as ordered.

• Wash skin surrounding the wound with soap and water, and pat dry using a sterile 4″ × 4″ gauze pad. Avoid oil-based soap because it may interfere with pouch adherence. Apply any prescribed topical medication.

• Apply a skin protectant if needed.

• If ordered, pack the wound with gauze pads or strips folded to fit. Avoid using cotton-lined gauze pads *because cotton fibers can adhere to the wound surface and cause complications.* Pack the wound using the wet-to-damp method. Soaking the packing material in solution and wringing it out so it's slightly moist provides a moist wound environment that absorbs debris and drainage. But removing the packing won't disrupt new tissue.

Applying a fresh gauze dressing

• Gently place sterile 4″ × 4″ gauze pads at the center of the wound, and move progressively outward to the edges of the wound site. Extend the gauze at least 1″ (2.5 cm) beyond the incision in each direction, and cover the wound evenly with enough sterile dressings (usually two or three layers) to absorb all drainage until the next dressing change. Use ABD pads to form outer layers, if needed, *to provide greater absorbency.*

• Secure the dressing's edges to the patient's skin with strips of tape *to maintain the sterility of the wound site.* Or secure the dressing with a T-binder or Montgomery straps *to prevent skin excoriation, which may occur with repeated tape removal necessitated by frequent dressing changes.* (See *How to make Montgomery straps.*)

• Make sure that the patient is comfortable.

• Properly dispose of the solutions and trash bag, and clean or discard soiled equipment and supplies according to your hospital's policy. If your patient's wound has purulent drainage, don't return unopened sterile supplies to the sterile supply cabi-

How to make Montgomery straps

An abdominal dressing requiring frequent changes can be secured with Montgomery straps to promote the patient's comfort. If ready-made straps aren't available, follow these steps to make your own:

• Cut four to six strips of 2″ or 3″ (5 cm to 7.5 cm) wide hypoallergenic tape of sufficient length to allow the tape to extend about 6″ (15 cm) beyond the wound on each side.

• Fold one end of each strip 2″ or 3″ back on itself to form a nonadhesive tab. Then cut a small hole in the folded tab's center, close to its top edge. Make as many pairs of straps as you'll need to snugly secure the dressing.

• Clean the patient's skin to prevent irritation. After the skin dries, apply a skin protectant. Then apply the sticky side of each tape to a skin barrier sheet composed of opaque hydrocolloidal or nonhydrocolloidal materials, and apply the sheet directly to the skin near the dressing. Next, thread a separate piece of gauze ties, umbilical tape, or twill tape (about 12″ [31 cm]) through each pair of holes in the straps and fasten each tie as you would a shoelace. Don't stress the surrounding skin by securing the ties too tightly.

• Repeat this procedure according to the number of Montgomery straps needed.

• Replace Montgomery straps whenever they become soiled (every 2 to 3 days). If skin maceration occurs, place new tapes about 1″ (2.5 cm) away from any irritation.

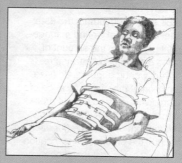

net *because this could cause cross-contamination of other equipment.*

Dressing a wound with a drain

• Prepare a drain dressing by using sterile scissors to cut a slit in a sterile 4″ × 4″ gauze pad. Fold the pad in half; then cut inward from the center of the folded edge. Don't use a cotton-lined gauze pad because cutting the gauze opens the lining and releases cotton fibers into the wound. Prepare a second pad the same way.

• Gently press one folded pad close to the skin around the drain so that the tubing fits into the slit. Press the second folded pad around the drain from the opposite direction so that the two pads encircle the tubing.

• Layer as many uncut sterile 4″ × 4″ gauze pads or ABD pads around the tubing as needed *to absorb expected drainage.* Tape the dressing in place, or use a T-binder or Montgomery straps.

Pouching a wound

• If your patient's wound is draining heavily or if drainage may damage surrounding skin, you'll need to apply a pouch.

BETTER CHARTING

Documenting surgical incision care

Besides documenting vital signs and level of consciousness when the patient returns from surgery, pay particular attention to maintaining records pertaining to the surgical incision and drains and the care you provide. Read the records that travel with the patient from the postanesthesia care unit. Look for a doctor's order directing whether you or the doctor will perform the first dressing change.

Be sure to document the date, time, and type of wound management procedure; the amount of soiled dressing and packing removed; wound appearance (size, condition of margins, presence of necrotic tissue) and odor (if present); the type, color, consistency, and amount of drainage (for each wound); the presence and location of drains; any additional procedures, such as irrigation, packing, or application of a topical medication; the type and amount of new dressing or pouch applied; and the patient's tolerance of the procedure.

• Measure the wound. Cut an opening ⅛″ (0.3 cm) larger than the wound in the facing of the collection pouch.
• Apply a skin protectant as needed. (Some protectants are incorporated within the collection pouch and also provide adhesion.)
• Make sure that the drainage port at the bottom of the pouch is firmly closed *to prevent leaks.* Then gently press the contoured pouch opening around the wound, starting at its lower edge, *to catch any drainage* .
• To empty the pouch, put on gloves, insert the pouch's bottom half into a graduated biohazard container, and open the drainage port. Note the color, consistency, odor, and amount of fluid. If ordered, obtain a culture specimen, and send it to the laboratory immediately. Remember to follow isolation precautions when handling infectious drainage.
• Wipe the bottom of the pouch and the drainage port with a gauze pad *to remove any drainage that could irritate the patient's skin or cause an odor.* Then reseal the port. Change the pouch only if it leaks or fails to adhere to the skin. More frequent changes are unnecessary and only irritate the patient's skin.

Complications
• A major complication of a dressing change is an allergic reaction to an antiseptic cleaning agent, a prescribed topical medication, or adhesive tape. This reaction may lead to skin redness, rash, excoriation, or infection.

Nursing considerations
• If the patient has two wounds in the same area, cover each wound separately with layers of sterile 4″ × 4″ gauze pads. Then cover both sites with an ABD pad secured to the patient's skin with tape. Don't use only an ABD pad to cover both sites because drainage quickly saturates a single pad, promoting cross-contamination.
• When packing a wound, don't pack it too tightly because this compresses adjacent capillaries and may prevent the wound edges from contracting. Avoid using overly damp packing

because it slows wound closure from within and increases the risk of infection.

• *To save time when dressing a wound with a drain,* use precut tracheostomy pads or drain dressings instead of custom-cutting gauze pads to fit around the drain. If your patient is sensitive to adhesive tape, use paper or silk tape because these are less likely to cause a skin reaction and will peel off more easily than adhesive tape. Use a surgical mask to cradle a chin or jawline dressing; this provides a secure dressing and avoids the need to shave the patient's hair.

• If ordered, use a collodion spray or similar topical protectant instead of a gauze dressing. Moisture- and contaminant-proof, this covering dries in a clear, impermeable film that leaves the wound visible for observation and avoids the friction caused by a dressing.

• If a sump drain isn't adequately collecting wound secretions, reinforce it with an ostomy pouch or another collection bag. Use waterproof tape to strengthen a spot on the front of the pouch near the adhesive opening; then cut a small X in the tape. Feed the drain catheter into the pouch through the X cut. Seal the cut around the tubing with more waterproof tape; then connect the tubing to the suction pump. *This method frees the drainage port at the bottom of the pouch so you don't have to remove the tubing to empty the pouch.* If you use more than one collection pouch for a wound or wounds, record drainage volume separately for each pouch. Avoid using waterproof material over the dressing *because it reduces air circulation and promotes infection from accumulated heat and moisture.*

• Because many doctors prefer to change the first postoperative dressing themselves to check the incision, don't change the first dressing unless you have specific instructions to do so. If you have no such order and drainage seeps through the dressings, reinforce the dressing with fresh sterile gauze. Request an order to change the dressing, or ask the doctor to change it as soon as possible. *A reinforced dressing should not remain in place longer than 24 hours because it's an excellent medium for bacterial growth.*

• For the recent postoperative patient or a patient with complications, check the dressing every 30 minutes or as ordered. For the patient with a properly healing wound, check the dressing at least once every 8 hours.

• If the dressing becomes wet from the outside (for example, from spilled drinking water), replace it as soon as possible *to prevent wound contamination.*

• If your patient will need wound care after discharge, provide appropriate teaching. If he'll be caring for the wound himself, stress the importance of using aseptic technique and teach him how to examine the wound for signs of infection and other complications. Also show him how to change dressings, and give him written instructions for all procedures to be performed at home.

Documentation

• Document special or detailed wound care instructions and pain management steps on the nursing care plan.

• Record the color and amount of measurable drainage on the intake and output sheet. (See *Documenting surgical incision care.*)

Wound management, traumatic

Traumatic wounds include abrasions, lacerations, puncture wounds, and amputations. In an abrasion, the skin is scraped, with partial loss of the skin surface. In a laceration, the skin is torn, causing jagged, irregular edges; the severity of a laceration depends on its size, depth, and location. A puncture wound occurs when a pointed object, such as a knife or glass fragment, penetrates the skin. Traumatic amputation refers to removal of a part of the body or a limb or part of a limb.

When caring for a patient with a traumatic wound, first assess his ABCs — airway, breathing, and circulation. It may seem natural to focus on a gruesome injury, but a patent airway and pumping heart take first priority. Once the patient's ABCs are stabilized, you can turn your attention to the traumatic wound. Initial management concentrates on controlling bleeding — usually by applying firm, direct pressure and elevating the extremity. If bleeding continues, you may need to compress a pressure point. Assess the condition of the wound. Management and cleaning technique usually depend on the specific type of wound and degree of contamination.

≫ Key nursing diagnoses and patient outcomes

Use these nursing diagnoses as a guide when developing your plan of care for a patient who has a traumatic wound.

Fluid volume deficit related to active loss
Based on this nursing diagnosis, you'll establish the following patient outcomes. The patient will:
• have vital signs remain stable.
• have fluid and blood volume return to normal.

Altered (specify type) tissue perfusion related to decreased cellular exchange
Based on this nursing diagnosis, you'll establish the following patient outcomes. The patient will:
• attain hemodynamic stability: Pulse not more than (specify) and not less than (specify); blood pressure not more than (specify) and not less than (specify).
• not exhibit arrhythmias.

Equipment

♦ sterile basin ♦ normal saline solution ♦ sterile 4″ ×4″ gauze pads ♦ sterile gloves ♦ clean gloves ♦ sterile cotton-tipped applicators ♦ dry sterile dressing, nonadherent pad, or petroleum gauze ♦ linen-saver pad ♦ optional: scissors, goggles, towel, mask, gown, 50-ml catheter-tip syringe, surgical scrub brush, antibacterial ointment, porous tape, sterile forceps, sutures and suture set, hydrogen peroxide.

Equipment preparation

• Place a linen-saver pad under the area to be cleaned. Remove any clothing covering the wound.
• If necessary, cut hair around the wound with scissors to promote cleaning and treatment.

• Assemble needed equipment at the patient's bedside. Fill a sterile basin with normal saline solution.

• Make sure the treatment area has enough light *to allow close observation of the wound.*

• Depending on the nature and location of the wound, wear sterile or clean gloves *to avoid spreading infection.*

Patient preparation

• Check the patient's medical history for previous tetanus immunization and, if needed and ordered, arrange for current immunization.

• Administer pain medication if ordered.

Implementation

• Wash your hands.

• Use appropriate protective equipment, such as a gown, mask, and goggles, if spraying or splashing of body fluids is possible.

For an abrasion

• Flush the scraped skin with normal saline solution.

• Remove dirt or gravel with a sterile 4″ × 4″ gauze pad moistened with normal saline solution. Rub in the opposite direction from which the dirt or gravel became embedded.

• If the wound is extremely dirty, you may use a surgical brush to scrub it.

• With a small wound, allow it to dry and form a scab. With a larger wound, you may need to cover it with a nonadherent pad or petroleum gauze and a light dressing. Apply antibacterial ointment if ordered.

For a laceration

• Moisten a sterile 4″ × 4″ gauze pad with normal saline solution. Clean the wound gently, working outward from its center to approximately 2″ (5 cm) beyond its edges. Discard the soiled gauze pad, and use a fresh one as necessary. Continue until the wound appears clean.

• If the wound is dirty, you may irrigate it with a 50-ml catheter-tip syringe and normal saline solution.

• Assist the doctor in suturing the wound edges using the suture kit, or apply sterile strips of porous tape.

• Apply the ordered antibacterial ointment *to help prevent infection.*

• Apply a dry sterile dressing over the wound *to absorb drainage and help prevent bacterial contamination.*

For a puncture wound

• If the wound is minor, allow it to bleed for a few minutes before cleaning it.

• For a larger puncture wound, you may need to irrigate it before applying a dry dressing.

• Stabilize any embedded foreign object until the doctor can remove it. After he removes the object and bleeding is stabilized, clean the wound as you'd clean a laceration or deep puncture wound.

For an amputation

• Apply a gauze pad moistened with normal saline solution to the amputation site. Elevate the affected part and immobilize it for surgery.

• Recover the amputated part and prepare it for transport to a facility where microvascular surgery is performed.

Complications

• Cleaning and care of traumatic wounds may temporarily increase the patient's pain. Excessive, vigorous cleaning may further disrupt tissue integrity.

Nursing considerations

• When irrigating a traumatic wound, avoid using more than 8 psi of pressure. *High-pressure irrigation can seriously interfere with healing, kill healthy cells, and allow bacteria to infiltrate the tissue.*

• To clean the wound, you may use hydrogen peroxide, whose foaming action facilitates debris removal. However, peroxide should *never* be instilled into a deep wound *because of the risk of embolism from the evolving gases.* Be sure to rinse your hands well after using hydrogen peroxide.

• Avoid cleaning a traumatic wound with alcohol *because it causes pain and tissue dehydration.* Also, avoid using antiseptics for wound cleaning because *they can impede healing.* In addition, never use a cotton ball or cotton-filled gauze pad to clean a wound *because cotton fibers left in the wound may cause contamination.*

• After a wound has been cleaned, the doctor may want to debride it *to remove dead tissue and reduce the risk of infection and scarring.* If this is necessary, pack the wound with gauze pads soaked in normal saline solution until debridement.

• Observe for signs and symptoms of infection, such as warm red skin at the site or purulent discharge. Be aware that infection of a traumatic wound can delay healing, increase scar formation, and trigger systemic infection such as septicemia.

• Observe all dressings. If edema is present, adjust the dressing *to avoid impairing circulation to the area.*

Documentation

• Document the date and time of the procedure, wound size and condition, medication administration, specific wound care measures, and patient teaching.

APPENDICES

Appendix A: **Guidelines for minimizing infection**
Appendix B: **Normal labratory test values**
Appendix C: **Sources of information**

Appendix A: Guidelines for minimizing infection

The table below lists the minimum requirements for using gloves, gowns, masks, and eye protection to avoid contacting and spreading pathogens. It assumes that thorough hand washing is performed in all cases.

PROCEDURE	GLOVES
Bathing, for patient with open lesions	✔
Bedding, changing visibly soiled	✔
Bleeding or pressure application to control it	✔
Blood glucose (capillary) testing	✔
Breathing treatment, routine	If soiling likely
Cardiopulmonary resuscitation	✔
Central venous line insertion and venesection	✔
Central venous pressure measurement	✔
Cervical cauterization	✔
Chest drainage system change	✔
Chest tube insertion	✔
Chest tube removal	✔
Cleaning, anal	✔
Cleaning (feces, spilled blood or body substances, or surfaces contaminated by blood or body fluids)	✔
Cleaning, urine	✔
Colonoscopy, flexible sigmoidoscope	✔
Coughing, frequent and forceful by patient; direct contact with secretions	✔
Dialysis, peritoneal	
Initiation of acute treatment	✔
Performing an exchange	✔
Termination of acute treatment	✔
Dismantling tubing from cycler	✔
Discarding peritoneal drainage	✔
Irrigating peritoneal catheter	✔
Specimen collection	✔
Tubing change	✔

Note: ✔ indicates that barrier is necessary; — indicates that barrier typically is not necessary.

Refer to your hospital's guidelines and use your own judgment when assessing the need for barrier protection in specific situations.

GOWN	MASK	EYE WEAR
If soiling likely	—	—
If soiling likely	—	—
If soiling likely	If splattering likely	If splattering likely
—	—	—
—	—	—
If soiling, splattering likely	If soiling, splattering likely	If soiling, splattering likely
—	If splattering likely	If splattering likely
—	—	—
—	—	—
If splattering likely	If splattering likely	If splattering likely
If soiling likely	If splattering likely	If splattering likely
If soiling likely	If splattering likely	If splattering likely
—	—	—
If soiling likely	If soiling likely	If soiling likely
—	—	—
✔	✔	✔
—	✔	✔
✔	If splattering likely	If splattering likely
✔	If splatteirng likely	If splattering likely
✔	If splattering likely	If splattering likely
✔	✔	✔
✔	✔	✔
✔	If splattering likely	If splattering likely
—	—	—
✔	If splattering likely	If splattering likely

(continued)

Appendix A: Guidelines for minimizing infection *(continued)*

PROCEDURE	GLOVES
Dialysis, peritoneal (continued) Skin care (catheter site)	✔
Assisting with insertion of acute peritoneal catheter (outside sterile field)	✔
Dressing change for burns	✔
Dressing removal or change for wounds with little or no drainage	✔
Dressing removal or change for wounds with large amount of drainage	✔
Emptying drainage receptacles, including suction containers, urine receptacles, bedpans, emesis basins	✔
Emptying wastebaskets	✔
Enema	✔
Fecal impaction, removal of	✔
Fecal incontinence, placement of indwelling urinary catheter for, and emptying bag	✔
Gastric lavage	✔
Incision and drainage of abscess	✔

Intravenous or intra-arterial line
  Insertion
  Removal
  Tubing change at catheter hub
	✔
	✔
	✔

Intubation or extubation	✔
Invasive procedures (lumbar puncture, bone marrow aspiration, paracentesis, liver biopsy) outside sterile field	✔

Irrigation
  Indwelling urinary catheter
  Vaginal
  Wound
	✔
	✔
	✔

Joint or nerve injection	✔
Lesion biopsy or removal	✔

Note: ✔ indicates that barrier is necessary; − indicates that barrier typically is not necessary.

GOWN	MASK	EYE WEAR
✔	✔	✔
✔	✔	✔
✔	–	–
–	–	–
If soiling likely	If soiling likely	If soiling likely
If soiling likely	If splattering likely	If splattering likely
–	–	–
If soiling likely	–	–
–	–	–
If splattering likely	–	–
If soiling likely	–	–
If splattering likely	If splattering likely	If splattering likely
If splattering likely	If splattering likely	If splattering likely
–	–	–
If splattering likely	If splattering likely	If splattering likely
✔	✔	✔
–	–	–
If soiling likely	–	–
If soiling likely	If splattering likely	If splattering likely
–	–	–
–	–	–

(continued)

Appendix A: Guidelines for minimizing infection *(continued)*

PROCEDURE	GLOVES
Medication administration	
Eye, ear, and nose drops	✔
I.M. or S.C.	✔
I.V. (direct or into hub of catheter or heparin lock)	✔
Oral	✔
Rectal or vaginal suppository	✔
Topical medication for lesion	✔
Nasogastric tube, insertion or irrigation	✔
Oral and nasal care	✔
Ostomy care, irrigation, and teaching	✔
Oxygen tubing, drainage of condensate	✔
Pelvic exam and Pap test	✔
Perineal cleaning	✔
Postmortem care	✔
Pressure ulcer care	✔
Shaving	✔
Specimen collection (blood, stool, urine, sputum, wound)	✔
Suctioning	
Nasotracheal or endotracheal	✔
Oral or nasal	✔
Temperature, rectal	✔
Tracheostomy suctioning and cannula cleaning	✔
Tracheostomy tube change	✔
Urine and stool testing	✔
Wound packing	✔

Note: ✔ indicates that barrier is necessary; — indicates that barrier typically is not necessary.

GOWN	MASK	EYE WEAR
–	–	–
–	–	–
–	–	–
–	–	–
–	–	–
–	–	–
If soiling likely	If splattering likely	If splattering likely
–	–	–
If soiling likely	If soiling likely	If soiling likely
–	–	–
–	–	–
–	–	–
If soiling likely	–	–
–	–	–
–	–	–
–	–	–
If soiling likely	If splattering likely	If splattering likely
–	–	–
–	–	–
If soiling likely	If splattering likely	If splattering likely
–	If splattering likely	If splattering likely
–	–	–
If soiling likely	–	–

Adapted from Pugliese, G., ed. *Universal Precautions: Policies, Procedures, and Resources.* Chicago: American Hospital Publishing, Inc., 1991.

Appendix B: Normal laboratory test values

HEMATOLOGY

Activated partial thromboplastin time
  25 to 36 seconds

Bleeding time
  Template: 2 to 8 minutes
  Ivy: 1 to 7 minutes
  Duke: 1 to 3 minutes

Clot retraction
  50%

Erythrocyte sedimentation rate
  Males: 0 to 10 mm/hour
  Females: 0 to 20 mm/hour

Fibrin split products
  Screening assay: < 10 µg/ml
  Quantitative assay: < 3 µg/ml

Fibrinogen, plasma
  195 to 365 mg/dl

Hematocrit
  Men: 42% to 54%
  Women: 38% to 46%

Hemoglobin, total
  Men: 14 to 18 g/dl
  Women: 12 to 16 g/dl

Platelet aggregation
  3 to 5 minutes

Platelet count
  130,000 to 370,000/mm^3

Platelet survival
  50% tagged platelets disappear within 84 to 116 hours
  100% disappear within 8 to 10 days

Prothrombin consumption time
  20 seconds

Prothrombin time
  10 to 14 seconds

Red blood cell count
  Men: 4.5 to 6.2 million/µl venous blood
  Women: 4.2 to 5.4 million/µl venous blood

Red cell indices
  MCV: 84 to 99 fl
  MCH: 26 to 32 fl
  MCHC: 30 to 36 g/dl

Reticulocyte count
  0.5% to 2% of total RBC count

Sickle cell test
  Negative

Thrombin time, plasma
  10 to 15 seconds

White blood cell count, blood
  4,100 to 10,900/µl

White blood cell differential, blood
  Neutrophils: 47.6% to 76.8%
  Lymphocytes: 16.2% to 43%
  Monocytes: 0.6% to 9.6%
  Eosinophils: 0.3% to 7%
  Basophils: 0.3% to 2 %

Whole blood clotting time
  5 to 15 minutes

BLOOD CHEMISTRY

Acid phosphatase
  0.5 to 1.9 U/L

Alanine aminotransferase
  Men: 10 to 32 U/L
  Women: 9 to 24 U/L

Alkaline phosphatase, serum
  1.5 to 4 Bodansky units/dl
  4 to 13.5 King-Armstrong units/dl
  Chemical inhibition method:
    Men, 90 to 239 U/L
    Women < age 45, 76 to 196 U/L; age 45, 87 to 250 U/L

Amylase, serum
  30 to 220 U/L

Arterial blood gases
  pH: 7.35 to 7.42 mm Hg
  Pao$_2$: 75 to 100 mm Hg
  Paco$_2$: 35 to 45 mm Hg
  O$_2$CT: 15% to 23%
  O$_2$Sat: 94% to 100%
  HCO$_3$–: 22 to 26 mEq/L

Appendix B: Normal laboratory test values *(continued)*

Aspartate aminotransferase
   8 to 20 U/L
Bilirubin, serum
   Adult: direct, < 0.5 mg/dl;
      indirect, ≤ 1.1 mg/dl
Blood urea nitrogen
   8 to 20 mg/dl
C-reactive protein, serum
   Negative
Calcium, serum
   4.5 to 5.5 mEq/L
   Atomic absorption: 8.9 to
      10.1 mg/dl
Carbon dioxide, total, blood
   22 to 34 mEq/L
Catecholamines, plasma
   Supine: Epinephrine, 0 to
      110 pg/ml; norepinephrine, 70
      to 750 pg/ml; dopamine, 0 to
      30 pg/ml
   Standing: Epinephrine, 0 to
      140 pg/ml; norepinephrine,
      200 to 1,700 pg/ml; dopamine,
      0 to 30 pg/ml
Chloride, serum
   100 to 108 mEq/L
Cholesterol, total, serum
   0 to 240 mg/dl
   CK-BB: None
   CK-MB: 0 to 7 IU/L
   CK-MM: 5 to 70 IU/L
Creatine
   Males: 0.2 to 0.6 mg/dl
   Females: 0.6 to 1.0 mg/dl
Creatine kinase
   Total: Men, 25 to 130 U/L;
   women, 10 to 150 U/L
Creatinine, serum
   Males: 0.8 to 1.2 mg/dl
   Females: 0.6 to 0.9 mg/dl
Free thyroxine, serum
   0.8 to 3.3 ng/dl
Free triiodothyronine
   0.2 to 0.6 ng/dl
Gamma glutamyl transferase
   Males: 8 to 37 U/L

   Females: $<$ age 45, 5 to 27 U/L;
      $>$ age 45, 6 to 37 U/L
Glucose, plasma, fasting
   70 to 100 mg/dl
Glucose, plasma, oral tolerance
   Peak at 160 to 180 mg/dl, 30 to
      60 minutes after challenge dose
Glucose, plasma, 2-hour post-prandial
   < 145 mg/dl
Hydroxybutyric dehydrogenase
   Serum HBD: 114 to 290 U/ml
   LD/HBD ratio: 1.2 to 1.6:1
Iron, serum
   Men: 70 to 150 μg/dl
   Women: 80 to 150 μg/dl
Lactic acid, blood
   0.93 to 1.65 mEq/L
Lactate dehydrogenase
   Total: 48 to 115 IU/L
   LD_1: 14% to 26%
   LD_2: 29% to 39%
   LD_3: 20% to 26%
   LD_4: 8% to 16%
   LD_5: 6% to 16%
Lipase
   < 300 U/L
Lipoproteins, serum
   HDL-cholesterol: 29 to 77 mg/dl
   LDL-cholesterol: 62 to 185 mg/dl
Magnesium, serum
   1.5 to 2.5 mEq/L
   Atomic absorption: 1.7 to
      2.1 mg/dl
Phosphates, serum
   1.8 to 2.6 mEq/L
   Atomic absorption: 2.5 to
      4.5 mg/dl
Potassium, serum
   3.8 to 5.5 mEq/L

Appendix B: Normal laboratory test values *(continued)*

Protein, total, serum
6.6 to 7.9 g/dl
Albumin fraction: 3.3 to 4.5 g/dl
Globulin level: alpha$_1$-globulin,
0.1 to 0.4 g/dl; alpha$_2$-globulin,
0.5 to 1 g/dl; beta globulin, 0.7
to 1.2 g/dl; and gamma globulin, 0.5 to 1.6 g/dl

Sodium, serum
135 to 145 mEq/L

Thyroxine, total, serum
5 to 13.5 µg/dl

Triglycerides, serum
Men: 40 to 160 mg/dl
Women: 35 to 135 mg/dl

Uric acid, serum
Men: 4.3 to 8 mg/dl
Women: 2.3 to 6 mg/dl

URINE CHEMISTRY

Amylase, urine
10 to 80 amylase units/hour

Bence Jones protein, urine
Negative

Bilirubin, urine
Negative

Calcium, urine
Males: < 275 mg/24 hours
Females: < 250 mg/24 hours

Calculi, urine
None

Catecholamines, urine
24-hour specimen: 0 to 135 µg
Random specimen: 0 to 18 µg/dl

Creatinine clearance
Men: 107 to 139 ml/minute
Women: 87 to 107 ml/minute

Creatinine, urine
Men: 1.0 to 1.9 g/24 hours
Women: 0.8 to 1.7 g/24 hours

Glucose, urine
Negative

17-Hydroxycorticosteroids, urine
Men: 4.5 to 12 mg/24 hours
Women: 2.5 to 10 mg/24 hours

17-Ketogenic steroids, urine
Men: 4 to 14 mg/24 hours
Women: 2 to 12 mg/24 hours

Ketones, urine
Negative

17-Ketosteroids, urine
Men: 6 to 21 mg/24 hours
Women: 4 to 17 mg/24 hours

Phenolsulfonphthalein excretion, urine
15 minutes: 25% of dose
excreted
30 minutes: 50% to 60% of
dose excreted
1 hour: 60% to 79% of dose
excreted
2 hours: 70% to 80% of dose
excreted

Protein, urine
≤ 150 mg/24 hours

Red blood cells, urine
0 to 3 per high-power field

Sodium, urine
30 to 280 mEq/24 hours

Sodium chloride, urine
5 to 20 g/24 hours

Urea, urine
Maximal clearance: 64 to
99 ml/minute

Uric acid, urine
250 to 750 mg/24 hours

Urinalysis, routine
Color: Straw
Odor: Slightly aromatic
Appearance: Clear
Specific gravity: 1.005 to 1.035
pH: 4.5 to 8.0
Sugars: None
Epithelial cells: Few
Casts: None, except occasional
hyaline casts
Crystals: Present
Yeast cells: None

Appendix B: Normal laboratory test values (continued)

Urine concentration
  Specific gravity: 1.025 to 1.032
  Osmolality: > 800 mOsm/kg
    water
Urine dilution
  Specific gravity: < 1.003
  Osmolality: < 100 mOsm/kg
  80% of water excreted in
    4 hours
Urobilinogen, urine
  Men: 0.3 to 2.1 Ehrlich units/
  2 hours
  Women: 0.1 to 1.1 Ehrlich
    units/2 hours
Vanillylmandelic acid, urine
  0.7 to 6.8 mg/24 hours
White blood cell count, urine
  0 to 4 per high-power field

MISCELLANEOUS
Cerebrospinal fluid
  Pressure: 50 to 180 mm water
**Lupus erythematosus cell
preparation**
  Negative
Occult blood, fecal
  < 2.5 mg/24 hours
Rheumatoid factor, serum
  Negative
Urobilinogen, fecal
  50 to 300 mg/24 hours
VDRL, serum
  Negative

Appendix C: Sources of information and help

ALCOHOLISM
Al-Anon Family Group Headquarters, P.O. Box 862, Midtown Station, New York, NY 10018
(212) 302-7240; (800) 356-9996

Alateen Family Group Headquarters, P.O. Box 862, Midtown Station, New York, NY 10018
(212) 302-7240; (800) 356-9996

Alcoholics Anonymous (AA) World Services, 475 Riverside Dr., New York, NY 10163
(212) 870-3400

ANOREXIA NERVOSA
Anorexia Nervosa and Related Eating Disorders, P.O. Box 5102, Eugene, OR 97405
(503) 344-1144

ARTHRITIS
Arthritis Foundation, 1314 Spring St., N.W., Atlanta, GA 30309
(404) 872-7100; (800) 283-7800

American College of Rheumatology, 60 Executive Park S., Suite 150, Atlanta, GA 30329
(404) 633-3777

AUTISM
Autism Society of America, 7910 Woodmont Ave., Suite 650, Bethesda, MD 20814
(301) 657-0881

BIRTH DEFECTS
March of Dimes Birth Defects Foundation, 1275 Mamaroneck Ave., White Plains, NY 10605
(914) 428-7100

BLINDNESS
American Foundation for the Blind, 11 Penn Plaza, Suite 300, New York, NY 10001
(212) 502-7600

CANCER
American Cancer Society, 1599 Clifton Rd., N.E., Atlanta, GA 30329
(404) 320-3333; (800) 227-2345

International Association of Laryngectomees, c/o American Cancer Society, 1599 Clifton Rd., N.E., Atlanta GA 30329
(404) 320-3333; (800) 227-2345

Reach to Recovery Foundation, c/o American Cancer Society, 1599 Clifton Rd., N.E., Atlanta GA 30329
(404) 320-3333; (800) 227-2345

CEREBRAL PALSY
United Cerebral Palsy Association, 1522 K St., N.W., Suite 1112, Washington, DC 20005
(202) 842-1266

CYSTIC FIBROSIS
Cystic Fibrosis Foundation, 6931 Arlington Rd., Suite 200, Bethesda, MD 20814
(301) 951-4422; (800) 344-4823

DIABETES
American Association of Diabetes Educators, 444 N. Michigan Ave., Suite 1240, Chicago, IL 60611-3901
(312) 644-2233; (800) 338-3633

American Diabetes Association, P.O. Box 2575, 1660 Duke St., Alexandria, VA 22314
(703) 549-1500; (800) 232-3472

Juvenile Diabetes Foundation International, 432 Park Ave. S., New York, NY 10016-8013
(212) 889-7557; (800) 233-1138

EPILEPSY
Epilepsy Foundation of America, 4351 Garden City Dr., Landover, MD 20785
(301) 459-3700; (800) 332-1000

Appendix C: Sources of information and help *(continued)*

HEMOPHILIA
National Hemophilia Foundation, 110 Greene St., Suite 303, New York, NY 10012
(212) 219-8180; (800) 424-2634

HUNTINGTON'S DISEASE
Huntington's Disease Society of America, 140 W. 22nd St., 6th Floor, New York, NY 10011-2420
(212) 242-1968; (800) 345-4372

INFECTIOUS DISEASES
Centers for Disease Control and Prevention, 1600 Clifton Rd., N.E., Atlanta, GA 30333
(404) 639-3534 or 639-3535

LUPUS ERYTHEMATOSUS
Lupus Foundation of America, 4 Research Pl., Suite 180, Rockville, MD 20850-3226
(301) 670-9292; (800) 558-0121

MENTAL RETARDATION
Association for Children with Retarded Mental Development, 345 Hudson St., New York, NY 10014
(212) 741-0100; (800) 969-2276

MULTIPLE SCLEROSIS
National Multiple Sclerosis Society, 733 Third Ave., 6th Floor, New York, NY 10017
(212) 986-3240; (800) 344-4867

MUSCULAR DYSTROPHY
Muscular Dystrophy Association, 3300 E. Sunrise Dr., Tucson, AZ 85718
(602) 529-2000

MYASTHENIA GRAVIS
Myasthenia Gravis Foundation, 53 W. Jackson Blvd., Suite 660, Chicago, IL 60604
(312) 427-6252; (800) 541-5454

NEUROFIBROMATOSIS
Neurofibromatosis, Inc., 8855 Annapolis Rd., Suite 110, Lanham, MD 20706-2924
(301) 577-8984; (800) 942-6825

PARKINSON'S DISEASE
National Parkinson Foundation, 1501 N.W. Ninth Ave., Miami, FL 33136
(305) 547-6666; (800) 327-4545

United Parkinson Foundation, 833 W. Washington Blvd., Chicago, IL 60607
(312) 733-1893

PSORIASIS
National Psoriasis Foundation, 6600 S.W. 92nd Ave., Suite 300, Portland, OR 97223
(503) 244-7404

RAPE TRAUMA SYNDROME
Women Against Rape, Box 02084, Columbus, OH 43202
(614) 291-9751

REYE'S SYNDROME
National Reye's Syndrome Foundation, 426 N. Lewis, P.O. Box 829, Bryan, OH 43506
(419) 636-2679; (800) 233-7393

RETINITIS PIGMENTOSA
The Foundation Fighting Blindness (RPFFB), 1401 Mt. Royal Ave., 4th Floor, Baltimore, MD 21217-4245
(410) 225-9400; (800) 638-5555

SEXUAL DYSFUNCTION
Sex Information and Education Counsel of the U.S., 130 W. 42nd St., Suite 350, New York, NY 10036
(212) 819-9770

Herpes Resource Center-American Social Health Association, P.O. Box 13827, Research Triangle Park, NC 27709
(919) 361-8488

SPEECH AND HEARING IMPAIRMENT
American Speech-Language-Hearing Association, 10801 Rockville Pike, Rockville, MD 20852
(310) 897-5700; (800) 638-8255

(continued)

Appendix C: Sources of information and help *(continued)*

SPINA BIFIDA
Spina Bifida Association of America,
4590 MacArthur Blvd., N.W., Suite 250,
Washington, DC 20007-4226
(202) 944-3285; (800) 621-3141

SUDDEN INFANT DEATH SYNDROME
SIDS Alliance, 10500 Little Patuxent
Parkway, Suite 420, Columbia, MD 21044
(410) 964-8000; (800) 221-SIDS

TAY-SACHS DISEASE
National Tay-Sachs and Allied Diseases
Association, 2001 Beacon St., Brookline,
MA 02146
(617) 277-4463

MISCELLANEOUS
American Red Cross, 430 17th St., N.W.,
Washington, DC 20006
(202) 737-8300

National AIDS Hotline (sponsored by
CDC)
(800) 342-AIDS; Spanish: (800) 344-
7432; Hearing Impaired: (800) 243-7889

INDEX

i refers to an illustration; t, to a table

i refers to an illustration; t, to a table

i refers to an illustration; t, to a table